AMA
AMERICAN MEDICAL ASSOCIATION

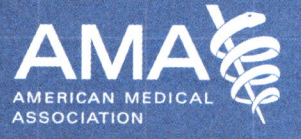

ICD-10-PCS 2025
The Complete Official Codebook

AMA publications fund initiatives that drive improvements in patient health, practice innovation and medical education.

Notice

ICD-10-PCS: The Complete Official Codebook is designed to be an accurate and authoritative source regarding coding and every reasonable effort has been made to ensure accuracy and completeness of the content. However, the American Medical Association (AMA) makes no guarantee, warranty, or representation that this publication is accurate, complete, or without errors. It is understood that the AMA is not rendering any legal or other professional services or advice in this publication and that the AMA bears no liability for any results or consequences that may arise from the use of this book.

Our Commitment to Accuracy

The AMA is committed to producing accurate and reliable materials. To report corrections, please call the AMA Unified Service Center at (800) 621-8335.

To purchase additional copies, visit the AMA store at amastore.com. Refer to product number OP201125.

Copyright

© 2024 Optum360, LLC
Made in the USA
OP201125
BQ50:8/24

Acknowledgments

Marianne Randall, CPC, *Senior Product Manager*
Anita Schmidt, BS, RHIA, AHIMA-approved ICD-10-CM/PCS Trainer, *Subject Matter Expert*
Laura M. Anderson, RN, BSN, CCDS, *Subject Matter Expert*
Stacy Perry, *Manager, Desktop Publishing*
Tracy Betzler, *Senior Desktop Publishing Specialist*
Hope M. Dunn, *Senior Desktop Publishing Specialist*
Katie Russell, *Desktop Publishing Specialist*
Kate Holden, *Editor*

Anita Schmidt, BS, RHIA, AHIMA-approved ICD-10-CM/PCS Trainer

Ms. Schmidt has expertise in ICD-10-CM/PCS, DRG, and CPT with more than 20 years' experience in coding in multiple settings, including inpatient, observation, and same-day surgery. Her experience includes analysis of medical record documentation, assignment of ICD-10-CM and PCS codes, and DRG validation. She has collaborated with clinical documentation specialists to identify documentation needs and potential areas for physician education. Most recently she has been developing content for resource and educational products related to ICD-10-CM, ICD-10-PCS, DRG, and CPT. Ms. Schmidt is an AHIMA-approved ICD-10-CM/PCS trainer and is an active member of the American Health Information Management Association (AHIMA) and the Minnesota Health Information Management Association (MHIMA).

Laura M. Anderson, RN, BSN, CCDS

Ms. Anderson is a Registered Nurse and CDI Specialist/Educator with more than 20 years of experience in the healthcare profession. She obtained her BSN at the University of Minnesota and spent most of her bedside nursing career on Medical-Surgical care units. Her clinical documentation experience began in 2007, covering CDI specialist training, education development, and physician engagement. She has served as a CDI Team Lead and consultant, working with senior leadership to incorporate CDI work into documentation compliance and quality metrics. Ms. Anderson also has a BS degree in Biology (Winthrop University), with research experience in liver cancer and radiation-induced leukemia. She has presented at the state and national levels for the Association of Clinical Documentation Integrity Specialists (ACDIS) and has served as a co-lead for the Minnesota state chapter.

Product Updates

Any changes and updates for this codebook, including the updates for April 1, 2025, will be provided on the AMA's product-updates page at ama-assn.org/product-updates.

Contents

What's New for 2025 iii

Introduction 1
    ICD-10-PCS Manual 1
    Medical and Surgical Section (Ø) 4
    Obstetrics Section (1) 7
    Placement Section (2) 8
    Administration Section (3) 8
    Measurement and Monitoring Section (4) 9
    Extracorporeal or Systemic Assistance and
        Performance Section (5) 9
    Extracorporeal or Systemic Therapies Section (6) 10
    Osteopathic Section (7) 11
    Other Procedures Section (8) 11
    Chiropractic Section (9) 11
    Imaging Section (B) 12
    Nuclear Medicine Section (C) 12
    Radiation Therapy Section (D) 13
    Physical Rehabilitation and Diagnostic Audiology Section (F) 14
    Mental Health Section (G) 15
    Substance Abuse Treatment Section (H) 15
    New Technology Section (X) 16

ICD-10-PCS Index and Tabular Format 17
    Index 17
    Code Tables 17

ICD-10-PCS Additional Features 19
    Use of Official Sources 19
    Table Notations 19
    Appendixes 20

**ICD-10-PCS Official Guidelines for Coding
and Reporting 2025** 23
    Conventions 23
    Medical and Surgical Section Guidelines (section Ø) 24
    Obstetric Section Guidelines (section 1) 29
    Radiation Therapy Section Guidelines (section D) 29
    New Technology Section Guidelines (section X) 30

ICD-10-PCS Index 31

ICD-10-PCS Tables 133
    Central Nervous System and Cranial Nerves 133
    Peripheral Nervous System 155
    Heart and Great Vessels 173
    Upper Arteries 195
    Lower Arteries 221
    Upper Veins 247
    Lower Veins 267
    Lymphatic and Hemic Systems 287
    Eye 305
    Ear, Nose, Sinus 323
    Respiratory System 343
    Mouth and Throat 359

    Gastrointestinal System 377
    Hepatobiliary System and Pancreas 405
    Endocrine System 419
    Skin and Breast 431
    Subcutaneous Tissue and Fascia 449
    Muscles 469
    Tendons 491
    Bursae and Ligaments 505
    Head and Facial Bones 527
    Upper Bones 547
    Lower Bones 567
    Upper Joints 587
    Lower Joints 607
    Urinary System 631
    Female Reproductive System 647
    Male Reproductive System 667
    Anatomical Regions, General 683
    Anatomical Regions, Upper Extremities 695
    Anatomical Regions, Lower Extremities 705
    Obstetrics 715
    Placement 719
    Administration 725
    Measurement and Monitoring 739
    Extracorporeal or Systemic Assistance and Performance 743
    Extracorporeal or Systemic Therapies 745
    Osteopathic 747
    Other Procedures 749
    Chiropractic 751
    Imaging 753
    Nuclear Medicine 783
    Radiation Therapy 793
    Physical Rehabilitation and Diagnostic Audiology 811
    Mental Health 823
    Substance Abuse Treatment 825
    New Technology 827

Appendixes 841
    Appendix A: Components of the Medical and Surgical
        Approach Definitions 841
    Appendix B: Root Operation Definitions 844
    Appendix C: Comparison of Medical and Surgical
        Root Operations 849
    Appendix D: Body Part Key 851
    Appendix E: Body Part Definitions 866
    Appendix F: Device Classification 876
    Appendix G: Device Key and Aggregation Table 878
    Appendix H: Device Definitions 887
    Appendix I: Substance Key/Substance Definitions 893
    Appendix J: Sections B–H Character Definitions 899
    Appendix K: Hospital Acquired Conditions 907
    Appendix L: Procedure Combination Tables 927
    Appendix M: Coding Exercises and Answers 943
    Answers to Coding Exercises 949

What's New for 2025

The Centers for Medicare and Medicaid Services is the agency charged with maintaining and updating ICD-10-PCS. CMS released the most current revisions, a summary of which may be found on the CMS website at https://www.cms.gov/medicare/coding-billing/icd-10-codes/2025-icd-10-pcs.

Due to the unique structure of ICD-10-PCS, a change in a character value may affect individual codes and several code tables.

Change Summary Table

2024 Total	New Codes	Revised Titles	Deleted Codes	2025 Total
78,638	371	0	61	78,948

ICD-10-PCS Code Totals, By Section

Section	Count
Medical and Surgical	68,367
Obstetrics	304
Placement	861
Administration	1,272
Measurement and Monitoring	422
Extracorporeal or Systemic Assistance and Performance	55
Extracorporeal or Systemic Therapies	46
Osteopathic	100
Other Procedures	89
Chiropractic	90
Imaging	2,978
Nuclear Medicine	463
Radiation Therapy	2,056
Physical Rehabilitation and Diagnostic Audiology	1,380
Mental Health	28
Substance Abuse Treatment	59
New Technology	378
Total	78,948

Table Addenda Highlights

- Qualifier value Sustained Release was added to root operation table Dilation in the Lower Arteries body system (047) to complement any device value of drug-eluting intraluminal device
- New root operation table Bypass in Lymphatic and Hemic Systems body system (071)
- Qualifier value Lumbar Artery Perforator added to root operation table Replacement in the Skin and Breast body system (0HR) for breast body parts
- Method value Fiber Optic 3D Guided Procedure added to root operation table Other Procedures in the Physiological Systems and Anatomical Regions body system (8E0)
- Device value Intraluminal Device, Everolimus-eluting Resorbable Scaffold(s) added to root operation table Dilation in the New Technology section (X27) for the body parts anterior and posterior tibial artery and peroneal artery
- New root operation table Division added to New Technology section for Cardiovascular System (X28)
- New root operation table Assistance added to New Technology section for Physiological Systems (XXA)

Definitions Addenda

Section 0 – Medical and Surgical Body Part Definitions

ICD-10-PCS Value		Definition
Hand Muscle, Right Hand Muscle, Left	Add	Adductor pollicis muscle
Hip Muscle, Right Hip Muscle, Left	Add	Iliopsoas muscle
Add Knee Region, Right Add Knee Region, Left	Add	Popliteal fossa
Lower Arm and Wrist Muscle, Right Lower Arm and Wrist Muscle, Left	Add	Anconeus muscle
Lower Leg Muscle, Right Lower Leg Muscle, Left	Add	Plantaris muscle
Pelvic Cavity	Add	Prevesical space
Thoracic Aorta, Ascending/Arch	Add Add	Aortic Isthmus Juxtaductal aorta
Temporal Bone, Right Temporal Bone, Left	Revised Revised	Petrous part of temporal bone Tympanic part of temporal bone
Upper Leg Muscle, Right Upper Leg Muscle, Left	Add	Hamstring muscle

Section 0 – Medical and Surgical Device Definitions

ICD-10-PCS Value		Definition
Cardiac Resynchronization Pacemaker Pulse Generator for Insertion in Subcutaneous Tissue and Fascia	Revised	Syncra CRT-P
Internal Fixation Device, Sustained Compression for Fusion in Lower Joints	Revised	DynaNail® (Delta) (Forte) (Quattro)
Internal Fixation Device, Sustained Compression for Fusion in Upper Joints	Revised	DynaNail® (Delta) (Forte) (Quattro)
Intraluminal Device	Add	Innova™ stent
Intraluminal Device, Drug-eluting in Lower Arteries	Add Add	Eluvia™ Drug-Eluting Vascular Stent System SAVAL below-the-knee (BTK) drug-eluting stent system
Intraluminal Device, Drug-eluting, Four or More in Lower Arteries	Add Add	Eluvia™ Drug-Eluting Vascular Stent System SAVAL below-the-knee (BTK) drug-eluting stent system
Intraluminal Device, Drug-eluting, Three in Lower Arteries	Add Add	Eluvia™ Drug-Eluting Vascular Stent System SAVAL below-the-knee (BTK) drug-eluting stent system
Intraluminal Device, Drug-eluting, Two in Lower Arteries	Add Add	Eluvia™ Drug-Eluting Vascular Stent System SAVAL below-the-knee (BTK) drug-eluting stent system

Section Ø – Medical and Surgical Device Definitions (continued)

ICD-10-PCS Value	Definition		
Nonautologous Tissue Substitute	Add	Fish skin	
	Add	Kerecis® (GraftGuide) (MariGen) (SurgiBind) (SurgiClose)	
	Add	Piscine Skin	
Add — Radioactive Element Palladium-103 Collagen Implant for Insertion in Central Nervous System and Cranial Nerves	Add	GammaTile™	
	Add	Palladium-103 Collagen Implant	
Synthetic Substitute	Add	LimFlow™ Transcatheter Arterialization of the Deep Veins (TADV) System	
Zooplastic Tissue in Heart and Great Vessels	Add	Inspiris Resilia valve	

Section 3 – Administration Substance Definitions

ICD-10-PCS Value	Definition	
Other Anti-infective	Add	CONTEPO™ (Fosfomycin Anti-infective)
	Add	Fosfomycin Anti-infective
	Add	IMI/REL
	Add	Imipenem-cilastatin-relebactam Anti-infective
	Add	Meropenem-vaborbactam Anti-infective
	Add	RECARBRIO™ (Imipenem-cilastatin-relebactam Anti-infective)
	Add	VABOMERE™ (Meropenem-vaborbactam Anti-infective)
Other Antineoplastic	Add	Apalutamide Antineoplastic
	Add	Balversa™ (Erdafitinib Antineoplastic)
	Add	Erdafitinib Antineoplastic
	Add	ERLEADA™ (Apalutamide Antineoplastic)
	Add	Gilteritinib
	Add	Venclexta® (Venetoclax Antineoplastic tablets)
	Add	Venetoclax Antineoplastic (tablets)
	Add	XOSPATA® (Gilteritinib)
Other Substance	Add	Dnase (Deoxyribonulcease)
	Add	Esketamine Hydrochloride
	Add	JAKAFI(R) (Ruxolitinib)
	Add	Ruxolitinib
	Add	SPRAVATO™ (Esketamine Hydrochloride)

Section X – New Technology Root Operation Definitions

ICD-10-PCS Value	Definition
Division	Definition: Cutting into a body part, without draining fluids and/or gases from the body part, in order to separate or transect a body part Explanation: All or a portion of the body part is separated into two or more portions

Section X – New Technology Device/Substance/Technology Definitions

ICD-10-PCS Value	Definition		
Add	AGN1 Bone Void Filler	Add	OSSURE™ implant material
Delete	Apalutamide Antineoplastic	Delete	ERLEADA™
Add	Bioengineered Human Acellular Vessel in New Technology	Add	HAV™ (Human Acellular Vessel)
		Add	Human Acellular Vessel™ (HAV)
Add	Branched Intraluminal Device, Manufactured Integrated System, Four or More Arteries in New Technology	Add	GORE® EXCLUDER® TAMBE Device (Thoracoabdominal Branch Endoprosthesis)
		Add	TAMBE Device (Thoracoabdominal Branch Endoprosthesis), GORE® EXCLUDER®
Add	Carbon/PEEK Spinal Stabilization Device, Pedicle Based in New Technology	Add	BlackArmor® Carbon/PEEK fixation system
		Add	VADER® Pedicle System
Add	Donislecel-jujn Allogeneic Pancreatic Islet Cellular Suspension	Add	Lantidra™
Add	Elranatamab Antineoplastic		ELREXFIO™
Add	Epcoritamab Monoclonal Antibody	Add	EPKINLY™
Delete	Esketamine Hydrochloride	Delete	SPRAVATO™
	Exagamglogene Autotemcel	Add	CASGEVY™
Add	Facet Joint Fusion Device, Paired Titanium Cages in New Technology	Add	Facet FiXation implant
		Add	FFX® (Facet FiXation) implant
Delete	Fosfomycin Anti-infective	Delete	CONTEPO™
		Delete	fosfomycin injection
Delete	Gilteritinib Antineoplastic	Delete	XOSPATA®
Add	Glofitamab Antineoplastic	Add	Columvi™
Delete	Imipenem-cilastatin-relebactam Anti-infective	Delete	IMI/REL
Add	Intraluminal Device, Everolimus-eluting Resorbable Scaffold(s) in New Technology	Add	Drug-eluting resorbable scaffold intraluminal device
		Add	Esprit™ BTK (scaffold) (stent)
		Add	Everolimus Eluting Resorbable Scaffold System
Delete	Intraluminal Device, Sustained Release Drug-eluting in New Technology	Delete	Eluvia™ Drug-Eluting Vascular Stent System
		Delete	SAVAL below-the-knee (BTK) drug-eluting stent system
Delete	Intraluminal Device, Sustained Release Drug-eluting, Four or More in New Technology	Delete	Eluvia™ Drug-Eluting Vascular Stent System
		Delete	SAVAL below-the-knee (BTK) drug-eluting stent system
Delete	Intraluminal Device, Sustained Release Drug-eluting, Three in New Technology	Delete	Eluvia™ Drug-Eluting Vascular Stent System
		Delete	SAVAL below-the-knee (BTK) drug-eluting stent system
Delete	Intraluminal Device, Sustained Release Drug-eluting, Two in New Technology	Delete	Eluvia™ Drug-Eluting Vascular Stent System
		Delete	SAVAL below-the-knee (BTK) drug-eluting stent system

ICD-10-PCS 2025

Section X – New Technology
Device/Substance/Technology Definition (continued)

ICD-10-PCS Value		Definition	
Add	Internal Fixation Device, Gyroid-Sheet Lattice Design in New Technology	Add	restor3d TIDAL™ Fusion Cage
	Lifileucel Immunotherapy	Add	AMTAGVI™
Add	Lovotibeglogene Autotemcel	Add	LYFGENIA™
Add	Marnetegragene Autotemcel	Add	RP-L201
Delete	Meropenem-vaborbactam Anti-infective	Delete	Vabomere™
Add	Multi-plane Flex Technology Bioprosthetic Valve in New Technology	Add	Edwards EVOQUE tricuspid valve replacement system
Add	Non-Chimeric Antigen Receptor T-cell Immune Effector Cell Therapy	Add	T-cell Antigen Coupler T-cell (TAC-T) Therapy
		Add	T-cell Receptor-Engineered T-cell (TCR-T) Therapy
		Add	Tumor-Infiltrating Lymphocyte (TIL) Therapy
Add	Obecabtagene Autoleucel	Add	obe-cel
Add	Omidubicel	Add	Omisirge®
Add	Prademagene Zamikeracel, Genetically Engineered Autologous Cell Therapy in New Technology	Add	EB-101 gene-corrected autologous cell therapy
		Add	EB-101 gene-corrected keratinocyte sheets
		Add	LZRSE-COL7A1 engineered autologous epidermal sheets
		Add	pz-cel
Delete	Ruxolitinib	Delete	Jakafi®
Add	SER-109	Add	VOWST™
Add	Spesolimab Monoclonal Antibody	Add	SPEVIGO®
	Sulbactam-Durlobactam	Add	Xacduro®
	Tabelecleucel Immunotherapy	Add	EBVALLO™
Add	Talquetamab Antineoplastic	Add	TALVEY™
Add	Teclistamab Antineoplastic	Add	TECVAYLI™
Delete	Venetoclax Antineoplastic	Delete	Venclexta®
Add	Vancomycin Hydrochloride and Tobramycin Sulfate Anti-Infective, Temporary Irrigation Spacer System	Add	VT-X7 (Irrigation System) (Spacer)

List of Updated Files

2025 Official ICD-10-PCS Coding Guidelines
- No changes were made to the Guidelines for October 1, 2024.

2025 ICD-10-PCS Code Tables and Index (Zip file)
- Code tables for use beginning October 1, 2024.
- Downloadable PDF, file name is pcs_2025.pdf
- Downloadable xml files for developers, file names are icd10pcs_tables_2025.xml, icd10pcs_index_2025.xml, icd10pcs_definitions_2025.xml
- Accompanying schema for developers, file names are icd10pcs_tables.xsd, icd10pcs_index.xsd, icd10pcs_definitions.xsd

2025 ICD-10-PCS Codes File (Zip file)
- ICD-10-PCS Codes file is a simple format for non-technical uses, containing the valid FY 2025 ICD-10-PCS codes and their long titles.
- File is in text file format, file name is icd10pcs_codes_2025.txt
- Accompanying documentation for codes file, file name is icd10pcsCodesFile.pdf
- Codes file addenda in text format, file name is codes_addenda_2025.txt

2025 ICD-10-PCS Order File (Long and Abbreviated Titles) (Zip file)
- ICD-10-PCS order file is for developers, provides a unique five-digit "order number" for each ICD-10-PCS table and code, as well as a long and abbreviated code title.
- ICD-10-PCS order file name is icd10pcs_order_2025.txt
- Accompanying documentation for tabular order file, file name is icd10pcsOrderFile.pdf
- Tabular order file addenda in text format, file name is order_addenda_2025.txt

2025 ICD-10-PCS Final Addenda (Zip file)
- Addenda files in downloadable PDF, file names are tables_addenda_2025.pdf, index_addenda_2025.pdf, definitions_addenda_2025.pdf
- Addenda files also in machine readable text format for developers, file names are tables_addenda_2025.txt, index_addenda_2025.txt, definitions_addenda_2025.txt

2025 ICD-10-PCS Conversion Table (Zip file)
- ICD-10-PCS code conversion table is provided to assist users in data retrieval, in downloadable Excel spreadsheet, file name is icd10pcs_conversion_table_2025.xlsx
- Conversion table also in machine readable text format for developers, file name is icd10pcs_conversion_table_2025.txt
- Accompanying documentation for code conversion table, file name is icd10pcsConversionTable.pdf

Introduction

ICD-10-PCS: The Complete Official Code Set is your definitive coding resource for procedure coding in acute inpatient hospitals. In addition to the official ICD-10-PCS Coding System Files, revised and distributed by the Centers for Medicare and Medicaid Services (CMS), Optum's coding experts have incorporated Medicare-related coding edits and proprietary features, such as coding tools and appendixes, into a comprehensive and easy-to-use reference.

This manual provides the most current information that was available at the time of publication. For updates to official source documents that may have occurred after this manual was published, please refer to the following:

- **CMS International Classification of Disease, 10th Revision, Procedural Coding System (ICD-10-PCS):**

    https://www.cms.gov/medicare/coding-billing/icd-10-codes/2025-icd-10-pcs

- **CMS Inpatient Prospective Payment System (IPPS) and v42 MS-DRG Data Files, FY 2025**

    https://www.cms.gov/medicare/payment/prospective-payment-systems/acute-inpatient-pps/fy-2025-ipps-proposed-rule-home-page

    https://www.cms.gov/medicare/payment/prospective-payment-systems/acute-inpatient-pps/ms-drg-classifications-and-software

- **American Hospital Association (AHA) Coding Clinics**

    https://www.codingclinicadvisor.com/

ICD-10-PCS Code Structure

All codes in ICD-10-PCS are seven characters long. Each character in the seven-character code represents an aspect of the procedure, as shown in the following diagram of characters from the main section of ICD-10-PCS, called the Medical and Surgical section.

Characters:	1	2	3	4	5	6	7
	Section	Body System	Root Operation	Body Part	Approach	Device	Qualifier

One of 34 possible alphanumeric values—using the digits 0–9 and letters A–H, J–N, and P–Z—can be assigned to each character in a code. The letters O and I are not used so as to avoid confusion with the digits 0 and 1. A code is derived by choosing a specific value for each of the seven characters, based on details about the procedure performed. Because the definition of each character is a function of its physical position in the code, the same value placed in a different position means something different; the value 0 as the first character means something different from 0 as the second character or as the third character, and so on.

The first character always determines the broad procedure category, or section. The second through seventh characters have the same meaning within a specific section, but these meanings can change in a different section. For example, the sixth character means "device" in the Medical and Surgical section but "qualifier" in the Imaging section.

ICD-10-PCS Manual

Index

Codes may be found in the index based on the general type of procedure (e.g., resection, transfusion, fluoroscopy), or a more commonly used term (e.g., appendectomy). For example, the code for percutaneous intraluminal dilation of the coronary arteries with an intraluminal device can be found in the Index under *Dilation*, or a synonym of *Dilation* (e.g., angioplasty). The Index then specifies the first three or four values of the code or directs the user to see another term.

Example:

> **Dilation**
> > Artery
> > > Coronary
> > > > One Artery 0270

Based on the first three values of the code provided in the Index, the corresponding table can be located. In the example above, the first three values indicate table 027 is to be referenced for code completion.

The tables and characters are arranged first by number and then by letter for each character (tables for 00-, 01-, 02-, etc., are followed by those for 0B-, 0C-, 0D-, etc., followed by 0B1, 0B2, etc., followed by 0BB, 0BC, 0BD, etc.).

Note: The Tables section must be used to construct a complete and valid code by specifying the last three or four values.

Tables

The tables in ICD-10-PCS provide the valid combination of character values needed to build a unique procedure code. Each table is preceded by the first three characters of the code, along with their descriptions. In the Medical and Surgical section, for example, the first three characters contain the name of the section (character 1), the body system (character 2), and the root operation performed (character 3).

Listed underneath the first three characters is a table comprising four columns and one or more rows. The four columns in the table specify the last four characters needed to complete the ICD-10-PCS code. Depending on the section, the labels for each column may be different. In the Medical and Surgical section, they are labeled body part (character 4), approach (character 5), device (character 6), and qualifier (character 7). Each row in the table specifies the valid combination of values for characters 4 through 7.

Introduction

Table 1: Row from table 027

0 Medical and Surgical
2 Heart and Great Vessels
7 Dilation   **Definition:** Expanding an orifice or the lumen of a tubular body part
                        Explanation: The orifice can be a natural orifice or an artificially created orifice. Accomplished by stretching a tubular body part using intraluminal pressure or by cutting part of the orifice or wall of the tubular body part.

Body Part Character 4	Approach Character 5	Device Character 6	Qualifier Character 7
0 Coronary Artery, One Artery 1 Coronary Artery, Two Arteries 2 Coronary Artery, Three Arteries 3 Coronary Artery, Four or More Arteries	0 Open 3 Percutaneous 4 Percutaneous Endoscopic	4 Intraluminal Device, Drug-eluting 5 Intraluminal Device, Drug-eluting, Two 6 Intraluminal Device, Drug-eluting, Three 7 Intraluminal Device, Drug-eluting, Four or More D Intraluminal Device E Intraluminal Device, Two F Intraluminal Device, Three G Intraluminal Device, Four or More T Intraluminal Device, Radioactive Z No Device	6 Bifurcation Z No Qualifier

For instance, table 1 above shows the first row from table 027 in ICD-10-PCS. The values 027 specify the section *Medical and Surgical (0)*, the body system *Heart and Great Vessels (2)*, and the root operation *Dilation (7)*. As shown, the root operation (Dilation) is also accompanied by its corresponding definition and explanation. Note, a definition of the root operation is provided for every table in ICD-10-PCS; however, an explanation may not always be applicable.

In total, this single row can be used to construct 240 unique procedure codes. The valid codes shown in table 2 (below) are constructed using the body part (character 4) value of 0, Coronary artery, one artery, combined with all valid approach (character 5) values, device (character 6) values, and a qualifier (character 7) value of Z, No Qualifier.

Table 2: Code titles for dilation of one coronary artery (0270)

Code	Title
027004Z	Dilation of Coronary Artery, One Artery with Drug-eluting Intraluminal Device, Open Approach
027005Z	Dilation of Coronary Artery, One Artery with Two Drug-eluting Intraluminal Devices, Open Approach
027006Z	Dilation of Coronary Artery, One Artery with Three Drug-eluting Intraluminal Devices, Open Approach
027007Z	Dilation of Coronary Artery, One Artery with Four or More Drug-eluting Intraluminal Devices, Open Approach
02700DZ	Dilation of Coronary Artery, One Artery with Intraluminal Device, Open Approach
02700EZ	Dilation of Coronary Artery, One Artery with Two Intraluminal Devices, Open Approach
02700FZ	Dilation of Coronary Artery, One Artery with Three Intraluminal Devices, Open Approach
02700GZ	Dilation of Coronary Artery, One Artery with Four or More Intraluminal Devices, Open Approach
02700TZ	Dilation of Coronary Artery, One Artery with Radioactive Intraluminal Device, Open Approach
02700ZZ	Dilation of Coronary Artery, One Artery, Open Approach
027034Z	Dilation of Coronary Artery, One Artery with Drug-eluting Intraluminal Device, Percutaneous Approach
027035Z	Dilation of Coronary Artery, One Artery with Two Drug-eluting Intraluminal Devices, Percutaneous Approach
027036Z	Dilation of Coronary Artery, One Artery with Three Drug-eluting Intraluminal Devices, Percutaneous Approach
027037Z	Dilation of Coronary Artery, One Artery with Four or More Drug-eluting Intraluminal Devices, Percutaneous Approach
02703DZ	Dilation of Coronary Artery, One Artery with Intraluminal Device, Percutaneous Approach
02703EZ	Dilation of Coronary Artery, One Artery with Two Intraluminal Devices, Percutaneous Approach
02703FZ	Dilation of Coronary Artery, One Artery with Three Intraluminal Devices, Percutaneous Approach
02703GZ	Dilation of Coronary Artery, One Artery with Four or More Intraluminal Devices, Percutaneous Approach
02703TZ	Dilation of Coronary Artery, One Artery with Radioactive Intraluminal Device, Percutaneous Approach
02703ZZ	Dilation of Coronary Artery, One Artery, Percutaneous Approach
027044Z	Dilation of Coronary Artery, One Artery with Drug-eluting Intraluminal Device, Percutaneous Endoscopic Approach
027045Z	Dilation of Coronary Artery, One Artery with Two Drug-eluting Intraluminal Devices, Percutaneous Endoscopic Approach
027046Z	Dilation of Coronary Artery, One Artery with Three Drug-eluting Intraluminal Devices, Percutaneous Endoscopic Approach
027047Z	Dilation of Coronary Artery, One Artery with Four or More Drug-eluting Intraluminal Devices, Percutaneous Endoscopic Approach
02704DZ	Dilation of Coronary Artery, One Artery with Intraluminal Device, Percutaneous Endoscopic Approach
02704EZ	Dilation of Coronary Artery, One Artery with Two Intraluminal Devices, Percutaneous Endoscopic Approach
02704FZ	Dilation of Coronary Artery, One Artery with Three Intraluminal Devices, Percutaneous Endoscopic Approach
02704GZ	Dilation of Coronary Artery, One Artery with Four or More Intraluminal Devices, Percutaneous Endoscopic Approach
02704TZ	Dilation of Coronary Artery, One Artery with Radioactive Intraluminal Device, Percutaneous Endoscopic Approach
02704ZZ	Dilation of Coronary Artery, One Artery, Percutaneous Endoscopic Approach

Table 3: Rows from table 00H

0 Medical and Surgical
0 Central Nervous System and Cranial Nerves
H Insertion Definition: Putting in a nonbiological appliance that monitors, assists, performs, or prevents a physiological function but does not physically take the place of a body part
Explanation: None

Body Part Character 4	Approach Character 5	Device Character 6	Qualifier Character 7

0 Brain
  Cerebrum
  Corpus callosum
  Encephalon
	0 Open	**1** Radioactive Element
		2 Monitoring Device
		3 Infusion Device
		4 Radioactive Element, Cesium-131 Collagen Implant
		5 Radioactive Element Palladium-103 Collagen Implant
		M Neurostimulator Lead
		Y Other Device
			Z No Qualifier

0 Brain
  Cerebrum
  Corpus callosum
  Encephalon
	3 Percutaneous
	4 Percutaneous Endoscopic
		1 Radioactive Element
		2 Monitoring Device
		3 Infusion Device
		M Neurostimulator Lead
		Y Other Device
			Z No Qualifier

6 Cerebral Ventricle
  Aqueduct of Sylvius
  Cerebral aqueduct (Sylvius)
  Choroid plexus
  Ependyma
  Foramen of Monro (intraventricular)
  Fourth ventricle
  Interventricular foramen (Monro)
  Left lateral ventricle
  Right lateral ventricle
  Third ventricle
E Cranial Nerve
U Spinal Canal
  Epidural space, spinal
  Extradural space, spinal
  Subarachnoid space, spinal
  Subdural space, spinal
  Vertebral canal
V Spinal Cord
  Dorsal root ganglion
	0 Open
	3 Percutaneous
	4 Percutaneous Endoscopic
		1 Radioactive Element
		2 Monitoring Device
		3 Infusion Device
		M Neurostimulator Lead
		Y Other Device
			Z No Qualifier

Table 3 is split into three rows; values of characters must all be selected from within the same row of the table. Rows 1 and 2 have the same body part (character 4) value of 0 Brain and the same qualifier value (character 7) of Z No Qualifier. However, the approach (character 5) values and the device (character 6) values are not the same for these two rows. As shown in row 1, body part value Brain (0) with device value Radioactive Element, Cesium-131 Collagen Implant (4) can only be used with approach value Open (0). In other words, code 00H034Z would be invalid as the approach value 3 is only applicable to row 2 and the device value 4 is only applicable to row 1. It would be inappropriate to build a code for body part 0 if all of the values are not contained in its own row.

Note: In this manual, there are instances in which some tables due to length must be continued on the next page. Each section must be used separately and value selection must be made within the same row of the table.

Character Meanings

In each section, each character has a specific meaning, and this character meaning remains constant within that section. Character meaning tables have been provided at the beginning of each body system in the Medical and Surgical section (0) and the Obstetric section (1) to help the user identify the character members available within that section. These tables have purple headers, unlike the official code tables that have green headers and **SHOULD NOT** be used to build a PCS code. Table 4 provides an excerpt of a character meaning table.

Introduction

ICD-10-PCS 2025

Table 4: Rows from Central Nervous System and Cranial Nerves - Character Meanings Table

Operation–Character 3	Body Part–Character 4	Approach–Character 5	Device–Character 6	Qualifier–Character 7
1 Bypass	0 Brain	0 Open	0 Drainage Device	0 Nasopharynx
2 Change	1 Cerebral Meninges	3 Percutaneous	1 Radioactive Element	1 Mastoid Sinus
5 Destruction	2 Dura Mater	4 Percutaneous Endoscopic	2 Monitoring Device	2 Atrium
7 Dilation	3 Epidural Space, Intracranial	X External	3 Infusion Device	3 Blood Vessel
8 Division	4 Subdural Space, Intracranial		4 Radioactive Element, Cesium-131 Collagen Implant	4 Pleural Cavity
9 Drainage	5 Subarachnoid Space, Intracranial		5 Radioactive Element, Palladium-103 Collagen Implant	5 Intestine
B Excision	6 Cerebral Ventricle		7 Autologous Tissue Substitute	6 Peritoneal Cavity
C Extirpation	7 Cerebral Hemisphere		J Synthetic Substitute	7 Urinary Tract
D Extraction	8 Basal Ganglia		K Nonautologous Tissue Substitute	8 Bone Marrow
F Fragmentation	9 Thalamus		M Neurostimulator Lead	9 Fallopian Tube
H Insertion	A Hypothalamus		Y Other Device	A Subgaleal space
J Inspection	B Pons		Z No Device	B Cerebral Cisterns

Sections

The first character of the procedure code always specifies the section. There are 17 sections within the PCS manual, listed below.

Medical and Surgical Section
- 0   Medical and Surgical

Medical and Surgical-related Sections
- 1   Obstetrics
- 2   Placement
- 3   Administration
- 4   Measurement and Monitoring
- 5   Extracorporeal or Systemic Assistance and Performance
- 6   Extracorporeal or Systemic Therapies
- 7   Osteopathic
- 8   Other Procedures
- 9   Chiropractic

Ancillary Sections
- B   Imaging
- C   Nuclear Medicine
- D   Radiation Therapy
- F   Physical Rehabilitation and Diagnostic Audiology
- G   Mental Health
- H   Substance Abuse Treatment

New Technology Section
- X   New Technology

Medical and Surgical Section (0)

The Medical and Surgical section contains codes for the vast majority of procedures typically reported in an inpatient setting.

Character Meaning

The seven characters for Medical and Surgical procedures have the following meaning:

Character	Meaning
1	Section
2	Body System
3	Root Operation
4	Body Part
5	Approach
6	Device
7	Qualifier

Section (Character 1)

Medical and Surgical procedure codes all have a first character value of 0.

Body Systems (Character 2)

The second character represents the body system—the general physiological system or anatomical region where the procedure is being performed.

Body Systems
- 0   Central Nervous System and Cranial Nerves
- 1   Peripheral Nervous System
- 2   Heart and Great Vessels
- 3   Upper Arteries
- 4   Lower Arteries
- 5   Upper Veins
- 6   Lower Veins
- 7   Lymphatic and Hemic Systems
- 8   Eye
- 9   Ear, Nose, Sinus

B	Respiratory System
C	Mouth and Throat
D	Gastrointestinal System
F	Hepatobiliary System and Pancreas
G	Endocrine System
H	Skin and Breast
J	Subcutaneous Tissue and Fascia
K	Muscles
L	Tendons
M	Bursae and Ligaments
N	Head and Facial Bones
P	Upper Bones
Q	Lower Bones
R	Upper Joints
S	Lower Joints
T	Urinary System
U	Female Reproductive System
V	Male Reproductive System
W	Anatomical Regions, General
X	Anatomical Regions, Upper Extremities
Y	Anatomical Regions, Lower Extremities

Root Operations (Character 3)

The third character represents the root operation, or the primary objective, of the procedure. There are 31 different root operations in this section, each with its own precise definition.

- *Alteration:* Modifying the natural anatomic structure of a body part without affecting the function of the body part
- *Bypass:* Altering the route of passage of the contents of a tubular body part
- *Change:* Taking out or off a device from a body part and putting back an identical or similar device in or on the same body part without cutting or puncturing the skin or a mucous membrane
- *Control:* Stopping, or attempting to stop, postprocedural or other acute bleeding
- *Creation:* Putting in or on biological or synthetic material to form a new body part that to the extent possible replicates the anatomic structure or function of an absent body part
- *Destruction:* Physical eradication of all or a portion of a body part by the direct use of energy, force, or a destructive agent
- *Detachment:* Cutting off all or a portion of the upper or lower extremities
- *Dilation:* Expanding an orifice or the lumen of a tubular body part
- *Division:* Cutting into a body part without draining fluids and/or gases from the body part in order to separate or transect a body part
- *Drainage:* Taking or letting out fluids and/or gases from a body part
- *Excision:* Cutting out or off, without replacement, a portion of a body part
- *Extirpation:* Taking or cutting out solid matter from a body part

- *Extraction:* Pulling or stripping out or off all or a portion of a body part by the use of force
- *Fragmentation:* Breaking solid matter in a body part into pieces
- *Fusion:* Joining together portions of an articular body part rendering the articular body part immobile
- *Insertion:* Putting in a nonbiological appliance that monitors, assists, performs, or prevents a physiological function but does not physically take the place of a body part
- *Inspection:* Visually and/or manually exploring a body part
- *Map:* Locating the route of passage of electrical impulses and/or locating functional areas in a body part
- *Occlusion:* Completely closing an orifice or lumen of a tubular body part
- *Reattachment:* Putting back in or on all or a portion of a separated body part to its normal location or other suitable location
- *Release:* Freeing a body part from an abnormal physical constraint by cutting or by use of force
- *Removal:* Taking out or off a device from a body part
- *Repair:* Restoring, to the extent possible, a body part to its normal anatomic structure and function
- *Replacement:* Putting in or on biological or synthetic material that physically takes the place and/or function of all or a portion of a body part
- *Reposition:* Moving to its normal location or other suitable location all or a portion of a body part
- *Resection:* Cutting out or off, without replacement, all of a body part
- *Restriction:* Partially closing an orifice or lumen of a tubular body part
- *Revision:* Correcting, to the extent possible, a portion of a malfunctioning device or the position of a displaced device
- *Supplement:* Putting in or on biological or synthetic material that physically reinforces and/or augments the function of a portion of a body part
- *Transfer:* Moving, without taking out, all or a portion of a body part to another location to take over the function of all or a portion of a body part
- *Transplantation:* Putting in or on all or a portion of a living body part taken from another individual or animal to physically take the place and/or function of all or a portion of a similar body part

The standardized level of specificity designed into ICD-10-PCS restricts the use of broadly applicable "not otherwise specified (NOS)" or "unspecified code" options in the system. A minimal level of specificity is required to construct a valid code. "Not elsewhere classified (NEC)" options are provided in ICD-10-PCS but only for specific, limited use. The root operation Repair in the Medical and Surgical section functions as a "not elsewhere classified" option. Repair is used only when the procedure performed is not one of the other specific root operations in the Medical and Surgical section.

Appendixes B and C provide additional subcategorization, explanations, and representative examples of the Medical and Surgical section root operations.

Body Part (Character 4)
The fourth character represents the body part, or specific anatomical site where the procedure was performed. The body system (second character) provides only a general indication of the procedure site. The body part and body system values, together, provide a precise description of the procedure site.

Approach (Character 5)
The fifth character represents the approach, or the technique used to reach the procedure site. There are seven different approach values in this section.

- *Open*: Cutting through the skin or mucous membrane and any other body layers necessary to expose the site of the procedure
- *Percutaneous*: Entry, by puncture or minor incision, of instrumentation through the skin or mucous membrane and any other body layers necessary to reach the site of the procedure
- *Percutaneous Endoscopic*: Entry, by puncture or minor incision, of instrumentation through the skin or mucous membrane and any other body layers necessary to reach and visualize the site of the procedure
- *Via Natural or Artificial Opening*: Entry of instrumentation through a natural or artificial external opening to reach the site of the procedure
- *Via Natural or Artificial Opening Endoscopic*: Entry of instrumentation through a natural or artificial external opening to reach and visualize the site of the procedure
- *Via Natural or Artificial Opening with Percutaneous Endoscopic Assistance:* Entry of instrumentation through a natural or artificial external opening and entry, by puncture or minor incision, of instrumentation through the skin or mucous membrane and any other body layers necessary to aid in the performance of the procedure
- *External*: Procedures performed directly on the skin or mucous membrane and procedures performed indirectly by the application of external force through the skin or mucous membrane

Appendix A provides definitions and comparisons of the components (access location, method, and type of instrumentation) for each approach and provides an example and illustration.

Device (Character 6)
The sixth character represents a device. Broad categories of devices found in this section include:

- Grafts (e.g., skin)
- Prostheses (e.g., hip joint)
- Implants (e.g., internal fixation device, mesh)
- Simple or Mechanical Appliances (e.g., drainage device, IUD)
- Electronic Appliances (e.g., pacemaker, monitoring device)

Depending on the procedure performed, there may or may not be a device left in place at the end of the procedure. For procedures that do not utilize a device, the value of *No Device* is available. For devices that cannot be categorized into one of the current values, many tables also have a device value of *Other Device*. This value is intended to be used temporarily until a more specific value can be added to the classification. No categories of medical or surgical devices are permanently classified to *Other Device*.

Instruments used to visualize the procedure site are specified in the fifth-character approach, not the sixth-character device value. Materials that are incidental to a procedure such as clips, ligatures, and sutures are not specified in the device character.

Appendix F compares the general device types and provides examples of each.

Appendix G provides an aggregation table that crosswalks specific device character values used for specific root operations to more general device character values used when the root operation represents an entire family of devices.

Qualifier (Character 7)
The seventh character is a qualifier that captures additional attributes of the procedure, where applicable.

Medical and Surgical Section Principles
In developing the Medical and Surgical procedure codes, several specific principles were followed.

Composite Terms Are Not Root Operations
Composite terms such as colonoscopy, sigmoidectomy, or appendectomy do not describe root operations, but they do specify multiple components of a specific root operation. In ICD-10-PCS, the components of a procedure are defined separately by the characters making up the complete code. The only component of a procedure specified in the root operation is the objective of the procedure. With each complete code the underlying objective of the procedure is specified by the root operation (third character), the precise part is specified by the body part (fourth character), and the method used to reach and visualize the procedure site is specified by the approach (fifth character). While colonoscopy, sigmoidectomy, and appendectomy are included in the Index, they do not constitute root operations in the Tables section. The objective of colonoscopy is the visualization of the colon and the root operation (character 3) is *Inspection*. Character 4 specifies the body part, which in this case is part of the colon. These composite terms, like colonoscopy or appendectomy, are included as cross-reference only. The index provides the correct root operation reference. Examples of other types of composite terms not representative of root operations are *partial* sigmoidectomy, *total* hysterectomy, and *partial* hip replacement. Always refer to the correct root operation in the Index and Tables section.

Root Operation Based on Objective of Procedure
The root operation is based on the objective of the procedure, such as *Resection* of transverse colon or *Dilation* of an artery. The assignment of the root operation is based on the procedure actually performed, which may or may not have been the intended procedure. If the intended procedure is modified or discontinued (e.g., excision instead of resection is performed), the root operation is determined by the procedure actually performed. If the desired result is not attained after completing the procedure (i.e., the artery does not remain expanded after the dilation procedure), the root operation is still determined by the procedure actually performed.

Examples:

- Dilating the urethra is coded as *Dilation* since the objective of the procedure is to dilate the urethra. If dilation of the urethra includes putting in an intraluminal stent, the root operation remains *Dilation* and not *Insertion* of the intraluminal device because the underlying objective of the procedure is dilation of the urethra. The stent is identified by the intraluminal device value in the sixth character of the dilation procedure code.

- If the objective is solely to put a radioactive element in the urethra, then the procedure is coded to the root operation *Insertion*, with the radioactive element identified in the sixth character of the code.
- If the objective of the procedure is to correct a malfunctioning or displaced device, then the procedure is coded to the root operation *Revision*. In the root operation *Revision*, the original device being revised is identified in the device character. *Revision* is typically performed on mechanical appliances (e.g., pacemaker) or materials used in replacement procedures (e.g., synthetic substitute). Typical revision procedures include adjustment of pacemaker position and correction of malfunctioning knee prosthesis.

Combination Procedures Are Coded Separately

If multiple procedures as defined by distinct objectives are performed during an operative episode, then multiple codes are used. For example, obtaining the vein graft used for coronary bypass surgery is coded as a separate procedure from the bypass itself.

Redo of Procedures

The complete or partial redo of the original procedure is coded to the root operation that identifies the procedure performed rather than *Revision*.

Example:

> A complete redo of a hip replacement procedure that requires putting in a new prosthesis is coded to the root operation *Replacement* rather than *Revision*.

The correction of complications arising from the original procedure, other than device complications, is coded to the procedure performed. Correction of a malfunctioning or displaced device would be coded to the root operation *Revision*.

Example:

> A procedure to control hemorrhage arising from the original procedure is coded to *Control* rather than *Revision*.

Examples of Procedures Coded in the Medical Surgical Section

The following are examples of procedures from the Medical and Surgical section, coded in ICD-10-PCS.

- Suture of skin laceration, left lower arm: 0HQEXZZ
- Laparoscopic appendectomy: 0DTJ4ZZ
- Sigmoidoscopy with biopsy: 0DBN8ZX
- Tracheostomy with tracheostomy tube: 0B110F4

Obstetrics Section (1)

The Obstetrics section includes codes for procedures performed on the products of conception only. Procedures on pregnant females are coded in the Medical and Surgical section (e.g., episiotomy). The term "products of conception" refers to all physical components of a pregnancy, including the fetus, amnion, umbilical cord, and placenta. There is no differentiation of the products of conception based on gestational age. Thus, the diagnosis code, not the procedure code, specifies the products of conception as a zygote, embryo, or fetus, or of the trimester of the pregnancy.

Character Meanings

The seven characters in the Obstetrics section have the same meaning as in the Medical and Surgical section.

Character	Meaning
1	Section
2	Body System
3	Root Operation
4	Body Part
5	Approach
6	Device
7	Qualifier

Section (Character 1)
Obstetrics procedure codes have a first character value of *1*.

Body System (Character 2)
The second character represents the body system. There is only one value used in this section: *Pregnancy*.

Root Operation (Character 3)
The third character represents the root operation, or the primary objective, of the procedure. There are 12 values available in this section. Ten of these values specify root operations as defined in the Medical and Surgical section and include *Change, Drainage, Extraction, Insertion, Inspection, Removal, Repair, Reposition, Resection,* and *Transplantation*. The other two values are specific to this section only and are defined as follows:

- *Abortion*: Artificially terminating a pregnancy
- *Delivery*: Assisting the passage of the products of conception from the genital canal

A cesarean section is not a separate root operation because the underlying objective is *Extraction* (i.e., pulling out all or a portion of a body part).

Body Part (Character 4)
The fourth character represents the body part, which in this section is specific to the products of conception. The three values available are as follows:

- *Products of conception*
- *Products of conception, retained*
- *Products of conception, ectopic*

Approach (Character 5)
The fifth character represents the approach, as defined in the Medical and Surgical section.

Device (Character 6)
The sixth character represents a device used during the procedure, where applicable.

Qualifier (Character 7)
The seventh character is a qualifier that captures additional attributes of the procedure, where applicable.

Placement Section (2)

The Placement section includes codes for procedures that put a device in an orifice or on a body region, without making an incision or a puncture.

Character Meanings

The seven characters in the Placement section have the following meaning:

Character	Meaning
1	Section
2	Body System
3	Root Operation
4	Body Region
5	Approach
6	Device
7	Qualifier

Section (Character 1)

Placement procedure codes have a first character value of *2*.

Body System (Character 2)

The second character contains two values specifying either *Anatomical Regions* or *Anatomical Orifices*.

Root Operation (Character 3)

The third character represents the root operation, or the primary objective, of the procedure. There are seven values available in this section. Two of the values specify root operations as defined in the Medical and Surgical section and include *Change* and *Removal*. The other five values are specific to this section only and are defined as follows:

- *Compression*: Putting pressure on a body region
- *Dressing*: Putting material on a body region for protection
- *Immobilization*: Limiting or preventing motion of an external body region
- *Packing*: Putting material in a body region or orifice
- *Traction*: Exerting a pulling force on a body region in a distal direction

Body Region (Character 4)

The fourth character represents the specific body region or orifice. The body system (second character) provides only a general indication of the procedure site. The body region values and body system values, together, precisely describe the procedure site.

Approach (Character 5)

The fifth character represents the approach. Since all placement procedures are performed directly or indirectly on the skin or mucous membrane, the approach value is always *External*.

Device (Character 6)

The sixth character represents a device placed during the procedure, where applicable.

Except for devices used for fractures and dislocations, devices in this section are off the shelf and do not require any extensive design, fabrication, or fitting.

Qualifier (Character 7)

The seventh character is a qualifier. Because there are currently no specific qualifier values in this section, the value is always *No Qualifier*.

Administration Section (3)

The Administration section includes infusions, injections, and transfusions, as well as other related procedures, such as irrigation and tattooing. All codes in this section define procedures in which a diagnostic or therapeutic substance is given to the patient.

Character Meanings

The seven characters in the Administration section have the following meaning:

Character	Meaning
1	Section
2	Body System
3	Root Operation
4	Body System/Region
5	Approach
6	Substance
7	Qualifier

Section (Character 1)

Administration procedure codes have a first character value of *3*.

Body System (Character 2)

The second character can represent the general physiological system, anatomical region, or device to which a substance is being administered. The three values available in this section are *Indwelling Device, Physiological Systems and Anatomical Regions,* and *Circulatory System*.

Root Operation (Character 3)

The third character represents the root operation, or the primary objective, of the procedure. There are three values available in this section.

- *Introduction*: Putting in or on a therapeutic, diagnostic, nutritional, physiological, or prophylactic substance except blood or blood products
- *Irrigation*: Putting in or on a cleansing substance
- *Transfusion*: Putting in blood or blood products

Body/System Region (Character 4)

The fourth character represents the body system/region. The fourth character identifies the site where the substance is administered, not the site where the substance administered takes effect. Sites include *Skin and Mucous Membranes, Subcutaneous Tissue,* and *Muscle*. These differentiate intradermal, subcutaneous, and intramuscular injections, respectively. Other sites include *Eye, Respiratory Tract, Peritoneal Cavity,* and *Epidural Space*.

The body systems/regions for arteries and veins are *Peripheral Artery, Central Artery, Peripheral Vein,* and *Central Vein*. The *Peripheral Artery* or *Vein* is typically used when a substance is introduced locally into an artery or vein. For example, chemotherapy is the introduction of an antineoplastic substance into a peripheral artery or vein by a percutaneous approach. In general, the substance introduced into a peripheral artery or vein has a systemic effect.

The *Central Artery* or *Vein* is typically used when the site where the substance is introduced is distant from the point of entry into the artery or vein. For example, the introduction of a substance directly at the site of a clot within an artery or vein using a catheter is coded as an introduction of a thrombolytic substance into a central artery or vein by a percutaneous approach. In general, the substance introduced into a central artery or vein has a local effect.

Approach (Character 5)
The fifth character represents the approach, as defined in the Medical and Surgical section. The approach for intradermal, subcutaneous, and intramuscular introductions (i.e., injections) is *Percutaneous*. If a catheter is placed to introduce a substance into an internal site within the circulatory system, then the approach is also *Percutaneous*. For example, if a catheter is used to introduce contrast directly into the heart for angiography, then the procedure would be coded as a percutaneous introduction of contrast into the heart.

Substance (Character 6)
The sixth character represents the substance being introduced. Most of the values capture broad categories of substances to which several specific substances may be categorized.

Qualifier (Character 7)
The seventh character is a qualifier. The substance value (second character) provides the broad category to which a substance is classified. The qualifier and substance values, together, precisely describe the substance administered. Not every substance administered has its own unique qualifier.

Measurement and Monitoring Section (4)
The Measurement and Monitoring section represents procedures for determining the level of a physiological or physical function.

Character Meanings
The seven characters in the Measurement and Monitoring section have the following meaning:

Character	Meaning
1	Section
2	Body System
3	Root Operation
4	Body System
5	Approach
6	Function/Device
7	Qualifier

Section (Character 1)
Measurement and Monitoring procedure codes have a first character value of *4*.

Body System (Character 2)
The second character represents the body system or device being measured or monitored. There are two values available in this section, *Physiological Systems* and *Physiological Devices*.

Root Operation (Character 3)
The third character represents the root operation, or the primary objective, of the procedure. There are two values available in this section.

- *Measurement*: Determining the level of a physiological or physical function at a point in time
- *Monitoring*: Determining the level of a physiological or physical function repetitively over a period of time

Body System (Character 4)
The fourth character represents the specific body system measured or monitored.

Approach (Character 5)
The fifth character represents the approach, as defined in the Medical and Surgical section.

Function/Device (Character 6)
The sixth character represents the physiological or physical function, or the device function being measured or monitored.

Qualifier (Character 7)
The seventh character is a qualifier, which captures additional attributes of the procedure, where applicable.

Extracorporeal or Systemic Assistance and Performance Section (5)
The Extracorporeal or Systemic Assistance and Performance section describes procedures performed in a critical care setting, such as mechanical ventilation and cardioversion. It also includes other procedures, such as hemodialysis and hyperbaric oxygen treatment.

The procedures described in this section are meant to be temporary; that is, the equipment is used only for the duration of the procedure. The equipment resides primarily outside the body, though it may interface with the body via a tube or other means. Although parts of the equipment may be attached or inserted into the patient, such as lines or catheters, these are not coded as separate device insertion procedures.

Character Meanings
The seven characters in the Extracorporeal or Systemic Assistance and Performance section have the following meaning:

Character	Meaning
1	Section
2	Body System
3	Root Operation
4	Body System
5	Duration
6	Function
7	Qualifier

Section (Character 1)
Extracorporeal or Systemic Assistance and Performance procedure codes have a first character value of *5*.

Body System (Character 2)
The second character represents the body system. There is one value available in this section, *Physiological Systems*.

Root Operation (Character 3)
The third character represents the root operation, or the primary objective, of the procedure. There are three values available in this section.

- *Assistance*: Taking over a portion of a physiological function by extracorporeal means
- *Performance*: Completely taking over a physiological function by extracorporeal means
- *Restoration*: Returning, or attempting to return, a physiological function to its natural state by extracorporeal means

The root operation *Restoration* contains a single procedure code that identifies extracorporeal cardioversion.

Body System (Character 4)
The fourth character represents the body system for which support of a physiological function is required.

Duration (Character 5)
The fifth character specifies the duration of the procedure.

Function (Character 6)
The sixth character represents the physiological function assisted or performed (e.g., oxygenation, ventilation) during the procedure.

Qualifier (Character 7)
The seventh character is a qualifier, which captures additional attributes of the procedure, where applicable, such as the type of equipment used to support or assist a physiological function.

Extracorporeal or Systemic Therapies Section (6)
The Extracorporeal or Systemic Therapies section describes procedures in which equipment outside the body is used for a therapeutic purpose that does not involve the assistance or performance of a physiological function. For procedures such as hypothermia, for which the therapy is not applied to a specific body system but the entire body, a fourth character for *None* is used.

Character Meanings
The seven characters in the Extracorporeal or Systemic Therapies section have the following meaning:

Character	Meaning
1	Section
2	Body System
3	Root Operation
4	Body System
5	Duration
6	Qualifier
7	Qualifier

Section (Character 1)
Extracorporeal or Systemic Therapy procedure codes have a first character value of *6*.

Body System (Character 2)
The second character represents the body system. There is one value available in this section, *Physiological Systems*.

Root Operation (Character 3)
The third character represents the root operation, or the primary objective, of the procedure. There are 11 values available in this section.

- *Atmospheric Control*: Extracorporeal control of atmospheric pressure and composition
- *Decompression*: Extracorporeal elimination of undissolved gas from body fluids

  Decompression involves only one type of procedure: treatment for decompression sickness (the bends) in a hyperbaric chamber.

- *Electromagnetic Therapy*: Extracorporeal treatment by electromagnetic rays
- *Hyperthermia*: Extracorporeal raising of body temperature

  The term hyperthermia is used to describe both a temperature imbalance treatment and also as an adjunct radiation treatment for cancer. When treating the temperature imbalance, it is coded to this section; for the cancer treatment, it is coded in the Radiation Therapy section.

- *Hypothermia*: Extracorporeal lowering of body temperature
- *Perfusion*: Extracorporeal treatment by diffusion of therapeutic fluid
- *Pheresis*: Extracorporeal separation of blood products

  Pheresis may be used for two main purposes: to treat diseases when too much of a blood component is produced (e.g., leukemia) and to remove a blood product such as platelets from a donor, for transfusion into another patient.

- *Phototherapy*: Extracorporeal treatment by light rays

  Phototherapy involves using a machine that exposes the blood to light rays outside the body, recirculates it, and then returns it to the body.

- *Shock Wave Therapy*: Extracorporeal treatment by shock waves
- *Ultrasound Therapy*: Extracorporeal treatment by ultrasound
- *Ultraviolet Light Therapy*: Extracorporeal treatment by ultraviolet light

Body System (Character 4)
The fourth character represents the body system on which the extracorporeal or systemic therapy is performed (e.g., skin, circulatory).

Duration (Character 5)
The fifth character specifies the duration of the procedure. There are two values available in this section, *Single* or *Multiple*.

Qualifier (Characters 6 and 7)
The sixth and seventh characters are qualifiers. The qualifier captures additional attributes of the procedure, where applicable.

Osteopathic Section (7)

Character Meanings
The seven characters in the Osteopathic section have the following meaning:

Character	Meaning
1	Section
2	Body System
3	Root Operation
4	Body Region
5	Approach
6	Method
7	Qualifier

Section (Character 1)
Osteopathic procedure codes have a first character value of *7*.

Body System (Character 2)
The second character represents the body system. There is one value available in this section, *Anatomical Regions*.

Root Operation (Character 3)
The third character represents the root operation, or the primary objective, of the procedure. There is one value available in this section.

- *Treatment*: Manual treatment to eliminate or alleviate somatic dysfunction and related disorders

Body Region (Character 4)
The fourth character represents the body region. The body system (second character) indicates only the anatomical region involved in the procedure. The body region values and body system value, together, precisely describe the procedure site.

Approach (Character 5)
The fifth character represents the approach. There is only one value available in this section, *External*.

Method (Character 6)
The sixth character represents the method used to carry out the osteopathic treatment.

Qualifier (Character 7)
The seventh character is a qualifier. Because there are currently no specific qualifier values in this section, the value is always *None*.

Other Procedures Section (8)
The Other Procedures section contains codes for procedures not included in the other medical and surgical-related sections, including computer- and robotic-assisted procedures.

Character Meanings
The seven characters in the Other Procedures section have the following meaning:

Character	Meaning
1	Section
2	Body System
3	Root Operation
4	Body Region
5	Approach
6	Method
7	Qualifier

Section (Character 1)
Other Procedures section codes have a first character value of *8*.

Body System (Character 2)
The second character represents the body system/region or a device. There are two values available in this section, *Physiological Systems and Anatomical Regions* and *Indwelling Device*.

Root Operation (Character 3)
The third character represents the root operation, or the primary objective, of the procedure. There is one value available in this section.

- *Other Procedures*: Methodologies that attempt to remediate or cure a disorder or disease.

Body Region (Character 4)
The fourth character contains specified body-region values, and also the body-region value *None*.

Approach (Character 5)
The fifth character represents the approach, as defined in the Medical and Surgical section.

Method (Character 6)
The sixth character specifies the method (e.g., *Acupuncture, Therapeutic Massage*).

Qualifier (Character 7)
The seventh character is a qualifier. The qualifier is used to capture additional attributes of the procedure, where applicable.

Chiropractic Section (9)

Character Meanings
The seven characters in the Chiropractic section have the following meaning:

Character	Meaning
1	Section
2	Body System
3	Root Operation
4	Body Region
5	Approach
6	Method
7	Qualifier

Introduction

Section (Character 1)
Chiropractic section procedure codes have a first character value of 9.

Body System (Character 2)
The second character represents the body region. There is one value available in this section, *Anatomical Regions*.

Root Operation (Character 3)
The third character represents the root operation, or the primary objective, of the procedure. There is one value available in this section.

- *Manipulation:* Manual procedure that involves a directed thrust to move a joint past the physiological range of motion, without exceeding the anatomical limit.

Body Region (Character 4)
The fourth character represents the body region on which the chiropractic manipulation is performed.

Approach (Character 5)
The fifth character represents the approach. There is only one value available in this section, *External*.

Method (Character 6)
The sixth character represents the method by which the manipulation is accomplished.

Qualifier (Character 7)
The seventh character is a qualifier. Because there are currently no specific qualifier values in this section, the value is always *None*.

Imaging Section (B)
The Imaging section contains codes for procedures such as plain radiography, fluoroscopy, CT, MRI, and ultrasound.

Procedures such as PET, uptakes, and scans are in the Nuclear Medicine section. Therapeutic radiation, for the treatment of cancer, is in the Radiation Therapy section.

Character Meanings
The seven characters in Imaging procedures have the following meaning:

Character	Meaning
1	Section
2	Body System
3	Root Type
4	Body Part
5	Contrast
6	Qualifier
7	Qualifier

Section (Character 1)
Imaging procedure codes have a first character value of *B*.

Body System (Character 2)
The second character represents the general body system where the imaging is being performed. The available values mimic those that are found in the Medical and Surgical section but may not be exact matches.

Root Type (Character 3)
The third character represents the root type. The section title, *Imaging*, essentially identifies the root operation, while the values for the third character describe the type of imaging being performed. There are six root types in this section.

- *Computerized Tomography (CT Scan)*: Computer reformatted digital display of multiplanar images developed from the capture of multiple exposures of external ionizing radiation
- *Fluoroscopy*: Single plane or bi-plane real time display of an image developed from the capture of external ionizing radiation on a fluorescent screen. The image may also be stored by either digital or analog means
- *Magnetic Resonance Imaging (MRI)*: Computer reformatted digital display of multiplanar images developed from the capture of radiofrequency signals emitted by nuclei in a body site excited within a magnetic field
- *Other Imaging:* Other specified modality for visualizing a body part
- *Plain Radiography*: Planar display of an image developed from the capture of external ionizing radiation on photographic or photoconductive plate
- *Ultrasonography*: Real time display of images of anatomy or flow information developed from the capture of reflected and attenuated high frequency sound waves

Body Part (Character 4)
The fourth character represents the body part, or specific anatomical site where the procedure was performed. The body system (second character) provides only a general indication of the procedure site. The body part and body system values, together, precisely describe the procedure site.

Contrast (Character 5)
The fifth character represents the type of contrast or enhancing material utilized to facilitate the procedure, when applicable.

Qualifier (Character 6)
The sixth character is a qualifier. The most common qualifier, *Unenhanced and Enhanced,* describes an image taken without contrast (unenhanced) followed by an image with contrast (enhanced). Other qualifier values describe other noncontrast material or technology used to facilitate the imaging.

Qualifier (Character 7)
The seventh character is a qualifier. The qualifier is used to capture additional attributes of the procedure, where applicable.

Nuclear Medicine Section (C)
The Nuclear Medicine section is organized like the Imaging section. Procedures captured in this section describe the introduction of radioactive material into the body to create an image, to diagnose or treat pathological conditions, or to assess metabolic functions.

The introduction of encapsulated radioactive material for the treatment of cancer is included in the Radiation Therapy section.

Character Meanings
The seven characters in the Nuclear Medicine section have the following meaning:

Character	Meaning
1	Section
2	Body System
3	Root Type
4	Body Part
5	Radionuclide
6	Qualifier
7	Qualifier

Section (Character 1)
Nuclear Medicine procedure codes have a first character value of *C*.

Body System (Character 2)
The second character represents the general body system or anatomical region to which the nuclear medicine procedure is performed.

Root Type (Character 3)
The third character represents the root type. The section title, *Nuclear Medicine*, essentially identifies the root operation, while the third character value describes the type of nuclear medicine being performed. There are seven root types available in this section.

- *Nonimaging Nuclear Medicine Assay:* Introduction of radioactive materials into the body for the study of body fluids and blood elements, by the detection of radioactive emissions
- *Nonimaging Nuclear Medicine Probe:* Introduction of radioactive materials into the body for the study of distribution and fate of certain substances by the detection of radioactive emissions; or alternatively, measurement of absorption of radioactive emissions from an external source
- *Nonimaging Nuclear Medicine Uptake:* Introduction of radioactive materials into the body for measurements of organ function, from the detection of radioactive emissions
- *Planar Nuclear Medicine Imaging*: Introduction of radioactive materials into the body for single-plane display of images developed from the capture of radioactive emissions
- *Positron Emission Tomography (PET) Imaging:* Introduction of radioactive materials into the body for three dimensional display of images developed from the simultaneous capture, 180 degrees apart, of radioactive emissions
- *Systemic Nuclear Medicine Therapy:* Introduction of unsealed radioactive materials into the body for treatment
- *Tomographic (Tomo) Nuclear Medicine Imaging*: Introduction of radioactive materials into the body for three dimensional display of images developed from the capture of radioactive emissions

Body Part (Character 4)
The fourth character represents the specific body part or region being studied, imaged, or treated. The body system (second character) provides only a general indication of the procedure site. The body part and body system values, together, provide a precise description of the procedure site.

Radionuclide (Character 5)
The fifth character represents the type of radioactive material utilized to facilitate the procedure, when applicable. The *Other Radionuclide* value is used for radioactive material that has been newly approved but does not yet have its own unique value in the coding system.

If more than one radioactive material is given to perform the procedure, more than one code is used.

Qualifier (Characters 6 and 7)
The sixth and seventh characters are qualifiers. Because there are currently no specific qualifier values in this section, the value is always *None*.

Radiation Therapy Section (D)
The Radiation Therapy section contains procedures performed for cancer treatment.

Character Meanings
The seven characters in the Radiation Therapy section have the following meaning:

Character	Meaning
1	Section
2	Body System
3	Modality
4	Treatment Site
5	Modality Qualifier
6	Isotope
7	Qualifier

Section (Character 1)
Radiation therapy procedure codes have a first character value of *D*.

Body System (Character 2)
The second character represents the general body system or anatomical region to which radiation therapy is being applied.

Modality (Character 3)
The third character represents the type of radiation, or modality, being used. There are four values available in this section.

- *Beam Radiation*
- *Brachytherapy*
- *Stereotactic Radiosurgery*
- *Other Radiation*

Treatment Site (Character 4)
The fourth character represents the specific body part or region being irradiated. The body system (second character) provides only a general indication of the procedure site. The treatment site and body system values, together, precisely describe the procedure site.

Modality Qualifier (Character 5)
The fifth character represents specific methods or materials unique to a particular type of radiation therapy. The modality (third character) and modality qualifier values, together, precisely describe the therapy performed.

Isotope (Character 6)
The sixth character represents the specific radioactive isotope introduced into the body, if applicable.

Qualifier (Character 7)
The seventh character is a qualifier. Besides the value of *None*, this section contains two other values, *Intraoperative* and *Unidirectional Source*.

Physical Rehabilitation and Diagnostic Audiology Section (F)

Character Meanings
The seven characters in the Physical Rehabilitation and Diagnostic Audiology section have the following meaning:

Character	Meaning
1	Section
2	Section Qualifier
3	Root Type
4	Body System/Region
5	Type Qualifier
6	Equipment
7	Qualifier

Section (Character 1)
Physical Rehabilitation and Diagnostic Audiology procedure codes have a first character value of *F*.

Section Qualifier (Character 2)
The second character qualifies which of the two services described in the section (character 1) is being represented. Therefore, only two values are available, *Rehabilitation* or *Diagnostic Audiology*.

Root Type (Character 3)
The third character represents the root type. The section qualifier (second character) identifies the root operation, while the third-character value describes the type of rehabilitation or diagnostic audiology being performed. There are 14 root types available in this section, each classified into four general categories.

Assessment: Used to evaluate a patient's level of function to determine the type and timing of treatment required. Assessment procedures focus on the faculties of hearing and speech, on various aspects of body function, and on the patient's quality of life, such as muscle performance, neuromotor development, and reintegration skills.

There are six root type values available for assessment.

- *Speech Assessment:* Measurement of speech and related functions
- *Motor and/or Nerve Function Assessment:* Measurement of motor, nerve, and related functions
- *Activities of Daily Living Assessment:* Measurement of functional level for activities of daily living
- *Hearing Assessment:* Measurement of hearing and related functions
- *Hearing Aid Assessment:* Measurement of the appropriateness and/or effectiveness of a hearing device
- *Vestibular Assessment:* Measurement of the vestibular system and related functions

Treatment: Use of specific activities or methods to develop, improve, and/or restore the performance of necessary functions, compensate for dysfunction and/or minimize debilitation. Procedures include swallowing dysfunction exercises, bathing and showering techniques, wound management, gait training, and a host of activities typically associated with rehabilitation.

There are six root type values available for treatment.

- *Speech Treatment:* Application of techniques to improve, augment, or compensate for speech and related functional impairment
- *Motor Treatment:* Exercise or activities to increase or facilitate motor function
- *Activities of Daily Living Treatment:* Exercise or activities to facilitate functional competence for activities of daily living
- *Hearing Treatment:* Application of techniques to improve, augment, or compensate for hearing and related functional impairment
- *Cochlear Implant Treatment:* Application of techniques to improve the communication abilities of individuals with cochlear implant
- *Vestibular Treatment:* Application of techniques to improve, augment, or compensate for vestibular and related functional impairment

Caregiver Training: Educating a caregiver with the skills and knowledge needed to interact with and assist the patient.

There is only one root type value available for caregiver training.

- *Caregiver Training:* Training in activities to support patient's optimal level of function

Fitting(s): Design, fabrication, modification, selection, and/or application of splint, orthosis, prosthesis, hearing aids, and/or other rehabilitation device. The fifth character used in Device Fitting procedures describes the device being fitted rather than the method used to fit the device. Definitions of devices, when provided, are in the definitions portion of the ICD-10-PCS tables and index, under section F, character 5.

There is only one root type value available for fittings.

- *Device Fitting:* Fitting of a device designed to facilitate or support achievement of a higher level of function

Body System/Region (Character 4)
The fourth character represents the body system and body region, where applicable, that requires rehabilitation. For diagnostic audiology procedures, this value is always *None*.

Type Qualifier (Character 5)
The fifth character represents a type qualifier. The root type (third character) and type qualifier values, together, precisely describe the procedure performed.

Equipment (Character 6)
The sixth character represents any equipment used to facilitate the procedure. The values provided are broad categories that may capture several specific types of equipment.

Qualifier (Character 7)
The seventh character is a qualifier. As there are currently no specific qualifier values in this section, the value is always *None*.

Mental Health Section (G)

Character Meanings
The seven characters in the Mental Health section have the following meaning:

Character	Meaning
1	Section
2	Body System
3	Type
4	Qualifier
5	Qualifier
6	Qualifier
7	Qualifier

Section (Character 1)
Mental health procedure codes have a first character value of *G*.

Body System (Character 2)
The second character is always represented by the value of *None*. As mental health care manages the psychological aspects of a patient's health, there is no specific body system or region that can be represented in this section.

Type (Character 3)
The third character represents the type of procedure. There are 12 values available in this section.

- *Psychological Tests:* The administration and interpretation of standardized psychological tests and measurement instruments for the assessment of psychological function
- *Crisis Intervention:* Treatment of a traumatized, acutely disturbed, or distressed individual for the purpose of short-term stabilization
- *Medication Management:* Monitoring and adjusting the use of medications for the treatment of a mental health disorder
- *Individual Psychotherapy:* Treatment of an individual with a mental health disorder by behavioral, cognitive, psychoanalytic, psychodynamic, or psychophysiological means to improve functioning or well-being
- *Counseling:* The application of psychological methods to treat an individual with normal developmental issues and psychological problems in order to increase function, improve well-being, alleviate distress, maladjustment, or resolve crises
- *Family Psychotherapy:* Treatment that includes one or more family members of an individual with a mental health disorder by behavioral, cognitive, psychoanalytic, psychodynamic, or psychophysiological means to improve functioning or well-being
- *Electroconvulsive Therapy:* The application of controlled electrical voltages to treat a mental health disorder
- *Biofeedback:* Provision of information from the monitoring and regulating of physiological processes in conjunction with cognitive-behavioral techniques to improve patient functioning or well-being
- *Hypnosis:* Induction of a state of heightened suggestibility by auditory, visual, and tactile techniques to elicit an emotional or behavioral response
- *Narcosynthesis:* Administration of intravenous barbiturates in order to release suppressed or repressed thoughts
- *Group Psychotherapy:* Treatment of two or more individuals with a mental health disorder by behavioral, cognitive, psychoanalytic, psychodynamic, or psychophysiological means to improve functioning or well-being
- *Light Therapy:* Application of specialized light treatments to improve functioning or well-being

Qualifier (Character 4)
The fourth character is a qualifier. This value represents the specific technique used to evaluate or treat a patient's mental health. In conjunction with the type (third character), the qualifier value precisely describes the procedure.

Qualifier (Characters 5, 6, and 7)
The fifth, sixth, and seventh characters are qualifiers. As there are currently no specific qualifier values in this section, the value is always *None*.

Substance Abuse Treatment Section (H)

Character Meanings
The seven characters in the Substance Abuse Treatment section have the following meaning:

Character	Meaning
1	Section
2	Body System
3	Type
4	Qualifier
5	Qualifier
6	Qualifier
7	Qualifier

Section (Character 1)
Substance Abuse Treatment codes have a first character value of *H*.

Body System (Character 2)
The second character is always represented by the value of *None*. As the substance abuse treatment section describes management of the psychological aspects of a patient's health, there is no specific body system or region that can be represented in this section.

Type (Character 3)
The third character represents the specific type of treatment. There are seven values available in this section.

- *Detoxification Services:* Detoxification from alcohol and/or drugs
- *Individual Counseling:* The application of psychological methods to treat an individual with addictive behavior
- *Group Counseling:* The application of psychological methods to treat two or more individuals with addictive behavior
- *Individual Psychotherapy:* Treatment of an individual with addictive behavior by behavioral, cognitive, psychoanalytic, psychodynamic, or psychophysiological means

- *Family Counseling:* The application of psychological methods that includes one or more family members to treat an individual with addictive behavior
- *Medication Management:* Monitoring and adjusting the use of replacement medications for the treatment of addiction
- *Pharmacotherapy:* The use of replacement medications for the treatment of addiction

Qualifier (Character 4)
The fourth character is a qualifier. The qualifier value further characterizes the type (character 3) of treatment being rendered, where applicable.

Qualifier (Characters 5, 6, and 7)
The fifth, sixth, and seventh characters are qualifiers. As there are currently no specific qualifier values in this section, the value is always *None*.

New Technology Section (X)

General Information
Section X New Technology is a section added to ICD-10-PCS beginning October 1, 2015. The new section provides a place for codes that uniquely identify procedures requested via the New Technology Application Process or that capture other new technologies not currently classified in ICD-10-PCS.

Section X does not introduce any new coding concepts or unusual guidelines for correct coding. In fact, Section X codes maintain continuity with the other sections in ICD-10-PCS by using the same root operation and body part values as their closest counterparts in other sections of ICD-10-PCS. For example, the codes for the infusion of Sarilumab, use the same root operation (Introduction) and body part values (Central Vein and Peripheral Vein) in section X as the infusion codes in section 3 Administration, which are their closest counterparts in the other sections of ICD-10-PCS.

Character Meanings
The seven characters in the new technology section have the following meaning:

Character	Meaning
1	Section
2	Body System
3	Root Operation
4	Body Part
5	Approach
6	Device/Substance/Technology
7	Qualifier

Section (Character 1)
New technology procedure codes have a first character value of *X*.

Body System (Character 2)
The second character values for body system combine the uses of body system, body region, and physiological system as specified in other sections in ICD-10-PCS.

Root Operation (Character 3)
The third character utilizes the same root operation values as their counterparts in other sections of ICD-10-PCS.

Body Part (Character 4)
The fourth character represents the same body part values as their closest counterparts in other sections of ICD-10-PCS.

Approach (Character 5)
The fifth character represents the approach, as defined in the Medical and Surgical section.

Device/Substance/Technology (Character 6)
The sixth character represents the key feature of the new technology procedure. It may be specified as a new device, a new substance, or other new technology. Examples of sixth character values are *Single-use Duodenoscope, Reduction Device,* and *Mosunetuzumab Antineoplastic*.

Qualifier (Character 7)
The seventh character qualifier is used exclusively to specify the new technology group, a number or letter that changes each year that new technology codes are added to the system. For example, Section X codes added for the first year have the seventh character value 1, *New Technology Group 1*, and the next year that Section X codes are added have the seventh character value 2, *New Technology Group 2*, and so on. Changing the seventh character value to a unique letter or number every year that there are new codes in the new technology section allows the ICD-10-PCS to "recycle" the values in the third, fourth, and sixth characters as needed.

ICD-10-PCS Index and Tabular Format

The *ICD-10-PCS: The Complete Official Code Set* is based on the official version of the International Classification of Diseases, 10th Revision, Procedure Classification System, issued by the U.S. Department of Health and Human Services, Centers for Medicare and Medicaid Services. This book is consistent with the content of the government's version of ICD-10-PCS and follows their official format.

Index

The Alphabetic Index can be used to locate the appropriate table containing all the information necessary to construct a procedure code, however, the PCS tables should always be consulted to find the most appropriate valid code. Users may choose a valid code directly from the tables—he or she need not consult the index before proceeding to the tables to complete the code.

Main Terms

The Alphabetic Index reflects the structure of the tables. Therefore, the index is organized as an alphabetic listing. The index:

- Is based on the value of the third character
- Contains common procedure terms
- Lists anatomic sites
- Uses device terms

The main terms in the Alphabetic Index are root operations, root procedure types, or common procedure names. In addition, anatomic sites from the Body Part Key and device terms from the Device Key have been added for ease of use.

Examples:

> *Resection* (root operation)
>
> *Fluoroscopy* (root type)
>
> *Prostatectomy* (common procedure name)
>
> *Brachiocephalic artery* (body part)
>
> *Bard® Dulex™ mesh* (device)

The index provides at least the first three or four values of the code, and some entries may provide complete valid codes. However, the user should always consult the appropriate table to verify that the most appropriate valid code has been selected.

Root Operation and Procedure Type Main Terms

For the *Medical and Surgical* and related sections, the root operation values are used as main terms in the index. The subterms under the root operation main terms are body parts. For the Ancillary section of the tables, the main terms in the index are the general type of procedure performed.

Examples:

> **Biofeedback** GZC9ZZZ
> **Destruction**
>   Acetabulum
>   Left 0Q55
>   Right 0Q54
>   Adenoids 0C5Q
>   Ampulla of Vater 0F5C

Planar Nuclear Medicine Imaging
    Abdomen CW10

See Reference

The second type of term in the index uses common procedure names, such as "appendectomy" or "fundoplication." These common terms are listed as main terms with a "see" reference noting the PCS root operations that are possible valid code tables based on the objective of the procedure.

Examples:

> **Tendonectomy**
>   *see* Excision, Tendons 0LB
>   *see* Resection, Tendons 0LT

Use Reference

The index also lists anatomic sites from the Body Part Key and device terms from the Device Key. These terms are listed with a "use" reference. The purpose of these references is to act as an additional reference to the terms located in the Appendix Keys. The term provided is the Body Part value or Device value to be selected when constructing a procedure code using the code tables. This type of index reference is not intended to direct the user to another term in the index, but to provide guidance regarding character value selection. Therefore, "use" references generally do not refer to specific valid code tables.

Examples:

> **CoAxia NeuroFlo catheter**
>   *use* Intraluminal Device
> **Epitrochlear lymph node**
>   *use* Lymphatic, Left Upper Extremity
>   *use* Lymphatic, Right Upper Extremity
> **SynCardia Total Artificial Heart**
>   *use* Synthetic Substitute

Code Tables

ICD-10-PCS contains 17 sections of Code Tables organized by general type of procedure. The first three characters of a procedure code define each table. The tables consist of columns providing the possible last four characters of codes and rows providing valid values for each character. Within a PCS table, valid codes include all combinations of choices in characters 4 through 7 contained in the same row of the table. All seven characters must be specified to form a valid code.

There are three main sections of tables:

- Medical and Surgical section:
  - *Medical and Surgical* (0)
- Medical and Surgical-related sections:
  - *Obstetrics* (1)
  - *Placement* (2)
  - *Administration* (3)
  - *Measurement and Monitoring* (4)
  - *Extracorporeal or Systemic Assistance and Performance* (5)
  - *Extracorporeal or Systemic Therapies* (6)
  - *Osteopathic* (7)

- — *Other Procedures* (8)
- — *Chiropractic* (9)
- Ancillary sections:
  - — *Imaging* (B)
  - — *Nuclear Medicine* (C)
  - — *Radiation Therapy* (D)
  - — *Physical Rehabilitation and Diagnostic Audiology* (F)
  - — *Mental Health* (G)
  - — *Substance Abuse Treatment* (H)
- New Technology section:
  - — *New Technology* (X)

The first three character values define each table. The root operation or root type designated for each table is accompanied by its official definition.

Example:

Table 00F provides codes for procedures on the central nervous system that involve breaking up of solid matter into pieces:

Character 1, Section	0: Medical and Surgical
Character 2, Body System	0: Central Nervous System and Cranial Nerves
Character 3, Root Operation	F: Fragmentation: Breaking solid matter in a body part into pieces

Tables are arranged numerically, then alphabetically.

When reviewing tables, the user should keep in mind that:

- Some tables may cover multiple pages in the code book—to ensure maximum clarity about character choices, valid entries do not split rows between pages. For instance, the entire table of valid characters completing a code beginning with 4A1 is split between two pages, but the split is between, not within, rows. This means that all the valid sixth and seventh characters for, say, body system *Arterial* (3) and approach *External* (X) are contained on one page.
- Individual entries may be listed in several horizontal "selection" lines.
- When a table is continued onto another page, a note to this effect has been added in red.

Body Part Definitions:

An exclusive Optum feature in the tables is the incorporation of the body part definitions provided in appendix E into the Medical and Surgical section (0) tables under their appropriate body part characters in the first column (character 4). This provides the user a direct reference to all anatomical descriptions, terms, and sites that could be coded to that particular body part value.

Paired body parts typically have values for the right and left side and in some cases a value for bilateral. These paired body parts often have the same list of inclusive body part definitions. When there are paired body parts with the same body part definitions, the first listed body part (usually the right side) contains the list of body part definitions while the second listed body part (usually the left side) contains a *See* instruction. This *See* instruction references the body part value that contains the body part definitions. In the table below, body part value P – Upper Eyelid, Left is followed by a *See* instruction that states *See N Upper Eyelid, Right*. All body part descriptions under value N also apply to body part value P.

Example:

0   Medical and Surgical
8   Eye
M   Reattachment   Definition: Putting back in or on all or a portion of a separated body part to its normal location or other suitable location
Explanation: Vascular circulation and nervous pathways may or may not be reestablished

Body Part Character 4	Approach Character 5	Device Character 6	Qualifier Character 7

N Upper Eyelid, Right
    Lateral canthus
    Levator palpebrae superioris muscle
    Orbicularis oculi muscle
    Superior tarsal plate
P Upper Eyelid, Left
    See N Upper Eyelid, Right
Q Lower Eyelid, Right
    Inferior tarsal plate
    Medial canthus
R Lower Eyelid, Left
    See Q Lower Eyelid, Right
	X External	Z No Device	Z No Qualifier

ICD-10-PCS Additional Features

Use of Official Sources

Color-coding, icons, and other annotations in this manual identify coding and reimbursement edits derived from the inpatient prospective payment system (IPPS) official tables and data files and from the MS-DRG Grouper software.

In most instances, FY 2025 data from the above sources were not available at the time this book was printed. In an effort to make available the most current source information, Optum has provided a document identifying FY 2025 changes to edit designations for ICD-10-PCS codes. Edit changes identified in this document may include:

- Hospital-acquired condition
- Noncovered procedures
- Limited coverage procedures
- Valid operating room procedures
- DRG nonoperating room procedures
- Nonoperating room procedures
- New-technology add-on payment

This document can be accessed at the following:

https://www.optumcoding.com/ProductUpdates/
Title: "2025 ICD-10-PCS Edit Changes"
Password: PCS25

Table Notations

Many tables in ICD-10-PCS contain color or symbol annotations that may aid in code selection, provide clinical or coding information, or alert the coder to reimbursement issues affected by the PCS code assignment. These annotations may be displayed on or next to a character 4, character 6, or character 7 value. Please note that some values may have more than one annotation; this is true most often with the character 4 value.

Refer to the color/symbol legend at the bottom of each page in the tables section for an abridged description of each color and symbol.

Annotation Box

An annotation box has been appended to all tables that contain color-coding or symbol annotations. The color bar or symbol attached to a character value is provided in the box, as well as a list of the valid PCS code(s) to which that edit applies. The box may also list conditional criteria that must be met to satisfy the edit.

For example, see Table 00F. Four character 4 body part values have a gray color bar. In the annotation box below the table, the gray color bar is defined as "Non-OR," or a nonoperating room procedure edit. Following the Non-OR annotation are the PCS codes that are considered nonoperating room procedures from that row of Table 00F.

Bracketed Code Notation

The use of bracketed codes is an efficient convention to provide all valid character value alternatives for a specific set of circumstances. The character values in the brackets correspond to the valid values for the character in the position the bracket appears.

Examples:

In the annotation box for Table 00F the Noncovered Procedure edit (NC) applies to codes represented in the bracketed code 00F[3,4,5,6]XZZ.

00F[3,4,5,6]XZZ   Fragmentation in (Central Nervous System and Cranial Nerves), External Approach

The valid fourth character values (body part) that may be selected for this specific circumstance are as follows:

  3   Epidural Space, Intracranial
  4   Subdural Space, Intracranial
  5   Subarachnoid Space, Intracranial
  6   Cerebral Ventricle

The fragmentation of matter in the spinal canal, Body Part value U, is not included in the noncovered procedure code edit.

Color-Coding/Symbols

New and Revised Text

Changes within the ICD-10-PCS tables, since the last published edition of this manual, are highlighted in two ways:

- **Red font** identifies new or revised text effective April 1, 2024.
- **Green font** identifies new or revised text effective October 1, 2024.

Medicare Code Edits

Medicare administrative contractors (MACs) and many payers use Medicare code edits to check the coding accuracy on claims. The coding edits provided in this manual include only those directly related to ICD-10-PCS codes used for acute care hospital inpatient admissions.

Sex Edit Symbols

Effective October 1, 2024, the Medicare Code Editor (MCE), a program used to detect and report errors in coding claims data, has deactivated the sex conflict edit. There is no longer a female or male edit restriction for ICD-10-PCS codes.

QA **Questionable Obstetric Admission**

An inpatient admission is considered questionable when a vaginal or cesarean delivery code is assigned without a corresponding secondary diagnosis code describing the outcome of delivery. Both a delivery (ICD-10-PCS) code and an outcome-of-delivery (ICD-10-CM) code must be present to avoid errors in MS-DRG assignment. This symbol is found only in the Obstetrics Section, appearing to the right of the body part (character 4) value.

NC **Noncovered Procedure**

Medicare does not cover all procedures. However, some noncovered procedures, due to the presence of certain diagnoses, are reimbursed.

LC **Limited Coverage**

For certain procedures whose medical complexity and serious nature incur extraordinary associated costs, Medicare limits coverage to a portion of the cost. The limited coverage edit indicates the type of limited coverage.

ICD-10 MS-DRG Definitions Manual Edits

An MS-DRG is assigned based on specific patient attributes, such as principal diagnosis, secondary diagnoses, procedures, and discharge status. The attributes (edits) provided in this manual include only those directly related to ICD-10-PCS codes used for acute care hospital inpatient admissions.

Non-Operating Room Procedures Not Affecting MS-DRG Assignment

In the Medical and Surgical section (001-0YW) and the Obstetric section (102-10Y) tables **only,** ICD-10-PCS procedures codes that DO NOT affect MS-DRG assignment are identified by a gray color bar over the body part (character 4) value and are considered non-operating room (non-OR) procedures.

Note: The majority of the ICD-10-PCS codes in the Medical and Surgical-Related, Ancillary and New Technology section tables are non-operating room procedures that do not typically affect MS-DRG assignment. Only the Valid Operating Room and DRG Non-Operating Room procedures are highlighted in these sections, *see* Non-Operating Room Procedures Affecting MS-DRG Assignment and Valid OR Procedure description below.

Non-Operating Room Procedures Affecting MS-DRG Assignment

Some ICD-10-PCS procedure codes, although considered non-operating room procedures, may still affect MS-DRG assignment. In all sections of the ICD-10-PCS book, these procedures are identified by a purple color bar over the body part (character 4) value.

Valid OR Procedure

In the Medical and Surgical-Related (2W0-9WB), Ancillary (B00-HZ9) and New Technology (X2A-XY0) section tables **only**, any codes that are considered a valid operating room procedure are identified with a blue color bar over the body part (character 4) value and will affect MS-DRG assignment. All codes without a color bar (blue or purple) are considered non-operating room procedures.

Hospital-Acquired Condition Related Procedures

Procedures associated with hospital-acquired conditions (HAC) are identified with the yellow color bar over the body part (character 4) value. Appendix K provides each specific HAC category and its associated ICD-10-CM and ICD-10-PCS codes.

Combination Only

Some ICD-10-PCS procedure codes that describe non-operating room procedures can group to a specific MS-DRG but only when used in combination with certain other ICD-10-PCS procedure codes. Such codes are designated by a red color bar over the body part (character 4) value.

⊞ Combination Member

A combination member, which can be either a valid operating room procedure or a non-operating room procedure, is an ICD-10-PCS procedure code that can influence MS-DRG assignment either on its own or in combination with other specific ICD-10-PCS procedure codes. Combination member codes are designated by a plus sign (⊞) to the right of the body part (character 4) value.

Note: In the few instances when a code is both a combination member and a non-operating room procedure affecting the MS-DRG assignment, the body part (character 4) value will have a purple color bar and the combination member icon.

See Appendix L for Procedure Combinations

Under certain circumstances, more than one procedure code is needed in order to group to a specific MS-DRG. When codes within a table have been identified as a Combination Only (red color bar) or Combination Member (⊞) code, there is also a footnote instructing the coder to *see Appendix L*. Appendix L contains tables that identify the other procedure codes needed in the combination and the title and number of the MS-DRG to which the combination will group.

Other Table Notations

AHA Coding Clinic:

Official citations from AHA's *Coding Clinic for ICD-10-CM/PCS* have been provided at the beginning of each section, when applicable. Each specific citation is listed below a header identifying the table to which that particular *Coding Clinic* citation applies. The citations appear in purple type with the year, quarter, and page of the reference as well as the title of the question as it appears in that *Coding Clinic's* table of contents. *Coding Clinic* citations included in this edition have been updated through second quarter 2024.

NT New Technology Add-on Payment

This symbol identifies procedure codes that involve new technologies or medical services that have qualified for a new technology add-on payment (NTAP). CMS provides incremental payment, in addition to the DRG payment, for technologies that have received the NTAP designation. This symbol appears to the right of the sixth character value.

Note: Only specific brand or trade named devices, substances, or technologies receive NTAP approval. The sixth character value in the PCS table provides a generalized description that may be applicable to several brand or trade names. Unless otherwise specified in the annotation box, refer to appendix H or I to determine the specific brand or trade name of the device, substance, or technology that is applicable to the new technology add-on payment. New technology add-on payments are not exclusive to the New Technology (X) section.

Appendixes

The resources described below have been included as appendixes for *ICD-10-PCS The Complete Official Code Set*. These resources further instruct the coder on the appropriate application of the ICD-10-PCS code set.

Appendix A: Components of the Medical and Surgical Approach Definitions

This resource further defines the approach characters used in the Medical and Surgical (0) section. Complementing the detailed definition of the approach, additional information includes whether or not instrumentation is a part of the approach, the typical access location, the method used to initiate the approach, related procedural examples, and illustrations all of which will help the user determine the appropriate approach value.

Appendix B: Root Operation Definitions

This resource is a compilation of all root operations found in the Medical and Surgical-related sections (0-9) of this PCS manual. It provides a definition and in some cases a more detailed explanation of the root operation, to better reflect the purpose or objective. Examples of related procedure(s) may also be provided.

Appendix C: Comparison of Medical and Surgical Root Operations
The Medical and Surgical (Ø) section root operations are divided into groups that share similar attributes. These groups, and the root operations in each group, are listed in this resource along with information identifying the target of the root operation, the action used to perform the root operation, any clarification or further explanation on the objective of the root operation, and procedure examples.

Appendix D: Body Part Key
When an anatomical term or description is provided in the documentation but does not have a specific body part character within a table, the user can reference this resource to search for the anatomical description or site noted in the documentation to determine if there is a specific PCS body part character (character 4) to which the anatomical description or site could be coded.

Appendix E: Body Part Definitions
This resource is the reverse look-up of the Body Part Key. Each table in the Medical and Surgical section (Ø) of the PCS manual contains anatomical terms linked to a body part character or value, for example, in Table ØBB the Body Part (character 4) of 1 is Trachea. The body part Trachea may have anatomical structures or descriptions that may be used in procedure documentation instead of the term trachea. The Body Part Definitions list other anatomical structures or synonyms that are included in specific ICD-10-PCS body part values. According to the body part definitions, in the example above, cricoid cartilage is included in the Trachea (character 1) body part.

Appendix F: Device Classification
This resource provides an explanation of how a device is defined in the ICD-10-PCS classification along with two tables. The first table groups devices used in the ICD-10-PCS tables into general categories, including a definition of each device type and related examples. The second table provides definitions of transplant and grafting tissue types and associated terminology that may be found in the documentation.

Appendix G: Device Key and Aggregation Table
The Device Key helps users code the appropriate PCS sixth character for device. Devices are listed alphabetically by brand name or commonly used medical terminology and are translated to the appropriate PCS language or value. The key also reflects the body system where the device is located. For example, a SAPIEN valve used for transaortic valve replacement translates to Zooplastic Tissue in Heart and Great Vessels.

The Aggregation Table crosswalks specific device character value definitions for specific root operations in a specific body system to the more general device character value to be used when the root operation covers a wide range of body parts and the device character represents an entire family of devices.

Appendix H: Device Definitions
This resource is a reverse look-up to the Device Key. The user may reference this resource to see all the specific devices that may be grouped to a particular device character (character 6).

Example:
The operative report states, "An internal fixation device was used to repair a fractured femur. Kirschner wire, bone screws and neutralization plate all used and left in the bone at the end of the procedure. "

Although PCS requires all devices left in the body to be coded and the operative report lists three different devices, a check in the device definitions shows that all of these devices are included in the PCS value "Internal Fixation Device" and require only one code.

Appendix I: Substance Key/Substance Definitions
The Substance Key lists substances by trade name or synonym and relates them to a PCS character in the Administration (3) or New Technology (X) section in the Substance (sixth character) or Qualifier (seventh character) column.

The Substance Definitions table is the reverse look-up of the substance key, relating all substance categories, the sixth- or seventh character values, to all trade name or synonyms that may be classified to that particular character.

Appendix J: Sections B-H Character Definitions
In each ancillary section (B-H) the characters in a particular column may have different meanings depending on which section the user is working from. This resource provides the values for the characters in these sections as well as a definition of the character value.

Appendix K: Hospital Acquired Conditions
Hospital acquired conditions (HACs) are conditions that are considered reasonably preventable when occurring during the hospital admission and may prevent a case from grouping to a higher-paying MS-DRG. In certain instances the HACs are conditional, requiring a specific ICD-10-CM diagnosis code in combination with a specific ICD-10-PCS procedure code. This resource identifies these conditional HACs, listing the diagnosis and procedure codes that, in combination, may trigger a HAC edit. All codes, ICD-10-CM and ICD-10-PCS, are listed with their full descriptions.

Appendix L: Procedure Combination Tables
The procedure combination tables provided in this resource illustrate certain procedure combinations that must occur in order to assign a specific MS-DRG.

Appendix M: Coding Exercises and Answers
This resource provides the coding exercises with answers, and in some cases a brief explanation as to the reason that particular code was used.

ICD-10-PCS Official Guidelines for Coding and Reporting 2025

Narrative changes effective October 1, 2024 appear in **bold** text.

Narrative changes effective April 1, 2024 appear in shaded text.

The Centers for Medicare and Medicaid Services (CMS) and the National Center for Health Statistics (NCHS), two departments within the U.S. Federal Government's Department of Health and Human Services (DHHS) provide the following guidelines for coding and reporting using the International Classification of Diseases, 10th Revision, Procedure Coding System (ICD-10-PCS). These guidelines should be used as a companion document to the official version of the ICD-10-PCS as published on the CMS website. The ICD-10-PCS is a procedure classification published by the United States for classifying procedures performed in hospital inpatient health care settings.

These guidelines have been approved by the four organizations that make up the Cooperating Parties for the ICD-10-PCS: the American Hospital Association (AHA), the American Health Information Management Association (AHIMA), CMS, and NCHS.

These guidelines are a set of rules that have been developed to accompany and complement the official conventions and instructions provided within the ICD-10-PCS itself. They are intended to provide direction that is applicable in most circumstances. However, there may be unique circumstances where exceptions are applied. The instructions and conventions of the classification take precedence over guidelines. These guidelines are based on the coding and sequencing instructions in the Tables, Index and Definitions of ICD-10-PCS, but provide additional instruction. Adherence to these guidelines when assigning ICD-10-PCS procedure codes is required under the Health Insurance Portability and Accountability Act (HIPAA). The procedure codes have been adopted under HIPAA for hospital inpatient healthcare settings. A joint effort between the healthcare provider and the coder is essential to achieve complete and accurate documentation, code assignment, and reporting of diagnoses and procedures. These guidelines have been developed to assist both the healthcare provider and the coder in identifying those procedures that are to be reported. The importance of consistent, complete documentation in the medical record cannot be overemphasized. Without such documentation accurate coding cannot be achieved.

Conventions

A1. ICD-10-PCS codes are composed of seven characters. Each character is an axis of classification that specifies information about the procedure performed. Within a defined code range, a character specifies the same type of information in that axis of classification.

Example:
The fifth axis of classification specifies the approach in sections Ø through 4 and 7 through 9 of the system.

A2. One of 34 possible values can be assigned to each axis of classification in the seven-character code: they are the numbers Ø through 9 and the alphabet (except I and O because they are easily confused with the numbers 1 and Ø). The number of unique values used in an axis of classification differs as needed.

Example:
Where the fifth axis of classification specifies the approach, seven different approach values are currently used to specify the approach.

A3. The valid values for an axis of classification can be added to as needed.

Example:
If a significantly distinct type of device is used in a new procedure, a new device value can be added to the system.

A4. As with words in their context, the meaning of any single value is a combination of its axis of classification and any preceding values on which it may be dependent.

Example:
The meaning of a body part value in the Medical and Surgical section is always dependent on the body system value. The body part value Ø in the Central Nervous body system specifies Brain and the body part value Ø in the Peripheral Nervous body system specifies Cervical Plexus.

A5. As the system is expanded to become increasingly detailed, over time more values will depend on preceding values for their meaning.

Example:
In the Lower Joints body system, the device value 3 in the root operation Insertion specifies Infusion Device and the device value 3 in the root operation Replacement specifies Ceramic Synthetic Substitute.

A6. The purpose of the alphabetic index is to locate the appropriate table that contains all information necessary to construct a procedure code. The PCS Tables should always be consulted to find the most appropriate valid code.

A7. It is not required to consult the index first before proceeding to the tables to complete the code. A valid code may be chosen directly from the tables.

A8. All seven characters must be specified to be a valid code. If the documentation is incomplete for coding purposes, the physician should be queried for the necessary information.

A9. Within a PCS table, valid codes include all combinations of choices in characters 4 through 7 contained in the same row of the table. In the example below, ØJHT3VZ is a valid code, and ØJHW3VZ is *not* a valid code.

Section: Ø Medical and Surgical
Body System: J Subcutaneous Tissue and Fascia
Operation: H Insertion Putting in a nonbiological appliance that monitors, assists, performs, or prevents a physiological function but does not physically take the place of a body part

Body Part	Approach	Device	Qualifier
S Subcutaneous Tissue and Fascia, Head and Neck V Subcutaneous Tissue and Fascia, Upper Extremity W Subcutaneous Tissue and Fascia, Lower Extremity	Ø Open 3 Percutaneous	1 Radioactive Element 3 Infusion Device Y Other Device	Z No Qualifier
T Subcutaneous Tissue and Fascia, Trunk	Ø Open 3 Percutaneous	1 Radioactive Element 3 Infusion Device V Infusion Pump Y Other Device	Z No Qualifier

ICD-10-PCS 2025

A10. "And," when used in a code description, means "and/or," except when used to describe a combination of multiple body parts for which separate values exist for each body part (e.g., Skin and Subcutaneous Tissue used as a qualifier, where there are separate body part values for "Skin" and "Subcutaneous Tissue").

Example:
Lower Arm and Wrist Muscle means lower arm and/or wrist muscle.

A11. Many of the terms used to construct PCS codes are defined within the system. It is the coder's responsibility to determine what the documentation in the medical record equates to in the PCS definitions. The physician is not expected to use the terms used in PCS code descriptions, nor is the coder required to query the physician when the correlation between the documentation and the defined PCS terms is clear.

Example:
When the physician documents "partial resection" the coder can independently correlate "partial resection" to the root operation Excision without querying the physician for clarification.

Medical and Surgical Section Guidelines (section 0)

B2. Body System

General guidelines

B2.1a. The procedure codes in Anatomical Regions, General, Anatomical Regions, Upper Extremities and Anatomical Regions, Lower Extremities can be used when the procedure is performed on an anatomical region rather than a specific body part, or on the rare occasion when no information is available to support assignment of a code to a specific body part.

Examples:
Chest tube drainage of the pleural cavity is coded to the root operation Drainage found in the body system Anatomical Regions, General.

Suture repair of the abdominal wall is coded to the root operation Repair in the body system Anatomical Regions, General.

Amputation of the foot is coded to the root operation Detachment in the body system Anatomical Regions, Lower Extremities.

B2.1b. Where the general body part values "upper" and "lower" are provided as an option in the Upper Arteries, Lower Arteries, Upper Veins, Lower Veins, Muscles and Tendons body systems, "upper" or "lower" specifies body parts located above or below the diaphragm respectively.

Example:
Vein body parts above the diaphragm are found in the Upper Veins body system; vein body parts below the diaphragm are found in the Lower Veins body system.

B3. Root Operation

General guidelines

B3.1a. In order to determine the appropriate root operation, the full definition of the root operation as contained in the PCS Tables must be applied.

B3.1b. Components of a procedure specified in the root operation definition or explanation as integral to that root operation are not coded separately. Procedural steps necessary to reach the operative site and close the operative site, including anastomosis of a tubular body part, are also not coded separately.

Examples:
Resection of a joint as part of a joint replacement procedure is included in the root operation definition of Replacement and is not coded separately.

Laparotomy performed to reach the site of an open liver biopsy is not coded separately.

In a resection of sigmoid colon with anastomosis of descending colon to rectum, the anastomosis is not coded separately.

Multiple procedures

B3.2. During the same operative episode, multiple procedures are coded if:

a. The same root operation is performed on different body parts as defined by distinct values of the body part character.

   Examples:
   Diagnostic excision of liver and pancreas are coded separately.

   Excision of lesion in the ascending colon and excision of lesion in the transverse colon are coded separately.

b. The same root operation is repeated in multiple body parts, and those body parts are separate and distinct body parts classified to a single ICD-10-PCS body part value.

   Examples:
   Excision of the sartorius muscle and excision of the gracilis muscle are both included in the upper leg muscle body part value, and multiple procedures are coded.

   Extraction of multiple toenails are coded separately.

c. Multiple root operations with distinct objectives are performed on the same body part.

   Example:
   Destruction of sigmoid lesion and bypass of sigmoid colon are coded separately.

d. The intended root operation is attempted using one approach but is converted to a different approach.

   Example:
   Laparoscopic cholecystectomy converted to an open cholecystectomy is coded as percutaneous endoscopic Inspection and open Resection.

Discontinued or incomplete procedures

B3.3. If the intended procedure is discontinued or otherwise not completed, code the procedure to the root operation performed. If a procedure is discontinued before any other root operation is performed, code the root operation Inspection of the body part or anatomical region inspected.

Example:
A planned aortic valve replacement procedure is discontinued after the initial thoracotomy and before any incision is made in the heart muscle, when the patient becomes hemodynamically unstable. This procedure is coded as an open Inspection of the mediastinum.

Biopsy procedures

B3.4a. Biopsy procedures are coded using the root operations Excision, Extraction, or Drainage and the qualifier Diagnostic.

Examples:
Fine needle aspiration biopsy of fluid in the lung is coded to the root operation Drainage with the qualifier Diagnostic.

Biopsy of bone marrow is coded to the root operation Extraction with the qualifier Diagnostic.

Lymph node sampling for biopsy is coded to the root operation Excision with the qualifier Diagnostic.

Biopsy followed by more definitive treatment

B3.4b. If a diagnostic Excision, Extraction, or Drainage procedure (biopsy) is followed by a more definitive procedure, such as Destruction, Excision or Resection at the same procedure site, both the biopsy and the more definitive treatment are coded.

> *Example:*
> Biopsy of breast followed by partial mastectomy at the same procedure site, both the biopsy and the partial mastectomy procedure are coded.

Overlapping body layers

B3.5. If root operations such as Excision, Extraction, Repair or Inspection are performed on overlapping layers of the musculoskeletal system, the body part specifying the deepest layer is coded.

> *Example:*
> Excisional debridement that includes skin and subcutaneous tissue and muscle is coded to the muscle body part.

Bypass procedures

B3.6a. Bypass procedures are coded by identifying the body part bypassed "from" and the body part bypassed "to." The fourth character body part specifies the body part bypassed from, and the qualifier specifies the body part bypassed to.

> *Example:*
> Bypass from stomach to jejunum, stomach is the body part and jejunum is the qualifier.

B3.6b. Coronary artery bypass procedures are coded differently than other bypass procedures as described in the previous guideline. Rather than identifying the body part bypassed from, the body part identifies the number of coronary arteries bypassed to, and the qualifier specifies the vessel bypassed from.

> *Example:*
> Aortocoronary artery bypass of the left anterior descending coronary artery and the obtuse marginal coronary artery is classified in the body part axis of classification as two coronary arteries, and the qualifier specifies the aorta as the body part bypassed from.

B3.6c. If multiple coronary arteries are bypassed, a separate procedure is coded for each coronary artery that uses a different device and/or qualifier.

> *Example:*
> Aortocoronary artery bypass and internal mammary coronary artery bypass are coded separately.

Control vs. more specific root operations

B3.7. The root operation Control is defined as, "Stopping, or attempting to stop, postprocedural or other acute bleeding." Control is the root operation coded when the procedure performed to achieve hemostasis, beyond what would be considered integral to a procedure, utilizes techniques (e.g. cautery, application of substances or pressure, suturing or ligation or clipping of bleeding points at the site) that are not described by a more specific root operation definition, such as Bypass, Detachment, Excision, Extraction, Reposition, Replacement, or Resection. If a more specific root operation definition applies to the procedure performed, then the more specific root operation is coded instead of Control.

> *Example:*
> Silver nitrate cautery to treat acute nasal bleeding is coded to the root operation Control.

> *Example:*
> Liquid embolization of the right internal iliac artery to treat acute hematoma by stopping blood flow is coded to the root operation Occlusion.

> *Example:*
> Suctioning of residual blood to achieve hemostasis during a transbronchial cryobiopsy is considered integral to the cryobiopsy procedure and is not coded separately.

Excision vs. Resection

B3.8. PCS contains specific body parts for anatomical subdivisions of a body part, such as lobes of the lungs or liver and regions of the intestine. Resection of the specific body part is coded whenever all of the body part is cut out or off, rather than coding Excision of a less specific body part.

> *Example:*
> Left upper lung lobectomy is coded to Resection of Upper Lung Lobe, Left rather than Excision of Lung, Left.

Excision for graft

B3.9. If an autograft is obtained from a different procedure site in order to complete the objective of the procedure, a separate procedure is coded, except when the seventh character qualifier value in the ICD-10-PCS table fully specifies the site from which the autograft was obtained.

> *Examples:*
> Coronary bypass with excision of saphenous vein graft, excision of saphenous vein is coded separately.
>
> Replacement of breast with autologous deep inferior epigastric artery perforator (DIEP) flap, excision of the DIEP flap is not coded separately. The seventh character qualifier value Deep Inferior Epigastric Artery Perforator Flap in the Replacement table fully specifies the site of the autograft harvest.

Fusion procedures of the spine

B3.10a. The body part coded for a spinal vertebral joint(s) rendered immobile by a spinal fusion procedure is classified by the level of the spine (e.g. thoracic). There are distinct body part values for a single vertebral joint and for multiple vertebral joints at each spinal level.

> *Example:*
> Body part values specify Lumbar Vertebral Joint, Lumbar Vertebral Joints, 2 or More and Lumbosacral Vertebral Joint.

B3.10b. If multiple vertebral joints are fused, a separate procedure is coded for each vertebral joint that uses a different device and/or qualifier.

> *Example:*
> Fusion of lumbar vertebral joint, posterior approach, anterior column and fusion of lumbar vertebral joint, posterior approach, posterior column are coded separately.

B3.10c. Combinations of devices and materials are often used on a vertebral joint to render the joint immobile. When combinations of devices are used on the same vertebral joint, the device value coded for the procedure is as follows:

- If an interbody fusion device is used to render the joint immobile (containing bone graft or bone graft substitute), the procedure is coded with the device value Interbody Fusion Device
- If bone graft is the *only* device used to render the joint immobile, the procedure is coded with the device value Nonautologous Tissue Substitute or Autologous Tissue Substitute
- If a mixture of autologous and nonautologous bone graft (with or without biological or synthetic extenders or binders) is used to render the joint immobile, code the procedure with the device value Autologous Tissue Substitute

Examples:
Fusion of a vertebral joint using a cage style interbody fusion device containing morsellized bone graft is coded to the device Interbody Fusion Device.

Fusion of a vertebral joint using a bone dowel interbody fusion device made of cadaver bone and packed with a mixture of local morsellized bone and demineralized bone matrix is coded to the device Interbody Fusion Device.

Fusion of a vertebral joint using both autologous bone graft and bone bank bone graft is coded to the device Autologous Tissue Substitute.

Inspection procedures

B3.11a. Inspection of a body part(s) performed in order to achieve the objective of a procedure is not coded separately.

Example:
Fiberoptic bronchoscopy performed for irrigation of bronchus, only the irrigation procedure is coded.

B3.11b. If multiple tubular body parts are inspected, the most distal body part (the body part furthest from the starting point of the inspection) is coded. If multiple non-tubular body parts in a region are inspected, the body part that specifies the entire area inspected is coded.

Examples:
Cystoureteroscopy with inspection of bladder and ureters is coded to the ureter body part value.

Exploratory laparotomy with general inspection of abdominal contents is coded to the peritoneal cavity body part value.

B3.11c. When both an Inspection procedure and another procedure are performed on the same body part during the same episode, if the Inspection procedure is performed using a different approach than the other procedure, the Inspection procedure is coded separately.

Example:
Endoscopic Inspection of the duodenum is coded separately when open Excision of the duodenum is performed during the same procedural episode.

Occlusion vs. Restriction for vessel embolization procedures

B3.12. If the objective of an embolization procedure is to completely close a vessel, the root operation Occlusion is coded. If the objective of an embolization procedure is to narrow the lumen of a vessel, the root operation Restriction is coded.

Examples:
Tumor embolization is coded to the root operation Occlusion, because the objective of the procedure is to cut off the blood supply to the vessel.

Embolization of a cerebral aneurysm is coded to the root operation Restriction, because the objective of the procedure is not to close off the vessel entirely, but to narrow the lumen of the vessel at the site of the aneurysm where it is abnormally wide.

Release procedures

B3.13. In the root operation Release, the body part value coded is the body part being freed and not the tissue being manipulated or cut to free the body part.

Example:
Lysis of intestinal adhesions is coded to the specific intestine body part value.

Release vs. Division

B3.14. If the sole objective of the procedure is freeing a body part without cutting the body part, the root operation is Release. If the sole objective of the procedure is separating or transecting a body part, the root operation is Division.

Examples:
Freeing a nerve root from surrounding scar tissue to relieve pain is coded to the root operation Release.

Severing a nerve root to relieve pain is coded to the root operation Division.

Reposition for fracture treatment

B3.15. Reduction of a displaced fracture is coded to the root operation Reposition and the application of a cast or splint in conjunction with the Reposition procedure is not coded separately. Treatment of a nondisplaced fracture is coded to the procedure performed.

Examples:
Casting of a nondisplaced fracture is coded to the root operation Immobilization in the Placement section.

Putting a pin in a nondisplaced fracture is coded to the root operation Insertion.

Transplantation vs. Administration

B3.16. Putting in a mature and functioning living body part taken from another individual or animal is coded to the root operation Transplantation. Putting in autologous or nonautologous cells is coded to the Administration section.

Example:
Putting in autologous or nonautologous bone marrow, pancreatic islet cells or stem cells is coded to the Administration section.

Transfer procedures using multiple tissue layers

B3.17. The root operation Transfer contains qualifiers that can be used to specify when a transfer flap is composed of more than one tissue layer, such as a musculocutaneous flap. For procedures involving transfer of multiple tissue layers including skin, subcutaneous tissue, fascia or muscle, the procedure is coded to the body part value that describes the deepest tissue layer in the flap, and the qualifier can be used to describe the other tissue layer(s) in the transfer flap.

Example:
A musculocutaneous flap transfer is coded to the appropriate body part value in the body system Muscles, and the qualifier is used to describe the additional tissue layer(s) in the transfer flap.

Excision/Resection followed by replacement

B3.18. If an excision or resection of a body part is followed by a replacement procedure, code both procedures to identify each distinct objective, except when the excision or resection is considered integral and preparatory for the replacement procedure.

Examples:
Mastectomy followed by reconstruction, both resection and replacement of the breast are coded to fully capture the distinct objectives of the procedures performed.

Maxillectomy with obturator reconstruction, both excision and replacement of the maxilla are coded to fully capture the distinct objectives of the procedures performed.

Excisional debridement of tendon with skin graft, both the excision of the tendon and the replacement of the skin with a graft are coded to fully capture the distinct objectives of the procedures performed.

Esophagectomy followed by reconstruction with colonic interposition, both the resection and the transfer of the large intestine to function as the esophagus are coded to fully capture the distinct objectives of the procedures performed.

Examples:
Resection of a joint as part of a joint replacement procedure is considered integral and preparatory for the replacement of the joint and the resection is not coded separately.

Resection of a valve as part of a valve replacement procedure is considered integral and preparatory for the valve replacement and the resection is not coded separately.

Detachment procedures of extremities

B3.19. The root operation Detachment contains qualifiers that can be used to specify the level where the extremity was amputated. These qualifiers are dependent on the body part value in the "upper extremities" and "lower extremities" body systems. For procedures involving the detachment of all or part of the upper or lower extremities, the procedure is coded to the body part value that describes the site of the detachment.

Example:
An amputation at the proximal portion of the shaft of the tibia and fibula is coded to the Lower leg body part value in the body system Anatomical Regions, Lower Extremities, and the qualifier High is used to specify the level where the extremity was detached.

The following definitions were developed for the Detachment qualifiers

Body Part	Qualifier	Definition
Upper arm and upper leg	1	High: Amputation at the proximal portion of the shaft of the humerus or femur
	2	Mid: Amputation at the middle portion of the shaft of the humerus or femur
	3	Low: Amputation at the distal portion of the shaft of the humerus or femur
Lower arm and lower leg	1	High: Amputation at the proximal portion of the shaft of the radius/ulna or tibia/fibula
	2	Mid: Amputation at the middle portion of the shaft of the radius/ulna or tibia/fibula
	3	Low: Amputation at the distal portion of the shaft of the radius/ulna or tibia/fibula
Hand and Foot	0	Complete*
	4	Complete 1st Ray
	5	Complete 2nd Ray
	6	Complete 3rd Ray
	7	Complete 4th Ray
	8	Complete 5th Ray
	9	Partial 1st Ray
	B	Partial 2nd Ray
	C	Partial 3rd Ray
	D	Partial 4th Ray
	F	Partial 5th Ray

Body Part	Qualifier	Definition
Thumb, finger, or toe	0	Complete: Amputation at the metacarpophalangeal/metatarsal-phalangeal joint
	1	High: Amputation anywhere along the proximal phalanx
	2	Mid: Amputation through the proximal interphalangeal joint or anywhere along the middle phalanx
	3	Low: Amputation through the distal interphalangeal joint or anywhere along the distal phalanx

*When coding amputation of Hand and Foot, the following definitions are followed:

- Complete: Amputation through the carpometacarpal joint of the hand, or through the tarsal-metatarsal joint of the foot.
- Partial: Amputation anywhere along the shaft or head of the metacarpal bone of the hand, or of the metatarsal bone of the foot.

B4. Body Part

General guidelines

B4.1a. If a procedure is performed on a portion of a body part that does not have a separate body part value, code the body part value corresponding to the whole body part.

Example:
A procedure performed on the alveolar process of the mandible is coded to the mandible body part.

B4.1b. If the prefix "peri" is combined with a body part to identify the site of the procedure, and the site of the procedure is not further specified, then the procedure is coded to the body part named. This guideline applies only when a more specific body part value is not available.

Examples:
A procedure site identified as perirenal is coded to the kidney body part when the site of the procedure is not further specified.

A procedure site described in the documentation as peri-urethral, and the documentation also indicates that it is the vulvar tissue and not the urethral tissue that is the site of the procedure, then the procedure is coded to the vulva body part.

A procedure site documented as involving the periosteum is coded to the corresponding bone body part.

B4.1c. If a single vascular procedure is performed on a continuous section of an arterial or venous body part, code the body part value corresponding to the anatomically most proximal (closest to the heart) portion of the arterial or venous body part.

Example:
A procedure performed on a continuous section of artery from the femoral artery to the external iliac artery with the point of entry at the femoral artery is coded to the external iliac body part.

A procedure performed on a continuous section of artery from the femoral artery to the external iliac artery with the point of entry at the external iliac artery is also coded to the external iliac artery body part.

Branches of body parts

B4.2. Where a specific branch of a body part does not have its own body part value in PCS, the body part is typically coded to the closest proximal branch that has a specific body part value. In the cardiovascular body systems, if a general body part is available in the correct root operation table, and coding to a proximal branch would require assigning a code in a different body system, the procedure is coded using the general body part value.

Examples:
A procedure performed on the mandibular branch of the trigeminal nerve is coded to the trigeminal nerve body part value.

Occlusion of the bronchial artery is coded to the body part value Upper Artery in the body system Upper Arteries, and not to the body part value Thoracic Aorta, Descending in the body system Heart and Great Vessels.

Bilateral body part values

B4.3. Bilateral body part values are available for a limited number of body parts. If the identical procedure is performed on contralateral body parts, and a bilateral body part value exists for that body part, a single procedure is coded using the bilateral body part value. If no bilateral body part value exists, each procedure is coded separately using the appropriate body part value.

Examples:
The identical procedure performed on both fallopian tubes is coded once using the body part value Fallopian Tube, Bilateral.

The identical procedure performed on both knee joints is coded twice using the body part values Knee Joint, Right and Knee Joint, Left.

Coronary arteries

B4.4. The coronary arteries are classified as a single body part that is further specified by number of arteries treated. One procedure code specifying multiple arteries is used when the same procedure is performed, including the same device and qualifier values.

Examples:
Angioplasty of two distinct coronary arteries with placement of two stents is coded as Dilation of Coronary Artery, Two Arteries with Two Intraluminal Devices.

Angioplasty of two distinct coronary arteries, one with stent placed and one without, is coded separately as Dilation of Coronary Artery, One Artery with Intraluminal Device, and Dilation of Coronary Artery, One Artery with no device.

Tendons, ligaments, bursae and fascia near a joint

B4.5. Procedures performed on tendons, ligaments, bursae and fascia supporting a joint are coded to the body part in the respective body system that is the focus of the procedure. Procedures performed on joint structures themselves are coded to the body part in the joint body systems.

Examples:
Repair of the anterior cruciate ligament of the knee is coded to the knee bursa and ligament body part in the bursae and ligaments body system.

Knee arthroscopy with shaving of articular cartilage is coded to the knee joint body part in the Lower Joints body system.

Skin, subcutaneous tissue and fascia overlying a joint

B4.6. If a procedure is performed on the skin, subcutaneous tissue or fascia overlying a joint, the procedure is coded to the following body part:

- Shoulder is coded to Upper Arm
- Elbow is coded to Lower Arm
- Wrist is coded to Lower Arm
- Hip is coded to Upper Leg
- Knee is coded to Lower Leg
- Ankle is coded to Foot

Fingers and toes

B4.7. If a body system does not contain a separate body part value for fingers, procedures performed on the fingers are coded to the body part value for the hand. If a body system does not contain a separate body part value for toes, procedures performed on the toes are coded to the body part value for the foot.

Example:
Excision of finger muscle is coded to one of the hand muscle body part values in the Muscles body system.

Upper and lower intestinal tract

B4.8. In the Gastrointestinal body system, the general body part values Upper Intestinal Tract and Lower Intestinal Tract are provided as an option for the root operations such as Change, Insertion, Inspection, Removal and Revision. Upper Intestinal Tract includes the portion of the gastrointestinal tract from the esophagus down to and including the duodenum, and Lower Intestinal Tract includes the portion of the gastrointestinal tract from the jejunum down to and including the rectum and anus.

Example:
In the root operation Change table, change of a device in the jejunum is coded using the body part Lower Intestinal Tract.

B5. Approach

Open approach with percutaneous endoscopic assistance

B5.2a. Procedures performed using the open approach with percutaneous endoscopic assistance are coded to the approach Open.

Example:
Laparoscopic-assisted sigmoidectomy is coded to the approach Open.

Percutaneous endoscopic approach with hand-assistance or extension of incision

B5.2b. Procedures performed using the percutaneous endoscopic approach, with hand-assistance, or with an incision or extension of an incision to assist in the removal of all or a portion of a body part, or to anastomose a tubular body part with or without the temporary exteriorization of a body structure, are coded to the approach value Percutaneous Endoscopic.

Examples:
Hand-assisted laparoscopic sigmoid colon resection with exteriorization of a segment of the colon for removal of specimen with return of colon back into abdominal cavity is coded to the approach value percutaneous endoscopic.

Laparoscopic sigmoid colectomy with extension of stapling port for removal of specimen and direct anastomosis is coded to the approach value percutaneous endoscopic.

Laparoscopic nephrectomy with midline incision for removing the resected kidney is coded to the approach value percutaneous endoscopic.

Robotic-assisted laparoscopic prostatectomy with extension of incision for removal of the resected prostate is coded to the approach value percutaneous endoscopic.

External approach

B5.3a. Procedures performed within an orifice on structures that are visible without the aid of any instrumentation are coded to the approach External.

Example:
Resection of tonsils is coded to the approach External.

B5.3b. Procedures performed indirectly by the application of external force through the intervening body layers are coded to the approach External.

Example:
Closed reduction of fracture is coded to the approach External.

Percutaneous procedure via device

B5.4. Procedures performed percutaneously via a device placed for the procedure are coded to the approach Percutaneous.

Example:
Fragmentation of kidney stone performed via percutaneous nephrostomy is coded to the approach Percutaneous.

B6. Device

General guidelines

B6.1a. A device is coded only if a device remains after the procedure is completed. If no device remains, the device value No Device is coded. In limited root operations, the classification provides the qualifier values Temporary and Intraoperative, for specific procedures involving clinically significant devices, where the purpose of the device is to be utilized for a brief duration during the procedure or current inpatient stay. If a device that is intended to remain after the procedure is completed requires removal before the end of the operative episode in which it was inserted, both the insertion and removal of the device should be coded.

B6.1b. Materials such as sutures, ligatures, radiological markers and temporary post-operative wound drains are considered integral to the performance of a procedure and are not coded as devices.

B6.1c. Procedures performed on a device only and not on a body part are specified in the root operations Change, Irrigation, Removal and Revision, and are coded to the procedure performed.

Example:
Irrigation of percutaneous nephrostomy tube is coded to the root operation Irrigation of indwelling device in the Administration section.

Drainage device

B6.2. A separate procedure to put in a drainage device is coded to the root operation Drainage with the device value Drainage Device.

Obstetric Section Guidelines (section 1)

C. Obstetrics Section

Products of conception

C1. Procedures performed on the products of conception are coded to the Obstetrics section. Procedures performed on the pregnant female other than the products of conception are coded to the appropriate root operation in the Medical and Surgical section.

Examples:
Amniocentesis is coded to the products of conception body part in the Obstetrics section.

Repair of obstetric urethral laceration is coded to the urethra body part in the Medical and Surgical section.

Procedures following delivery or abortion

C2. Procedures performed following a delivery or abortion for curettage of the endometrium or evacuation of retained products of conception are all coded in the Obstetrics section, to the root operation Extraction and the body part Products of Conception, Retained.

Diagnostic or therapeutic dilation and curettage performed during times other than the postpartum or post-abortion period are all coded in the Medical and Surgical section, to the root operation Extraction and the body part Endometrium.

Radiation Therapy Section Guidelines (section D)

D. Radiation Therapy Section

Brachytherapy

D1.a. Brachytherapy is coded to the modality Brachytherapy in the Radiation Therapy section. When a radioactive brachytherapy source is left in the body at the end of the procedure, it is coded separately to the root operation Insertion with the device value Radioactive Element.

Example:
Brachytherapy with implantation of a low dose rate brachytherapy source left in the body at the end of the procedure is coded to the applicable treatment site in section D, Radiation Therapy, with the modality Brachytherapy, the modality qualifier value Low Dose Rate, and the applicable isotope value and qualifier value. The implantation of the brachytherapy source is coded separately to the device value Radioactive Element in the appropriate Insertion table of the Medical and Surgical section. The Radiation Therapy section code identifies the specific modality and isotope of the brachytherapy, and the root operation Insertion code identifies the implantation of the brachytherapy source that remains in the body at the end of the procedure.

Exceptions:
Implantation of Cesium-131 brachytherapy seeds embedded in a collagen matrix to the treatment site after resection of brain tumor is coded to the root operation Insertion with the device value Radioactive Element, Cesium-131 Collagen Implant. Similarly, implantation of Palladium-103 brachytherapy seeds embedded in a collagen matrix to the treatment site after resection of brain tumor is coded to the root operation Insertion with the device value Radioactive Element, Palladium-103 Collagen Implant. These procedures are coded to the root operation Insertion only, because the device value identifies both the implantation of the radioactive element and a specific brachytherapy isotope.

D1.b. A separate procedure to place a temporary applicator for delivering the brachytherapy is coded to the root operation Insertion and the device value Other Device.

Examples:
Intrauterine brachytherapy applicator placed as a separate procedure from the brachytherapy procedure is coded to Insertion of Other Device, and the brachytherapy is coded separately using the modality Brachytherapy in the Radiation Therapy section.

Intrauterine brachytherapy applicator placed concomitantly with delivery of the brachytherapy dose is coded with a single code using the modality Brachytherapy in the Radiation Therapy section.

New Technology Section Guidelines (section X)

E. New Technology Section

General guidelines

E1.a. Section X codes fully represent the specific procedure described in the code title, and do not require additional codes from other sections of ICD-10-PCS. When section X contains a code title which fully describes a specific new technology procedure, and it is the only procedure performed, only the section X code is reported for the procedure. There is no need to report an additional code in another section of ICD-10-PCS.

Example:
XW043A6 Introduction of Cefiderocol Anti-infective into Central Vein, Percutaneous Approach, New Technology Group 6, can be coded to indicate that Cefiderocol Anti-infective was administered via a central vein. A separate code from table 3E0 in the Administration section of ICD-10-PCS is not coded in addition to this code.

E1.b. When multiple procedures are performed, New Technology section X codes are coded following the multiple procedures guideline.

Examples:
Dual filter cerebral embolic filtration used during transcatheter aortic valve replacement (TAVR), X2A5312 Cerebral Embolic Filtration, Dual Filter in Innominate Artery and Left Common Carotid Artery, Percutaneous Approach, New Technology Group 2, is coded for the cerebral embolic filtration, along with an ICD-10-PCS code for the TAVR procedure.

An extracorporeal flow reversal circuit for embolic neuroprotection placed during a transcarotid arterial revascularization procedure, a code from table X2A, Assistance of the Cardiovascular System is coded for the use of the extracorporeal flow reversal circuit, along with an ICD-10-PCS code for the transcarotid arterial revascularization procedure.

F. Selection of Principal Procedure

The following instructions should be applied in the selection of principal procedure and clarification on the importance of the relation to the principal diagnosis when more than one procedure is performed:

1. Procedure performed for definitive treatment of both principal diagnosis and secondary diagnosis

   a. Sequence procedure performed for definitive treatment most related to principal diagnosis as principal procedure.

2. Procedure performed for definitive treatment and diagnostic procedures performed for both principal diagnosis and secondary diagnosis.

   a. Sequence procedure performed for definitive treatment most related to principal diagnosis as principal procedure

3. A diagnostic procedure was performed for the principal diagnosis and a procedure is performed for definitive treatment of a secondary diagnosis.

   a. Sequence diagnostic procedure as principal procedure, since the procedure most related to the principal diagnosis takes precedence.

4. No procedures performed that are related to principal diagnosis; procedures performed for definitive treatment and diagnostic procedures were performed for secondary diagnosis

   a. Sequence procedure performed for definitive treatment of secondary diagnosis as principal procedure, since there are no procedures (definitive or nondefinitive treatment) related to principal diagnosis.

# #

3f (Aortic) Bioprosthesis valve *use* Zooplastic Tissue in Heart and Great Vessels

A

Abdominal aortic plexus *use* Abdominal Sympathetic Nerve
Abdominal cavity *use* Peritoneal Cavity
Abdominal esophagus *use* Esophagus, Lower
Abdominohysterectomy *see* Resection, Uterus 0UT9
Abdominoplasty
  see Alteration, Abdominal Wall 0W0F
  see Repair, Abdominal Wall 0WQF
  see Supplement, Abdominal Wall 0WUF
Abductor hallucis muscle
  use Foot Muscle, Left
  use Foot Muscle, Right
ABECMA® *use* Idecabtagene Vicleucel Immunotherapy
AbioCor® Total Replacement Heart *use* Synthetic Substitute
Ablation
  see Control bleeding in
  see Destruction
Abortion
  Abortifacient 10A07ZX
  Laminaria 10A07ZW
  Products of Conception 10A0
  Vacuum 10A07Z6
Abrasion *see* Extraction
Absolute Pro Vascular (OTW) Self-Expanding Stent System *use* Intraluminal Device
Accelerate PhenoTest™ BC XXE5XN6
Accessory cephalic vein
  use Cephalic Vein, Left
  use Cephalic Vein, Right
Accessory obturator nerve *use* Lumbar Plexus
Accessory phrenic nerve *use* Phrenic Nerve
Accessory spleen *use* Spleen
Acculink (RX) Carotid Stent System *use* Intraluminal Device
Acellular Hydrated Dermis *use* Nonautologous Tissue Substitute
Acetabular cup *use* Liner in Lower Joints
Acetabulectomy
  see Excision, Lower Bones 0QB
  see Resection, Lower Bones 0QT
Acetabulofemoral joint
  use Hip Joint, Left
  use Hip Joint, Right
Acetabuloplasty
  see Repair, Lower Bones 0QQ
  see Replacement, Lower Bones 0QR
  see Supplement, Lower Bones 0QU
Achilles tendon
  use Lower Leg Tendon, Left
  use Lower Leg Tendon, Right
Achillorrhaphy *see* Repair, Tendons 0LQ
Achillotenotomy, achillotomy
  see Division, Tendons 0L8
  see Drainage, Tendons 0L9
Acoustic Pulse Thrombolysis *see* Fragmentation, Artery
Acromioclavicular ligament
  use Shoulder Bursa and Ligament, Left
  use Shoulder Bursa and Ligament, Right
Acromion (process)
  use Scapula, Left
  use Scapula, Right
Acromionectomy
  see Excision, Upper Joints 0RB
  see Resection, Upper Joints 0RT
Acromioplasty
  see Repair, Upper Joints 0RQ
  see Replacement, Upper Joints 0RR
  see Supplement, Upper Joints 0RU
ACTEMRA® *use* Tocilizumab
Activa PC neurostimulator *use* Stimulator Generator, Multiple Array in 0JH
Activa RC neurostimulator *use* Stimulator Generator, Multiple Array Rechargeable in 0JH
Activa SC neurostimulator *use* Stimulator Generator, Single Array in 0JH
Activities of Daily Living Assessment F02
Activities of Daily Living Treatment F08
ACUITY™ Steerable Lead
  use Cardiac Lead, Defibrillator in 02H
  use Cardiac Lead, Pacemaker in 02H
Acupuncture
  Breast
    Anesthesia 8E0H300
    No Qualifier 8E0H30Z
  Integumentary System
    Anesthesia 8E0H300
    No Qualifier 8E0H30Z
Adductor brevis muscle
  use Upper Leg Muscle, Left
  use Upper Leg Muscle, Right
Adductor hallucis muscle
  use Foot Muscle, Left
  use Foot Muscle, Right
Adductor longus muscle
  use Upper Leg Muscle, Left
  use Upper Leg Muscle, Right
Adductor magnus muscle
  use Upper Leg Muscle, Left
  use Upper Leg Muscle, Right
Adductor pollicis muscle
  use Hand Muscle, Left
  use Hand Muscle, Right
Adenohypophysis *use* Pituitary Gland
Adenoidectomy
  see Excision, Adenoids 0CBQ
  see Resection, Adenoids 0CTQ
Adenoidotomy *see* Drainage, Adenoids 0C9Q
Adhesiolysis *see* Release
Adhesive Ultrasound Patch Technology, Blood Flow XX25X0A
Administration
  Blood products *see* Transfusion
  Other substance *see* Introduction of substance in or on
Adrenalectomy
  see Excision, Endocrine System 0GB
  see Resection, Endocrine System 0GT
Adrenalorrhaphy *see* Repair, Endocrine System 0GQ
Adrenalotomy *see* Drainage, Endocrine System 0G9
Advancement
  see Reposition
  see Transfer
Advisa (MRI) *use* Pacemaker, Dual Chamber in 0JH
afami-cel *use* Afamitresgene Autoleucel Immunotherapy
Afamitresgene Autoleucel Immunotherapy XW0
AFX® Endovascular AAA System *use* Intraluminal Device
AGENT™ Paclitaxel-Coated Balloon *see* New Technology, Anatomical Regions XW0
AGN1 Bone Void Filler XW0V3WA
Aidoc Briefcase for PE (pulmonary embolism) XXE3X27
AIGISRx Antibacterial Envelope *use* Anti-Infective Envelope
Alar ligament of axis *use* Head and Neck Bursa and Ligament
Alfapump® system *use* Other Device
Alfieri Stitch Valvuloplasty *see* Restriction, Valve, Mitral 02VG
Alimentation *see* Introduction of substance in or on
ALPPS (Associating liver partition and portal vein ligation)
  see Division, Hepatobiliary System and Pancreas 0F8
  see Resection, Hepatobiliary System and Pancreas 0FT
Alteration
  Abdominal Wall 0W0F
  Ankle Region
    Left 0Y0L
    Right 0Y0K
  Arm
    Lower
      Left 0X0F
      Right 0X0D
    Upper
      Left 0X09
      Right 0X08
  Axilla
    Left 0X05
    Right 0X04
Alteration — *continued*
  Back
    Lower 0W0L
    Upper 0W0K
  Breast
    Bilateral 0H0V
    Left 0H0U
    Right 0H0T
  Buttock
    Left 0Y01
    Right 0Y00
  Chest Wall 0W08
  Ear
    Bilateral 0902
    Left 0901
    Right 0900
  Elbow Region
    Left 0X0C
    Right 0X0B
  Extremity
    Lower
      Left 0Y0B
      Right 0Y09
    Upper
      Left 0X07
      Right 0X06
  Eyelid
    Lower
      Left 080R
      Right 080Q
    Upper
      Left 080P
      Right 080N
  Face 0W02
  Head 0W00
  Jaw
    Lower 0W05
    Upper 0W04
  Knee Region
    Left 0Y0G
    Right 0Y0F
  Leg
    Lower
      Left 0Y0J
      Right 0Y0H
    Upper
      Left 0Y0D
      Right 0Y0C
  Lip
    Lower 0C01X
    Upper 0C00X
  Nasal Mucosa and Soft Tissue 090K
  Neck 0W06
  Perineum
    Female 0W0N
    Male 0W0M
  Shoulder Region
    Left 0X03
    Right 0X02
  Subcutaneous Tissue and Fascia
    Abdomen 0J08
    Back 0J07
    Buttock 0J09
    Chest 0J06
    Face 0J01
    Lower Arm
      Left 0J0H
      Right 0J0G
    Lower Leg
      Left 0J0P
      Right 0J0N
    Neck
      Left 0J05
      Right 0J04
    Upper Arm
      Left 0J0F
      Right 0J0D
    Upper Leg
      Left 0J0M
      Right 0J0L
  Wrist Region
    Left 0X0H
    Right 0X0G
Alveolar process of mandible
  use Mandible, Left
  use Mandible, Right
Alveolar process of maxilla *use* Maxilla
Alveolectomy
  see Excision, Head and Facial Bones 0NB

▽ Subterms under main terms may continue to next column or page

Alveolectomy — continued
see Resection, Head and Facial Bones 0NT
Alveoloplasty
see Repair, Head and Facial Bones 0NQ
see Replacement, Head and Facial Bones 0NR
see Supplement, Head and Facial Bones 0NU
Alveolotomy
see Division, Head and Facial Bones 0N8
see Drainage, Head and Facial Bones 0N9
Ambulatory cardiac monitoring 4A12X45
Amivantamab Monoclonal Antibody XW0
Amniocentesis see Drainage, Products of Conception 10902
Amnioinfusion see Introduction of substance in or on, Products of Conception 3E0E
Amnioscopy 10J08ZZ
Amniotomy see Drainage, Products of Conception 10902
AMPLATZER® Muscular VSD Occluder use Synthetic Substitute
Amputation see Detachment
AMS 800® Urinary Control System use Artificial Sphincter in Urinary System
AMTAGVI™ use Lifileucel Immunotherapy
Anacaulase-bcdb XW0
Anal orifice use Anus
Analog radiography see Plain Radiography
Analog radiology see Plain Radiography
Anastomosis see Bypass
Anatomical snuffbox
use Lower Arm and Wrist Muscle, Left
use Lower Arm and Wrist Muscle, Right
Anconeus muscle
use Lower Arm and Wrist Muscle, Left
use Lower Arm and Wrist Muscle, Right
Andexanet Alfa, Factor Xa Inhibitor Reversal Agent use Coagulation Factor Xa, Inactivated
Andexxa use Coagulation Factor Xa, Inactivated
AneuRx® AAA Advantage® use Intraluminal Device
Angiectomy
see Excision, Heart and Great Vessels 02B
see Excision, Lower Arteries 04B
see Excision, Lower Veins 06B
see Excision, Upper Arteries 03B
see Excision, Upper Veins 05B
Angio Vac System, for extracorporeal filtration during percutaneous thrombectomy 5A05A0L
Angiocardiography
Combined right and left heart see Fluoroscopy, Heart, Right and Left B216
Left Heart see Fluoroscopy, Heart, Left B215
Right Heart see Fluoroscopy, Heart, Right B214
SPY system intravascular fluorescence see Monitoring, Physiological Systems 4A1
Angiography
see Computerized Tomography (CT Scan), Artery
see Fluoroscopy, Artery
see Magnetic Resonance Imaging (MRI), Artery
see Plain Radiography, Artery
Angioplasty
see Dilation, Heart and Great Vessels 027
see Dilation, Lower Arteries 047
see Dilation, Upper Arteries 037
see Repair, Heart and Great Vessels 02Q
see Repair, Lower Arteries 04Q
see Repair, Upper Arteries 03Q
see Replacement, Heart and Great Vessels 02R
see Replacement, Lower Arteries 04R
see Replacement, Upper Arteries 03R
see Supplement, Heart and Great Vessels 02U
see Supplement, Lower Arteries 04U
see Supplement, Upper Arteries 03U
Angiorrhaphy
see Repair, Heart and Great Vessels 02Q
see Repair, Lower Arteries 04Q
see Repair, Upper Arteries 03Q
Angioscopy 02JY4ZZ, 03JY4ZZ, 04JY4ZZ
Angiotensin II use Vasopressor
Angiotripsy
see Occlusion, Lower Arteries 04L
see Occlusion, Upper Arteries 03L
Angular artery use Face Artery
Angular vein
use Face Vein, Left
use Face Vein, Right
Ankle Truss System™ (ATS) use Internal Fixation Device, Open-truss Design in New Technology

Annalise Enterprise CTB Triage software (Measurement of Intracranial Cerebrospinal Fluid Flow) XXE0X1A
Annular ligament
use Elbow Bursa and Ligament, Left
use Elbow Bursa and Ligament, Right
Annuloplasty
see Repair, Heart and Great Vessels 02Q
see Restriction, Heart and Great Vessels 02V
see Supplement, Heart and Great Vessels 02U
Annuloplasty ring use Synthetic Substitute
Anoplasty
see Repair, Anus 0DQQ
see Supplement, Anus 0DUQ
Anorectal junction use Rectum
Anoscopy 0DJD8ZZ
Ansa cervicalis use Cervical Plexus
Antabuse therapy HZ93ZZZ
Antebrachial fascia
use Subcutaneous Tissue and Fascia, Left Lower Arm
use Subcutaneous Tissue and Fascia, Right Lower Arm
Anterior cerebral artery use Intracranial Artery
Anterior cerebral vein use Intracranial Vein
Anterior choroidal artery use Intracranial Artery
Anterior circumflex humeral artery
use Axillary Artery, Left
use Axillary Artery, Right
Anterior communicating artery use Intracranial Artery
Anterior cruciate ligament (ACL)
use Knee Bursa and Ligament, Left
use Knee Bursa and Ligament, Right
Anterior crural nerve use Femoral Nerve
Anterior facial vein
use Face Vein, Left
use Face Vein, Right
Anterior intercostal artery
use Internal Mammary Artery, Left
use Internal Mammary Artery, Right
Anterior interosseous nerve use Median Nerve
Anterior lateral malleolar artery
use Anterior Tibial Artery, Left
use Anterior Tibial Artery, Right
Anterior lingual gland use Minor Salivary Gland
Anterior (pectoral) lymph node
use Lymphatic, Left Axillary
use Lymphatic, Right Axillary
Anterior medial malleolar artery
use Anterior Tibial Artery, Left
use Anterior Tibial Artery, Right
Anterior spinal artery
use Vertebral Artery, Left
use Vertebral Artery, Right
Anterior tibial recurrent artery
use Anterior Tibial Artery, Left
use Anterior Tibial Artery, Right
Anterior ulnar recurrent artery
use Ulnar Artery, Left
use Ulnar Artery, Right
Anterior vagal trunk use Vagus Nerve
Anterior vertebral muscle
use Neck Muscle, Left
use Neck Muscle, Right
Antibacterial Envelope (TYRX) (AIGISRx) use Anti-Infective Envelope
Antibiotic-eluting Bone Void Filler XW0V0P7
Antigen-free air conditioning see Atmospheric Control, Physiological Systems 6A0
Antihelix
use External Ear, Bilateral
use External Ear, Left
use External Ear, Right
Antimicrobial envelope use Anti-Infective Envelope
Anti-SARS-CoV-2 hyperimmune globulin use Hyperimmune Globulin
Antitragus
use External Ear, Bilateral
use External Ear, Left
use External Ear, Right
Antrostomy see Drainage, Ear, Nose, Sinus 099
Antrotomy see Drainage, Ear, Nose, Sinus 099
Antrum of Highmore
use Maxillary Sinus, Left
use Maxillary Sinus, Right

Aortic annulus use Aortic Valve
Aortic arch use Thoracic Aorta, Ascending/Arch
Aortic intercostal artery use Upper Artery
Aortic isthmus use Thoracic Aorta, Ascending/Arch
Aortix™ System use Short-term External Heart Assist System in Heart and Great Vessels
Aortography
see Fluoroscopy, Lower Arteries B41
see Fluoroscopy, Upper Arteries B31
see Plain Radiography, Lower Arteries B40
see Plain Radiography, Upper Arteries B30
Aortoplasty
see Repair, Aorta, Abdominal 04Q0
see Repair, Aorta, Thoracic, Ascending/Arch 02QX
see Repair, Aorta, Thoracic, Descending 02QW
see Replacement, Aorta, Abdominal 04R0
see Replacement, Aorta, Thoracic, Ascending/Arch 02RX
see Replacement, Aorta, Thoracic, Descending 02RW
see Supplement, Aorta, Abdominal 04U0
see Supplement, Aorta, Thoracic, Ascending/Arch 02UX
see Supplement, Aorta, Thoracic, Descending 02UW
Apalutamide Antineoplastic use Other Antineoplastic
Apical (subclavicular) lymph node
use Lymphatic, Left Axillary
use Lymphatic, Right Axillary
ApiFix® Minimally Invasive Deformity Correction (MID-C) System use Posterior (Dynamic) Distraction Device in New Technology
Apneustic center use Pons
Appendectomy
see Excision, Appendix 0DBJ
see Resection, Appendix 0DTJ
Appendiceal orifice use Appendix
Appendicolysis see Release, Appendix 0DNJ
Appendicotomy see Drainage, Appendix 0D9J
Application see Introduction of substance in or on
aprevo™ use Interbody Fusion Device, Custom-Made Anatomically Designed in New Technology
Aquablation therapy, prostate 0V508ZZ
Aquapheresis 6A550Z3
Aqueduct of Sylvius use Cerebral Ventricle
Aqueous humour
use Anterior Chamber, Left
use Anterior Chamber, Right
Arachnoid mater, intracranial use Cerebral Meninges
Arachnoid mater, spinal use Spinal Meninges
Arcuate artery
use Foot Artery, Left
use Foot Artery, Right
Areola
use Nipple, Left
use Nipple, Right
AROM (artificial rupture of membranes) 10907ZC
Arterial canal (duct) use Pulmonary Artery, Left
Arterial pulse tracing see Measurement, Arterial 4A03
Arteriectomy
see Excision, Heart and Great Vessels 02B
see Excision, Lower Arteries 04B
see Excision, Upper Arteries 03B
Arteriography
see Fluoroscopy, Heart B21
see Fluoroscopy, Lower Arteries B41
see Fluoroscopy, Upper Arteries B31
see Plain Radiography, Heart B20
see Plain Radiography, Lower Arteries B40
see Plain Radiography, Upper Arteries B30
Arterioplasty
see Repair, Heart and Great Vessels 02Q
see Repair, Lower Arteries 04Q
see Repair, Upper Arteries 03Q
see Replacement, Heart and Great Vessels 02R
see Replacement, Lower Arteries 04R
see Replacement, Upper Arteries 03R
see Supplement, Heart and Great Vessels 02U
see Supplement, Lower Arteries 04U
see Supplement, Upper Arteries 03U
Arteriorrhaphy
see Repair, Heart and Great Vessels 02Q
see Repair, Lower Arteries 04Q
see Repair, Upper Arteries 03Q
Arterioscopy
see Inspection, Artery, Lower 04JY

Arterioscopy — *continued*
   see Inspection, Artery, Upper 03JY
   see Inspection, Great Vessel 02JY
Arteriovenous Fistula, Extraluminal Support Device, Supplement X2U
Arthrectomy
   see Excision, Lower Joints 0SB
   see Excision, Upper Joints 0RB
   see Resection, Lower Joints 0ST
   see Resection, Upper Joints 0RT
Arthrocentesis
   see Drainage, Lower Joints 0S9
   see Drainage, Upper Joints 0R9
Arthrodesis
   see Fusion, Lower Joints 0SG
   see Fusion, Upper Joints 0RG
Arthrography
   see Plain Radiography, Non-Axial Lower Bones BQ0
   see Plain Radiography, Non-Axial Upper Bones BP0
   see Plain Radiography, Skull and Facial Bones BN0
Arthrolysis
   see Release, Lower Joints 0SN
   see Release, Upper Joints 0RN
Arthropexy
   see Repair, Lower Joints 0SQ
   see Repair, Upper Joints 0RQ
   see Reposition, Lower Joints 0SS
   see Reposition, Upper Joints 0RS
Arthroplasty
   see Repair, Lower Joints 0SQ
   see Repair, Upper Joints 0RQ
   see Replacement, Lower Joints 0SR
   see Replacement, Upper Joints 0RR
   see Supplement, Lower Joints 0SU
   see Supplement, Upper Joints 0RU
Arthroplasty, radial head
   see Replacement, Radius, Left 0PRJ
   see Replacement, Radius, Right 0PRH
Arthroscopy
   see Inspection, Lower Joints 0SJ
   see Inspection, Upper Joints 0RJ
Arthrotomy
   see Drainage, Lower Joints 0S9
   see Drainage, Upper Joints 0R9
Articulating Spacer (Antibiotic) use Articulating Spacer in Lower Joints
Artificial anal sphincter (AAS) use Artificial Sphincter in Gastrointestinal System
Artificial bowel sphincter (neosphincter) use Artificial Sphincter in Gastrointestinal System
Artificial Sphincter
   Insertion of device in
     Anus 0DHQ
     Bladder 0THB
     Bladder Neck 0THC
     Urethra 0THD
   Removal of device from
     Anus 0DPQ
     Bladder 0TPB
     Urethra 0TPD
   Revision of device in
     Anus 0DWQ
     Bladder 0TWB
     Urethra 0TWD
Artificial urinary sphincter (AUS) use Artificial Sphincter in Urinary System
Aryepiglottic fold use Larynx
Arytenoid cartilage use Larynx
Arytenoid muscle
   use Neck Muscle, Left
   use Neck Muscle, Right
Arytenoidectomy see Excision, Larynx 0CBS
Arytenoidopexy see Repair, Larynx 0CQS
Ascenda Intrathecal Catheter use Infusion Device
Ascending aorta use Thoracic Aorta, Ascending/Arch
Ascending palatine artery use Face Artery
Ascending pharyngeal artery
   use External Carotid Artery, Left
   use External Carotid Artery, Right
aScope™ Duodeno see New Technology, Hepatobiliary System and Pancreas XFJ
Aspiration, fine needle
   Fluid or gas see Drainage
   Tissue biopsy
     see Excision
     see Extraction

Assessment
   Activities of daily living see Activities of Daily Living Assessment, Rehabilitation F02
   Hearing see Hearing Assessment, Diagnostic Audiology F13
   Hearing aid see Hearing Aid Assessment, Diagnostic Audiology F14
   Intravascular perfusion, using indocyanine green (ICG) dye see Monitoring, Physiological Systems 4A1
   Motor function see Motor Function Assessment, Rehabilitation F01
   Nerve function see Motor Function Assessment, Rehabilitation F01
   Speech see Speech Assessment, Rehabilitation F00
   Vestibular see Vestibular Assessment, Diagnostic Audiology F15
   Vocational see Activities of Daily Living Treatment, Rehabilitation F08
Assistance
   Cardiac
     Continuous
       Output
         Balloon Pump 5A02210
         Impeller Pump 5A0221D
         Other Pump 5A02216
         Pulsatile Compression 5A02215
       Oxygenation, Supersaturated 5A0222C
     Intermittent
       Balloon Pump 5A02110
       Impeller Pump 5A0211D
       Other Pump 5A02116
       Pulsatile Compression 5A02115
   Circulatory
     Continuous, Oxygenation, Hyperbaric 5A05221
     Intermittent, Oxygenation, Hyperbaric 5A05121
     Intraoperative, Filtration, Peripheral Venovenous 5A05A0L
   Respiratory
     24-96 Consecutive Hours
       Continuous Negative Airway Pressure 5A09459
       Continuous Positive Airway Pressure 5A09457
       High Flow/Velocity Cannula 5A0945A
       Intermittent Negative Airway Pressure 5A0945B
       Intermittent Positive Airway Pressure 5A09458
       No Qualifier 5A0945Z
     8-24 Consecutive Hours, Ventilation, Intubated Prone Positioning 5A09C5K
     Continuous, Filtration 5A0920Z
     Greater than 24 Consecutive Hours, Ventilation, Intubated Prone Positioning 5A09D5K
     Greater than 96 Consecutive Hours
       Continuous Negative Airway Pressure 5A09559
       Continuous Positive Airway Pressure 5A09557
       High Flow/Velocity Cannula 5A0955A
       Intermittent Negative Airway Pressure 5A0955B
       Intermittent Positive Airway Pressure 5A09558
       No Qualifier 5A0955Z
     Less than 24 Consecutive Hours
       Continuous Negative Airway Pressure 5A09359
       Continuous Positive Airway Pressure 5A09357
       High Flow/Velocity Cannula 5A0935A
       Intermittent Negative Airway Pressure 5A0935B
       Intermittent Positive Airway Pressure 5A09358
       No Qualifier 5A0935Z
     Less than 8 Consecutive Hours, Ventilation, Intubated Prone Positioning 5A09B5K
Associating liver partition and portal vein ligation (ALPPS)
   see Division, Hepatobiliary System and Pancreas 0F8
   see Resection, Hepatobiliary System and Pancreas 0FT

Assurant (Cobalt) stent use Intraluminal Device
ASTar® XXE5X2A
Atezolizumab Antineoplastic XW0
Atherectomy
   see Extirpation, Heart and Great Vessels 02C
   see Extirpation, Lower Arteries 04C
   see Extirpation, Upper Arteries 03C
Atlantoaxial joint use Cervical Vertebral Joint
Atmospheric Control 6A0Z
AtriClip LAA Exclusion System use Extraluminal Device
Atrioseptoplasty
   see Repair, Heart and Great Vessels 02Q
   see Replacement, Heart and Great Vessels 02R
   see Supplement, Heart and Great Vessels 02U
Atrioventricular node use Conduction Mechanism
Atrium dextrum cordis use Atrium, Right
Atrium pulmonale use Atrium, Left
Attain Ability® lead 02H
   use Cardiac Lead, Defibrillator in 02H
   use Cardiac Lead, Pacemaker in 02H
Attain StarFix® (OTW) lead
   use Cardiac Lead, Defibrillator in 02H
   use Cardiac Lead, Pacemaker in 02H
Audiology, diagnostic
   see Hearing Aid Assessment, Diagnostic Audiology F14
   see Hearing Assessment, Diagnostic Audiology F13
   see Vestibular Assessment, Diagnostic Audiology F15
Audiometry see Hearing Assessment, Diagnostic Audiology F13
Auditory tube
   use Eustachian Tube, Left
   use Eustachian Tube, Right
Auerbach's (myenteric) plexus use Abdominal Sympathetic Nerve
Auricle
   use External Ear, Bilateral
   use External Ear, Left
   use External Ear, Right
Auricularis muscle use Head Muscle
Autograft use Autologous Tissue Substitute
AutoLITT® System see Destruction
Autologous artery graft
   use Autologous Arterial Tissue in Heart and Great Vessels
   use Autologous Arterial Tissue in Lower Arteries
   use Autologous Arterial Tissue in Lower Veins
   use Autologous Arterial Tissue in Upper Arteries
   use Autologous Arterial Tissue in Upper Veins
Autologous vein graft
   use Autologous Venous Tissue in Heart and Great Vessels
   use Autologous Venous Tissue in Lower Arteries
   use Autologous Venous Tissue in Lower Veins
   use Autologous Venous Tissue in Upper Arteries
   use Autologous Venous Tissue in Upper Veins
Automated Chest Compression (ACC) 5A1221J
AutoPulse® Resuscitation System 5A1221J
Autotransfusion see Transfusion
Autotransplant
   Adrenal tissue see Reposition, Endocrine System 0GS
   Kidney see Reposition, Urinary System 0TS
   Pancreatic tissue see Reposition, Pancreas 0FSG
   Parathyroid tissue see Reposition, Endocrine System 0GS
   Thyroid tissue see Reposition, Endocrine System 0GS
   Tooth see Reattachment, Mouth and Throat 0CM
Aveir™ AR, as dual chamber use Intracardiac Pacemaker, Dual-Chamber in New Technology
Aveir™ DR, dual chamber use Intracardiac Pacemaker, Dual-Chamber in New Technology
Aveir™ VR, as single chamber use Intracardiac Pacemaker in Heart and Great Vessels
Avulsion see Extraction
AVYCAZ® (ceftazidime-avibactam) use Other Anti-infective
Axial Lumbar Interbody Fusion System use Interbody Fusion Device in Lower Joints
AxiaLIF® System use Interbody Fusion Device in Lower Joints
Axicabtagene Ciloleucel use Axicabtagene Ciloleucel Immunotherapy

Axicabtagene Ciloleucel Immunotherapy XW0
Axillary fascia
  use Subcutaneous Tissue and Fascia, Left Upper Arm
  use Subcutaneous Tissue and Fascia, Right Upper Arm
Axillary nerve use Brachial Plexus
AZEDRA® use Iobenguane I-131 Antineoplastic

B

BAK/C® Interbody Cervical Fusion System use Interbody Fusion Device in Upper Joints
BAL (bronchial alveolar lavage), diagnostic see Drainage, Respiratory System 0B9
Balanoplasty
  see Repair, Penis 0VQS
  see Supplement, Penis 0VUS
Balloon atrial septostomy (BAS) 02163Z7
Balloon Pump
  Continuous, Output 5A02210
  Intermittent, Output 5A02110
Balversa™ (Erdafitinib Antineoplastic) use Other Antineoplastic
Bamlanivimab Monoclonal Antibody XW0
Bandage, Elastic see Compression
Banding
  see Occlusion
  see Restriction
Banding, esophageal varices see Occlusion, Vein, Esophageal 06L3
Banding, laparoscopic (adjustable) gastric
  Initial procedure 0DV64CZ
  Surgical correction see Revision of device in, Stomach 0DW6
Bard® Composix® Kugel® patch use Synthetic Substitute
Bard® Composix® (E/X) (LP) mesh use Synthetic Substitute
Bard® Dulex™ mesh use Synthetic Substitute
Bard® Ventralex™ hernia patch use Synthetic Substitute
Baricitinib XW0
Barium swallow see Fluoroscopy, Gastrointestinal System BD1
Baroreflex Activation Therapy® (BAT®)
  use Stimulator Generator in Subcutaneous Tissue and Fascia
  use Stimulator Lead in Upper Arteries
Barricaid® Annular Closure Device (ACD) use Synthetic Substitute
Bartholin's (greater vestibular) gland use Vestibular Gland
Basal (internal) cerebral vein use Intracranial Vein
Basal metabolic rate (BMR) see Measurement, Physiological Systems 4A0Z
Basal nuclei use Basal Ganglia
Base of Tongue use Pharynx
Basilar artery use Intracranial Artery
Basis pontis use Pons
Beam Radiation
  Abdomen DW03
    Intraoperative DW033Z0
  Adrenal Gland DG02
    Intraoperative DG023Z0
  Bile Ducts DF02
    Intraoperative DF023Z0
  Bladder DT02
    Intraoperative DT023Z0
  Bone
    Intraoperative DP0C3Z0
    Other DP0C
  Bone Marrow D700
    Intraoperative D7003Z0
  Brain D000
    Intraoperative D0003Z0
  Brain Stem D001
    Intraoperative D0013Z0
  Breast
    Left DM00
      Intraoperative DM003Z0
    Right DM01
      Intraoperative DM013Z0
  Bronchus DB01
    Intraoperative DB013Z0
  Cervix DU01
    Intraoperative DU013Z0

Beam Radiation — continued
  Chest DW02
    Intraoperative DW023Z0
  Chest Wall DB07
    Intraoperative DB073Z0
  Colon DD05
    Intraoperative DD053Z0
  Diaphragm DB08
    Intraoperative DB083Z0
  Duodenum DD02
    Intraoperative DD023Z0
  Ear D900
    Intraoperative D9003Z0
  Esophagus DD00
    Intraoperative DD003Z0
  Eye D800
    Intraoperative D8003Z0
  Femur DP09
    Intraoperative DP093Z0
  Fibula DP0B
    Intraoperative DP0B3Z0
  Gallbladder DF01
    Intraoperative DF013Z0
  Gland
    Adrenal DG02
      Intraoperative DG023Z0
    Parathyroid DG04
      Intraoperative DG043Z0
    Pituitary DG00
      Intraoperative DG003Z0
    Thyroid DG05
      Intraoperative DG053Z0
  Glands
    Intraoperative D9063Z0
    Salivary D906
  Head and Neck DW01
    Intraoperative DW013Z0
  Hemibody DW04
    Intraoperative DW043Z0
  Humerus DP06
    Intraoperative DP063Z0
  Hypopharynx D903
    Intraoperative D9033Z0
  Ileum DD04
    Intraoperative DD043Z0
  Jejunum DD03
    Intraoperative DD033Z0
  Kidney DT00
    Intraoperative DT003Z0
  Larynx D90B
    Intraoperative D90B3Z0
  Liver DF00
    Intraoperative DF003Z0
  Lung DB02
    Intraoperative DB023Z0
  Lymphatics
    Abdomen D706
      Intraoperative D7063Z0
    Axillary D704
      Intraoperative D7043Z0
    Inguinal D708
      Intraoperative D7083Z0
    Neck D703
      Intraoperative D7033Z0
    Pelvis D707
      Intraoperative D7073Z0
    Thorax D705
      Intraoperative D7053Z0
  Mandible DP03
    Intraoperative DP033Z0
  Maxilla DP02
    Intraoperative DP023Z0
  Mediastinum DB06
    Intraoperative DB063Z0
  Mouth D904
    Intraoperative D9043Z0
  Nasopharynx D90D
    Intraoperative D90D3Z0
  Neck and Head DW01
    Intraoperative DW013Z0
  Nerve
    Intraoperative D0073Z0
    Peripheral D007
  Nose D901
    Intraoperative D9013Z0
  Oropharynx D90F
    Intraoperative D90F3Z0
  Ovary DU00
    Intraoperative DU003Z0

Beam Radiation — continued
  Palate
    Hard D908
      Intraoperative D9083Z0
    Soft D909
      Intraoperative D9093Z0
  Pancreas DF03
    Intraoperative DF033Z0
  Parathyroid Gland DG04
    Intraoperative DG043Z0
  Pelvic Bones DP08
    Intraoperative DP083Z0
  Pelvic Region DW06
    Intraoperative DW063Z0
  Pineal Body DG01
    Intraoperative DG013Z0
  Pituitary Gland DG00
    Intraoperative DG003Z0
  Pleura DB05
    Intraoperative DB053Z0
  Prostate DV00
    Intraoperative DV003Z0
  Radius DP07
    Intraoperative DP073Z0
  Rectum DD07
    Intraoperative DD073Z0
  Rib DP05
    Intraoperative DP053Z0
  Sinuses D907
    Intraoperative D9073Z0
  Skin
    Abdomen DH08
      Intraoperative DH083Z0
    Arm DH04
      Intraoperative DH043Z0
    Back DH07
      Intraoperative DH073Z0
    Buttock DH09
      Intraoperative DH093Z0
    Chest DH06
      Intraoperative DH063Z0
    Face DH02
      Intraoperative DH023Z0
    Leg DH0B
      Intraoperative DH0B3Z0
    Neck DH03
      Intraoperative DH033Z0
  Skull DP00
    Intraoperative DP003Z0
  Spinal Cord D006
    Intraoperative D0063Z0
  Spleen D702
    Intraoperative D7023Z0
  Sternum DP04
    Intraoperative DP043Z0
  Stomach DD01
    Intraoperative DD013Z0
  Testis DV01
    Intraoperative DV013Z0
  Thymus D701
    Intraoperative D7013Z0
  Thyroid Gland DG05
    Intraoperative DG053Z0
  Tibia DP0B
    Intraoperative DP0B3Z0
  Tongue D905
    Intraoperative D9053Z0
  Trachea DB00
    Intraoperative DB003Z0
  Ulna DP07
    Intraoperative DP073Z0
  Ureter DT01
    Intraoperative DT013Z0
  Urethra DT03
    Intraoperative DT033Z0
  Uterus DU02
    Intraoperative DU023Z0
  Whole Body DW05
    Intraoperative DW053Z0
Bedside swallow F00ZJWZ
Bentracimab, Ticagrelor Reversal Agent XW0
Berlin Heart Ventricular Assist Device use Implantable Heart Assist System in Heart and Great Vessels
Betibeglogene Autotemcel XW1
beti-cel use Betibeglogene Autotemcel
Bezlotoxumab infusion see Introduction with qualifier Other Therapeutic Monoclonal Antibody

Biceps brachii muscle
　use Upper Arm Muscle, Left
　use Upper Arm Muscle, Right
Biceps femoris muscle
　use Upper Leg Muscle, Left
　use Upper Leg Muscle, Right
Bicipital aponeurosis
　use Subcutaneous Tissue and Fascia, Left Lower Arm
　use Subcutaneous Tissue and Fascia, Right Lower Arm
Bicuspid valve use Mitral Valve
Bili light therapy see Phototherapy, Skin 6A60
Bioactive embolization coil(s) use Intraluminal Device, Bioactive in Upper Arteries
Bioengineered Allogeneic Construct, Skin XHRPXF7
Bioengineered Human Acellular Vessel X2R
Biofeedback GZC9ZZZ
BioFire® FilmArray® Pneumonia Panel XXEBXQ6
Biopsy
　see Drainage with qualifier Diagnostic
　see Excision with qualifier Diagnostic
　see Extraction with qualifier Diagnostic
BiPAP see Assistance, Respiratory 5A09
Bisection see Division
Biventricular external heart assist system use Short-term External Heart Assist System in Heart and Great Vessels
BlackArmor® Carbon/PEEK fixation system use Carbon/PEEK Spinal Stabilization Device, Pedicle Based in New Technology
Blepharectomy
　see Excision, Eye 08B
　see Resection, Eye 08T
Blepharoplasty
　see Repair, Eye 08Q
　see Replacement, Eye 08R
　see Reposition, Eye 08S
　see Supplement, Eye 08U
Blepharorrhaphy see Repair, Eye 08Q
Blepharotomy see Drainage, Eye 089
Blinatumomab use Other Antineoplastic
BLINCYTO® (blinatumomab) use Other Antineoplastic
Block, Nerve, anesthetic injection 3E0T3BZ
Blood glucose monitoring system use Monitoring Device
Blood pressure see Measurement, Arterial 4A03
BMR (basal metabolic rate) see Measurement, Physiological Systems 4A0Z
Body of femur
　use Femoral Shaft, Left
　use Femoral Shaft, Right
Body of fibula
　use Fibula, Left
　use Fibula, Right
Bone anchored hearing device
　use Hearing Device, Bone Conduction in 09H
　use Hearing Device in Head and Facial Bones
Bone bank bone graft use Nonautologous Tissue Substitute
Bone Growth Stimulator
　Insertion of device in
　　Bone
　　　Facial 0NHW
　　　Lower 0QHY
　　　Nasal 0NHB
　　　Upper 0PHY
　　　Skull 0NH0
　Removal of device from
　　Bone
　　　Facial 0NPW
　　　Lower 0QPY
　　　Nasal 0NPB
　　　Upper 0PPY
　　　Skull 0NP0
　Revision of device in
　　Bone
　　　Facial 0NWW
　　　Lower 0QWY
　　　Nasal 0NWB
　　　Upper 0PWY
　　　Skull 0NW0
Bone marrow transplant see Transfusion, Circulatory 302
Bone morphogenetic protein 2 (BMP 2) use Recombinant Bone Morphogenetic Protein

Bone screw (interlocking) (lag) (pedicle) (recessed)
　use Internal Fixation Device in Head and Facial Bones
　use Internal Fixation Device in Lower Bones
　use Internal Fixation Device in Upper Bones
Bony labyrinth
　use Inner Ear, Left
　use Inner Ear, Right
Bony orbit
　use Orbit, Left
　use Orbit, Right
Bony vestibule
　use Inner Ear, Left
　use Inner Ear, Right
Botallo's duct use Pulmonary Artery, Left
Bovine pericardial valve use Zooplastic Tissue in Heart and Great Vessels
Bovine pericardium graft use Zooplastic Tissue in Heart and Great Vessels
BP (blood pressure) see Measurement, Arterial 4A03
Brachial (lateral) lymph node
　use Lymphatic, Left Axillary
　use Lymphatic, Right Axillary
Brachialis muscle
　use Upper Arm Muscle, Left
　use Upper Arm Muscle, Right
Brachiocephalic artery use Innominate Artery
Brachiocephalic trunk use Innominate Artery
Brachiocephalic vein
　use Innominate Vein, Left
　use Innominate Vein, Right
Brachioradialis muscle
　use Lower Arm and Wrist Muscle, Left
　use Lower Arm and Wrist Muscle, Right
Brachytherapy
　Abdomen DW13
　Adrenal Gland DG12
　Back
　　Lower DW1LBB
　　Upper DW1KBB
　Bile Ducts DF12
　Bladder DT12
　Bone Marrow D710
　Brain D010
　Brain Stem D011
　Breast
　　Left DM10
　　Right DM11
　Bronchus DB11
　Cervix DU11
　Chest DW12
　Chest Wall DB17
　Colon DD15
　Cranial Cavity DW10BB
　Diaphragm DB18
　Duodenum DD12
　Ear D910
　Esophagus DD10
　Extremity
　　Lower DW1YBB
　　Upper DW1XBB
　Eye D810
　Gallbladder DF11
　Gastrointestinal Tract DW1PBB
　Genitourinary Tract DW1RBB
　Gland
　　Adrenal DG12
　　Parathyroid DG14
　　Pituitary DG10
　　Thyroid DG15
　Glands, Salivary D916
　Head and Neck DW11
　Hypopharynx D913
　Ileum DD14
　Jejunum DD13
　Kidney DT10
　Larynx D91B
　Liver DF10
　Lung DB12
　Lymphatics
　　Abdomen D716
　　Axillary D714
　　Inguinal D718
　　Neck D713
　　Pelvis D717
　　Thorax D715
　Mediastinum DB16
　Mouth D914

Brachytherapy — continued
　Nasopharynx D91D
　Neck and Head DW11
　Nerve, Peripheral D017
　Nose D911
　Oropharynx D91F
　Ovary DU10
　Palate
　　Hard D918
　　Soft D919
　Pancreas DF13
　Parathyroid Gland DG14
　Pelvic Region DW16
　Pineal Body DG11
　Pituitary Gland DG10
　Pleura DB15
　Prostate DV10
　Rectum DD17
　Respiratory Tract DW1QBB
　Sinuses D917
　Spinal Cord D016
　Spleen D712
　Stomach DD11
　Testis DV11
　Thymus D711
　Thyroid Gland DG15
　Tongue D915
　Trachea DB10
　Ureter DT11
　Urethra DT13
　Uterus DU12
Brachytherapy, CivaSheet®
　see Brachytherapy with qualifier Unidirectional Source
　see Insertion with device Radioactive Element
Brachytherapy seeds use Radioactive Element
Brain Connectomic Analysis Mapping 00K0XZ1
Brain Electrical Activity
　Computer-aided Detection and Notification XX20X89
　Computer-aided Semiologic Analysis XXE0X48
Branched Intraluminal Device, Manufactured Integrated System, Four or More Arteries, Aorta, Thoracodominal X2VE3SA
Breast procedures, skin only use Skin, Chest
Brexanolone XW0
Brexucabtagene Autoleucel use Brexucabtagene Autoleucel Immunotherapy
Brexucabtagene Autoleucel Immunotherapy XW0
Breyanzi® use Lisocabtagene Maraleucel Immunotherapy
Broad Consortium Microbiota-based Live Biotherapeutic Suspension XW0H7X8
Broad ligament use Uterine Supporting Structure
Bromelain-enriched Proteolytic Enzyme use Anacaulase-bcdb
Bronchial artery use Upper Artery
Bronchography
　see Fluoroscopy, Respiratory System BB1
　see Plain Radiography, Respiratory System BB0
Bronchoplasty
　see Repair, Respiratory System 0BQ
　see Supplement, Respiratory System 0BU
Bronchorrhaphy see Repair, Respiratory System 0BQ
Bronchoscopy 0BJ08ZZ
Bronchotomy see Drainage, Respiratory System 0B9
Bronchus Intermedius use Main Bronchus, Right
BRYAN® Cervical Disc System use Synthetic Substitute
Buccal gland use Buccal Mucosa
Buccinator lymph node use Lymphatic, Head
Buccinator muscle use Facial Muscle
Buckling, scleral with implant see Supplement, Eye 08U
Bulbospongiosus muscle use Perineum Muscle
Bulbourethral (Cowper's) gland use Urethra
Bundle of His use Conduction Mechanism
Bundle of Kent use Conduction Mechanism
Bunionectomy see Excision, Lower Bones 0QB
Bursectomy
　see Excision, Bursae and Ligaments 0MB
　see Resection, Bursae and Ligaments 0MT
Bursocentesis see Drainage, Bursae and Ligaments 0M9
Bursography
　see Plain Radiography, Non-Axial Lower Bones BQ0
　see Plain Radiography, Non-Axial Upper Bones BP0

Bursotomy
see Division, Bursae and Ligaments 0M8
see Drainage, Bursae and Ligaments 0M9
BVS 5000 Ventricular Assist Device use Short-term External Heart Assist System in Heart and Great Vessels

Bypass
Anterior Chamber
  Left 08133
  Right 08123
Aorta
  Abdominal 0410
  Thoracic
    Ascending/Arch 021X
    Descending 021W
Artery
  Anterior Tibial
    Left 041Q
    Right 041P
  Axillary
    Left 03160
    Right 03150
  Brachial
    Left 0318
    Right 0317
  Common Carotid
    Left 031J0
    Right 031H0
  Common Iliac
    Left 041D
    Right 041C
  Coronary
    Four or More Arteries 0213
    One Artery 0210
    Three Arteries 0212
    Two Arteries 0211
  External Carotid
    Left 031N0
    Right 031M0
  External Iliac
    Left 041J
    Right 041H
  Femoral
    Left 041L
    Right 041K
  Foot
    Left 041W
    Right 041V
  Hepatic 0413
  Innominate 03120
  Internal Carotid
    Left 031L0
    Right 031K0
  Internal Iliac
    Left 041F
    Right 041E
  Intracranial 031G0
  Peroneal
    Left 041U
    Right 041T
  Popliteal
    Left 041N
    Right 041M
  Posterior Tibial
    Left 041S
    Right 041R
  Pulmonary
    Left 021R
    Right 021Q
  Pulmonary Trunk 021P
  Radial
    Left 031C
    Right 031B
  Splenic 0414
  Subclavian
    Left 03140
    Right 03130
  Temporal
    Left 031T0
    Right 031S0
  Ulnar
    Left 031A
    Right 0319
Atrium
  Left 0217
  Right 0216
Bladder 0T1B
Cavity, Cranial 0W110J
Cecum 0D1H

Bypass — continued
Cerebral Ventricle 0016
Cisterna Chyli 071L
Colon
  Ascending 0D1K
  Descending 0D1M
  Sigmoid 0D1N
  Transverse 0D1L
Conduit through Femoral Vein to Popliteal Artery X2K
Conduit through Femoral Vein to Superficial Femoral Artery X2K
Duct
  Common Bile 0F19
  Cystic 0F18
  Hepatic
    Common 0F17
    Left 0F16
    Right 0F15
  Lacrimal
    Left 081Y
    Right 081X
  Pancreatic 0F1D
    Accessory 0F1F
Duodenum 0D19
Ear
  Left 091E0
  Right 091D0
Esophagus 0D15
  Lower 0D13
  Middle 0D12
  Upper 0D11
Fallopian Tube
  Left 0U16
  Right 0U15
Gallbladder 0F14
Ileum 0D1B
Intestine
  Large 0D1E
  Small 0D18
Jejunum 0D1A
Kidney Pelvis
  Left 0T14
  Right 0T13
Lymphatic
  Aortic 071D
  Axillary
    Left 0716
    Right 0715
  Head 0710
  Inguinal
    Left 071J
    Right 071H
  Internal Mammary
    Left 0719
    Right 0718
  Lower Extremity
    Left 071G
    Right 071F
  Mesenteric 071B
  Neck
    Left 0712
    Right 0711
  Pelvis 071C
  Thoracic Duct 071K
  Thorax 0717
  Upper Extremity
    Left 0714
    Right 0713
Pancreas 0F1G
Pelvic Cavity 0W1J
Peritoneal Cavity 0W1G
Pleural Cavity
  Left 0W1B
  Right 0W19
Spinal Canal 001U
Stomach 0D16
Trachea 0B11
Ureter
  Left 0T17
  Right 0T16
Ureters, Bilateral 0T18
Vas Deferens
  Bilateral 0V1Q
  Left 0V1P
  Right 0V1N
Vein
  Axillary
    Left 0518

Bypass — continued
Vein — continued
  Axillary — continued
    Right 0517
  Azygos 0510
  Basilic
    Left 051C
    Right 051B
  Brachial
    Left 051A
    Right 0519
  Cephalic
    Left 051F
    Right 051D
  Colic 0617
  Common Iliac
    Left 061D
    Right 061C
  Esophageal 0613
  External Iliac
    Left 061G
    Right 061F
  External Jugular
    Left 051Q
    Right 051P
  Face
    Left 051V
    Right 051T
  Femoral
    Left 061N
    Right 061M
  Foot
    Left 061V
    Right 061T
  Gastric 0612
  Hand
    Left 051H
    Right 051G
  Hemiazygos 0511
  Hepatic 0614
  Hypogastric
    Left 061J
    Right 061H
  Inferior Mesenteric 0616
  Innominate
    Left 0514
    Right 0513
  Internal Jugular
    Left 051N
    Right 051M
  Intracranial 051L
  Portal 0618
  Renal
    Left 061B
    Right 0619
  Saphenous
    Left 061Q
    Right 061P
  Splenic 0611
  Subclavian
    Left 0516
    Right 0515
  Superior Mesenteric 0615
  Vertebral
    Left 051S
    Right 051R
Vena Cava
  Inferior 0610
  Superior 021V
Ventricle
  Left 021L
  Right 021K
Bypass, cardiopulmonary 5A1221Z

C

Caesarean section see Extraction, Products of Conception 10D0
Calcaneocuboid joint
  use Tarsal Joint, Left
  use Tarsal Joint, Right
Calcaneocuboid ligament
  use Foot Bursa and Ligament, Left
  use Foot Bursa and Ligament, Right
Calcaneofibular ligament
  use Ankle Bursa and Ligament, Left
  use Ankle Bursa and Ligament, Right

Calcaneus
  use Tarsal, Left
  use Tarsal, Right
Cannulation
  see Bypass
  see Dilation
  see Drainage
  see Irrigation
Canthorrhaphy see Repair, Eye 08Q
Canthotomy see Release, Eye 08N
Canturio™ te (Tibial Extension) use Tibial Extension with Motion Sensors in New Technology
Capitate bone
  use Carpal, Left
  use Carpal, Right
Caplacizumab XW0
Capsulectomy, lens see Excision, Eye 08B
Capsulorrhaphy, joint
  see Repair, Lower Joints 0SQ
  see Repair, Upper Joints 0RQ
Caption Guidance system X2JAX47
Carbon/PEEK Spinal Stabilization Device, Pedicle Based
  Lumbar Vertebral XRHB
    2 or more XRHC
  Lumbosacral XRHD
  Thoracic Vertebral XRH6
    2 to 7 XRH7
    8 or more XRH8
  Thoracolumbar Vertebral XRHA
Cardia use Esophagogastric Junction
Cardiac contractility modulation lead use Cardiac Lead in Heart and Great Vessels
Cardiac event recorder use Monitoring Device
Cardiac Lead
  Defibrillator
    Atrium
      Left 02H7
      Right 02H6
    Pericardium 02HN
    Vein, Coronary 02H4
    Ventricle
      Left 02HL
      Right 02HK
  Insertion of device in
    Atrium
      Left 02H7
      Right 02H6
    Pericardium 02HN
    Vein, Coronary 02H4
    Ventricle
      Left 02HL
      Right 02HK
  Pacemaker
    Atrium
      Left 02H7
      Right 02H6
    Pericardium 02HN
    Vein, Coronary 02H4
    Ventricle
      Left 02HL
      Right 02HK
  Removal of device from, Heart 02PA
  Revision of device in, Heart 02WA
Cardiac plexus use Thoracic Sympathetic Nerve
Cardiac Resynchronization Defibrillator Pulse Generator
  Abdomen 0JH8
  Chest 0JH6
Cardiac Resynchronization Pacemaker Pulse Generator
  Abdomen 0JH8
  Chest 0JH6
Cardiac resynchronization therapy (CRT) lead
  use Cardiac Lead, Defibrillator in 02H
  use Cardiac Lead, Pacemaker in 02H
Cardiac Rhythm Related Device
  Insertion of device in
    Abdomen 0JH8
    Chest 0JH6
  Removal of device from, Subcutaneous Tissue and Fascia, Trunk 0JPT
  Revision of device in, Subcutaneous Tissue and Fascia, Trunk 0JWT
Cardiocentesis see Drainage, Pericardial Cavity 0W9D
Cardioesophageal junction use Esophagogastric Junction
Cardiolysis see Release, Heart and Great Vessels 02N

CardioMEMS® pressure sensor use Monitoring Device, Pressure Sensor in 02H
Cardiomyotomy see Division, Esophagogastric Junction 0D84
Cardioplegia see Introduction of substance in or on, Heart 3E08
Cardiorrhaphy see Repair, Heart and Great Vessels 02Q
Cardioversion 5A2204Z
Caregiver Training F0FZ
Carmat total artificial heart (TAH) use Biologic with Synthetic Substitute, Autoregulated Electrohydraulic in 02R
Caroticotympanic artery
  use Internal Carotid Artery, Left
  use Internal Carotid Artery, Right
Carotid glomus
  use Carotid Bodies, Bilateral
  use Carotid Body, Left
  use Carotid Body, Right
Carotid sinus
  use Internal Carotid Artery, Left
  use Internal Carotid Artery, Right
Carotid (artery) sinus (baroreceptor) lead use Stimulator Lead in Upper Arteries
Carotid sinus nerve use Glossopharyngeal Nerve
Carotid WALLSTENT® Monorail® Endoprosthesis use Intraluminal Device
Carpectomy
  see Excision, Upper Bones 0PB
  see Resection, Upper Bones 0PT
Carpometacarpal ligament
  use Hand Bursa and Ligament, Left
  use Hand Bursa and Ligament, Right
CARVYKTI™ use Ciltacabtagene Autoleucel
CASGEVY™ use Exagamglogene Autotemcel
Casirivimab (REGN10933) and Imdevimab (REGN10987) use REGN-COV2 Monoclonal Antibody
Casting see Immobilization
CAT scan see Computerized Tomography (CT Scan)
Catheterization
  see Dilation
  see Drainage
  see Insertion of device in
  see Irrigation
  Heart see Measurement, Cardiac 4A02
  Umbilical vein, for infusion 06H33T
Cauda equina use Lumbar Spinal Cord
Cauterization
  see Destruction
  see Repair
Cavernous plexus use Head and Neck Sympathetic Nerve
Cavoatrial junction use Superior Vena Cava
CBMA (Concentrated Bone Marrow Aspirate) use Other Substance
CBMA (Concentrated Bone Marrow Aspirate) injection see Introduction of substance in or on, Muscle 3E02
CD24Fc Immunomodulator XW0
Cecectomy
  see Excision, Cecum 0DBH
  see Resection, Cecum 0DTH
Cecocolostomy
  see Bypass, Gastrointestinal System 0D1
  see Drainage, Gastrointestinal System 0D9
Cecopexy
  see Repair, Cecum 0DQH
  see Reposition, Cecum 0DSH
Cecoplication see Restriction, Cecum 0DVH
Cecorrhaphy see Repair, Cecum 0DQH
Cecostomy
  see Bypass, Cecum 0D1H
  see Drainage, Cecum 0D9H
Cecotomy see Drainage, Cecum 0D9H
Cefepime-taniborbactam Anti-infective XW0
Cefiderocol Anti-infective XW0
Ceftazidime-avibactam use Other Anti-infective
Ceftobiprole Medocaril Anti-infective XW0
Ceftolozane/Tazobactam Anti-infective XW0
Celiac ganglion use Abdominal Sympathetic Nerve
Celiac lymph node use Lymphatic, Aortic
Celiac (solar) plexus use Abdominal Sympathetic Nerve
Celiac trunk use Celiac Artery

Central axillary lymph node
  use Lymphatic, Left Axillary
  use Lymphatic, Right Axillary
Central venous pressure see Measurement, Venous 4A04
Centrimag® Blood Pump use Short-term External Heart Assist System in Heart and Great Vessels
Cephalogram BN00ZZZ
CERAMENT® G use Antibiotic-eluting Bone Void Filler
Ceramic on ceramic bearing surface use Synthetic Substitute, Ceramic in 0SR
Cerclage see Restriction
Cerebral aqueduct (Sylvius) use Cerebral Ventricle
Cerebral Embolic Filtration
  Dual Filter X2A5312
  Extracorporeal Flow Reversal Circuit X2A
  Single Deflection Filter X2A6325
Cerebrum use Brain
Ceribell® Monitor XX20X89
Cervical esophagus use Esophagus, Upper
Cervical facet joint
  use Cervical Vertebral Joint
  use Cervical Vertebral Joint, 2 or more
Cervical ganglion use Head and Neck Sympathetic Nerve
Cervical interspinous ligament use Head and Neck Bursa and Ligament
Cervical intertransverse ligament use Head and Neck Bursa and Ligament
Cervical Ligamentum Flavum use Head and Neck Bursa and Ligament
Cervical Lymph Node
  use Lymphatic, Left Neck
  use Lymphatic, Right Neck
Cervicectomy
  see Excision, Cervix 0UBC
  see Resection, Cervix 0UTC
Cervicothoracic facet joint use Cervicothoracic Vertebral Joint
Cesarean section see Extraction, Products of Conception 10D0
Cesium-131 Collagen Implant use Radioactive Element, Cesium-131 Collagen Implant in 00H
Change Device in
  Abdominal Wall 0W2FX
  Back
    Lower 0W2LX
    Upper 0W2KX
  Bladder 0T2BX
  Bone
    Facial 0N2WX
    Lower 0Q2YX
    Nasal 0N2BX
    Upper 0P2YX
  Bone Marrow 072TX
  Brain 0020X
  Breast
    Left 0H2UX
    Right 0H2TX
  Bursa and Ligament
    Lower 0M2YX
    Upper 0M2XX
  Cavity, Cranial 0W21X
  Chest Wall 0W28X
  Cisterna Chyli 072LX
  Diaphragm 0B2TX
  Duct
    Hepatobiliary 0F2BX
    Pancreatic 0F2DX
  Ear
    Left 092JX
    Right 092HX
  Epididymis and Spermatic Cord 0V2MX
  Extremity
    Lower
      Left 0Y2BX
      Right 0Y29X
    Upper
      Left 0X27X
      Right 0X26X
  Eye
    Left 0821X
    Right 0820X
  Face 0W22X
  Fallopian Tube 0U28X
  Gallbladder 0F24X
  Gland
    Adrenal 0G25X

Change Device in — continued
Gland — continued
Endocrine 0G2SX
Pituitary 0G20X
Salivary 0C2AX
Head 0W20X
Intestinal Tract
Lower Intestinal Tract 0D2DXUZ
Upper Intestinal Tract 0D20XUZ
Jaw
Lower 0W25X
Upper 0W24X
Joint
Lower 0S2YX
Upper 0R2YX
Kidney 0T25X
Larynx 0C2SX
Liver 0F20X
Lung
Left 0B2LX
Right 0B2KX
Lymphatic 072NX
Thoracic Duct 072KX
Mediastinum 0W2CX
Mesentery 0D2VX
Mouth and Throat 0C2YX
Muscle
Lower 0K2YX
Upper 0K2XX
Nasal Mucosa and Soft Tissue 092KX
Neck 0W26X
Nerve
Cranial 002EX
Peripheral 012YX
Omentum 0D2UX
Ovary 0U23X
Pancreas 0F2GX
Parathyroid Gland 0G2RX
Pelvic Cavity 0W2JX
Penis 0V2SX
Pericardial Cavity 0W2DX
Perineum
Female 0W2NX
Male 0W2MX
Peritoneal Cavity 0W2GX
Peritoneum 0D2WX
Pineal Body 0G21X
Pleura 0B2QX
Pleural Cavity
Left 0W2BX
Right 0W29X
Products of Conception 10207
Prostate and Seminal Vesicles 0V24X
Retroperitoneum 0W2HX
Scrotum and Tunica Vaginalis 0V28X
Sinus 092YX
Skin 0H2PX
Skull 0N20X
Spinal Canal 002UX
Spleen 072PX
Subcutaneous Tissue and Fascia
Head and Neck 0J2SX
Lower Extremity 0J2WX
Trunk 0J2TX
Upper Extremity 0J2VX
Tendon
Lower 0L2YX
Upper 0L2XX
Testis 0V2DX
Thymus 072MX
Thyroid Gland 0G2KX
Trachea 0B21
Tracheobronchial Tree 0B20X
Ureter 0T29X
Urethra 0T2DX
Uterus and Cervix 0U2DXHZ
Vagina and Cul-de-sac 0U2HXGZ
Vas Deferens 0V2RX
Vulva 0U2MX
Change Device in or on
Abdominal Wall 2W03X
Anorectal 2Y03X5Z
Arm
Lower
Left 2W0DX
Right 2W0CX
Upper
Left 2W0BX
Right 2W0AX

Change Device in or on — continued
Back 2W05X
Chest Wall 2W04X
Ear 2Y02X5Z
Extremity
Lower
Left 2W0MX
Right 2W0LX
Upper
Left 2W09X
Right 2W08X
Face 2W01X
Finger
Left 2W0KX
Right 2W0JX
Foot
Left 2W0TX
Right 2W0SX
Genital Tract, Female 2Y04X5Z
Hand
Left 2W0FX
Right 2W0EX
Head 2W00X
Inguinal Region
Left 2W07X
Right 2W06X
Leg
Lower
Left 2W0RX
Right 2W0QX
Upper
Left 2W0PX
Right 2W0NX
Mouth and Pharynx 2Y00X5Z
Nasal 2Y01X5Z
Neck 2W02X
Thumb
Left 2W0HX
Right 2W0GX
Toe
Left 2W0VX
Right 2W0UX
Urethra 2Y05X5Z
Chemoembolization see Introduction of substance in or on
Chemosurgery, Skin 3E00XTZ
Chemothalamectomy see Destruction, Thalamus 0059
Chemotherapy, Infusion for Cancer see Introduction of substance in or on
Chest compression (CPR), external
Manual 5A12012
Mechanical 5A1221J
Chest x-ray see Plain Radiography, Chest BW03
Chin use Subcutaneous Tissue and Fascia, Face
Chiropractic Manipulation
Abdomen 9WB9X
Cervical 9WB1X
Extremities
Lower 9WB6X
Upper 9WB7X
Head 9WB0X
Lumbar 9WB3X
Pelvis 9WB5X
Rib Cage 9WB8X
Sacrum 9WB4X
Thoracic 9WB2X
Choana use Nasopharynx
Cholangiogram
see Fluoroscopy, Hepatobiliary System and Pancreas BF1
see Plain Radiography, Hepatobiliary System and Pancreas BF0
Cholecystectomy
see Excision, Gallbladder 0FB4
see Resection, Gallbladder 0FT4
Cholecystojejunostomy
see Bypass, Hepatobiliary System and Pancreas 0F1
see Drainage, Hepatobiliary System and Pancreas 0F9
Cholecystopexy
see Repair, Gallbladder 0FQ4
see Reposition, Gallbladder 0FS4
Cholecystoscopy 0FJ44ZZ
Cholecystostomy
see Bypass, Gallbladder 0F14
see Drainage, Gallbladder 0F94
Cholecystotomy see Drainage, Gallbladder 0F94

Choledochectomy
see Excision, Hepatobiliary System and Pancreas 0FB
see Resection, Hepatobiliary System and Pancreas 0FT
Choledocholithotomy see Extirpation, Duct, Common Bile 0FC9
Choledochoplasty
see Repair, Hepatobiliary System and Pancreas 0FQ
see Replacement, Hepatobiliary System and Pancreas 0FR
see Supplement, Hepatobiliary System and Pancreas 0FU
Choledochoscopy 0FJB8ZZ
Choledochotomy see Drainage, Hepatobiliary System and Pancreas 0F9
Cholelithotomy see Extirpation, Hepatobiliary System and Pancreas 0FC
Chondrectomy
see Excision, Lower Joints 0SB
see Excision, Upper Joints 0RB
Knee see Excision, Lower Joints 0SB
Semilunar cartilage see Excision, Lower Joints 0SB
Chondroglossus muscle use Tongue, Palate, Pharynx Muscle
Chorda tympani use Facial Nerve
Chordotomy see Division, Central Nervous System and Cranial Nerves 008
Choroid plexus use Cerebral Ventricle
Choroidectomy
see Excision, Eye 08B
see Resection, Eye 08T
Ciliary body
use Eye, Left
use Eye, Right
Ciliary ganglion use Head and Neck Sympathetic Nerve
Ciltacabtagene Autoleucel XW0
cilta-cel use Ciltacabtagene Autoleucel
Circle of Willis use Intracranial Artery
Circumcision 0VTTXZZ
Circumflex iliac artery
use Femoral Artery, Left
use Femoral Artery, Right
CivaSheet® use Radioactive Element
CivaSheet® Brachytherapy
see Brachytherapy with qualifier Unidirectional Source
see Insertion with device Radioactive Element
Clamp and rod internal fixation system (CRIF)
use Internal Fixation Device in Lower Bones
use Internal Fixation Device in Upper Bones
Clamping see Occlusion
Claustrum use Basal Ganglia
Claviculectomy
see Excision, Upper Bones 0PB
see Resection, Upper Bones 0PT
Claviculotomy
see Division, Upper Bones 0P8
see Drainage, Upper Bones 0P9
Clipping, aneurysm
see Occlusion using Extraluminal Device
see Restriction using Extraluminal Device
Clitorectomy, clitoridectomy
see Excision, Clitoris 0UBJ
see Resection, Clitoris 0UTJ
Clolar use Clofarabine
Closure
see Occlusion
see Repair
Clysis see Introduction of substance in or on
Coagulation see Destruction
Coagulation Factor Xa, Inactivated XW0
Coagulation Factor Xa, (Recombinant) Inactivated use Coagulation Factor Xa, Inactivated
COALESCE® radiolucent interbody fusion device
use Interbody Fusion Device in Lower Joints
use Interbody Fusion Device in Upper Joints
CoAxia NeuroFlo catheter use Intraluminal Device
Cobalt/chromium head and polyethylene socket
use Synthetic Substitute, Metal on Polyethylene in 0SR
Cobalt/chromium head and socket use Synthetic Substitute, Metal in 0SR
Coccygeal body use Coccygeal Glomus
Coccygeus muscle
use Trunk Muscle, Left

Coccygeus muscle — continued
    use Trunk Muscle, Right
Cochlea
    use Inner Ear, Left
    use Inner Ear, Right
Cochlear implant (CI), multiple channel (electrode)
    use Hearing Device, Multiple Channel Cochlear Prosthesis in 09H
Cochlear implant (CI), single channel (electrode)
    use Hearing Device, Single Channel Cochlear Prosthesis in 09H
Cochlear Implant Treatment F0BZ0
Cochlear nerve use Acoustic Nerve
COGNIS® CRT-D use Cardiac Resynchronization Defibrillator Pulse Generator in 0JH
COHERE® radiolucent interbody fusion device
    use Interbody Fusion Device in Lower Joints
    use Interbody Fusion Device in Upper Joints
Colectomy
    see Excision, Gastrointestinal System 0DB
    see Resection, Gastrointestinal System 0DT
Collapse see Occlusion
Collection from
    Breast, Breast Milk 8E0HX62
    Indwelling Device
        Circulatory System
            Blood 8C02X6K
            Other Fluid 8C02X6L
        Nervous System
            Cerebrospinal Fluid 8C01X6J
            Other Fluid 8C01X6L
    Integumentary System, Breast Milk 8E0HX62
    Reproductive System, Male, Sperm 8E0VX63
Colocentesis see Drainage, Gastrointestinal System 0D9
Colofixation
    see Repair, Gastrointestinal System 0DQ
    see Reposition, Gastrointestinal System 0DS
Cololysis see Release, Gastrointestinal System 0DN
Colonic Z-Stent® use Intraluminal Device
Colonoscopy 0DJD8ZZ
Colopexy
    see Repair, Gastrointestinal System 0DQ
    see Reposition, Gastrointestinal System 0DS
Coloplication see Restriction, Gastrointestinal System 0DV
Coloproctectomy
    see Excision, Gastrointestinal System 0DB
    see Resection, Gastrointestinal System 0DT
Coloproctostomy
    see Bypass, Gastrointestinal System 0D1
    see Drainage, Gastrointestinal System 0D9
Colopuncture see Drainage, Gastrointestinal System 0D9
Colorrhaphy see Repair, Gastrointestinal System 0DQ
Colostomy
    see Bypass, Gastrointestinal System 0D1
    see Drainage, Gastrointestinal System 0D9
Colpectomy
    see Excision, Vagina 0UBG
    see Resection, Vagina 0UTG
Colpocentesis see Drainage, Vagina 0U9G
Colpopexy
    see Repair, Vagina 0UQG
    see Reposition, Vagina 0USG
Colpoplasty
    see Repair, Vagina 0UQG
    see Supplement, Vagina 0UUG
Colporrhaphy see Repair, Vagina 0UQG
Colposcopy 0UJH8ZZ
Columella use Nasal Mucosa and Soft Tissue
Columvi™ use Glofitamab Antineoplastic
COMIRNATY®
    use COVID-19 Vaccine
    use COVID-19 Vaccine Booster
    use COVID-19 Vaccine Dose 1
    use COVID-19 Vaccine Dose 2
    use COVID-19 Vaccine Dose 3
Common digital vein
    use Foot Vein, Left
    use Foot Vein, Right
Common facial vein
    use Face Vein, Left
    use Face Vein, Right
Common fibular nerve use Peroneal Nerve
Common hepatic artery use Hepatic Artery

Common iliac (subaortic) lymph node use Lymphatic, Pelvis
Common interosseous artery
    use Ulnar Artery, Left
    use Ulnar Artery, Right
Common peroneal nerve use Peroneal Nerve
Complete (SE) stent use Intraluminal Device
Compression
    see Restriction
    Abdominal Wall 2W13X
    Arm
        Lower
            Left 2W1DX
            Right 2W1CX
        Upper
            Left 2W1BX
            Right 2W1AX
    Back 2W15X
    Chest Wall 2W14X
    Extremity
        Lower
            Left 2W1MX
            Right 2W1LX
        Upper
            Left 2W19X
            Right 2W18X
    Face 2W11X
    Finger
        Left 2W1KX
        Right 2W1JX
    Foot
        Left 2W1TX
        Right 2W1SX
    Hand
        Left 2W1FX
        Right 2W1EX
    Head 2W10X
    Inguinal Region
        Left 2W17X
        Right 2W16X
    Leg
        Lower
            Left 2W1RX
            Right 2W1QX
        Upper
            Left 2W1PX
            Right 2W1NX
    Neck 2W12X
    Thumb
        Left 2W1HX
        Right 2W1GX
    Toe
        Left 2W1VX
        Right 2W1UX
Computer Assisted Procedure
    Extremity
        Lower
            No Qualifier 8E0YXBZ
            With Computerized Tomography 8E0YXBG
            With Fluoroscopy 8E0YXBF
            With Magnetic Resonance Imaging 8E0YXBH
        Upper
            No Qualifier 8E0XXBZ
            With Computerized Tomography 8E0XXBG
            With Fluoroscopy 8E0XXBF
            With Magnetic Resonance Imaging 8E0XXBH
    Head and Neck Region
        No Qualifier 8E09XBZ
        With Computerized Tomography 8E09XBG
        With Fluoroscopy 8E09XBF
        With Magnetic Resonance Imaging 8E09XBH
    Trunk Region
        No Qualifier 8E0WXBZ
        With Computerized Tomography 8E0WXBG
        With Fluoroscopy 8E0WXBF
        With Magnetic Resonance Imaging 8E0WXBH
Computer-aided Assessment
    Cardiac Output XXE2X19
    Intracranial Vascular Activity XXE0X07
Computer-aided Guidance, Transthoracic Echocardiography X2JAX47
Computer-aided Mechanical Aspiration X2C
Computer-aided Triage and Notification, Pulmonary Artery Flow XXE3X27

Computer-aided Valve Modeling and Notification, Coronary Artery Flow XXE3X68
Computer-assisted Intermittent Aspiration see New Technology, Cardiovascular System X2C
Computer-assisted Transcranial Magnetic Stimulation X0Z0X18
Computerized Tomography (CT Scan)
    Abdomen BW20
        Chest and Pelvis BW25
    Abdomen and Chest BW24
    Abdomen and Pelvis BW21
    Airway, Trachea BB2F
    Ankle
        Left BQ2H
        Right BQ2G
    Aorta
        Abdominal B420
            Intravascular Optical Coherence B420Z2Z
        Thoracic B320
            Intravascular Optical Coherence B320Z2Z
    Arm
        Left BP2F
        Right BP2E
    Artery
        Celiac B421
            Intravascular Optical Coherence B421Z2Z
        Common Carotid
            Bilateral B325
            Intravascular Optical Coherence B325Z2Z
        Coronary
            Bypass Graft
                Intravascular Optical Coherence B223Z2Z
                Multiple B223
            Multiple B221
                Intravascular Optical Coherence B221Z2Z
        Internal Carotid
            Bilateral B328
            Intravascular Optical Coherence B328Z2Z
        Intracranial B32R
            Intravascular Optical Coherence B32RZ2Z
        Lower Extremity
            Bilateral B42H
                Intravascular Optical Coherence B42HZ2Z
            Left B42G
                Intravascular Optical Coherence B42GZ2Z
            Right B42F
                Intravascular Optical Coherence B42FZ2Z
        Pelvic B42C
            Intravascular Optical Coherence B42CZ2Z
        Pulmonary
            Left B32T
                Intravascular Optical Coherence B32TZ2Z
            Right B32S
                Intravascular Optical Coherence B32SZ2Z
        Renal
            Bilateral B428
                Intravascular Optical Coherence B428Z2Z
            Transplant B42M
                Intravascular Optical Coherence B42MZ2Z
        Superior Mesenteric B424
            Intravascular Optical Coherence B424Z2Z
        Vertebral
            Bilateral B32G
                Intravascular Optical Coherence B32GZ2Z
    Bladder BT20
    Bone
        Facial BN25
        Temporal BN2F
    Brain B020
    Calcaneus
        Left BQ2K

Computerized Tomography (CT Scan) — continued
- Calcaneus — continued
  - Right BQ2J
- Cerebral Ventricle B028
- Chest, Abdomen and Pelvis BW25
- Chest and Abdomen BW24
- Cisterna B027
- Clavicle
  - Left BP25
  - Right BP24
- Coccyx BR2F
- Colon BD24
- Ear B920
- Elbow
  - Left BP2H
  - Right BP2G
- Extremity
  - Lower
    - Left BQ2S
    - Right BQ2R
  - Upper
    - Bilateral BP2V
    - Left BP2U
    - Right BP2T
- Eye
  - Bilateral B827
  - Left B826
  - Right B825
- Femur
  - Left BQ24
  - Right BQ23
- Fibula
  - Left BQ2C
  - Right BQ2B
- Finger
  - Left BP2S
  - Right BP2R
- Foot
  - Left BQ2M
  - Right BQ2L
- Forearm
  - Left BP2K
  - Right BP2J
- Gland
  - Adrenal, Bilateral BG22
  - Parathyroid BG23
  - Parotid, Bilateral B926
  - Salivary, Bilateral B92D
  - Submandibular, Bilateral B929
  - Thyroid BG24
- Hand
  - Left BP2P
  - Right BP2N
- Hands and Wrists, Bilateral BP2Q
- Head BW28
- Head and Neck BW29
- Heart
  - Intravascular Optical Coherence B226Z2Z
  - Right and Left B226
- Hepatobiliary System, All BF2C
- Hip
  - Left BQ21
  - Right BQ20
- Humerus
  - Left BP2B
  - Right BP2A
- Intracranial Sinus B522
  - Intravascular Optical Coherence B522Z2Z
- Joint
  - Acromioclavicular, Bilateral BP23
  - Finger
    - Left BP2DZZZ
    - Right BP2CZZZ
  - Foot
    - Left BQ2Y
    - Right BQ2X
  - Hand
    - Left BP2DZZZ
    - Right BP2CZZZ
  - Sacroiliac BR2D
  - Sternoclavicular
    - Bilateral BP22
    - Left BP21
    - Right BP20
  - Temporomandibular, Bilateral BN29
  - Toe
    - Left BQ2Y
    - Right BQ2X

Computerized Tomography (CT Scan) — continued
- Kidney
  - Bilateral BT23
  - Left BT22
  - Right BT21
  - Transplant BT29
- Knee
  - Left BQ28
  - Right BQ27
- Larynx B92J
- Leg
  - Left BQ2F
  - Right BQ2D
- Liver BF25
- Liver and Spleen BF26
- Lung, Bilateral BB24
- Mandible BN26
- Nasopharynx B92F
- Neck BW2F
- Neck and Head BW29
- Orbit, Bilateral BN23
- Oropharynx B92F
- Pancreas BF27
- Patella
  - Left BQ2W
  - Right BQ2V
- Pelvic Region BW2G
- Pelvis BR2C
  - Chest and Abdomen BW25
- Pelvis and Abdomen BW21
- Pituitary Gland B029
- Prostate BV23
- Ribs
  - Left BP2Y
  - Right BP2X
- Sacrum BR2F
- Scapula
  - Left BP27
  - Right BP26
- Sella Turcica B029
- Shoulder
  - Left BP29
  - Right BP28
- Sinus
  - Intracranial B522
    - Intravascular Optical Coherence B522Z2Z
  - Paranasal B922
- Skull BN20
- Spinal Cord B02B
- Spine
  - Cervical BR20
  - Lumbar BR29
  - Thoracic BR27
- Spleen and Liver BF26
- Thorax BP2W
- Tibia
  - Left BQ2C
  - Right BQ2B
- Toe
  - Left BQ2Q
  - Right BQ2P
- Trachea BB2F
- Tracheobronchial Tree
  - Bilateral BB29
  - Left BB28
  - Right BB27
- Vein
  - Pelvic (Iliac)
    - Left B52G
      - Intravascular Optical Coherence B52GZ2Z
    - Right B52F
      - Intravascular Optical Coherence B52FZ2Z
  - Pelvic (Iliac) Bilateral B52H
    - Intravascular Optical Coherence B52HZ2Z
  - Portal B52T
    - Intravascular Optical Coherence B52TZ2Z
  - Pulmonary
    - Bilateral B52S
      - Intravascular Optical Coherence B52SZ2Z
    - Left B52R
      - Intravascular Optical Coherence B52RZ2Z
    - Right B52Q

Computerized Tomography (CT Scan) — continued
- Vein — continued
  - Pulmonary — continued
    - Right — continued
      - Intravascular Optical Coherence B52QZ2Z
  - Renal
    - Bilateral B52L
      - Intravascular Optical Coherence B52LZ2Z
    - Left B52K
      - Intravascular Optical Coherence B52KZ2Z
    - Right B52J
      - Intravascular Optical Coherence B52JZ2Z
  - Splanchnic B52T
    - Intravascular Optical Coherence B52TZ2Z
  - Vena Cava
    - Inferior B529
      - Intravascular Optical Coherence B529Z2Z
    - Superior B528
      - Intravascular Optical Coherence B528Z2Z
- Ventricle, Cerebral B028
- Wrist
  - Left BP2M
  - Right BP2L

Concerto II CRT-D use Cardiac Resynchronization Defibrillator Pulse Generator in 0JH

Conduit through Femoral Vein to Popliteal Artery, Bypass X2K

Conduit through Femoral Vein to Superficial Femoral Artery, Bypass X2K

Conduit to Short-term External Heart Assist System, Insertion X2H

Condylectomy
- see Excision, Head and Facial Bones 0NB
- see Excision, Lower Bones 0QB
- see Excision, Upper Bones 0PB

Condyloid process
- use Mandible, Left
- use Mandible, Right

Condylotomy
- see Division, Head and Facial Bones 0N8
- see Division, Lower Bones 0Q8
- see Division, Upper Bones 0P8
- see Drainage, Head and Facial Bones 0N9
- see Drainage, Lower Bones 0Q9
- see Drainage, Upper Bones 0P9

Condylysis
- see Release, Head and Facial Bones 0NN
- see Release, Lower Bones 0QN
- see Release, Upper Bones 0PN

Conization, cervix see Excision, Cervix 0UBC

Conjunctivoplasty
- see Repair, Eye 08Q
- see Replacement, Eye 08R

Connectomic Analysis (Brain) Mapping 00K0XZ1

CONSERVE® PLUS Total Resurfacing Hip System
- use Resurfacing Device in Lower Joints

Construction
- Auricle, ear see Replacement, Ear, Nose, Sinus 09R
- Ileal conduit see Bypass, Urinary System 0T1

Consulta CRT-D use Cardiac Resynchronization Defibrillator Pulse Generator in 0JH

Consulta CRT-P use Cardiac Resynchronization Pacemaker Pulse Generator in 0JH

Contact Radiation
- Abdomen DWY37ZZ
- Adrenal Gland DGY27ZZ
- Bile Ducts DFY27ZZ
- Bladder DTY27ZZ
- Bone, Other DPYC7ZZ
- Brain D0Y07ZZ
- Brain Stem D0Y17ZZ
- Breast
  - Left DMY07ZZ
  - Right DMY17ZZ
- Bronchus DBY17ZZ
- Cervix DUY17ZZ
- Chest DWY27ZZ
- Chest Wall DBY77ZZ
- Colon DDY57ZZ
- Diaphragm DBY87ZZ
- Duodenum DDY27ZZ

Contact Radiation — *continued*
  Ear D9Y07ZZ
  Esophagus DDY07ZZ
  Eye D8Y07ZZ
  Femur DPY97ZZ
  Fibula DPYB7ZZ
  Gallbladder DFY17ZZ
  Gland
    Adrenal DGY27ZZ
    Parathyroid DGY47ZZ
    Pituitary DGY07ZZ
    Thyroid DGY57ZZ
  Glands, Salivary D9Y67ZZ
  Head and Neck DWY17ZZ
  Hemibody DWY47ZZ
  Humerus DPY67ZZ
  Hypopharynx D9Y37ZZ
  Ileum DDY47ZZ
  Jejunum DDY37ZZ
  Kidney DTY07ZZ
  Larynx D9YB7ZZ
  Liver DFY07ZZ
  Lung DBY27ZZ
  Mandible DPY37ZZ
  Maxilla DPY27ZZ
  Mediastinum DBY67ZZ
  Mouth D9Y47ZZ
  Nasopharynx D9YD7ZZ
  Neck and Head DWY17ZZ
  Nerve, Peripheral D0Y77ZZ
  Nose D9Y17ZZ
  Oropharynx D9YF7ZZ
  Ovary DUY07ZZ
  Palate
    Hard D9Y87ZZ
    Soft D9Y97ZZ
  Pancreas DFY37ZZ
  Parathyroid Gland DGY47ZZ
  Pelvic Bones DPY87ZZ
  Pelvic Region DWY67ZZ
  Pineal Body DGY17ZZ
  Pituitary Gland DGY07ZZ
  Pleura DBY57ZZ
  Prostate DVY07ZZ
  Radius DPY77ZZ
  Rectum DDY77ZZ
  Rib DPY57ZZ
  Sinuses D9Y77ZZ
  Skin
    Abdomen DHY87ZZ
    Arm DHY47ZZ
    Back DHY77ZZ
    Buttock DHY97ZZ
    Chest DHY67ZZ
    Face DHY27ZZ
    Leg DHYB7ZZ
    Neck DHY37ZZ
  Skull DPY07ZZ
  Spinal Cord D0Y67ZZ
  Sternum DPY47ZZ
  Stomach DDY17ZZ
  Testis DVY17ZZ
  Thyroid Gland DGY57ZZ
  Tibia DPYB7ZZ
  Tongue D9Y57ZZ
  Trachea DBY07ZZ
  Ulna DPY77ZZ
  Ureter DTY17ZZ
  Urethra DTY37ZZ
  Uterus DUY27ZZ
  Whole Body DWY57ZZ
ContaCT software (Measurement of intracranial arterial flow) 4A03X5D
CONTAK RENEWAL® 3 RF (HE) CRT-D *use* Cardiac Resynchronization Defibrillator Pulse Generator in 0JH
Contegra Pulmonary Valved Conduit *use* Zooplastic Tissue in Heart and Great Vessels
CONTEPO™ (Fosfomycin Anti-infective) *use* Other Anti-infective
Continent ileostomy *see* Bypass, Ileum 0D1B
Continuous Glucose Monitoring (CGM) device *use* Monitoring Device
Continuous Negative Airway Pressure
  24-96 Consecutive Hours, Ventilation 5A09459
  Greater than 96 Consecutive Hours, Ventilation 5A09559

Continuous Negative Airway Pressure — *continued*
  Less than 24 Consecutive Hours, Ventilation 5A09359
Continuous Positive Airway Pressure
  24-96 Consecutive Hours, Ventilation 5A09457
  Greater than 96 Consecutive Hours, Ventilation 5A09557
  Less than 24 Consecutive Hours, Ventilation 5A09357
Continuous renal replacement therapy (CRRT) 5A1D90Z
Contraceptive Device
  Change device in, Uterus and Cervix 0U2DXHZ
  Insertion of device in
    Cervix 0UHC
    Subcutaneous Tissue and Fascia
      Abdomen 0JH8
      Chest 0JH6
      Lower Arm
        Left 0JHH
        Right 0JHG
      Lower Leg
        Left 0JHP
        Right 0JHN
      Upper Arm
        Left 0JHF
        Right 0JHD
      Upper Leg
        Left 0JHM
        Right 0JHL
    Uterus 0UH9
  Removal of device from
    Subcutaneous Tissue and Fascia
      Lower Extremity 0JPW
      Trunk 0JPT
      Upper Extremity 0JPV
    Uterus and Cervix 0UPD
  Revision of device in
    Subcutaneous Tissue and Fascia
      Lower Extremity 0JWW
      Trunk 0JWT
      Upper Extremity 0JWV
    Uterus and Cervix 0UWD
Contractility Modulation Device
  Abdomen 0JH8
  Chest 0JH6
Control bleeding in
  Abdominal Wall 0W3F
  Ankle Region
    Left 0Y3L
    Right 0Y3K
  Arm
    Lower
      Left 0X3F
      Right 0X3D
    Upper
      Left 0X39
      Right 0X38
  Axilla
    Left 0X35
    Right 0X34
  Back
    Lower 0W3L
    Upper 0W3K
  Buttock
    Left 0Y31
    Right 0Y30
  Cavity, Cranial 0W31
  Chest Wall 0W38
  Elbow Region
    Left 0X3C
    Right 0X3B
  Extremity
    Lower
      Left 0Y3B
      Right 0Y39
    Upper
      Left 0X37
      Right 0X36
  Face 0W32
  Femoral Region
    Left 0Y38
    Right 0Y37
  Foot
    Left 0Y3N
    Right 0Y3M
  Gastrointestinal Tract 0W3P
  Genitourinary Tract 0W3R

Control bleeding in — *continued*
  Hand
    Left 0X3K
    Right 0X3J
  Head 0W30
  Inguinal Region
    Left 0Y36
    Right 0Y35
  Jaw
    Lower 0W35
    Upper 0W34
  Knee Region
    Left 0Y3G
    Right 0Y3F
  Leg
    Lower
      Left 0Y3J
      Right 0Y3H
    Upper
      Left 0Y3D
      Right 0Y3C
  Mediastinum 0W3C
  Nasal Mucosa and Soft Tissue 093K
  Neck 0W36
  Oral Cavity and Throat 0W33
  Pelvic Cavity 0W3J
  Pericardial Cavity 0W3D
  Perineum
    Female 0W3N
    Male 0W3M
  Peritoneal Cavity 0W3G
  Pleural Cavity
    Left 0W3B
    Right 0W39
  Respiratory Tract 0W3Q
  Retroperitoneum 0W3H
  Shoulder Region
    Left 0X33
    Right 0X32
  Wrist Region
    Left 0X3H
    Right 0X3G
Control bleeding using Tourniquet, External *see* Compression, Anatomical Regions 2W1
Control, Epistaxis *see* Control bleeding in, Nasal Mucosa and Soft Tissue 093K
Conus arteriosus *use* Ventricle, Right
Conus medullaris *use* Lumbar Spinal Cord
Convalescent Plasma (Nonautologous) *see* New Technology, Anatomical Regions XW1
Conversion
  Cardiac rhythm 5A2204Z
  Gastrostomy to jejunostomy feeding device *see* Insertion of device in, Jejunum 0DHA
Cook Biodesign® Fistula Plug(s) *use* Nonautologous Tissue Substitute
Cook Biodesign® Hernia Graft(s) *use* Nonautologous Tissue Substitute
Cook Biodesign® Layered Graft(s) *use* Nonautologous Tissue Substitute
Cook Zenapro™ Layered Graft(s) *use* Nonautologous Tissue Substitute
Cook Zenith AAA Endovascular Graft *use* Intraluminal Device
Cook Zenith® Fenestrated AAA Endovascular Graft
  use Intraluminal Device, Branched or Fenestrated, One or Two Arteries in 04V
  use Intraluminal Device, Branched or Fenestrated, Three or More Arteries in 04V
Coracoacromial ligament
  use Shoulder Bursa and Ligament, Left
  use Shoulder Bursa and Ligament, Right
Coracobrachialis muscle
  use Upper Arm Muscle, Left
  use Upper Arm Muscle, Right
Coracoclavicular ligament
  use Shoulder Bursa and Ligament, Left
  use Shoulder Bursa and Ligament, Right
Coracohumeral ligament
  use Shoulder Bursa and Ligament, Left
  use Shoulder Bursa and Ligament, Right
Coracoid process
  use Scapula, Left
  use Scapula, Right
Cordotomy *see* Division, Central Nervous System and Cranial Nerves 008
Core needle biopsy *see* Biopsy

CoreValve transcatheter aortic valve use Zooplastic Tissue in Heart and Great Vessels
Cormet Hip Resurfacing System use Resurfacing Device in Lower Joints
Corniculate cartilage use Larynx
CoRoent® XL use Interbody Fusion Device in Lower Joints
Coronary arteriography
   see Fluoroscopy, Heart B21
   see Plain Radiography, Heart B20
Corox (OTW) Bipolar Lead
   use Cardiac Lead, Defibrillator in 02H
   use Cardiac Lead, Pacemaker in 02H
Corpus callosum use Brain
Corpus cavernosum use Penis
Corpus spongiosum use Penis
Corpus striatum use Basal Ganglia
Corrugator supercilii muscle use Facial Muscle
Cortical strip neurostimulator lead use Neurostimulator Lead in Central Nervous System and Cranial Nerves
Corvia IASD® use Synthetic Substitute
COSELA™ use Trilaciclib
Costatectomy
   see Excision, Upper Bones 0PB
   see Resection, Upper Bones 0PT
Costectomy
   see Excision, Upper Bones 0PB
   see Resection, Upper Bones 0PT
Costocervical trunk
   use Subclavian Artery, Left
   use Subclavian Artery, Right
Costochondrectomy
   see Excision, Upper Bones 0PB
   see Resection, Upper Bones 0PT
Costoclavicular ligament
   use Shoulder Bursa and Ligament, Left
   use Shoulder Bursa and Ligament, Right
Costosternoplasty
   see Repair, Upper Bones 0PQ
   see Replacement, Upper Bones 0PR
   see Supplement, Upper Bones 0PU
Costotomy
   see Division, Upper Bones 0P8
   see Drainage, Upper Bones 0P9
Costotransverse joint use Thoracic Vertebral Joint
Costotransverse ligament use Rib(s) Bursa and Ligament
Costovertebral joint use Thoracic Vertebral Joint
Costoxiphoid ligament use Sternum Bursa and Ligament
Counseling
   Family, for substance abuse, Other Family Counseling HZ63ZZZ
   Group
     12-Step HZ43ZZZ
     Behavioral HZ41ZZZ
     Cognitive HZ40ZZZ
     Cognitive-Behavioral HZ42ZZZ
     Confrontational HZ48ZZZ
     Continuing Care HZ49ZZZ
     Infectious Disease
       Post-Test HZ4CZZZ
       Pre-Test HZ4CZZZ
     Interpersonal HZ44ZZZ
     Motivational Enhancement HZ47ZZZ
     Psychoeducation HZ46ZZZ
     Spiritual HZ4BZZZ
     Vocational HZ45ZZZ
   Individual
     12-Step HZ33ZZZ
     Behavioral HZ31ZZZ
     Cognitive HZ30ZZZ
     Cognitive-Behavioral HZ32ZZZ
     Confrontational HZ38ZZZ
     Continuing Care HZ39ZZZ
     Infectious Disease
       Post-Test HZ3CZZZ
       Pre-Test HZ3CZZZ
     Interpersonal HZ34ZZZ
     Motivational Enhancement HZ37ZZZ
     Psychoeducation HZ36ZZZ
     Spiritual HZ3BZZZ
     Vocational HZ35ZZZ
   Mental Health Services
     Educational GZ60ZZZ
     Other Counseling GZ63ZZZ

Counseling — continued
   Mental Health Services — continued
     Vocational GZ61ZZZ
Countershock, cardiac 5A2204Z
COVID-19 Vaccine XW0
COVID-19 Vaccine Booster XW0
COVID-19 Vaccine Dose 1 XW0
COVID-19 Vaccine Dose 2 XW0
COVID-19 Vaccine Dose 3 XW0
Cowper's (bulbourethral) gland use Urethra
CPAP (continuous positive airway pressure) see Assistance, Respiratory 5A09
Craniectomy
   see Excision, Head and Facial Bones 0NB
   see Resection, Head and Facial Bones 0NT
Cranioplasty
   see Repair, Head and Facial Bones 0NQ
   see Replacement, Head and Facial Bones 0NR
   see Supplement, Head and Facial Bones 0NU
Craniotomy
   see Division, Head and Facial Bones 0N8
   see Drainage, Central Nervous System and Cranial Nerves 009
   see Drainage, Head and Facial Bones 0N9
Creation
   Perineum
     Female 0W4N0
     Male 0W4M0
   Valve
     Aortic 024F0
     Mitral 024G0
     Tricuspid 024J0
Cremaster muscle use Perineum Muscle
CRESEMBA® (isavuconazonium sulfate) use Other Anti-infective
Cribriform plate
   use Ethmoid Bone, Left
   use Ethmoid Bone, Right
Cricoid cartilage use Trachea
Cricoidectomy see Excision, Larynx 0CBS
Cricothyroid artery
   use Thyroid Artery, Left
   use Thyroid Artery, Right
Cricothyroid muscle
   use Neck Muscle, Left
   use Neck Muscle, Right
Crisis Intervention GZ2ZZZZ
CRRT (Continuous renal replacement therapy) 5A1D90Z
Crural fascia
   use Subcutaneous Tissue and Fascia, Left Upper Leg
   use Subcutaneous Tissue and Fascia, Right Upper Leg
Crushing, nerve
   Cranial see Destruction, Central Nervous System and Cranial Nerves 005
   Peripheral see Destruction, Peripheral Nervous System 015
Cryoablation see Destruction
Cryoanalgesia see Destruction, Peripheral Nervous System 015
CryoICE® cryo-ablation probe (Cryo2)
   see Destruction, Conduction Mechanism 0258
   see Destruction, Peripheral Nervous System 015
CryoICE® CryoSPHERE® cryoablation probe (CryoS, CryoS-L) see Destruction, Peripheral Nervous System 015
Cryotherapy see Destruction
Cryptorchidectomy
   see Excision, Male Reproductive System 0VB
   see Resection, Male Reproductive System 0VT
Cryptorchiectomy
   see Excision, Male Reproductive System 0VB
   see Resection, Male Reproductive System 0VT
Cryptotomy
   see Division, Gastrointestinal System 0D8
   see Drainage, Gastrointestinal System 0D9
CT scan see Computerized Tomography (CT Scan)
CT sialogram see Computerized Tomography (CT Scan), Ear, Nose, Mouth and Throat B92
CTX001™ use Exagamglogene Autotemcel
Cubital lymph node
   use Lymphatic, Left Upper Extremity
   use Lymphatic, Right Upper Extremity
Cubital nerve use Ulnar Nerve

Cuboid bone
   use Tarsal, Left
   use Tarsal, Right
Cuboideonavicular joint
   use Tarsal Joint, Left
   use Tarsal Joint, Right
Culdocentesis see Drainage, Cul-de-sac 0U9F
Culdoplasty
   see Repair, Cul-de-sac 0UQF
   see Supplement, Cul-de-sac 0UUF
Culdoscopy 0UJH8ZZ
Culdotomy see Drainage, Cul-de-sac 0U9F
Culmen use Cerebellum
Cultured epidermal cell autograft use Autologous Tissue Substitute
Cuneiform cartilage use Larynx
Cuneonavicular joint
   use Joint, Tarsal, Left
   use Joint, Tarsal, Right
Cuneonavicular ligament
   use Foot Bursa and Ligament, Left
   use Foot Bursa and Ligament, Right
Curettage
   see Excision
   see Extraction
Cutaneous (transverse) cervical nerve use Cervical Plexus
CVP (central venous pressure) see Measurement, Venous 4A04
Cyclodiathermy see Destruction, Eye 085
Cyclophotocoagulation see Destruction, Eye 085
CYPHER® Stent use Intraluminal Device, Drug-eluting in Heart and Great Vessels
Cystectomy
   see Excision, Bladder 0TBB
   see Resection, Bladder 0TTB
Cystocele repair see Repair, Subcutaneous Tissue and Fascia, Pelvic Region 0JQC
Cystography
   see Fluoroscopy, Urinary System BT1
   see Plain Radiography, Urinary System BT0
Cystolithotomy see Extirpation, Bladder 0TCB
Cystopexy
   see Repair, Bladder 0TQB
   see Reposition, Bladder 0TSB
Cystoplasty
   see Repair, Bladder 0TQB
   see Replacement, Bladder 0TRB
   see Supplement, Bladder 0TUB
Cystorrhaphy see Repair, Bladder 0TQB
Cystoscopy 0TJB8ZZ
Cystostomy see Bypass, Bladder 0T1B
Cystostomy Tube use Drainage Device
Cystotomy see Drainage, Bladder 0T9B
Cystourethrography
   see Fluoroscopy, Urinary System BT1
   see Plain Radiography, Urinary System BT0
Cystourethroplasty
   see Repair, Urinary System 0TQ
   see Replacement, Urinary System 0TR
   see Supplement, Urinary System 0TU
CYTALUX® (Pafolacianine), in Fluorescence Guided Procedure see Fluorescence Guided Procedure
Cytarabine and Daunorubicin Liposome Antineoplastic XW0

D

Daratumumab and Hyaluronidase-fihj XW01318
Darzalex Faspro® use Daratumumab and Hyaluronidase-fihj
Dasiglucagon XW0136A
DBS lead use Neurostimulator Lead in Central Nervous System and Cranial Nerves
DeBakey Left Ventricular Assist Device use Implantable Heart Assist System in Heart and Great Vessels
Debridement
   Excisional see Excision
   Non-excisional see Extraction
Debris collection circuit, during percutaneous thrombectomy 5A05A0L
Decompression, Circulatory 6A15
Decortication, lung
   see Extirpation, Respiratory System 0BC
   see Release, Respiratory System 0BN

Deep brain neurostimulator lead use Neurostimulator Lead in Central Nervous System and Cranial Nerves
Deep cervical fascia
 use Subcutaneous Tissue and Fascia, Left Neck
 use Subcutaneous Tissue and Fascia, Right Neck
Deep cervical vein
 use Vertebral Vein, Left
 use Vertebral Vein, Right
Deep circumflex iliac artery
 use External Iliac Artery, Left
 use External Iliac Artery, Right
Deep facial vein
 use Face Vein, Left
 use Face Vein, Right
Deep femoral artery
 use Femoral Artery, Left
 use Femoral Artery, Right
Deep femoral (profunda femoris) vein
 use Femoral Vein, Left
 use Femoral Vein, Right
Deep Inferior Epigastric Artery Perforator Flap
 Replacement
  Bilateral 0HRV077
  Left 0HRU077
  Right 0HRT077
 Transfer
  Left 0KXG
  Right 0KXF
Deep palmar arch
 use Hand Artery, Left
 use Hand Artery, Right
Deep transverse perineal muscle use Perineum Muscle
DefenCath™ use Taurolidine Anti-infective and Heparin Anticoagulant
Deferential artery
 use Internal Iliac Artery, Left
 use Internal Iliac Artery, Right
Defibrillator Generator
 Abdomen 0JH8
 Chest 0JH6
Defibrillator Lead
 Insertion of device in, Mediastinum 0WHC
 Removal of device from, Mediastinum 0WPC
 Revision of device in, Mediastinum 0WWC
Defibtech Automated Chest Compression (ACC) device 5A1221J
Defitelio use Other Substance
Defitelio® infusion see Introduction of substance in or on, Physiological Systems and Anatomical Regions 3E0
Delivery
 Cesarean see Extraction, Products of Conception 10D0
 Forceps see Extraction, Products of Conception 10D0
 Manually assisted 10E0XZZ
 Products of Conception 10E0XZZ
 Vacuum assisted see Extraction, Products of Conception 10D0
Delta frame external fixator
 use External Fixation Device, Hybrid in 0PH
 use External Fixation Device, Hybrid in 0PS
 use External Fixation Device, Hybrid in 0QH
 use External Fixation Device, Hybrid in 0QS
Delta III Reverse shoulder prosthesis use Synthetic Substitute, Reverse Ball and Socket in 0RR
Deltoid fascia
 use Subcutaneous Tissue and Fascia, Left Upper Arm
 use Subcutaneous Tissue and Fascia, Right Upper Arm
Deltoid ligament
 use Ankle Bursa and Ligament, Left
 use Ankle Bursa and Ligament, Right
Deltoid muscle
 use Shoulder Muscle, Left
 use Shoulder Muscle, Right
Deltopectoral (infraclavicular) lymph node
 use Lymphatic, Left Upper Extremity
 use Lymphatic, Right Upper Extremity
Denervation
 Cranial nerve see Destruction, Central Nervous System and Cranial Nerves 005
 Peripheral nerve see Destruction, Peripheral Nervous System 015

Dens use Cervical Vertebra
Densitometry
 Plain Radiography
  Femur
   Left BQ04ZZ1
   Right BQ03ZZ1
  Hip
   Left BQ01ZZ1
   Right BQ00ZZ1
  Spine
   Cervical BR00ZZ1
   Lumbar BR09ZZ1
   Thoracic BR07ZZ1
   Whole BR0GZZ1
 Ultrasonography
  Elbow
   Left BP4HZZ1
   Right BP4GZZ1
  Hand
   Left BP4PZZ1
   Right BP4NZZ1
  Shoulder
   Left BP49ZZ1
   Right BP48ZZ1
  Wrist
   Left BP4MZZ1
   Right BP4LZZ1
Denticulate (dentate) ligament use Spinal Meninges
Depressor anguli oris muscle use Facial Muscle
Depressor labii inferioris muscle use Facial Muscle
Depressor septi nasi muscle use Facial Muscle
Depressor supercilii muscle use Facial Muscle
Dermabrasion see Extraction, Skin and Breast 0HD
Dermis use Skin
Descending genicular artery
 use Femoral Artery, Left
 use Femoral Artery, Right
Destruction
 Acetabulum
  Left 0Q55
  Right 0Q54
 Adenoids 0C5Q
 Ampulla of Vater 0F5C
 Anal Sphincter 0D5R
 Anterior Chamber
  Left 08533ZZ
  Right 08523ZZ
 Anus 0D5Q
 Aorta
  Abdominal
  Thoracic
   Ascending/Arch 025X
   Descending 025W
 Aortic Body 0G5D
 Appendix 0D5J
 Artery
  Anterior Tibial
   Left 045Q
   Right 045P
  Axillary
   Left 0356
   Right 0355
  Brachial
   Left 0358
   Right 0357
  Celiac 0451
  Colic
   Left 0457
   Middle 0458
   Right 0456
  Common Carotid
   Left 035J
   Right 035H
  Common Iliac
   Left 045D
   Right 045C
  External Carotid
   Left 035N
   Right 035M
  External Iliac
   Left 045J
   Right 045H
  Face 035R
  Femoral
   Left 045L
   Right 045K
  Foot
   Left 045W

Destruction — continued
 Artery — continued
  Foot — continued
   Right 045V
  Gastric 0452
  Hand
   Left 035F
   Right 035D
  Hepatic 0453
  Inferior Mesenteric 045B
  Innominate 0352
  Internal Carotid
   Left 035L
   Right 035K
  Internal Iliac
   Left 045F
   Right 045E
  Internal Mammary
   Left 0351
   Right 0350
  Intracranial 035G
  Lower 045Y
  Peroneal
   Left 045U
   Right 045T
  Popliteal
   Left 045N
   Right 045M
  Posterior Tibial
   Left 045S
   Right 045R
  Pulmonary
   Left 025R
   Right 025Q
  Pulmonary Trunk 025P
  Radial
   Left 035C
   Right 035B
  Renal
   Left 045A
   Right 0459
  Splenic 0454
  Subclavian
   Left 0354
   Right 0353
  Superior Mesenteric 0455
  Temporal
   Left 035T
   Right 035S
  Thyroid
   Left 035V
   Right 035U
  Ulnar
   Left 035A
   Right 0359
  Upper 035Y
  Vertebral
   Left 035Q
   Right 035P
 Atrium
  Left 0257
  Right 0256
 Auditory Ossicle
  Left 095A
  Right 0959
 Basal Ganglia 0058
 Bladder 0T5B
 Bladder Neck 0T5C
 Bone
  Ethmoid
   Left 0N5G
   Right 0N5F
  Frontal 0N51
  Hyoid 0N5X
  Lacrimal
   Left 0N5J
   Right 0N5H
  Nasal 0N5B
  Occipital 0N57
  Palatine
   Left 0N5L
   Right 0N5K
  Parietal
   Left 0N54
   Right 0N53
  Pelvic
   Left 0Q53
   Right 0Q52
  Sphenoid 0N5C

Destruction

Destruction — *continued*
- Bone — *continued*
  - Temporal
    - Left 0N56
    - Right 0N55
  - Zygomatic
    - Left 0N5N
    - Right 0N5M
- Brain 0050
  - Stereoelectroencephalographic Radiofrequency Ablation 00503Z4
- Breast
  - Bilateral 0H5V
  - Left 0H5U
  - Right 0H5T
- Bronchus
  - Lingula 0B59
  - Lower Lobe
    - Left 0B5B
    - Right 0B56
  - Main
    - Left 0B57
    - Right 0B53
  - Middle Lobe, Right 0B55
  - Upper Lobe
    - Left 0B58
    - Right 0B54
- Buccal Mucosa 0C54
- Bursa and Ligament
  - Abdomen
    - Left 0M5J
    - Right 0M5H
  - Ankle
    - Left 0M5R
    - Right 0M5Q
  - Elbow
    - Left 0M54
    - Right 0M53
  - Foot
    - Left 0M5T
    - Right 0M5S
  - Hand
    - Left 0M58
    - Right 0M57
  - Head and Neck 0M50
  - Hip
    - Left 0M5M
    - Right 0M5L
  - Knee
    - Left 0M5P
    - Right 0M5N
  - Lower Extremity
    - Left 0M5W
    - Right 0M5V
  - Perineum 0M5K
  - Rib(s) 0M5G
  - Shoulder
    - Left 0M52
    - Right 0M51
  - Spine
    - Lower 0M5D
    - Upper 0M5C
  - Sternum 0M5F
  - Upper Extremity
    - Left 0M5B
    - Right 0M59
  - Wrist
    - Left 0M56
    - Right 0M55
- Carina 0B52
- Carotid Bodies, Bilateral 0G58
- Carotid Body
  - Left 0G56
  - Right 0G57
- Carpal
  - Left 0P5N
  - Right 0P5M
- Cecum 0D5H
- Cerebellum 005C
- Cerebral Hemisphere 0057
- Cerebral Meninges 0051
- Cerebral Ventricle 0056
- Cervix 0U5C
- Chordae Tendineae 0259
- Choroid
  - Left 085B
  - Right 085A
- Cisterna Chyli 075L

Destruction — *continued*
- Clavicle
  - Left 0P5B
  - Right 0P59
- Clitoris 0U5J
- Coccygeal Glomus 0G5B
- Coccyx 0Q5S
- Colon
  - Ascending 0D5K
  - Descending 0D5M
  - Sigmoid 0D5N
  - Transverse 0D5L
- Conduction Mechanism 0258
- Conjunctiva
  - Left 085TXZZ
  - Right 085SXZZ
- Cord
  - Bilateral 0V5H
  - Left 0V5G
  - Right 0V5F
- Cornea
  - Left 0859XZZ
  - Right 0858XZZ
- Cul-de-sac 0U5F
- Diaphragm 0B5T
- Disc
  - Cervical Vertebral 0R53
  - Cervicothoracic Vertebral 0R55
  - Lumbar Vertebral 0S52
  - Lumbosacral 0S54
  - Thoracic Vertebral 0R59
  - Thoracolumbar Vertebral 0R5B
- Duct
  - Common Bile 0F59
  - Cystic 0F58
  - Hepatic
    - Common 0F57
    - Left 0F56
    - Right 0F55
  - Lacrimal
    - Left 085Y
    - Right 085X
  - Pancreatic 0F5D
    - Accessory 0F5F
  - Parotid
    - Left 0C5C
    - Right 0C5B
- Duodenum 0D59
- Dura Mater 0052
- Ear
  - External
    - Left 0951
    - Right 0950
  - External Auditory Canal
    - Left 0954
    - Right 0953
  - Inner
    - Left 095E
    - Right 095D
  - Middle
    - Left 0956
    - Right 0955
- Endometrium 0U5B
- Epididymis
  - Bilateral 0V5L
  - Left 0V5K
  - Right 0V5J
- Epiglottis 0C5R
- Esophagogastric Junction 0D54
- Esophagus 0D55
  - Lower 0D53
  - Middle 0D52
  - Upper 0D51
- Eustachian Tube
  - Left 095G
  - Right 095F
- Eye
  - Left 0851XZZ
  - Right 0850XZZ
- Eyelid
  - Lower
    - Left 085R
    - Right 085Q
  - Upper
    - Left 085P
    - Right 085N
- Fallopian Tube
  - Left 0U56
  - Right 0U55

Destruction — *continued*
- Fallopian Tubes, Bilateral 0U57
- Femoral Shaft
  - Left 0Q59
  - Right 0Q58
- Femur
  - Lower
    - Left 0Q5C
    - Right 0Q5B
  - Upper
    - Left 0Q57
    - Right 0Q56
- Fibula
  - Left 0Q5K
  - Right 0Q5J
- Finger Nail 0H5QXZZ
- Gallbladder 0F54
- Gingiva
  - Lower 0C56
  - Upper 0C55
- Gland
  - Adrenal
    - Bilateral 0G54
    - Left 0G52
    - Right 0G53
  - Lacrimal
    - Left 085W
    - Right 085V
  - Minor Salivary 0C5J
  - Parotid
    - Left 0C59
    - Right 0C58
  - Pituitary 0G50
  - Sublingual
    - Left 0C5F
    - Right 0C5D
  - Submaxillary
    - Left 0C5H
    - Right 0C5G
  - Vestibular 0U5L
- Glenoid Cavity
  - Left 0P58
  - Right 0P57
- Glomus Jugulare 0G5C
- Humeral Head
  - Left 0P5D
  - Right 0P5C
- Humeral Shaft
  - Left 0P5G
  - Right 0P5F
- Hymen 0U5K
- Hypothalamus 005A
- Ileocecal Valve 0D5C
- Ileum 0D5B
- Intestine
  - Large 0D5E
    - Left 0D5G
    - Right 0D5F
  - Small 0D58
- Iris
  - Left 085D3ZZ
  - Right 085C3ZZ
- Jejunum 0D5A
- Joint
  - Acromioclavicular
    - Left 0R5H
    - Right 0R5G
  - Ankle
    - Left 0S5G
    - Right 0S5F
  - Carpal
    - Left 0R5R
    - Right 0R5Q
  - Carpometacarpal
    - Left 0R5T
    - Right 0R5S
  - Cervical Vertebral 0R51
  - Cervicothoracic Vertebral 0R54
  - Coccygeal 0S56
  - Elbow
    - Left 0R5M
    - Right 0R5L
  - Finger Phalangeal
    - Left 0R5X
    - Right 0R5W
  - Hip
    - Left 0S5B
    - Right 0S59

Destruction — *continued*
  Joint — *continued*
    Knee
      Left 0S5D
      Right 0S5C
    Lumbar Vertebral 0S50
    Lumbosacral 0S53
    Metacarpophalangeal
      Left 0R5V
      Right 0R5U
    Metatarsal-Phalangeal
      Left 0S5N
      Right 0S5M
    Occipital-cervical 0R50
    Sacrococcygeal 0S55
    Sacroiliac
      Left 0S58
      Right 0S57
    Shoulder
      Left 0R5K
      Right 0R5J
    Sternoclavicular
      Left 0R5F
      Right 0R5E
    Tarsal
      Left 0S5J
      Right 0S5H
    Tarsometatarsal
      Left 0S5L
      Right 0S5K
    Temporomandibular
      Left 0R5D
      Right 0R5C
    Thoracic Vertebral 0R56
    Thoracolumbar Vertebral 0R5A
    Toe Phalangeal
      Left 0S5Q
      Right 0S5P
    Wrist
      Left 0R5P
      Right 0R5N
  Kidney
    Left 0T51
    Right 0T50
  Kidney Pelvis
    Left 0T54
    Right 0T53
  Larynx 0C5S
  Lens
    Left 085K3ZZ
    Right 085J3ZZ
  Lip
    Lower 0C51
    Upper 0C50
  Liver 0F50
    Left Lobe 0F52
    Right Lobe 0F51
    Ultrasound-guided Cavitation XF5
  Lung
    Bilateral 0B5M
    Left 0B5L
    Lower Lobe
      Left 0B5J
      Right 0B5F
    Middle Lobe, Right 0B5D
    Right 0B5K
    Upper Lobe
      Left 0B5G
      Right 0B5C
  Lung Lingula 0B5H
  Lymphatic
    Aortic 075D
    Axillary
      Left 0756
      Right 0755
    Head 0750
    Inguinal
      Left 075J
      Right 075H
    Internal Mammary
      Left 0759
      Right 0758
    Lower Extremity
      Left 075G
      Right 075F
    Mesenteric 075B
    Neck
      Left 0752
      Right 0751

Destruction — *continued*
  Lymphatic — *continued*
    Pelvis 075C
    Thoracic Duct 075K
    Thorax 0757
    Upper Extremity
      Left 0754
      Right 0753
  Mandible
    Left 0N5V
    Right 0N5T
  Maxilla 0N5R
  Medulla Oblongata 005D
  Mesentery 0D5V
  Metacarpal
    Left 0P5Q
    Right 0P5P
  Metatarsal
    Left 0Q5P
    Right 0Q5N
  Muscle
    Abdomen
      Left 0K5L
      Right 0K5K
    Extraocular
      Left 085M
      Right 085L
    Facial 0K51
    Foot
      Left 0K5W
      Right 0K5V
    Hand
      Left 0K5D
      Right 0K5C
    Head 0K50
    Hip
      Left 0K5P
      Right 0K5N
    Lower Arm and Wrist
      Left 0K5B
      Right 0K59
    Lower Leg
      Left 0K5T
      Right 0K5S
    Neck
      Left 0K53
      Right 0K52
    Papillary 025D
    Perineum 0K5M
    Shoulder
      Left 0K56
      Right 0K55
    Thorax
      Left 0K5J
      Right 0K5H
    Tongue, Palate, Pharynx 0K54
    Trunk
      Left 0K5G
      Right 0K5F
    Upper Arm
      Left 0K58
      Right 0K57
    Upper Leg
      Left 0K5R
      Right 0K5Q
  Nasal Mucosa and Soft Tissue 095K
  Nasopharynx 095N
  Nerve
    Abdominal Sympathetic 015M
    Abducens 005L
    Accessory 005R
    Acoustic 005N
    Brachial Plexus 0153
    Cervical 0151
    Cervical Plexus 0150
    Facial 005M
    Femoral 015D
    Glossopharyngeal 005P
    Head and Neck Sympathetic 015K
    Hypoglossal 005S
    Lumbar 015B
    Lumbar Plexus 0159
    Lumbar Sympathetic 015N
    Lumbosacral Plexus 015A
    Median 0155
    Oculomotor 005H
    Olfactory 005F
    Optic 005G
    Peroneal 015H

Destruction — *continued*
  Nerve — *continued*
    Phrenic 0152
    Pudendal 015C
    Radial 0156
    Sacral 015R
    Sacral Plexus 015Q
    Sacral Sympathetic 015P
    Sciatic 015F
    Thoracic 0158
    Thoracic Sympathetic 015L
    Tibial 015G
    Trigeminal 005K
    Trochlear 005J
    Ulnar 0154
    Vagus 005Q
  Nipple
    Left 0H5X
    Right 0H5W
  Omentum 0D5U
  Orbit
    Left 0N5Q
    Right 0N5P
  Ovary
    Bilateral 0U52
    Left 0U51
    Right 0U50
  Palate
    Hard 0C52
    Soft 0C53
  Pancreas 0F5G
  Para-aortic Body 0G59
  Paraganglion Extremity 0G5F
  Parathyroid Gland 0G5R
    Inferior
      Left 0G5P
      Right 0G5N
    Multiple 0G5Q
    Superior
      Left 0G5M
      Right 0G5L
  Patella
    Left 0Q5F
    Right 0Q5D
  Penis 0V5S
  Pericardium 025N
  Peritoneum 0D5W
  Phalanx
    Finger
      Left 0P5V
      Right 0P5T
    Thumb
      Left 0P5S
      Right 0P5R
    Toe
      Left 0Q5R
      Right 0Q5Q
  Pharynx 0C5M
  Pineal Body 0G51
  Pleura
    Left 0B5P
    Right 0B5N
  Pons 005B
  Prepuce 0V5T
  Prostate 0V50
  Radius
    Left 0P5J
    Right 0P5H
  Rectum 0D5P
  Renal Sympathetic Nerve(s)
    Radiofrequency Ablation X05133A
    Ultrasound Ablation X051329
  Retina
    Left 085F3ZZ
    Right 085E3ZZ
  Retinal Vessel
    Left 085H3ZZ
    Right 085G3ZZ
  Ribs
    1 to 2 0P51
    3 or More 0P52
  Sacrum 0Q51
  Scapula
    Left 0P56
    Right 0P55
  Sclera
    Left 0857XZZ
    Right 0856XZZ
  Scrotum 0V55

Destruction — *continued*
- Septum
  - Atrial 0255
  - Nasal 095M
  - Ventricular 025M
- Sinus
  - Accessory 095P
  - Ethmoid
    - Left 095V
    - Right 095U
  - Frontal
    - Left 095T
    - Right 095S
  - Mastoid
    - Left 095C
    - Right 095B
  - Maxillary
    - Left 095R
    - Right 095Q
  - Sphenoid
    - Left 095X
    - Right 095W
- Skin
  - Abdomen 0H57XZ
  - Back 0H56XZ
  - Buttock 0H58XZ
  - Chest 0H55XZ
  - Ear
    - Left 0H53XZ
    - Right 0H52XZ
  - Face 0H51XZ
  - Foot
    - Left 0H5NXZ
    - Right 0H5MXZ
  - Hand
    - Left 0H5GXZ
    - Right 0H5FXZ
  - Inguinal 0H5AXZ
  - Lower Arm
    - Left 0H5EXZ
    - Right 0H5DXZ
  - Lower Leg
    - Left 0H5LXZ
    - Right 0H5KXZ
  - Neck 0H54XZ
  - Perineum 0H59XZ
  - Scalp 0H50XZ
  - Upper Arm
    - Left 0H5CXZ
    - Right 0H5BXZ
  - Upper Leg
    - Left 0H5JXZ
    - Right 0H5HXZ
- Skull 0N50
- Spinal Cord
  - Cervical 005W
  - Lumbar 005Y
  - Thoracic 005X
- Spinal Meninges 005T
- Spleen 075P
- Sternum 0P50
- Stomach 0D56
  - Pylorus 0D57
- Subcutaneous Tissue and Fascia
  - Abdomen 0J58
  - Back 0J57
  - Buttock 0J59
  - Chest 0J56
  - Face 0J51
  - Foot
    - Left 0J5R
    - Right 0J5Q
  - Hand
    - Left 0J5K
    - Right 0J5J
  - Lower Arm
    - Left 0J5H
    - Right 0J5G
  - Lower Leg
    - Left 0J5P
    - Right 0J5N
  - Neck
    - Left 0J55
    - Right 0J54
  - Pelvic Region 0J5C
  - Perineum 0J5B
  - Scalp 0J50
  - Upper Arm
    - Left 0J5F

Destruction — *continued*
- Subcutaneous Tissue and Fascia — *continued*
  - Upper Arm — *continued*
    - Right 0J5D
  - Upper Leg
    - Left 0J5M
    - Right 0J5L
- Tarsal
  - Left 0Q5M
  - Right 0Q5L
- Tendon
  - Abdomen
    - Left 0L5G
    - Right 0L5F
  - Ankle
    - Left 0L5T
    - Right 0L5S
  - Foot
    - Left 0L5W
    - Right 0L5V
  - Hand
    - Left 0L58
    - Right 0L57
  - Head and Neck 0L50
  - Hip
    - Left 0L5K
    - Right 0L5J
  - Knee
    - Left 0L5R
    - Right 0L5Q
  - Lower Arm and Wrist
    - Left 0L56
    - Right 0L55
  - Lower Leg
    - Left 0L5P
    - Right 0L5N
  - Perineum 0L5H
  - Shoulder
    - Left 0L52
    - Right 0L51
  - Thorax
    - Left 0L5D
    - Right 0L5C
  - Trunk
    - Left 0L5B
    - Right 0L59
  - Upper Arm
    - Left 0L54
    - Right 0L53
  - Upper Leg
    - Left 0L5M
    - Right 0L5L
- Testis
  - Bilateral 0V5C
  - Left 0V5B
  - Right 0V59
- Thalamus 0059
- Thymus 075M
- Thyroid Gland 0G5K
  - Left Lobe 0G5G
  - Right Lobe 0G5H
- Tibia
  - Left 0Q5H
  - Right 0Q5G
- Toe Nail 0H5RXZZ
- Tongue 0C57
- Tonsils 0C5P
- Tooth
  - Lower 0C5X
  - Upper 0C5W
- Trachea 0B51
- Tunica Vaginalis
  - Left 0V57
  - Right 0V56
- Turbinate, Nasal 095L
- Tympanic Membrane
  - Left 0958
  - Right 0957
- Ulna
  - Left 0P5L
  - Right 0P5K
- Ureter
  - Left 0T57
  - Right 0T56
- Urethra 0T5D
- Uterine Supporting Structure 0U54
- Uterus 0U59
- Uvula 0C5N
- Vagina 0U5G

Destruction — *continued*
- Valve
  - Aortic 025F
  - Mitral 025G
  - Pulmonary 025H
  - Tricuspid 025J
- Vas Deferens
  - Bilateral 0V5Q
  - Left 0V5P
  - Right 0V5N
- Vein
  - Axillary
    - Left 0558
    - Right 0557
  - Azygos 0550
  - Basilic
    - Left 055C
    - Right 055B
  - Brachial
    - Left 055A
    - Right 0559
  - Cephalic
    - Left 055F
    - Right 055D
  - Colic 0657
  - Common Iliac
    - Left 065D
    - Right 065C
  - Coronary 0254
  - Esophageal 0653
  - External Iliac
    - Left 065G
    - Right 065F
  - External Jugular
    - Left 055Q
    - Right 055P
  - Face
    - Left 055V
    - Right 055T
  - Femoral
    - Left 065N
    - Right 065M
  - Foot
    - Left 065V
    - Right 065T
  - Gastric 0652
  - Hand
    - Left 055H
    - Right 055G
  - Hemiazygos 0551
  - Hepatic 0654
  - Hypogastric
    - Left 065J
    - Right 065H
  - Inferior Mesenteric 0656
  - Innominate
    - Left 0554
    - Right 0553
  - Internal Jugular
    - Left 055N
    - Right 055M
  - Intracranial 055L
  - Lower 065Y
  - Portal 0658
  - Pulmonary
    - Left 025T
    - Right 025S
  - Renal
    - Left 065B
    - Right 0659
  - Saphenous
    - Left 065Q
    - Right 065P
  - Splenic 0651
  - Subclavian
    - Left 0556
    - Right 0555
  - Superior Mesenteric 0655
  - Upper 055Y
  - Vertebral
    - Left 055S
    - Right 055R
- Vena Cava
  - Inferior 0650
  - Superior 025V
- Ventricle
  - Left 025L
  - Right 025K

Destruction — continued
  Vertebra
    Cervical 0P53
    Lumbar 0Q50
    Thoracic 0P54
  Vesicle
    Bilateral 0V53
    Left 0V52
    Right 0V51
  Vitreous
    Left 08553ZZ
    Right 08543ZZ
  Vocal Cord
    Left 0C5V
    Right 0C5T
  Vulva 0U5M
Detachment
  Arm
    Lower
      Left 0X6F0Z
      Right 0X6D0Z
    Upper
      Left 0X690Z
      Right 0X680Z
  Elbow Region
    Left 0X6C0ZZ
    Right 0X6B0ZZ
  Femoral Region
    Left 0Y680ZZ
    Right 0Y670ZZ
  Finger
    Index
      Left 0X6P0Z
      Right 0X6N0Z
    Little
      Left 0X6W0Z
      Right 0X6V0Z
    Middle
      Left 0X6R0Z
      Right 0X6Q0Z
    Ring
      Left 0X6T0Z
      Right 0X6S0Z
  Foot
    Left 0Y6N0Z
    Right 0Y6M0Z
  Forequarter
    Left 0X610ZZ
    Right 0X600ZZ
  Hand
    Left 0X6K0Z
    Right 0X6J0Z
  Hindquarter
    Bilateral 0Y640ZZ
    Left 0Y630ZZ
    Right 0Y620ZZ
  Knee Region
    Left 0Y6G0ZZ
    Right 0Y6F0ZZ
  Leg
    Lower
      Left 0Y6J0Z
      Right 0Y6H0Z
    Upper
      Left 0Y6D0Z
      Right 0Y6C0Z
  Shoulder Region
    Left 0X630ZZ
    Right 0X620ZZ
  Thumb
    Left 0X6M0Z
    Right 0X6L0Z
  Toe
    1st
      Left 0Y6Q0Z
      Right 0Y6P0Z
    2nd
      Left 0Y6S0Z
      Right 0Y6R0Z
    3rd
      Left 0Y6U0Z
      Right 0Y6T0Z
    4th
      Left 0Y6W0Z
      Right 0Y6V0Z
    5th
      Left 0Y6Y0Z
      Right 0Y6X0Z
Determination, Mental status GZ14ZZZ

Detorsion
  see Release
  see Reposition
DETOUR® System
  use Conduit through Femoral Vein to Popliteal Artery in New Technology
  use Conduit through Femoral Vein to Superficial Femoral Artery in New Technology
Detoxification Services, for substance abuse
  HZ2ZZZZ
Device Fitting F0DZ
Diagnostic Audiology see Audiology, Diagnostic
Diagnostic imaging see Imaging, Diagnostic
Diagnostic radiology see Imaging, Diagnostic
Dialysis
  Hemodialysis see Performance, Urinary 5A1D
  Peritoneal 3E1M39Z
Diaphragma sellae use Dura Mater
Diaphragmatic pacemaker generator use Stimulator Generator in Subcutaneous Tissue and Fascia
Diaphragmatic Pacemaker Lead
  Insertion of device in, Diaphragm 0BHT
  Removal of device from, Diaphragm 0BPT
  Revision of device in, Diaphragm 0BWT
Digital radiography, plain see Plain Radiography
Dilation
  Ampulla of Vater 0F7C
  Anus 0D7Q
  Aorta
    Abdominal
    Thoracic
      Ascending/Arch 027X
      Descending 027W
  Artery
    Anterior Tibial
      Left 047Q
        Intraluminal Device, Everolimus-eluting Resorbable Scaffold(s) X27Q3TA
      Right 047P
        Intraluminal Device, Everolimus-eluting Resorbable Scaffold(s) X27P3TA
    Axillary
      Left 0376
      Right 0375
    Brachial
      Left 0378
      Right 0377
    Celiac 0471
    Colic
      Left 0477
      Middle 0478
      Right 0476
    Common Carotid
      Left 037J
      Right 037H
    Common Iliac
      Left 047D
      Right 047C
    Coronary
      Four or More Arteries 0273
      One Artery 0270
      Three Arteries 0272
      Two Arteries 0271
    External Carotid
      Left 037N
      Right 037M
    External Iliac
      Left 047J
      Right 047H
    Face 037R
    Femoral
      Left 047L
      Right 047K
    Foot
      Left 047W
      Right 047V
    Gastric 0472
    Hand
      Left 037F
      Right 037D
    Hepatic 0473
    Inferior Mesenteric 047B
    Innominate 0372
    Internal Carotid
      Left 037L
      Right 037K

Dilation — continued
  Artery — continued
    Internal Iliac
      Left 047F
      Right 047E
    Internal Mammary
      Left 0371
      Right 0370
    Intracranial 037G
    Lower 047Y
    Peroneal
      Left 047U
        Intraluminal Device, Everolimus-eluting Resorbable Scaffold(s) X27U3TA
      Right 047T
        Intraluminal Device, Everolimus-eluting Resorbable Scaffold(s) X27T3TA
    Popliteal
      Left 047N
      Right 047M
    Posterior Tibial
      Left 047S
        Intraluminal Device Everolimus-eluting Resorbable Scaffold(s) X27S3TA
      Right 047R
        Intraluminal Device Everolimus-eluting Resorbable Scaffold(s) X27R3TA
    Pulmonary
      Left 027R
      Right 027Q
    Pulmonary Trunk 027P
    Radial
      Left 037C
      Right 037B
    Renal
      Left 047A
      Right 0479
    Splenic 0474
    Subclavian
      Left 0374
      Right 0373
    Superior Mesenteric 0475
    Temporal
      Left 037T
      Right 037S
    Thyroid
      Left 037V
      Right 037U
    Ulnar
      Left 037A
      Right 0379
    Upper 037Y
    Vertebral
      Left 037Q
      Right 037P
  Bladder 0T7B
  Bladder Neck 0T7C
  Bronchus
    Lingula 0B79
    Lower Lobe
      Left 0B7B
      Right 0B76
    Main
      Left 0B77
      Right 0B73
    Middle Lobe, Right 0B75
    Upper Lobe
      Left 0B78
      Right 0B74
  Carina 0B72
  Cecum 0D7H
  Cerebral Ventricle 0076
  Cervix 0U7C
  Colon
    Ascending 0D7K
    Descending 0D7M
    Sigmoid 0D7N
    Transverse 0D7L
  Duct
    Common Bile 0F79
    Cystic 0F78
    Hepatic
      Common 0F77
      Left 0F76
      Right 0F75

Dilation

Dilation — continued
  Duct — continued
    Lacrimal
      Left 087Y
      Right 087X
    Pancreatic 0F7D
      Accessory 0F7F
    Parotid
      Left 0C7C
      Right 0C7B
  Duodenum 0D79
  Esophagogastric Junction 0D74
  Esophagus 0D75
    Lower 0D73
    Middle 0D72
    Upper 0D71
  Eustachian Tube
    Left 097G
    Right 097F
  Fallopian Tube
    Left 0U76
    Right 0U75
  Fallopian Tubes, Bilateral 0U77
  Hymen 0U7K
  Ileocecal Valve 0D7C
  Ileum 0D7B
  Intestine
    Large 0D7E
      Left 0D7G
      Right 0D7F
    Small 0D78
  Jejunum 0D7A
  Kidney Pelvis
    Left 0T74
    Right 0T73
  Larynx 0C7S
  Nasopharynx 097N
  Pharynx 0C7M
  Rectum 0D7P
  Stomach 0D76
    Pylorus 0D77
  Trachea 0B71
  Ureter
    Left 0T77
    Right 0T76
  Ureters, Bilateral 0T78
  Urethra 0T7D
  Uterus 0U79
  Vagina 0U7G
  Valve
    Aortic 027F
    Mitral 027G
    Pulmonary 027H
    Tricuspid 027J
  Vas Deferens
    Bilateral 0V7Q
    Left 0V7P
    Right 0V7N
  Vein
    Axillary
      Left 0578
      Right 0577
    Azygos 0570
    Basilic
      Left 057C
      Right 057B
    Brachial
      Left 057A
      Right 0579
    Cephalic
      Left 057F
      Right 057D
    Colic 0677
    Common Iliac
      Left 067D
      Right 067C
    Esophageal 0673
    External Iliac
      Left 067G
      Right 067F
    External Jugular
      Left 057Q
      Right 057P
    Face
      Left 057V
      Right 057T
    Femoral
      Left 067N
      Right 067M

Dilation — continued
  Vein — continued
    Foot
      Left 067V
      Right 067T
    Gastric 0672
    Hand
      Left 057H
      Right 057G
    Hemiazygos 0571
    Hepatic 0674
    Hypogastric
      Left 067J
      Right 067H
    Inferior Mesenteric 0676
    Innominate
      Left 0574
      Right 0573
    Internal Jugular
      Left 057N
      Right 057M
    Intracranial 057L
    Lower 067Y
    Portal 0678
    Pulmonary
      Left 027T
      Right 027S
    Renal
      Left 067B
      Right 0679
    Saphenous
      Left 067Q
      Right 067P
    Splenic 0671
    Subclavian
      Left 0576
      Right 0575
    Superior Mesenteric 0675
    Upper 057Y
    Vertebral
      Left 057S
      Right 057R
    Vena Cava
      Inferior 0670
      Superior 027V
    Ventricle
      Left 027L
      Right 027K
Direct Lateral Interbody Fusion (DLIF) device use
  Interbody Fusion Device in Lower Joints
Disarticulation see Detachment
Discectomy, diskectomy
  see Excision, Lower Joints 0SB
  see Excision, Upper Joints 0RB
  see Resection, Lower Joints 0ST
  see Resection, Upper Joints 0RT
Discography
  see Fluoroscopy, Axial Skeleton, Except Skull and Facial Bones BR1
  see Plain Radiography, Axial Skeleton, Except Skull and Facial Bones BR0
Dismembered pyeloplasty see Repair, Kidney Pelvis
Distal humerus
  use Humeral Shaft, Left
  use Humeral Shaft, Right
Distal humerus, involving joint
  use Elbow Joint, Left
  use Elbow Joint, Right
Distal radioulnar joint
  use Wrist Joint, Left
  use Wrist Joint, Right
Diversion see Bypass
Diverticulectomy see Excision, Gastrointestinal System 0DB
Division
  Acetabulum
    Left 0Q85
    Right 0Q84
  Anal Sphincter 0D8R
  Basal Ganglia 0088
  Bladder Neck 0T8C
  Bone
    Ethmoid
      Left 0N8G
      Right 0N8F
    Frontal 0N81
    Hyoid 0N8X

Division — continued
  Bone — continued
    Lacrimal
      Left 0N8J
      Right 0N8H
    Nasal 0N8B
    Occipital 0N87
    Palatine
      Left 0N8L
      Right 0N8K
    Parietal
      Left 0N84
      Right 0N83
    Pelvic
      Left 0Q83
      Right 0Q82
    Sphenoid 0N8C
    Temporal
      Left 0N86
      Right 0N85
    Zygomatic
      Left 0N8N
      Right 0N8M
  Brain 0080
  Bursa and Ligament
    Abdomen
      Left 0M8J
      Right 0M8H
    Ankle
      Left 0M8R
      Right 0M8Q
    Elbow
      Left 0M84
      Right 0M83
    Foot
      Left 0M8T
      Right 0M8S
    Hand
      Left 0M88
      Right 0M87
    Head and Neck 0M80
    Hip
      Left 0M8M
      Right 0M8L
    Knee
      Left 0M8P
      Right 0M8N
    Lower Extremity
      Left 0M8W
      Right 0M8V
    Perineum 0M8K
    Rib(s) 0M8G
    Shoulder
      Left 0M82
      Right 0M81
    Spine
      Lower 0M8D
      Upper 0M8C
    Sternum 0M8F
    Upper Extremity
      Left 0M8B
      Right 0M89
    Wrist
      Left 0M86
      Right 0M85
  Carpal
    Left 0P8N
    Right 0P8M
  Cerebral Hemisphere 0087
  Chordae Tendineae 0289
  Clavicle
    Left 0P8B
    Right 0P89
  Coccyx 0Q8S
  Conduction Mechanism 0288
  Esophagogastric Junction 0D84
  Femoral Shaft
    Left 0Q89
    Right 0Q88
  Femur
    Lower
      Left 0Q8C
      Right 0Q8B
    Upper
      Left 0Q87
      Right 0Q86
  Fibula
    Left 0Q8K
    Right 0Q8J

Division — *continued*
- Gland, Pituitary 0G80
- Glenoid Cavity
  - Left 0P88
  - Right 0P87
- Humeral Head
  - Left 0P8D
  - Right 0P8C
- Humeral Shaft
  - Left 0P8G
  - Right 0P8F
- Hymen 0U8K
- Intraluminal Bioprosthetic Valve Leaflet Splitting Technology in Existing Valve X28F3VA
- Kidneys, Bilateral 0T82
- Liver 0F80
  - Left Lobe 0F82
  - Right Lobe 0F81
- Mandible
  - Left 0N8V
  - Right 0N8T
- Maxilla 0N8R
- Metacarpal
  - Left 0P8Q
  - Right 0P8P
- Metatarsal
  - Left 0Q8P
  - Right 0Q8N
- Muscle
  - Abdomen
    - Left 0K8L
    - Right 0K8K
  - Facial 0K81
  - Foot
    - Left 0K8W
    - Right 0K8V
  - Hand
    - Left 0K8D
    - Right 0K8C
  - Head 0K80
  - Hip
    - Left 0K8P
    - Right 0K8N
  - Lower Arm and Wrist
    - Left 0K8B
    - Right 0K89
  - Lower Leg
    - Left 0K8T
    - Right 0K8S
  - Neck
    - Left 0K83
    - Right 0K82
  - Papillary 028D
  - Perineum 0K8M
  - Shoulder
    - Left 0K86
    - Right 0K85
  - Thorax
    - Left 0K8J
    - Right 0K8H
  - Tongue, Palate, Pharynx 0K84
  - Trunk
    - Left 0K8G
    - Right 0K8F
  - Upper Arm
    - Left 0K88
    - Right 0K87
  - Upper Leg
    - Left 0K8R
    - Right 0K8Q
- Nerve
  - Abdominal Sympathetic 018M
  - Abducens 008L
  - Accessory 008R
  - Acoustic 008N
  - Brachial Plexus 0183
  - Cervical 0181
  - Cervical Plexus 0180
  - Facial 008M
  - Femoral 018D
  - Glossopharyngeal 008P
  - Head and Neck Sympathetic 018K
  - Hypoglossal 008S
  - Lumbar 018B
  - Lumbar Plexus 0189
  - Lumbar Sympathetic 018N
  - Lumbosacral Plexus 018A
  - Median 0185
  - Oculomotor 008H

Division — *continued*
- Nerve — *continued*
  - Olfactory 008F
  - Optic 008G
  - Peroneal 018H
  - Phrenic 0182
  - Pudendal 018C
  - Radial 0186
  - Sacral 018R
  - Sacral Plexus 018Q
  - Sacral Sympathetic 018P
  - Sciatic 018F
  - Thoracic 0188
  - Thoracic Sympathetic 018L
  - Tibial 018G
  - Trigeminal 008K
  - Trochlear 008J
  - Ulnar 0184
  - Vagus 008Q
- Orbit
  - Left 0N8Q
  - Right 0N8P
- Ovary
  - Bilateral 0U82
  - Left 0U81
  - Right 0U80
- Pancreas 0F8G
- Patella
  - Left 0Q8F
  - Right 0Q8D
- Perineum, Female 0W8NXZZ
- Phalanx
  - Finger
    - Left 0P8V
    - Right 0P8T
  - Thumb
    - Left 0P8S
    - Right 0P8R
  - Toe
    - Left 0Q8R
    - Right 0Q8Q
- Radius
  - Left 0P8J
  - Right 0P8H
- Ribs
  - 1 to 2 0P81
  - 3 or More 0P82
- Sacrum 0Q81
- Scapula
  - Left 0P86
  - Right 0P85
- Skin
  - Abdomen 0H87XZZ
  - Back 0H86XZZ
  - Buttock 0H88XZZ
  - Chest 0H85XZZ
  - Ear
    - Left 0H83XZZ
    - Right 0H82XZZ
  - Face 0H81XZZ
  - Foot
    - Left 0H8NXZZ
    - Right 0H8MXZZ
  - Hand
    - Left 0H8GXZZ
    - Right 0H8FXZZ
  - Inguinal 0H8AXZZ
  - Lower Arm
    - Left 0H8EXZZ
    - Right 0H8DXZZ
  - Lower Leg
    - Left 0H8LXZZ
    - Right 0H8KXZZ
  - Neck 0H84XZZ
  - Perineum 0H89XZZ
  - Scalp 0H80XZZ
  - Upper Arm
    - Left 0H8CXZZ
    - Right 0H8BXZZ
  - Upper Leg
    - Left 0H8JXZZ
    - Right 0H8HXZZ
- Skull 0N80
- Spinal Cord
  - Cervical 008W
  - Lumbar 008Y
  - Thoracic 008X
- Sternum 0P80
- Stomach, Pylorus 0D87

Division — *continued*
- Subcutaneous Tissue and Fascia
  - Abdomen 0J88
  - Back 0J87
  - Buttock 0J89
  - Chest 0J86
  - Face 0J81
  - Foot
    - Left 0J8R
    - Right 0J8Q
  - Hand
    - Left 0J8K
    - Right 0J8J
  - Head and Neck 0J8S
  - Lower Arm
    - Left 0J8H
    - Right 0J8G
  - Lower Extremity 0J8W
  - Lower Leg
    - Left 0J8P
    - Right 0J8N
  - Neck
    - Left 0J85
    - Right 0J84
  - Pelvic Region 0J8C
  - Perineum 0J8B
  - Scalp 0J80
  - Trunk 0J8T
  - Upper Arm
    - Left 0J8F
    - Right 0J8D
  - Upper Extremity 0J8V
  - Upper Leg
    - Left 0J8M
    - Right 0J8L
- Tarsal
  - Left 0Q8M
  - Right 0Q8L
- Tendon
  - Abdomen
    - Left 0L8G
    - Right 0L8F
  - Ankle
    - Left 0L8T
    - Right 0L8S
  - Foot
    - Left 0L8W
    - Right 0L8V
  - Hand
    - Left 0L88
    - Right 0L87
  - Head and Neck 0L80
  - Hip
    - Left 0L8K
    - Right 0L8J
  - Knee
    - Left 0L8R
    - Right 0L8Q
  - Lower Arm and Wrist
    - Left 0L86
    - Right 0L85
  - Lower Leg
    - Left 0L8P
    - Right 0L8N
  - Perineum 0L8H
  - Shoulder
    - Left 0L82
    - Right 0L81
  - Thorax
    - Left 0L8D
    - Right 0L8C
  - Trunk
    - Left 0L8B
    - Right 0L89
  - Upper Arm
    - Left 0L84
    - Right 0L83
  - Upper Leg
    - Left 0L8M
    - Right 0L8L
- Thyroid Gland Isthmus 0G8J
- Tibia
  - Left 0Q8H
  - Right 0Q8G
- Turbinate, Nasal 098L
- Ulna
  - Left 0P8L
  - Right 0P8K
- Uterine Supporting Structure 0U84

Division — *continued*
- Vertebra
  - Cervical 0P83
  - Lumbar 0Q80
  - Thoracic 0P84

DNase (Deoxyribonuclease) *use* Other Substance

Donislecel-jujn Allogeneic Pancreatic Islet Cellular Suspension XW033DA

Doppler study *see* Ultrasonography

Dorsal digital nerve *use* Radial Nerve

Dorsal metacarpal vein
- *use* Hand Vein, Left
- *use* Hand Vein, Right

Dorsal metatarsal artery
- *use* Foot Artery, Left
- *use* Foot Artery, Right

Dorsal metatarsal vein
- *use* Foot Vein, Left
- *use* Foot Vein, Right

Dorsal root ganglion
- *use* Cervical Spinal Cord
- *use* Lumbar Spinal Cord
- *use* Spinal Cord
- *use* Thoracic Spinal Cord

Dorsal scapular artery
- *use* Subclavian Artery, Left
- *use* Subclavian Artery, Right

Dorsal scapular nerve *use* Brachial Plexus

Dorsal venous arch
- *use* Foot Vein, Left
- *use* Foot Vein, Right

Dorsalis pedis artery
- *use* Anterior Tibial Artery, Left
- *use* Anterior Tibial Artery, Right

DownStream® System 5A0512C, 5A0522C

Drainage
- Abdominal Wall 0W9F
- Acetabulum
  - Left 0Q95
  - Right 0Q94
- Adenoids 0C9Q
- Ampulla of Vater 0F9C
- Anal Sphincter 0D9R
- Ankle Region
  - Left 0Y9L
  - Right 0Y9K
- Anterior Chamber
  - Left 0893
  - Right 0892
- Anus 0D9Q
- Aorta, Abdominal 0490
- Aortic Body 0G9D
- Appendix 0D9J
- Arm
  - Lower
    - Left 0X9F
    - Right 0X9D
  - Upper
    - Left 0X99
    - Right 0X98
- Artery
  - Anterior Tibial
    - Left 049Q
    - Right 049P
  - Axillary
    - Left 0396
    - Right 0395
  - Brachial
    - Left 0398
    - Right 0397
  - Celiac 0491
  - Colic
    - Left 0497
    - Middle 0498
    - Right 0496
  - Common Carotid
    - Left 039J
    - Right 039H
  - Common Iliac
    - Left 049D
    - Right 049C
  - External Carotid
    - Left 039N
    - Right 039M
  - External Iliac
    - Left 049J
    - Right 049H
  - Face 039R

Drainage — *continued*
- Artery — *continued*
  - Femoral
    - Left 049L
    - Right 049K
  - Foot
    - Left 049W
    - Right 049V
  - Gastric 0492
  - Hand
    - Left 039F
    - Right 039D
  - Hepatic 0493
  - Inferior Mesenteric 049B
  - Innominate 0392
  - Internal Carotid
    - Left 039L
    - Right 039K
  - Internal Iliac
    - Left 049F
    - Right 049E
  - Internal Mammary
    - Left 0391
    - Right 0390
  - Intracranial 039G
  - Lower 049Y
  - Peroneal
    - Left 049U
    - Right 049T
  - Popliteal
    - Left 049N
    - Right 049M
  - Posterior Tibial
    - Left 049S
    - Right 049R
  - Radial
    - Left 039C
    - Right 039B
  - Renal
    - Left 049A
    - Right 0499
  - Splenic 0494
  - Subclavian
    - Left 0394
    - Right 0393
  - Superior Mesenteric 0495
  - Temporal
    - Left 039T
    - Right 039S
  - Thyroid
    - Left 039V
    - Right 039U
  - Ulnar
    - Left 039A
    - Right 0399
  - Upper 039Y
  - Vertebral
    - Left 039Q
    - Right 039P
- Auditory Ossicle
  - Left 099A
  - Right 0999
- Axilla
  - Left 0X95
  - Right 0X94
- Back
  - Lower 0W9L
  - Upper 0W9K
- Basal Ganglia 0098
- Bladder 0T9B
- Bladder Neck 0T9C
- Bone
  - Ethmoid
    - Left 0N9G
    - Right 0N9F
  - Frontal 0N91
  - Hyoid 0N9X
  - Lacrimal
    - Left 0N9J
    - Right 0N9H
  - Nasal 0N9B
  - Occipital 0N97
  - Palatine
    - Left 0N9L
    - Right 0N9K
  - Parietal
    - Left 0N94
    - Right 0N93

Drainage — *continued*
- Bone — *continued*
  - Pelvic
    - Left 0Q93
    - Right 0Q92
  - Sphenoid 0N9C
  - Temporal
    - Left 0N96
    - Right 0N95
  - Zygomatic
    - Left 0N9N
    - Right 0N9M
- Bone Marrow 079T
- Brain 0090
- Breast
  - Bilateral 0H9V
  - Left 0H9U
  - Right 0H9T
- Bronchus
  - Lingula 0B99
  - Lower Lobe
    - Left 0B9B
    - Right 0B96
  - Main
    - Left 0B97
    - Right 0B93
  - Middle Lobe, Right 0B95
  - Upper Lobe
    - Left 0B98
    - Right 0B94
- Buccal Mucosa 0C94
- Bursa and Ligament
  - Abdomen
    - Left 0M9J
    - Right 0M9H
  - Ankle
    - Left 0M9R
    - Right 0M9Q
  - Elbow
    - Left 0M94
    - Right 0M93
  - Foot
    - Left 0M9T
    - Right 0M9S
  - Hand
    - Left 0M98
    - Right 0M97
  - Head and Neck 0M90
  - Hip
    - Left 0M9M
    - Right 0M9L
  - Knee
    - Left 0M9P
    - Right 0M9N
  - Lower Extremity
    - Left 0M9W
    - Right 0M9V
  - Perineum 0M9K
  - Rib(s) 0M9G
  - Shoulder
    - Left 0M92
    - Right 0M91
  - Spine
    - Lower 0M9D
    - Upper 0M9C
  - Sternum 0M9F
  - Upper Extremity
    - Left 0M9B
    - Right 0M99
  - Wrist
    - Left 0M96
    - Right 0M95
- Buttock
  - Left 0Y91
  - Right 0Y90
- Carina 0B92
- Carotid Bodies, Bilateral 0G98
- Carotid Body
  - Left 0G96
  - Right 0G97
- Carpal
  - Left 0P9N
  - Right 0P9M
- Cavity, Cranial 0W91
- Cecum 0D9H
- Cerebellum 009C
- Cerebral Hemisphere 0097
- Cerebral Meninges 0091
- Cerebral Ventricle 0096

Drainage — continued
- Cervix 0U9C
- Chest Wall 0W98
- Choroid
  - Left 089B
  - Right 089A
- Cisterna Chyli 079L
- Clavicle
  - Left 0P9B
  - Right 0P99
- Clitoris 0U9J
- Coccygeal Glomus 0G9B
- Coccyx 0Q9S
- Colon
  - Ascending 0D9K
  - Descending 0D9M
  - Sigmoid 0D9N
  - Transverse 0D9L
- Conjunctiva
  - Left 089T
  - Right 089S
- Cord
  - Bilateral 0V9H
  - Left 0V9G
  - Right 0V9F
- Cornea
  - Left 0899
  - Right 0898
- Cul-de-sac 0U9F
- Diaphragm 0B9T
- Disc
  - Cervical Vertebral 0R93
  - Cervicothoracic Vertebral 0R95
  - Lumbar Vertebral 0S92
  - Lumbosacral 0S94
  - Thoracic Vertebral 0R99
  - Thoracolumbar Vertebral 0R9B
- Duct
  - Common Bile 0F99
  - Cystic 0F98
  - Hepatic
    - Common 0F97
    - Left 0F96
    - Right 0F95
  - Lacrimal
    - Left 089Y
    - Right 089X
  - Pancreatic 0F9D
    - Accessory 0F9F
  - Parotid
    - Left 0C9C
    - Right 0C9B
- Duodenum 0D99
- Dura Mater 0092
- Ear
  - External
    - Left 0991
    - Right 0990
  - External Auditory Canal
    - Left 0994
    - Right 0993
  - Inner
    - Left 099E
    - Right 099D
  - Middle
    - Left 0996
    - Right 0995
- Elbow Region
  - Left 0X9C
  - Right 0X9B
- Epididymis
  - Bilateral 0V9L
  - Left 0V9K
  - Right 0V9J
- Epidural Space, Intracranial 0093
- Epiglottis 0C9R
- Esophagogastric Junction 0D94
- Esophagus 0D95
  - Lower 0D93
  - Middle 0D92
  - Upper 0D91
- Eustachian Tube
  - Left 099G
  - Right 099F
- Extremity
  - Lower
    - Left 0Y9B
    - Right 0Y99

Drainage — continued
- Extremity — continued
  - Upper
    - Left 0X97
    - Right 0X96
- Eye
  - Left 0891
  - Right 0890
- Eyelid
  - Lower
    - Left 089R
    - Right 089Q
  - Upper
    - Left 089P
    - Right 089N
- Face 0W92
- Fallopian Tube
  - Left 0U96
  - Right 0U95
- Fallopian Tubes, Bilateral 0U97
- Femoral Region
  - Left 0Y98
  - Right 0Y97
- Femoral Shaft
  - Left 0Q99
  - Right 0Q98
- Femur
  - Lower
    - Left 0Q9C
    - Right 0Q9B
  - Upper
    - Left 0Q97
    - Right 0Q96
- Fibula
  - Left 0Q9K
  - Right 0Q9J
- Finger Nail 0H9Q
- Foot
  - Left 0Y9N
  - Right 0Y9M
- Gallbladder 0F94
- Gingiva
  - Lower 0C96
  - Upper 0C95
- Gland
  - Adrenal
    - Bilateral 0G94
    - Left 0G92
    - Right 0G93
  - Lacrimal
    - Left 089W
    - Right 089V
  - Minor Salivary 0C9J
  - Parotid
    - Left 0C99
    - Right 0C98
  - Pituitary 0G90
  - Sublingual
    - Left 0C9F
    - Right 0C9D
  - Submaxillary
    - Left 0C9H
    - Right 0C9G
  - Vestibular 0U9L
- Glenoid Cavity
  - Left 0P98
  - Right 0P97
- Glomus Jugulare 0G9C
- Hand
  - Left 0X9K
  - Right 0X9J
- Head 0W90
- Humeral Head
  - Left 0P9D
  - Right 0P9C
- Humeral Shaft
  - Left 0P9G
  - Right 0P9F
- Hymen 0U9K
- Hypothalamus 009A
- Ileocecal Valve 0D9C
- Ileum 0D9B
- Inguinal Region
  - Left 0Y96
  - Right 0Y95
- Intestine
  - Large 0D9E
    - Left 0D9G
    - Right 0D9F

Drainage — continued
- Intestine — continued
  - Small 0D98
- Iris
  - Left 089D
  - Right 089C
- Jaw
  - Lower 0W95
  - Upper 0W94
- Jejunum 0D9A
- Joint
  - Acromioclavicular
    - Left 0R9H
    - Right 0R9G
  - Ankle
    - Left 0S9G
    - Right 0S9F
  - Carpal
    - Left 0R9R
    - Right 0R9Q
  - Carpometacarpal
    - Left 0R9T
    - Right 0R9S
  - Cervical Vertebral 0R91
  - Cervicothoracic Vertebral 0R94
  - Coccygeal 0S96
  - Elbow
    - Left 0R9M
    - Right 0R9L
  - Finger Phalangeal
    - Left 0R9X
    - Right 0R9W
  - Hip
    - Left 0S9B
    - Right 0S99
  - Knee
    - Left 0S9D
    - Right 0S9C
  - Lumbar Vertebral 0S90
  - Lumbosacral 0S93
  - Metacarpophalangeal
    - Left 0R9V
    - Right 0R9U
  - Metatarsal-Phalangeal
    - Left 0S9N
    - Right 0S9M
  - Occipital-cervical 0R90
  - Sacrococcygeal 0S95
  - Sacroiliac
    - Left 0S98
    - Right 0S97
  - Shoulder
    - Left 0R9K
    - Right 0R9J
  - Sternoclavicular
    - Left 0R9F
    - Right 0R9E
  - Tarsal
    - Left 0S9J
    - Right 0S9H
  - Tarsometatarsal
    - Left 0S9L
    - Right 0S9K
  - Temporomandibular
    - Left 0R9D
    - Right 0R9C
  - Thoracic Vertebral 0R96
  - Thoracolumbar Vertebral 0R9A
  - Toe Phalangeal
    - Left 0S9Q
    - Right 0S9P
  - Wrist
    - Left 0R9P
    - Right 0R9N
- Kidney
  - Left 0T91
  - Right 0T90
- Kidney Pelvis
  - Left 0T94
  - Right 0T93
- Knee Region
  - Left 0Y9G
  - Right 0Y9F
- Larynx 0C9S
- Leg
  - Lower
    - Left 0Y9J
    - Right 0Y9H

▼ Subterms under main terms may continue to next column or page

Drainage — continued
  Leg — continued
    Upper
      Left 0Y9D
      Right 0Y9C
  Lens
    Left 089K
    Right 089J
  Lip
    Lower 0C91
    Upper 0C90
  Liver 0F90
    Left Lobe 0F92
    Right Lobe 0F91
  Lung
    Bilateral 0B9M
    Left 0B9L
    Lower Lobe
      Left 0B9J
      Right 0B9F
    Middle Lobe, Right 0B9D
    Right 0B9K
    Upper Lobe
      Left 0B9G
      Right 0B9C
  Lung Lingula 0B9H
  Lymphatic
    Aortic 079D
    Axillary
      Left 0796
      Right 0795
    Head 0790
    Inguinal
      Left 079J
      Right 079H
    Internal Mammary
      Left 0799
      Right 0798
    Lower Extremity
      Left 079G
      Right 079F
    Mesenteric 079B
    Neck
      Left 0792
      Right 0791
    Pelvis 079C
    Thoracic Duct 079K
    Thorax 0797
    Upper Extremity
      Left 0794
      Right 0793
  Mandible
    Left 0N9V
    Right 0N9T
  Maxilla 0N9R
  Mediastinum 0W9C
  Medulla Oblongata 009D
  Mesentery 0D9V
  Metacarpal
    Left 0P9Q
    Right 0P9P
  Metatarsal
    Left 0Q9P
    Right 0Q9N
  Muscle
    Abdomen
      Left 0K9L
      Right 0K9K
    Extraocular
      Left 089M
      Right 089L
    Facial 0K91
    Foot
      Left 0K9W
      Right 0K9V
    Hand
      Left 0K9D
      Right 0K9C
    Head 0K90
    Hip
      Left 0K9P
      Right 0K9N
    Lower Arm and Wrist
      Left 0K9B
      Right 0K99
    Lower Leg
      Left 0K9T
      Right 0K9S

Drainage — continued
  Muscle — continued
    Neck
      Left 0K93
      Right 0K92
    Perineum 0K9M
    Shoulder
      Left 0K96
      Right 0K95
    Thorax
      Left 0K9J
      Right 0K9H
    Tongue, Palate, Pharynx 0K94
    Trunk
      Left 0K9G
      Right 0K9F
    Upper Arm
      Left 0K98
      Right 0K97
    Upper Leg
      Left 0K9R
      Right 0K9Q
  Nasal Mucosa and Soft Tissue 099K
  Nasopharynx 099N
  Neck 0W96
  Nerve
    Abdominal Sympathetic 019M
    Abducens 009L
    Accessory 009R
    Acoustic 009N
    Brachial Plexus 0193
    Cervical 0191
    Cervical Plexus 0190
    Facial 009M
    Femoral 019D
    Glossopharyngeal 009P
    Head and Neck Sympathetic 019K
    Hypoglossal 009S
    Lumbar 019B
    Lumbar Plexus 0199
    Lumbar Sympathetic 019N
    Lumbosacral Plexus 019A
    Median 0195
    Oculomotor 009H
    Olfactory 009F
    Optic 009G
    Peroneal 019H
    Phrenic 0192
    Pudendal 019C
    Radial 0196
    Sacral 019R
    Sacral Plexus 019Q
    Sacral Sympathetic 019P
    Sciatic 019F
    Thoracic 0198
    Thoracic Sympathetic 019L
    Tibial 019G
    Trigeminal 009K
    Trochlear 009J
    Ulnar 0194
    Vagus 009Q
  Nipple
    Left 0H9X
    Right 0H9W
  Omentum 0D9U
  Oral Cavity and Throat 0W93
  Orbit
    Left 0N9Q
    Right 0N9P
  Ovary
    Bilateral 0U92
    Left 0U91
    Right 0U90
  Palate
    Hard 0C92
    Soft 0C93
  Pancreas 0F9G
  Para-aortic Body 0G99
  Paraganglion Extremity 0G9F
  Parathyroid Gland 0G9R
    Inferior
      Left 0G9P
      Right 0G9N
    Multiple 0G9Q
    Superior
      Left 0G9M
      Right 0G9L
  Patella
    Left 0Q9F

Drainage — continued
  Patella — continued
    Right 0Q9D
  Pelvic Cavity 0W9J
  Penis 0V9S
  Pericardial Cavity 0W9D
  Perineum
    Female 0W9N
    Male 0W9M
  Peritoneal Cavity 0W9G
  Peritoneum 0D9W
  Phalanx
    Finger
      Left 0P9V
      Right 0P9T
    Thumb
      Left 0P9S
      Right 0P9R
    Toe
      Left 0Q9R
      Right 0Q9Q
  Pharynx 0C9M
  Pineal Body 0G91
  Pleura
    Left 0B9P
    Right 0B9N
  Pleural Cavity
    Left 0W9B
    Right 0W99
  Pons 009B
  Prepuce 0V9T
  Products of Conception
    Amniotic Fluid
      Diagnostic 1090
      Therapeutic 1090
    Fetal Blood 1090
    Fetal Cerebrospinal Fluid 1090
    Fetal Fluid, Other 1090
    Fluid, Other 1090
  Prostate 0V90
  Radius
    Left 0P9J
    Right 0P9H
  Rectum 0D9P
  Retina
    Left 089F
    Right 089E
  Retinal Vessel
    Left 089H
    Right 089G
  Retroperitoneum 0W9H
  Ribs
    1 to 2 0P91
    3 or More 0P92
  Sacrum 0Q91
  Scapula
    Left 0P96
    Right 0P95
  Sclera
    Left 0897
    Right 0896
  Scrotum 0V95
  Septum, Nasal 099M
  Shoulder Region
    Left 0X93
    Right 0X92
  Sinus
    Accessory 099P
    Ethmoid
      Left 099V
      Right 099U
    Frontal
      Left 099T
      Right 099S
    Mastoid
      Left 099C
      Right 099B
    Maxillary
      Left 099R
      Right 099Q
    Sphenoid
      Left 099X
      Right 099W
  Skin
    Abdomen 0H97
    Back 0H96
    Buttock 0H98
    Chest 0H95

Drainage — *continued*
  Skin — *continued*
    Ear
      Left 0H93
      Right 0H92
    Face 0H91
    Foot
      Left 0H9N
      Right 0H9M
    Hand
      Left 0H9G
      Right 0H9F
    Inguinal 0H9A
    Lower Arm
      Left 0H9E
      Right 0H9D
    Lower Leg
      Left 0H9L
      Right 0H9K
    Neck 0H94
    Perineum 0H99
    Scalp 0H90
    Upper Arm
      Left 0H9C
      Right 0H9B
    Upper Leg
      Left 0H9J
      Right 0H9H
  Skull 0N90
  Spinal Canal 009U
  Spinal Cord
    Cervical 009W
    Lumbar 009Y
    Thoracic 009X
  Spinal Meninges 009T
  Spleen 079P
  Sternum 0P90
  Stomach 0D96
    Pylorus 0D97
  Subarachnoid Space, Intracranial 0095
  Subcutaneous Tissue and Fascia
    Abdomen 0J98
    Back 0J97
    Buttock 0J99
    Chest 0J96
    Face 0J91
    Foot
      Left 0J9R
      Right 0J9Q
    Hand
      Left 0J9K
      Right 0J9J
    Lower Arm
      Left 0J9H
      Right 0J9G
    Lower Leg
      Left 0J9P
      Right 0J9N
    Neck
      Left 0J95
      Right 0J94
    Pelvic Region 0J9C
    Perineum 0J9B
    Scalp 0J90
    Upper Arm
      Left 0J9F
      Right 0J9D
    Upper Leg
      Left 0J9M
      Right 0J9L
  Subdural Space, Intracranial 0094
  Tarsal
    Left 0Q9M
    Right 0Q9L
  Tendon
    Abdomen
      Left 0L9G
      Right 0L9F
    Ankle
      Left 0L9T
      Right 0L9S
    Foot
      Left 0L9W
      Right 0L9V
    Hand
      Left 0L98
      Right 0L97
    Head and Neck 0L90

Drainage — *continued*
  Tendon — *continued*
    Hip
      Left 0L9K
      Right 0L9J
    Knee
      Left 0L9R
      Right 0L9Q
    Lower Arm and Wrist
      Left 0L96
      Right 0L95
    Lower Leg
      Left 0L9P
      Right 0L9N
    Perineum 0L9H
    Shoulder
      Left 0L92
      Right 0L91
    Thorax
      Left 0L9D
      Right 0L9C
    Trunk
      Left 0L9B
      Right 0L99
    Upper Arm
      Left 0L94
      Right 0L93
    Upper Leg
      Left 0L9M
      Right 0L9L
  Testis
    Bilateral 0V9C
    Left 0V9B
    Right 0V99
  Thalamus 0099
  Thymus 079M
  Thyroid Gland 0G9K
    Left Lobe 0G9G
    Right Lobe 0G9H
  Tibia
    Left 0Q9H
    Right 0Q9G
  Toe Nail 0H9R
  Tongue 0C97
  Tonsils 0C9P
  Tooth
    Lower 0C9X
    Upper 0C9W
  Trachea 0B91
  Tunica Vaginalis
    Left 0V97
    Right 0V96
  Turbinate, Nasal 099L
  Tympanic Membrane
    Left 0998
    Right 0997
  Ulna
    Left 0P9L
    Right 0P9K
  Ureter
    Left 0T97
    Right 0T96
  Ureters, Bilateral 0T98
  Urethra 0T9D
  Uterine Supporting Structure 0U94
  Uterus 0U99
  Uvula 0C9N
  Vagina 0U9G
  Vas Deferens
    Bilateral 0V9Q
    Left 0V9P
    Right 0V9N
  Vein
    Axillary
      Left 0598
      Right 0597
    Azygos 0590
    Basilic
      Left 059C
      Right 059B
    Brachial
      Left 059A
      Right 0599
    Cephalic
      Left 059F
      Right 059D
    Colic 0697
    Common Iliac
      Left 069D

Drainage — *continued*
  Vein — *continued*
    Common Iliac — *continued*
      Right 069C
    Esophageal 0693
    External Iliac
      Left 069G
      Right 069F
    External Jugular
      Left 059Q
      Right 059P
    Face
      Left 059V
      Right 059T
    Femoral
      Left 069N
      Right 069M
    Foot
      Left 069V
      Right 069T
    Gastric 0692
    Hand
      Left 059H
      Right 059G
    Hemiazygos 0591
    Hepatic 0694
    Hypogastric
      Left 069J
      Right 069H
    Inferior Mesenteric 0696
    Innominate
      Left 0594
      Right 0593
    Internal Jugular
      Left 059N
      Right 059M
    Intracranial 059L
    Lower 069Y
    Portal 0698
    Renal
      Left 069B
      Right 0699
    Saphenous
      Left 069Q
      Right 069P
    Splenic 0691
    Subclavian
      Left 0596
      Right 0595
    Superior Mesenteric 0695
    Upper 059Y
    Vertebral
      Left 059S
      Right 059R
  Vena Cava, Inferior 0690
  Vertebra
    Cervical 0P93
    Lumbar 0Q90
    Thoracic 0P94
  Vesicle
    Bilateral 0V93
    Left 0V92
    Right 0V91
  Vitreous
    Left 0895
    Right 0894
  Vocal Cord
    Left 0C9V
    Right 0C9T
  Vulva 0U9M
  Wrist Region
    Left 0X9H
    Right 0X9G
Dressing
  Abdominal Wall 2W23X4Z
  Arm
    Lower
      Left 2W2DX4Z
      Right 2W2CX4Z
    Upper
      Left 2W2BX4Z
      Right 2W2AX4Z
  Back 2W25X4Z
  Chest Wall 2W24X4Z
  Extremity
    Lower
      Left 2W2MX4Z
      Right 2W2LX4Z

Dressing — continued
Extremity — continued
Upper
Left 2W29X4Z
Right 2W28X4Z
Face 2W21X4Z
Finger
Left 2W2KX4Z
Right 2W2JX4Z
Foot
Left 2W2TX4Z
Right 2W2SX4Z
Hand
Left 2W2FX4Z
Right 2W2EX4Z
Head 2W20X4Z
Inguinal Region
Left 2W27X4Z
Right 2W26X4Z
Leg
Lower
Left 2W2RX4Z
Right 2W2QX4Z
Upper
Left 2W2PX4Z
Right 2W2NX4Z
Neck 2W22X4Z
Thumb
Left 2W2HX4Z
Right 2W2GX4Z
Toe
Left 2W2VX4Z
Right 2W2UX4Z
Driver stent (RX) (OTW) use Intraluminal Device
Drotrecogin alfa, infusion see Introduction of Recombinant Human-activated Protein C
Drug-eluting resorbable scaffold intraluminal device use Intraluminal Device, Everolimus-eluting Resorbable Scaffold(s) in New Technology
Duct of Santorini use Pancreatic Duct, Accessory
Duct of Wirsung use Pancreatic Duct
Ductogram, mammary see Plain Radiography, Skin, Subcutaneous Tissue and Breast BH0
Ductography, mammary see Plain Radiography, Skin, Subcutaneous Tissue and Breast BH0
Ductus deferens
use Vas Deferens
use Vas Deferens, Bilateral
use Vas Deferens, Left
use Vas Deferens, Right
Duodenal ampulla use Ampulla of Vater
Duodenectomy
see Excision, Duodenum 0DB9
see Resection, Duodenum 0DT9
Duodenocholedochotomy see Drainage, Gallbladder 0F94
Duodenocystostomy
see Bypass, Gallbladder 0F14
see Drainage, Gallbladder 0F94
Duodenoenterostomy
see Bypass, Gastrointestinal System 0D1
see Drainage, Gastrointestinal System 0D9
Duodenojejunal flexure use Jejunum
Duodenolysis see Release, Duodenum 0DN9
Duodenorrhaphy see Repair, Duodenum 0DQ9
Duodenoscopy, single-use (aScope™ Duodeno) (EXALT™ Model D) see New Technology, Hepatobiliary System and Pancreas XFJ
Duodenostomy
see Bypass, Duodenum 0D19
see Drainage, Duodenum 0D99
Duodenotomy see Drainage, Duodenum 0D99
Dura mater, intracranial use Dura Mater
Dura mater, spinal use Spinal Meninges
DuraGraft® Endothelial Damage Inhibitor use Endothelial Damage Inhibitor
DuraHeart Left Ventricular Assist System use Implantable Heart Assist System in Heart and Great Vessels
Dural venous sinus use Intracranial Vein
Durata® Defibrillation Lead use Cardiac Lead, Defibrillator in 02H
Durvalumab Antineoplastic XW0
DynaClip® (Delta) (Forte) (Quattro)
use Internal Fixation Device, Sustained Compression in 0RG

DynaClip® (Delta) (Forte) (Quattro) — continued
use Internal Fixation Device, Sustained Compression in 0SG
DynaNail® (Helix) (Hybrid) (Mini)
use Internal Fixation Device, Sustained Compression in 0RG
use Internal Fixation Device, Sustained Compression in 0SG
Dynesys® Dynamic Stabilization System
use Spinal Stabilization Device, Pedicle-Based in 0RH
use Spinal Stabilization Device, Pedicle-Based in 0SH

E

Earlobe
use Ear, External, Bilateral
use Ear, External, Left
use Ear, External, Right
EB-101 gene-corrected autologous cell therapy use Prademagene Zamikeracel, Genetically Engineered Autologous Cell Therapy in New Technology
EB-101 gene-corrected keratinocyte sheets use Prademagene Zamikeracel, Genetically Engineered Autologous Cell Therapy in New Technology
EBVALLO™ use Tabelecleucel Immunotherapy
ECCO2R (Extracorporeal Carbon Dioxide Removal) 5A0920Z
Echocardiogram see Ultrasonography, Heart B24
EchoGo Heart Failure 1.0 software XXE2X19
Echography see Ultrasonography
EchoTip® Insight™ Portosystemic Pressure Gradient Measurement System 4A044B2
ECMO see Performance, Circulatory 5A15
ECMO, intraoperative see Performance, Circulatory 5A15A
Eculizumab XW0
Edwards EVOQUE tricuspid valve replacement system use Multi-plane Flex Technology Bioprosthetic Valve in New Technology
EDWARDS INTUITY Elite valve system (rapid deployment technique) see Replacement, Valve, Aortic 02RF
EEG (electroencephalogram) see Measurement, Central Nervous 4A00
EGD (esophagogastroduodenoscopy) 0DJ08ZZ
Eighth cranial nerve use Acoustic Nerve
Ejaculatory duct
use Vas Deferens
use Vas Deferens, Bilateral
use Vas Deferens, Left
use Vas Deferens, Right
EKG (electrocardiogram) see Measurement, Cardiac 4A02
EKOS™ EkoSonic® Endovascular System see Fragmentation, Artery
Eladocagene exuparvovec XW0Q316
Electrical bone growth stimulator (EBGS)
use Bone Growth Stimulator in Head and Facial Bones
use Bone Growth Stimulator in Lower Bones
use Bone Growth Stimulator in Upper Bones
Electrical muscle stimulation (EMS) lead use Stimulator Lead in Muscles
Electrocautery
Destruction see Destruction
Repair see Repair
Electroconvulsive Therapy
Bilateral-Single Seizure GZB2ZZZ
Electroconvulsive Therapy, Other GZB4ZZZ
Unilateral-Single Seizure GZB0ZZZ
Electroencephalogram (EEG) see Measurement, Central Nervous 4A00
Electromagnetic Therapy
Central Nervous 6A22
Urinary 6A21
Electronic muscle stimulator lead use Stimulator Lead in Muscles
Electrophysiologic stimulation (EPS) see Measurement, Cardiac 4A02
Electroshock therapy see Electroconvulsive Therapy
Elevation, bone fragments, skull see Reposition, Head and Facial Bones 0NS

Eleventh cranial nerve use Accessory Nerve
Ellipsys® vascular access system see New Technology, Cardiovascular System X2K
Elranatamab Antineoplastic XW013L9
ELREXFIO™ use Elranatamab Antineoplastic
E-Luminexx™ (Biliary) (Vascular) Stent use Intraluminal Device
Eluvia™ Drug-Eluting Vascular Stent System
use Intraluminal Device, Drug-eluting in Lower Arteries
use Intraluminal Device, Drug-eluting, Two in Lower Arteries
use Intraluminal Device, Drug-eluting, Three in Lower Arteries
use Intraluminal Device, Drug-eluting, Four or More in Lower Arteries
ELZONRIS™ use Tagraxofusp-erzs Antineoplastic
Embolectomy see Extirpation
Emboli trap circuit, during percutaneous thrombectomy 5A05A0L
Embolization
see Occlusion
see Restriction
Embolization coil(s) use Intraluminal Device
EMG (electromyogram) see Measurement, Musculoskeletal 4A0F
Encephalon use Brain
Endarterectomy
see Extirpation, Lower Arteries 04C
see Extirpation, Upper Arteries 03C
Endeavor® (III) (IV) (Sprint) Zotarolimus-eluting Coronary Stent System use Intraluminal Device, Drug-eluting in Heart and Great Vessels
EndoAVF procedure, using magnetic-guided radiofrequency see Bypass, Upper Arteries 031
EndoAVF procedure, using thermal resistance energy see New Technology, Cardiovascular System X2K
Endologix AFX® Endovascular AAA System use Intraluminal Device
EndoSure® sensor use Monitoring Device, Pressure Sensor in 02H
ENDOTAK RELIANCE® (G) Defibrillation Lead use Cardiac Lead, Defibrillator in 02H
Endothelial damage inhibitor, applied to vein graft XY0VX83
Endotracheal tube (cuffed) (double-lumen) use Intraluminal Device, Endotracheal Airway in Respiratory System
Endovascular fistula creation, using magnetic-guided radiofrequency see Bypass, Upper Arteries 031
Endovascular fistula creation, using thermal resistance energy see New Technology, Cardiovascular System X2K
Endurant® Endovascular Stent Graft use Intraluminal Device
Endurant® II AAA Stent Graft System use Intraluminal Device
Engineered Allogeneic Thymus Tissue XW020D8
Engineered Chimeric Antigen Receptor T-cell Immunotherapy
Allogeneic XW0
Autologous XW0
Enlargement
see Dilation
see Repair
EnRhythm use Pacemaker, Dual Chamber in 0JH
ENROUTE® Transcarotid Neuroprotection System see New Technology, Cardiovascular System X2A
ENSPRYNG™ use Satralizumab-mwge
Enterorrhaphy see Repair, Gastrointestinal System 0DQ
Enterra gastric neurostimulator use Stimulator Generator, Multiple Array in 0JH
Enucleation
Eyeball see Resection, Eye 08T
Eyeball with prosthetic implant see Replacement, Eye 08R
Epcoritamab Monoclonal Antibody XW013S9
Ependyma use Cerebral Ventricle
Epicel® cultured epidermal autograft use Autologous Tissue Substitute
Epic™ Stented Tissue Valve (aortic) use Zooplastic Tissue in Heart and Great Vessels
Epidermis use Skin

ICD-10-PCS 2025 — Excision Index

Epididymectomy
 see Excision, Male Reproductive System 0VB
 see Resection, Male Reproductive System 0VT
Epididymoplasty
 see Repair, Male Reproductive System 0VQ
 see Supplement, Male Reproductive System 0VU
Epididymorrhaphy see Repair, Male Reproductive System 0VQ
Epididymotomy see Drainage, Male Reproductive System 0V9
Epidural space, spinal use Spinal Canal
Epiphysiodesis
 see Insertion of device in, Lower Bones 0QH
 see Insertion of device in, Upper Bones 0PH
 see Repair, Lower Bones 0QQ
 see Repair, Upper Bones 0PQ
Epiploic foramen use Peritoneum
Epiretinal Visual Prosthesis
 Left 08H105Z
 Right 08H005Z
Episiorrhaphy see Repair, Perineum, Female 0WQN
Episiotomy see Division, Perineum, Female 0W8N
Epithalamus use Thalamus
Epitrochlear lymph node
 use Lymphatic, Left Upper Extremity
 use Lymphatic, Right Upper Extremity
EPKINLY™ use Epcoritamab Monoclonal Antibody
EPS (electrophysiologic stimulation) see Measurement, Cardiac 4A02
Eptifibatide, infusion see Introduction of Platelet Inhibitor
ERCP (endoscopic retrograde cholangiopancreatography) see Fluoroscopy, Hepatobiliary System and Pancreas BF1
Erdafitinib Antineoplastic use Other Antineoplastic
Erector spinae muscle
 use Trunk Muscle, Left
 use Trunk Muscle, Right
ERLEADA™ (Apalutamide Antineoplastic) use Other Antineoplastic
Esketamine Hydrochloride use Other Substance
Esophageal artery use Upper Artery
Esophageal obturator airway (EOA) use Intraluminal Device, Airway in Gastrointestinal System
Esophageal plexus use Thoracic Sympathetic Nerve
Esophagectomy
 see Excision, Gastrointestinal System 0DB
 see Resection, Gastrointestinal System 0DT
Esophagocoloplasty
 see Repair, Gastrointestinal System 0DQ
 see Supplement, Gastrointestinal System 0DU
Esophagoenterostomy
 see Bypass, Gastrointestinal System 0D1
 see Drainage, Gastrointestinal System 0D9
Esophagoesophagostomy
 see Bypass, Gastrointestinal System 0D1
 see Drainage, Gastrointestinal System 0D9
Esophagogastrectomy
 see Excision, Gastrointestinal System 0DB
 see Resection, Gastrointestinal System 0DT
Esophagogastroduodenoscopy (EGD) 0DJ08ZZ
Esophagogastroplasty
 see Repair, Gastrointestinal System 0DQ
 see Supplement, Gastrointestinal System 0DU
Esophagogastroscopy 0DJ68ZZ
Esophagogastrostomy
 see Bypass, Gastrointestinal System 0D1
 see Drainage, Gastrointestinal System 0D9
Esophagojejunoplasty see Supplement, Gastrointestinal System 0DU
Esophagojejunostomy
 see Bypass, Gastrointestinal System 0D1
 see Drainage, Gastrointestinal System 0D9
Esophagomyotomy see Division, Esophagogastric Junction 0D84
Esophagoplasty
 see Repair, Gastrointestinal System 0DQ
 see Replacement, Esophagus 0DR5
 see Supplement, Gastrointestinal System 0DU
Esophagoplication see Restriction, Gastrointestinal System 0DV
Esophagorrhaphy see Repair, Gastrointestinal System 0DQ
Esophagoscopy 0DJ08ZZ
Esophagotomy see Drainage, Gastrointestinal System 0D9

Esprit™ BTK (scaffold) (stent) use Intraluminal Device, Everolimus-eluting Resorbable Scaffold(s) in New Technology
Esteem® implantable hearing system use Hearing Device in Ear, Nose, Sinus
ESWL (extracorporeal shock wave lithotripsy) see Fragmentation
Etesevimab Monoclonal Antibody XW0
Ethmoidal air cell
 use Ethmoid Sinus, Left
 use Ethmoid Sinus, Right
Ethmoidectomy
 see Excision, Ear, Nose, Sinus 09B
 see Excision, Head and Facial Bones 0NB
 see Resection, Ear, Nose, Sinus 09T
 see Resection, Head and Facial Bones 0NT
Ethmoidotomy see Drainage, Ear, Nose, Sinus 099
EV ICD System (Extravascular implantable defibrillator lead) use Defibrillator Lead in Anatomical Regions, General
Evacuation
 Hematoma see Extirpation
 Other Fluid see Drainage
Evera (XT) (S) (DR/VR) use Defibrillator Generator in 0JH
Everolimus Eluting Resorbable Scaffold System use Intraluminal Device, Everolimus-eluting Resorbable Scaffold(s) in New Technology
Everolimus-eluting coronary stent use Intraluminal Device, Drug-eluting in Heart and Great Vessels
Evisceration
 Eyeball see Resection, Eye 08T
 Eyeball with prosthetic implant see Replacement, Eye 08R
Evo® sEEG-RF probes (for radiofrequency ablation of brain tissue) 00503Z4
EVUSHELD™ use Tixagevimab and Cilgavimab Monoclonal Antibody
Exagamglogene Autotemcel XW1
EXALT™ Model D Single-Use Duodenoscope see New Technology, Hepatobiliary System and Pancreas XFJ
Examination see Inspection
Exchange see Change device in
Excision
 Abdominal Wall 0WBF
 Acetabulum
  Left 0QB5
  Right 0QB4
 Adenoids 0CBQ
 Ampulla of Vater 0FBC
 Anal Sphincter 0DBR
 Ankle Region
  Left 0YBL
  Right 0YBK
 Anus 0DBQ
 Aorta
  Abdominal
  Thoracic
   Ascending/Arch 02BX
   Descending 02BW
 Aortic Body 0GBD
 Appendix 0DBJ
 Arm
  Lower
   Left 0XBF
   Right 0XBD
  Upper
   Left 0XB9
   Right 0XB8
 Artery
  Anterior Tibial
   Left 04BQ
   Right 04BP
  Axillary
   Left 03B6
   Right 03B5
  Brachial
   Left 03B8
   Right 03B7
  Celiac 04B1
  Colic
   Left 04B7
   Middle 04B8
   Right 04B6
  Common Carotid
   Left 03BJ
   Right 03BH

Excision — continued
 Artery — continued
  Common Iliac
   Left 04BD
   Right 04BC
  External Carotid
   Left 03BN
   Right 03BM
  External Iliac
   Left 04BJ
   Right 04BH
  Face 03BR
  Femoral
   Left 04BL
   Right 04BK
  Foot
   Left 04BW
   Right 04BV
  Gastric 04B2
  Hand
   Left 03BF
   Right 03BD
  Hepatic 04B3
  Inferior Mesenteric 04BB
  Innominate 03B2
  Internal Carotid
   Left 03BL
   Right 03BK
  Internal Iliac
   Left 04BF
   Right 04BE
  Internal Mammary
   Left 03B1
   Right 03B0
  Intracranial 03BG
  Lower 04BY
  Peroneal
   Left 04BU
   Right 04BT
  Popliteal
   Left 04BN
   Right 04BM
  Posterior Tibial
   Left 04BS
   Right 04BR
  Pulmonary
   Left 02BR
   Right 02BQ
  Pulmonary Trunk 02BP
  Radial
   Left 03BC
   Right 03BB
  Renal
   Left 04BA
   Right 04B9
  Splenic 04B4
  Subclavian
   Left 03B4
   Right 03B3
  Superior Mesenteric 04B5
  Temporal
   Left 03BT
   Right 03BS
  Thyroid
   Left 03BV
   Right 03BU
  Ulnar
   Left 03BA
   Right 03B9
  Upper 03BY
  Vertebral
   Left 03BQ
   Right 03BP
 Atrium
  Left 02B7
  Right 02B6
 Auditory Ossicle
  Left 09BA
  Right 09B9
 Axilla
  Left 0XB5
  Right 0XB4
 Back
  Lower 0WBL
  Upper 0WBK
 Basal Ganglia 00B8
 Bladder 0TBB
 Bladder Neck 0TBC

Excision

Excision — *continued*
- Bone
  - Ethmoid
    - Left ØNBG
    - Right ØNBF
  - Frontal ØNB1
  - Hyoid ØNBX
  - Lacrimal
    - Left ØNBJ
    - Right ØNBH
  - Nasal ØNBB
  - Occipital ØNB7
  - Palatine
    - Left ØNBL
    - Right ØNBK
  - Parietal
    - Left ØNB4
    - Right ØNB3
  - Pelvic
    - Left ØQB3
    - Right ØQB2
  - Sphenoid ØNBC
  - Temporal
    - Left ØNB6
    - Right ØNB5
  - Zygomatic
    - Left ØNBN
    - Right ØNBM
- Brain ØØBØ
- Breast
  - Bilateral ØHBV
  - Left ØHBU
  - Right ØHBT
  - Supernumerary ØHBY
- Bronchus
  - Lingula ØBB9
  - Lower Lobe
    - Left ØBBB
    - Right ØBB6
  - Main
    - Left ØBB7
    - Right ØBB3
  - Middle Lobe, Right ØBB5
  - Upper Lobe
    - Left ØBB8
    - Right ØBB4
- Buccal Mucosa ØCB4
- Bursa and Ligament
  - Abdomen
    - Left ØMBJ
    - Right ØMBH
  - Ankle
    - Left ØMBR
    - Right ØMBQ
  - Elbow
    - Left ØMB4
    - Right ØMB3
  - Foot
    - Left ØMBT
    - Right ØMBS
  - Hand
    - Left ØMB8
    - Right ØMB7
  - Head and Neck ØMBØ
  - Hip
    - Left ØMBM
    - Right ØMBL
  - Knee
    - Left ØMBP
    - Right ØMBN
  - Lower Extremity
    - Left ØMBW
    - Right ØMBV
  - Perineum ØMBK
  - Rib(s) ØMBG
  - Shoulder
    - Left ØMB2
    - Right ØMB1
  - Spine
    - Lower ØMBD
    - Upper ØMBC
  - Sternum ØMBF
  - Upper Extremity
    - Left ØMBB
    - Right ØMB9
  - Wrist
    - Left ØMB6
    - Right ØMB5

Excision — *continued*
- Buttock
  - Left ØYB1
  - Right ØYBØ
- Carina ØBB2
- Carotid Bodies, Bilateral ØGB8
- Carotid Body
  - Left ØGB6
  - Right ØGB7
- Carpal
  - Left ØPBN
  - Right ØPBM
- Cecum ØDBH
- Cerebellum ØØBC
- Cerebral Hemisphere ØØB7
- Cerebral Meninges ØØB1
- Cerebral Ventricle ØØB6
- Cervix ØUBC
- Chest Wall ØWB8
- Chordae Tendineae Ø2B9
- Choroid
  - Left Ø8BB
  - Right Ø8BA
- Cisterna Chyli Ø7BL
- Clavicle
  - Left ØPBB
  - Right ØPB9
- Clitoris ØUBJ
- Coccygeal Glomus ØGBB
- Coccyx ØQBS
- Colon
  - Ascending ØDBK
  - Descending ØDBM
  - Sigmoid ØDBN
  - Transverse ØDBL
- Conduction Mechanism Ø2B8
- Conjunctiva
  - Left Ø8BTXZ
  - Right Ø8BSXZ
- Cord
  - Bilateral ØVBH
  - Left ØVBG
  - Right ØVBF
- Cornea
  - Left Ø8B9XZ
  - Right Ø8B8XZ
- Cul-de-sac ØUBF
- Diaphragm ØBBT
- Disc
  - Cervical Vertebral ØRB3
  - Cervicothoracic Vertebral ØRB5
  - Lumbar Vertebral ØSB2
  - Lumbosacral ØSB4
  - Thoracic Vertebral ØRB9
  - Thoracolumbar Vertebral ØRBB
- Duct
  - Common Bile ØFB9
  - Cystic ØFB8
  - Hepatic
    - Common ØFB7
    - Left ØFB6
    - Right ØFB5
  - Lacrimal
    - Left Ø8BY
    - Right Ø8BX
  - Pancreatic ØFBD
    - Accessory ØFBF
  - Parotid
    - Left ØCBC
    - Right ØCBB
- Duodenum ØDB9
- Dura Mater ØØB2
- Ear
  - External
    - Left Ø9B1
    - Right Ø9BØ
  - External Auditory Canal
    - Left Ø9B4
    - Right Ø9B3
  - Inner
    - Left Ø9BE
    - Right Ø9BD
  - Middle
    - Left Ø9B6
    - Right Ø9B5
- Elbow Region
  - Left ØXBC
  - Right ØXBB

Excision — *continued*
- Epididymis
  - Bilateral ØVBL
  - Left ØVBK
  - Right ØVBJ
- Epiglottis ØCBR
- Esophagogastric Junction ØDB4
- Esophagus ØDB5
  - Lower ØDB3
  - Middle ØDB2
  - Upper ØDB1
- Eustachian Tube
  - Left Ø9BG
  - Right Ø9BF
- Extremity
  - Lower
    - Left ØYBB
    - Right ØYB9
  - Upper
    - Left ØXB7
    - Right ØXB6
- Eye
  - Left Ø8B1
  - Right Ø8BØ
- Eyelid
  - Lower
    - Left Ø8BR
    - Right Ø8BQ
  - Upper
    - Left Ø8BP
    - Right Ø8BN
- Face ØWB2
- Fallopian Tube
  - Left ØUB6
  - Right ØUB5
- Fallopian Tubes, Bilateral ØUB7
- Femoral Region
  - Left ØYB8
  - Right ØYB7
- Femoral Shaft
  - Left ØQB9
  - Right ØQB8
- Femur
  - Lower
    - Left ØQBC
    - Right ØQBB
  - Upper
    - Left ØQB7
    - Right ØQB6
- Fibula
  - Left ØQBK
  - Right ØQBJ
- Finger Nail ØHBQXZ
- Floor of mouth *see* Excision, Oral Cavity and Throat ØWB3
- Foot
  - Left ØYBN
  - Right ØYBM
- Gallbladder ØFB4
- Gingiva
  - Lower ØCB6
  - Upper ØCB5
- Gland
  - Adrenal
    - Bilateral ØGB4
    - Left ØGB2
    - Right ØGB3
  - Lacrimal
    - Left Ø8BW
    - Right Ø8BV
  - Minor Salivary ØCBJ
  - Parotid
    - Left ØCB9
    - Right ØCB8
  - Pituitary ØGBØ
  - Sublingual
    - Left ØCBF
    - Right ØCBD
  - Submaxillary
    - Left ØCBH
    - Right ØCBG
  - Vestibular ØUBL
- Glenoid Cavity
  - Left ØPB8
  - Right ØPB7
- Glomus Jugulare ØGBC
- Hand
  - Left ØXBK
  - Right ØXBJ

Excision — continued
  Head 0WB0
  Humeral Head
    Left 0PBD
    Right 0PBC
  Humeral Shaft
    Left 0PBG
    Right 0PBF
  Hymen 0UBK
  Hypothalamus 00BA
  Ileocecal Valve 0DBC
  Ileum 0DBB
  Inguinal Region
    Left 0YB6
    Right 0YB5
  Intestine
    Large 0DBE
      Left 0DBG
      Right 0DBF
    Small 0DB8
  Iris
    Left 08BD3Z
    Right 08BC3Z
  Jaw
    Lower 0WB5
    Upper 0WB4
  Jejunum 0DBA
  Joint
    Acromioclavicular
      Left 0RBH
      Right 0RBG
    Ankle
      Left 0SBG
      Right 0SBF
    Carpal
      Left 0RBR
      Right 0RBQ
    Carpometacarpal
      Left 0RBT
      Right 0RBS
    Cervical Vertebral 0RB1
    Cervicothoracic Vertebral 0RB4
    Coccygeal 0SB6
    Elbow
      Left 0RBM
      Right 0RBL
    Finger Phalangeal
      Left 0RBX
      Right 0RBW
    Hip
      Left 0SBB
      Right 0SB9
    Knee
      Left 0SBD
      Right 0SBC
    Lumbar Vertebral 0SB0
    Lumbosacral 0SB3
    Metacarpophalangeal
      Left 0RBV
      Right 0RBU
    Metatarsal-Phalangeal
      Left 0SBN
      Right 0SBM
    Occipital-cervical 0RB0
    Sacrococcygeal 0SB5
    Sacroiliac
      Left 0SB8
      Right 0SB7
    Shoulder
      Left 0RBK
      Right 0RBJ
    Sternoclavicular
      Left 0RBF
      Right 0RBE
    Tarsal
      Left 0SBJ
      Right 0SBH
    Tarsometatarsal
      Left 0SBL
      Right 0SBK
    Temporomandibular
      Left 0RBD
      Right 0RBC
    Thoracic Vertebral 0RB6
    Thoracolumbar Vertebral 0RBA
    Toe Phalangeal
      Left 0SBQ
      Right 0SBP

Excision — continued
  Joint — continued
    Wrist
      Left 0RBP
      Right 0RBN
  Kidney
    Left 0TB1
    Right 0TB0
  Kidney Pelvis
    Left 0TB4
    Right 0TB3
  Knee Region
    Left 0YBG
    Right 0YBF
  Larynx 0CBS
  Leg
    Lower
      Left 0YBJ
      Right 0YBH
    Upper
      Left 0YBD
      Right 0YBC
  Lens
    Left 08BK3Z
    Right 08BJ3Z
  Lip
    Lower 0CB1
    Upper 0CB0
  Liver 0FB0
    Left Lobe 0FB2
    Right Lobe 0FB1
  Lung
    Bilateral 0BBM
    Left 0BBL
    Lower Lobe
      Left 0BBJ
      Right 0BBF
    Middle Lobe, Right 0BBD
    Right 0BBK
    Upper Lobe
      Left 0BBG
      Right 0BBC
  Lung Lingula 0BBH
  Lymphatic
    Aortic 07BD
    Axillary
      Left 07B6
      Right 07B5
    Head 07B0
    Inguinal
      Left 07BJ
      Right 07BH
    Internal Mammary
      Left 07B9
      Right 07B8
    Lower Extremity
      Left 07BG
      Right 07BF
    Mesenteric 07BB
    Neck
      Left 07B2
      Right 07B1
    Pelvis 07BC
    Thoracic Duct 07BK
    Thorax 07B7
    Upper Extremity
      Left 07B4
      Right 07B3
  Mandible
    Left 0NBV
    Right 0NBT
  Maxilla 0NBR
  Mediastinum 0WBC
  Medulla Oblongata 00BD
  Mesentery 0DBV
  Metacarpal
    Left 0PBQ
    Right 0PBP
  Metatarsal
    Left 0QBP
    Right 0QBN
  Muscle
    Abdomen
      Left 0KBL
      Right 0KBK
    Extraocular
      Left 08BM
      Right 08BL
    Facial 0KB1

Excision — continued
  Muscle — continued
    Foot
      Left 0KBW
      Right 0KBV
    Hand
      Left 0KBD
      Right 0KBC
    Head 0KB0
    Hip
      Left 0KBP
      Right 0KBN
    Lower Arm and Wrist
      Left 0KBB
      Right 0KB9
    Lower Leg
      Left 0KBT
      Right 0KBS
    Neck
      Left 0KB3
      Right 0KB2
    Papillary 02BD
    Perineum 0KBM
    Shoulder
      Left 0KB6
      Right 0KB5
    Thorax
      Left 0KBJ
      Right 0KBH
    Tongue, Palate, Pharynx 0KB4
    Trunk
      Left 0KBG
      Right 0KBF
    Upper Arm
      Left 0KB8
      Right 0KB7
    Upper Leg
      Left 0KBR
      Right 0KBQ
  Nasal Mucosa and Soft Tissue 09BK
  Nasopharynx 09BN
  Neck 0WB6
  Nerve
    Abdominal Sympathetic 01BM
    Abducens 00BL
    Accessory 00BR
    Acoustic 00BN
    Brachial Plexus 01B3
    Cervical 01B1
    Cervical Plexus 01B0
    Facial 00BM
    Femoral 01BD
    Glossopharyngeal 00BP
    Head and Neck Sympathetic 01BK
    Hypoglossal 00BS
    Lumbar 01BB
    Lumbar Plexus 01B9
    Lumbar Sympathetic 01BN
    Lumbosacral Plexus 01BA
    Median 01B5
    Oculomotor 00BH
    Olfactory 00BF
    Optic 00BG
    Peroneal 01BH
    Phrenic 01B2
    Pudendal 01BC
    Radial 01B6
    Sacral 01BR
    Sacral Plexus 01BQ
    Sacral Sympathetic 01BP
    Sciatic 01BF
    Thoracic 01B8
    Thoracic Sympathetic 01BL
    Tibial 01BG
    Trigeminal 00BK
    Trochlear 00BJ
    Ulnar 01B4
    Vagus 00BQ
  Nipple
    Left 0HBX
    Right 0HBW
  Omentum 0DBU
  Oral Cavity and Throat 0WB3
  Orbit
    Left 0NBQ
    Right 0NBP
  Ovary
    Bilateral 0UB2
    Left 0UB1

Excision

Excision — *continued*
- Ovary — *continued*
  - Right 0UB0
- Palate
  - Hard 0CB2
  - Soft 0CB3
- Pancreas 0FBG
- Para-aortic Body 0GB9
- Paraganglion Extremity 0GBF
- Parathyroid Gland 0GBR
  - Inferior
    - Left 0GBP
    - Right 0GBN
  - Multiple 0GBQ
  - Superior
    - Left 0GBM
    - Right 0GBL
- Patella
  - Left 0QBF
  - Right 0QBD
- Penis 0VBS
- Pericardium 02BN
- Perineum
  - Female 0WBN
  - Male 0WBM
- Peritoneum 0DBW
- Phalanx
  - Finger
    - Left 0PBV
    - Right 0PBT
  - Thumb
    - Left 0PBS
    - Right 0PBR
  - Toe
    - Left 0QBR
    - Right 0QBQ
- Pharynx 0CBM
- Pineal Body 0GB1
- Pleura
  - Left 0BBP
  - Right 0BBN
- Pons 00BB
- Prepuce 0VBT
- Prostate 0VB0
- Radius
  - Left 0PBJ
  - Right 0PBH
- Rectum 0DBP
- Retina
  - Left 08BF3Z
  - Right 08BE3Z
- Retroperitoneum 0WBH
- Ribs
  - 1 to 2 0PB1
  - 3 or More 0PB2
- Sacrum 0QB1
- Scapula
  - Left 0PB6
  - Right 0PB5
- Sclera
  - Left 08B7XZ
  - Right 08B6XZ
- Scrotum 0VB5
- Septum
  - Atrial 02B5
  - Nasal 09BM
  - Ventricular 02BM
- Shoulder Region
  - Left 0XB3
  - Right 0XB2
- Sinus
  - Accessory 09BP
  - Ethmoid
    - Left 09BV
    - Right 09BU
  - Frontal
    - Left 09BT
    - Right 09BS
  - Mastoid
    - Left 09BC
    - Right 09BB
  - Maxillary
    - Left 09BR
    - Right 09BQ
  - Sphenoid
    - Left 09BX
    - Right 09BW
- Skin
  - Abdomen 0HB7XZ

Excision — *continued*
- Skin — *continued*
  - Back 0HB6XZ
  - Buttock 0HB8XZ
  - Chest 0HB5XZ
  - Ear
    - Left 0HB3XZ
    - Right 0HB2XZ
  - Face 0HB1XZ
  - Foot
    - Left 0HBNXZ
    - Right 0HBMXZ
  - Hand
    - Left 0HBGXZ
    - Right 0HBFXZ
  - Inguinal 0HBAXZ
  - Lower Arm
    - Left 0HBEXZ
    - Right 0HBDXZ
  - Lower Leg
    - Left 0HBLXZ
    - Right 0HBKXZ
  - Neck 0HB4XZ
  - Perineum 0HB9XZ
  - Scalp 0HB0XZ
  - Upper Arm
    - Left 0HBCXZ
    - Right 0HBBXZ
  - Upper Leg
    - Left 0HBJXZ
    - Right 0HBHXZ
- Skull 0NB0
- Spinal Cord
  - Cervical 00BW
  - Lumbar 00BY
  - Thoracic 00BX
- Spinal Meninges 00BT
- Spleen 07BP
- Sternum 0PB0
- Stomach 0DB6
  - Pylorus 0DB7
- Subcutaneous Tissue and Fascia
  - Abdomen 0JB8
  - Back 0JB7
  - Buttock 0JB9
  - Chest 0JB6
  - Face 0JB1
  - Foot
    - Left 0JBR
    - Right 0JBQ
  - Hand
    - Left 0JBK
    - Right 0JBJ
  - Lower Arm
    - Left 0JBH
    - Right 0JBG
  - Lower Leg
    - Left 0JBP
    - Right 0JBN
  - Neck
    - Left 0JB5
    - Right 0JB4
  - Pelvic Region 0JBC
  - Perineum 0JBB
  - Scalp 0JB0
  - Upper Arm
    - Left 0JBF
    - Right 0JBD
  - Upper Leg
    - Left 0JBM
    - Right 0JBL
- Tarsal
  - Left 0QBM
  - Right 0QBL
- Tendon
  - Abdomen
    - Left 0LBG
    - Right 0LBF
  - Ankle
    - Left 0LBT
    - Right 0LBS
  - Foot
    - Left 0LBW
    - Right 0LBV
  - Hand
    - Left 0LB8
    - Right 0LB7
  - Head and Neck 0LB0

Excision — *continued*
- Tendon — *continued*
  - Hip
    - Left 0LBK
    - Right 0LBJ
  - Knee
    - Left 0LBR
    - Right 0LBQ
  - Lower Arm and Wrist
    - Left 0LB6
    - Right 0LB5
  - Lower Leg
    - Left 0LBP
    - Right 0LBN
  - Perineum 0LBH
  - Shoulder
    - Left 0LB2
    - Right 0LB1
  - Thorax
    - Left 0LBD
    - Right 0LBC
  - Trunk
    - Left 0LBB
    - Right 0LB9
  - Upper Arm
    - Left 0LB4
    - Right 0LB3
  - Upper Leg
    - Left 0LBM
    - Right 0LBL
- Testis
  - Bilateral 0VBC
  - Left 0VBB
  - Right 0VB9
- Thalamus 00B9
- Thymus 07BM
- Thyroid Gland
  - Left Lobe 0GBG
  - Right Lobe 0GBH
- Thyroid Gland Isthmus 0GBJ
- Tibia
  - Left 0QBH
  - Right 0QBG
- Toe Nail 0HBRXZ
- Tongue 0CB7
- Tonsils 0CBP
- Tooth
  - Lower 0CBX
  - Upper 0CBW
- Trachea 0BB1
- Tunica Vaginalis
  - Left 0VB7
  - Right 0VB6
- Turbinate, Nasal 09BL
- Tympanic Membrane
  - Left 09B8
  - Right 09B7
- Ulna
  - Left 0PBL
  - Right 0PBK
- Ureter
  - Left 0TB7
  - Right 0TB6
- Urethra 0TBD
- Uterine Supporting Structure 0UB4
- Uterus 0UB9
- Uvula 0CBN
- Vagina 0UBG
- Valve
  - Aortic 02BF
  - Mitral 02BG
  - Pulmonary 02BH
  - Tricuspid 02BJ
- Vas Deferens
  - Bilateral 0VBQ
  - Left 0VBP
  - Right 0VBN
- Vein
  - Axillary
    - Left 05B8
    - Right 05B7
  - Azygos 05B0
  - Basilic
    - Left 05BC
    - Right 05BB
  - Brachial
    - Left 05BA
    - Right 05B9

Excision — *continued*
  Vein — *continued*
    Cephalic
      Left 05BF
      Right 05BD
    Colic 06B7
    Common Iliac
      Left 06BD
      Right 06BC
    Coronary 02B4
    Esophageal 06B3
    External Iliac
      Left 06BG
      Right 06BF
    External Jugular
      Left 05BQ
      Right 05BP
    Face
      Left 05BV
      Right 05BT
    Femoral
      Left 06BN
      Right 06BM
    Foot
      Left 06BV
      Right 06BT
    Gastric 06B2
    Hand
      Left 05BH
      Right 05BG
    Hemiazygos 05B1
    Hepatic 06B4
    Hypogastric
      Left 06BJ
      Right 06BH
    Inferior Mesenteric 06B6
    Innominate
      Left 05B4
      Right 05B3
    Internal Jugular
      Left 05BN
      Right 05BM
    Intracranial 05BL
    Lower 06BY
    Portal 06B8
    Pulmonary
      Left 02BT
      Right 02BS
    Renal
      Left 06BB
      Right 06B9
    Saphenous
      Left 06BQ
      Right 06BP
    Splenic 06B1
    Subclavian
      Left 05B6
      Right 05B5
    Superior Mesenteric 06B5
    Upper 05BY
    Vertebral
      Left 05BS
      Right 05BR
  Vena Cava
    Inferior 06B0
    Superior 02BV
  Ventricle
    Left 02BL
    Right 02BK
  Vertebra
    Cervical 0PB3
    Lumbar 0QB0
    Thoracic 0PB4
  Vesicle
    Bilateral 0VB3
    Left 0VB2
    Right 0VB1
  Vitreous
    Left 08B53Z
    Right 08B43Z
  Vocal Cord
    Left 0CBV
    Right 0CBT
  Vulva 0UBM
  Wrist Region
    Left 0XBH
    Right 0XBG
EXCLUDER® AAA Endoprosthesis
  use Intraluminal Device

EXCLUDER® AAA Endoprosthesis — *continued*
  use Intraluminal Device, Branched or Fenestrated, One or Two Arteries in 04V
  use Intraluminal Device, Branched or Fenestrated, Three or More Arteries in 04V
EXCLUDER® IBE Endoprosthesis *use* Intraluminal Device, Branched or Fenestrated, One or Two Arteries in 04V
Exclusion, Left atrial appendage (LAA) *see* Occlusion, Atrium, Left 02L7
Exercise, rehabilitation *see* Motor Treatment, Rehabilitation F07
Exploration *see* Inspection
Exploratory
  see Inspection, Anatomical Regions, General 0WJ
  see Laparotomy
  see Thoracotomy
Express® Biliary SD Monorail® Premounted Stent System *use* Intraluminal Device
Express® (LD) Premounted Stent System *use* Intraluminal Device
Express® SD Renal Monorail® Premounted Stent System *use* Intraluminal Device
Ex-PRESS™ mini glaucoma shunt *use* Synthetic Substitute
Extensor carpi radialis muscle
  use Lower Arm and Wrist Muscle, Left
  use Lower Arm and Wrist Muscle, Right
Extensor carpi ulnaris muscle
  use Lower Arm and Wrist Muscle, Left
  use Lower Arm and Wrist Muscle, Right
Extensor digitorum brevis muscle
  use Foot Muscle, Left
  use Foot Muscle, Right
Extensor digitorum longus muscle
  use Lower Leg Muscle, Left
  use Lower Leg Muscle, Right
Extensor hallucis brevis muscle
  use Foot Muscle, Left
  use Foot Muscle, Right
Extensor hallucis longus muscle
  use Lower Leg Muscle, Left
  use Lower Leg Muscle, Right
External anal sphincter *use* Anal Sphincter
External auditory meatus
  use External Auditory Canal, Left
  use External Auditory Canal, Right
External fixator
  use External Fixation Device in Head and Facial Bones
  use External Fixation Device in Lower Bones
  use External Fixation Device in Lower Joints
  use External Fixation Device in Upper Bones
  use External Fixation Device in Upper Joints
External maxillary artery *use* Face Artery
External naris *use* Nasal Mucosa and Soft Tissue
External oblique aponeurosis *use* Subcutaneous Tissue and Fascia, Trunk
External oblique muscle
  use Abdomen Muscle, Left
  use Abdomen Muscle, Right
External popliteal nerve *use* Peroneal Nerve
External pudendal artery
  use Femoral Artery, Left
  use Femoral Artery, Right
External pudendal vein
  use Saphenous Vein, Left
  use Saphenous Vein, Right
External urethral sphincter *use* Urethra
Extirpation
  Acetabulum
    Left 0QC5
    Right 0QC4
  Adenoids 0CCQ
  Ampulla of Vater 0FCC
  Anal Sphincter 0DCR
  Anterior Chamber
    Left 08C3
    Right 08C2
  Anus 0DCQ
  Aorta
    Abdominal 04C0
    Thoracic
      Ascending/Arch 02CX
      Descending 02CW
  Aortic Body 0GCD
  Appendix 0DCJ

Extirpation — *continued*
  Artery
    Anterior Tibial
      Left 04CQ
      Right 04CP
    Axillary
      Left 03C6
      Right 03C5
    Brachial
      Left 03C8
      Right 03C7
    Celiac 04C1
    Colic
      Left 04C7
      Middle 04C8
      Right 04C6
    Common Carotid
      Left 03CJ
      Right 03CH
    Common Iliac
      Left 04CD
      Right 04CC
    Coronary
      Four or More Arteries 02C3
      One Artery 02C0
      Three Arteries 02C2
      Two Arteries 02C1
    External Carotid
      Left 03CN
      Right 03CM
    External Iliac
      Left 04CJ
      Right 04CH
    Face 03CR
    Femoral
      Left 04CL
      Right 04CK
    Foot
      Left 04CW
      Right 04CV
    Gastric 04C2
    Hand
      Left 03CF
      Right 03CD
    Hepatic 04C3
    Inferior Mesenteric 04CB
    Innominate 03C2
    Internal Carotid
      Left 03CL
      Right 03CK
    Internal Iliac
      Left 04CF
      Right 04CE
    Internal Mammary
      Left 03C1
      Right 03C0
    Intracranial 03CG
    Lower 04CY
    Peroneal
      Left 04CU
      Right 04CT
    Popliteal
      Left 04CN
      Right 04CM
    Posterior Tibial
      Left 04CS
      Right 04CR
    Pulmonary
      Left 02CR
      Right 02CQ
    Pulmonary Trunk 02CP
    Radial
      Left 03CC
      Right 03CB
    Renal
      Left 04CA
      Right 04C9
    Splenic 04C4
    Subclavian
      Left 03C4
      Right 03C3
    Superior Mesenteric 04C5
    Temporal
      Left 03CT
      Right 03CS
    Thyroid
      Left 03CV
      Right 03CU

Extirpation

Extirpation — continued
- Artery — continued
  - Ulnar
    - Left 03CA
    - Right 03C9
  - Upper 03CY
  - Vertebral
    - Left 03CQ
    - Right 03CP
- Atrium
  - Left 02C7
  - Right 02C6
- Auditory Ossicle
  - Left 09CA
  - Right 09C9
- Basal Ganglia 00C8
- Bladder 0TCB
- Bladder Neck 0TCC
- Bone
  - Ethmoid
    - Left 0NCG
    - Right 0NCF
  - Frontal 0NC1
  - Hyoid 0NCX
  - Lacrimal
    - Left 0NCJ
    - Right 0NCH
  - Nasal 0NCB
  - Occipital 0NC7
  - Palatine
    - Left 0NCL
    - Right 0NCK
  - Parietal
    - Left 0NC4
    - Right 0NC3
  - Pelvic
    - Left 0QC3
    - Right 0QC2
  - Sphenoid 0NCC
  - Temporal
    - Left 0NC6
    - Right 0NC5
  - Zygomatic
    - Left 0NCN
    - Right 0NCM
- Brain 00C0
- Breast
  - Bilateral 0HCV
  - Left 0HCU
  - Right 0HCT
- Bronchus
  - Lingula 0BC9
  - Lower Lobe
    - Left 0BCB
    - Right 0BC6
  - Main
    - Left 0BC7
    - Right 0BC3
  - Middle Lobe, Right 0BC5
  - Upper Lobe
    - Left 0BC8
    - Right 0BC4
- Buccal Mucosa 0CC4
- Bursa and Ligament
  - Abdomen
    - Left 0MCJ
    - Right 0MCH
  - Ankle
    - Left 0MCR
    - Right 0MCQ
  - Elbow
    - Left 0MC4
    - Right 0MC3
  - Foot
    - Left 0MCT
    - Right 0MCS
  - Hand
    - Left 0MC8
    - Right 0MC7
  - Head and Neck 0MC0
  - Hip
    - Left 0MCM
    - Right 0MCL
  - Knee
    - Left 0MCP
    - Right 0MCN
  - Lower Extremity
    - Left 0MCW
    - Right 0MCV

Extirpation — continued
- Bursa and Ligament — continued
  - Perineum 0MCK
  - Rib(s) 0MCG
  - Shoulder
    - Left 0MC2
    - Right 0MC1
  - Spine
    - Lower 0MCD
    - Upper 0MCC
  - Sternum 0MCF
  - Upper Extremity
    - Left 0MCB
    - Right 0MC9
  - Wrist
    - Left 0MC6
    - Right 0MC5
- Carina 0BC2
- Carotid Bodies, Bilateral 0GC8
- Carotid Body
  - Left 0GC6
  - Right 0GC7
- Carpal
  - Left 0PCN
  - Right 0PCM
- Cavity, Cranial 0WC1
- Cecum 0DCH
- Cerebellum 00CC
- Cerebral Hemisphere 00C7
- Cerebral Meninges 00C1
- Cerebral Ventricle 00C6
- Cervix 0UCC
- Chordae Tendineae 02C9
- Choroid
  - Left 08CB
  - Right 08CA
- Cisterna Chyli 07CL
- Clavicle
  - Left 0PCB
  - Right 0PC9
- Clitoris 0UCJ
- Coccygeal Glomus 0GCB
- Coccyx 0QCS
- Colon
  - Ascending 0DCK
  - Descending 0DCM
  - Sigmoid 0DCN
  - Transverse 0DCL
- Computer-aided Mechanical Aspiration X2C
- Conduction Mechanism 02C8
- Conjunctiva
  - Left 08CTXZZ
  - Right 08CSXZZ
- Cord
  - Bilateral 0VCH
  - Left 0VCG
  - Right 0VCF
- Cornea
  - Left 08C9XZZ
  - Right 08C8XZZ
- Cul-de-sac 0UCF
- Diaphragm 0BCT
- Disc
  - Cervical Vertebral 0RC3
  - Cervicothoracic Vertebral 0RC5
  - Lumbar Vertebral 0SC2
  - Lumbosacral 0SC4
  - Thoracic Vertebral 0RC9
  - Thoracolumbar Vertebral 0RCB
- Duct
  - Common Bile 0FC9
  - Cystic 0FC8
  - Hepatic
    - Common 0FC7
    - Left 0FC6
    - Right 0FC5
  - Lacrimal
    - Left 08CY
    - Right 08CX
  - Pancreatic 0FCD
    - Accessory 0FCF
  - Parotid
    - Left 0CCC
    - Right 0CCB
- Duodenum 0DC9
- Dura Mater 00C2
- Ear
  - External
    - Left 09C1

Extirpation — continued
- Ear — continued
  - External — continued
    - Right 09C0
  - External Auditory Canal
    - Left 09C4
    - Right 09C3
  - Inner
    - Left 09CE
    - Right 09CD
  - Middle
    - Left 09C6
    - Right 09C5
- Endometrium 0UCB
- Epididymis
  - Bilateral 0VCL
  - Left 0VCK
  - Right 0VCJ
- Epidural Space, Intracranial 00C3
- Epiglottis 0CCR
- Esophagogastric Junction 0DC4
- Esophagus 0DC5
  - Lower 0DC3
  - Middle 0DC2
  - Upper 0DC1
- Eustachian Tube
  - Left 09CG
  - Right 09CF
- Eye
  - Left 08C1XZZ
  - Right 08C0XZZ
- Eyelid
  - Lower
    - Left 08CR
    - Right 08CQ
  - Upper
    - Left 08CP
    - Right 08CN
- Fallopian Tube
  - Left 0UC6
  - Right 0UC5
- Fallopian Tubes, Bilateral 0UC7
- Femoral Shaft
  - Left 0QC9
  - Right 0QC8
- Femur
  - Lower
    - Left 0QCC
    - Right 0QCB
  - Upper
    - Left 0QC7
    - Right 0QC6
- Fibula
  - Left 0QCK
  - Right 0QCJ
- Finger Nail 0HCQXZZ
- Gallbladder 0FC4
- Gastrointestinal Tract 0WCP
- Genitourinary Tract 0WCR
- Gingiva
  - Lower 0CC6
  - Upper 0CC5
- Gland
  - Adrenal
    - Bilateral 0GC4
    - Left 0GC2
    - Right 0GC3
  - Lacrimal
    - Left 08CW
    - Right 08CV
  - Minor Salivary 0CCJ
  - Parotid
    - Left 0CC9
    - Right 0CC8
  - Pituitary 0GC0
  - Sublingual
    - Left 0CCF
    - Right 0CCD
  - Submaxillary
    - Left 0CCH
    - Right 0CCG
  - Vestibular 0UCL
- Glenoid Cavity
  - Left 0PC8
  - Right 0PC7
- Glomus Jugulare 0GCC
- Humeral Head
  - Left 0PCD
  - Right 0PCC

Extirpation — continued
  Humeral Shaft
    Left 0PCG
    Right 0PCF
  Hymen 0UCK
  Hypothalamus 00CA
  Ileocecal Valve 0DCC
  Ileum 0DCB
  Intestine
    Large 0DCE
      Left 0DCG
      Right 0DCF
    Small 0DC8
  Iris
    Left 08CD
    Right 08CC
  Jaw
    Lower 0WC5
    Upper 0WC4
  Jejunum 0DCA
  Joint
    Acromioclavicular
      Left 0RCH
      Right 0RCG
    Ankle
      Left 0SCG
      Right 0SCF
    Carpal
      Left 0RCR
      Right 0RCQ
    Carpometacarpal
      Left 0RCT
      Right 0RCS
    Cervical Vertebral 0RC1
    Cervicothoracic Vertebral 0RC4
    Coccygeal 0SC6
    Elbow
      Left 0RCM
      Right 0RCL
    Finger Phalangeal
      Left 0RCX
      Right 0RCW
    Hip
      Left 0SCB
      Right 0SC9
    Knee
      Left 0SCD
      Right 0SCC
    Lumbar Vertebral 0SC0
    Lumbosacral 0SC3
    Metacarpophalangeal
      Left 0RCV
      Right 0RCU
    Metatarsal-Phalangeal
      Left 0SCN
      Right 0SCM
    Occipital-cervical 0RC0
    Sacrococcygeal 0SC5
    Sacroiliac
      Left 0SC8
      Right 0SC7
    Shoulder
      Left 0RCK
      Right 0RCJ
    Sternoclavicular
      Left 0RCF
      Right 0RCE
    Tarsal
      Left 0SCJ
      Right 0SCH
    Tarsometatarsal
      Left 0SCL
      Right 0SCK
    Temporomandibular
      Left 0RCD
      Right 0RCC
    Thoracic Vertebral 0RC6
    Thoracolumbar Vertebral 0RCA
    Toe Phalangeal
      Left 0SCQ
      Right 0SCP
    Wrist
      Left 0RCP
      Right 0RCN
  Kidney
    Left 0TC1
    Right 0TC0
  Kidney Pelvis
    Left 0TC4

Extirpation — continued
  Kidney Pelvis — continued
    Right 0TC3
  Larynx 0CCS
  Lens
    Left 08CK
    Right 08CJ
  Lip
    Lower 0CC1
    Upper 0CC0
  Liver 0FC0
    Left Lobe 0FC2
    Right Lobe 0FC1
  Lung
    Bilateral 0BCM
    Left 0BCL
    Lower Lobe
      Left 0BCJ
      Right 0BCF
    Middle Lobe, Right 0BCD
    Right 0BCK
    Upper Lobe
      Left 0BCG
      Right 0BCC
  Lung Lingula 0BCH
  Lymphatic
    Aortic 07CD
    Axillary
      Left 07C6
      Right 07C5
    Head 07C0
    Inguinal
      Left 07CJ
      Right 07CH
    Internal Mammary
      Left 07C9
      Right 07C8
    Lower Extremity
      Left 07CG
      Right 07CF
    Mesenteric 07CB
    Neck
      Left 07C2
      Right 07C1
    Pelvis 07CC
    Thoracic Duct 07CK
    Thorax 07C7
    Upper Extremity
      Left 07C4
      Right 07C3
  Mandible
    Left 0NCV
    Right 0NCT
  Maxilla 0NCR
  Mediastinum 0WCC
  Medulla Oblongata 00CD
  Mesentery 0DCV
  Metacarpal
    Left 0PCQ
    Right 0PCP
  Metatarsal
    Left 0QCP
    Right 0QCN
  Muscle
    Abdomen
      Left 0KCL
      Right 0KCK
    Extraocular
      Left 08CM
      Right 08CL
    Facial 0KC1
    Foot
      Left 0KCW
      Right 0KCV
    Hand
      Left 0KCD
      Right 0KCC
    Head 0KC0
    Hip
      Left 0KCP
      Right 0KCN
    Lower Arm and Wrist
      Left 0KCB
      Right 0KC9
    Lower Leg
      Left 0KCT
      Right 0KCS
    Neck
      Left 0KC3

Extirpation — continued
  Muscle — continued
    Neck — continued
      Right 0KC2
    Papillary 02CD
    Perineum 0KCM
    Shoulder
      Left 0KC6
      Right 0KC5
    Thorax
      Left 0KCJ
      Right 0KCH
    Tongue, Palate, Pharynx 0KC4
    Trunk
      Left 0KCG
      Right 0KCF
    Upper Arm
      Left 0KC8
      Right 0KC7
    Upper Leg
      Left 0KCR
      Right 0KCQ
  Nasal Mucosa and Soft Tissue 09CK
  Nasopharynx 09CN
  Nerve
    Abdominal Sympathetic 01CM
    Abducens 00CL
    Accessory 00CR
    Acoustic 00CN
    Brachial Plexus 01C3
    Cervical 01C1
    Cervical Plexus 01C0
    Facial 00CM
    Femoral 01CD
    Glossopharyngeal 00CP
    Head and Neck Sympathetic 01CK
    Hypoglossal 00CS
    Lumbar 01CB
    Lumbar Plexus 01C9
    Lumbar Sympathetic 01CN
    Lumbosacral Plexus 01CA
    Median 01C5
    Oculomotor 00CH
    Olfactory 00CF
    Optic 00CG
    Peroneal 01CH
    Phrenic 01C2
    Pudendal 01CC
    Radial 01C6
    Sacral 01CR
    Sacral Plexus 01CQ
    Sacral Sympathetic 01CP
    Sciatic 01CF
    Thoracic 01C8
    Thoracic Sympathetic 01CL
    Tibial 01CG
    Trigeminal 00CK
    Trochlear 00CJ
    Ulnar 01C4
    Vagus 00CQ
  Nipple
    Left 0HCX
    Right 0HCW
  Omentum 0DCU
  Oral Cavity and Throat 0WC3
  Orbit
    Left 0NCQ
    Right 0NCP
  Orbital Atherectomy *see* Extirpation, Heart and Great Vessels 02C
  Ovary
    Bilateral 0UC2
    Left 0UC1
    Right 0UC0
  Palate
    Hard 0CC2
    Soft 0CC3
  Pancreas 0FCG
  Para-aortic Body 0GC9
  Paraganglion Extremity 0GCF
  Parathyroid Gland 0GCR
    Inferior
      Left 0GCP
      Right 0GCN
    Multiple 0GCQ
    Superior
      Left 0GCM
      Right 0GCL

▽ Subterms under main terms may continue to next column or page

Extirpation — continued
  Patella
    Left 0QCF
    Right 0QCD
  Pelvic Cavity 0WCJ
  Penis 0VCS
  Pericardial Cavity 0WCD
  Pericardium 02CN
  Peritoneal Cavity 0WCG
  Peritoneum 0DCW
  Phalanx
    Finger
      Left 0PCV
      Right 0PCT
    Thumb
      Left 0PCS
      Right 0PCR
    Toe
      Left 0QCR
      Right 0QCQ
  Pharynx 0CCM
  Pineal Body 0GC1
  Pleura
    Left 0BCP
    Right 0BCN
  Pleural Cavity
    Left 0WCB
    Right 0WC9
  Pons 00CB
  Prepuce 0VCT
  Prostate 0VC0
  Radius
    Left 0PCJ
    Right 0PCH
  Rectum 0DCP
  Respiratory Tract 0WCQ
  Retina
    Left 08CF
    Right 08CE
  Retinal Vessel
    Left 08CH
    Right 08CG
  Retroperitoneum 0WCH
  Ribs
    1 to 2 0PC1
    3 or More 0PC2
  Sacrum 0QC1
  Scapula
    Left 0PC6
    Right 0PC5
  Sclera
    Left 08C7XZZ
    Right 08C6XZZ
  Scrotum 0VC5
  Septum
    Atrial 02C5
    Nasal 09CM
    Ventricular 02CM
  Sinus
    Accessory 09CP
    Ethmoid
      Left 09CV
      Right 09CU
    Frontal
      Left 09CT
      Right 09CS
    Mastoid
      Left 09CC
      Right 09CB
    Maxillary
      Left 09CR
      Right 09CQ
    Sphenoid
      Left 09CX
      Right 09CW
  Skin
    Abdomen 0HC7XZZ
    Back 0HC6XZZ
    Buttock 0HC8XZZ
    Chest 0HC5XZZ
    Ear
      Left 0HC3XZZ
      Right 0HC2XZZ
    Face 0HC1XZZ
    Foot
      Left 0HCNXZZ
      Right 0HCMXZZ
    Hand
      Left 0HCGXZZ

Extirpation — continued
  Skin — continued
    Hand — continued
      Right 0HCFXZZ
    Inguinal 0HCAXZZ
    Lower Arm
      Left 0HCEXZZ
      Right 0HCDXZZ
    Lower Leg
      Left 0HCLXZZ
      Right 0HCKXZZ
    Neck 0HC4XZZ
    Perineum 0HC9XZZ
    Scalp 0HC0XZZ
    Upper Arm
      Left 0HCCXZZ
      Right 0HCBXZZ
    Upper Leg
      Left 0HCJXZZ
      Right 0HCHXZZ
  Spinal Canal 00CU
  Spinal Cord
    Cervical 00CW
    Lumbar 00CY
    Thoracic 00CX
  Spinal Meninges 00CT
  Spleen 07CP
  Sternum 0PC0
  Stomach 0DC6
    Pylorus 0DC7
  Subarachnoid Space, Intracranial 00C5
  Subcutaneous Tissue and Fascia
    Abdomen 0JC8
    Back 0JC7
    Buttock 0JC9
    Chest 0JC6
    Face 0JC1
    Foot
      Left 0JCR
      Right 0JCQ
    Hand
      Left 0JCK
      Right 0JCJ
    Lower Arm
      Left 0JCH
      Right 0JCG
    Lower Leg
      Left 0JCP
      Right 0JCN
    Neck
      Left 0JC5
      Right 0JC4
    Pelvic Region 0JCC
    Perineum 0JCB
    Scalp 0JC0
    Upper Arm
      Left 0JCF
      Right 0JCD
    Upper Leg
      Left 0JCM
      Right 0JCL
  Subdural Space, Intracranial 00C4
  Tarsal
    Left 0QCM
    Right 0QCL
  Tendon
    Abdomen
      Left 0LCG
      Right 0LCF
    Ankle
      Left 0LCT
      Right 0LCS
    Foot
      Left 0LCW
      Right 0LCV
    Hand
      Left 0LC8
      Right 0LC7
    Head and Neck 0LC0
    Hip
      Left 0LCK
      Right 0LCJ
    Knee
      Left 0LCR
      Right 0LCQ
    Lower Arm and Wrist
      Left 0LC6
      Right 0LC5

Extirpation — continued
  Tendon — continued
    Lower Leg
      Left 0LCP
      Right 0LCN
    Perineum 0LCH
    Shoulder
      Left 0LC2
      Right 0LC1
    Thorax
      Left 0LCD
      Right 0LCC
    Trunk
      Left 0LCB
      Right 0LC9
    Upper Arm
      Left 0LC4
      Right 0LC3
    Upper Leg
      Left 0LCM
      Right 0LCL
  Testis
    Bilateral 0VCC
    Left 0VCB
    Right 0VC9
  Thalamus 00C9
  Thymus 07CM
  Thyroid Gland 0GCK
    Left Lobe 0GCG
    Right Lobe 0GCH
  Tibia
    Left 0QCH
    Right 0QCG
  Toe Nail 0HCRXZZ
  Tongue 0CC7
  Tonsils 0CCP
  Tooth
    Lower 0CCX
    Upper 0CCW
  Trachea 0BC1
  Tunica Vaginalis
    Left 0VC7
    Right 0VC6
  Turbinate, Nasal 09CL
  Tympanic Membrane
    Left 09C8
    Right 09C7
  Ulna
    Left 0PCL
    Right 0PCK
  Ureter
    Left 0TC7
    Right 0TC6
  Urethra 0TCD
  Uterine Supporting Structure 0UC4
  Uterus 0UC9
  Uvula 0CCN
  Vagina 0UCG
  Valve
    Aortic 02CF
    Mitral 02CG
    Pulmonary 02CH
    Tricuspid 02CJ
  Vas Deferens
    Bilateral 0VCQ
    Left 0VCP
    Right 0VCN
  Vein
    Axillary
      Left 05C8
      Right 05C7
    Azygos 05C0
    Basilic
      Left 05CC
      Right 05CB
    Brachial
      Left 05CA
      Right 05C9
    Cephalic
      Left 05CF
      Right 05CD
    Colic 06C7
    Common Iliac
      Left 06CD
      Right 06CC
    Coronary 02C4
    Esophageal 06C3
    External Iliac
      Left 06CG

Extirpation — continued
  Vein — continued
    External Iliac — continued
      Right 06CF
    External Jugular
      Left 05CQ
      Right 05CP
    Face
      Left 05CV
      Right 05CT
    Femoral
      Left 06CN
      Right 06CM
    Foot
      Left 06CV
      Right 06CT
    Gastric 06C2
    Hand
      Left 05CH
      Right 05CG
    Hemiazygos 05C1
    Hepatic 06C4
    Hypogastric
      Left 06CJ
      Right 06CH
    Inferior Mesenteric 06C6
    Innominate
      Left 05C4
      Right 05C3
    Internal Jugular
      Left 05CN
      Right 05CM
    Intracranial 05CL
    Lower 06CY
    Portal 06C8
    Pulmonary
      Left 02CT
      Right 02CS
    Renal
      Left 06CB
      Right 06C9
    Saphenous
      Left 06CQ
      Right 06CP
    Splenic 06C1
    Subclavian
      Left 05C6
      Right 05C5
    Superior Mesenteric 06C5
    Upper 05CY
    Vertebral
      Left 05CS
      Right 05CR
  Vena Cava
    Inferior 06C0
    Superior 02CV
  Ventricle
    Left 02CL
    Right 02CK
  Vertebra
    Cervical 0PC3
    Lumbar 0QC0
    Thoracic 0PC4
  Vesicle
    Bilateral 0VC3
    Left 0VC2
    Right 0VC1
  Vitreous
    Left 08C5
    Right 08C4
  Vocal Cord
    Left 0CCV
    Right 0CCT
  Vulva 0UCM
Extracorporeal Carbon Dioxide Removal (ECCO2R) 5A0920Z
Extracorporeal filter circuit, during percutaneous thrombectomy 5A05A0L
Extracorporeal Pathogen Removal Procedure XXA536A
Extracorporeal return, during percutaneous thrombectomy 5A05A0L
Extracorporeal shock wave lithotripsy see Fragmentation
Extracranial-intracranial bypass (EC-IC) see Bypass, Upper Arteries 031

Extraction
  Acetabulum
    Left 0QD50ZZ
    Right 0QD40ZZ
  Ampulla of Vater 0FDC
  Anus 0DDQ
  Appendix 0DDJ
  Auditory Ossicle
    Left 09DA0ZZ
    Right 09D90ZZ
  Bone
    Ethmoid
      Left 0NDG0ZZ
      Right 0NDF0ZZ
    Frontal 0ND10ZZ
    Hyoid 0NDX0ZZ
    Lacrimal
      Left 0NDJ0ZZ
      Right 0NDH0ZZ
    Nasal 0NDB0ZZ
    Occipital 0ND70ZZ
    Palatine
      Left 0NDL0ZZ
      Right 0NDK0ZZ
    Parietal
      Left 0ND40ZZ
      Right 0ND30ZZ
    Pelvic
      Left 0QD30ZZ
      Right 0QD20ZZ
    Sphenoid 0NDC0ZZ
    Temporal
      Left 0ND60ZZ
      Right 0ND50ZZ
    Zygomatic
      Left 0NDN0ZZ
      Right 0NDM0ZZ
  Bone Marrow 07DT
    Iliac 07DR
    Sternum 07DQ
    Vertebral 07DS
  Brain 00D0
  Breast
    Bilateral 0HDV0ZZ
    Left 0HDU0ZZ
    Right 0HDT0ZZ
    Supernumerary 0HDY0ZZ
  Bronchus
    Lingula 0BD9
    Lower Lobe
      Left 0BDB
      Right 0BD6
    Main
      Left 0BD7
      Right 0BD3
    Middle Lobe, Right 0BD5
    Upper Lobe
      Left 0BD8
      Right 0BD4
  Bursa and Ligament
    Abdomen
      Left 0MDJ
      Right 0MDH
    Ankle
      Left 0MDR
      Right 0MDQ
    Elbow
      Left 0MD4
      Right 0MD3
    Foot
      Left 0MDT
      Right 0MDS
    Hand
      Left 0MD8
      Right 0MD7
    Head and Neck 0MD0
    Hip
      Left 0MDM
      Right 0MDL
    Knee
      Left 0MDP
      Right 0MDN
    Lower Extremity
      Left 0MDW
      Right 0MDV
    Perineum 0MDK
    Rib(s) 0MDG
    Shoulder
      Left 0MD2

Extraction — continued
  Bursa and Ligament — continued
    Shoulder — continued
      Right 0MD1
    Spine
      Lower 0MDD
      Upper 0MDC
    Sternum 0MDF
    Upper Extremity
      Left 0MDB
      Right 0MD9
    Wrist
      Left 0MD6
      Right 0MD5
  Carina 0BD2
  Carpal
    Left 0PDN0ZZ
    Right 0PDM0ZZ
  Cecum 0DDH
  Cerebellum 00DC
  Cerebral Hemisphere 00D7
  Cerebral Meninges 00D1
  Cisterna Chyli 07DL
  Clavicle
    Left 0PDB0ZZ
    Right 0PD90ZZ
  Coccyx 0QDS0ZZ
  Colon
    Ascending 0DDK
    Descending 0DDM
    Sigmoid 0DDN
    Transverse 0DDL
  Cornea
    Left 08D9XZ
    Right 08D8XZ
  Duct
    Common Bile 0FD9
    Cystic 0FD8
    Hepatic
      Common 0FD7
      Left 0FD6
      Right 0FD5
    Pancreatic 0FDD
      Accessory 0FDF
  Duodenum 0DD9
  Dura Mater 00D2
  Endometrium 0UDB
  Esophagogastric Junction 0DD4
  Esophagus 0DD5
    Lower 0DD3
    Middle 0DD2
    Upper 0DD1
  Femoral Shaft
    Left 0QD90ZZ
    Right 0QD80ZZ
  Femur
    Lower
      Left 0QDC0ZZ
      Right 0QDB0ZZ
    Upper
      Left 0QD70ZZ
      Right 0QD60ZZ
  Fibula
    Left 0QDK0ZZ
    Right 0QDJ0ZZ
  Finger Nail 0HDQXZZ
  Gallbladder 0FD4
  Glenoid Cavity
    Left 0PD80ZZ
    Right 0PD70ZZ
  Hair 0HDSXZZ
  Humeral Head
    Left 0PDD0ZZ
    Right 0PDC0ZZ
  Humeral Shaft
    Left 0PDG0ZZ
    Right 0PDF0ZZ
  Ileocecal Valve 0DDC
  Ileum 0DDB
  Intestine
    Large 0DDE
      Left 0DDG
      Right 0DDF
    Small 0DD8
  Jejunum 0DDA
  Kidney
    Left 0TD1
    Right 0TD0

Extraction

Extraction — *continued*
- Lens
  - Left 08DK3ZZ
  - Right 08DJ3ZZ
- Liver 0FD0
  - Left Lobe 0FD2
  - Right Lobe 0FD1
- Lung
  - Bilateral 0BDM
  - Left 0BDL
  - Lower Lobe
    - Left 0BDJ
    - Right 0BDF
  - Middle Lobe, Right 0BDD
  - Right 0BDK
  - Upper Lobe
    - Left 0BDG
    - Right 0BDC
- Lung Lingula 0BDH
- Lymphatic
  - Aortic 07DD
  - Axillary
    - Left 07D6
    - Right 07D5
  - Head 07D0
  - Inguinal
    - Left 07DJ
    - Right 07DH
  - Internal Mammary
    - Left 07D9
    - Right 07D8
  - Lower Extremity
    - Left 07DG
    - Right 07DF
  - Mesenteric 07DB
  - Neck
    - Left 07D2
    - Right 07D1
  - Pelvis 07DC
  - Thoracic Duct 07DK
  - Thorax 07D7
  - Upper Extremity
    - Left 07D4
    - Right 07D3
- Mandible
  - Left 0NDV0ZZ
  - Right 0NDT0ZZ
- Maxilla 0NDR0ZZ
- Metacarpal
  - Left 0PDQ0ZZ
  - Right 0PDP0ZZ
- Metatarsal
  - Left 0QDP0ZZ
  - Right 0QDN0ZZ
- Muscle
  - Abdomen
    - Left 0KDL0ZZ
    - Right 0KDK0ZZ
  - Facial 0KD10ZZ
  - Foot
    - Left 0KDW0ZZ
    - Right 0KDV0ZZ
  - Hand
    - Left 0KDD0ZZ
    - Right 0KDC0ZZ
  - Head 0KD00ZZ
  - Hip
    - Left 0KDP0ZZ
    - Right 0KDN0ZZ
  - Lower Arm and Wrist
    - Left 0KDB0ZZ
    - Right 0KD90ZZ
  - Lower Leg
    - Left 0KDT0ZZ
    - Right 0KDS0ZZ
  - Neck
    - Left 0KD30ZZ
    - Right 0KD20ZZ
  - Perineum 0KDM0ZZ
  - Shoulder
    - Left 0KD60ZZ
    - Right 0KD50ZZ
  - Thorax
    - Left 0KDJ0ZZ
    - Right 0KDH0ZZ
  - Tongue, Palate, Pharynx 0KD40ZZ
  - Trunk
    - Left 0KDG0ZZ
    - Right 0KDF0ZZ

Extraction — *continued*
- Muscle — *continued*
  - Upper Arm
    - Left 0KD80ZZ
    - Right 0KD70ZZ
  - Upper Leg
    - Left 0KDR0ZZ
    - Right 0KDQ0ZZ
- Nerve
  - Abdominal Sympathetic 01DM
  - Abducens 00DL
  - Accessory 00DR
  - Acoustic 00DN
  - Brachial Plexus 01D3
  - Cervical 01D1
  - Cervical Plexus 01D0
  - Facial 00DM
  - Femoral 01DD
  - Glossopharyngeal 00DP
  - Head and Neck Sympathetic 01DK
  - Hypoglossal 00DS
  - Lumbar 01DB
  - Lumbar Plexus 01D9
  - Lumbar Sympathetic 01DN
  - Lumbosacral Plexus 01DA
  - Median 01D5
  - Oculomotor 00DH
  - Olfactory 00DF
  - Optic 00DG
  - Peroneal 01DH
  - Phrenic 01D2
  - Pudendal 01DC
  - Radial 01D6
  - Sacral 01DR
  - Sacral Plexus 01DQ
  - Sacral Sympathetic 01DP
  - Sciatic 01DF
  - Thoracic 01D8
  - Thoracic Sympathetic 01DL
  - Tibial 01DG
  - Trigeminal 00DK
  - Trochlear 00DJ
  - Ulnar 01D4
  - Vagus 00DQ
- Orbit
  - Left 0NDQ0ZZ
  - Right 0NDP0ZZ
- Ova 0UDN
- Pancreas 0FDG
- Patella
  - Left 0QDF0ZZ
  - Right 0QDD0ZZ
- Phalanx
  - Finger
    - Left 0PDV0ZZ
    - Right 0PDT0ZZ
  - Thumb
    - Left 0PDS0ZZ
    - Right 0PDR0ZZ
  - Toe
    - Left 0QDR0ZZ
    - Right 0QDQ0ZZ
- Pleura
  - Left 0BDP
  - Right 0BDN
- Products of Conception
  - Ectopic 10D2
  - Extraperitoneal 10D00Z2
  - High 10D00Z0
  - High Forceps 10D07Z5
  - Internal Version 10D07Z7
  - Low 10D00Z1
  - Low Forceps 10D07Z3
  - Mid Forceps 10D07Z4
  - Other 10D07Z8
  - Retained 10D1
  - Vacuum 10D07Z6
- Radius
  - Left 0PDJ0ZZ
  - Right 0PDH0ZZ
- Rectum 0DDP
- Ribs
  - 1 to 2 0PD10ZZ
  - 3 or More 0PD20ZZ
- Sacrum 0QD10ZZ
- Scapula
  - Left 0PD60ZZ
  - Right 0PD50ZZ
- Septum, Nasal 09DM

Extraction — *continued*
- Sinus
  - Accessory 09DP
  - Ethmoid
    - Left 09DV
    - Right 09DU
  - Frontal
    - Left 09DT
    - Right 09DS
  - Mastoid
    - Left 09DC
    - Right 09DB
  - Maxillary
    - Left 09DR
    - Right 09DQ
  - Sphenoid
    - Left 09DX
    - Right 09DW
- Skin
  - Abdomen 0HD7XZZ
  - Back 0HD6XZZ
  - Buttock 0HD8XZZ
  - Chest 0HD5XZZ
  - Ear
    - Left 0HD3XZZ
    - Right 0HD2XZZ
  - Face 0HD1XZZ
  - Foot
    - Left 0HDNXZZ
    - Right 0HDMXZZ
  - Hand
    - Left 0HDGXZZ
    - Right 0HDFXZZ
  - Inguinal 0HDAXZZ
  - Lower Arm
    - Left 0HDEXZZ
    - Right 0HDDXZZ
  - Lower Leg
    - Left 0HDLXZZ
    - Right 0HDKXZZ
  - Neck 0HD4XZZ
  - Perineum 0HD9XZZ
  - Scalp 0HD0XZZ
  - Upper Arm
    - Left 0HDCXZZ
    - Right 0HDBXZZ
  - Upper Leg
    - Left 0HDJXZZ
    - Right 0HDHXZZ
- Skull 0ND00ZZ
- Spinal Meninges 00DT
- Spleen 07DP
- Sternum 0PD00ZZ
- Stomach 0DD6
  - Pylorus 0DD7
- Subcutaneous Tissue and Fascia
  - Abdomen 0JD8
  - Back 0JD7
  - Buttock 0JD9
  - Chest 0JD6
  - Face 0JD1
  - Foot
    - Left 0JDR
    - Right 0JDQ
  - Hand
    - Left 0JDK
    - Right 0JDJ
  - Lower Arm
    - Left 0JDH
    - Right 0JDG
  - Lower Leg
    - Left 0JDP
    - Right 0JDN
  - Neck
    - Left 0JD5
    - Right 0JD4
  - Pelvic Region 0JDC
  - Perineum 0JDB
  - Scalp 0JD0
  - Upper Arm
    - Left 0JDF
    - Right 0JDD
  - Upper Leg
    - Left 0JDM
    - Right 0JDL
- Tarsal
  - Left 0QDM0ZZ
  - Right 0QDL0ZZ

Extraction — *continued*
  Tendon
    Abdomen
      Left ØLDGØZZ
      Right ØLDFØZZ
    Ankle
      Left ØLDTØZZ
      Right ØLDSØZZ
    Foot
      Left ØLDWØZZ
      Right ØLDVØZZ
    Hand
      Left ØLD8ØZZ
      Right ØLD7ØZZ
    Head and Neck ØLDØØZZ
    Hip
      Left ØLDKØZZ
      Right ØLDJØZZ
    Knee
      Left ØLDRØZZ
      Right ØLDQØZZ
    Lower Arm and Wrist
      Left ØLD6ØZZ
      Right ØLD5ØZZ
    Lower Leg
      Left ØLDPØZZ
      Right ØLDNØZZ
    Perineum ØLDHØZZ
    Shoulder
      Left ØLD2ØZZ
      Right ØLD1ØZZ
    Thorax
      Left ØLDDØZZ
      Right ØLDCØZZ
    Trunk
      Left ØLDBØZZ
      Right ØLD9ØZZ
    Upper Arm
      Left ØLD4ØZZ
      Right ØLD3ØZZ
    Upper Leg
      Left ØLDMØZZ
      Right ØLDLØZZ
  Thymus Ø7DM
  Tibia
    Left ØQDHØZZ
    Right ØQDGØZZ
  Toe Nail ØHDRXZZ
  Tooth
    Lower ØCDXXZ
    Upper ØCDWXZ
  Trachea ØBD1
  Turbinate, Nasal Ø9DL
  Tympanic Membrane
    Left Ø9D8
    Right Ø9D7
  Ulna
    Left ØPDLØZZ
    Right ØPDKØZZ
  Vein
    Basilic
      Left Ø5DC
      Right Ø5DB
    Brachial
      Left Ø5DA
      Right Ø5D9
    Cephalic
      Left Ø5DF
      Right Ø5DD
    Femoral
      Left Ø6DN
      Right Ø6DM
    Foot
      Left Ø6DV
      Right Ø6DT
    Hand
      Left Ø5DH
      Right Ø5DG
    Lower Ø6DY
    Saphenous
      Left Ø6DQ
      Right Ø6DP
    Upper Ø5DY
  Vertebra
    Cervical ØPD3ØZZ
    Lumbar ØQDØØZZ
    Thoracic ØPD4ØZZ
  Vocal Cord
    Left ØCDV

Extraction — *continued*
  Vocal Cord — *continued*
    Right ØCDT
Extradural space, intracranial *use* Epidural Space, Intracranial
Extradural space, spinal *use* Spinal Canal
EXtreme Lateral Interbody Fusion (XLIF) device *use* Interbody Fusion Device in Lower Joints

F

Face lift *see* Alteration, Face ØWØ2
Facet FiXation implant *use* Facet Joint Fusion Device, Paired Titanium Cages in New Technology
Facet Joint Fusion Device, Paired Titanium Cages
  Lumbar Vertebral XRGBØEA
    2 or more XRGCØEA
  Lumbosacral XRGDØEA
  Thoracolumbar Vertebral XRGAØEA
Facet replacement spinal stabilization device
  use Spinal Stabilization Device, Facet Replacement in ØRH
  use Spinal Stabilization Device, Facet Replacement in ØSH
Facial artery *use* Face Artery
Factor Xa Inhibitor Reversal Agent, Andexanet Alfa *use* Coagulation Factor Xa, Inactivated
False vocal cord *use* Larynx
Falx cerebri *use* Dura Mater
Fascia lata
  use Subcutaneous Tissue and Fascia, Left Upper Leg
  use Subcutaneous Tissue and Fascia, Right Upper Leg
Fasciaplasty, fascioplasty
  see Repair, Subcutaneous Tissue and Fascia ØJQ
  see Replacement, Subcutaneous Tissue and Fascia ØJR
Fasciectomy *see* Excision, Subcutaneous Tissue and Fascia ØJB
Fasciorrhaphy *see* Repair, Subcutaneous Tissue and Fascia ØJQ
Fasciotomy
  see Division, Subcutaneous Tissue and Fascia ØJ8
  see Drainage, Subcutaneous Tissue and Fascia ØJ9
  see Release
Feeding Device
  Change device in
    Lower Intestinal Tract ØD2DXUZ
    Upper Intestinal Tract ØD2ØXUZ
  Insertion of device in
    Duodenum ØDH9
    Esophagus ØDH5
    Ileum ØDHB
    Intestine, Small ØDH8
    Jejunum ØDHA
    Stomach ØDH6
  Removal of device from
    Esophagus ØDP5
    Intestinal Tract
      Lower Intestinal Tract ØDPD
      Upper Intestinal Tract ØDPØ
    Stomach ØDP6
  Revision of device in
    Intestinal Tract
      Lower Intestinal Tract ØDWD
      Upper Intestinal Tract ØDWØ
    Stomach ØDW6
    Upper Intestinal Tract ØDWØ
Femoral head
  use Upper Femur, Left
  use Upper Femur, Right
Femoral lymph node
  use Lymphatic, Left Lower Extremity
  use Lymphatic, Right Lower Extremity
Femoropatellar joint
  use Knee Joint, Left
  use Knee Joint, Left, Tibial Surface
  use Knee Joint, Right
  use Knee Joint, Right, Femoral Surface
Femorotibial joint
  use Knee Joint, Left
  use Knee Joint, Left, Tibial Surface
  use Knee Joint, Right
  use Knee Joint, Right, Tibial Surface
FETROJA® *use* Cefiderocol Anti-infective

FFX® (Facet FiXation) implant *use* Facet Joint Fusion Device, Paired Titanium Cages in New Technology
FGS (fluorescence-guided surgery) *see* Fluorescence Guided Procedure
Fiber Optic 3D Guided Procedure, Circulatory System 8EØ23FZ
Fibular artery
  use Peroneal Artery, Left
  use Peroneal Artery, Right
Fibular sesamoid
  use Metatarsal, Left
  use Metatarsal, Right
Fibularis brevis muscle
  use Lower Leg Muscle, Left
  use Lower Leg Muscle, Right
Fibularis longus muscle
  use Lower Leg Muscle, Left
  use Lower Leg Muscle, Right
Fifth cranial nerve *use* Trigeminal Nerve
Filtration, Blood Pathogens XXA536A
Filtration circuit, during percutaneous thrombectomy 5AØ5AØL
Filum terminale *use* Spinal Meninges
Fimbriectomy
  see Excision, Female Reproductive System ØUB
  see Resection, Female Reproductive System ØUT
Fine needle aspiration
  Fluid or gas *see* Drainage
  Tissue biopsy
    see Excision
    see Extraction
First cranial nerve *use* Olfactory Nerve
First intercostal nerve *use* Brachial Plexus
Fish skin *use* Nonautologous Tissue Substitute
Fistulization
  see Bypass
  see Drainage
  see Repair
Fistulization, Tracheoesophageal ØB11ØD6
Fitting
  Arch bars, for fracture reduction *see* Reposition, Mouth and Throat ØCS
  Arch bars, for immobilization *see* Immobilization, Face 2W31
  Artificial limb *see* Device Fitting, Rehabilitation FØD
  Hearing aid *see* Device Fitting, Rehabilitation FØD
  Ocular prosthesis FØDZ8UZ
  Prosthesis, limb *see* Device Fitting, Rehabilitation FØD
  Prosthesis, ocular FØDZ8UZ
Fixation, bone
  External, with fracture reduction *see* Reposition
  External, without fracture reduction *see* Insertion
  Internal, with fracture reduction *see* Reposition
  Internal, without fracture reduction *see* Insertion
FLAIR® Endovascular Stent Graft *use* Intraluminal Device
Flexible Composite Mesh *use* Synthetic Substitute
Flexor carpi radialis muscle
  use Lower Arm and Wrist Muscle, Left
  use Lower Arm and Wrist Muscle, Right
Flexor carpi ulnaris muscle
  use Lower Arm and Wrist Muscle, Left
  use Lower Arm and Wrist Muscle, Right
Flexor digitorum brevis muscle
  use Foot Muscle, Left
  use Foot Muscle, Right
Flexor digitorum longus muscle
  use Lower Leg Muscle, Left
  use Lower Leg Muscle, Right
Flexor hallucis brevis muscle
  use Foot Muscle, Left
  use Foot Muscle, Right
Flexor hallucis longus muscle
  use Lower Leg Muscle, Left
  use Lower Leg Muscle, Right
Flexor pollicis longus muscle
  use Lower Arm and Wrist Muscle, Left
  use Lower Arm and Wrist Muscle, Right
FloPatch FP12Ø XX25XØA
Flourish® Pediatric Esophageal Atresia Device *use* Magnetic Lengthening Device in Gastrointestinal System
Flow Diverter embolization device *use* Intraluminal Device, Flow Diverter in Ø3V

▽ **Subterms under main terms may continue to next column or page**

FlowSense Noninvasive Thermal Sensor 4B00XW0
Fluorescence Guided Procedure
  Extremity
    Lower 8E0Y
    Upper 8E0X
  Head and Neck Region 8E09
    Aminolevulinic Acid 8E090EM
    No Qualifier 8E090EZ
    Reproductive System, Female, Pafolacianine (CY-TALUX®) 8E0U
  Trunk Region
    No Qualifier 8E0W
    Pafolacianine (CYTALUX®) 8E0W
Fluorescent Pyrazine, Kidney XT25XE5
Fluoroscopy
  Abdomen and Pelvis BW11
  Airway, Upper BB1DZZZ
  Ankle
    Left BQ1H
    Right BQ1G
  Aorta
    Abdominal B410
      Laser, Intraoperative B410
    Thoracic B310
      Laser, Intraoperative B310
    Thoraco-Abdominal B31P
      Laser, Intraoperative B31P
  Aorta and Bilateral Lower Extremity Arteries B41D
    Laser, Intraoperative B41D
  Arm
    Left BP1FZZZ
    Right BP1EZZZ
  Artery
    Brachiocephalic-Subclavian
      Laser, Intraoperative B311
      Right B311
    Bronchial B31L
      Laser, Intraoperative B31L
    Bypass Graft, Other B21F
    Cervico-Cerebral Arch B31Q
      Laser, Intraoperative B31Q
    Common Carotid
      Bilateral B315
        Laser, Intraoperative B315
      Left B314
        Laser, Intraoperative B314
      Right B313
        Laser, Intraoperative B313
    Coronary
      Bypass Graft
        Multiple B213
          Laser, Intraoperative B213
        Single B212
          Laser, Intraoperative B212
      Multiple B211
        Laser, Intraoperative B211
      Single B210
        Laser, Intraoperative B210
    External Carotid
      Bilateral B31C
        Laser, Intraoperative B31C
      Left B31B
        Laser, Intraoperative B31B
      Right B319
        Laser, Intraoperative B319
    Hepatic B412
      Laser, Intraoperative B412
    Inferior Mesenteric B415
      Laser, Intraoperative B415
    Intercostal B31L
      Laser, Intraoperative B31L
    Internal Carotid
      Bilateral B318
        Laser, Intraoperative B318
      Left B317
        Laser, Intraoperative B317
      Right B316
        Laser, Intraoperative B316
    Internal Mammary Bypass Graft
      Left B218
      Right B217
    Intra-Abdominal
      Laser, Intraoperative B41B
      Other B41B
    Intracranial B31R
      Laser, Intraoperative B31R
    Lower
      Laser, Intraoperative B41J
      Other B41J

Fluoroscopy — continued
  Artery — continued
    Lower Extremity
      Bilateral and Aorta B41D
        Laser, Intraoperative B41D
      Left B41G
        Laser, Intraoperative B41G
      Right B41F
        Laser, Intraoperative B41F
    Lumbar B419
      Laser, Intraoperative B419
    Pelvic B41C
      Laser, Intraoperative B41C
    Pulmonary
      Left B31T
        Laser, Intraoperative B31T
      Right B31S
        Laser, Intraoperative B31S
    Pulmonary Trunk B31U
      Laser, Intraoperative B31U
    Renal
      Bilateral B418
        Laser, Intraoperative B418
      Left B417
        Laser, Intraoperative B417
      Right B416
        Laser, Intraoperative B416
    Spinal B31M
      Laser, Intraoperative B31M
    Splenic B413
      Laser, Intraoperative B413
    Subclavian
      Laser, Intraoperative B312
      Left B312
    Superior Mesenteric B414
      Laser, Intraoperative B414
    Upper
      Laser, Intraoperative B31N
      Other B31N
    Upper Extremity
      Bilateral B31K
        Laser, Intraoperative B31K
      Left B31J
        Laser, Intraoperative B31J
      Right B31H
        Laser, Intraoperative B31H
    Vertebral
      Bilateral B31G
        Laser, Intraoperative B31G
      Left B31F
        Laser, Intraoperative B31F
      Right B31D
        Laser, Intraoperative B31D
  Bile Duct BF10
    Pancreatic Duct and Gallbladder BF14
  Bile Duct and Gallbladder BF13
  Biliary Duct BF11
  Bladder BT10
    Kidney and Ureter BT14
    Left BT1F
    Right BT1D
  Bladder and Urethra BT1B
  Bowel, Small BD1
  Calcaneus
    Left BQ1KZZZ
    Right BQ1JZZZ
  Clavicle
    Left BP15ZZZ
    Right BP14ZZZ
  Coccyx BR1F
  Colon BD14
  Corpora Cavernosa BV10
  Dialysis Fistula B51W
  Dialysis Shunt B51W
  Diaphragm BB16ZZZ
  Disc
    Cervical BR11
    Lumbar BR13
    Thoracic BR12
  Duodenum BD19
  Elbow
    Left BP1H
    Right BP1G
  Epiglottis B91G
  Esophagus BD11
  Extremity
    Lower BW1C
    Upper BW1J

Fluoroscopy — continued
  Facet Joint
    Cervical BR14
    Lumbar BR16
    Thoracic BR15
  Fallopian Tube
    Bilateral BU12
    Left BU11
    Right BU10
  Fallopian Tube and Uterus BU18
  Femur
    Left BQ14ZZZ
    Right BQ13ZZZ
  Finger
    Left BP1SZZZ
    Right BP1RZZZ
  Foot
    Left BQ1MZZZ
    Right BQ1LZZZ
  Forearm
    Left BP1KZZZ
    Right BP1JZZZ
  Gallbladder BF12
    Bile Duct and Pancreatic Duct BF14
  Gallbladder and Bile Duct BF13
  Gastrointestinal, Upper BD1
  Hand
    Left BP1PZZZ
    Right BP1NZZZ
  Head and Neck BW19
  Heart
    Left B215
    Right B214
    Right and Left B216
  Hip
    Left BQ11
    Right BQ10
  Humerus
    Left BP1BZZZ
    Right BP1AZZZ
  Ileal Diversion Loop BT1C
  Ileal Loop, Ureters and Kidney BT1G
  Intracranial Sinus B512
  Joint
    Acromioclavicular, Bilateral BP13ZZZ
    Finger
      Left BP1D
      Right BP1C
    Foot
      Left BQ1Y
      Right BQ1X
    Hand
      Left BP1D
      Right BP1C
    Lumbosacral BR1B
    Sacroiliac BR1D
    Sternoclavicular
      Bilateral BP12ZZZ
      Left BP11ZZZ
      Right BP10ZZZ
    Temporomandibular
      Bilateral BN19
      Left BN18
      Right BN17
    Thoracolumbar BR18
    Toe
      Left BQ1Y
      Right BQ1X
  Kidney
    Bilateral BT13
    Ileal Loop and Ureter BT1G
    Left BT12
    Right BT11
    Ureter and Bladder BT14
      Left BT1F
      Right BT1D
  Knee
    Left BQ18
    Right BQ17
  Larynx B91J
  Leg
    Left BQ1FZZZ
    Right BQ1DZZZ
  Liver BF15
  Lung
    Bilateral BB14ZZZ
    Left BB13ZZZ
    Right BB12ZZZ
  Mediastinum BB1CZZZ

Fluoroscopy — continued
  Mouth BD1B
  Neck and Head BW19
  Oropharynx BD1B
  Pancreatic Duct BF1
    Gallbladder and Bile Duct BF14
  Patella
    Left BQ1WZZZ
    Right BQ1VZZZ
  Pelvis BR1C
  Pelvis and Abdomen BW11
  Pharynx B91G
  Ribs
    Left BP1YZZZ
    Right BP1XZZZ
  Sacrum BR1F
  Scapula
    Left BP17ZZZ
    Right BP16ZZZ
  Shoulder
    Left BP19
    Right BP18
  Sinus, Intracranial B512
  Spinal Cord B01B
  Spine
    Cervical BR10
    Lumbar BR19
    Thoracic BR17
    Whole BR1G
  Sternum BR1H
  Stomach BD12
  Toe
    Left BQ1QZZZ
    Right BQ1PZZZ
  Tracheobronchial Tree
    Bilateral BB19YZZ
    Left BB18YZZ
    Right BB17YZZ
  Ureter
    Ileal Loop and Kidney BT1G
    Kidney and Bladder BT14
    Left BT1F
    Right BT1D
  Left BT17
  Right BT16
  Urethra BT15
  Urethra and Bladder BT1B
  Uterus BU16
  Uterus and Fallopian Tube BU18
  Vagina BU19
  Vasa Vasorum BV18
  Vein
    Cerebellar B511
    Cerebral B511
    Epidural B510
    Jugular
      Bilateral B515
      Left B514
      Right B513
    Lower Extremity
      Bilateral B51D
      Left B51C
      Right B51B
    Other B51V
    Pelvic (Iliac)
      Left B51G
      Right B51F
    Pelvic (Iliac) Bilateral B51H
    Portal B51T
    Pulmonary
      Bilateral B51S
      Left B51R
      Right B51Q
    Renal
      Bilateral B51L
      Left B51K
      Right B51J
    Splanchnic B51T
    Subclavian
      Left B517
      Right B516
    Upper Extremity
      Bilateral B51P
      Left B51N
      Right B51M
  Vena Cava
    Inferior B519
    Superior B518

Fluoroscopy — continued
  Wrist
    Left BP1M
    Right BP1L
Fluoroscopy, laser intraoperative
  see Fluoroscopy, Heart B21
  see Fluoroscopy, Lower Arteries B41
  see Fluoroscopy, Upper Arteries B31
Flushing see Irrigation
Foley catheter use Drainage Device
Fontan completion procedure Stage II see Bypass, Vena Cava, Inferior 0610
Foramen magnum use Occipital Bone
Foramen of Monro (intraventricular) use Cerebral Ventricle
Foreskin use Prepuce
Formula™ Balloon-Expandable Renal Stent System use Intraluminal Device
Fosfomycin Anti-infective use Other Anti-infective
Fossa of Rosenmuller use Nasopharynx
Fostamatinib XW0
Fourth cranial nerve use Trochlear Nerve
Fourth ventricle use Cerebral Ventricle
Fovea
  use Retina, Left
  use Retina, Right
Fragmentation
  Ampulla of Vater 0FFC
  Anus 0DFQ
  Appendix 0DFJ
  Artery
    Anterior Tibial
      Left 04FQ3Z
      Right 04FP3Z
    Axillary
      Left 03F63Z
      Right 03F53Z
    Brachial
      Left 03F83Z
      Right 03F73Z
    Common Iliac
      Left 04FD3Z
      Right 04FC3Z
    Coronary
      Four or More Arteries 02F33ZZ
      One Artery 02F03ZZ
      Three Arteries 02F23ZZ
      Two Arteries 02F13ZZ
    External Iliac
      Left 04FJ3Z
      Right 04FH3Z
    Femoral
      Left 04FL3Z
      Right 04FK3Z
    Innominate 03F23Z
    Internal Iliac
      Left 04FF3Z
      Right 04FE3Z
    Intracranial 03FG3Z
    Lower 04FY3Z
    Peroneal
      Left 04FU3Z
      Right 04FT3Z
    Popliteal
      Left 04FN3Z
      Right 04FM3Z
    Posterior Tibial
      Left 04FS3Z
      Right 04FR3Z
    Pulmonary
      Left 02FR3Z
      Right 02FQ3Z
    Pulmonary Trunk 02FP3Z
    Radial
      Left 03FC3Z
      Right 03FB3Z
    Subclavian
      Left 03F43Z
      Right 03F33Z
    Ulnar
      Left 03FA3Z
      Right 03F93Z
    Upper 03FY3Z
  Bladder 0TFB
  Bladder Neck 0TFC
  Bronchus
    Lingula 0BF9

Fragmentation — continued
  Bronchus — continued
    Lower Lobe
      Left 0BFB
      Right 0BF6
    Main
      Left 0BF7
      Right 0BF3
    Middle Lobe, Right 0BF5
    Upper Lobe
      Left 0BF8
      Right 0BF4
  Carina 0BF2
  Cavity, Cranial 0WF1
  Cecum 0DFH
  Cerebral Ventricle 00F6
  Colon
    Ascending 0DFK
    Descending 0DFM
    Sigmoid 0DFN
    Transverse 0DFL
  Duct
    Common Bile 0FF9
    Cystic 0FF8
    Hepatic
      Common 0FF7
      Left 0FF6
      Right 0FF5
    Pancreatic 0FFD
      Accessory 0FFF
    Parotid
      Left 0CFC
      Right 0CFB
  Duodenum 0DF9
  Epidural Space, Intracranial 00F3
  Esophagus 0DF5
  Fallopian Tube
    Left 0UF6
    Right 0UF5
  Fallopian Tubes, Bilateral 0UF7
  Gallbladder 0FF4
  Gastrointestinal Tract 0WFP
  Genitourinary Tract 0WFR
  Ileum 0DFB
  Intestine
    Large 0DFE
      Left 0DFG
      Right 0DFF
    Small 0DF8
  Jejunum 0DFA
  Kidney Pelvis
    Left 0TF4
    Right 0TF3
  Mediastinum 0WFC
  Oral Cavity and Throat 0WF3
  Pelvic Cavity 0WFJ
  Pericardial Cavity 0WFD
  Pericardium 02FN
  Peritoneal Cavity 0WFG
  Pleural Cavity
    Left 0WFB
    Right 0WF9
  Rectum 0DFP
  Respiratory Tract 0WFQ
  Spinal Canal 00FU
  Stomach 0DF6
  Subarachnoid Space, Intracranial 00F5
  Subdural Space, Intracranial 00F4
  Trachea 0BF1
  Ureter
    Left 0TF7
    Right 0TF6
  Urethra 0TFD
  Uterus 0UF9
  Vein
    Axillary
      Left 05F83Z
      Right 05F73Z
    Basilic
      Left 05FC3Z
      Right 05FB3Z
    Brachial
      Left 05FA3Z
      Right 05F93Z
    Cephalic
      Left 05FF3Z
      Right 05FD3Z
    Common Iliac
      Left 06FD3Z

Fragmentation
- **Fragmentation** — *continued*
  - Vein — *continued*
    - Common Iliac — *continued*
      - Right 06FC3Z
    - External Iliac
      - Left 06FG3Z
      - Right 06FF3Z
    - Femoral
      - Left 06FN3Z
      - Right 06FM3Z
    - Hypogastric
      - Left 06FJ3Z
      - Right 06FH3Z
    - Innominate
      - Left 05F43Z
      - Right 05F33Z
    - Lower 06FY3Z
    - Pulmonary
      - Left 02FT3Z
      - Right 02FS3Z
    - Saphenous
      - Left 06FQ3Z
      - Right 06FP3Z
    - Subclavian
      - Left 05F63Z
      - Right 05F53Z
    - Upper 05FY3Z
  - Vitreous
    - Left 08F5
    - Right 08F4
- **Fragmentation, Ultrasonic** *see* Fragmentation, Artery
- **Freestyle (Stentless) Aortic Root Bioprosthesis** *use* Zooplastic Tissue in Heart and Great Vessels
- **Frenectomy**
  - *see* Excision, Mouth and Throat 0CB
  - *see* Resection, Mouth and Throat 0CT
- **Frenoplasty, frenuloplasty**
  - *see* Repair, Mouth and Throat 0CQ
  - *see* Replacement, Mouth and Throat 0CR
  - *see* Supplement, Mouth and Throat 0CU
- **Frenotomy**
  - *see* Drainage, Mouth and Throat 0C9
  - *see* Release, Mouth and Throat 0CN
- **Frenulotomy**
  - *see* Drainage, Mouth and Throat 0C9
  - *see* Release, Mouth and Throat 0CN
- **Frenulum labii inferioris** *use* Lower Lip
- **Frenulum labii superioris** *use* Upper Lip
- **Frenulum linguae** *use* Tongue
- **Frenulumectomy**
  - *see* Excision, Mouth and Throat 0CB
  - *see* Resection, Mouth and Throat 0CT
- **Frontal lobe** *use* Cerebral Hemisphere
- **Frontal vein**
  - *use* Face Vein, Left
  - *use* Face Vein, Right
- **Frozen elephant trunk (FET) technique, aortic arch replacement**
  - *see* New Technology, Cardiovascular System X2R
  - *see* Replacement, Heart and Great Vessels 02R
- **Frozen elephant trunk (FET) technique, thoracic aorta restriction**
  - *see* New Technology, Cardiovascular System X2V
  - *see* Restriction, Heart and Great Vessels 02V
- **FUJIFILM EP-7000X System for Oxygen Saturation Endoscopic Imaging (OXEI)** *see* New Technology, Gastrointestinal System XD2
- **Fulguration** *see* Destruction
- **Fundoplication, gastroesophageal** *see* Restriction, Esophagogastric Junction 0DV4
- **Fundus uteri** *use* Uterus
- **Fusion**
  - Acromioclavicular
    - Left 0RGH
    - Right 0RGG
  - Ankle
    - Left 0SGG
      - Gyroid-Sheet Lattice Design Internal Fixation Device XRGK0CA
      - Open-truss Design Internal Fixation Device XRGK0B9
    - Right 0SGF
      - Gyroid-Sheet Lattice Design Internal Fixation Device XRGJ0CA
      - Open-truss Design Internal Fixation Device XRGJ0B9

Fusion — *continued*
- Carpal
  - Left 0RGR
  - Right 0RGQ
- Carpometacarpal
  - Left 0RGT
  - Right 0RGS
- Cervical Vertebral 0RG1
  - 2 or more 0RG2
- Cervicothoracic Vertebral 0RG4
- Coccygeal 0SG6
- Elbow
  - Left 0RGM
  - Right 0RGL
- Finger Phalangeal
  - Left 0RGX
  - Right 0RGW
- Hip
  - Left 0SGB
  - Right 0SG9
- Knee
  - Left 0SGD
  - Right 0SGC
- Lumbar Vertebral 0SG0
  - 2 or more 0SG1
    - Facet Joint Fusion Device, Paired Titanium Cages XRGC0EA
    - Interbody Fusion Device, Custom-Made Anatomically Designed XRGC
  - Facet Joint Fusion Device, Paired Titanium Cages XRGB0EA
  - Interbody Fusion Device, Custom-Made Anatomically Designed XRGB
- Lumbosacral 0SG3
  - Facet Joint Fusion Device, Paired Titanium Cages XRGD0EA
  - Interbody Fusion Device, Custom-Made Anatomically Designed XRGD
- Metacarpophalangeal
  - Left 0RGV
  - Right 0RGU
- Metatarsal-Phalangeal
  - Left 0SGN
  - Right 0SGM
- Occipital-cervical 0RG0
- Sacrococcygeal 0SG5
- Sacroiliac
  - Internal Fixation Device with Tulip Connector XRG
  - Left 0SG8
  - Right 0SG7
- Shoulder
  - Left 0RGK
  - Right 0RGJ
- Sternoclavicular
  - Left 0RGF
  - Right 0RGE
- Tarsal
  - Left 0SGJ
    - Gyroid-Sheet Lattice Design Internal Fixation Device XRGM0CA
    - Open-truss Design Internal Fixation Device XRGM0B9
  - Right 0SGH
    - Gyroid-Sheet Lattice Design Internal Fixation Device XRGL0CA
    - Open-truss Design Internal Fixation Device XRGL0B9
- Tarsometatarsal
  - Left 0SGL
  - Right 0SGK
- Temporomandibular
  - Left 0RGD
  - Right 0RGC
- Thoracic Vertebral 0RG6
  - 2 to 7 0RG7
  - 8 or more 0RG8
- Thoracolumbar Vertebral 0RGA
  - Facet Joint Fusion Device, Paired Titanium Cages XRGA0EA
  - Interbody Fusion Device, Custom-Made Anatomically Designed XRGA
- Toe Phalangeal
  - Left 0SGQ
  - Right 0SGP
- Wrist
  - Left 0RGP
  - Right 0RGN

Fusion screw (compression) (lag) (locking)
- *use* Internal Fixation Device in Lower Joints
- *use* Internal Fixation Device in Upper Joints

G

- **Gait training** *see* Motor Treatment, Rehabilitation F07
- **Galea aponeurotica** *use* Subcutaneous Tissue and Fascia, Scalp
- **Gammaglobulin** *use* Globulin
- **GammaTile™**
  - *use* Radioactive Element, Cesium-131 Collagen Implant in 00H
  - *use* Radioactive Element, Palladium-103 Collagen Implant in 00H
- **GAMUNEX-C, for COVID-19 treatment** *use* High-Dose Intravenous Immune Globulin
- **Ganglion impar (ganglion of Walther)** *use* Sacral Sympathetic Nerve
- **Ganglionectomy**
  - Destruction of lesion *see* Destruction
  - Excision of lesion *see* Excision
- **Gasserian ganglion** *use* Trigeminal Nerve
- **Gastrectomy**
  - Partial *see* Excision, Stomach 0DB6
  - Total *see* Resection, Stomach 0DT6
  - Vertical (sleeve) *see* Excision, Stomach 0DB6
- **Gastric electrical stimulation (GES) lead** *use* Stimulator Lead in Gastrointestinal System
- **Gastric lymph node** *use* Lymphatic, Aortic
- **Gastric pacemaker lead** *use* Stimulator Lead in Gastrointestinal System
- **Gastric plexus** *use* Abdominal Sympathetic Nerve
- **Gastrocnemius muscle**
  - *use* Lower Leg Muscle, Left
  - *use* Lower Leg Muscle, Right
- **Gastrocolic ligament** *use* Omentum
- **Gastrocolic omentum** *use* Omentum
- **Gastrocolostomy**
  - *see* Bypass, Gastrointestinal System 0D1
  - *see* Drainage, Gastrointestinal System 0D9
- **Gastroduodenal artery** *use* Hepatic Artery
- **Gastroduodenectomy**
  - *see* Excision, Gastrointestinal System 0DB
  - *see* Resection, Gastrointestinal System 0DT
- **Gastroduodenoscopy** 0DJ08ZZ
- **Gastroenteroplasty**
  - *see* Repair, Gastrointestinal System 0DQ
  - *see* Supplement, Gastrointestinal System 0DU
- **Gastroenterostomy**
  - *see* Bypass, Gastrointestinal System 0D1
  - *see* Drainage, Gastrointestinal System 0D9
- **Gastroesophageal (GE) junction** *use* Esophagogastric Junction
- **Gastrogastrostomy**
  - *see* Bypass, Stomach 0D16
  - *see* Drainage, Stomach 0D96
- **Gastrohepatic omentum** *use* Omentum
- **Gastrojejunostomy**
  - *see* Bypass, Stomach 0D16
  - *see* Drainage, Stomach 0D96
- **Gastrolysis** *see* Release, Stomach 0DN6
- **Gastropexy**
  - *see* Repair, Stomach 0DQ6
  - *see* Reposition, Stomach 0DS6
- **Gastrophrenic ligament** *use* Omentum
- **Gastroplasty**
  - *see* Repair, Stomach 0DQ6
  - *see* Supplement, Stomach 0DU6
- **Gastroplication** *see* Restriction, Stomach 0DV6
- **Gastropylorectomy** *see* Excision, Gastrointestinal System 0DB
- **Gastrorrhaphy** *see* Repair, Stomach 0DQ6
- **Gastroscopy** 0DJ68ZZ
- **Gastrosplenic ligament** *use* Omentum
- **Gastrostomy**
  - *see* Bypass, Stomach 0D16
  - *see* Drainage, Stomach 0D96
- **Gastrotomy** *see* Drainage, Stomach 0D96
- **Gemellus muscle**
  - *use* Hip Muscle, Left
  - *use* Hip Muscle, Right
- **Geniculate ganglion** *use* Facial Nerve
- **Geniculate nucleus** *use* Thalamus
- **Genioglossus muscle** *use* Tongue, Palate, Pharynx Muscle

Genioplasty see Alteration, Jaw, Lower 0W05
Genitofemoral nerve use Lumbar Plexus
GIAPREZA™ use Vasopressor
Gilteritinib use Other Antineoplastic
Gingivectomy see Excision, Mouth and Throat 0CB
Gingivoplasty
  see Repair, Mouth and Throat 0CQ
  see Replacement, Mouth and Throat 0CR
  see Supplement, Mouth and Throat 0CU
Glans penis use Prepuce
Glenohumeral joint
  use Shoulder Joint, Left
  use Shoulder Joint, Right
Glenohumeral ligament
  use Shoulder Bursa and Ligament, Left
  use Shoulder Bursa and Ligament, Right
Glenoid fossa (of scapula)
  use Glenoid Cavity, Left
  use Glenoid Cavity, Right
Glenoid ligament (labrum)
  use Shoulder Joint, Left
  use Shoulder Joint, Right
Globus pallidus use Basal Ganglia
Glofitamab Antineoplastic XW0
Glomectomy
  see Excision, Endocrine System 0GB
  see Resection, Endocrine System 0GT
Glossectomy
  see Excision, Tongue 0CB7
  see Resection, Tongue 0CT7
Glossoepiglottic fold use Epiglottis
Glossopexy
  see Repair, Tongue 0CQ7
  see Reposition, Tongue 0CS7
Glossoplasty
  see Repair, Tongue 0CQ7
  see Replacement, Tongue 0CR7
  see Supplement, Tongue 0CU7
Glossorrhaphy see Repair, Tongue 0CQ7
Glossotomy see Drainage, Tongue 0C97
Glottis use Larynx
Gluteal Artery Perforator Flap
  Replacement
    Bilateral 0HRV079
    Left 0HRU079
    Right 0HRT079
  Transfer
    Left 0KXG
    Right 0KXF
Gluteal lymph node use Lymphatic, Pelvis
Gluteal vein
  use Hypogastric Vein, Left
  use Hypogastric Vein, Right
Gluteus maximus muscle
  use Hip Muscle, Left
  use Hip Muscle, Right
Gluteus medius muscle
  use Hip Muscle, Left
  use Hip Muscle, Right
Gluteus minimus muscle
  use Hip Muscle, Left
  use Hip Muscle, Right
GORE EXCLUDER® AAA Endoprosthesis
  use Intraluminal Device
  use Intraluminal Device, Branched or Fenestrated, One or Two Arteries in 04V
  use Intraluminal Device, Branched or Fenestrated, Three or More Arteries in 04V
GORE EXCLUDER® IBE Endoprosthesis use Intraluminal Device, Branched or Fenestrated, One or Two Arteries in 04V
GORE TAG® Thoracic Endoprosthesis use Intraluminal Device
GORE® DUALMESH® use Synthetic Substitute
GORE® EXCLUDER® TAMBE Device (Thoracoabdominal Branch Endoprosthesis) use Branched Intraluminal Device, Manufactured Integrated System, Four or More Arteries in New Technology
Gracilis muscle
  use Upper Leg Muscle, Left
  use Upper Leg Muscle, Right
Graft
  see Replacement
  see Supplement
Great auricular nerve use Cervical Plexus
Great cerebral vein use Intracranial Vein

Great(er) saphenous vein
  use Saphenous Vein, Left
  use Saphenous Vein, Right
Greater alar cartilage use Nasal Mucosa and Soft Tissue
Greater occipital nerve use Cervical Nerve
Greater Omentum use Omentum
Greater splanchnic nerve use Thoracic Sympathetic Nerve
Greater superficial petrosal nerve use Facial Nerve
Greater trochanter
  use Upper Femur, Left
  use Upper Femur, Right
Greater tuberosity
  use Humeral Head, Left
  use Humeral Head, Right
Greater vestibular (Bartholin's) gland use Vestibular Gland
Greater wing use Sphenoid Bone
GS-5734 use Remdesivir Anti-infective
Guedel airway use Intraluminal Device, Airway in Mouth and Throat
Guidance, catheter placement
  EKG see Measurement, Physiological Systems 4A0
  Fluoroscopy see Fluoroscopy, Veins B51
  Ultrasound see Ultrasonography, Veins B54
Gyroid-Sheet Lattice Design Internal Fixation Device
  Ankle
    Left XRGK0CA
    Right XRGJ0CA
  Tarsal
    Left XRGM0CA
    Right XRGL0CA

H

Hallux
  use 1st Toe, Left
  use 1st Toe, Right
Hamate bone
  use Carpal, Left
  use Carpal, Right
Hamstring muscle
  use Upper Leg Muscle, Left
  use Upper Leg Muscle, Right
Hancock Bioprosthesis (aortic) (mitral) valve use Zooplastic Tissue in Heart and Great Vessels
Hancock Bioprosthetic Valved Conduit use Zooplastic Tissue in Heart and Great Vessels
Harmony™ transcatheter pulmonary valve (TPV) placement 02RH38M
Harvesting, Stem Cells see Pheresis, Circulatory 6A55
HAV™ (Human Acellular Vessel) use Bioengineered Human Acellular Vessel in New Technology
hdIVIG (high-dose intravenous immunoglobulin), for COVID-19 treatment use High-Dose Intravenous Immune Globulin
Head of fibula
  use Fibula, Left
  use Fibula, Right
Hearing Aid Assessment F14Z
Hearing Assessment F13Z
Hearing Device
  Bone Conduction
    Left 09HE
    Right 09HD
  Insertion of device in
    Left 0NH6
    Right 0NH5
  Multiple Channel Cochlear Prosthesis
    Left 09HE
    Right 09HD
  Removal of device from, Skull 0NP0
  Revision of device in, Skull 0NW0
  Single Channel Cochlear Prosthesis
    Left 09HE
    Right 09HD
Hearing Treatment F09Z
Heart Assist System
  Implantable
    Insertion of device in, Heart 02HA
    Removal of device from, Heart 02PA
    Revision of device in, Heart 02WA

Heart Assist System — continued
  Short-term External
    Insertion of device in
      Aorta, Thoracic, Descending 02HW3RZ
      Heart 02HA
    Removal of device from
      Aorta, Thoracic, Descending 02PW3RZ
      Heart 02PA
    Revision of device in
      Aorta, Thoracic, Descending 02WW3RZ
      Heart 02WA
HeartMate 3™ LVAS use Implantable Heart Assist System in Heart and Great Vessels
HeartMate II® Left Ventricular Assist Device (LVAD) use Implantable Heart Assist System in Heart and Great Vessels
HeartMate XVE® Left Ventricular Assist Device (LVAD) use Implantable Heart Assist System in Heart and Great Vessels
HeartMate® implantable heart assist system see Insertion of device in, Heart 02HA
Helix
  use Ear, External, Bilateral
  use Ear, External, Left
  use Ear, External, Right
Hematopoietic cell transplant (HCT) see Transfusion, Circulatory 302
Hemicolectomy see Resection, Gastrointestinal System 0DT
Hemicystectomy see Excision, Urinary System 0TB
Hemigastrectomy see Excision, Gastrointestinal System 0DB
Hemiglossectomy see Excision, Mouth and Throat 0CB
Hemilaminectomy
  see Excision, Lower Bones 0QB
  see Excision, Upper Bones 0PB
Hemilaminotomy
  see Drainage, Lower Bones 0Q9
  see Drainage, Upper Bones 0P9
  see Excision, Lower Bones 0QB
  see Excision, Upper Bones 0PB
  see Release, Central Nervous System and Cranial Nerves 00N
  see Release, Lower Bones 0QN
  see Release, Peripheral Nervous System 01N
  see Release, Upper Bones 0PN
Hemilaryngectomy see Excision, Larynx 0CBS
Hemimandibulectomy see Excision, Head and Facial Bones 0NB
Hemimaxillectomy see Excision, Head and Facial Bones 0NB
Hemipylorectomy see Excision, Gastrointestinal System 0DB
Hemispherectomy
  see Excision, Central Nervous System and Cranial Nerves 00B
  see Resection, Central Nervous System and Cranial Nerves 00T
Hemithyroidectomy
  see Excision, Endocrine System 0GB
  see Resection, Endocrine System 0GT
Hemodialysis see Performance, Urinary 5A1D
Hemolung® Respiratory Assist System (RAS) 5A0920Z
Hemospray® Endoscopic Hemostat use Mineral-based Topical Hemostatic Agent
Hepatectomy
  see Excision, Hepatobiliary System and Pancreas 0FB
  see Resection, Hepatobiliary System and Pancreas 0FT
Hepatic artery proper use Hepatic Artery
Hepatic flexure use Transverse Colon
Hepatic lymph node use Lymphatic, Aortic
Hepatic plexus use Abdominal Sympathetic Nerve
Hepatic portal vein use Portal Vein
Hepaticoduodenostomy
  see Bypass, Hepatobiliary System and Pancreas 0F1
  see Drainage, Hepatobiliary System and Pancreas 0F9
Hepaticotomy see Drainage, Hepatobiliary System and Pancreas 0F9
Hepatocholedochostomy see Drainage, Duct, Common Bile 0F99
Hepatogastric ligament use Omentum
Hepatopancreatic ampulla use Ampulla of Vater

Hepatopexy
  see Repair, Hepatobiliary System and Pancreas 0FQ
  see Reposition, Hepatobiliary System and Pancreas 0FS

Hepatorrhaphy see Repair, Hepatobiliary System and Pancreas 0FQ

Hepatotomy see Drainage, Hepatobiliary System and Pancreas 0F9

HEPZATO™ KIT (melphalan hydrochloride Hepatic Delivery System) use Melphalan Hydrochloride Antineoplastic

Herculink (RX) Elite Renal Stent System use Intraluminal Device

Herniorrhaphy
  see Repair, Anatomical Regions, General 0WQ
  see Repair, Anatomical Regions, Lower Extremities 0YQ
  With synthetic substitute
    see Supplement, Anatomical Regions, General 0WU
    see Supplement, Anatomical Regions, Lower Extremities 0YU

HIG (hyperimmune globulin), for COVID-19 treatment use Hyperimmune Globulin

High-Dose Intravenous Immune Globulin, for COVID-19 treatment XW1

High-dose intravenous immunoglobulin (hdIVIG), for COVID-19 treatment use High-Dose Intravenous Immune Globulin

Hip (joint) liner use Liner in Lower Joints

HIPEC (hyperthermic intraperitoneal chemotherapy) 3E0M30Y

HistoSonics® System see New Technology, Hepatobiliary System and Pancreas XF5

Histotripsy, liver see New Technology, Hepatobiliary System and Pancreas XF5

hIVIG (hyperimmune intravenous immunoglobulin), for COVID-19 treatment use Hyperimmune Globulin

Holter Monitoring 4A12X45

Holter valve ventricular shunt use Synthetic Substitute

Human Acellular Vessel™ (HAV) use Bioengineered Human Acellular Vessel in New Technology

Human angiotensin II, synthetic use Vasopressor

Humeroradial joint
  use Elbow Joint, Left
  use Elbow Joint, Right

Humeroulnar joint
  use Elbow Joint, Left
  use Elbow Joint, Right

Humerus, distal
  use Humeral Shaft, Left
  use Humeral Shaft, Right

Hydrocelectomy see Excision, Male Reproductive System 0VB

Hydrotherapy
  Assisted exercise in pool see Motor Treatment, Rehabilitation F07
  Whirlpool see Activities of Daily Living Treatment, Rehabilitation F08

Hymenectomy
  see Excision, Hymen 0UBK
  see Resection, Hymen 0UTK

Hymenoplasty
  see Repair, Hymen 0UQK
  see Supplement, Hymen 0UUK

Hymenorrhaphy see Repair, Hymen 0UQK

Hymenotomy
  see Division, Hymen 0U8K
  see Drainage, Hymen 0U9K

Hyoglossus muscle use Tongue, Palate, Pharynx Muscle

Hyoid artery
  use Thyroid Artery, Left
  use Thyroid Artery, Right

Hyperalimentation see Introduction of substance in or on

Hyperbaric oxygenation
  Decompression sickness treatment see Decompression, Circulatory 6A15
  Other treatment see Assistance, Circulatory 5A05

Hyperimmune globulin use Globulin

Hyperimmune Globulin, for COVID-19 treatment XW1

Hyperimmune intravenous immunoglobulin (hIVIG), for COVID-19 treatment use Hyperimmune Globulin

Hyperthermia
  Radiation Therapy
    Abdomen DWY38ZZ
    Adrenal Gland DGY28ZZ
    Bile Ducts DFY28ZZ
    Bladder DTY28ZZ
    Bone Marrow D7Y08ZZ
    Bone, Other DPYC8ZZ
    Brain D0Y08ZZ
    Brain Stem D0Y18ZZ
    Breast
      Left DMY08ZZ
      Right DMY18ZZ
    Bronchus DBY18ZZ
    Cervix DUY18ZZ
    Chest DWY28ZZ
    Chest Wall DBY78ZZ
    Colon DDY58ZZ
    Diaphragm DBY88ZZ
    Duodenum DDY28ZZ
    Ear D9Y08ZZ
    Esophagus DDY08ZZ
    Eye D8Y08ZZ
    Femur DPY98ZZ
    Fibula DPYB8ZZ
    Gallbladder DFY18ZZ
    Gland
      Adrenal DGY28ZZ
      Parathyroid DGY48ZZ
      Pituitary DGY08ZZ
      Thyroid DGY58ZZ
    Glands, Salivary D9Y68ZZ
    Head and Neck DWY18ZZ
    Hemibody DWY48ZZ
    Humerus DPY68ZZ
    Hypopharynx D9Y38ZZ
    Ileum DDY48ZZ
    Jejunum DDY38ZZ
    Kidney DTY08ZZ
    Larynx D9YB8ZZ
    Liver DFY08ZZ
    Lung DBY28ZZ
    Lymphatics
      Abdomen D7Y68ZZ
      Axillary D7Y48ZZ
      Inguinal D7Y88ZZ
      Neck D7Y38ZZ
      Pelvis D7Y78ZZ
      Thorax D7Y58ZZ
    Mandible DPY38ZZ
    Maxilla DPY28ZZ
    Mediastinum DBY68ZZ
    Mouth D9Y48ZZ
    Nasopharynx D9YD8ZZ
    Neck and Head DWY18ZZ
    Nerve, Peripheral D0Y78ZZ
    Nose D9Y18ZZ
    Oropharynx D9YF8ZZ
    Ovary DUY08ZZ
    Palate
      Hard D9Y88ZZ
      Soft D9Y98ZZ
    Pancreas DFY38ZZ
    Parathyroid Gland DGY48ZZ
    Pelvic Bones DPY88ZZ
    Pelvic Region DWY68ZZ
    Pineal Body DGY18ZZ
    Pituitary Gland DGY08ZZ
    Pleura DBY58ZZ
    Prostate DVY08ZZ
    Radius DPY78ZZ
    Rectum DDY78ZZ
    Rib DPY58ZZ
    Sinuses D9Y78ZZ
    Skin
      Abdomen DHY88ZZ
      Arm DHY48ZZ
      Back DHY78ZZ
      Buttock DHY98ZZ
      Chest DHY68ZZ
      Face DHY28ZZ
      Leg DHYB8ZZ
      Neck DHY38ZZ
    Skull DPY08ZZ
    Spinal Cord D0Y68ZZ
    Spleen D7Y28ZZ

Hyperthermia — continued
  Radiation Therapy — continued
    Sternum DPY48ZZ
    Stomach DDY18ZZ
    Testis DVY18ZZ
    Thymus D7Y18ZZ
    Thyroid Gland DGY58ZZ
    Tibia DPYB8ZZ
    Tongue D9Y58ZZ
    Trachea DBY08ZZ
    Ulna DPY78ZZ
    Ureter DTY18ZZ
    Urethra DTY38ZZ
    Uterus DUY28ZZ
    Whole Body DWY58ZZ
  Whole Body 6A3Z

Hyperthermic Intraperitoneal Chemotherapy (HIPEC) 3E0M30Y

Hypnosis GZFZZZZ

Hypogastric artery
  use Internal Iliac Artery, Left
  use Internal Iliac Artery, Right

Hypopharynx use Pharynx

Hypophysectomy
  see Excision, Gland, Pituitary 0GB0
  see Resection, Gland, Pituitary 0GT0

Hypophysis use Pituitary Gland

Hypothalamotomy see Destruction, Thalamus 0059

Hypothenar muscle
  use Hand Muscle, Left
  use Hand Muscle, Right

Hypothermia, Whole Body 6A4Z

Hysterectomy
  Supracervical see Resection, Uterus 0UT9
  Total see Resection, Uterus 0UT9

Hysterolysis see Release, Uterus 0UN9

Hysteropexy
  see Repair, Uterus 0UQ9
  see Reposition, Uterus 0US9

Hysteroplasty see Repair, Uterus 0UQ9

Hysterorrhaphy see Repair, Uterus 0UQ9

Hysteroscopy 0UJD8ZZ

Hysterotomy see Drainage, Uterus 0U99

Hysterotrachelectomy
  see Resection, Cervix 0UTC
  see Resection, Uterus 0UT9

Hysterotracheloplasty see Repair, Uterus 0UQ9

Hysterotrachelorrhaphy see Repair, Uterus 0UQ9

I

IABP (Intra-aortic balloon pump) see Assistance, Cardiac 5A02

IAEMT (Intraoperative anesthetic effect monitoring and titration) see Monitoring, Central Nervous 4A10

IASD® (InterAtrial Shunt Device), Corvia use Synthetic Substitute

Idarucizumab, Pradaxa® (dabigatran) reversal agent use Other Therapeutic Substance

Idecabtagene Vicleucel use Idecabtagene Vicleucel Immunotherapy

Idecabtagene Vicleucel Immunotherapy XW0

Ide-cel use Idecabtagene Vicleucel Immunotherapy

iFuse Bedrock™ Granite Implant System use Internal Fixation Device with Tulip Connector in New Technology

IGIV-C, for COVID-19 treatment use Hyperimmune Globulin

IHD (Intermittent hemodialysis) 5A1D70Z

Ileal artery use Superior Mesenteric Artery

Ileectomy
  see Excision, Ileum 0DBB
  see Resection, Ileum 0DTB

Ileocolic artery use Superior Mesenteric Artery

Ileocolic vein use Colic Vein

Ileopexy
  see Repair, Ileum 0DQB
  see Reposition, Ileum 0DSB

Ileorrhaphy see Repair, Ileum 0DQB

Ileoscopy 0DJD8ZZ

Ileostomy
  see Bypass, Ileum 0D1B
  see Drainage, Ileum 0D9B

Ileotomy see Drainage, Ileum 0D9B

Ileoureterostomy see Bypass, Urinary System 0T1

Iliac crest
   use Pelvic Bone, Left
   use Pelvic Bone, Right
Iliac fascia
   use Subcutaneous Tissue and Fascia, Left Upper Leg
   use Subcutaneous Tissue and Fascia, Right Upper Leg
Iliac lymph node use Lymphatic, Pelvis
Iliacus muscle
   use Hip Muscle, Left
   use Hip Muscle, Right
Iliofemoral ligament
   use Hip Bursa and Ligament, Left
   use Hip Bursa and Ligament, Right
Iliohypogastric nerve use Lumbar Plexus
Ilioinguinal nerve use Lumbar Plexus
Iliolumbar artery
   use Internal Iliac Artery, Left
   use Internal Iliac Artery, Right
Iliolumbar ligament use Lower Spine Bursa and Ligament
Iliopsoas muscle
   use Hip Muscle, Left
   use Hip Muscle, Right
Iliotibial tract (band)
   use Subcutaneous Tissue and Fascia, Left Upper Leg
   use Subcutaneous Tissue and Fascia, Right Upper Leg
Ilium
   use Pelvic Bone, Left
   use Pelvic Bone, Right
Ilizarov external fixator
   use External Fixation Device, Ring in 0PH
   use External Fixation Device, Ring in 0PS
   use External Fixation Device, Ring in 0QH
   use External Fixation Device, Ring in 0QS
Ilizarov-Vecklich device
   use External Fixation Device, Limb Lengthening in 0PH
   use External Fixation Device, Limb Lengthening in 0QH
Imaging, diagnostic
   see Computerized Tomography (CT Scan)
   see Fluoroscopy
   see Magnetic Resonance Imaging (MRI)
   see Plain Radiography
   see Ultrasonography
Imdevimab (REGN10987) and Casirivimab (REGN10933) use REGN-COV2 Monoclonal Antibody
IMFINZI® use Durvalumab Antineoplastic
Imipenem-cilastatin-relebactam Anti-infective use Other Anti-infective
IMI/REL use Other Anti-infective
Immobilization
   Abdominal Wall 2W33X
   Arm
      Lower
         Left 2W3DX
         Right 2W3CX
      Upper
         Left 2W3BX
         Right 2W3AX
   Back 2W35X
   Chest Wall 2W34X
   Extremity
      Lower
         Left 2W3MX
         Right 2W3LX
      Upper
         Left 2W39X
         Right 2W38X
   Face 2W31X
   Finger
      Left 2W3KX
      Right 2W3JX
   Foot
      Left 2W3TX
      Right 2W3SX
   Hand
      Left 2W3FX
      Right 2W3EX
   Head 2W30X
   Inguinal Region
      Left 2W37X

Immobilization — continued
   Inguinal Region — continued
      Right 2W36X
   Leg
      Lower
         Left 2W3RX
         Right 2W3QX
      Upper
         Left 2W3PX
         Right 2W3NX
   Neck 2W32X
   Thumb
      Left 2W3HX
      Right 2W3GX
   Toe
      Left 2W3VX
      Right 2W3UX
Immunization see Introduction of Serum, Toxoid, and Vaccine
Immunoglobulin use Globulin
Immunotherapy see Introduction of Immunotherapeutic Substance
Immunotherapy, antineoplastic
   Interferon see Introduction of Low-dose Interleukin-2
   Interleukin-2, high-dose see Introduction of High-dose Interleukin-2
   Interleukin-2, low-dose see Introduction of Low-dose Interleukin-2
   Monoclonal antibody see Introduction of Monoclonal Antibody
   Proleukin, high-dose see Introduction of High-dose Interleukin-2
   Proleukin, low-dose see Introduction of Low-dose Interleukin-2
Impella® 5.5 with SmartAssist® System use Conduit to Short-term External Heart Assist System in New Technology
Impella® heart pump use Short-term External Heart Assist System in Heart and Great Vessels
Impeller Pump
   Continuous, Output 5A0221D
   Intermittent, Output 5A0211D
Implantable cardioverter-defibrillator (ICD) use Defibrillator Generator in 0JH
Implantable drug infusion pump (anti-spasmodic) (chemotherapy) (pain) use Infusion Device, Pump in Subcutaneous Tissue and Fascia
Implantable glucose monitoring device use Monitoring Device
Implantable hemodynamic monitor (IHM) use Monitoring Device, Hemodynamic in 0JH
Implantable hemodynamic monitoring system (IHMS) use Monitoring Device, Hemodynamic in 0JH
Implantable Miniature Telescope™ (IMT) use Synthetic Substitute, Intraocular Telescope in 08R
Implantation
   see Insertion
   see Replacement
Implanted (venous)(access) port use Vascular Access Device, Totally Implantable in Subcutaneous Tissue and Fascia
IMV (intermittent mandatory ventilation) see Assistance, Respiratory 5A09
In Vitro Fertilization 8E0ZXY1
Incision, abscess see Drainage
Incudectomy
   see Excision, Ear, Nose, Sinus 09B
   see Resection, Ear, Nose, Sinus 09T
Incudopexy
   see Repair, Ear, Nose, Sinus 09Q
   see Reposition, Ear, Nose, Sinus 09S
Incus
   use Auditory Ossicle, Left
   use Auditory Ossicle, Right
Induction of labor
   Artificial rupture of membranes see Drainage, Pregnancy 109
   Oxytocin see Introduction of Hormone
InDura, intrathecal catheter (1P) (spinal) use Infusion Device
Inebilizumab-cdon XW0
Inferior cardiac nerve use Thoracic Sympathetic Nerve
Inferior cerebellar vein use Intracranial Vein
Inferior cerebral vein use Intracranial Vein

Inferior epigastric artery
   use External Iliac Artery, Left
   use External Iliac Artery, Right
Inferior epigastric lymph node use Lymphatic, Pelvis
Inferior genicular artery
   use Popliteal Artery, Left
   use Popliteal Artery, Right
Inferior gluteal artery
   use Internal Iliac Artery, Left
   use Internal Iliac Artery, Right
Inferior gluteal nerve use Sacral Plexus
Inferior hypogastric plexus use Abdominal Sympathetic Nerve
Inferior labial artery use Face Artery
Inferior longitudinal muscle use Tongue, Palate, Pharynx Muscle
Inferior mesenteric ganglion use Abdominal Sympathetic Nerve
Inferior mesenteric lymph node use Lymphatic, Mesenteric
Inferior mesenteric plexus use Abdominal Sympathetic Nerve
Inferior oblique muscle
   use Extraocular Muscle, Left
   use Extraocular Muscle, Right
Inferior pancreaticoduodenal artery use Superior Mesenteric Artery
Inferior phrenic artery use Abdominal Aorta
Inferior rectus muscle
   use Extraocular Muscle, Left
   use Extraocular Muscle, Right
Inferior suprarenal artery
   use Renal Artery, Left
   use Renal Artery, Right
Inferior tarsal plate
   use Lower Eyelid, Left
   use Lower Eyelid, Right
Inferior thyroid vein
   use Innominate Vein, Left
   use Innominate Vein, Right
Inferior tibiofibular joint
   use Ankle Joint, Left
   use Ankle Joint, Right
Inferior turbinate use Nasal Turbinate
Inferior ulnar collateral artery
   use Brachial Artery, Left
   use Brachial Artery, Right
Inferior vesical artery
   use Internal Iliac Artery, Left
   use Internal Iliac Artery, Right
Infraauricular lymph node use Lymphatic, Head
Infraclavicular (deltopectoral) lymph node
   use Lymphatic, Left Upper Extremity
   use Lymphatic, Right Upper Extremity
Infrahyoid muscle
   use Neck Muscle, Left
   use Neck Muscle, Right
Infraparotid lymph node use Lymphatic, Head
Infraspinatus fascia
   use Subcutaneous Tissue and Fascia, Left Upper Arm
   use Subcutaneous Tissue and Fascia, Right Upper Arm
Infraspinatus muscle
   use Shoulder Muscle, Left
   use Shoulder Muscle, Right
Infundibulopelvic ligament use Uterine Supporting Structure
Infusion see Introduction of substance in or on
Infusion Device, Pump
   Insertion of device in
      Abdomen 0JH8
      Back 0JH7
      Chest 0JH6
      Lower Arm
         Left 0JHH
         Right 0JHG
      Lower Leg
         Left 0JHP
         Right 0JHN
      Trunk 0JHT
      Upper Arm
         Left 0JHF
         Right 0JHD
      Upper Leg
         Left 0JHM
         Right 0JHL

▽ **Subterms under main terms may continue to next column or page**

Infusion Device, Pump — *continued*
  Removal of device from
    Lower Extremity 0JPW
    Trunk 0JPT
    Upper Extremity 0JPV
  Revision of device in
    Lower Extremity 0JWW
    Trunk 0JWT
    Upper Extremity 0JWV
Infusion, glucarpidase
  Central Vein 3E043GQ
  Peripheral Vein 3E033GQ
Inguinal canal
  use Inguinal Region, Bilateral
  use Inguinal Region, Left
  use Inguinal Region, Right
Inguinal triangle
  use Inguinal Region, Bilateral
  use Inguinal Region, Left
  use Inguinal Region, Right
Injection *see* Introduction of substance in or on
Injection reservoir, port *use* Vascular Access Device, Totally Implantable in Subcutaneous Tissue and Fascia
Injection reservoir, pump *use* Infusion Device, Pump in Subcutaneous Tissue and Fascia
Innova™ stent *use* Intraluminal Device
Insemination, artificial 3E0P7LZ
Insertion
  Antimicrobial envelope *see* Introduction of Anti-infective
  Aqueous drainage shunt
    see Bypass, Eye 081
    see Drainage, Eye 089
  Bone, Pelvic, Internal Fixation Device with Tulip Connector XNH
  Conduit to Short-term External Heart Assist System X2H
  Intracardiac Pacemaker, Dual-Chamber X2H
  Intraluminal Device, Bioprosthetic Valve X2H
  Joint
    Lumbar Vertebral
      2 or more, Carbon/PEEK Spinal Stabilization Device, Pedicle Based XRHC
      Carbon/PEEK Spinal Stabilization Device, Pedicle Based XRHB
      Posterior Spinal Motion Preservation Device XRHB018
    Lumbosacral
      Carbon/PEEK Spinal Stabilization Device, Pedicle Based XRHD
      Posterior Spinal Motion Preservation Device XRHD018
    Thoracic Vertebral
      2 to 7, Carbon/PEEK Spinal Stabilization Device, Pedicle Based XRH7
      8 or more, Carbon/PEEK Spinal Stabilization Device, Pedicle Based XRH8
      Carbon/PEEK Spinal Stabilization Device, Pedicle Based XRH6
    Thoracolumbar Vertebral, Carbon/PEEK Spinal Stabilization Device, Pedicle Based XRHA
  Neurostimulator Lead, Sphenopalatine Ganglion X0HK3Q8
  Neurostimulator Lead with Paired Stimulation System X0HQ3R8
  Products of Conception 10H0
  Spinal Stabilization Device
    see Insertion of device in, Lower Joints 0SH
    see Insertion of device in, Upper Joints 0RH
  Tibial Extension with Motion Sensors XNH
Insertion of device in
  Abdominal Wall 0WHF
  Acetabulum
    Left 0QH5
    Right 0QH4
  Anal Sphincter 0DHR
  Ankle Region
    Left 0YHL
    Right 0YHK
  Anus 0DHQ
  Aorta
    Abdominal 04H0
    Thoracic
      Ascending/Arch 02HX
      Descending 02HW

Insertion of device in — *continued*
  Arm
    Lower
      Left 0XHF
      Right 0XHD
    Upper
      Left 0XH9
      Right 0XH8
  Artery
    Anterior Tibial
      Left 04HQ
      Right 04HP
    Axillary
      Left 03H6
      Right 03H5
    Brachial
      Left 03H8
      Right 03H7
    Celiac 04H1
    Colic
      Left 04H7
      Middle 04H8
      Right 04H6
    Common Carotid
      Left 03HJ
      Right 03HH
    Common Iliac
      Left 04HD
      Right 04HC
    Coronary
      Four or More Arteries 02H3
      One Artery 02H0
      Three Arteries 02H2
      Two Arteries 02H1
    External Carotid
      Left 03HN
      Right 03HM
    External Iliac
      Left 04HJ
      Right 04HH
    Face 03HR
    Femoral
      Left 04HL
      Right 04HK
    Foot
      Left 04HW
      Right 04HV
    Gastric 04H2
    Hand
      Left 03HF
      Right 03HD
    Hepatic 04H3
    Inferior Mesenteric 04HB
    Innominate 03H2
    Internal Carotid
      Left 03HL
      Right 03HK
    Internal Iliac
      Left 04HF
      Right 04HE
    Internal Mammary
      Left 03H1
      Right 03H0
    Intracranial 03HG
    Lower 04HY
    Peroneal
      Left 04HU
      Right 04HT
    Popliteal
      Left 04HN
      Right 04HM
    Posterior Tibial
      Left 04HS
      Right 04HR
    Pulmonary
      Left 02HR
      Right 02HQ
    Pulmonary Trunk 02HP
    Radial
      Left 03HC
      Right 03HB
    Renal
      Left 04HA
      Right 04H9
    Splenic 04H4
    Subclavian
      Left 03H4
      Right 03H3
    Superior Mesenteric 04H5

Insertion of device in — *continued*
  Artery — *continued*
    Temporal
      Left 03HT
      Right 03HS
    Thyroid
      Left 03HV
      Right 03HU
    Ulnar
      Left 03HA
      Right 03H9
    Upper 03HY
    Vertebral
      Left 03HQ
      Right 03HP
  Atrium
    Left 02H7
    Right 02H6
  Axilla
    Left 0XH5
    Right 0XH4
  Back
    Lower 0WHL
    Upper 0WHK
  Bladder 0THB
  Bladder Neck 0THC
  Bone
    Ethmoid
      Left 0NHG
      Right 0NHF
    Facial 0NHW
    Frontal 0NH1
    Hyoid 0NHX
    Lacrimal
      Left 0NHJ
      Right 0NHH
    Lower 0QHY
    Nasal 0NHB
    Occipital 0NH7
    Palatine
      Left 0NHL
      Right 0NHK
    Parietal
      Left 0NH4
      Right 0NH3
    Pelvic
      Left 0QH3
      Right 0QH2
    Sphenoid 0NHC
    Temporal
      Left 0NH6
      Right 0NH5
    Upper 0PHY
    Zygomatic
      Left 0NHN
      Right 0NHM
  Bone Marrow 07HT
  Brain 00H0
  Breast
    Bilateral 0HHV
    Left 0HHU
    Right 0HHT
  Bronchus
    Lingula 0BH9
    Lower Lobe
      Left 0BHB
      Right 0BH6
    Main
      Left 0BH7
      Right 0BH3
    Middle Lobe, Right 0BH5
    Upper Lobe
      Left 0BH8
      Right 0BH4
  Bursa and Ligament
    Lower 0MHY
    Upper 0MHX
  Buttock
    Left 0YH1
    Right 0YH0
  Carpal
    Left 0PHN
    Right 0PHM
  Cavity, Cranial 0WH1
  Cerebral Ventricle 00H6
  Cervix 0UHC
  Chest Wall 0WH8
  Cisterna Chyli 07HL

Insertion of device in — *continued*
- Clavicle
  - Left 0PHB
  - Right 0PH9
- Coccyx 0QHS
- Cul-de-sac 0UHF
- Diaphragm 0BHT
- Disc
  - Cervical Vertebral 0RH3
  - Cervicothoracic Vertebral 0RH5
  - Lumbar Vertebral 0SH2
  - Lumbosacral 0SH4
  - Thoracic Vertebral 0RH9
  - Thoracolumbar Vertebral 0RHB
- Duct
  - Hepatobiliary 0FHB
  - Pancreatic 0FHD
- Duodenum 0DH9
- Ear
  - Inner
    - Left 09HE
    - Right 09HD
  - Left 09HJ
  - Right 09HH
- Elbow Region
  - Left 0XHC
  - Right 0XHB
- Epididymis and Spermatic Cord 0VHM
- Esophagus 0DH5
  - Lower, Magnetic Lengthening Device 0DH37JZ
  - Middle, Magnetic Lengthening Device 0DH27JZ
  - Upper, Magnetic Lengthening Device 0DH17JZ
- Extremity
  - Lower
    - Left 0YHB
    - Right 0YH9
  - Upper
    - Left 0XH7
    - Right 0XH6
- Eye
  - Left 08H1
  - Right 08H0
- Face 0WH2
- Fallopian Tube 0UH8
- Femoral Region
  - Left 0YH8
  - Right 0YH7
- Femoral Shaft
  - Left 0QH9
  - Right 0QH8
- Femur
  - Lower
    - Left 0QHC
    - Right 0QHB
  - Upper
    - Left 0QH7
    - Right 0QH6
- Fibula
  - Left 0QHK
  - Right 0QHJ
- Foot
  - Left 0YHN
  - Right 0YHM
- Gallbladder 0FH4
- Gastrointestinal Tract 0WHP
- Genitourinary Tract 0WHR
- Gland
  - Endocrine 0GHS
  - Salivary 0CHA
- Glenoid Cavity
  - Left 0PH8
  - Right 0PH7
- Hand
  - Left 0XHK
  - Right 0XHJ
- Head 0WH0
- Heart 02HA
- Humeral Head
  - Left 0PHD
  - Right 0PHC
- Humeral Shaft
  - Left 0PHG
  - Right 0PHF
- Ileum 0DHB
- Inguinal Region
  - Left 0YH6

Insertion of device in — *continued*
- Inguinal Region — *continued*
  - Right 0YH5
- Intestinal Tract
  - Lower Intestinal Tract 0DHD
  - Upper Intestinal Tract 0DH0
- Intestine
  - Large 0DHE
  - Small 0DH8
- Jaw
  - Lower 0WH5
  - Upper 0WH4
- Jejunum 0DHA
- Joint
  - Acromioclavicular
    - Left 0RHH
    - Right 0RHG
  - Ankle
    - Left 0SHG
    - Right 0SHF
  - Carpal
    - Left 0RHR
    - Right 0RHQ
  - Carpometacarpal
    - Left 0RHT
    - Right 0RHS
  - Cervical Vertebral 0RH1
  - Cervicothoracic Vertebral 0RH4
  - Coccygeal 0SH6
  - Elbow
    - Left 0RHM
    - Right 0RHL
  - Finger Phalangeal
    - Left 0RHX
    - Right 0RHW
  - Hip
    - Left 0SHB
    - Right 0SH9
  - Knee
    - Left 0SHD
    - Right 0SHC
  - Lumbar Vertebral 0SH0
  - Lumbosacral 0SH3
  - Metacarpophalangeal
    - Left 0RHV
    - Right 0RHU
  - Metatarsal-Phalangeal
    - Left 0SHN
    - Right 0SHM
  - Occipital-cervical 0RH0
  - Sacrococcygeal 0SH5
  - Sacroiliac
    - Left 0SH8
    - Right 0SH7
  - Shoulder
    - Left 0RHK
    - Right 0RHJ
  - Sternoclavicular
    - Left 0RHF
    - Right 0RHE
  - Tarsal
    - Left 0SHJ
    - Right 0SHH
  - Tarsometatarsal
    - Left 0SHL
    - Right 0SHK
  - Temporomandibular
    - Left 0RHD
    - Right 0RHC
  - Thoracic Vertebral 0RH6
  - Thoracolumbar Vertebral 0RHA
  - Toe Phalangeal
    - Left 0SHQ
    - Right 0SHP
  - Wrist
    - Left 0RHP
    - Right 0RHN
- Kidney 0TH5
- Knee Region
  - Left 0YHG
  - Right 0YHF
- Larynx 0CHS
- Leg
  - Lower
    - Left 0YHJ
    - Right 0YHH
  - Upper
    - Left 0YHD
    - Right 0YHC

Insertion of device in — *continued*
- Liver 0FH0
  - Left Lobe 0FH2
  - Right Lobe 0FH1
- Lung
  - Left 0BHL
  - Right 0BHK
- Lymphatic 07HN
  - Thoracic Duct 07HK
- Mandible
  - Left 0NHV
  - Right 0NHT
- Maxilla 0NHR
- Mediastinum 0WHC
- Metacarpal
  - Left 0PHQ
  - Right 0PHP
- Metatarsal
  - Left 0QHP
  - Right 0QHN
- Mouth and Throat 0CHY
- Muscle
  - Lower 0KHY
  - Upper 0KHX
- Nasal Mucosa and Soft Tissue 09HK
- Nasopharynx 09HN
- Neck 0WH6
- Nerve
  - Cranial 00HE
  - Peripheral 01HY
- Nipple
  - Left 0HHX
  - Right 0HHW
- Oral Cavity and Throat 0WH3
- Orbit
  - Left 0NHQ
  - Right 0NHP
- Ovary 0UH3
- Pancreas 0FHG
- Patella
  - Left 0QHF
  - Right 0QHD
- Pelvic Cavity 0WHJ
- Penis 0VHS
- Pericardial Cavity 0WHD
- Pericardium 02HN
- Perineum
  - Female 0WHN
  - Male 0WHM
- Peritoneal Cavity 0WHG
- Phalanx
  - Finger
    - Left 0PHV
    - Right 0PHT
  - Thumb
    - Left 0PHS
    - Right 0PHR
  - Toe
    - Left 0QHR
    - Right 0QHQ
- Pleura 0BHQ
- Pleural Cavity
  - Left 0WHB
  - Right 0WH9
- Prostate 0VH0
- Prostate and Seminal Vesicles 0VH4
- Radius
  - Left 0PHJ
  - Right 0PHH
- Rectum 0DHP
- Respiratory Tract 0WHQ
- Retroperitoneum 0WHH
- Ribs
  - 1 to 2 0PH1
  - 3 or More 0PH2
- Sacrum 0QH1
- Scapula
  - Left 0PH6
  - Right 0PH5
- Scrotum and Tunica Vaginalis 0VH8
- Shoulder Region
  - Left 0XH3
  - Right 0XH2
- Sinus 09HY
- Skin 0HHPXYZ
- Skull 0NH0
- Spinal Canal 00HU
- Spinal Cord 00HV
- Spleen 07HP

Insertion of device in — continued
- Sternum 0PH0
- Stomach 0DH6
- Subcutaneous Tissue and Fascia
  - Abdomen 0JH8
  - Back 0JH7
  - Buttock 0JH9
  - Chest 0JH6
  - Face 0JH1
  - Foot
    - Left 0JHR
    - Right 0JHQ
  - Hand
    - Left 0JHK
    - Right 0JHJ
  - Head and Neck 0JHS
  - Lower Arm
    - Left 0JHH
    - Right 0JHG
  - Lower Extremity 0JHW
  - Lower Leg
    - Left 0JHP
    - Right 0JHN
  - Neck
    - Left 0JH5
    - Right 0JH4
  - Pelvic Region 0JHC
  - Perineum 0JHB
  - Scalp 0JH0
  - Trunk 0JHT
  - Upper Arm
    - Left 0JHF
    - Right 0JHD
  - Upper Extremity 0JHV
  - Upper Leg
    - Left 0JHM
    - Right 0JHL
- Tarsal
  - Left 0QHM
  - Right 0QHL
- Tendon
  - Lower 0LHY
  - Upper 0LHX
- Testis 0VHD
- Thymus 07HM
- Tibia
  - Left 0QHH
  - Right 0QHG
- Tongue 0CH7
- Trachea 0BH1
- Tracheobronchial Tree 0BH0
- Ulna
  - Left 0PHL
  - Right 0PHK
- Ureter 0TH9
- Urethra 0THD
- Uterus 0UH9
- Uterus and Cervix 0UHD
- Vagina 0UHG
- Vagina and Cul-de-sac 0UHH
- Vas Deferens 0VHR
- Vein
  - Axillary
    - Left 05H8
    - Right 05H7
  - Azygos 05H0
  - Basilic
    - Left 05HC
    - Right 05HB
  - Brachial
    - Left 05HA
    - Right 05H9
  - Cephalic
    - Left 05HF
    - Right 05HD
  - Colic 06H7
  - Common Iliac
    - Left 06HD
    - Right 06HC
  - Coronary 02H4
  - Esophageal 06H3
  - External Iliac
    - Left 06HG
    - Right 06HF
  - External Jugular
    - Left 05HQ
    - Right 05HP
  - Face
    - Left 05HV

Insertion of device in — continued
- Vein — continued
  - Face — continued
    - Right 05HT
  - Femoral
    - Left 06HN
    - Right 06HM
  - Foot
    - Left 06HV
    - Right 06HT
  - Gastric 06H2
  - Hand
    - Left 05HH
    - Right 05HG
  - Hemiazygos 05H1
  - Hepatic 06H4
  - Hypogastric
    - Left 06HJ
    - Right 06HH
  - Inferior Mesenteric 06H6
  - Innominate
    - Left 05H4
    - Right 05H3
  - Internal Jugular
    - Left 05HN
    - Right 05HM
  - Intracranial 05HL
  - Lower 06HY
  - Portal 06H8
  - Pulmonary
    - Left 02HT
    - Right 02HS
  - Renal
    - Left 06HB
    - Right 06H9
  - Saphenous
    - Left 06HQ
    - Right 06HP
  - Splenic 06H1
  - Subclavian
    - Left 05H6
    - Right 05H5
  - Superior Mesenteric 06H5
  - Upper 05HY
  - Vertebral
    - Left 05HS
    - Right 05HR
- Vena Cava
  - Inferior 06H0
  - Superior 02HV
- Ventricle
  - Left 02HL
  - Right 02HK
- Vertebra
  - Cervical 0PH3
  - Lumbar 0QH0
  - Thoracic 0PH4
- Wrist Region
  - Left 0XHH
  - Right 0XHG

Inspection
- Abdominal Wall 0WJF
- Ankle Region
  - Left 0YJL
  - Right 0YJK
- Arm
  - Lower
    - Left 0XJF
    - Right 0XJD
  - Upper
    - Left 0XJ9
    - Right 0XJ8
- Artery
  - Lower 04JY
  - Upper 03JY
- Axilla
  - Left 0XJ5
  - Right 0XJ4
- Back
  - Lower 0WJL
  - Upper 0WJK
- Bladder 0TJB
- Bone
  - Facial 0NJW
  - Lower 0QJY
  - Nasal 0NJB
  - Upper 0PJY
- Bone Marrow 07JT
- Brain 00J0

Inspection — continued
- Breast
  - Left 0HJU
  - Right 0HJT
- Bursa and Ligament
  - Lower 0MJY
  - Upper 0MJX
- Buttock
  - Left 0YJ1
  - Right 0YJ0
- Cavity, Cranial 0WJ1
- Chest Wall 0WJ8
- Cisterna Chyli 07JL
- Diaphragm 0BJT
- Disc
  - Cervical Vertebral 0RJ3
  - Cervicothoracic Vertebral 0RJ5
  - Lumbar Vertebral 0SJ2
  - Lumbosacral 0SJ4
  - Thoracic Vertebral 0RJ9
  - Thoracolumbar Vertebral 0RJB
- Duct
  - Hepatobiliary 0FJB
  - Pancreatic 0FJD
- Ear
  - Inner
    - Left 09JE
    - Right 09JD
  - Left 09JJ
  - Right 09JH
- Elbow Region
  - Left 0XJC
  - Right 0XJB
- Epididymis and Spermatic Cord 0VJM
- Extremity
  - Lower
    - Left 0YJB
    - Right 0YJ9
  - Upper
    - Left 0XJ7
    - Right 0XJ6
- Eye
  - Left 08J1XZZ
  - Right 08J0XZZ
- Face 0WJ2
- Fallopian Tube 0UJ8
- Femoral Region
  - Bilateral 0YJE
  - Left 0YJ8
  - Right 0YJ7
- Finger Nail 0HJQXZZ
- Foot
  - Left 0YJN
  - Right 0YJM
- Gallbladder 0FJ4
- Gastrointestinal Tract 0WJP
- Genitourinary Tract 0WJR
- Gland
  - Adrenal 0GJ5
  - Endocrine 0GJS
  - Pituitary 0GJ0
  - Salivary 0CJA
- Great Vessel 02JY
- Hand
  - Left 0XJK
  - Right 0XJJ
- Head 0WJ0
- Heart 02JA
- Inguinal Region
  - Bilateral 0YJA
  - Left 0YJ6
  - Right 0YJ5
- Intestinal Tract
  - Lower Intestinal Tract 0DJD
  - Upper Intestinal Tract 0DJ0
- Jaw
  - Lower 0WJ5
  - Upper 0WJ4
- Joint
  - Acromioclavicular
    - Left 0RJH
    - Right 0RJG
  - Ankle
    - Left 0SJG
    - Right 0SJF
  - Carpal
    - Left 0RJR
    - Right 0RJQ

Inspection — *continued*
  Joint — *continued*
    Carpometacarpal
      Left ØRJT
      Right ØRJS
    Cervical Vertebral ØRJ1
    Cervicothoracic Vertebral ØRJ4
    Coccygeal ØSJ6
    Elbow
      Left ØRJM
      Right ØRJL
    Finger Phalangeal
      Left ØRJX
      Right ØRJW
    Hip
      Left ØSJB
      Right ØSJ9
    Knee
      Left ØSJD
      Right ØSJC
    Lumbar Vertebral ØSJØ
    Lumbosacral ØSJ3
    Metacarpophalangeal
      Left ØRJV
      Right ØRJU
    Metatarsal-Phalangeal
      Left ØSJN
      Right ØSJM
    Occipital-cervical ØRJØ
    Sacrococcygeal ØSJ5
    Sacroiliac
      Left ØSJ8
      Right ØSJ7
    Shoulder
      Left ØRJK
      Right ØRJJ
    Sternoclavicular
      Left ØRJF
      Right ØRJE
    Tarsal
      Left ØSJJ
      Right ØSJH
    Tarsometatarsal
      Left ØSJL
      Right ØSJK
    Temporomandibular
      Left ØRJD
      Right ØRJC
    Thoracic Vertebral ØRJ6
    Thoracolumbar Vertebral ØRJA
    Toe Phalangeal
      Left ØSJQ
      Right ØSJP
    Wrist
      Left ØRJP
      Right ØRJN
  Kidney ØTJ5
  Knee Region
    Left ØYJG
    Right ØYJF
  Larynx ØCJS
  Leg
    Lower
      Left ØYJJ
      Right ØYJH
    Upper
      Left ØYJD
      Right ØYJC
  Lens
    Left Ø8JKXZZ
    Right Ø8JJXZZ
  Liver ØFJØ
  Lung
    Left ØBJL
    Right ØBJK
  Lymphatic Ø7JN
    Thoracic Duct Ø7JK
  Mediastinum ØWJC
  Mesentery ØDJV
  Mouth and Throat ØCJY
  Muscle
    Extraocular
      Left Ø8JM
      Right Ø8JL
    Lower ØKJY
    Upper ØKJX
  Nasal Mucosa and Soft Tissue Ø9JK
  Neck ØWJ6

Inspection — *continued*
  Nerve
    Cranial ØØJE
    Peripheral Ø1JY
  Omentum ØDJU
  Oral Cavity and Throat ØWJ3
  Ovary ØUJ3
  Pancreas ØFJG
  Parathyroid Gland ØGJR
  Pelvic Cavity ØWJJ
  Penis ØVJS
  Pericardial Cavity ØWJD
  Perineum
    Female ØWJN
    Male ØWJM
  Peritoneal Cavity ØWJG
  Peritoneum ØDJW
  Pineal Body ØGJ1
  Pleura ØBJQ
  Pleural Cavity
    Left ØWJB
    Right ØWJ9
  Products of Conception 10JØ
    Ectopic 10J2
    Retained 10J1
  Prostate and Seminal Vesicles ØVJ4
  Respiratory Tract ØWJQ
  Retroperitoneum ØWJH
  Scrotum and Tunica Vaginalis ØVJ8
  Shoulder Region
    Left ØXJ3
    Right ØXJ2
  Sinus Ø9JY
  Skin ØHJPXZZ
  Skull ØNJØ
  Spinal Canal ØØJU
  Spinal Cord ØØJV
  Spleen Ø7JP
  Stomach ØDJ6
  Subcutaneous Tissue and Fascia
    Head and Neck ØJJS
    Lower Extremity ØJJW
    Trunk ØJJT
    Upper Extremity ØJJV
  Tendon
    Lower ØLJY
    Upper ØLJX
  Testis ØVJD
  Thymus Ø7JM
  Thyroid Gland ØGJK
  Toe Nail ØHJRXZZ
  Trachea ØBJ1
  Tracheobronchial Tree ØBJØ
  Tympanic Membrane
    Left Ø9J8
    Right Ø9J7
  Ureter ØTJ9
  Urethra ØTJD
  Uterus and Cervix ØUJD
  Vagina and Cul-de-sac ØUJH
  Vas Deferens ØVJR
  Vein
    Lower Ø6JY
    Upper Ø5JY
  Vulva ØUJM
  Wrist Region
    Left ØXJH
    Right ØXJG
Inspiris Resilia valve *use* Zooplastic Tissue in Heart and Great Vessels
Instillation *see* Introduction of substance in or on
Insufflation *see* Introduction of substance in or on
Intellis™ neurostimulator *use* Stimulator Generator, Multiple Array Rechargeable in ØJH
Interatrial septum *use* Atrial Septum
InterAtrial Shunt Device IASD®, Corvia *use* Synthetic Substitute
Interbody fusion (spine) cage
  use Interbody Fusion Device in Lower Joints
  use Interbody Fusion Device in Upper Joints
Interbody Fusion Device, Custom-Made Anatomically Designed
  Lumbar Vertebral XRGB
    2 or more XRGC
  Lumbosacral XRGD
  Thoracolumbar Vertebral XRGA
Intercarpal joint
  use Carpal Joint, Left

Intercarpal joint — *continued*
  use Carpal Joint, Right
Intercarpal ligament
  use Hand Bursa and Ligament, Left
  use Hand Bursa and Ligament, Right
INTERCEPT Blood System for Plasma Pathogen Reduced Cryoprecipitated Fibrinogen Complex *use* Pathogen Reduced Cryoprecipitated Fibrinogen Complex
INTERCEPT Fibrinogen Complex *use* Pathogen Reduced Cryoprecipitated Fibrinogen Complex
Interclavicular ligament
  use Shoulder Bursa and Ligament, Left
  use Shoulder Bursa and Ligament, Right
Intercostal lymph node *use* Lymphatic, Thorax
Intercostal muscle
  use Thorax Muscle, Left
  use Thorax Muscle, Right
Intercostal nerve *use* Thoracic Nerve
Intercostobrachial nerve *use* Thoracic Nerve
Intercuneiform joint
  use Tarsal Joint, Left
  use Tarsal Joint, Right
Intercuneiform ligament
  use Foot Bursa and Ligament, Left
  use Foot Bursa and Ligament, Right
Intermediate bronchus *use* Main Bronchus, Right
Intermediate cuneiform bone
  use Tarsal, Left
  use Tarsal, Right
Intermittent Coronary Sinus Occlusion X2A7358
Intermittent hemodialysis (IHD) 5A1D7ØZ
Intermittent mandatory ventilation *see* Assistance, Respiratory 5AØ9
Intermittent Negative Airway Pressure
  24-96 Consecutive Hours, Ventilation 5AØ945B
  Greater than 96 Consecutive Hours, Ventilation 5AØ955B
  Less than 24 Consecutive Hours, Ventilation 5AØ935B
Intermittent Positive Airway Pressure
  24-96 Consecutive Hours, Ventilation 5AØ9458
  Greater than 96 Consecutive Hours, Ventilation 5AØ9558
  Less than 24 Consecutive Hours, Ventilation 5AØ9358
Intermittent positive pressure breathing *see* Assistance, Respiratory 5AØ9
Internal anal sphincter *use* Anal Sphincter
Internal carotid artery, intracranial portion *use* Intracranial Artery
Internal carotid plexus *use* Head and Neck Sympathetic Nerve
Internal (basal) cerebral vein *use* Intracranial Vein
Internal Fixation Device with Tulip Connector
  Fusion, Joint, Sacroiliac XRG
  Insertion, Bone, Pelvic XNH
Internal iliac vein
  use Hypogastric Vein, Left
  use Hypogastric Vein, Right
Internal maxillary artery
  use External Carotid Artery, Left
  use External Carotid Artery, Right
Internal naris *use* Nasal Mucosa and Soft Tissue
Internal oblique muscle
  use Abdomen Muscle, Left
  use Abdomen Muscle, Right
Internal pudendal artery
  use Internal Iliac Artery, Left
  use Internal Iliac Artery, Right
Internal pudendal vein
  use Hypogastric Vein, Left
  use Hypogastric Vein, Right
Internal thoracic artery
  use Internal Mammary Artery, Left
  use Internal Mammary Artery, Right
  use Subclavian Artery, Left
  use Subclavian Artery, Right
Internal urethral sphincter *use* Urethra
Interphalangeal (IP) joint
  use Finger Phalangeal Joint, Left
  use Finger Phalangeal Joint, Right
  use Toe Phalangeal Joint, Left
  use Toe Phalangeal Joint, Right
Interphalangeal ligament
  use Foot Bursa and Ligament, Left
  use Foot Bursa and Ligament, Right

Interphalangeal ligament — continued
  use Hand Bursa and Ligament, Left
  use Hand Bursa and Ligament, Right
Interrogation, cardiac rhythm related device
  Interrogation only see Measurement, Cardiac 4B02
  With cardiac function testing see Measurement, Cardiac 4A02
Interruption see Occlusion
Interspinalis muscle
  use Trunk Muscle, Left
  use Trunk Muscle, Right
Interspinous ligament, cervical use Head and Neck Bursa and Ligament
Interspinous ligament, lumbar use Lower Spine Bursa and Ligament
Interspinous ligament, thoracic use Upper Spine Bursa and Ligament
Interspinous process spinal stabilization device
  use Spinal Stabilization Device, Interspinous Process in 0RH
  use Spinal Stabilization Device, Interspinous Process in 0SH
InterStim® Therapy lead use Neurostimulator Lead in Peripheral Nervous System
InterStim™ II Therapy neurostimulator use Stimulator Generator, Single Array in 0JH
InterStim™ Micro Therapy neurostimulator use Stimulator Generator, Single Array Rechargeable in 0JH
Interstitial Fluid Volume, Sub-Epidermal Moisture using Electrical Biocapacitance XX2KXP9
Intertransversarius muscle
  use Trunk Muscle, Left
  use Trunk Muscle, Right
Intertransverse ligament, cervical use Head and Neck Bursa and Ligament
Intertransverse ligament, lumbar use Lower Spine Bursa and Ligament
Intertransverse ligament, thoracic use Upper Spine Bursa and Ligament
Interventricular foramen (Monro) use Cerebral Ventricle
Interventricular septum use Ventricular Septum
Intestinal lymphatic trunk use Cisterna Chyli
Intracardiac Pacemaker, Dual-Chamber, Insertion X2H
Intracranial Arterial Flow, Whole Blood mRNA XXE5XT7
Intracranial Cerebrospinal Fluid Flow, Computer-aided Triage and Notification XXE0X1A
Intraluminal Bioprosthetic Valve Leaflet Splitting Technology in Existing Valve, Division X28F3VA
Intraluminal Device
  Airway
    Esophagus 0DH5
    Mouth and Throat 0CHY
    Nasopharynx 09HN
  Bioactive
    Occlusion
      Common Carotid
        Left 03LJ
        Right 03LH
      External Carotid
        Left 03LN
        Right 03LM
      Internal Carotid
        Left 03LL
        Right 03LK
      Intracranial 03LG
      Vertebral
        Left 03LQ
        Right 03LP
    Restriction
      Common Carotid
        Left 03VJ
        Right 03VH
      External Carotid
        Left 03VN
        Right 03VM
      Internal Carotid
        Left 03VL
        Right 03VK
      Intracranial 03VG
      Vertebral
        Left 03VQ
        Right 03VP
  Bioprosthetic Valve, Insertion X2H

Intraluminal Device — continued
  Endobronchial Valve
    Lingula 0BH9
    Lower Lobe
      Left 0BHB
      Right 0BH6
    Main
      Left 0BH7
      Right 0BH3
    Middle Lobe, Right 0BH5
    Upper Lobe
      Left 0BH8
      Right 0BH4
  Endotracheal Airway
    Change device in, Trachea 0B21XEZ
    Insertion of device in, Trachea 0BH1
  Everolimus-eluting Resorbable Scaffold(s)
    Anterior Tibial
      Left X27Q3TA
      Right X27P3TA
    Peroneal
      Left X27U3TA
      Right X27T3TA
    Posterior Tibial
      Left X27S3TA
      Right X27R3TA
  Pessary
    Change device in, Vagina and Cul-de-sac 0U2HXGZ
    Insertion of device in
      Cul-de-sac 0UHF
      Vagina 0UHG
Intramedullary (IM) rod (nail)
  use Internal Fixation Device, Intramedullary in Lower Bones
  use Internal Fixation Device, Intramedullary in Upper Bones
Intramedullary skeletal kinetic distractor (ISKD)
  use Internal Fixation Device, Intramedullary in Lower Bones
  use Internal Fixation Device, Intramedullary in Upper Bones
Intraocular Telescope
  Left 08RK30Z
  Right 08RJ30Z
Intraoperative Radiation Therapy (IORT)
  Anus DDY8CZZ
  Bile Ducts DFY2CZZ
  Bladder DTY2CZZ
  Brain D0Y0CZZ
  Brain Stem D0Y1CZZ
  Cervix DUY1CZZ
  Colon DDY5CZZ
  Duodenum DDY2CZZ
  Gallbladder DFY1CZZ
  Ileum DDY4CZZ
  Jejunum DDY3CZZ
  Kidney DTY0CZZ
  Larynx D9YBCZZ
  Liver DFY0CZZ
  Mouth D9Y4CZZ
  Nasopharynx D9YDCZZ
  Nerve, Peripheral D0Y7CZZ
  Ovary DUY0CZZ
  Pancreas DFY3CZZ
  Pharynx D9YCCZZ
  Prostate DVY0CZZ
  Rectum DDY7CZZ
  Spinal Cord D0Y6CZZ
  Stomach DDY1CZZ
  Ureter DTY1CZZ
  Urethra DTY3CZZ
  Uterus DUY2CZZ
Intra.OX 8E02XDZ
Intrauterine Device (IUD) use Contraceptive Device in Female Reproductive System
Intravascular fluorescence angiography (IFA) see Monitoring, Physiological Systems 4A1
Intravascular Lithotripsy (IVL) see Fragmentation
Intravascular ultrasound assisted thrombolysis see Fragmentation, Artery
Introduction of substance in or on
  Artery
    Central 3E06
      Analgesics 3E06
      Anesthetic, Intracirculatory 3E06
      Antiarrhythmic 3E06
      Anti-infective 3E06

Introduction of substance in or on — continued
  Artery — continued
    Central — continued
      Anti-inflammatory 3E06
      Antineoplastic 3E06
      Destructive Agent 3E06
      Diagnostic Substance, Other 3E06
      Electrolytic Substance 3E06
      Hormone 3E06
      Hypnotics 3E06
      Immunotherapeutic 3E06
      Nutritional Substance 3E06
      Platelet Inhibitor 3E06
      Radioactive Substance 3E06
      Sedatives 3E06
      Serum 3E06
      Thrombolytic 3E06
      Toxoid 3E06
      Vaccine 3E06
      Vasopressor 3E06
      Water Balance Substance 3E06
    Coronary 3E07
      Diagnostic Substance, Other 3E07
      Platelet Inhibitor 3E07
      Thrombolytic 3E07
    Peripheral 3E05
      Analgesics 3E05
      Anesthetic, Intracirculatory 3E05
      Antiarrhythmic 3E05
      Anti-infective 3E05
      Anti-inflammatory 3E05
      Antineoplastic 3E05
      Destructive Agent 3E05
      Diagnostic Substance, Other 3E05
      Electrolytic Substance 3E05
      Hormone 3E05
      Hypnotics 3E05
      Immunotherapeutic 3E05
      Nutritional Substance 3E05
      Platelet Inhibitor 3E05
      Radioactive Substance 3E05
      Sedatives 3E05
      Serum 3E05
      Thrombolytic 3E05
      Toxoid 3E05
      Vaccine 3E05
      Vasopressor 3E05
      Water Balance Substance 3E05
  Biliary Tract 3E0J
    Analgesics 3E0J
    Anesthetic Agent 3E0J
    Anti-infective 3E0J
    Anti-inflammatory 3E0J
    Antineoplastic 3E0J
    Destructive Agent 3E0J
    Diagnostic Substance, Other 3E0J
    Electrolytic Substance 3E0J
    Gas 3E0J
    Hypnotics 3E0J
    Islet Cells, Pancreatic 3E0J
    Nutritional Substance 3E0J
    Radioactive Substance 3E0J
    Sedatives 3E0J
    Water Balance Substance 3E0J
  Bone 3E0V
    Analgesics 3E0V3NZ
    Anesthetic Agent 3E0V3BZ
    Anti-infective 3E0V32
    Anti-inflammatory 3E0V33Z
    Antineoplastic 3E0V30
    Destructive Agent 3E0V3TZ
    Diagnostic Substance, Other 3E0V3KZ
    Electrolytic Substance 3E0V37Z
    Hypnotics 3E0V3NZ
    Nutritional Substance 3E0V36Z
    Radioactive Substance 3E0V3HZ
    Sedatives 3E0V3NZ
    Water Balance Substance 3E0V37Z
  Bone Marrow 3E0A3GC
    Antineoplastic 3E0A30
  Brain 3E0Q
    Analgesics 3E0Q
    Anesthetic Agent 3E0Q
    Anti-infective 3E0Q
    Anti-inflammatory 3E0Q
    Antineoplastic 3E0Q
    Destructive Agent 3E0Q
    Diagnostic Substance, Other 3E0Q
    Electrolytic Substance 3E0Q

Introduction of substance in or on — *continued*
   Brain — *continued*
     Gas 3E0Q
     Hypnotics 3E0Q
     Nutritional Substance 3E0Q
     Radioactive Substance 3E0Q
     Sedatives 3E0Q
     Stem Cells
       Embryonic 3E0Q
       Somatic 3E0Q
     Water Balance Substance 3E0Q
   Cranial Cavity 3E0Q
     Analgesics 3E0Q
     Anesthetic Agent 3E0Q
     Anti-infective 3E0Q
     Anti-inflammatory 3E0Q
     Antineoplastic 3E0Q
     Destructive Agent 3E0Q
     Diagnostic Substance, Other 3E0Q
     Electrolytic Substance 3E0Q
     Gas 3E0Q
     Hypnotics 3E0Q
     Nutritional Substance 3E0Q
     Radioactive Substance 3E0Q
     Sedatives 3E0Q
     Stem Cells
       Embryonic 3E0Q
       Somatic 3E0Q
     Water Balance Substance 3E0Q
   Ear 3E0B
     Analgesics 3E0B
     Anesthetic Agent 3E0B
     Anti-infective 3E0B
     Anti-inflammatory 3E0B
     Antineoplastic 3E0B
     Destructive Agent 3E0B
     Diagnostic Substance, Other 3E0B
     Hypnotics 3E0B
     Radioactive Substance 3E0B
     Sedatives 3E0B
   Epidural Space 3E0S3GC
     Analgesics 3E0S3NZ
     Anesthetic Agent 3E0S3BZ
     Anti-infective 3E0S32
     Anti-inflammatory 3E0S33Z
     Antineoplastic 3E0S30
     Destructive Agent 3E0S3TZ
     Diagnostic Substance, Other 3E0S3KZ
     Electrolytic Substance 3E0S37Z
     Gas 3E0S
     Hypnotics 3E0S3NZ
     Nutritional Substance 3E0S36Z
     Radioactive Substance 3E0S3HZ
     Sedatives 3E0S3NZ
     Water Balance Substance 3E0S37Z
   Eye 3E0C
     Analgesics 3E0C
     Anesthetic Agent 3E0C
     Anti-infective 3E0C
     Anti-inflammatory 3E0C
     Antineoplastic 3E0C
     Destructive Agent 3E0C
     Diagnostic Substance, Other 3E0C
     Gas 3E0C
     Hypnotics 3E0C
     Pigment 3E0C
     Radioactive Substance 3E0C
     Sedatives 3E0C
   Gastrointestinal Tract
     Lower 3E0H
       Analgesics 3E0H
       Anesthetic Agent 3E0H
       Anti-infective 3E0H
       Anti-inflammatory 3E0H
       Antineoplastic 3E0H
       Destructive Agent 3E0H
       Diagnostic Substance, Other 3E0H
       Electrolytic Substance 3E0H
       Gas 3E0H
       Hypnotics 3E0H
       Nutritional Substance 3E0H
       Radioactive Substance 3E0H
       Sedatives 3E0H
       Water Balance Substance 3E0H
     Upper 3E0G
       Analgesics 3E0G
       Anesthetic Agent 3E0G
       Anti-infective 3E0G
       Anti-inflammatory 3E0G

Introduction of substance in or on — *continued*
   Gastrointestinal Tract — *continued*
     Upper — *continued*
       Antineoplastic 3E0G
       Destructive Agent 3E0G
       Diagnostic Substance, Other 3E0G
       Electrolytic Substance 3E0G
       Gas 3E0G
       Hypnotics 3E0G
       Nutritional Substance 3E0G
       Radioactive Substance 3E0G
       Sedatives 3E0G
       Water Balance Substance 3E0G
   Genitourinary Tract 3E0K
     Analgesics 3E0K
     Anesthetic Agent 3E0K
     Anti-infective 3E0K
     Anti-inflammatory 3E0K
     Antineoplastic 3E0K
     Destructive Agent 3E0K
     Diagnostic Substance, Other 3E0K
     Electrolytic Substance 3E0K
     Gas 3E0K
     Hypnotics 3E0K
     Nutritional Substance 3E0K
     Radioactive Substance 3E0K
     Sedatives 3E0K
     Water Balance Substance 3E0K
   Heart 3E08
     Diagnostic Substance, Other 3E08
     Platelet Inhibitor 3E08
     Thrombolytic 3E08
   Joint 3E0U
     Analgesics 3E0U3NZ
     Anesthetic Agent 3E0U3BZ
     Anti-infective 3E0U
     Anti-inflammatory 3E0U33Z
     Antineoplastic 3E0U30
     Destructive Agent 3E0U3TZ
     Diagnostic Substance, Other 3E0U3KZ
     Electrolytic Substance 3E0U37Z
     Gas 3E0U3SF
     Hypnotics 3E0U3NZ
     Nutritional Substance 3E0U36Z
     Radioactive Substance 3E0U3HZ
     Sedatives 3E0U3NZ
     Water Balance Substance 3E0U37Z
   Lymphatic 3E0W3GC
     Analgesics 3E0W3NZ
     Anesthetic Agent 3E0W3BZ
     Anti-infective 3E0W32
     Anti-inflammatory 3E0W33Z
     Antineoplastic 3E0W30
     Destructive Agent 3E0W3TZ
     Diagnostic Substance, Other 3E0W3KZ
     Electrolytic Substance 3E0W37Z
     Hypnotics 3E0W3NZ
     Nutritional Substance 3E0W36Z
     Radioactive Substance 3E0W3HZ
     Sedatives 3E0W3NZ
     Water Balance Substance 3E0W37Z
   Mouth 3E0D
     Analgesics 3E0D
     Anesthetic Agent 3E0D
     Antiarrhythmic 3E0D
     Anti-infective 3E0D
     Anti-inflammatory 3E0D
     Antineoplastic 3E0D
     Destructive Agent 3E0D
     Diagnostic Substance, Other 3E0D
     Electrolytic Substance 3E0D
     Hypnotics 3E0D
     Nutritional Substance 3E0D
     Radioactive Substance 3E0D
     Sedatives 3E0D
     Serum 3E0D
     Toxoid 3E0D
     Vaccine 3E0D
     Water Balance Substance 3E0D
   Mucous Membrane 3E00XGC
     Analgesics 3E00XNZ
     Anesthetic Agent 3E00XBZ
     Anti-infective 3E00X2
     Anti-inflammatory 3E00X3Z
     Antineoplastic 3E00X0
     Destructive Agent 3E00XTZ
     Diagnostic Substance, Other 3E00XKZ
     Hypnotics 3E00XNZ
     Pigment 3E00XMZ

Introduction of substance in or on — *continued*
   Mucous Membrane — *continued*
     Sedatives 3E00XNZ
     Serum 3E00X4Z
     Toxoid 3E00X4Z
     Vaccine 3E00X4Z
   Muscle 3E023GC
     Analgesics 3E023NZ
     Anesthetic Agent 3E023BZ
     Anti-infective 3E0232
     Anti-inflammatory 3E0233Z
     Antineoplastic 3E0230
     Destructive Agent 3E023TZ
     Diagnostic Substance, Other 3E023KZ
     Electrolytic Substance 3E0237Z
     Hypnotics 3E023NZ
     Nutritional Substance 3E0236Z
     Radioactive Substance 3E023HZ
     Sedatives 3E023NZ
     Serum 3E0234Z
     Toxoid 3E0234Z
     Vaccine 3E0234Z
     Water Balance Substance 3E0237Z
   Nerve
     Cranial 3E0X3GC
       Anesthetic Agent 3E0X3BZ
       Anti-inflammatory 3E0X33Z
       Destructive Agent 3E0X3TZ
     Peripheral 3E0T3GC
       Anesthetic Agent 3E0T3BZ
       Anti-inflammatory 3E0T33Z
       Destructive Agent 3E0T3TZ
     Plexus 3E0T3GC
       Anesthetic Agent 3E0T3BZ
       Anti-inflammatory 3E0T33Z
       Destructive Agent 3E0T3TZ
   Nose 3E09
     Analgesics 3E09
     Anesthetic Agent 3E09
     Anti-infective 3E09
     Anti-inflammatory 3E09
     Antineoplastic 3E09
     Destructive Agent 3E09
     Diagnostic Substance, Other 3E09
     Hypnotics 3E09
     Radioactive Substance 3E09
     Sedatives 3E09
     Serum 3E09
     Toxoid 3E09
     Vaccine 3E09
   Pancreatic Tract 3E0J
     Analgesics 3E0J
     Anesthetic Agent 3E0J
     Anti-infective 3E0J
     Anti-inflammatory 3E0J
     Antineoplastic 3E0J
     Destructive Agent 3E0J
     Diagnostic Substance, Other 3E0J
     Electrolytic Substance 3E0J
     Gas 3E0J
     Hypnotics 3E0J
     Islet Cells, Pancreatic 3E0J
     Nutritional Substance 3E0J
     Radioactive Substance 3E0J
     Sedatives 3E0J
     Water Balance Substance 3E0J
   Pericardial Cavity 3E0Y
     Analgesics 3E0Y3NZ
     Anesthetic Agent 3E0Y3BZ
     Anti-infective 3E0Y32
     Anti-inflammatory 3E0Y33Z
     Antineoplastic 3E0Y
     Destructive Agent 3E0Y3TZ
     Diagnostic Substance, Other 3E0Y3KZ
     Electrolytic Substance 3E0Y37Z
     Gas 3E0Y
     Hypnotics 3E0Y3NZ
     Nutritional Substance 3E0Y36Z
     Radioactive Substance 3E0Y3HZ
     Sedatives 3E0Y3NZ
     Water Balance Substance 3E0Y37Z
   Peritoneal Cavity 3E0M
     Adhesion Barrier 3E0M
     Analgesics 3E0M3NZ
     Anesthetic Agent 3E0M3BZ
     Anti-infective 3E0M32
     Anti-inflammatory 3E0M33Z
     Antineoplastic 3E0M
     Destructive Agent 3E0M3TZ

Subterms under main terms may continue to next column or page

Introduction of substance in or on — *continued*
  Peritoneal Cavity — *continued*
    Diagnostic Substance, Other 3E0M3KZ
    Electrolytic Substance 3E0M37Z
    Gas 3E0M
    Hypnotics 3E0M3NZ
    Nutritional Substance 3E0M36Z
    Radioactive Substance 3E0M3HZ
    Sedatives 3E0M3NZ
    Water Balance Substance 3E0M37Z
  Pharynx 3E0D
    Analgesics 3E0D
    Anesthetic Agent 3E0D
    Antiarrhythmic 3E0D
    Anti-infective 3E0D
    Anti-inflammatory 3E0D
    Antineoplastic 3E0D
    Destructive Agent 3E0D
    Diagnostic Substance, Other 3E0D
    Electrolytic Substance 3E0D
    Hypnotics 3E0D
    Nutritional Substance 3E0D
    Radioactive Substance 3E0D
    Sedatives 3E0D
    Serum 3E0D
    Toxoid 3E0D
    Vaccine 3E0D
    Water Balance Substance 3E0D
  Pleural Cavity 3E0L
    Adhesion Barrier 3E0L
    Analgesics 3E0L3NZ
    Anesthetic Agent 3E0L3BZ
    Anti-infective 3E0L32
    Anti-inflammatory 3E0L33Z
    Antineoplastic 3E0L
    Destructive Agent 3E0L3TZ
    Diagnostic Substance, Other 3E0L3KZ
    Electrolytic Substance 3E0L37Z
    Gas 3E0L
    Hypnotics 3E0L3NZ
    Nutritional Substance 3E0L36Z
    Radioactive Substance 3E0L3HZ
    Sedatives 3E0L3NZ
    Thrombolytic 3E0L317
    Water Balance Substance 3E0L37Z
  Products of Conception 3E0E
    Analgesics 3E0E
    Anesthetic Agent 3E0E
    Anti-infective 3E0E
    Anti-inflammatory 3E0E
    Antineoplastic 3E0E
    Destructive Agent 3E0E
    Diagnostic Substance, Other 3E0E
    Electrolytic Substance 3E0E
    Gas 3E0E
    Hypnotics 3E0E
    Nutritional Substance 3E0E
    Radioactive Substance 3E0E
    Sedatives 3E0E
    Water Balance Substance 3E0E
  Reproductive
    Female 3E0P
      Adhesion Barrier 3E0P
      Analgesics 3E0P
      Anesthetic Agent 3E0P
      Anti-infective 3E0P
      Anti-inflammatory 3E0P
      Antineoplastic 3E0P
      Destructive Agent 3E0P
      Diagnostic Substance, Other 3E0P
      Electrolytic Substance 3E0P
      Gas 3E0P
      Hormone 3E0P
      Hypnotics 3E0P
      Nutritional Substance 3E0P
      Ovum, Fertilized 3E0P
      Radioactive Substance 3E0P
      Sedatives 3E0P
      Sperm 3E0P
      Water Balance Substance 3E0P
    Male 3E0N
      Analgesics 3E0N
      Anesthetic Agent 3E0N
      Anti-infective 3E0N
      Anti-inflammatory 3E0N
      Antineoplastic 3E0N
      Destructive Agent 3E0N
      Diagnostic Substance, Other 3E0N
      Electrolytic Substance 3E0N

Introduction of substance in or on — *continued*
  Reproductive
    Male — *continued*
      Gas 3E0N
      Hypnotics 3E0N
      Nutritional Substance 3E0N
      Radioactive Substance 3E0N
      Sedatives 3E0N
      Water Balance Substance 3E0N
  Respiratory Tract 3E0F
    Analgesics 3E0F
    Anesthetic Agent 3E0F
    Anti-infective 3E0F
    Anti-inflammatory 3E0F
    Antineoplastic 3E0F
    Destructive Agent 3E0F
    Diagnostic Substance, Other 3E0F
    Electrolytic Substance 3E0F
    Gas 3E0F
    Hypnotics 3E0F
    Nutritional Substance 3E0F
    Radioactive Substance 3E0F
    Sedatives 3E0F
    Water Balance Substance 3E0F
  Skin 3E00XGC
    Analgesics 3E00XNZ
    Anesthetic Agent 3E00XBZ
    Anti-infective 3E00X2
    Anti-inflammatory 3E00X3Z
    Antineoplastic 3E00X0
    Destructive Agent 3E00XTZ
    Diagnostic Substance, Other 3E00XKZ
    Hypnotics 3E00XNZ
    Pigment 3E00XMZ
    Sedatives 3E00XNZ
    Serum 3E00X4Z
    Toxoid 3E00X4Z
    Vaccine 3E00X4Z
  Spinal Canal 3E0R3GC
    Analgesics 3E0R3NZ
    Anesthetic Agent 3E0R3BZ
    Anti-infective 3E0R32
    Anti-inflammatory 3E0R33Z
    Antineoplastic 3E0R30
    Destructive Agent 3E0R3TZ
    Diagnostic Substance, Other 3E0R3KZ
    Electrolytic Substance 3E0R37Z
    Gas 3E0R
    Hypnotics 3E0R3NZ
    Nutritional Substance 3E0R36Z
    Radioactive Substance 3E0R3HZ
    Sedatives 3E0R3NZ
    Stem Cells
      Embryonic 3E0R
      Somatic 3E0R
    Water Balance Substance 3E0R37Z
  Subcutaneous Tissue 3E013GC
    Analgesics 3E013NZ
    Anesthetic Agent 3E013BZ
    Anti-infective 3E01
    Anti-inflammatory 3E0133Z
    Antineoplastic 3E0130
    Destructive Agent 3E013TZ
    Diagnostic Substance, Other 3E013KZ
    Electrolytic Substance 3E0137Z
    Hormone 3E013V
    Hypnotics 3E013NZ
    Nutritional Substance 3E0136Z
    Radioactive Substance 3E013HZ
    Sedatives 3E013NZ
    Serum 3E0134Z
    Toxoid 3E0134Z
    Vaccine 3E0134Z
    Water Balance Substance 3E0137Z
  Vein
    Central 3E04
      Analgesics 3E04
      Anesthetic, Intracirculatory 3E04
      Antiarrhythmic 3E04
      Anti-infective 3E04
      Anti-inflammatory 3E04
      Antineoplastic 3E04
      Destructive Agent 3E04
      Diagnostic Substance, Other 3E04
      Electrolytic Substance 3E04
      Hormone 3E04
      Hypnotics 3E04
      Immunotherapeutic 3E04
      Nutritional Substance 3E04

Introduction of substance in or on — *continued*
  Vein — *continued*
    Central — *continued*
      Platelet Inhibitor 3E04
      Radioactive Substance 3E04
      Sedatives 3E04
      Serum 3E04
      Thrombolytic 3E04
      Toxoid 3E04
      Vaccine 3E04
      Vasopressor 3E04
      Water Balance Substance 3E04
    Peripheral 3E03
      Analgesics 3E03
      Anesthetic, Intracirculatory 3E03
      Antiarrhythmic 3E03
      Anti-infective 3E03
      Anti-inflammatory 3E03
      Antineoplastic 3E03
      Destructive Agent 3E03
      Diagnostic Substance, Other 3E03
      Electrolytic Substance 3E03
      Hormone 3E03
      Hypnotics 3E03
      Immunotherapeutic 3E03
      Islet Cells, Pancreatic 3E03
      Nutritional Substance 3E03
      Platelet Inhibitor 3E03
      Radioactive Substance 3E03
      Sedatives 3E03
      Serum 3E03
      Thrombolytic 3E03
      Toxoid 3E03
      Vaccine 3E03
      Vasopressor 3E03
      Water Balance Substance 3E03

Intubated prone positioning *see* Assistance, Respiratory 5A09
Intubation
  Airway
    see Insertion of device in, Esophagus 0DH5
    see Insertion of device in, Mouth and Throat 0CHY
    see Insertion of device in, Trachea 0BH1
  Drainage device *see* Drainage
  Feeding Device *see* Insertion of device in, Gastrointestinal System 0DH
INTUITY Elite valve system, EDWARDS (rapid deployment technique) *see* Replacement, Valve, Aortic 02RF
Iobenguane I-131 Antineoplastic XW0
Iobenguane I-131, High Specific Activity (HSA) *use* Iobenguane I-131 Antineoplastic
IPPB (intermittent positive pressure breathing) *see* Assistance, Respiratory 5A09
IRE (Irreversible Electroporation) *see* Destruction, Hepatobiliary System and Pancreas 0F5
Iridectomy
  see Excision, Eye 08B
  see Resection, Eye 08T
Iridoplasty
  see Repair, Eye 08Q
  see Replacement, Eye 08R
  see Supplement, Eye 08U
Iridotomy *see* Drainage, Eye 089
Irreversible Electroporation (IRE)
  see Destruction, Heart and Great Vessels 025
  see Destruction, Hepatobiliary System and Pancreas 0F5
Irrigation
  Biliary Tract, Irrigating Substance 3E1J
  Brain, Irrigating Substance 3E1Q38Z
  Cranial Cavity, Irrigating Substance 3E1Q38Z
  Ear, Irrigating Substance 3E1B
  Epidural Space, Irrigating Substance 3E1S38Z
  Eye, Irrigating Substance 3E1C
  Gastrointestinal Tract
    Lower, Irrigating Substance 3E1H
    Upper, Irrigating Substance 3E1G
  Genitourinary Tract, Irrigating Substance 3E1K
  Irrigating Substance 3C1ZX8Z
  Joint, Irrigating Substance 3E1U
  Mucous Membrane, Irrigating Substance 3E10
  Nose, Irrigating Substance 3E19
  Pancreatic Tract, Irrigating Substance 3E1J
  Pericardial Cavity, Irrigating Substance 3E1Y38Z
  Peritoneal Cavity
    Dialysate 3E1M39Z

Irrigation — continued
Peritoneal Cavity — continued
Irrigating Substance 3E1M
Pleural Cavity, Irrigating Substance 3E1L38Z
Reproductive
Female, Irrigating Substance 3E1P
Male, Irrigating Substance 3E1N
Respiratory Tract, Irrigating Substance 3E1F
Skin, Irrigating Substance 3E10
Spinal Canal, Irrigating Substance 3E1R38Z
Isavuconazole (isavuconazonium sulfate) use Other Anti-infective
Ischemic Stroke System (ISS500) use Neurostimulator Lead in New Technology
Ischiatic nerve use Sciatic Nerve
Ischiocavernosus muscle use Perineum Muscle
Ischiofemoral ligament
use Hip Bursa and Ligament, Left
use Hip Bursa and Ligament, Right
Ischium
use Pelvic Bone, Left
use Pelvic Bone, Right
ISC-REST kit
ISCDx XXE5XT7
QIAGEN Access Anti-SARS-CoV-2 Total Test XXE5XV7
QIAstat-Dx Respiratory SARS-CoV-2 Panel XXE97U7
Isolation 8E0ZXY6
Isotope Administration, Other Radiation, Whole Body DWY5G
ISS500 (Ischemic Stroke System) use Neurostimulator Lead in New Technology
Itrel (3) (4) neurostimulator use Stimulator Generator, Single Array in 0JH

J

JAKAFI® (Ruxolitinib) use Other Substance
Jejunal artery use Superior Mesenteric Artery
Jejunectomy
see Excision, Jejunum 0DBA
see Resection, Jejunum 0DTA
Jejunocolostomy
see Bypass, Gastrointestinal System 0D1
see Drainage, Gastrointestinal System 0D9
Jejunopexy
see Repair, Jejunum 0DQA
see Reposition, Jejunum 0DSA
Jejunostomy
see Bypass, Jejunum 0D1A
see Drainage, Jejunum 0D9A
Jejunotomy see Drainage, Jejunum 0D9A
Joint fixation plate
use Internal Fixation Device in Lower Joints
use Internal Fixation Device in Upper Joints
Joint liner (insert) use Liner in Lower Joints
Joint spacer (antibiotic)
use Spacer in Lower Joints
use Spacer in Upper Joints
Jugular body use Glomus Jugulare
Jugular lymph node
use Lymphatic, Left Neck
use Lymphatic, Right Neck
Juxtaductal aorta use Thoracic Aorta, Ascending/Arch

K

Kappa use Pacemaker, Dual Chamber in 0JH
Kcentra use 4-Factor Prothrombin Complex Concentrate
Keratectomy, kerectomy
see Excision, Eye 08B
see Resection, Eye 08T
Keratocentesis see Drainage, Eye 089
Keratoplasty
see Repair, Eye 08Q
see Replacement, Eye 08R
see Supplement, Eye 08U
Keratotomy
see Drainage, Eye 089
see Repair, Eye 08Q
Kerecis® (GraftGuide) (MariGen) (SurgiBind) (SurgiClose) use Nonautologous Tissue Substitute
KEVZARA® use Sarilumab

Keystone Heart TriGuard 3™ CEPD (cerebral embolic protection device) X2A6325
Kirschner wire (K-wire)
use Internal Fixation Device in Head and Facial Bones
use Internal Fixation Device in Lower Bones
use Internal Fixation Device in Lower Joints
use Internal Fixation Device in Upper Bones
use Internal Fixation Device in Upper Joints
Knee (implant) insert use Liner in Lower Joints
KUB x-ray see Plain Radiography, Kidney, Ureter and Bladder BT04
Kuntscher nail
use Internal Fixation Device, Intramedullary in Lower Bones
use Internal Fixation Device, Intramedullary in Upper Bones
KYMRIAH® use Tisagenlecleucel Immunotherapy

L

Labia majora use Vulva
Labia minora use Vulva
Labial gland
use Lower Lip
use Upper Lip
Labiectomy
see Excision, Female Reproductive System 0UB
see Resection, Female Reproductive System 0UT
Lacrimal canaliculus
use Lacrimal Duct, Left
use Lacrimal Duct, Right
Lacrimal punctum
use Lacrimal Duct, Left
use Lacrimal Duct, Right
Lacrimal sac
use Lacrimal Duct, Left
use Lacrimal Duct, Right
LAGB (laparoscopic adjustable gastric banding)
Initial procedure 0DV64CZ
Surgical correction see Revision of device in, Stomach 0DW6
Laminectomy
see Excision, Lower Bones 0QB
see Excision, Upper Bones 0PB
see Release, Central Nervous System and Cranial Nerves 00N
see Release, Peripheral Nervous System 01N
Laminotomy
see Drainage, Lower Bones 0Q9
see Drainage, Upper Bones 0P9
see Excision, Lower Bones 0QB
see Excision, Upper Bones 0PB
see Release, Central Nervous System and Cranial Nerves 00N
see Release, Lower Bones 0QN
see Release, Peripheral Nervous System 01N
see Release, Upper Bones 0PN
Lantidra™ use Donislecel-jujn Allogeneic Pancreatic Islet Cellular Suspension
Laparoscopic-assisted transanal pull-through
see Excision, Gastrointestinal System 0DB
see Resection, Gastrointestinal System 0DT
Laparoscopy see Inspection
Laparotomy
Drainage see Drainage, Peritoneal Cavity 0W9G
Exploratory see Inspection, Peritoneal Cavity 0WJG
LAP-BAND® adjustable gastric banding system use Extraluminal Device
Laryngectomy
see Excision, Larynx 0CBS
see Resection, Larynx 0CTS
Laryngocentesis see Drainage, Larynx 0C9S
Laryngogram see Fluoroscopy, Larynx B91J
Laryngopexy see Repair, Larynx 0CQS
Laryngopharynx use Pharynx
Laryngoplasty
see Repair, Larynx 0CQS
see Replacement, Larynx 0CRS
see Supplement, Larynx 0CUS
Laryngorrhaphy see Repair, Larynx 0CQS
Laryngoscopy 0CJS8ZZ
Laryngotomy see Drainage, Larynx 0C9S
Laser Interstitial Thermal Therapy
Ampulla of Vater 0F5C
Anus 0D5Q

Laser Interstitial Thermal Therapy — continued
Aortic Body 0G5D
Appendix 0D5J
Brain 0050
Breast
Bilateral 0H5V
Left 0H5U
Right 0H5T
Carotid Bodies, Bilateral 0G58
Carotid Body
Left 0G56
Right 0G57
Cecum 0D5H
Coccygeal Glomus 0G5B
Colon
Ascending 0D5K
Descending 0D5M
Sigmoid 0D5N
Transverse 0D5L
Duct
Common Bile 0F59
Cystic 0F58
Hepatic
Common 0F57
Left 0F56
Right 0F55
Pancreatic 0F5D
Accessory 0F5F
Duodenum 0D59
Esophagogastric Junction 0D54
Esophagus 0D55
Lower 0D53
Middle 0D52
Upper 0D51
Gallbladder 0F54
Gland
Adrenal
Bilateral 0G54
Left 0G52
Right 0G53
Pituitary 0G50
Glomus Jugulare 0G5C
Ileocecal Valve 0D5C
Ileum 0D5B
Intestine
Large 0D5E
Left 0D5G
Right 0D5F
Small 0D58
Jejunum 0D5A
Liver 0F50
Left Lobe 0F52
Right Lobe 0F51
Lung
Bilateral 0B5M
Left 0B5L
Lower Lobe
Left 0B5J
Right 0B5F
Middle Lobe, Right 0B5D
Right 0B5K
Upper Lobe
Left 0B5G
Right 0B5C
Lung Lingula 0B5H
Pancreas 0F5G
Para-aortic Body 0G59
Paraganglion Extremity 0G5F
Parathyroid Gland 0G5R
Inferior
Left 0G5P
Right 0G5N
Multiple 0G5Q
Superior
Left 0G5M
Right 0G5L
Pineal Body 0G51
Prostate 0V50
Rectum 0D5P
Sacrum 0Q51
Spinal Cord
Cervical 005W
Lumbar 005Y
Thoracic 005X
Stomach 0D56
Pylorus 0D57
Thyroid Gland 0G5K
Left Lobe 0G5G
Right Lobe 0G5H

Laser Interstitial Thermal Therapy

Laser Interstitial Thermal Therapy — continued
  Vertebra
    Cervical 0P53
    Lumbar 0Q50
    Thoracic 0P54
Lateral canthus
  use Upper Eyelid, Left
  use Upper Eyelid, Right
Lateral collateral ligament (LCL)
  use Knee Bursa and Ligament, Left
  use Knee Bursa and Ligament, Right
Lateral condyle of femur
  use Lower Femur, Left
  use Lower Femur, Right
Lateral condyle of tibia
  use Tibia, Left
  use Tibia, Right
Lateral cuneiform bone
  use Tarsal, Left
  use Tarsal, Right
Lateral epicondyle of femur
  use Lower Femur, Left
  use Lower Femur, Right
Lateral epicondyle of humerus
  use Humeral Shaft, Left
  use Humeral Shaft, Right
Lateral femoral cutaneous nerve use Lumbar Plexus
Lateral (brachial) lymph node
  use Lymphatic, Left Axillary
  use Lymphatic, Right Axillary
Lateral malleolus
  use Fibula, Left
  use Fibula, Right
Lateral meniscus
  use Knee Joint, Left
  use Knee Joint, Right
Lateral nasal cartilage use Nasal Mucosa and Soft Tissue
Lateral plantar artery
  use Foot Artery, Left
  use Foot Artery, Right
Lateral plantar nerve use Tibial Nerve
Lateral rectus muscle
  use Extraocular Muscle, Left
  use Extraocular Muscle, Right
Lateral sacral artery
  use Internal Iliac Artery, Left
  use Internal Iliac Artery, Right
Lateral sacral vein
  use Hypogastric Vein, Left
  use Hypogastric Vein, Right
Lateral sural cutaneous nerve use Peroneal Nerve
Lateral tarsal artery
  use Foot Artery, Left
  use Foot Artery, Right
Lateral temporomandibular ligament use Head and Neck Bursa and Ligament
Lateral thoracic artery
  use Axillary Artery, Left
  use Axillary Artery, Right
Latissimus dorsi muscle
  use Trunk Muscle, Left
  use Trunk Muscle, Right
Latissimus Dorsi Myocutaneous Flap
  Replacement
    Bilateral 0HRV075
    Left 0HRU075
    Right 0HRT075
  Transfer
    Left 0KXG
    Right 0KXF
Lavage
  see Irrigation
  Bronchial alveolar, diagnostic see Drainage, Respiratory System 0B9
Leaflet laceration/division/modification/splitting device, used during transcatheter aortic valve replacement (TAVR) procedure X28F3VA
Least splanchnic nerve use Thoracic Sympathetic Nerve
Lefamulin Anti-infective XW0
Left ascending lumbar vein use Hemiazygos Vein
Left atrioventricular valve use Mitral Valve
Left auricular appendix use Atrium, Left
Left colic vein use Colic Vein
Left coronary sulcus use Heart, Left

Left gastric artery use Gastric Artery
Left gastroepiploic artery use Splenic Artery
Left gastroepiploic vein use Splenic Vein
Left inferior phrenic vein use Renal Vein, Left
Left inferior pulmonary vein use Pulmonary Vein, Left
Left jugular trunk use Thoracic Duct
Left lateral ventricle use Cerebral Ventricle
Left ovarian vein use Renal Vein, Left
Left second lumbar vein use Renal Vein, Left
Left subclavian trunk use Thoracic Duct
Left subcostal vein use Hemiazygos Vein
Left superior pulmonary vein use Pulmonary Vein, Left
Left suprarenal vein use Renal Vein, Left
Left testicular vein use Renal Vein, Left
Lengthening
  Bone, with device see Insertion of Limb Lengthening Device
  Muscle, by incision see Division, Muscles 0K8
  Tendon, by incision see Division, Tendons 0L8
Leptomeninges, intracranial use Cerebral Meninges
Leptomeninges, spinal use Spinal Meninges
Leronlimab Monoclonal Antibody XW013K6
Lesser alar cartilage use Nasal Mucosa and Soft Tissue
Lesser occipital nerve use Cervical Plexus
Lesser Omentum use Omentum
Lesser saphenous vein
  use Saphenous Vein, Left
  use Saphenous Vein, Right
Lesser splanchnic nerve use Thoracic Sympathetic Nerve
Lesser trochanter
  use Upper Femur, Left
  use Upper Femur, Right
Lesser tuberosity
  use Humeral Head, Left
  use Humeral Head, Right
Lesser wing use Sphenoid Bone
Leukopheresis, therapeutic see Pheresis, Circulatory 6A55
Levator anguli oris muscle use Facial Muscle
Levator ani muscle use Perineum Muscle
Levator labii superioris alaeque nasi muscle use Facial Muscle
Levator labii superioris muscle use Facial Muscle
Levator palpebrae superioris muscle
  use Upper Eyelid, Left
  use Upper Eyelid, Right
Levator scapulae muscle
  use Neck Muscle, Left
  use Neck Muscle, Right
Levator veli palatini muscle use Tongue, Palate, Pharynx Muscle
Levatores costarum muscle
  use Thorax Muscle, Left
  use Thorax Muscle, Right
Lifeline ARM Automated Chest Compression (ACC) device 5A1221J
LifeStent® (Flexstar) (XL) Vascular Stent System use Intraluminal Device
Lifileucel use Lifileucel Immunotherapy
Lifileucel Immunotherapy XW0
Ligament of head of fibula
  use Knee Bursa and Ligament, Left
  use Knee Bursa and Ligament, Right
Ligament of the lateral malleolus
  use Ankle Bursa and Ligament, Left
  use Ankle Bursa and Ligament, Right
Ligamentum flavum, cervical use Head and Neck Bursa and Ligament
Ligamentum flavum, lumbar use Lower Spine Bursa and Ligament
Ligamentum flavum, thoracic use Upper Spine Bursa and Ligament
LigaPASS 2.0™ PJK Prevention System use Posterior Vertebral Tether in New Technology
Ligation see Occlusion
Ligation, hemorrhoid see Occlusion, Lower Veins, Hemorrhoidal Plexus
Light Therapy GZJZZZZ
LimFlow™ TADV (Transcatheter Arterialization of the Deep Veins) Procedure see Bypass, Lower Arteries 041

LimFlow™ Transcatheter Arterialization of the Deep Veins (TADV) System use Synthetic Substitute
Liner
  Removal of device from
    Hip
      Left 0SPB09Z
      Right 0SP909Z
    Knee
      Left 0SPD09Z
      Right 0SPC09Z
  Revision of device in
    Hip
      Left 0SWB09Z
      Right 0SW909Z
    Knee
      Left 0SWD09Z
      Right 0SWC09Z
  Supplement
    Hip
      Left 0SUB09Z
        Acetabular Surface 0SUE09Z
        Femoral Surface 0SUS09Z
      Right 0SU909Z
        Acetabular Surface 0SUA09Z
        Femoral Surface 0SUR09Z
    Knee
      Left 0SUD09
        Femoral Surface 0SUU09Z
        Tibial Surface 0SUW09Z
      Right 0SUC09
        Femoral Surface 0SUT09Z
        Tibial Surface 0SUV09Z
Lingual artery
  use External Carotid Artery, Left
  use External Carotid Artery, Right
Lingual tonsil use Pharynx
Lingulectomy, lung
  see Excision, Lung Lingula 0BBH
  see Resection, Lung Lingula 0BTH
Lisocabtagene Maraleucel use Lisocabtagene Maraleucel Immunotherapy
Lisocabtagene Maraleucel Immunotherapy XW0
Lithoplasty see Fragmentation
Lithotripsy
  see Fragmentation
  With removal of fragments see Extirpation
LITT (laser interstitial thermal therapy)
  see Destruction
  see Laser Interstitial Thermal Therapy
LIVIAN™ CRT-D use Cardiac Resynchronization Defibrillator Pulse Generator in 0JH
LIVTENCITY™ use Maribavir Anti-infective
Lobectomy
  see Excision, Central Nervous System and Cranial Nerves 00B
  see Excision, Endocrine System 0GB
  see Excision, Hepatobiliary System and Pancreas 0FB
  see Excision, Respiratory System 0BB
  see Resection, Endocrine System 0GT
  see Resection, Hepatobiliary System and Pancreas 0FT
  see Resection, Respiratory System 0BT
Lobotomy see Division, Brain 0080
Localization
  see Imaging
  see Map
Locus ceruleus use Pons
LOEP® (Local Osteo-Enhancement Procedure) XW0V3WA
Long thoracic nerve use Brachial Plexus
Longeviti ClearFit® Cranial Implant use Synthetic Substitute, Ultrasound Penetrable in New Technology
Longeviti ClearFit® OTS Cranial Implant use Synthetic Substitute, Ultrasound Penetrable in New Technology
Loop ileostomy see Bypass, Ileum 0D1B
Loop recorder, implantable use Monitoring Device
Lovotibeglogene Autotemcel XW1
Lower GI series see Fluoroscopy, Colon BD14
Lower Respiratory Fluid Nucleic Acid-base Microbial Detection XXEBXQ6
LTX Regional Anticoagulant use Nafamostat Anticoagulant
LUCAS® Chest Compression System 5A1221J

Lumbar artery use Abdominal Aorta
Lumbar Artery Perforator Flap
   Bilateral ØHRVØ7B
   Left ØHRUØ7B
   Right ØHRTØ7B
Lumbar facet joint use Lumbar Vertebral Joint
Lumbar ganglion use Lumbar Sympathetic Nerve
Lumbar lymph node use Lymphatic, Aortic
Lumbar lymphatic trunk use Cisterna Chyli
Lumbar splanchnic nerve use Lumbar Sympathetic Nerve
Lumbosacral facet joint use Lumbosacral Joint
Lumbosacral trunk use Lumbar Nerve
LumiGuide (Fiber optic 3D guidance for endovascular procedures) 8E023FZ
Lumpectomy see Excision
Lunate bone
   use Carpal, Left
   use Carpal, Right
Lunotriquetral ligament
   use Hand Bursa and Ligament, Left
   use Hand Bursa and Ligament, Right
LUNSUMIO™ use Mosunetuzumab Antineoplastic
Lurbinectedin XWØ
LVA (Lymphovenous Anastomosis) see Bypass, Lymphatic and Hemic Systems Ø71
LVB (Lymphovenous Bypass) see Bypass, Lymphatic and Hemic Systems Ø71
LYFGENIA™ use Lovotibeglogene Autotemcel
Lymphadenectomy
   see Excision, Lymphatic and Hemic Systems Ø7B
   see Resection, Lymphatic and Hemic Systems Ø7T
Lymphadenotomy see Drainage, Lymphatic and Hemic Systems Ø79
Lymphangiectomy
   see Excision, Lymphatic and Hemic Systems Ø7B
   see Resection, Lymphatic and Hemic Systems Ø7T
Lymphangiogram see Plain Radiography, Lymphatic System B7Ø
Lymphangioplasty
   see Repair, Lymphatic and Hemic Systems Ø7Q
   see Supplement, Lymphatic and Hemic Systems Ø7U
Lymphangiorrhaphy see Repair, Lymphatic and Hemic Systems Ø7Q
Lymphangiotomy see Drainage, Lymphatic and Hemic Systems Ø79
Lymphaticovenular Anastomosis see Bypass, Lymphatic and Hemic Systems Ø71
Lymphovenous Anastomosis (LVA) see Bypass, Lymphatic and Hemic Systems Ø71
Lymphovenous Bypass (LVB) see Bypass, Lymphatic and Hemic Systems Ø71
Lymphovenous Shunt see Bypass, Lymphatic and Hemic Systems Ø71
Lysis see Release
LZRSE-COL7A1 engineered autologous epidermal sheets use Prademagene Zamikeracel, Genetically Engineered Autologous Cell Therapy in New Technology

M

Macula XXE5XR7
   use Retina, Left
   use Retina, Right
MAGEC® Spinal Bracing and Distraction System use Magnetically Controlled Growth Rod(s) in New Technology
Magnet extraction, ocular foreign body see Extirpation, Eye Ø8C
Magnetic Resonance Imaging (MRI)
   Abdomen BW3Ø
   Ankle
     Left BQ3H
     Right BQ3G
   Aorta
     Abdominal B43Ø
     Thoracic B33Ø
   Arm
     Left BP3F
     Right BP3E
   Artery
     Celiac B431
     Cervico-Cerebral Arch B33Q
     Common Carotid, Bilateral B335

Magnetic Resonance Imaging (MRI) — continued
   Artery — continued
     Coronary
       Bypass Graft, Multiple B233
       Multiple B231
     Internal Carotid, Bilateral B338
     Intracranial B33R
     Lower Extremity
       Bilateral B43H
       Left B43G
       Right B43F
     Pelvic B43C
     Renal, Bilateral B438
     Spinal B33M
     Superior Mesenteric B434
     Upper Extremity
       Bilateral B33K
       Left B33J
       Right B33H
     Vertebral, Bilateral B33G
   Bladder BT3Ø
   Brachial Plexus BW3P
   Brain BØ3Ø
   Breast
     Bilateral BH32
     Left BH31
     Right BH3Ø
   Calcaneus
     Left BQ3K
     Right BQ3J
   Chest BW33Y
   Coccyx BR3F
   Connective Tissue
     Lower Extremity BL31
     Upper Extremity BL3Ø
   Corpora Cavernosa BV3Ø
   Disc
     Cervical BR31
     Lumbar BR33
     Thoracic BR32
   Ear B93Ø
   Elbow
     Left BP3H
     Right BP3G
   Eye
     Bilateral B837
     Left B836
     Right B835
   Femur
     Left BQ34
     Right BQ33
   Fetal Abdomen BY33
   Fetal Extremity BY35
   Fetal Head BY3Ø
   Fetal Heart BY31
   Fetal Spine BY34
   Fetal Thorax BY32
   Fetus, Whole BY36
   Foot
     Left BQ3M
     Right BQ3L
   Forearm
     Left BP3K
     Right BP3J
   Gland
     Adrenal, Bilateral BG32
     Parathyroid BG33
     Parotid, Bilateral B936
     Salivary, Bilateral B93D
     Submandibular, Bilateral B939
     Thyroid BG34
   Head BW38
   Heart, Right and Left B236
   Hip
     Left BQ31
     Right BQ3Ø
   Intracranial Sinus B532
   Joint
     Finger
       Left BP3D
       Right BP3C
     Hand
       Left BP3D
       Right BP3C
     Temporomandibular, Bilateral BN39
   Kidney
     Bilateral BT33
     Left BT32
     Right BT31

Magnetic Resonance Imaging (MRI) — continued
   Kidney — continued
     Transplant BT39
   Knee
     Left BQ38
     Right BQ37
   Larynx B93J
   Leg
     Left BQ3F
     Right BQ3D
   Liver BF35
   Liver and Spleen BF36
   Lung Apices BB3G
   Lung, Bilateral, Hyperpolarized Xenon 129 (Xe-129) BB34Z3Z
   Nasopharynx B93F
   Neck BW3F
   Nerve
     Acoustic BØ3C
     Brachial Plexus BW3P
   Oropharynx B93F
   Ovary
     Bilateral BU35
     Left BU34
     Right BU33
   Ovary and Uterus BU3C
   Pancreas BF37
   Patella
     Left BQ3W
     Right BQ3V
   Pelvic Region BW3G
   Pelvis BR3C
   Pituitary Gland BØ39
   Plexus, Brachial BW3P
   Prostate BV33
   Retroperitoneum BW3H
   Sacrum BR3F
   Scrotum BV34
   Sella Turcica BØ39
   Shoulder
     Left BP39
     Right BP38
   Sinus
     Intracranial B532
     Paranasal B932
   Spinal Cord BØ3B
   Spine
     Cervical BR3Ø
     Lumbar BR39
     Thoracic BR37
   Spleen and Liver BF36
   Subcutaneous Tissue
     Abdomen BH3H
     Extremity
       Lower BH3J
       Upper BH3F
     Head BH3D
     Neck BH3D
     Pelvis BH3H
     Thorax BH3G
   Tendon
     Lower Extremity BL33
     Upper Extremity BL32
   Testicle
     Bilateral BV37
     Left BV36
     Right BV35
   Toe
     Left BQ3Q
     Right BQ3P
   Uterus BU36
     Pregnant BU3B
   Uterus and Ovary BU3C
   Vagina BU39
   Vein
     Cerebellar B531
     Cerebral B531
     Jugular, Bilateral B535
     Lower Extremity
       Bilateral B53D
       Left B53C
       Right B53B
     Other B53V
     Pelvic (Iliac) Bilateral B53H
     Portal B53T
     Pulmonary, Bilateral B53S
     Renal, Bilateral B53L
     Splanchnic B53T

Magnetic Resonance Imaging (MRI) — continued
  Vein — continued
    Upper Extremity
      Bilateral B53P
      Left B53N
      Right B53M
    Vena Cava
      Inferior B539
      Superior B538
    Wrist
      Left BP3M
      Right BP3L
Magnetically Controlled Growth Rod(s)
  Cervical XNS3
  Lumbar XNS0
  Thoracic XNS4
Magnetic-guided radiofrequency endovascular fistula
  Radial Artery, Left 031C3ZF
  Radial Artery, Right 031B3ZF
  Ulnar Artery, Left 031A3ZF
  Ulnar Artery, Right 03193ZF
Magnus Neuromodulation System (MNS) X0Z0X18
Malleotomy see Drainage, Ear, Nose, Sinus 099
Malleus
  use Auditory Ossicle, Left
  use Auditory Ossicle, Right
Mammaplasty, mammoplasty
  see Alteration, Skin and Breast 0H0
  see Repair, Skin and Breast 0HQ
  see Replacement, Skin and Breast 0HR
  see Supplement, Skin and Breast 0HU
Mammary duct
  use Breast, Bilateral
  use Breast, Left
  use Breast, Right
Mammary gland
  use Breast, Bilateral
  use Breast, Left
  use Breast, Right
Mammectomy
  see Excision, Skin and Breast 0HB
  see Resection, Skin and Breast 0HT
Mammillary body use Hypothalamus
Mammography see Plain Radiography, Skin, Subcutaneous Tissue and Breast BH0
Mammotomy see Drainage, Skin and Breast 0H9
Mandibular nerve use Trigeminal Nerve
Mandibular notch
  use Mandible, Left
  use Mandible, Right
Mandibulectomy
  see Excision, Head and Facial Bones 0NB
  see Resection, Head and Facial Bones 0NT
Manipulation
  Adhesions see Release
  Chiropractic see Chiropractic Manipulation
Manual removal, retained placenta see Extraction, Products of Conception, Retained 10D1
Manubrium use Sternum
Map
  Basal Ganglia 00K8
  Brain 00K0
    Connectomic Analysis 00K0XZ1
  Cerebellum 00KC
  Cerebral Hemisphere 00K7
  Conduction Mechanism 02K8
  Hypothalamus 00KA
  Medulla Oblongata 00KD
  Pons 00KB
  Thalamus 00K9
Mapping
  Connectomic Analysis (Brain) 00K0XZ1
  Doppler ultrasound see Ultrasonography
  Electrocardiogram only see Measurement, Cardiac 4A02
Maribavir Anti-infective XW0
Mark IV Breathing Pacemaker System use Stimulator Generator in Subcutaneous Tissue and Fascia
Marnetegragene Autotemcel XW1
MarrowStim™ PAD Kit for CBMA (Concentrated Bone Marrow Aspirate) use Other Substance
MarrowStim™ PAD Kit, for injection of concentrated bone marrow aspirate see Introduction of substance in or on, Muscle 3E02
Marsupialization
  see Drainage

Marsupialization — continued
  see Excision
Massage, cardiac
  External 5A12012
  Open 02QA0ZZ
Masseter muscle use Head Muscle
Masseteric fascia use Subcutaneous Tissue and Fascia, Face
Mastectomy
  see Excision, Skin and Breast 0HB
  see Resection, Skin and Breast 0HT
Mastoid air cells
  use Mastoid Sinus, Left
  use Mastoid Sinus, Right
Mastoid (postauricular) lymph node
  use Lymphatic, Left Neck
  use Lymphatic, Right Neck
Mastoid process
  use Temporal Bone, Left
  use Temporal Bone, Right
Mastoidectomy
  see Excision, Ear, Nose, Sinus 09B
  see Resection, Ear, Nose, Sinus 09T
Mastoidotomy see Drainage, Ear, Nose, Sinus 099
Mastopexy
  see Repair, Skin and Breast 0HQ
  see Reposition, Skin and Breast 0HS
Mastorrhaphy see Repair, Skin and Breast 0HQ
Mastotomy see Drainage, Skin and Breast 0H9
Maxillary artery
  use External Carotid Artery, Left
  use External Carotid Artery, Right
Maxillary nerve use Trigeminal Nerve
Maximo II DR (VR) use Defibrillator Generator in 0JH
Maximo II DR CRT-D use Cardiac Resynchronization Defibrillator Pulse Generator in 0JH
Measurement
  Arterial
    Flow
      Coronary 4A03
      Intracranial 4A03X5D
      Peripheral 4A03
      Pulmonary 4A03
    Pressure
      Coronary 4A03
      Peripheral 4A03
      Pulmonary 4A03
      Thoracic, Other 4A03
    Pulse
      Coronary 4A03
      Peripheral 4A03
      Pulmonary 4A03
    Saturation, Peripheral 4A03
    Sound, Peripheral 4A03
  Biliary
    Flow 4A0C
    Pressure 4A0C
  Cardiac
    Action Currents 4A02
    Defibrillator 4B02XTZ
    Electrical Activity 4A02
      Guidance 4A02X4A
      No Qualifier 4A02X4Z
    Output 4A02
    Pacemaker 4B02XSZ
    Rate 4A02
    Rhythm 4A02
    Sampling and Pressure
      Bilateral 4A02
      Left Heart 4A02
      Right Heart 4A02
    Sound 4A02
    Total Activity, Stress 4A02XM4
  Central Nervous
    Cerebrospinal Fluid Shunt, Wireless Sensor 4B00XW0
    Conductivity 4A00
    Electrical Activity 4A00
    Pressure 4A000BZ
      Intracranial 4A00
    Saturation, Intracranial 4A00
    Stimulator 4B00XVZ
    Temperature, Intracranial 4A00
  Circulatory, Volume 4A05XLZ
  Gastrointestinal
    Motility 4A0B
    Pressure 4A0B
    Secretion 4A0B

Measurement — continued
  Intracranial Cerebrospinal Fluid Flow, Computer-aided Triage and Notification XXE0X1A
  Lower Respiratory Fluid Nucleic Acid-base Microbial Detection XXEBXQ6
  Lymphatic
    Flow 4A06
    Pressure 4A06
  Metabolism 4A0Z
  Musculoskeletal
    Contractility 4A0F
    Pressure 4A0F3BE
    Stimulator 4B0FXVZ
  Olfactory, Acuity 4A08X0Z
  Peripheral Nervous
    Conductivity
      Motor 4A01
      Sensory 4A01
    Electrical Activity 4A01
    Stimulator 4B01XVZ
  Phenotypic Fully Automated Rapid Susceptibility Technology with Controlled Inoculum XXE5X2A
  Positive Blood Culture Fluorescence Hybridization for Organism Identification, Concentration and Susceptibility XXE5XN6
  Positive Blood Culture Small Molecule Sensor Array Technology XXE5X4A
  Products of Conception
    Cardiac
      Electrical Activity 4A0H
      Rate 4A0H
      Rhythm 4A0H
      Sound 4A0H
    Nervous
      Conductivity 4A0J
      Electrical Activity 4A0J
      Pressure 4A0J
  Respiratory
    Capacity 4A09
    Flow 4A09
    Pacemaker 4B09XSZ
    Rate 4A09
    Resistance 4A09
    Total Activity 4A09
    Volume 4A09
  Sleep 4A0ZXQZ
  Temperature 4A0Z
  Urinary
    Contractility 4A0D
    Flow 4A0D
    Pressure 4A0D
    Resistance 4A0D
    Volume 4A0D
  Venous
    Flow
      Central 4A04
      Peripheral 4A04
      Portal 4A04
      Pulmonary 4A04
    Pressure
      Central 4A04
      Peripheral 4A04
      Portal 4A04
      Pulmonary 4A04
    Pulse
      Central 4A04
      Peripheral 4A04
      Portal 4A04
      Pulmonary 4A04
    Saturation, Peripheral 4A04
  Visual
    Acuity 4A07X0Z
    Mobility 4A07X7Z
    Pressure 4A07XBZ
Meatoplasty, urethra see Repair, Urethra 0TQD
Meatotomy see Drainage, Urinary System 0T9
Mechanical chest compression (mCPR) 5A1221J
Mechanical Initial Specimen Diversion Technique Using Active Negative Pressure (blood collection) XXE5XR7
Mechanical ventilation see Performance, Respiratory 5A19
Medial canthus
  use Lower Eyelid, Left
  use Lower Eyelid, Right
Medial collateral ligament (MCL)
  use Knee Bursa and Ligament, Left

Medial collateral ligament (MCL) — continued
  use Knee Bursa and Ligament, Right
Medial condyle of femur
  use Lower Femur, Left
  use Lower Femur, Right
Medial condyle of tibia
  use Tibia, Left
  use Tibia, Right
Medial cuneiform bone
  use Tarsal, Left
  use Tarsal, Right
Medial epicondyle of femur
  use Lower Femur, Left
  use Lower Femur, Right
Medial epicondyle of humerus
  use Humeral Shaft, Left
  use Humeral Shaft, Right
Medial malleolus
  use Tibia, Left
  use Tibia, Right
Medial meniscus
  use Knee Joint, Left
  use Knee Joint, Right
Medial plantar artery
  use Foot Artery, Left
  use Foot Artery, Right
Medial plantar nerve use Tibial Nerve
Medial popliteal nerve use Tibial Nerve
Medial rectus muscle
  use Extraocular Muscle, Left
  use Extraocular Muscle, Right
Medial sural cutaneous nerve use Tibial Nerve
Median antebrachial vein
  use Basilic Vein, Left
  use Basilic Vein, Right
Median cubital vein
  use Basilic Vein, Left
  use Basilic Vein, Right
Median sacral artery use Abdominal Aorta
Mediastinal cavity use Mediastinum
Mediastinal lymph node use Lymphatic, Thorax
Mediastinal space use Mediastinum
Mediastinoscopy 0WJC4ZZ
Medication Management GZ3ZZZZ
  for substance abuse
    Antabuse HZ83ZZZ
    Bupropion HZ87ZZZ
    Clonidine HZ86ZZZ
    Levo-alpha-acetyl-methadol (LAAM) HZ82ZZZ
    Methadone Maintenance HZ81ZZZ
    Naloxone HZ85ZZZ
    Naltrexone HZ84ZZZ
    Nicotine Replacement HZ80ZZZ
    Other Replacement Medication HZ89ZZZ
    Psychiatric Medication HZ88ZZZ
Meditation 8E0ZXY5
Medtronic Endurant® II AAA stent graft system use Intraluminal Device
Meissner's (submucous) plexus use Abdominal Sympathetic Nerve
Melody® transcatheter pulmonary valve use Zooplastic Tissue in Heart and Great Vessels
Melphalan Hydrochloride Antineoplastic XW053T9
Membranous urethra use Urethra
Meningeorrhaphy
  see Repair, Cerebral Meninges 00Q1
  see Repair, Spinal Meninges 00QT
Meniscectomy, knee
  see Excision, Joint, Knee, Left 0SBD
  see Excision, Joint, Knee, Right 0SBC
Mental foramen
  use Mandible, Left
  use Mandible, Right
Mentalis muscle use Facial Muscle
Mentoplasty see Alteration, Jaw, Lower 0W05
Meropenem-vaborbactam Anti-infective use Other Anti-infective
Mesenterectomy see Excision, Mesentery 0DBV
Mesenteriorrhaphy, mesenterorrhaphy see Repair, Mesentery 0DQV
Mesenteriplication see Repair, Mesentery 0DQV
Mesoappendix use Mesentery
Mesocolon use Mesentery
Metacarpal ligament
  use Hand Bursa and Ligament, Left
  use Hand Bursa and Ligament, Right

Metacarpophalangeal ligament
  use Hand Bursa and Ligament, Left
  use Hand Bursa and Ligament, Right
Metal on metal bearing surface use Synthetic Substitute, Metal in 0SR
Metatarsal Ligament
  use Foot Bursa and Ligament, Left
  use Foot Bursa and Ligament, Right
Metatarsectomy
  see Excision, Lower Bones 0QB
  see Resection, Lower Bones 0QT
Metatarsophalangeal (MTP) joint
  use Metatarsal-Phalangeal Joint, Left
  use Metatarsal-Phalangeal Joint, Right
Metatarsophalangeal Ligament
  use Foot Bursa and Ligament, Left
  use Foot Bursa and Ligament, Right
Metathalamus use Thalamus
Micro-Driver stent (RX) (OTW) use Intraluminal Device
MicroMed HeartAssist use Implantable Heart Assist System in Heart and Great Vessels
Microsurgical Lymph Bypass see Bypass, Lymphatic and Hemic Systems 071
Micrus CERECYTE Microcoil use Intraluminal Device, Bioactive in Upper Arteries
Midcarpal joint
  use Carpal Joint, Left
  use Carpal Joint, Right
Middle cardiac nerve use Thoracic Sympathetic Nerve
Middle cerebral artery use Intracranial Artery
Middle cerebral vein use Intracranial Vein
Middle colic vein use Colic Vein
Middle genicular artery
  use Popliteal Artery, Left
  use Popliteal Artery, Right
Middle hemorrhoidal vein
  use Hypogastric Vein, Left
  use Hypogastric Vein, Right
Middle meningeal artery, intracranial portion use Intracranial Artery
Middle rectal artery
  use Internal Iliac Artery, Left
  use Internal Iliac Artery, Right
Middle suprarenal artery use Abdominal Aorta
Middle temporal artery
  use Temporal Artery, Left
  use Temporal Artery, Right
Middle turbinate use Nasal Turbinate
Mineral-based Topical Hemostatic Agent XW0
MIRODERM™ Biologic Wound Matrix use Nonautologous Tissue Substitute
MIRODERM™ skin graft see Replacement, Skin and Breast 0HR
MitraClip valve repair system use Synthetic Substitute
Mitral annulus use Mitral Valve
Mitroflow® Aortic Pericardial Heart Valve use Zooplastic Tissue in Heart and Great Vessels
MNS (Magnus Neuromodulation System) X0Z0X18
Mobilization, adhesions see Release
Molar gland use Buccal Mucosa
MolecuLight i:X® wound imaging see Other Imaging, Anatomical Regions BW5
Monitoring
  Adhesive Ultrasound Patch Technology, Blood Flow XX25X0A
  Arterial
    Flow
      Coronary 4A13
      Peripheral 4A13
      Pulmonary 4A13
    Pressure
      Coronary 4A13
      Peripheral 4A13
      Pulmonary 4A13
    Pulse
      Coronary 4A13
      Peripheral 4A13
      Pulmonary 4A13
    Saturation, Peripheral 4A13
    Sound, Peripheral 4A13
  Brain Electrical Activity, Computer-aided Detection and Notification XX20X89
  Cardiac
    Electrical Activity 4A12
      Ambulatory 4A12X45
      No Qualifier 4A12X4Z

Monitoring — continued
  Cardiac — continued
    Output 4A12
    Rate 4A12
    Rhythm 4A12
    Sound 4A12
    Total Activity, Stress 4A12XM4
    Vascular Perfusion, Indocyanine Green Dye 4A12XSH
  Central Nervous
    Conductivity 4A10
    Electrical Activity
      Intraoperative 4A10
      No Qualifier 4A10
    Pressure 4A100BZ
      Intracranial 4A10
    Saturation, Intracranial 4A10
    Temperature, Intracranial 4A10
  Gastrointestinal
    Motility 4A1B
    Pressure 4A1B
    Secretion 4A1B
    Vascular Perfusion, Indocyanine Green Dye 4A1BXSH
  Interstitial Fluid Volume, Sub-Epidermal Moisture using Electrical Biocapacitance XX2KXP9
  Kidney, Fluorescent Pyrazine XT25XE5
  Lymphatic
    Flow
      Indocyanine Green Dye 4A16
      No Qualifier 4A16
    Pressure 4A16
  Muscle Compartment Pressure, Micro-Electro-Mechanical System XX2F3W9
  Oxygen Saturation Endoscopic Imaging (OXEI) XD2
  Peripheral Nervous
    Conductivity
      Motor 4A11
      Sensory 4A11
    Electrical Activity
      Intraoperative 4A11
      No Qualifier 4A11
  Products of Conception
    Cardiac
      Electrical Activity 4A1H
      Rate 4A1H
      Rhythm 4A1H
      Sound 4A1H
    Nervous
      Conductivity 4A1J
      Electrical Activity 4A1J
      Pressure 4A1J
  Respiratory
    Capacity 4A19
    Flow 4A19
    Rate 4A19
    Resistance 4A19
    Volume 4A19
  Skin and Breast, Vascular Perfusion, Indocyanine Green Dye 4A1GXSH
  Sleep 4A1ZXQZ
  Temperature 4A1Z
  Urinary
    Contractility 4A1D
    Flow 4A1D
    Pressure 4A1D
    Resistance 4A1D
    Volume 4A1D
  Venous
    Flow
      Central 4A14
      Peripheral 4A14
      Portal 4A14
      Pulmonary 4A14
    Pressure
      Central 4A14
      Peripheral 4A14
      Portal 4A14
      Pulmonary 4A14
    Pulse
      Central 4A14
      Peripheral 4A14
      Portal 4A14
      Pulmonary 4A14
    Saturation
      Central 4A14
      Portal 4A14
      Pulmonary 4A14

Monitoring Device, Hemodynamic
  Abdomen 0JH8
  Chest 0JH6
Mosaic Bioprosthesis (aortic) (mitral) valve use Zooplastic Tissue in Heart and Great Vessels
Mosunetuzumab Antineoplastic XW0
Motor Function Assessment F01
Motor Treatment F07
MR Angiography
  see Magnetic Resonance Imaging (MRI), Heart B23
  see Magnetic Resonance Imaging (MRI), Lower Arteries B43
  see Magnetic Resonance Imaging (MRI), Upper Arteries B33
MULTI-LINK (VISION) (MINI-VISION) (ULTRA) Coronary Stent System use Intraluminal Device
Multi-plane Flex Technology Bioprosthetic Valve X2RJ3RA
Multiple sleep latency test 4A0ZXQZ
Muscle Compartment Pressure, Micro-Electro-Mechanical System XX2F3W9
Musculocutaneous nerve use Brachial Plexus
Musculopexy
  see Repair, Muscles 0KQ
  see Reposition, Muscles 0KS
Musculophrenic artery
  use Internal Mammary Artery, Left
  use Internal Mammary Artery, Right
Musculoplasty
  see Repair, Muscles 0KQ
  see Supplement, Muscles 0KU
Musculorrhaphy see Repair, Muscles 0KQ
Musculospiral nerve use Radial Nerve
MY01 Continuous Compartmental Pressure Monitor XX2F3W9
Myectomy
  see Excision, Muscles 0KB
  see Resection, Muscles 0KT
Myelencephalon use Medulla Oblongata
Myelogram
  CT see Computerized Tomography (CT Scan), Central Nervous System B02
  MRI see Magnetic Resonance Imaging (MRI), Central Nervous System B03
Myenteric (Auerbach's) plexus use Abdominal Sympathetic Nerve
Myocardial Bridge Release see Release, Artery, Coronary
Myomectomy see Excision, Female Reproductive System 0UB
Myometrium use Uterus
Myopexy
  see Repair, Muscles 0KQ
  see Reposition, Muscles 0KS
Myoplasty
  see Repair, Muscles 0KQ
  see Supplement, Muscles 0KU
Myorrhaphy see Repair, Muscles 0KQ
Myoscopy see Inspection, Muscles 0KJ
Myotomy
  see Division, Muscles 0K8
  see Drainage, Muscles 0K9
Myringectomy
  see Excision, Ear, Nose, Sinus 09B
  see Resection, Ear, Nose, Sinus 09T
Myringoplasty
  see Repair, Ear, Nose, Sinus 09Q
  see Replacement, Ear, Nose, Sinus 09R
  see Supplement, Ear, Nose, Sinus 09U
Myringostomy see Drainage, Ear, Nose, Sinus 099
Myringotomy see Drainage, Ear, Nose, Sinus 099

N

NA-1 (Nerinitide) use Nerinitide
Nafamostat Anticoagulant XY0YX37
Nail bed
  use Finger Nail
  use Toe Nail
Nail plate
  use Finger Nail
  use Toe Nail
nanoLOCK™ interbody fusion device
  use Interbody Fusion Device in Lower Joints
  use Interbody Fusion Device in Upper Joints
Narcosynthesis GZGZZZZZ

Narsoplimab Monoclonal Antibody XW0
Nasal cavity use Nasal Mucosa and Soft Tissue
Nasal concha use Nasal Turbinate
Nasalis muscle use Facial Muscle
Nasolacrimal duct
  use Lacrimal Duct, Left
  use Lacrimal Duct, Right
Nasopharyngeal airway (NPA) use Intraluminal Device, Airway in Ear, Nose, Sinus
Navicular bone
  use Tarsal, Left
  use Tarsal, Right
Near Infrared Spectroscopy, Circulatory System 8E02
Neck of femur
  use Upper Femur, Left
  use Upper Femur, Right
Neck of humerus (anatomical) (surgical)
  use Humeral Head, Left
  use Humeral Head, Right
Nelli® Seizure Monitoring System XXE0X48
Neovasc Reducer™ use Reduction Device in New Technology
Nephrectomy
  see Excision, Urinary System 0TB
  see Resection, Urinary System 0TT
Nephrolithotomy see Extirpation, Urinary System 0TC
Nephrolysis see Release, Urinary System 0TN
Nephropexy
  see Repair, Urinary System 0TQ
  see Reposition, Urinary System 0TS
Nephroplasty
  see Repair, Urinary System 0TQ
  see Supplement, Urinary System 0TU
Nephropyeloureterostomy
  see Bypass, Urinary System 0T1
  see Drainage, Urinary System 0T9
Nephrorrhaphy see Repair, Urinary System 0TQ
Nephroscopy, transurethral 0TJ58ZZ
Nephrostomy
  see Bypass, Urinary System 0T1
  see Drainage, Urinary System 0T9
Nephrotomography
  see Fluoroscopy, Urinary System BT1
  see Plain Radiography, Urinary System BT0
Nephrotomy
  see Division, Urinary System 0T8
  see Drainage, Urinary System 0T9
Nerinitide XW0
Nerve conduction study
  see Measurement, Central Nervous 4A00
  see Measurement, Peripheral Nervous 4A01
Nerve Function Assessment F01
Nerve to the stapedius use Facial Nerve
Nesiritide use Human B-Type Natriuretic Peptide
Neurectomy
  see Excision, Central Nervous System and Cranial Nerves 00B
  see Excision, Peripheral Nervous System 01B
Neurexeresis
  see Extraction, Central Nervous System and Cranial Nerves 00D
  see Extraction, Peripheral Nervous System 01D
NeuroBlate™ System see Destruction
Neurohypophysis use Pituitary Gland
Neurolysis
  see Release, Central Nervous System and Cranial Nerves 00N
  see Release, Peripheral Nervous System 01N
Neuromuscular electrical stimulation (NEMS) lead use Stimulator Lead in Muscles
Neurophysiologic monitoring see Monitoring, Central Nervous 4A10
Neuroplasty
  see Repair, Central Nervous System and Cranial Nerves 00Q
  see Repair, Peripheral Nervous System 01Q
  see Supplement, Central Nervous System and Cranial Nerves 00U
  see Supplement, Peripheral Nervous System 01U
Neurorrhaphy
  see Repair, Central Nervous System and Cranial Nerves 00Q
  see Repair, Peripheral Nervous System 01Q
Neurostimulator Generator
  Insertion of device in, Skull 0NH00NZ

Neurostimulator Generator — continued
  Removal of device from, Skull 0NP00NZ
  Revision of device in, Skull 0NW00NZ
Neurostimulator generator, multiple channel use Stimulator Generator, Multiple Array in 0JH
Neurostimulator generator, multiple channel rechargeable use Stimulator Generator, Multiple Array Rechargeable in 0JH
Neurostimulator generator, single channel use Stimulator Generator, Single Array in 0JH
Neurostimulator generator, single channel rechargeable use Stimulator Generator, Single Array Rechargeable in 0JH
Neurostimulator Lead
  Insertion of device in
    Brain 00H0
    Cerebral Ventricle 00H6
    Nerve
      Cranial 00HE
      Peripheral 01HY
    Spinal Canal 00HU
    Spinal Cord 00HV
    Vein
      Azygos 05H0
      Innominate
        Left 05H4
        Right 05H3
  Removal of device from
    Brain 00P0
    Cerebral Ventricle 00P6
    Nerve
      Cranial 00PE
      Peripheral 01PY
    Spinal Canal 00PU
    Spinal Cord 00PV
    Vein
      Azygos 05P0
      Innominate
        Left 05P4
        Right 05P3
  Revision of device in
    Brain 00W0
    Cerebral Ventricle 00W6
    Nerve
      Cranial 00WE
      Peripheral 01WY
    Spinal Canal 00WU
    Spinal Cord 00WV
    Vein
      Azygos 05W0
      Innominate
        Left 05W4
        Right 05W3
  Sphenopalatine Ganglion, Insertion X0HK3Q8
Neurostimulator Lead in Oropharynx XWHD7Q7
Neurostimulator Lead with Paired Stimulation System, Insertion X0HQ3R8
Neurotomy
  see Division, Central Nervous System and Cranial Nerves 008
  see Division, Peripheral Nervous System 018
Neurotripsy
  see Destruction, Central Nervous System and Cranial Nerves 005
  see Destruction, Peripheral Nervous System 015
Neutralization plate
  use Internal Fixation Device in Head and Facial Bones
  use Internal Fixation Device in Lower Bones
  use Internal Fixation Device in Upper Bones
New Technology
  Adhesive Ultrasound Patch Technology, Blood Flow XX25X0A
  Afamitresgene Autoleucel Immunotherapy XW0
  AGN1 Bone Void Filler XW0V3WA
  Amivantamab Monoclonal Antibody XW0
  Anacaulase-bcdb XW0
  Antibiotic-eluting Bone Void Filler XW0V0P7
  Aorta
    Thoracic Arch using Branched Synthetic Substitute with Intraluminal Device X2RX0N7
    Thoracic Descending using Branched Synthetic Substitute with Intraluminal Device X2VW0N7
    Thoracodominal, Branched Intraluminal Device, Manufactured Integrated System, Four or More Arteries X2VE3SA

New Technology — continued
  Atezolizumab Antineoplastic XWØ
  Axicabtagene Ciloleucel Immunotherapy XWØ
  Bamlanivimab Monoclonal Antibody XWØ
  Baricitinib XWØ
  Bentracimab, Ticagrelor Reversal Agent XWØ
  Betibeglogene Autotemcel XW1
  Bioengineered Allogeneic Construct, Skin XHRPXF7
  Bioengineered Human Acellular Vessel X2R
  Brain Electrical Activity
    Computer-aided Detection and Notification XX20X89
    Computer-aided Semiologic Analysis XXEØX48
  Brexanolone XWØ
  Brexucabtagene Autoleucel Immunotherapy XWØ
  Broad Consortium Microbiota-based Live Biotherapeutic Suspension XWØH7X8
  Bypass
    Conduit through Femoral Vein to Popliteal Artery X2K
    Conduit through Femoral Vein to Superficial Femoral Artery X2K
  Caplacizumab XWØ
  CD24Fc Immunomodulator XWØ
  Cefepime-taniborbactam Anti-infective XWØ
  Cefiderocol Anti-infective XWØ
  Ceftobiprole Medocaril Anti-infective XWØ
  Ceftolozane/Tazobactam Anti-infective XWØ
  Cerebral Embolic Filtration
    Dual Filter X2A5312
    Extracorporeal Flow Reversal Circuit X2A
    Single Deflection Filter X2A6325
  Ciltacabtagene Autoleucel XWØ
  Coagulation Factor Xa, Inactivated XWØ
  Computer-aided Assessment
    Cardiac Output XXE2X19
    Intracranial Vascular Activity XXEØX07
  Computer-aided Guidance, Transthoracic Echocardiography X2JAX47
  Computer-aided Mechanical Aspiration X2C
  Computer-aided Triage and Notification, Pulmonary Artery Flow XXE3X27
  Computer-aided Valve Modeling and Notification, Coronary Artery Flow XXE3X68
  Computer-assisted Transcranial Magnetic Stimulation XØZØX18
  Coronary Sinus, Reduction Device X2V73Q7
  COVID-19 Vaccine XWØ
  COVID-19 Vaccine Booster XWØ
  COVID-19 Vaccine Dose 1 XWØ
  COVID-19 Vaccine Dose 2 XWØ
  COVID-19 Vaccine Dose 3 XWØ
  Cytarabine and Daunorubicin Liposome Antineoplastic XWØ
  Daratumumab and Hyaluronidase-fihj XWØ1318
  Dasiglucagon XWØ136A
  Destruction
    Liver, Ultrasound-guided Cavitation XF5
    Renal Sympathetic Nerve(s), Ultrasound Ablation XØ51329
  Dilation
    Anterior Tibial
      Left, Intraluminal Device, Everolimus-eluting Resorbable Scaffold(s) X27Q3TA
      Right, Intraluminal Device, Everolimus-eluting Resorbable Scaffold(s) X27P3TA
    Peroneal
      Left, Intraluminal Device, Everolimus-eluting Resorbable Scaffold(s) X27U3TA
      Right, Intraluminal Device, Everolimus-eluting Resorbable Scaffold(s) X27T3TA
    Posterior Tibial
      Left, Intraluminal Device, Everolimus-eluting Resorbable Scaffold(s) X27S3TA
      Right, Intraluminal Device, Everolimus-eluting Resorbable Scaffold(s) X27R3TA
  Division, Intraluminal Bioprosthetic Valve Leaflet Splitting Technology in Existing Valve X28F3VA
  Donislecel-jujn Allogeneic Pancreatic Islet Cellular Suspension XWØ33DA
  Durvalumab Antineoplastic XWØ

New Technology — continued
  Eculizumab XWØ
  Eladocagene exuparvovec XWØQ316
  Elranatamab Antineoplastic XWØ13L9
  Endothelial Damage Inhibitor XYØVX83
  Engineered Allogeneic Thymus Tissue XWØ20D8
  Engineered Chimeric Antigen Receptor T-cell Immunotherapy
    Allogeneic XWØ
    Autologous XWØ
  Epcoritamab Monoclonal Antibody XWØ13S9
  Etesevimab Monoclonal Antibody XWØ
  Exagamglogene Autotemcel XW1
  Filtration, Blood Pathogens XXA536A
  Fostamatinib XWØ
  Fusion
    Ankle
      Left
        Gyroid-Sheet Lattice Design Internal Fixation Device XRGKØCA
        Open-truss Design Internal Fixation Device XRGKØB9
      Right
        Gyroid-Sheet Lattice Design Internal Fixation Device XRGJØCA
        Open-truss Design Internal Fixation Device XRGJØB9
    Lumbar Vertebral
      2 or more
        Facet Joint Fusion Device, Paired Titanium Cages XRGCØEA
        Interbody Fusion Device, Custom-Made Anatomically Designed XRGC
      Facet Joint Fusion Device, Paired Titanium Cages XRGBØEA
      Interbody Fusion Device, Custom-Made Anatomically Designed XRGB
    Lumbosacral
      Facet Joint Fusion Device, Paired Titanium Cages XRGDØEA
      Interbody Fusion Device, Custom-Made Anatomically Designed XRGD
    Sacroiliac, Internal Fixation Device with Tulip Connector XRG
    Tarsal
      Left
        Gyroid-Sheet Lattice Design Internal Fixation Device XRGMØCA
        Open-truss Design Internal Fixation Device XRGMØB9
      Right
        Gyroid-Sheet Lattice Design Internal Fixation Device XRGLØCA
        Open-truss Design Internal Fixation Device XRGLØB9
    Thoracolumbar Vertebral
      Facet Joint Fusion Device, Paired Titanium Cages XRGAØEA
      Interbody Fusion Device, Custom-Made Anatomically Designed XRGA
  Glofitamab Antineoplastic XWØ
  High-Dose Intravenous Immune Globulin, for COVID-19 treatment XW1
  Hyperimmune Globulin, for COVID-19 treatment XW1
  Idecabtagene Vicleucel Immunotherapy XWØ
  Inebilizumab-cdon XWØ
  Insertion
    Bone, Pelvic, Internal Fixation Device with Tulip Connector XNH
    Conduit to Short-term External Heart Assist System X2H
    Intracardiac Pacemaker, Dual-Chamber X2H
    Intraluminal Device, Bioprosthetic Valve X2H
    Joint
      Lumbar Vertebral
        2 or more, Carbon/PEEK Spinal Stabilization Device, Pedicle Based XRHC
        Carbon/PEEK Spinal Stabilization Device, Pedicle Based XRHB
        Posterior Spinal Motion Preservation Device XRHBØ18

New Technology — continued
  Insertion — continued
    Joint — continued
      Lumbosacral
        Carbon/PEEK Spinal Stabilization Device, Pedicle Based XRHD
        Posterior Spinal Motion Preservation Device XRHDØ18
      Thoracic Vertebral
        2 to 7, Carbon/PEEK Spinal Stabilization Device, Pedicle Based XRH7
        8 or more, Carbon/PEEK Spinal Stabilization Device, Pedicle Based XRH8
        Carbon/PEEK Spinal Stabilization Device, Pedicle Based XRH6
      Thoracolumbar Vertebral, Carbon/PEEK Spinal Stabilization Device, Pedicle Based XRHA
    Neurostimulator Lead, Sphenopalatine Ganglion XØHK3Q8
    Neurostimulator Lead with Paired Stimulation System XØHQ3R8
    Tibial Extension with Motion Sensors XNH
  Intermittent Coronary Sinus Occlusion X2A7358
  Interstitial Fluid Volume, Sub-Epidermal Moisture using Electrical Biocapacitance XX2KXP9
  Intracranial Arterial Flow, Whole Blood mRNA XXE5XT7
  Intracranial Cerebrospinal Fluid Flow, Computer-aided Triage and Notification XXEØX1A
  Iobenguane I-131 Antineoplastic XWØ
  Kidney, Fluorescent Pyrazine XT25XE5
  Lefamulin Anti-infective XWØ
  Leronlimab Monoclonal Antibody XWØ13K6
  Lifileucel Immunotherapy XWØ
  Lisocabtagene Maraleucel Immunotherapy XWØ
  Lovotibeglogene Autotemcel XW1
  Lower Respiratory Fluid Nucleic Acid-base Microbial Detection XXEBXQ6
  Lurbinectedin XWØ
  Maribavir Anti-infective XWØ
  Marnetegragene Autotemcel XW1
  Mechanical Initial Specimen Diversion Technique Using Active Negative Pressure (blood collection) XXE5XR7
  Melphalan Hydrochloride Antineoplastic XWØ53T9
  Mineral-based Topical Hemostatic Agent XWØ
  Mosunetuzumab Antineoplastic XWØ
  Multi-plane Flex Technology Bioprosthetic Valve X2RJ3RA
  Muscle Compartment Pressure, Micro-Electro-Mechanical System XX2F3W9
  Nafamostat Anticoagulant XYØYX37
  Narsoplimab Monoclonal Antibody XWØ
  Nerinitide XWØ
  Neurostimulator Lead in Oropharynx XWHD7Q7
  Non-Chimeric Antigen Receptor T-cell Immune Effector Cell Therapy XWØ
  Obecabtagene Autoleucel XWØ
  Odronextamab Antineoplastic XWØ
  Omadacycline Anti-infective XWØ
  Omidubicel XW1
  Orca-T Allogeneic T-cell Immunotherapy XWØ
  Other New Technology Monoclonal Antibody XWØ
  Other New Technology Therapeutic Substance XWØ
  Other Positive Blood/Isolated Colonies Bimodal Phenotypic Susceptibility Technology XXE5XY9
  OTL-103 XW1
  OTL-200 XW1
  Oxygen Saturation Endoscopic Imaging (OXEI) XD2
  Paclitaxel-Coated Balloon Technology XWØ
  Phenotypic Fully Automated Rapid Susceptibility Technology with Controlled Inoculum XXE5X2A
  Plasma, Convalescent (Nonautologous) XW1
  Positive Blood Culture Fluorescence Hybridization for Organism Identification, Concentration and Susceptibility XXE5XN6
  Positive Blood Culture Small Molecule Sensor Array Technology XXE5X4A
  Posoleucel XWØ
  Quantitative Flow Ratio Analysis, Coronary Artery Flow XXE3X58
  Quizartinib Antineoplastic XWØDXJ9

▽ Subterms under main terms may continue to next column or page

New Technology

New Technology — *continued*
- Radial artery arteriovenous fistula, using Thermal Resistance Energy X2K
- REGN-COV2 Monoclonal Antibody XW0
- Remdesivir Anti-infective XW0
- Renal Sympathetic Nerve(s), Radiofrequency Ablation X05133Z
- Replacement
  - Lateral Meniscus Synthetic Substitute XRR
  - Medial Meniscus Synthetic Substitute XRR
- Reposition
  - Cervical, Magnetically Controlled Growth Rod(s) XNS3
  - Lumbar
    - Magnetically Controlled Growth Rod(s) XNS0
    - Posterior (Dynamic) Distraction Device XNS0
  - Thoracic
    - Magnetically Controlled Growth Rod(s) XNS4
    - Posterior (Dynamic) Distraction Device XNS4
- Rezafungin XW0
- Sabizabulin XW0
- Sarilumab XW0
- SARS-CoV-2 Antibody Detection, Serum/Plasma Nanoparticle Fluorescence XXE5XV7
- SARS-CoV-2 Polymerase Chain Reaction, Nasopharyngeal Fluid XXE97U7
- Satralizumab-mwge XW01397
- SER-109 XW0DXN9
- Single-use Duodenoscope XFJ
- Single-use Oversleeve with Intraoperative Colonic Irrigation XDPH8K7
- Skin
  - Abdomen, Prademagene Zamikeracel, Genetically Engineered Autologous Cell Therapy XHR2XGA
  - Back, Prademagene Zamikeracel, Genetically Engineered Autologous Cell Therapy XHR3XGA
  - Chest, Prademagene Zamikeracel, Genetically Engineered Autologous Cell Therapy XHR1XGA
  - Head and Neck, Prademagene Zamikeracel, Genetically Engineered Autologous Cell Therapy XHR0XGA
  - Lower Extremity
    - Left, Prademagene Zamikeracel, Genetically Engineered Autologous Cell Therapy XHR7XGA
    - Right, Prademagene Zamikeracel, Genetically Engineered Autologous Cell Therapy XHR6XGA
  - Upper Extremity
    - Left, Prademagene Zamikeracel, Genetically Engineered Autologous Cell Therapy XHR5XGA
    - Right, Prademagene Zamikeracel, Genetically Engineered Autologous Cell Therapy XHR4XGA
- Spesolimab Monoclonal Antibody XW0
- Sulbactam-Durlobactam XW0
- Supplement
  - Arteriovenous Fistula, Extraluminal Support Device X2U
  - Bursa and Ligament, Spine, Posterior Vertebral Tether XKU
  - Coronary Artery/Arteries, Vein Graft Extraluminal Support Device(s) X2U4079
  - Vertebra
    - Lumbar, Mechanically Expandable (Paired) Synthetic Substitute XNU0356
    - Thoracic, Mechanically Expandable (Paired) Synthetic Substitute XNU4356
- Tabelecleucel Immunotherapy XW0
- Tagraxofusp-erzs Antineoplastic XW0
- Talar Prosthesis Synthetic Substitute XNR
- Talquetamab Antineoplastic XW01329
- Taurolidine Anti-infective and Heparin Anticoagulant XY0YX28
- Teclistamab Antineoplastic XW01348
- Terlipressin XW0
- Tisagenlecleucel Immunotherapy XW0
- Tixagevimab and Cilgavimab Monoclonal Antibody XW023X7

New Technology — *continued*
- Tocilizumab XW0
- Treosulfan XW0
- Trilaciclib XW0
- Ultrasound Penetrable Synthetic Substitute, Skull XNR80D9
- Uridine Triacetate XW0DX82
- Vancomycin Hydrochloride and Tobramycin Sulfate Anti-infective, Temporary Irrigation Spacer System XW0U0GA
- Whole Blood Reverse Transcription and Quantitative Real-time Polymerase Chain Reaction XXE5X38
- Zanidatamab Antineoplastic XW0

NexoBrid™ *use* Anacaulase-bcdb
Ninth cranial nerve *use* Glossopharyngeal Nerve
NIRS (Near Infrared Spectroscopy) *see* Physiological Systems and Anatomical Regions 8E0
Nitinol framed polymer mesh *use* Synthetic Substitute
Niyad™ *use* Nafamostat Anticoagulant
Non-Chimeric Antigen Receptor T-cell Immune Effector Cell Therapy XW0
Nonimaging Nuclear Medicine Assay
- Bladder, Kidneys and Ureters CT63
- Blood C763
- Kidneys, Ureters and Bladder CT63
- Lymphatics and Hematologic System C76YYZZ
- Ureters, Kidneys and Bladder CT63
- Urinary System CT6YYZZ

Nonimaging Nuclear Medicine Probe
- Abdomen CW50
- Abdomen and Chest CW54
- Abdomen and Pelvis CW51
- Brain C050
- Central Nervous System C05YYZZ
- Chest CW53
- Chest and Abdomen CW54
- Chest and Neck CW56
- Extremity
  - Lower CP5PZZZ
  - Upper CP5NZZZ
- Head and Neck CW5B
- Heart C25YYZZ
  - Right and Left C256
- Lymphatics
  - Head C75J
  - Head and Neck C755
  - Lower Extremity C75P
  - Neck C75K
  - Pelvic C75D
  - Trunk C75M
  - Upper Chest C75L
  - Upper Extremity C75N
- Lymphatics and Hematologic System C75YYZZ
- Musculoskeletal System, Other CP5YYZZ
- Neck and Chest CW56
- Neck and Head CW5B
- Pelvic Region CW5J
- Pelvis and Abdomen CW51
- Spine CP55ZZZ

Nonimaging Nuclear Medicine Uptake
- Endocrine System CG4YYZZ
- Gland, Thyroid CG42

Non-tunneled central venous catheter *use* Infusion Device
Nostril *use* Nasal Mucosa and Soft Tissue
Novacor Left Ventricular Assist Device *use* Implantable Heart Assist System in Heart and Great Vessels
Novation® Ceramic AHS® (Articulation Hip System) *use* Synthetic Substitute, Ceramic in 0SR
Nuclear medicine
- *see* Nonimaging Nuclear Medicine Assay
- *see* Nonimaging Nuclear Medicine Probe
- *see* Nonimaging Nuclear Medicine Uptake
- *see* Planar Nuclear Medicine Imaging
- *see* Positron Emission Tomographic (PET) Imaging
- *see* Systemic Nuclear Medicine Therapy
- *see* Tomographic (Tomo) Nuclear Medicine Imaging

Nuclear scintigraphy *see* Nuclear Medicine
NUsurface® Meniscus Implant
- *use* Synthetic Substitute, Lateral Meniscus in New Technology
- *use* Synthetic Substitute, Medial Meniscus in New Technology

Nutrition, concentrated substances
- Enteral infusion 3E0G36Z
- Parenteral (peripheral) infusion *see* Introduction of Nutritional Substance

NUZYRA™ *use* Omadacycline Anti-infective

O

Obecabtagene Autoleucel XW0
obe-cel *use* Obecabtagene Autoleucel
Obliteration *see* Destruction
Obturator artery
- *use* Internal Iliac Artery, Left
- *use* Internal Iliac Artery, Right

Obturator lymph node *use* Lymphatic, Pelvis
Obturator muscle
- *use* Hip Muscle, Left
- *use* Hip Muscle, Right

Obturator nerve *use* Lumbar Plexus
Obturator vein
- *use* Hypogastric Vein, Left
- *use* Hypogastric Vein, Right

Obtuse margin *use* Heart, Left
Occipital artery
- *use* External Carotid Artery, Left
- *use* External Carotid Artery, Right

Occipital lobe *use* Cerebral Hemisphere
Occipital lymph node
- *use* Lymphatic, Left Neck
- *use* Lymphatic, Right Neck

Occipitofrontalis muscle *use* Facial Muscle
Occlusion
- Ampulla of Vater 0FLC
- Anus 0DLQ
- Aorta
  - Abdominal 04L0
  - Thoracic, Descending 02LW
- Artery
  - Anterior Tibial
    - Left 04LQ
    - Right 04LP
  - Axillary
    - Left 03L6
    - Right 03L5
  - Brachial
    - Left 03L8
    - Right 03L7
  - Celiac 04L1
  - Colic
    - Left 04L7
    - Middle 04L8
    - Right 04L6
  - Common Carotid
    - Left 03LJ
    - Right 03LH
  - Common Iliac
    - Left 04LD
    - Right 04LC
  - External Carotid
    - Left 03LN
    - Right 03LM
  - External Iliac
    - Left 04LJ
    - Right 04LH
  - Face 03LR
  - Femoral
    - Left 04LL
    - Right 04LK
  - Foot
    - Left 04LW
    - Right 04LV
  - Gastric 04L2
  - Hand
    - Left 03LF
    - Right 03LD
  - Hepatic 04L3
  - Inferior Mesenteric 04LB
  - Innominate 03L2
  - Internal Carotid
    - Left 03LL
    - Right 03LK
  - Internal Iliac
    - Left 04LF
    - Right 04LE
  - Internal Mammary
    - Left 03L1
    - Right 03L0

Occlusion — continued
- Artery — continued
  - Intracranial 03LG
  - Lower 04LY
  - Peroneal
    - Left 04LU
    - Right 04LT
  - Popliteal
    - Left 04LN
    - Right 04LM
  - Posterior Tibial
    - Left 04LS
    - Right 04LR
  - Pulmonary
    - Left 02LR
    - Right 02LQ
  - Pulmonary Trunk 02LP
  - Radial
    - Left 03LC
    - Right 03LB
  - Renal
    - Left 04LA
    - Right 04L9
  - Splenic 04L4
  - Subclavian
    - Left 03L4
    - Right 03L3
  - Superior Mesenteric 04L5
  - Temporal
    - Left 03LT
    - Right 03LS
  - Thyroid
    - Left 03LV
    - Right 03LU
  - Ulnar
    - Left 03LA
    - Right 03L9
  - Upper 03LY
  - Vertebral
    - Left 03LQ
    - Right 03LP
- Atrium, Left 02L7
- Bladder 0TLB
- Bladder Neck 0TLC
- Bronchus
  - Lingula 0BL9
  - Lower Lobe
    - Left 0BLB
    - Right 0BL6
  - Main
    - Left 0BL7
    - Right 0BL3
  - Middle Lobe, Right 0BL5
  - Upper Lobe
    - Left 0BL8
    - Right 0BL4
- Carina 0BL2
- Cecum 0DLH
- Cisterna Chyli 07LL
- Colon
  - Ascending 0DLK
  - Descending 0DLM
  - Sigmoid 0DLN
  - Transverse 0DLL
- Cord
  - Bilateral 0VLH
  - Left 0VLG
  - Right 0VLF
- Cul-de-sac 0ULF
- Duct
  - Common Bile 0FL9
  - Cystic 0FL8
  - Hepatic
    - Common 0FL7
    - Left 0FL6
    - Right 0FL5
  - Lacrimal
    - Left 08LY
    - Right 08LX
  - Pancreatic 0FLD
    - Accessory 0FLF
  - Parotid
    - Left 0CLC
    - Right 0CLB
- Duodenum 0DL9
- Esophagogastric Junction 0DL4
- Esophagus 0DL5
  - Lower 0DL3
  - Middle 0DL2

Occlusion — continued
- Esophagus — continued
  - Upper 0DL1
- Fallopian Tube
  - Left 0UL6
  - Right 0UL5
- Fallopian Tubes, Bilateral 0UL7
- Ileocecal Valve 0DLC
- Ileum 0DLB
- Intestine
  - Large 0DLE
    - Left 0DLG
    - Right 0DLF
  - Small 0DL8
- Jejunum 0DLA
- Kidney Pelvis
  - Left 0TL4
  - Right 0TL3
- Left atrial appendage (LAA) see Occlusion, Atrium, Left 02L7
- Lymphatic
  - Aortic 07LD
  - Axillary
    - Left 07L6
    - Right 07L5
  - Head 07L0
  - Inguinal
    - Left 07LJ
    - Right 07LH
  - Internal Mammary
    - Left 07L9
    - Right 07L8
  - Lower Extremity
    - Left 07LG
    - Right 07LF
  - Mesenteric 07LB
  - Neck
    - Left 07L2
    - Right 07L1
  - Pelvis 07LC
  - Thoracic Duct 07LK
  - Thorax 07L7
  - Upper Extremity
    - Left 07L4
    - Right 07L3
- Rectum 0DLP
- Stomach 0DL6
  - Pylorus 0DL7
- Trachea 0BL1
- Ureter
  - Left 0TL7
  - Right 0TL6
- Urethra 0TLD
- Vagina 0ULG
- Valve, Pulmonary 02LH
- Vas Deferens
  - Bilateral 0VLQ
  - Left 0VLP
  - Right 0VLN
- Vein
  - Axillary
    - Left 05L8
    - Right 05L7
  - Azygos 05L0
  - Basilic
    - Left 05LC
    - Right 05LB
  - Brachial
    - Left 05LA
    - Right 05L9
  - Cephalic
    - Left 05LF
    - Right 05LD
  - Colic 06L7
  - Common Iliac
    - Left 06LD
    - Right 06LC
  - Esophageal 06L3
  - External Iliac
    - Left 06LG
    - Right 06LF
  - External Jugular
    - Left 05LQ
    - Right 05LP
  - Face
    - Left 05LV
    - Right 05LT
  - Femoral
    - Left 06LN

Occlusion — continued
- Vein — continued
  - Femoral — continued
    - Right 06LM
  - Foot
    - Left 06LV
    - Right 06LT
  - Gastric 06L2
  - Hand
    - Left 05LH
    - Right 05LG
  - Hemiazygos 05L1
  - Hepatic 06L4
  - Hypogastric
    - Left 06LJ
    - Right 06LH
  - Inferior Mesenteric 06L6
  - Innominate
    - Left 05L4
    - Right 05L3
  - Internal Jugular
    - Left 05LN
    - Right 05LM
  - Intracranial 05LL
  - Lower 06LY
  - Portal 06L8
  - Pulmonary
    - Left 02LT
    - Right 02LS
  - Renal
    - Left 06LB
    - Right 06L9
  - Saphenous
    - Left 06LQ
    - Right 06LP
  - Splenic 06L1
  - Subclavian
    - Left 05L6
    - Right 05L5
  - Superior Mesenteric 06L5
  - Upper 05LY
  - Vertebral
    - Left 05LS
    - Right 05LR
- Vena Cava
  - Inferior 06L0
  - Superior 02LV

Occlusion, REBOA (resuscitative endovascular balloon occlusion of the aorta)
- 02LW3DJ
- 04L03DJ

Occupational therapy see Activities of Daily Living Treatment, Rehabilitation F08

Octagam 10%, for COVID-19 treatment use High-Dose Intravenous Immune Globulin

Odentectomy
- see Excision, Mouth and Throat 0CB
- see Resection, Mouth and Throat 0CT

Odontoid process use Cervical Vertebra

Odronextamab Antineoplastic XW0

Olecranon bursa
- use Elbow Bursa and Ligament, Left
- use Elbow Bursa and Ligament, Right

Olecranon process
- use Ulna, Left
- use Ulna, Right

Olfactory bulb use Olfactory Nerve

Olumiant® use Baricitinib

Omadacycline Anti-infective XW0

Omentectomy, omentumectomy
- see Excision, Gastrointestinal System 0DB
- see Resection, Gastrointestinal System 0DT

Omentofixation see Repair, Gastrointestinal System 0DQ

Omentoplasty
- see Repair, Gastrointestinal System 0DQ
- see Replacement, Gastrointestinal System 0DR
- see Supplement, Gastrointestinal System 0DU

Omentoplasty, pedicled see Transfer, Omentum 0DXU

Omentorrhaphy see Repair, Gastrointestinal System 0DQ

Omentotomy see Drainage, Gastrointestinal System 0D9

Omidubicel XW1

Omisirge® use Omidubicel

Omnilink Elite Vascular Balloon Expandable Stent System use Intraluminal Device

OneRF™ Ablation System 00503Z4

Onychectomy
see Excision, Skin and Breast 0HB
see Resection, Skin and Breast 0HT

Onychoplasty
see Repair, Skin and Breast 0HQ
see Replacement, Skin and Breast 0HR

Onychotomy see Drainage, Skin and Breast 0H9

Oophorectomy
see Excision, Female Reproductive System 0UB
see Resection, Female Reproductive System 0UT

Oophoropexy
see Repair, Female Reproductive System 0UQ
see Reposition, Female Reproductive System 0US

Oophoroplasty
see Repair, Female Reproductive System 0UQ
see Supplement, Female Reproductive System 0UU

Oophororrhaphy see Repair, Female Reproductive System 0UQ

Oophorostomy see Drainage, Female Reproductive System 0U9

Oophorotomy
see Division, Female Reproductive System 0U8
see Drainage, Female Reproductive System 0U9

Oophorrhaphy see Repair, Female Reproductive System 0UQ

Open Pivot Aortic Valve Graft (AVG) use Synthetic Substitute

Open Pivot (mechanical) Valve use Synthetic Substitute

Open-truss Design Internal Fixation Device
Ankle
Left XRGK0B9
Right XRGJ0B9
Tarsal
Left XRGM0B9
Right XRGL0B9

Ophthalmic artery use Intracranial Artery
Ophthalmic nerve use Trigeminal Nerve
Ophthalmic vein use Intracranial Vein

Opponensplasty
Tendon replacement see Replacement, Tendons 0LR
Tendon transfer see Transfer, Tendons 0LX

Optic chiasma use Optic Nerve

Optic disc
use Retina, Left
use Retina, Right

Optic foramen use Sphenoid Bone

Optical coherence tomography, intravascular see Computerized Tomography (CT Scan)

Optimizer™ III implantable pulse generator use Contractility Modulation Device in 0JH

Orbicularis oculi muscle
use Upper Eyelid, Left
use Upper Eyelid, Right

Orbicularis oris muscle use Facial Muscle

Orbital Atherectomy see Extirpation, Heart and Great Vessels 02C

Orbital fascia use Subcutaneous Tissue and Fascia, Face

Orbital portion of ethmoid bone
use Orbit, Left
use Orbit, Right

Orbital portion of frontal bone
use Orbit, Left
use Orbit, Right

Orbital portion of lacrimal bone
use Orbit, Left
use Orbit, Right

Orbital portion of maxilla
use Orbit, Left
use Orbit, Right

Orbital portion of palatine bone
use Orbit, Left
use Orbit, Right

Orbital portion of sphenoid bone
use Orbit, Left
use Orbit, Right

Orbital portion of zygomatic bone
use Orbit, Left
use Orbit, Right

Orca-T Allogeneic T-cell Immunotherapy XW0

Orchectomy, orchidectomy, orchiectomy
see Excision, Male Reproductive System 0VB
see Resection, Male Reproductive System 0VT

Orchidoplasty, orchioplasty
see Repair, Male Reproductive System 0VQ

Orchidoplasty, orchioplasty — continued
see Replacement, Male Reproductive System 0VR
see Supplement, Male Reproductive System 0VU

Orchidorrhaphy, orchiorrhaphy see Repair, Male Reproductive System 0VQ

Orchidotomy, orchiotomy, orchotomy see Drainage, Male Reproductive System 0V9

Orchiopexy
see Repair, Male Reproductive System 0VQ
see Reposition, Male Reproductive System 0VS

Oropharyngeal airway (OPA) use Intraluminal Device, Airway in Mouth and Throat

Oropharynx use Pharynx

Ossiculectomy
see Excision, Ear, Nose, Sinus 09B
see Resection, Ear, Nose, Sinus 09T

Ossiculotomy see Drainage, Ear, Nose, Sinus 099

OSSURE® XW0V3WA

OSSURE™ implant material use AGN1 Bone Void Filler

Ostectomy
see Excision, Head and Facial Bones 0NB
see Excision, Lower Bones 0QB
see Excision, Upper Bones 0PB
see Resection, Head and Facial Bones 0NT
see Resection, Lower Bones 0QT
see Resection, Upper Bones 0PT

Osteoclasis
see Division, Head and Facial Bones 0N8
see Division, Lower Bones 0Q8
see Division, Upper Bones 0P8

Osteolysis
see Release, Head and Facial Bones 0NN
see Release, Lower Bones 0QN
see Release, Upper Bones 0PN

Osteopathic Treatment
Abdomen 7W09X
Cervical 7W01X
Extremity
Lower 7W06X
Upper 7W07X
Head 7W00X
Lumbar 7W03X
Pelvis 7W05X
Rib Cage 7W08X
Sacrum 7W04X
Thoracic 7W02X

Osteopexy
see Repair, Head and Facial Bones 0NQ
see Repair, Lower Bones 0QQ
see Repair, Upper Bones 0PQ
see Reposition, Head and Facial Bones 0NS
see Reposition, Lower Bones 0QS
see Reposition, Upper Bones 0PS

Osteoplasty
see Repair, Head and Facial Bones 0NQ
see Repair, Lower Bones 0QQ
see Repair, Upper Bones 0PQ
see Replacement, Head and Facial Bones 0NR
see Replacement, Lower Bones 0QR
see Replacement, Upper Bones 0PR
see Supplement, Head and Facial Bones 0NU
see Supplement, Lower Bones 0QU
see Supplement, Upper Bones 0PU

Osteorrhaphy
see Repair, Head and Facial Bones 0NQ
see Repair, Lower Bones 0QQ
see Repair, Upper Bones 0PQ

Osteotomy, ostotomy
see Division, Head and Facial Bones 0N8
see Division, Lower Bones 0Q8
see Division, Upper Bones 0P8
see Drainage, Head and Facial Bones 0N9
see Drainage, Lower Bones 0Q9
see Drainage, Upper Bones 0P9

Other Imaging
Bile Duct and Gallbladder, Indocyanine Green Dye, Intraoperative BF53200
Bile Duct, Indocyanine Green Dye, Intraoperative BF50200
Extremity
Lower BW5CZ1Z
Upper BW5JZ1Z
Gallbladder and Bile Duct, Indocyanine Green Dye, Intraoperative BF53200
Gallbladder, Indocyanine Green Dye, Intraoperative BF52200
Head and Neck BW59Z1Z

Other Imaging — continued
Hepatobiliary System, All, Indocyanine Green Dye, Intraoperative BF5C200
Liver and Spleen, Indocyanine Green Dye, Intraoperative BF56200
Liver, Indocyanine Green Dye, Intraoperative BF55200
Neck and Head BW59Z1Z
Pancreas, Indocyanine Green Dye, Intraoperative BF57200
Spleen and Liver, Indocyanine Green Dye, Intraoperative BF56200
Trunk BW52Z1Z

Other New Technology Monoclonal Antibody XW0

Other New Technology Therapeutic Substance XW0

Other Positive Blood/Isolated Colonies Bimodal Phenotypic Susceptibility Technology XXE5XY9

Otic ganglion use Head and Neck Sympathetic Nerve

OTL-101 use Hematopoietic Stem/Progenitor Cells, Genetically Modified

OTL-103 XW1

OTL-200 XW1

Otoplasty
see Repair, Ear, Nose, Sinus 09Q
see Replacement, Ear, Nose, Sinus 09R
see Supplement, Ear, Nose, Sinus 09U

Otoscopy see Inspection, Ear, Nose, Sinus 09J

Oval window
use Middle Ear, Left
use Middle Ear, Right

Ovarian artery use Abdominal Aorta

Ovarian ligament use Uterine Supporting Structure

Ovariectomy
see Excision, Female Reproductive System 0UB
see Resection, Female Reproductive System 0UT

Ovariocentesis see Drainage, Female Reproductive System 0U9

Ovariopexy
see Repair, Female Reproductive System 0UQ
see Reposition, Female Reproductive System 0US

Ovariotomy
see Division, Female Reproductive System 0U8
see Drainage, Female Reproductive System 0U9

Ovatio™ CRT-D use Cardiac Resynchronization Defibrillator Pulse Generator in 0JH

Oversewing
Gastrointestinal ulcer see Repair, Gastrointestinal System 0DQ
Pleural bleb see Repair, Respiratory System 0BQ

Oviduct
use Fallopian Tube, Left
use Fallopian Tube, Right

Oximetry, Fetal pulse 10H073Z

OXINIUM use Synthetic Substitute, Oxidized Zirconium on Polyethylene in 0SR

Oxygen Saturation Endoscopic Imaging (OXEI) XD2

Oxygenation
Extracorporeal membrane (ECMO) see Performance, Circulatory 5A15
Hyperbaric see Assistance, Circulatory 5A05
Supersaturated see Assistance, Cardiac 5A02

P

Pacemaker
Dual Chamber
Abdomen 0JH8
Chest 0JH6
Intracardiac
Insertion of device in
Atrium
Left 02H7
Right 02H6
Vein, Coronary 02H4
Ventricle
Left 02HL
Right 02HK
Removal of device from, Heart 02PA
Revision of device in, Heart 02WA
Single Chamber
Abdomen 0JH8
Chest 0JH6
Single Chamber Rate Responsive
Abdomen 0JH8
Chest 0JH6

Packing
  Abdominal Wall 2W43X5Z
  Anorectal 2Y43X5Z
  Arm
    Lower
      Left 2W4DX5Z
      Right 2W4CX5Z
    Upper
      Left 2W4BX5Z
      Right 2W4AX5Z
  Back 2W45X5Z
  Chest Wall 2W44X5Z
  Ear 2Y42X5Z
  Extremity
    Lower
      Left 2W4MX5Z
      Right 2W4LX5Z
    Upper
      Left 2W49X5Z
      Right 2W48X5Z
  Face 2W41X5Z
  Finger
    Left 2W4KX5Z
    Right 2W4JX5Z
  Foot
    Left 2W4TX5Z
    Right 2W4SX5Z
  Genital Tract, Female 2Y44X5Z
  Hand
    Left 2W4FX5Z
    Right 2W4EX5Z
  Head 2W40X5Z
  Inguinal Region
    Left 2W47X5Z
    Right 2W46X5Z
  Leg
    Lower
      Left 2W4RX5Z
      Right 2W4QX5Z
    Upper
      Left 2W4PX5Z
      Right 2W4NX5Z
  Mouth and Pharynx 2Y40X5Z
  Nasal 2Y41X5Z
  Neck 2W42X5Z
  Thumb
    Left 2W4HX5Z
    Right 2W4GX5Z
  Toe
    Left 2W4VX5Z
    Right 2W4UX5Z
  Urethra 2Y45X5Z
Paclitaxel-Coated Balloon Technology XW0
Paclitaxel-eluting coronary stent use Intraluminal Device, Drug-eluting in Heart and Great Vessels
Paclitaxel-eluting peripheral stent
  use Intraluminal Device, Drug-eluting in Lower Arteries
  use Intraluminal Device, Drug-eluting in Upper Arteries
Palatine gland use Buccal Mucosa
Palatine tonsil use Tonsils
Palatine uvula use Uvula
Palatoglossal muscle use Tongue, Palate, Pharynx Muscle
Palatopharyngeal muscle use Tongue, Palate, Pharynx Muscle
Palatoplasty
  see Repair, Mouth and Throat 0CQ
  see Replacement, Mouth and Throat 0CR
  see Supplement, Mouth and Throat 0CU
Palatorrhaphy see Repair, Mouth and Throat 0CQ
Palladium-103 Collagen Implant use Radioactive Element, Palladium-103 Collagen Implant in 00H
Palmar cutaneous nerve
  use Median Nerve
  use Radial Nerve
Palmar (volar) digital vein
  use Hand Vein, Left
  use Hand Vein, Right
Palmar fascia (aponeurosis)
  use Subcutaneous Tissue and Fascia, Left Hand
  use Subcutaneous Tissue and Fascia, Right Hand
Palmar interosseous muscle
  use Hand Muscle, Left
  use Hand Muscle, Right
Palmar (volar) metacarpal vein
  use Hand Vein, Left

Palmar (volar) metacarpal vein — continued
  use Hand Vein, Right
Palmar ulnocarpal ligament
  use Wrist Bursa and Ligament, Left
  use Wrist Bursa and Ligament, Right
Palmaris longus muscle
  use Lower Arm and Wrist Muscle, Left
  use Lower Arm and Wrist Muscle, Right
Pancreatectomy
  see Excision, Pancreas 0FBG
  see Resection, Pancreas 0FTG
Pancreatic artery use Splenic Artery
Pancreatic plexus use Abdominal Sympathetic Nerve
Pancreatic vein use Splenic Vein
Pancreaticoduodenostomy see Bypass, Hepatobiliary System and Pancreas 0F1
Pancreaticosplenic lymph node use Lymphatic, Aortic
Pancreatogram, endoscopic retrograde see Fluoroscopy, Pancreatic Duct BF18
Pancreatolithotomy see Extirpation, Pancreas 0FCG
Pancreatotomy
  see Division, Pancreas 0F8G
  see Drainage, Pancreas 0F9G
Panniculectomy
  see Excision, Skin, Abdomen 0HB7
  see Excision, Subcutaneous Tissue and Fascia, Abdomen 0JB8
Paraaortic lymph node use Lymphatic, Aortic
Paracentesis
  Eye see Drainage, Eye 089
  Peritoneal Cavity see Drainage, Peritoneal Cavity 0W9G
  Tympanum see Drainage, Ear, Nose, Sinus 099
Paradise™ Ultrasound Renal Denervation System X051329
Parapharyngeal space use Neck
Pararectal lymph node use Lymphatic, Mesenteric
Parasternal lymph node use Lymphatic, Thorax
Parathyroidectomy
  see Excision, Endocrine System 0GB
  see Resection, Endocrine System 0GT
Paratracheal lymph node use Lymphatic, Thorax
Paraurethral (Skene's) gland use Vestibular Gland
Parenteral nutrition, total see Introduction of Nutritional Substance
Parietal lobe use Cerebral Hemisphere
Parotid lymph node use Lymphatic, Head
Parotid plexus use Facial Nerve
Parotidectomy
  see Excision, Mouth and Throat 0CB
  see Resection, Mouth and Throat 0CT
Pars flaccida
  use Tympanic Membrane, Left
  use Tympanic Membrane, Right
Partial joint replacement
  Hip see Replacement, Lower Joints 0SR
  Knee see Replacement, Lower Joints 0SR
  Shoulder see Replacement, Upper Joints 0RR
Partially absorbable mesh use Synthetic Substitute
Patch, blood, spinal 3E0R3GC
Patellapexy
  see Repair, Lower Bones 0QQ
  see Reposition, Lower Bones 0QS
Patellaplasty
  see Repair, Lower Bones 0QQ
  see Replacement, Lower Bones 0QR
  see Supplement, Lower Bones 0QU
Patellar ligament
  use Knee Bursa and Ligament, Left
  use Knee Bursa and Ligament, Right
Patellar tendon
  use Knee Tendon, Left
  use Knee Tendon, Right
Patellectomy
  see Excision, Lower Bones 0QB
  see Resection, Lower Bones 0QT
Patellofemoral joint
  use Knee Joint, Left
  use Knee Joint, Left, Femoral Surface
  use Knee Joint, Right
  use Knee Joint, Right, Femoral Surface
pAVF (percutaneous arteriovenous fistula), using magnetic-guided radiofrequency see Bypass, Upper Arteries 031

pAVF (percutaneous arteriovenous fistula), using thermal resistance energy see New Technology, Cardiovascular System X2K
Pectineus muscle
  use Upper Leg Muscle, Left
  use Upper Leg Muscle, Right
Pectoral fascia use Subcutaneous Tissue and Fascia, Chest
Pectoral (anterior) lymph node
  use Lymphatic Left, Axillary
  use Lymphatic Right, Axillary
Pectoralis major muscle
  use Thorax Muscle, Left
  use Thorax Muscle, Right
Pectoralis minor muscle
  use Thorax Muscle, Left
  use Thorax Muscle, Right
Pedicle-based dynamic stabilization device
  use Spinal Stabilization Device, Pedicle-Based in 0SH
  use Spinal Stabilization Device, Pedicle-Based in 0RH
PEEP (positive end expiratory pressure) see Assistance, Respiratory 5A09
PEG (percutaneous endoscopic gastrostomy) 0DH63UZ
PEJ (percutaneous endoscopic jejunostomy) 0DHA3UZ
Pelvic splanchnic nerve
  use Abdominal Sympathetic Nerve
  use Sacral Sympathetic Nerve
Penectomy
  see Excision, Male Reproductive System 0VB
  see Resection, Male Reproductive System 0VT
Penile urethra use Urethra
Penumbra Indigo® Aspiration System see New Technology, Cardiovascular System X2C
PERCEPT™ PC neurostimulator use Stimulator Generator, Multiple Array in 0JH
Perceval sutureless valve (rapid deployment technique) see Replacement, Valve, Aortic 02RF
Percutaneous endoscopic gastrojejunostomy (PEG/J) tube use Feeding Device in Gastrointestinal System
Percutaneous endoscopic gastrostomy (PEG) tube use Feeding Device in Gastrointestinal System
Percutaneous nephrostomy catheter use Drainage Device
Percutaneous transluminal coronary angioplasty (PTCA) see Dilation, Heart and Great Vessels 027
Percutaneous tricuspid valve replacement
  EVOQUE valve/system (Edwards) X2RJ3RA
  Other valve/system 02RJ38Z
Performance
  Biliary
    Multiple, Filtration 5A1C60Z
    Single, Filtration 5A1C00Z
  Cardiac
    Continuous
      Output 5A1221Z
      Pacing 5A1223Z
    Intermittent, Pacing 5A1213Z
    Single, Output, Manual 5A12012
  Circulatory
    Continuous
      Central Membrane 5A1522F
      Peripheral Veno-arterial Membrane 5A1522G
      Peripheral Veno-venous Membrane 5A1522H
    Intraoperative
      Central Membrane 5A15A2F
      Peripheral Veno-arterial Membrane 5A15A2G
      Peripheral Veno-venous Membrane 5A15A2H
  Respiratory
    24-96 Consecutive Hours, Ventilation 5A1945Z
    Greater than 96 Consecutive Hours, Ventilation 5A1955Z
    Less than 24 Consecutive Hours, Ventilation 5A1935Z
    Single, Ventilation, Nonmechanical 5A19054
  Urinary
    Continuous, Greater than 18 hours per day, Filtration 5A1D90Z

Performance — *continued*
  Urinary — *continued*
    Intermittent, Less than 6 Hours Per Day, Filtration 5A1D70Z
    Prolonged Intermittent, 6-18 hours per day, Filtration 5A1D80Z
Perfusion *see* Introduction of substance in or on
Perfusion, donor organ
  Heart 6AB50BZ
  Kidney(s) 6ABT0BZ
  Liver 6ABF0BZ
  Lung(s) 6ABB0BZ
Perianal skin *use* Skin, Perineum
Pericardiectomy
  see Excision, Pericardium 02BN
  see Resection, Pericardium 02TN
Pericardiocentesis *see* Drainage, Pericardial Cavity 0W9D
Pericardiolysis *see* Release, Pericardium 02NN
Pericardiophrenic artery
  use Internal Mammary Artery, Left
  use Internal Mammary Artery, Right
Pericardioplasty
  see Repair, Pericardium 02QN
  see Replacement, Pericardium 02RN
  see Supplement, Pericardium 02UN
Pericardiorrhaphy *see* Repair, Pericardium 02QN
Pericardiostomy *see* Drainage, Pericardial Cavity 0W9D
Pericardiotomy *see* Drainage, Pericardial Cavity 0W9D
Perimetrium *use* Uterus
Peripheral Intravascular Lithotripsy (Peripheral IVL) *see* Fragmentation
Peripheral parenteral nutrition *see* Introduction of Nutritional Substance
Peripherally inserted central catheter (PICC) *use* Infusion Device
Peritoneal dialysis 3E1M39Z
Peritoneocentesis
  see Drainage, Peritoneal Cavity 0W9G
  see Drainage, Peritoneum 0D9W
Peritoneoplasty
  see Repair, Peritoneum 0DQW
  see Replacement, Peritoneum 0DRW
  see Supplement, Peritoneum 0DUW
Peritoneoscopy 0DJW4ZZ
Peritoneotomy *see* Drainage, Peritoneum 0D9W
Peritoneumectomy *see* Excision, Peritoneum 0DBW
Peroneus brevis muscle
  use Lower Leg Muscle, Left
  use Lower Leg Muscle, Right
Peroneus longus muscle
  use Lower Leg Muscle, Left
  use Lower Leg Muscle, Right
Pessary ring *use* Intraluminal Device, Pessary in Female Reproductive System
PET scan *see* Positron Emission Tomographic (PET) Imaging
Petrous part of temporal bone
  use Temporal Bone, Left
  use Temporal Bone, Right
Phacoemulsification, lens
  With IOL implant *see* Replacement, Eye 08R
  Without IOL implant *see* Extraction, Eye 08D
Phagenyx® System XWHD7Q7
Phalangectomy
  see Excision, Lower Bones 0QB
  see Excision, Upper Bones 0PB
  see Resection, Lower Bones 0QT
  see Resection, Upper Bones 0PT
Phallectomy
  see Excision, Penis 0VBS
  see Resection, Penis 0VTS
Phalloplasty
  see Repair, Penis 0VQS
  see Supplement, Penis 0VUS
Phallotomy *see* Drainage, Penis 0V9S
Pharmacotherapy, for substance abuse
  Antabuse HZ93ZZZ
  Bupropion HZ97ZZZ
  Clonidine HZ96ZZZ
  Levo-alpha-acetyl-methadol (LAAM) HZ92ZZZ
  Methadone Maintenance HZ91ZZZ
  Naloxone HZ95ZZZ
  Naltrexone HZ94ZZZ
  Nicotine Replacement HZ90ZZZ
  Psychiatric Medication HZ98ZZZ
  Replacement Medication, Other HZ99ZZZ

Pharyngeal constrictor muscle *use* Tongue, Palate, Pharynx Muscle
Pharyngeal plexus *use* Vagus Nerve
Pharyngeal recess *use* Nasopharynx
Pharyngeal tonsil *use* Adenoids
Pharyngogram *see* Fluoroscopy, Pharynx B91G
Pharyngoplasty
  see Repair, Mouth and Throat 0CQ
  see Replacement, Mouth and Throat 0CR
  see Supplement, Mouth and Throat 0CU
Pharyngorrhaphy *see* Repair, Mouth and Throat 0CQ
Pharyngotomy *see* Drainage, Mouth and Throat 0C9
Pharyngotympanic tube
  use Eustachian Tube, Left
  use Eustachian Tube, Right
Phenotypic Fully Automated Rapid Susceptibility Technology with Controlled Inoculum XXE5X2A
Pheresis
  Erythrocytes 6A55
  Leukocytes 6A55
  Plasma 6A55
  Platelets 6A55
  Stem Cells
    Cord Blood 6A55
    Hematopoietic 6A55
Phlebectomy
  see Excision, Lower Veins 06B
  see Excision, Upper Veins 05B
  see Extraction, Lower Veins 06D
  see Extraction, Upper Veins 05D
Phlebography
  see Plain Radiography, Veins B50
  Impedance 4A04X51
Phleborrhaphy
  see Repair, Lower Veins 06Q
  see Repair, Upper Veins 05Q
Phlebotomy
  see Drainage, Lower Veins 069
  see Drainage, Upper Veins 059
Photocoagulation
  For Destruction *see* Destruction
  For Repair *see* Repair
Photopheresis, therapeutic *see* Phototherapy, Circulatory 6A65
Phototherapy
  Circulatory 6A65
  Skin 6A60
  Ultraviolet light *see* Ultraviolet Light Therapy, Physiological Systems 6A8
Phrenectomy, phrenoneurectomy *see* Excision, Nerve, Phrenic 01B2
Phrenemphraxis *see* Destruction, Nerve, Phrenic 0152
Phrenic nerve stimulator generator *use* Stimulator Generator in Subcutaneous Tissue and Fascia
Phrenic nerve stimulator lead *use* Diaphragmatic Pacemaker Lead in Respiratory System
Phreniclasis *see* Destruction, Nerve, Phrenic 0152
Phrenicoexeresis *see* Extraction, Nerve, Phrenic 01D2
Phrenicotomy *see* Division, Nerve, Phrenic 0182
Phrenicotripsy *see* Destruction, Nerve, Phrenic 0152
Phrenoplasty
  see Repair, Respiratory System 0BQ
  see Supplement, Respiratory System 0BU
Phrenotomy *see* Drainage, Respiratory System 0B9
Physiatry *see* Motor Treatment, Rehabilitation F07
Physical medicine *see* Motor Treatment, Rehabilitation F07
Physical therapy *see* Motor Treatment, Rehabilitation F07
PHYSIOMESH™ Flexible Composite Mesh *use* Synthetic Substitute
Pia mater, intracranial *use* Cerebral Meninges
Pia mater, spinal *use* Spinal Meninges
PiCSO® Impulse System X2A7358
Pinealectomy
  see Excision, Pineal Body 0GB1
  see Resection, Pineal Body 0GT1
Pinealoscopy 0GJ14ZZ
Pinealotomy *see* Drainage, Pineal Body 0G91
Pinna
  use External Ear, Bilateral
  use External Ear, Left
  use External Ear, Right
Pipeline™ (Flex) embolization device *use* Intraluminal Device, Flow Diverter in 03V
Piriform recess (sinus) *use* Pharynx

Piriformis muscle
  use Hip Muscle, Left
  use Hip Muscle, Right
PIRRT (Prolonged intermittent renal replacement therapy) 5A1D80Z
Piscine skin *use* Nonautologous Tissue Substitute
Pisiform bone
  use Carpal, Left
  use Carpal, Right
Pisohamate ligament
  use Hand Bursa and Ligament, Left
  use Hand Bursa and Ligament, Right
Pisometacarpal ligament
  use Hand Bursa and Ligament, Left
  use Hand Bursa and Ligament, Right
Pituitectomy
  see Excision, Gland, Pituitary 0GB0
  see Resection, Gland, Pituitary 0GT0
Plain film radiology *see* Plain Radiography
Plain Radiography
  Abdomen BW00ZZZ
  Abdomen and Pelvis BW01ZZZ
  Abdominal Lymphatic
    Bilateral B701
    Unilateral B700
  Airway, Upper BB0DZZZ
  Ankle
    Left BQ0H
    Right BQ0G
  Aorta
    Abdominal B400
    Thoracic B300
    Thoraco-Abdominal B30P
  Aorta and Bilateral Lower Extremity Arteries B40D
  Arch
    Bilateral BN0DZZZ
    Left BN0CZZZ
    Right BN0BZZZ
  Arm
    Left BP0FZZZ
    Right BP0EZZZ
  Artery
    Brachiocephalic-Subclavian, Right B301
    Bronchial B30L
    Bypass Graft, Other B20F
    Cervico-Cerebral Arch B30Q
    Common Carotid
      Bilateral B305
      Left B304
      Right B303
    Coronary
      Bypass Graft
        Multiple B203
        Single B202
      Multiple B201
      Single B200
    External Carotid
      Bilateral B30C
      Left B30B
      Right B309
    Hepatic B402
    Inferior Mesenteric B405
    Intercostal B30L
    Internal Carotid
      Bilateral B308
      Left B307
      Right B306
    Internal Mammary Bypass Graft
      Left B208
      Right B207
    Intra-Abdominal, Other B40B
    Intracranial B30R
    Lower Extremity
      Bilateral and Aorta B40D
      Left B40G
      Right B40F
    Lower, Other B40J
    Lumbar B409
    Pelvic B40C
    Pulmonary
      Left B30T
      Right B30S
    Renal
      Bilateral B408
      Left B407
      Right B406
      Transplant B40M
    Spinal B30M

Plain Radiography — continued
  Artery — continued
    Splenic B403
    Subclavian, Left B302
    Superior Mesenteric B404
    Upper Extremity
      Bilateral B30K
      Left B30J
      Right B30H
    Upper, Other B30N
    Vertebral
      Bilateral B30G
      Left B30F
      Right B30D
  Bile Duct BF00
  Bile Duct and Gallbladder BF03
  Bladder BT00
    Kidney and Ureter BT04
  Bladder and Urethra BT0B
  Bone
    Facial BN05ZZZ
    Nasal BN04ZZZ
  Bones, Long, All BW0BZZZ
  Breast
    Bilateral BH02ZZZ
    Left BH01ZZZ
    Right BH00ZZZ
  Calcaneus
    Left BQ0KZZZ
    Right BQ0JZZZ
  Chest BW03ZZZ
  Clavicle
    Left BP05ZZZ
    Right BP04ZZZ
  Coccyx BR0FZZZ
  Corpora Cavernosa BV00
  Dialysis Fistula B50W
  Dialysis Shunt B50W
  Disc
    Cervical BR01
    Lumbar BR03
    Thoracic BR02
  Duct
    Lacrimal
      Bilateral B802
      Left B801
      Right B800
    Mammary
      Multiple
        Left BH06
        Right BH05
      Single
        Left BH04
        Right BH03
  Elbow
    Left BP0H
    Right BP0G
  Epididymis
    Left BV02
    Right BV01
  Extremity
    Lower BW0CZZZ
    Upper BW0JZZZ
  Eye
    Bilateral B807ZZZ
    Left B806ZZZ
    Right B805ZZZ
  Facet Joint
    Cervical BR04
    Lumbar BR06
    Thoracic BR05
  Fallopian Tube
    Bilateral BU02
    Left BU01
    Right BU00
  Fallopian Tube and Uterus BU08
  Femur
    Left, Densitometry BQ04ZZ1
    Right, Densitometry BQ03ZZ1
  Finger
    Left BP0SZZZ
    Right BP0RZZZ
  Foot
    Left BQ0MZZZ
    Right BQ0LZZZ
  Forearm
    Left BP0KZZZ
    Right BP0JZZZ
  Gallbladder and Bile Duct BF03

Plain Radiography — continued
  Gland
    Parotid
      Bilateral B906
      Left B905
      Right B904
    Salivary
      Bilateral B90D
      Left B90C
      Right B90B
    Submandibular
      Bilateral B909
      Left B908
      Right B907
  Hand
    Left BP0PZZZ
    Right BP0NZZZ
  Heart
    Left B205
    Right B204
    Right and Left B206
  Hepatobiliary System, All BF0C
  Hip
    Left BQ01
      Densitometry BQ01ZZ1
    Right BQ00
      Densitometry BQ00ZZ1
  Humerus
    Left BP0BZZZ
    Right BP0AZZZ
  Ileal Diversion Loop BT0C
  Intracranial Sinus B502
  Joint
    Acromioclavicular, Bilateral BP03ZZZ
    Finger
      Left BP0D
      Right BP0C
    Foot
      Left BQ0Y
      Right BQ0X
    Hand
      Left BP0D
      Right BP0C
    Lumbosacral BR0BZZZ
    Sacroiliac BR0D
    Sternoclavicular
      Bilateral BP02ZZZ
      Left BP01ZZZ
      Right BP00ZZZ
    Temporomandibular
      Bilateral BN09
      Left BN08
      Right BN07
    Thoracolumbar BR08ZZZ
    Toe
      Left BQ0Y
      Right BQ0X
  Kidney
    Bilateral BT03
    Left BT02
    Right BT01
    Ureter and Bladder BT04
  Knee
    Left BQ08
    Right BQ07
  Leg
    Left BQ0FZZZ
    Right BQ0DZZZ
  Lymphatic
    Head B704
    Lower Extremity
      Bilateral B70B
      Left B709
      Right B708
    Neck B704
    Pelvic B70C
    Upper Extremity
      Bilateral B707
      Left B706
      Right B705
  Mandible BN06ZZZ
  Mastoid B90HZZZ
  Nasopharynx B90FZZZ
  Optic Foramina
    Left B804ZZZ
    Right B803ZZZ
  Orbit
    Bilateral BN03ZZZ
    Left BN02ZZZ

Plain Radiography — continued
  Orbit — continued
    Right BN01ZZZ
  Oropharynx B90FZZZ
  Patella
    Left BQ0WZZZ
    Right BQ0VZZZ
  Pelvis BR0CZZZ
  Pelvis and Abdomen BW01ZZZ
  Prostate BV03
  Retroperitoneal Lymphatic
    Bilateral B701
    Unilateral B700
  Ribs
    Left BP0YZZZ
    Right BP0XZZZ
  Sacrum BR0FZZZ
  Scapula
    Left BP07ZZZ
    Right BP06ZZZ
  Shoulder
    Left BP09
    Right BP08
  Sinus
    Intracranial B502
    Paranasal B902ZZZ
  Skull BN00ZZZ
  Spinal Cord B00B
  Spine
    Cervical, Densitometry BR00ZZ1
    Lumbar, Densitometry BR09ZZ1
    Thoracic, Densitometry BR07ZZ1
    Whole, Densitometry BR0GZZ1
  Sternum BR0HZZZ
  Teeth
    All BN0JZZZ
    Multiple BN0HZZZ
  Testicle
    Left BV06
    Right BV05
  Toe
    Left BQ0QZZZ
    Right BQ0PZZZ
  Tooth, Single BN0GZZZ
  Tracheobronchial Tree
    Bilateral BB09YZZ
    Left BB08YZZ
    Right BB07YZZ
  Ureter
    Bilateral BT08
    Kidney and Bladder BT04
    Left BT07
    Right BT06
  Urethra BT05
  Urethra and Bladder BT0B
  Uterus BU06
  Uterus and Fallopian Tube BU08
  Vagina BU09
  Vasa Vasorum BV08
  Vein
    Cerebellar B501
    Cerebral B501
    Epidural B500
    Jugular
      Bilateral B505
      Left B504
      Right B503
    Lower Extremity
      Bilateral B50D
      Left B50C
      Right B50B
    Other B50V
    Pelvic (Iliac)
      Left B50G
      Right B50F
    Pelvic (Iliac) Bilateral B50H
    Portal B50T
    Pulmonary
      Bilateral B50S
      Left B50R
      Right B50Q
    Renal
      Bilateral B50L
      Left B50K
      Right B50J
    Splanchnic B50T
    Subclavian
      Left B507
      Right B506

▽ **Subterms under main terms may continue to next column or page**

Plain Radiography

Plain Radiography — continued
Vein — continued
  Upper Extremity
    Bilateral B50P
    Left B50N
    Right B50M
  Vena Cava
    Inferior B509
    Superior B508
  Whole Body BW0KZZZ
    Infant BW0MZZZ
  Whole Skeleton BW0LZZZ
  Wrist
    Left BP0M
    Right BP0L
Planar Nuclear Medicine Imaging
  Abdomen CW10
  Abdomen and Chest CW14
  Abdomen and Pelvis CW11
  Anatomical Region, Other CW1ZZZZ
  Anatomical Regions, Multiple CW1YYZZ
  Bladder and Ureters CT1H
  Bladder, Kidneys and Ureters CT13
  Blood C713
  Bone Marrow C710
  Brain C010
  Breast CH1YYZZ
    Bilateral CH12
    Left CH11
    Right CH10
  Bronchi and Lungs CB12
  Central Nervous System C01YYZZ
  Cerebrospinal Fluid C015
  Chest CW13
  Chest and Abdomen CW14
  Chest and Neck CW16
  Digestive System CD1YYZZ
  Ducts, Lacrimal, Bilateral C819
  Ear, Nose, Mouth and Throat C91YYZZ
  Endocrine System CG1YYZZ
  Extremity
    Lower CW1D
      Bilateral CP1F
      Left CP1D
      Right CP1C
    Upper CW1M
      Bilateral CP1B
      Left CP19
      Right CP18
  Eye C81YYZZ
  Gallbladder CF14
  Gastrointestinal Tract CD17
    Upper CD15
  Gland
    Adrenal, Bilateral CG14
    Parathyroid CG11
    Thyroid CG12
  Glands, Salivary, Bilateral C91B
  Head and Neck CW1B
  Heart C21YYZZ
    Right and Left C216
  Hepatobiliary System, All CF1C
  Hepatobiliary System and Pancreas CF1YYZZ
  Kidneys, Ureters and Bladder CT13
  Liver CF15
  Liver and Spleen CF16
  Lungs and Bronchi CB12
  Lymphatics
    Head C71J
    Head and Neck C715
    Lower Extremity C71P
    Neck C71K
    Pelvic C71D
    Trunk C71M
    Upper Chest C71L
    Upper Extremity C71N
  Lymphatics and Hematologic System C71YYZZ
  Musculoskeletal System
    All CP1Z
    Other CP1YYZZ
  Myocardium C21G
  Neck and Chest CW16
  Neck and Head CW1B
  Pancreas and Hepatobiliary System CF1YYZZ
  Pelvic Region CW1J
  Pelvis CP16
  Pelvis and Abdomen CW11
  Pelvis and Spine CP17
  Reproductive System, Male CV1YYZZ

Planar Nuclear Medicine Imaging — continued
  Respiratory System CB1YYZZ
  Skin CH1YYZZ
  Skull CP11
  Spine CP15
  Spine and Pelvis CP17
  Spleen C712
  Spleen and Liver CF16
  Subcutaneous Tissue CH1YYZZ
  Testicles, Bilateral CV19
  Thorax CP14
  Ureters and Bladder CT1H
  Ureters, Kidneys and Bladder CT13
  Urinary System CT1YYZZ
  Veins C51YYZZ
    Central C51R
    Lower Extremity
      Bilateral C51D
      Left C51C
      Right C51B
    Upper Extremity
      Bilateral C51Q
      Left C51P
      Right C51N
  Whole Body CW1N
Plantar digital vein
  use Foot Vein, Left
  use Foot Vein, Right
Plantar fascia (aponeurosis)
  use Subcutaneous Tissue and Fascia, Left Foot
  use Subcutaneous Tissue and Fascia, Right Foot
Plantar metatarsal vein
  use Foot Vein, Left
  use Foot Vein, Right
Plantar venous arch
  use Foot Vein, Left
  use Foot Vein, Right
Plantaris muscle
  use Lower Leg Muscle, Left
  use Lower Leg Muscle, Right
Plaque Radiation
  Abdomen DWY3FZZ
  Adrenal Gland DGY2FZZ
  Anus DDY8FZZ
  Bile Ducts DFY2FZZ
  Bladder DTY2FZZ
  Bone Marrow D7Y0FZZ
  Bone, Other DPYCFZZ
  Brain D0Y0FZZ
  Brain Stem D0Y1FZZ
  Breast
    Left DMY0FZZ
    Right DMY1FZZ
  Bronchus DBY1FZZ
  Cervix DUY1FZZ
  Chest DWY2FZZ
  Chest Wall DBY7FZZ
  Colon DDY5FZZ
  Diaphragm DBY8FZZ
  Duodenum DDY2FZZ
  Ear D9Y0FZZ
  Esophagus DDY0FZZ
  Eye D8Y0FZZ
  Femur DPY9FZZ
  Fibula DPYBFZZ
  Gallbladder DFY1FZZ
  Gland
    Adrenal DGY2FZZ
    Parathyroid DGY4FZZ
    Pituitary DGY0FZZ
    Thyroid DGY5FZZ
  Glands, Salivary D9Y6FZZ
  Head and Neck DWY1FZZ
  Hemibody DWY4FZZ
  Humerus DPY6FZZ
  Ileum DDY4FZZ
  Jejunum DDY3FZZ
  Kidney DTY0FZZ
  Larynx D9YBFZZ
  Liver DFY0FZZ
  Lung DBY2FZZ
  Lymphatics
    Abdomen D7Y6FZZ
    Axillary D7Y4FZZ
    Inguinal D7Y8FZZ
    Neck D7Y3FZZ
    Pelvis D7Y7FZZ
    Thorax D7Y5FZZ

Plaque Radiation — continued
  Mandible DPY3FZZ
  Maxilla DPY2FZZ
  Mediastinum DBY6FZZ
  Mouth D9Y4FZZ
  Nasopharynx D9YDFZZ
  Neck and Head DWY1FZZ
  Nerve, Peripheral D0Y7FZZ
  Nose D9Y1FZZ
  Ovary DUY0FZZ
  Palate
    Hard D9Y8FZZ
    Soft D9Y9FZZ
  Pancreas DFY3FZZ
  Parathyroid Gland DGY4FZZ
  Pelvic Bones DPY8FZZ
  Pelvic Region DWY6FZZ
  Pharynx D9YCFZZ
  Pineal Body DGY1FZZ
  Pituitary Gland DGY0FZZ
  Pleura DBY5FZZ
  Prostate DVY0FZZ
  Radius DPY7FZZ
  Rectum DDY7FZZ
  Rib DPY5FZZ
  Sinuses D9Y7FZZ
  Skin
    Abdomen DHY8FZZ
    Arm DHY4FZZ
    Back DHY7FZZ
    Buttock DHY9FZZ
    Chest DHY6FZZ
    Face DHY2FZZ
    Foot DHYCFZZ
    Hand DHY5FZZ
    Leg DHYBFZZ
    Neck DHY3FZZ
  Skull DPY0FZZ
  Spinal Cord D0Y6FZZ
  Spleen D7Y2FZZ
  Sternum DPY4FZZ
  Stomach DDY1FZZ
  Testis DVY1FZZ
  Thymus D7Y1FZZ
  Thyroid Gland DGY5FZZ
  Tibia DPYBFZZ
  Tongue D9Y5FZZ
  Trachea DBY0FZZ
  Ulna DPY7FZZ
  Ureter DTY1FZZ
  Urethra DTY3FZZ
  Uterus DUY2FZZ
  Whole Body DWY5FZZ
Plasma, Convalescent (Nonautologous) XW1
Plasmapheresis, therapeutic see Pheresis, Physiological Systems 6A5
Plateletpheresis, therapeutic see Pheresis, Physiological Systems 6A5
Platysma muscle
  use Neck Muscle, Left
  use Neck Muscle, Right
Plazomicin use Other Anti-infective
Pleurectomy
  see Excision, Respiratory System 0BB
  see Resection, Respiratory System 0BT
Pleurocentesis see Drainage, Anatomical Regions, General 0W9
Pleurodesis, pleurosclerosis
  Chemical injection see Introduction of Substance in or on, Pleural Cavity 3E0L
  Surgical see Destruction, Respiratory System 0B5
Pleurolysis see Release, Respiratory System 0BN
Pleuroscopy 0BJQ4ZZ
Pleurotomy see Drainage, Respiratory System 0B9
Plica semilunaris
  use Conjunctiva, Left
  use Conjunctiva, Right
Plication see Restriction
Pneumectomy
  see Excision, Respiratory System 0BB
  see Resection, Respiratory System 0BT
Pneumocentesis see Drainage, Respiratory System 0B9
Pneumogastric nerve use Vagus Nerve
Pneumolysis see Release, Respiratory System 0BN
Pneumonectomy see Resection, Respiratory System 0BT
Pneumonolysis see Release, Respiratory System 0BN

Pneumonopexy
see Repair, Respiratory System ØBQ
see Reposition, Respiratory System ØBS
Pneumonorrhaphy see Repair, Respiratory System ØBQ
Pneumonotomy see Drainage, Respiratory System ØB9
Pneumotaxic center use Pons
Pneumotomy see Drainage, Respiratory System ØB9
Pollicization see Transfer, Anatomical Regions, Upper Extremities ØXX
Polyclonal hyperimmune globulin use Globulin
Polyethylene socket use Synthetic Substitute, Polyethylene in ØSR
Polymethylmethacrylate (PMMA) use Synthetic Substitute
Polypectomy, gastrointestinal see Excision, Gastrointestinal System ØDB
Polypropylene mesh use Synthetic Substitute
Polysomnogram 4A1ZXQZ
Pontine tegmentum use Pons
Popliteal fossa
use Knee Region, Left
use Knee Region, Right
Popliteal ligament
use Knee Bursa and Ligament, Left
use Knee Bursa and Ligament, Right
Popliteal lymph node
use Lymphatic, Left Lower Extremity
use Lymphatic, Right Lower Extremity
Popliteal vein
use Femoral Vein, Left
use Femoral Vein, Right
Popliteus muscle
use Lower Leg Muscle, Left
use Lower Leg Muscle, Right
Porcine (bioprosthetic) valve use Zooplastic Tissue in Heart and Great Vessels
Positive Blood Culture Fluorescence Hybridization for Organism Identification, Concentration and Susceptibility XXE5XN6
Positive Blood Culture Small Molecule Sensor Array Technology XXE5X4A
Positive end expiratory pressure see Performance, Respiratory 5A19
Positron Emission Tomographic (PET) Imaging
Brain CØ3Ø
Bronchi and Lungs CB32
Central Nervous System CØ3YYZZ
Heart C23YYZZ
Lungs and Bronchi CB32
Myocardium C23G
Respiratory System CB3YYZZ
Whole Body CW3NYZZ
Positron emission tomography see Positron Emission Tomographic (PET) Imaging
Posoleucel XWØ
Postauricular (mastoid) lymph node
use Lymphatic, Left Neck
use Lymphatic, Right Neck
Postcava use Inferior Vena Cava
Posterior auricular artery
use External Carotid Artery, Left
use External Carotid Artery, Right
Posterior auricular nerve use Facial Nerve
Posterior auricular vein
use External Jugular Vein, Left
use External Jugular Vein, Right
Posterior cerebral artery use Intracranial Artery
Posterior chamber
use Eye, Left
use Eye, Right
Posterior circumflex humeral artery
use Axillary Artery, Left
use Axillary Artery, Right
Posterior communicating artery use Intracranial Artery
Posterior cruciate ligament (PCL)
use Knee Bursa and Ligament, Left
use Knee Bursa and Ligament, Right
Posterior (Dynamic) Distraction Device
Lumbar XNSØ
Thoracic XNS4
Posterior facial (retromandibular) vein
use Face Vein, Left
use Face Vein, Right
Posterior femoral cutaneous nerve use Sacral Plexus

Posterior inferior cerebellar artery (PICA) use Intracranial Artery
Posterior interosseous nerve use Radial Nerve
Posterior labial nerve use Pudendal Nerve
Posterior (subscapular) lymph node
use Lymphatic, Left Axillary
use Lymphatic, Right Axillary
Posterior scrotal nerve use Pudendal Nerve
Posterior spinal artery
use Vertebral Artery, Left
use Vertebral Artery, Right
Posterior tibial recurrent artery
use Anterior Tibial Artery, Left
use Anterior Tibial Artery, Right
Posterior ulnar recurrent artery
use Ulnar Artery, Left
use Ulnar Artery, Right
Posterior vagal trunk use Vagus Nerve
PPN (peripheral parenteral nutrition) see Introduction of Nutritional Substance
Prademagene Zamikeracel, Genetically Engineered Autologous Cell Therapy
Abdomen XHR2XGA
Back XHR3XGA
Chest XHR1XGA
Head and Neck XHRØXGA
Lower Extremity
Left XHR7XGA
Right XHR6XGA
Upper Extremity
Left XHR5XGA
Right XHR4XGA
Praxbind® (idarucizumab), Pradaxa® (dabigatran) reversal agent use Other Therapeutic Substance
Preauricular lymph node use Lymphatic, Head
Precava use Superior Vena Cava
PRECICE intramedullary limb lengthening system
use Internal Fixation Device, Intramedullary Limb Lengthening in ØPH
use Internal Fixation Device, Intramedullary Limb Lengthening in ØQH
Precision TAVI™ Coronary Obstruction Module XXE3X68
Prepatellar bursa
use Knee Bursa and Ligament, Left
use Knee Bursa and Ligament, Right
Preputiotomy see Drainage, Male Reproductive System ØV9
Pressure support ventilation see Performance, Respiratory 5A19
PRESTIGE® Cervical Disc use Synthetic Substitute
Pretracheal fascia
use Subcutaneous Tissue and Fascia, Left Neck
use Subcutaneous Tissue and Fascia, Right Neck
Prevertebral fascia
use Subcutaneous Tissue and Fascia, Left Neck
use Subcutaneous Tissue and Fascia, Right Neck
Prevesical space use Pelvic Cavity
PrimeAdvanced neurostimulator (SureScan) (MRI Safe) use Stimulator Generator, Multiple Array in ØJH
Princeps pollicis artery
use Hand Artery, Left
use Hand Artery, Right
Probing, duct
Diagnostic see Inspection
Dilation see Dilation
PROCEED™ Ventral Patch use Synthetic Substitute
Procerus muscle use Facial Muscle
Proctectomy
see Excision, Rectum ØDBP
see Resection, Rectum ØDTP
Proctoclysis see Introduction of substance in or on, Gastrointestinal Tract, Lower 3EØH
Proctocolectomy
see Excision, Gastrointestinal System ØDB
see Resection, Gastrointestinal System ØDT
Proctocolpoplasty
see Repair, Gastrointestinal System ØDQ
see Supplement, Gastrointestinal System ØDU
Proctoperineoplasty
see Repair, Gastrointestinal System ØDQ
see Supplement, Gastrointestinal System ØDU
Proctoperineorrhaphy see Repair, Gastrointestinal System ØDQ
Proctopexy
see Repair, Rectum ØDQP

Proctopexy — continued
see Reposition, Rectum ØDSP
Proctoplasty
see Repair, Rectum ØDQP
see Supplement, Rectum ØDUP
Proctorrhaphy see Repair, Rectum ØDQP
Proctoscopy ØDJD8ZZ
Proctosigmoidectomy
see Excision, Gastrointestinal System ØDB
see Resection, Gastrointestinal System ØDT
Proctosigmoidoscopy ØDJD8ZZ
Proctostomy see Drainage, Rectum ØD9P
Proctotomy see Drainage, Rectum ØD9P
Prodisc-C use Synthetic Substitute
Prodisc-L use Synthetic Substitute
Production, atrial septal defect see Excision, Septum, Atrial Ø2B5
Profunda brachii
use Brachial Artery, Left
use Brachial Artery, Right
Profunda femoris (deep femoral) vein
use Femoral Vein, Left
use Femoral Vein, Right
PROLENE Polypropylene Hernia System (PHS) use Synthetic Substitute
Prolonged intermittent renal replacement therapy (PIRRT) 5A1D80Z
Pronator quadratus muscle
use Lower Arm and Wrist Muscle, Left
use Lower Arm and Wrist Muscle, Right
Pronator teres muscle
use Lower Arm and Wrist Muscle, Left
use Lower Arm and Wrist Muscle, Right
Prone positioning, intubated see Assistance, Respiratory 5A09
Prostatectomy
see Excision, Prostate ØVBØ
see Resection, Prostate ØVTØ
Prostatic artery
use Internal Iliac Artery, Left
use Internal Iliac Artery, Right
Prostatic urethra use Urethra
Prostatomy, prostatotomy see Drainage, Prostate ØV9Ø
Protecta XT CRT-D use Cardiac Resynchronization Defibrillator Pulse Generator in ØJH
Protecta XT DR (XT VR) use Defibrillator Generator in ØJH
Protege® RX Carotid Stent System use Intraluminal Device
Provizio® SEM Scanner XX2KXP9
Proximal radioulnar joint
use Elbow Joint, Left
use Elbow Joint, Right
Psoas muscle
use Hip Muscle, Left
use Hip Muscle, Right
PSV (pressure support ventilation) see Performance, Respiratory 5A19
Psychoanalysis GZ54ZZZ
Psychological Tests
Cognitive Status GZ14ZZZ
Developmental GZ10ZZZ
Intellectual and Psychoeducational GZ12ZZZ
Neurobehavioral Status GZ14ZZZ
Neuropsychological GZ13ZZZ
Personality and Behavioral GZ11ZZZ
Psychotherapy
Family, Mental Health Services GZ72ZZZ
Group GZHZZZZ
Mental Health Services GZHZZZZ
Individual
see Psychotherapy, Individual, Mental Health Services
for substance abuse
12-Step HZ53ZZZ
Behavioral HZ51ZZZ
Cognitive HZ50ZZZ
Cognitive-Behavioral HZ52ZZZ
Confrontational HZ58ZZZ
Interactive HZ55ZZZ
Interpersonal HZ54ZZZ
Motivational Enhancement HZ57ZZZ
Psychoanalysis HZ5BZZZ
Psychodynamic HZ5CZZZ
Psychoeducation HZ56ZZZ
Psychophysiological HZ5DZZZ

Psychotherapy — continued
  Individual — continued
    for substance abuse — continued
      Supportive HZ59ZZZ
    Mental Health Services
      Behavioral GZ51ZZZ
      Cognitive GZ52ZZZ
      Cognitive-Behavioral GZ58ZZZ
      Interactive GZ50ZZZ
      Interpersonal GZ53ZZZ
      Psychoanalysis GZ54ZZZ
      Psychodynamic GZ55ZZZ
      Psychophysiological GZ59ZZZ
      Supportive GZ56ZZZ
PTCA (percutaneous transluminal coronary angioplasty) see Dilation, Heart and Great Vessels 027
Pterygoid muscle use Head Muscle
Pterygoid process use Sphenoid Bone
Pterygopalatine (sphenopalatine) ganglion use Head and Neck Sympathetic Nerve
Pubis
  use Pelvic Bone, Left
  use Pelvic Bone, Right
Pubofemoral ligament
  use Hip Bursa and Ligament, Left
  use Hip Bursa and Ligament, Right
Pudendal nerve use Sacral Plexus
Pull-through, laparoscopic-assisted transanal
  see Excision, Gastrointestinal System 0DB
  see Resection, Gastrointestinal System 0DT
Pull-through, rectal see Resection, Rectum 0DTP
Pulmoaortic canal use Pulmonary Artery, Left
Pulmonary annulus use Pulmonary Valve
Pulmonary artery wedge monitoring see Monitoring, Arterial 4A13
Pulmonary plexus
  use Thoracic Sympathetic Nerve
  use Vagus Nerve
Pulmonic valve use Pulmonary Valve
Pulpectomy see Excision, Mouth and Throat 0CB
PulseSelect™ PFA System, for cardiac IRE (Irreversible Electroporation) 02583ZF
Pulverization see Fragmentation
Pulvinar use Thalamus
Pump reservoir use Infusion Device, Pump in Subcutaneous Tissue and Fascia
Punch biopsy see Excision with qualifier Diagnostic
Puncture see Drainage
Puncture, lumbar see Drainage, Spinal Canal 009U
Pure-Vu® System XDPH8K7
Pyelography
  see Fluoroscopy, Urinary System BT1
  see Plain Radiography, Urinary System BT0
Pyeloileostomy, urinary diversion see Bypass, Urinary System 0T1
Pyeloplasty
  see Repair, Urinary System 0TQ
  see Replacement, Urinary System 0TR
  see Supplement, Urinary System 0TU
Pyeloplasty, dismembered see Repair, Kidney Pelvis
Pyelorrhaphy see Repair, Urinary System 0TQ
Pyeloscopy 0TJ58ZZ
Pyelostomy
  see Bypass, Urinary System 0T1
  see Drainage, Urinary System 0T9
Pyelotomy see Drainage, Urinary System 0T9
Pylorectomy
  see Excision, Stomach, Pylorus 0DB7
  see Resection, Stomach, Pylorus 0DT7
Pyloric antrum use Stomach, Pylorus
Pyloric canal use Stomach, Pylorus
Pyloric sphincter use Stomach, Pylorus
Pylorodiosis see Dilation, Stomach, Pylorus 0D77
Pylorogastrectomy
  see Excision, Gastrointestinal System 0DB
  see Resection, Gastrointestinal System 0DT
Pyloroplasty
  see Repair, Stomach, Pylorus 0DQ7
  see Supplement, Stomach, Pylorus 0DU7
Pyloroscopy 0DJ68ZZ
Pylorotomy see Drainage, Stomach, Pylorus 0D97
Pyramidalis muscle
  use Abdomen Muscle, Left
  use Abdomen Muscle, Right
pz-cel use Prademagene Zamikeracel, Genetically Engineered Autologous Cell Therapy in New Technology

Q

QAngio XA® 3D XXE3X58
QFR® (Quantitative Flow Ratio) analysis of coronary angiography XXE3X58
Quadrangular cartilage use Nasal Septum
Quadrant resection of breast see Excision, Skin and Breast 0HB
Quadrate lobe use Liver
Quadratus femoris muscle
  use Hip Muscle, Left
  use Hip Muscle, Right
Quadratus lumborum muscle
  use Trunk Muscle, Left
  use Trunk Muscle, Right
Quadratus plantae muscle
  use Foot Muscle, Left
  use Foot Muscle, Right
Quadriceps (femoris)
  use Upper Leg Muscle, Left
  use Upper Leg Muscle, Right
Quantitative Flow Ratio Analysis, Coronary Artery Flow XXE3X58
Quarantine 8E0ZXY6
Quicktome 00K0XZ1
Quizartinib Antineoplastic XW0DXJ9

R

Radial artery arteriovenous fistula, using Thermal Resistance Energy X2K
Radial collateral carpal ligament
  use Wrist Bursa and Ligament, Left
  use Wrist Bursa and Ligament, Right
Radial collateral ligament
  use Elbow Bursa and Ligament, Left
  use Elbow Bursa and Ligament, Right
Radial notch
  use Ulna, Left
  use Ulna, Right
Radial recurrent artery
  use Radial Artery, Left
  use Radial Artery, Right
Radial vein
  use Brachial Vein, Left
  use Brachial Vein, Right
Radialis indicis
  use Hand Artery, Left
  use Hand Artery, Right
Radiation Therapy
  see Beam Radiation
  see Brachytherapy
  see Other Radiation
  see Stereotactic Radiosurgery
Radiation treatment see Radiation Therapy
Radiocarpal joint
  use Wrist Joint, Left
  use Wrist Joint, Right
Radiocarpal ligament
  use Wrist Bursa and Ligament, Left
  use Wrist Bursa and Ligament, Right
Radiofrequency Ablation
  see Destruction
  Brain, Stereoelectroencephalographic (sEEG) 00503Z4
  Renal Sympathetic Nerve(s) X05133A
Radiography see Plain Radiography
Radiology, analog see Plain Radiography
Radiology, diagnostic see Imaging, Diagnostic
Radioulnar ligament
  use Wrist Bursa and Ligament, Left
  use Wrist Bursa and Ligament, Right
Range of motion testing see Motor Function Assessment, Rehabilitation F01
Rapid ASPECTS XXE0X07
REALIZE® Adjustable Gastric Band use Extraluminal Device
Reattachment
  Abdominal Wall 0WMF0ZZ
  Ampulla of Vater 0FMC
  Ankle Region
    Left 0YML0ZZ
    Right 0YMK0ZZ

Reattachment — continued
  Arm
    Lower
      Left 0XMF0ZZ
      Right 0XMD0ZZ
    Upper
      Left 0XM90ZZ
      Right 0XM80ZZ
  Axilla
    Left 0XM50ZZ
    Right 0XM40ZZ
  Back
    Lower 0WML0ZZ
    Upper 0WMK0ZZ
  Bladder 0TMB
  Bladder Neck 0TMC
  Breast
    Bilateral 0HMVXZZ
    Left 0HMUXZZ
    Right 0HMTXZZ
  Bronchus
    Lingula 0BM90ZZ
    Lower Lobe
      Left 0BMB0ZZ
      Right 0BM60ZZ
    Main
      Left 0BM70ZZ
      Right 0BM30ZZ
    Middle Lobe, Right 0BM50ZZ
    Upper Lobe
      Left 0BM80ZZ
      Right 0BM40ZZ
  Bursa and Ligament
    Abdomen
      Left 0MMJ
      Right 0MMH
    Ankle
      Left 0MMR
      Right 0MMQ
    Elbow
      Left 0MM4
      Right 0MM3
    Foot
      Left 0MMT
      Right 0MMS
    Hand
      Left 0MM8
      Right 0MM7
    Head and Neck 0MM0
    Hip
      Left 0MMM
      Right 0MML
    Knee
      Left 0MMP
      Right 0MMN
    Lower Extremity
      Left 0MMW
      Right 0MMV
    Perineum 0MMK
    Rib(s) 0MMG
    Shoulder
      Left 0MM2
      Right 0MM1
    Spine
      Lower 0MMD
      Upper 0MMC
    Sternum 0MMF
    Upper Extremity
      Left 0MMB
      Right 0MM9
    Wrist
      Left 0MM6
      Right 0MM5
  Buttock
    Left 0YM10ZZ
    Right 0YM00ZZ
  Carina 0BM20ZZ
  Cecum 0DMH
  Cervix 0UMC
  Chest Wall 0WM80ZZ
  Clitoris 0UMJXZZ
  Colon
    Ascending 0DMK
    Descending 0DMM
    Sigmoid 0DMN
    Transverse 0DML
  Cord
    Bilateral 0VMH
    Left 0VMG

Reattachment — *continued*
   Cord — *continued*
      Right 0VMF
   Cul-de-sac 0UMF
   Diaphragm 0BMT0ZZ
   Duct
      Common Bile 0FM9
      Cystic 0FM8
      Hepatic
         Common 0FM7
         Left 0FM6
         Right 0FM5
      Pancreatic 0FMD
         Accessory 0FMF
   Duodenum 0DM9
   Ear
      Left 09M1XZZ
      Right 09M0XZZ
   Elbow Region
      Left 0XMC0ZZ
      Right 0XMB0ZZ
   Esophagus 0DM5
   Extremity
      Lower
         Left 0YMB0ZZ
         Right 0YM90ZZ
      Upper
         Left 0XM70ZZ
         Right 0XM60ZZ
   Eyelid
      Lower
         Left 08MRXZZ
         Right 08MQXZZ
      Upper
         Left 08MPXZZ
         Right 08MNXZZ
   Face 0WM20ZZ
   Fallopian Tube
      Left 0UM6
      Right 0UM5
   Fallopian Tubes, Bilateral 0UM7
   Femoral Region
      Left 0YM80ZZ
      Right 0YM70ZZ
   Finger
      Index
         Left 0XMP0ZZ
         Right 0XMN0ZZ
      Little
         Left 0XMW0ZZ
         Right 0XMV0ZZ
      Middle
         Left 0XMR0ZZ
         Right 0XMQ0ZZ
      Ring
         Left 0XMT0ZZ
         Right 0XMS0ZZ
   Foot
      Left 0YMN0ZZ
      Right 0YMM0ZZ
   Forequarter
      Left 0XM10ZZ
      Right 0XM00ZZ
   Gallbladder 0FM4
   Gland
      Left 0GM2
      Right 0GM3
   Hand
      Left 0XMK0ZZ
      Right 0XMJ0ZZ
   Hindquarter
      Bilateral 0YM40ZZ
      Left 0YM30ZZ
      Right 0YM20ZZ
   Hymen 0UMK
   Ileum 0DMB
   Inguinal Region
      Left 0YM60ZZ
      Right 0YM50ZZ
   Intestine
      Large 0DME
         Left 0DMG
         Right 0DMF
      Small 0DM8
   Jaw
      Lower 0WM50ZZ
      Upper 0WM40ZZ
   Jejunum 0DMA

Reattachment — *continued*
   Kidney
      Left 0TM1
      Right 0TM0
   Kidney Pelvis
      Left 0TM4
      Right 0TM3
   Kidneys, Bilateral 0TM2
   Knee Region
      Left 0YMG0ZZ
      Right 0YMF0ZZ
   Leg
      Lower
         Left 0YMJ0ZZ
         Right 0YMH0ZZ
      Upper
         Left 0YMD0ZZ
         Right 0YMC0ZZ
   Lip
      Lower 0CM10ZZ
      Upper 0CM00ZZ
   Liver 0FM0
      Left Lobe 0FM2
      Right Lobe 0FM1
   Lung
      Left 0BML0ZZ
      Lower Lobe
         Left 0BMJ0ZZ
         Right 0BMF0ZZ
      Middle Lobe, Right 0BMD0ZZ
      Right 0BMK0ZZ
      Upper Lobe
         Left 0BMG0ZZ
         Right 0BMC0ZZ
   Lung Lingula 0BMH0ZZ
   Muscle
      Abdomen
         Left 0KML
         Right 0KMK
      Facial 0KM1
      Foot
         Left 0KMW
         Right 0KMV
      Hand
         Left 0KMD
         Right 0KMC
      Head 0KM0
      Hip
         Left 0KMP
         Right 0KMN
      Lower Arm and Wrist
         Left 0KMB
         Right 0KM9
      Lower Leg
         Left 0KMT
         Right 0KMS
      Neck
         Left 0KM3
         Right 0KM2
      Perineum 0KMM
      Shoulder
         Left 0KM6
         Right 0KM5
      Thorax
         Left 0KMJ
         Right 0KMH
      Tongue, Palate, Pharynx 0KM4
      Trunk
         Left 0KMG
         Right 0KMF
      Upper Arm
         Left 0KM8
         Right 0KM7
      Upper Leg
         Left 0KMR
         Right 0KMQ
   Nasal Mucosa and Soft Tissue 09MKXZZ
   Neck 0WM60ZZ
   Nipple
      Left 0HMXXZZ
      Right 0HMWXZZ
   Ovary
      Bilateral 0UM2
      Left 0UM1
      Right 0UM0
   Palate, Soft 0CM30ZZ
   Pancreas 0FMG
   Parathyroid Gland 0GMR

Reattachment — *continued*
   Parathyroid Gland — *continued*
      Inferior
         Left 0GMP
         Right 0GMN
      Multiple 0GMQ
      Superior
         Left 0GMM
         Right 0GML
   Penis 0VMSXZZ
   Perineum
      Female 0WMN0ZZ
      Male 0WMM0ZZ
   Rectum 0DMP
   Scrotum 0VM5XZZ
   Shoulder Region
      Left 0XM30ZZ
      Right 0XM20ZZ
   Skin
      Abdomen 0HM7XZZ
      Back 0HM6XZZ
      Buttock 0HM8XZZ
      Chest 0HM5XZZ
      Ear
         Left 0HM3XZZ
         Right 0HM2XZZ
      Face 0HM1XZZ
      Foot
         Left 0HMNXZZ
         Right 0HMMXZZ
      Hand
         Left 0HMGXZZ
         Right 0HMFXZZ
      Inguinal 0HMAXZZ
      Lower Arm
         Left 0HMEXZZ
         Right 0HMDXZZ
      Lower Leg
         Left 0HMLXZZ
         Right 0HMKXZZ
      Neck 0HM4XZZ
      Perineum 0HM9XZZ
      Scalp 0HM0XZZ
      Upper Arm
         Left 0HMCXZZ
         Right 0HMBXZZ
      Upper Leg
         Left 0HMJXZZ
         Right 0HMHXZZ
   Stomach 0DM6
   Tendon
      Abdomen
         Left 0LMG
         Right 0LMF
      Ankle
         Left 0LMT
         Right 0LMS
      Foot
         Left 0LMW
         Right 0LMV
      Hand
         Left 0LM8
         Right 0LM7
      Head and Neck 0LM0
      Hip
         Left 0LMK
         Right 0LMJ
      Knee
         Left 0LMR
         Right 0LMQ
      Lower Arm and Wrist
         Left 0LM6
         Right 0LM5
      Lower Leg
         Left 0LMP
         Right 0LMN
      Perineum 0LMH
      Shoulder
         Left 0LM2
         Right 0LM1
      Thorax
         Left 0LMD
         Right 0LMC
      Trunk
         Left 0LMB
         Right 0LM9
      Upper Arm
         Left 0LM4
         Right 0LM3

Reattachment

Reattachment — *continued*
- Tendon — *continued*
  - Upper Leg
    - Left 0LMM
    - Right 0LML
- Testis
  - Bilateral 0VMC
  - Left 0VMB
  - Right 0VM9
- Thumb
  - Left 0XMM0ZZ
  - Right 0XML0ZZ
- Thyroid Gland
  - Left Lobe 0GMG
  - Right Lobe 0GMH
- Toe
  - 1st
    - Left 0YMQ0ZZ
    - Right 0YMP0ZZ
  - 2nd
    - Left 0YMS0ZZ
    - Right 0YMR0ZZ
  - 3rd
    - Left 0YMU0ZZ
    - Right 0YMT0ZZ
  - 4th
    - Left 0YMW0ZZ
    - Right 0YMV0ZZ
  - 5th
    - Left 0YMY0ZZ
    - Right 0YMX0ZZ
- Tongue 0CM70ZZ
- Tooth
  - Lower 0CMX
  - Upper 0CMW
- Trachea 0BM10ZZ
- Tunica Vaginalis
  - Left 0VM7
  - Right 0VM6
- Ureter
  - Left 0TM7
  - Right 0TM6
- Ureters, Bilateral 0TM8
- Urethra 0TMD
- Uterine Supporting Structure 0UM4
- Uterus 0UM9
- Uvula 0CMN0ZZ
- Vagina 0UMG
- Vulva 0UMMXZZ
- Wrist Region
  - Left 0XMH0ZZ
  - Right 0XMG0ZZ

REBOA (resuscitative endovascular balloon occlusion of the aorta)
- 02LW3DJ
- 04L03DJ

Rebound HRD® (Hernia Repair Device) *use* Synthetic Substitute

REBYOTA® *use* Broad Consortium Microbiota-based Live Biotherapeutic Suspension

RECARBRIO™ (Imipenem-cilastatin-relebactam Anti-infective) *use* Other Anti-infective

RECELL® cell suspension autograft *see* Replacement, Skin and Breast 0HR

Recession
- *see* Repair
- *see* Reposition

Reclosure, disrupted abdominal wall 0WQFXZZ

Reconstruction
- *see* Repair
- *see* Replacement
- *see* Supplement

Rectectomy
- *see* Excision, Rectum 0DBP
- *see* Resection, Rectum 0DTP

Rectocele repair *see* Repair, Subcutaneous Tissue and Fascia, Pelvic Region 0JQC

Rectopexy
- *see* Repair, Gastrointestinal System 0DQ
- *see* Reposition, Gastrointestinal System 0DS

Rectoplasty
- *see* Repair, Gastrointestinal System 0DQ
- *see* Supplement, Gastrointestinal System 0DU

Rectorrhaphy *see* Repair, Gastrointestinal System 0DQ

Rectoscopy 0DJD8ZZ

Rectosigmoid junction *use* Sigmoid Colon

Rectosigmoidectomy
- *see* Excision, Gastrointestinal System 0DB

Rectosigmoidectomy — *continued*
- *see* Resection, Gastrointestinal System 0DT

Rectostomy *see* Drainage, Rectum 0D9P

Rectotomy *see* Drainage, Rectum 0D9P

Rectus abdominis muscle
- *use* Abdomen Muscle, Left
- *use* Abdomen Muscle, Right

Rectus femoris muscle
- *use* Upper Leg Muscle, Left
- *use* Upper Leg Muscle, Right

Recurrent laryngeal nerve *use* Vagus Nerve

Reducer™ System *use* Reduction Device in New Technology

Reduction
- Dislocation *see* Reposition
- Fracture *see* Reposition
- Intussusception, intestinal *see* Reposition, Gastrointestinal System 0DS
- Mammoplasty *see* Excision, Skin and Breast 0HB
- Prolapse *see* Reposition
- Torsion *see* Reposition
- Volvulus, gastrointestinal *see* Reposition, Gastrointestinal System 0DS

Reduction Device, Coronary Sinus X2V73Q7

Refusion *see* Fusion

REGN-COV2 Monoclonal Antibody XW0

Rehabilitation
- *see* Activities of Daily Living Assessment, Rehabilitation F02
- *see* Activities of Daily Living Treatment, Rehabilitation F08
- *see* Caregiver Training, Rehabilitation F0F
- *see* Cochlear Implant Treatment, Rehabilitation F0B
- *see* Device Fitting, Rehabilitation F0D
- *see* Hearing Treatment, Rehabilitation F09
- *see* Motor Function Assessment, Rehabilitation F01
- *see* Motor Treatment, Rehabilitation F07
- *see* Speech Assessment, Rehabilitation F00
- *see* Speech Treatment, Rehabilitation F06
- *see* Vestibular Treatment, Rehabilitation F0C

Reimplantation
- *see* Reattachment
- *see* Reposition
- *see* Transfer

Reinforcement
- *see* Repair
- *see* Supplement

Relaxation, scar tissue *see* Release

Release
- Acetabulum
  - Left 0QN5
  - Right 0QN4
- Adenoids 0CNQ
- Ampulla of Vater 0FNC
- Anal Sphincter 0DNR
- Anterior Chamber
  - Left 08N33ZZ
  - Right 08N23ZZ
- Anus 0DNQ
- Aorta
  - Abdominal 04N0
  - Thoracic
    - Ascending/Arch 02NX
    - Descending 02NW
- Aortic Body 0GND
- Appendix 0DNJ
- Artery
  - Anterior Tibial
    - Left 04NQ
    - Right 04NP
  - Axillary
    - Left 03N6
    - Right 03N5
  - Brachial
    - Left 03N8
    - Right 03N7
  - Celiac 04N1
  - Colic
    - Left 04N7
    - Middle 04N8
    - Right 04N6
  - Common Carotid
    - Left 03NJ
    - Right 03NH

Release — *continued*
- Artery — *continued*
  - Common Iliac
    - Left 04ND
    - Right 04NC
  - Coronary
    - Four or More Arteries 02N3
    - One Artery 02N0
    - Three Arteries 02N2
    - Two Arteries 02N1
  - External Carotid
    - Left 03NN
    - Right 03NM
  - External Iliac
    - Left 04NJ
    - Right 04NH
  - Face 03NR
  - Femoral
    - Left 04NL
    - Right 04NK
  - Foot
    - Left 04NW
    - Right 04NV
  - Gastric 04N2
  - Hand
    - Left 03NF
    - Right 03ND
  - Hepatic 04N3
  - Inferior Mesenteric 04NB
  - Innominate 03N2
  - Internal Carotid
    - Left 03NL
    - Right 03NK
  - Internal Iliac
    - Left 04NF
    - Right 04NE
  - Internal Mammary
    - Left 03N1
    - Right 03N0
  - Intracranial 03NG
  - Lower 04NY
  - Peroneal
    - Left 04NU
    - Right 04NT
  - Popliteal
    - Left 04NN
    - Right 04NM
  - Posterior Tibial
    - Left 04NS
    - Right 04NR
  - Pulmonary
    - Left 02NR
    - Right 02NQ
  - Pulmonary Trunk 02NP
  - Radial
    - Left 03NC
    - Right 03NB
  - Renal
    - Left 04NA
    - Right 04N9
  - Splenic 04N4
  - Subclavian
    - Left 03N4
    - Right 03N3
  - Superior Mesenteric 04N5
  - Temporal
    - Left 03NT
    - Right 03NS
  - Thyroid
    - Left 03NV
    - Right 03NU
  - Ulnar
    - Left 03NA
    - Right 03N9
  - Upper 03NY
  - Vertebral
    - Left 03NQ
    - Right 03NP
- Atrium
  - Left 02N7
  - Right 02N6
- Auditory Ossicle
  - Left 09NA
  - Right 09N9
- Basal Ganglia 00N8
- Bladder 0TNB
- Bladder Neck 0TNC

Release — continued
  Bone
    Ethmoid
      Left ØNNG
      Right ØNNF
    Frontal ØNN1
    Hyoid ØNNX
    Lacrimal
      Left ØNNJ
      Right ØNNH
    Nasal ØNNB
    Occipital ØNN7
    Palatine
      Left ØNNL
      Right ØNNK
    Parietal
      Left ØNN4
      Right ØNN3
    Pelvic
      Left ØQN3
      Right ØQN2
    Sphenoid ØNNC
    Temporal
      Left ØNN6
      Right ØNN5
    Zygomatic
      Left ØNNN
      Right ØNNM
  Brain ØØNØ
  Breast
    Bilateral ØHNV
    Left ØHNU
    Right ØHNT
  Bronchus
    Lingula ØBN9
    Lower Lobe
      Left ØBNB
      Right ØBN6
    Main
      Left ØBN7
      Right ØBN3
    Middle Lobe, Right ØBN5
    Upper Lobe
      Left ØBN8
      Right ØBN4
  Buccal Mucosa ØCN4
  Bursa and Ligament
    Abdomen
      Left ØMNJ
      Right ØMNH
    Ankle
      Left ØMNR
      Right ØMNQ
    Elbow
      Left ØMN4
      Right ØMN3
    Foot
      Left ØMNT
      Right ØMNS
    Hand
      Left ØMN8
      Right ØMN7
    Head and Neck ØMNØ
    Hip
      Left ØMNM
      Right ØMNL
    Knee
      Left ØMNP
      Right ØMNN
    Lower Extremity
      Left ØMNW
      Right ØMNV
    Perineum ØMNK
    Rib(s) ØMNG
    Shoulder
      Left ØMN2
      Right ØMN1
    Spine
      Lower ØMND
      Upper ØMNC
    Sternum ØMNF
    Upper Extremity
      Left ØMNB
      Right ØMN9
    Wrist
      Left ØMN6
      Right ØMN5
  Carina ØBN2
  Carotid Bodies, Bilateral ØGN8

Release — continued
  Carotid Body
    Left ØGN6
    Right ØGN7
  Carpal
    Left ØPNN
    Right ØPNM
  Cecum ØDNH
  Cerebellum ØØNC
  Cerebral Hemisphere ØØN7
  Cerebral Meninges ØØN1
  Cerebral Ventricle ØØN6
  Cervix ØUNC
  Chordae Tendineae Ø2N9
  Choroid
    Left Ø8NB
    Right Ø8NA
  Cisterna Chyli Ø7NL
  Clavicle
    Left ØPNB
    Right ØPN9
  Clitoris ØUNJ
  Coccygeal Glomus ØGNB
  Coccyx ØQNS
  Colon
    Ascending ØDNK
    Descending ØDNM
    Sigmoid ØDNN
    Transverse ØDNL
  Conduction Mechanism Ø2N8
  Conjunctiva
    Left Ø8NTXZZ
    Right Ø8NSXZZ
  Cord
    Bilateral ØVNH
    Left ØVNG
    Right ØVNF
  Cornea
    Left Ø8N9XZZ
    Right Ø8N8XZZ
  Cul-de-sac ØUNF
  Diaphragm ØBNT
  Disc
    Cervical Vertebral ØRN3
    Cervicothoracic Vertebral ØRN5
    Lumbar Vertebral ØSN2
    Lumbosacral ØSN4
    Thoracic Vertebral ØRN9
    Thoracolumbar Vertebral ØRNB
  Duct
    Common Bile ØFN9
    Cystic ØFN8
    Hepatic
      Common ØFN7
      Left ØFN6
      Right ØFN5
    Lacrimal
      Left Ø8NY
      Right Ø8NX
    Pancreatic ØFND
      Accessory ØFNF
    Parotid
      Left ØCNC
      Right ØCNB
  Duodenum ØDN9
  Dura Mater ØØN2
  Ear
    External
      Left Ø9N1
      Right Ø9NØ
    External Auditory Canal
      Left Ø9N4
      Right Ø9N3
    Inner
      Left Ø9NE
      Right Ø9ND
    Middle
      Left Ø9N6
      Right Ø9N5
  Epididymis
    Bilateral ØVNL
    Left ØVNK
    Right ØVNJ
  Epiglottis ØCNR
  Esophagogastric Junction ØDN4
  Esophagus ØDN5
    Lower ØDN3
    Middle ØDN2
    Upper ØDN1

Release — continued
  Eustachian Tube
    Left Ø9NG
    Right Ø9NF
  Eye
    Left Ø8N1XZZ
    Right Ø8NØXZZ
  Eyelid
    Lower
      Left Ø8NR
      Right Ø8NQ
    Upper
      Left Ø8NP
      Right Ø8NN
  Fallopian Tube
    Left ØUN6
    Right ØUN5
  Fallopian Tubes, Bilateral ØUN7
  Femoral Shaft
    Left ØQN9
    Right ØQN8
  Femur
    Lower
      Left ØQNC
      Right ØQNB
    Upper
      Left ØQN7
      Right ØQN6
  Fibula
    Left ØQNK
    Right ØQNJ
  Finger Nail ØHNQXZZ
  Gallbladder ØFN4
  Gingiva
    Lower ØCN6
    Upper ØCN5
  Gland
    Adrenal
      Bilateral ØGN4
      Left ØGN2
      Right ØGN3
    Lacrimal
      Left Ø8NW
      Right Ø8NV
    Minor Salivary ØCNJ
    Parotid
      Left ØCN9
      Right ØCN8
    Pituitary ØGNØ
    Sublingual
      Left ØCNF
      Right ØCND
    Submaxillary
      Left ØCNH
      Right ØCNG
    Vestibular ØUNL
  Glenoid Cavity
    Left ØPN8
    Right ØPN7
  Glomus Jugulare ØGNC
  Humeral Head
    Left ØPND
    Right ØPNC
  Humeral Shaft
    Left ØPNG
    Right ØPNF
  Hymen ØUNK
  Hypothalamus ØØNA
  Ileocecal Valve ØDNC
  Ileum ØDNB
  Intestine
    Large ØDNE
      Left ØDNG
      Right ØDNF
    Small ØDN8
  Iris
    Left Ø8ND3ZZ
    Right Ø8NC3ZZ
  Jejunum ØDNA
  Joint
    Acromioclavicular
      Left ØRNH
      Right ØRNG
    Ankle
      Left ØSNG
      Right ØSNF
    Carpal
      Left ØRNR
      Right ØRNQ

Release — *continued*
   Joint — *continued*
      Carpometacarpal
         Left 0RNT
         Right 0RNS
      Cervical Vertebral 0RN1
      Cervicothoracic Vertebral 0RN4
      Coccygeal 0SN6
      Elbow
         Left 0RNM
         Right 0RNL
      Finger Phalangeal
         Left 0RNX
         Right 0RNW
      Hip
         Left 0SNB
         Right 0SN9
      Knee
         Left 0SND
         Right 0SNC
      Lumbar Vertebral 0SN0
      Lumbosacral 0SN3
      Metacarpophalangeal
         Left 0RNV
         Right 0RNU
      Metatarsal-Phalangeal
         Left 0SNN
         Right 0SNM
      Occipital-cervical 0RN0
      Sacrococcygeal 0SN5
      Sacroiliac
         Left 0SN8
         Right 0SN7
      Shoulder
         Left 0RNK
         Right 0RNJ
      Sternoclavicular
         Left 0RNF
         Right 0RNE
      Tarsal
         Left 0SNJ
         Right 0SNH
      Tarsometatarsal
         Left 0SNL
         Right 0SNK
      Temporomandibular
         Left 0RND
         Right 0RNC
      Thoracic Vertebral 0RN6
      Thoracolumbar Vertebral 0RNA
      Toe Phalangeal
         Left 0SNQ
         Right 0SNP
      Wrist
         Left 0RNP
         Right 0RNN
   Kidney
      Left 0TN1
      Right 0TN0
   Kidney Pelvis
      Left 0TN4
      Right 0TN3
   Larynx 0CNS
   Lens
      Left 08NK3ZZ
      Right 08NJ3ZZ
   Lip
      Lower 0CN1
      Upper 0CN0
   Liver 0FN0
      Left Lobe 0FN2
      Right Lobe 0FN1
   Lung
      Bilateral 0BNM
      Left 0BNL
      Lower Lobe
         Left 0BNJ
         Right 0BNF
      Middle Lobe, Right 0BND
      Right 0BNK
      Upper Lobe
         Left 0BNG
         Right 0BNC
   Lung Lingula 0BNH
   Lymphatic
      Aortic 07ND
      Axillary
         Left 07N6
         Right 07N5

Release — *continued*
   Lymphatic — *continued*
      Head 07N0
      Inguinal
         Left 07NJ
         Right 07NH
      Internal Mammary
         Left 07N9
         Right 07N8
      Lower Extremity
         Left 07NG
         Right 07NF
      Mesenteric 07NB
      Neck
         Left 07N2
         Right 07N1
      Pelvis 07NC
      Thoracic Duct 07NK
      Thorax 07N7
      Upper Extremity
         Left 07N4
         Right 07N3
   Mandible
      Left 0NNV
      Right 0NNT
   Maxilla 0NNR
   Medulla Oblongata 00ND
   Mesentery 0DNV
   Metacarpal
      Left 0PNQ
      Right 0PNP
   Metatarsal
      Left 0QNP
      Right 0QNN
   Muscle
      Abdomen
         Left 0KNL
         Right 0KNK
      Extraocular
         Left 08NM
         Right 08NL
      Facial 0KN1
      Foot
         Left 0KNW
         Right 0KNV
      Hand
         Left 0KND
         Right 0KNC
      Head 0KN0
      Hip
         Left 0KNP
         Right 0KNN
      Lower Arm and Wrist
         Left 0KNB
         Right 0KN9
      Lower Leg
         Left 0KNT
         Right 0KNS
      Neck
         Left 0KN3
         Right 0KN2
      Papillary 02ND
      Perineum 0KNM
      Shoulder
         Left 0KN6
         Right 0KN5
      Thorax
         Left 0KNJ
         Right 0KNH
      Tongue, Palate, Pharynx 0KN4
      Trunk
         Left 0KNG
         Right 0KNF
      Upper Arm
         Left 0KN8
         Right 0KN7
      Upper Leg
         Left 0KNR
         Right 0KNQ
   Myocardial Bridge *see* Release, Artery, Coronary
   Nasal Mucosa and Soft Tissue 09NK
   Nasopharynx 09NN
   Nerve
      Abdominal Sympathetic 01NM
      Abducens 00NL
      Accessory 00NR
      Acoustic 00NN
      Brachial Plexus 01N3
      Cervical 01N1

Release — *continued*
   Nerve — *continued*
      Cervical Plexus 01N0
      Facial 00NM
      Femoral 01ND
      Glossopharyngeal 00NP
      Head and Neck Sympathetic 01NK
      Hypoglossal 00NS
      Lumbar 01NB
      Lumbar Plexus 01N9
      Lumbar Sympathetic 01NN
      Lumbosacral Plexus 01NA
      Median 01N5
      Oculomotor 00NH
      Olfactory 00NF
      Optic 00NG
      Peroneal 01NH
      Phrenic 01N2
      Pudendal 01NC
      Radial 01N6
      Sacral 01NR
      Sacral Plexus 01NQ
      Sacral Sympathetic 01NP
      Sciatic 01NF
      Thoracic 01N8
      Thoracic Sympathetic 01NL
      Tibial 01NG
      Trigeminal 00NK
      Trochlear 00NJ
      Ulnar 01N4
      Vagus 00NQ
   Nipple
      Left 0HNX
      Right 0HNW
   Omentum 0DNU
   Orbit
      Left 0NNQ
      Right 0NNP
   Ovary
      Bilateral 0UN2
      Left 0UN1
      Right 0UN0
   Palate
      Hard 0CN2
      Soft 0CN3
   Pancreas 0FNG
   Para-aortic Body 0GN9
   Paraganglion Extremity 0GNF
   Parathyroid Gland 0GNR
      Inferior
         Left 0GNP
         Right 0GNN
      Multiple 0GNQ
      Superior
         Left 0GNM
         Right 0GNL
   Patella
      Left 0QNF
      Right 0QND
   Penis 0VNS
   Pericardium 02NN
   Peritoneum 0DNW
   Phalanx
      Finger
         Left 0PNV
         Right 0PNT
      Thumb
         Left 0PNS
         Right 0PNR
      Toe
         Left 0QNR
         Right 0QNQ
   Pharynx 0CNM
   Pineal Body 0GN1
   Pleura
      Left 0BNP
      Right 0BNN
   Pons 00NB
   Prepuce 0VNT
   Prostate 0VN0
   Radius
      Left 0PNJ
      Right 0PNH
   Rectum 0DNP
   Retina
      Left 08NF3ZZ
      Right 08NE3ZZ
   Retinal Vessel
      Left 08NH3ZZ

Release — continued
    Retinal Vessel — continued
        Right 08NG3ZZ
    Ribs
        1 to 2 0PN1
        3 or More 0PN2
    Sacrum 0QN1
    Scapula
        Left 0PN6
        Right 0PN5
    Sclera
        Left 08N7XZZ
        Right 08N6XZZ
    Scrotum 0VN5
    Septum
        Atrial 02N5
        Nasal 09NM
        Ventricular 02NM
    Sinus
        Accessory 09NP
        Ethmoid
            Left 09NV
            Right 09NU
        Frontal
            Left 09NT
            Right 09NS
        Mastoid
            Left 09NC
            Right 09NB
        Maxillary
            Left 09NR
            Right 09NQ
        Sphenoid
            Left 09NX
            Right 09NW
    Skin
        Abdomen 0HN7XZZ
        Back 0HN6XZZ
        Buttock 0HN8XZZ
        Chest 0HN5XZZ
        Ear
            Left 0HN3XZZ
            Right 0HN2XZZ
        Face 0HN1XZZ
        Foot
            Left 0HNNXZZ
            Right 0HNMXZZ
        Hand
            Left 0HNGXZZ
            Right 0HNFXZZ
        Inguinal 0HNAXZZ
        Lower Arm
            Left 0HNEXZZ
            Right 0HNDXZZ
        Lower Leg
            Left 0HNLXZZ
            Right 0HNKXZZ
        Neck 0HN4XZZ
        Perineum 0HN9XZZ
        Scalp 0HN0XZZ
        Upper Arm
            Left 0HNCXZZ
            Right 0HNBXZZ
        Upper Leg
            Left 0HNJXZZ
            Right 0HNHXZZ
    Spinal Cord
        Cervical 00NW
        Lumbar 00NY
        Thoracic 00NX
    Spinal Meninges 00NT
    Spleen 07NP
    Sternum 0PN0
    Stomach 0DN6
        Pylorus 0DN7
    Subcutaneous Tissue and Fascia
        Abdomen 0JN8
        Back 0JN7
        Buttock 0JN9
        Chest 0JN6
        Face 0JN1
        Foot
            Left 0JNR
            Right 0JNQ
        Hand
            Left 0JNK
            Right 0JNJ
        Lower Arm
            Left 0JNH

Release — continued
    Subcutaneous Tissue and Fascia — continued
        Lower Arm — continued
            Right 0JNG
        Lower Leg
            Left 0JNP
            Right 0JNN
        Neck
            Left 0JN5
            Right 0JN4
        Pelvic Region 0JNC
        Perineum 0JNB
        Scalp 0JN0
        Upper Arm
            Left 0JNF
            Right 0JND
        Upper Leg
            Left 0JNM
            Right 0JNL
    Tarsal
        Left 0QNM
        Right 0QNL
    Tendon
        Abdomen
            Left 0LNG
            Right 0LNF
        Ankle
            Left 0LNT
            Right 0LNS
        Foot
            Left 0LNW
            Right 0LNV
        Hand
            Left 0LN8
            Right 0LN7
        Head and Neck 0LN0
        Hip
            Left 0LNK
            Right 0LNJ
        Knee
            Left 0LNR
            Right 0LNQ
        Lower Arm and Wrist
            Left 0LN6
            Right 0LN5
        Lower Leg
            Left 0LNP
            Right 0LNN
        Perineum 0LNH
        Shoulder
            Left 0LN2
            Right 0LN1
        Thorax
            Left 0LND
            Right 0LNC
        Trunk
            Left 0LNB
            Right 0LN9
        Upper Arm
            Left 0LN4
            Right 0LN3
        Upper Leg
            Left 0LNM
            Right 0LNL
    Testis
        Bilateral 0VNC
        Left 0VNB
        Right 0VN9
    Thalamus 00N9
    Thymus 07NM
    Thyroid Gland 0GNK
        Left Lobe 0GNG
        Right Lobe 0GNH
    Tibia
        Left 0QNH
        Right 0QNG
    Toe Nail 0HNRXZZ
    Tongue 0CN7
    Tonsils 0CNP
    Tooth
        Lower 0CNX
        Upper 0CNW
    Trachea 0BN1
    Tunica Vaginalis
        Left 0VN7
        Right 0VN6
    Turbinate, Nasal 09NL
    Tympanic Membrane
        Left 09N8

Release — continued
    Tympanic Membrane — continued
        Right 09N7
    Ulna
        Left 0PNL
        Right 0PNK
    Ureter
        Left 0TN7
        Right 0TN6
    Urethra 0TND
    Uterine Supporting Structure 0UN4
    Uterus 0UN9
    Uvula 0CNN
    Vagina 0UNG
    Valve
        Aortic 02NF
        Mitral 02NG
        Pulmonary 02NH
        Tricuspid 02NJ
    Vas Deferens
        Bilateral 0VNQ
        Left 0VNP
        Right 0VNN
    Vein
        Axillary
            Left 05N8
            Right 05N7
        Azygos 05N0
        Basilic
            Left 05NC
            Right 05NB
        Brachial
            Left 05NA
            Right 05N9
        Cephalic
            Left 05NF
            Right 05ND
        Colic 06N7
        Common Iliac
            Left 06ND
            Right 06NC
        Coronary 02N4
        Esophageal 06N3
        External Iliac
            Left 06NG
            Right 06NF
        External Jugular
            Left 05NQ
            Right 05NP
        Face
            Left 05NV
            Right 05NT
        Femoral
            Left 06NN
            Right 06NM
        Foot
            Left 06NV
            Right 06NT
        Gastric 06N2
        Hand
            Left 05NH
            Right 05NG
        Hemiazygos 05N1
        Hepatic 06N4
        Hypogastric
            Left 06NJ
            Right 06NH
        Inferior Mesenteric 06N6
        Innominate
            Left 05N4
            Right 05N3
        Internal Jugular
            Left 05NN
            Right 05NM
        Intracranial 05NL
        Lower 06NY
        Portal 06N8
        Pulmonary
            Left 02NT
            Right 02NS
        Renal
            Left 06NB
            Right 06N9
        Saphenous
            Left 06NQ
            Right 06NP
        Splenic 06N1
        Subclavian
            Left 05N6

Subterms under main terms may continue to next column or page

Release

Release — continued
- **Vein** — continued
  - Subclavian — continued
    - Right 05N5
  - Superior Mesenteric 06N5
  - Upper 05NY
  - Vertebral
    - Left 05NS
    - Right 05NR
- **Vena Cava**
  - Inferior 06N0
  - Superior 02NV
- **Ventricle**
  - Left 02NL
  - Right 02NK
- **Vertebra**
  - Cervical 0PN3
  - Lumbar 0QN0
  - Thoracic 0PN4
- **Vesicle**
  - Bilateral 0VN3
  - Left 0VN2
  - Right 0VN1
- **Vitreous**
  - Left 08N53ZZ
  - Right 08N43ZZ
- **Vocal Cord**
  - Left 0CNV
  - Right 0CNT
- **Vulva** 0UNM

Relocation see Reposition
Remdesivir Anti-infective XW0
Removal
- Abdominal Wall 2W53X
- Anorectal 2Y53X5Z
- Arm
  - Lower
    - Left 2W5DX
    - Right 2W5CX
  - Upper
    - Left 2W5BX
    - Right 2W5AX
- Back 2W55X
- Chest Wall 2W54X
- Ear 2Y52X5Z
- Extremity
  - Lower
    - Left 2W5MX
    - Right 2W5LX
  - Upper
    - Left 2W59X
    - Right 2W58X
- Face 2W51X
- Finger
  - Left 2W5KX
  - Right 2W5JX
- Foot
  - Left 2W5TX
  - Right 2W5SX
- Genital Tract, Female 2Y54X5Z
- Hand
  - Left 2W5FX
  - Right 2W5EX
- Head 2W50X
- Inguinal Region
  - Left 2W57X
  - Right 2W56X
- Leg
  - Lower
    - Left 2W5RX
    - Right 2W5QX
  - Upper
    - Left 2W5PX
    - Right 2W5NX
- Mouth and Pharynx 2Y50X5Z
- Nasal 2Y51X5Z
- Neck 2W52X
- Thumb
  - Left 2W5HX
  - Right 2W5GX
- Toe
  - Left 2W5VX
  - Right 2W5UX
- Urethra 2Y55X5Z

Removal of device from
- Abdominal Wall 0WPF
- Acetabulum
  - Left 0QP5
  - Right 0QP4

Removal of device from — continued
- Anal Sphincter 0DPR
- Anus 0DPQ
- Aorta, Thoracic, Descending 02PW3RZ
- Artery
  - Lower 04PY
  - Upper 03PY
- Back
  - Lower 0WPL
  - Upper 0WPK
- Bladder 0TPB
- Bone
  - Facial 0NPW
  - Lower 0QPY
  - Nasal 0NPB
  - Pelvic
    - Left 0QP3
    - Right 0QP2
  - Upper 0PPY
- Bone Marrow 07PT
- Brain 00P0
- Breast
  - Left 0HPU
  - Right 0HPT
- Bursa and Ligament
  - Lower 0MPY
  - Upper 0MPX
- Carpal
  - Left 0PPN
  - Right 0PPM
- Cavity, Cranial 0WP1
- Cerebral Ventricle 00P6
- Chest Wall 0WP8
- Cisterna Chyli 07PL
- Clavicle
  - Left 0PPB
  - Right 0PP9
- Coccyx 0QPS
- Diaphragm 0BPT
- Disc
  - Cervical Vertebral 0RP3
  - Cervicothoracic Vertebral 0RP5
  - Lumbar Vertebral 0SP2
  - Lumbosacral 0SP4
  - Thoracic Vertebral 0RP9
  - Thoracolumbar Vertebral 0RPB
- Duct
  - Hepatobiliary 0FPB
  - Pancreatic 0FPD
- Ear
  - Inner
    - Left 09PJ
    - Right 09PD
  - Left 09PJ
  - Right 09PH
- Epididymis and Spermatic Cord 0VPM
- Esophagus 0DP5
- Extremity
  - Lower
    - Left 0YPB
    - Right 0YP9
  - Upper
    - Left 0XP7
    - Right 0XP6
- Eye
  - Left 08P1
  - Right 08P0
- Face 0WP2
- Fallopian Tube 0UP8
- Femoral Shaft
  - Left 0QP9
  - Right 0QP8
- Femur
  - Lower
    - Left 0QPC
    - Right 0QPB
  - Upper
    - Left 0QP7
    - Right 0QP6
- Fibula
  - Left 0QPK
  - Right 0QPJ
- Finger Nail 0HPQX
- Gallbladder 0FP4
- Gastrointestinal Tract 0WPP
- Genitourinary Tract 0WPR
- Gland
  - Adrenal 0GP5
  - Endocrine 0GPS

Removal of device from — continued
- Gland — continued
  - Pituitary 0GP0
  - Salivary 0CPA
- Glenoid Cavity
  - Left 0PP8
  - Right 0PP7
- Great Vessel 02PY
- Hair 0HPSX
- Head 0WP0
- Heart 02PA
- Humeral Head
  - Left 0PPD
  - Right 0PPC
- Humeral Shaft
  - Left 0PPG
  - Right 0PPF
- Intestinal Tract
  - Lower Intestinal Tract 0DPD
  - Upper Intestinal Tract 0DP0
- Jaw
  - Lower 0WP5
  - Upper 0WP4
- Joint
  - Acromioclavicular
    - Left 0RPH
    - Right 0RPG
  - Ankle
    - Left 0SPG
    - Right 0SPF
  - Carpal
    - Left 0RPR
    - Right 0RPQ
  - Carpometacarpal
    - Left 0RPT
    - Right 0RPS
  - Cervical Vertebral 0RP1
  - Cervicothoracic Vertebral 0RP4
  - Coccygeal 0SP6
  - Elbow
    - Left 0RPM
    - Right 0RPL
  - Finger Phalangeal
    - Left 0RPX
    - Right 0RPW
  - Hip
    - Left 0SPB
      - Acetabular Surface 0SPE
      - Femoral Surface 0SPS
    - Right 0SP9
      - Acetabular Surface 0SPA
      - Femoral Surface 0SPR
  - Knee
    - Left 0SPD
      - Femoral Surface 0SPU
      - Tibial Surface 0SPW
    - Right 0SPC
      - Femoral Surface 0SPT
      - Tibial Surface 0SPV
  - Lumbar Vertebral 0SP0
  - Lumbosacral 0SP3
  - Metacarpophalangeal
    - Left 0RPV
    - Right 0RPU
  - Metatarsal-Phalangeal
    - Left 0SPN
    - Right 0SPM
  - Occipital-cervical 0RP0
  - Sacrococcygeal 0SP5
  - Sacroiliac
    - Left 0SP8
    - Right 0SP7
  - Shoulder
    - Left 0RPK
    - Right 0RPJ
  - Sternoclavicular
    - Left 0RPF
    - Right 0RPE
  - Tarsal
    - Left 0SPJ
    - Right 0SPH
  - Tarsometatarsal
    - Left 0SPL
    - Right 0SPK
  - Temporomandibular
    - Left 0RPD
    - Right 0RPC
  - Thoracic Vertebral 0RP6
  - Thoracolumbar Vertebral 0RPA

Removal of device from — continued
Joint — continued
- Toe Phalangeal
  - Left 0SPQ
  - Right 0SPP
- Wrist
  - Left 0RPP
  - Right 0RPN
- Kidney 0TP5
- Larynx 0CPS
- Lens
  - Left 08PK3
  - Right 08PJ3
- Liver 0FP0
- Lung
  - Left 0BPL
  - Right 0BPK
- Lymphatic 07PN
  - Thoracic Duct 07PK
- Mediastinum 0WPC
- Mesentery 0DPV
- Metacarpal
  - Left 0PPQ
  - Right 0PPP
- Metatarsal
  - Left 0QPP
  - Right 0QPN
- Mouth and Throat 0CPY
- Muscle
  - Extraocular
    - Left 08PM
    - Right 08PL
  - Lower 0KPY
  - Upper 0KPX
- Nasal Mucosa and Soft Tissue 09PK
- Neck 0WP6
- Nerve
  - Cranial 00PE
  - Peripheral 01PY
- Omentum 0DPU
- Ovary 0UP3
- Pancreas 0FPG
- Parathyroid Gland 0GPR
- Patella
  - Left 0QPF
  - Right 0QPD
- Pelvic Cavity 0WPJ
- Penis 0VPS
- Pericardial Cavity 0WPD
- Perineum
  - Female 0WPN
  - Male 0WPM
- Peritoneal Cavity 0WPG
- Peritoneum 0DPW
- Phalanx
  - Finger
    - Left 0PPV
    - Right 0PPT
  - Thumb
    - Left 0PPS
    - Right 0PPR
  - Toe
    - Left 0QPR
    - Right 0QPQ
- Pineal Body 0GP1
- Pleura 0BPQ
- Pleural Cavity
  - Left 0WPB
  - Right 0WP9
- Products of Conception 10P0
- Prostate and Seminal Vesicles 0VP4
- Radius
  - Left 0PPJ
  - Right 0PPH
- Rectum 0DPP
- Respiratory Tract 0WPQ
- Retroperitoneum 0WPH
- Ribs
  - 1 to 2 0PP1
  - 3 or More 0PP2
- Sacrum 0QP1
- Scapula
  - Left 0PP6
  - Right 0PP5
- Scrotum and Tunica Vaginalis 0VP8
- Sinus 09PY
- Skin 0HPPX
- Skull 0NP0
- Spinal Canal 00PU

Removal of device from — continued
- Spinal Cord 00PV
- Spleen 07PP
- Sternum 0PP0
- Stomach 0DP6
- Subcutaneous Tissue and Fascia
  - Head and Neck 0JPS
  - Lower Extremity 0JPW
  - Trunk 0JPT
  - Upper Extremity 0JPV
- Tarsal
  - Left 0QPM
  - Right 0QPL
- Tendon
  - Lower 0LPY
  - Upper 0LPX
- Testis 0VPD
- Thymus 07PM
- Thyroid Gland 0GPK
- Tibia
  - Left 0QPH
  - Right 0QPG
- Toe Nail 0HPRX
- Trachea 0BP1
- Tracheobronchial Tree 0BP0
- Tympanic Membrane
  - Left 09P8
  - Right 09P7
- Ulna
  - Left 0PPL
  - Right 0PPK
- Ureter 0TP9
- Urethra 0TPD
- Uterus and Cervix 0UPD
- Vagina and Cul-de-sac 0UPH
- Vas Deferens 0VPR
- Vein
  - Azygos 05P0
  - Innominate
    - Left 05P4
    - Right 05P3
  - Lower 06PY
  - Upper 05PY
- Vertebra
  - Cervical 0PP3
  - Lumbar 0QP0
  - Thoracic 0PP4
- Vulva 0UPM

Renal calyx
- use Kidney
- use Kidney, Left
- use Kidney, Right
- use Kidneys, Bilateral

Renal capsule
- use Kidney
- use Kidney, Left
- use Kidney, Right
- use Kidneys, Bilateral

Renal cortex
- use Kidney
- use Kidney, Left
- use Kidney, Right
- use Kidneys, Bilateral

Renal dialysis see Performance, Urinary 5A1D
Renal nerve use Abdominal Sympathetic Nerve
Renal plexus use Abdominal Sympathetic Nerve

Renal segment
- use Kidney
- use Kidney, Left
- use Kidney, Right
- use Kidneys, Bilateral

Renal segmental artery
- use Renal Artery, Left
- use Renal Artery, Right

Reopening, operative site
Control of bleeding see Control bleeding in
Inspection only see Inspection

Repair
- Abdominal Wall 0WQF
- Acetabulum
  - Left 0QQ5
  - Right 0QQ4
- Adenoids 0CQQ
- Ampulla of Vater 0FQC
- Anal Sphincter 0DQR
- Ankle Region
  - Left 0YQL
  - Right 0YQK

Repair — continued
- Anterior Chamber
  - Left 08Q33ZZ
  - Right 08Q23ZZ
- Anus 0DQQ
- Aorta
  - Abdominal 04Q0
  - Thoracic
    - Ascending/Arch 02QX
    - Descending 02QW
- Aortic Body 0GQD
- Appendix 0DQJ
- Arm
  - Lower
    - Left 0XQF
    - Right 0XQD
  - Upper
    - Left 0XQ9
    - Right 0XQ8
- Artery
  - Anterior Tibial
    - Left 04QQ
    - Right 04QP
  - Axillary
    - Left 03Q6
    - Right 03Q5
  - Brachial
    - Left 03Q8
    - Right 03Q7
  - Celiac 04Q1
  - Colic
    - Left 04Q7
    - Middle 04Q8
    - Right 04Q6
  - Common Carotid
    - Left 03QJ
    - Right 03QH
  - Common Iliac
    - Left 04QD
    - Right 04QC
  - Coronary
    - Four or More Arteries 02Q3
    - One Artery 02Q0
    - Three Arteries 02Q2
    - Two Arteries 02Q1
  - External Carotid
    - Left 03QN
    - Right 03QM
  - External Iliac
    - Left 04QJ
    - Right 04QH
  - Face 03QR
  - Femoral
    - Left 04QL
    - Right 04QK
  - Foot
    - Left 04QW
    - Right 04QV
  - Gastric 04Q2
  - Hand
    - Left 03QF
    - Right 03QD
  - Hepatic 04Q3
  - Inferior Mesenteric 04QB
  - Innominate 03Q2
  - Internal Carotid
    - Left 03QL
    - Right 03QK
  - Internal Iliac
    - Left 04QF
    - Right 04QE
  - Internal Mammary
    - Left 03Q1
    - Right 03Q0
  - Intracranial 03QG
  - Lower 04QY
  - Peroneal
    - Left 04QU
    - Right 04QT
  - Popliteal
    - Left 04QN
    - Right 04QM
  - Posterior Tibial
    - Left 04QS
    - Right 04QR
  - Pulmonary
    - Left 02QR
    - Right 02QQ
  - Pulmonary Trunk 02QP

Repair

Repair — *continued*
- Artery — *continued*
  - Radial
    - Left 03QC
    - Right 03QB
  - Renal
    - Left 04QA
    - Right 04Q9
  - Splenic 04Q4
  - Subclavian
    - Left 03Q4
    - Right 03Q3
  - Superior Mesenteric 04Q5
  - Temporal
    - Left 03QT
    - Right 03QS
  - Thyroid
    - Left 03QV
    - Right 03QU
  - Ulnar
    - Left 03QA
    - Right 03Q9
  - Upper 03QY
  - Vertebral
    - Left 03QQ
    - Right 03QP
- Atrium
  - Left 02Q7
  - Right 02Q6
- Auditory Ossicle
  - Left 09QA
  - Right 09Q9
- Axilla
  - Left 0XQ5
  - Right 0XQ4
- Back
  - Lower 0WQL
  - Upper 0WQK
- Basal Ganglia 00Q8
- Bladder 0TQB
- Bladder Neck 0TQC
- Bone
  - Ethmoid
    - Left 0NQG
    - Right 0NQF
  - Frontal 0NQ1
  - Hyoid 0NQX
  - Lacrimal
    - Left 0NQJ
    - Right 0NQH
  - Nasal 0NQB
  - Occipital 0NQ7
  - Palatine
    - Left 0NQL
    - Right 0NQK
  - Parietal
    - Left 0NQ4
    - Right 0NQ3
  - Pelvic
    - Left 0QQ3
    - Right 0QQ2
  - Sphenoid 0NQC
  - Temporal
    - Left 0NQ6
    - Right 0NQ5
  - Zygomatic
    - Left 0NQN
    - Right 0NQM
- Brain 00Q0
- Breast
  - Bilateral 0HQV
  - Left 0HQU
  - Right 0HQT
  - Supernumerary 0HQY
- Bronchus
  - Lingula 0BQ9
  - Lower Lobe
    - Left 0BQB
    - Right 0BQ6
  - Main
    - Left 0BQ7
    - Right 0BQ3
  - Middle Lobe, Right 0BQ5
  - Upper Lobe
    - Left 0BQ8
    - Right 0BQ4
- Buccal Mucosa 0CQ4

Repair — *continued*
- Bursa and Ligament
  - Abdomen
    - Left 0MQJ
    - Right 0MQH
  - Ankle
    - Left 0MQR
    - Right 0MQQ
  - Elbow
    - Left 0MQ4
    - Right 0MQ3
  - Foot
    - Left 0MQT
    - Right 0MQS
  - Hand
    - Left 0MQ8
    - Right 0MQ7
  - Head and Neck 0MQ0
  - Hip
    - Left 0MQM
    - Right 0MQL
  - Knee
    - Left 0MQP
    - Right 0MQN
  - Lower Extremity
    - Left 0MQW
    - Right 0MQV
  - Perineum 0MQK
  - Rib(s) 0MQG
  - Shoulder
    - Left 0MQ2
    - Right 0MQ1
  - Spine
    - Lower 0MQD
    - Upper 0MQC
  - Sternum 0MQF
  - Upper Extremity
    - Left 0MQB
    - Right 0MQ9
  - Wrist
    - Left 0MQ6
    - Right 0MQ5
- Buttock
  - Left 0YQ1
  - Right 0YQ0
- Carina 0BQ2
- Carotid Bodies, Bilateral 0GQ8
- Carotid Body
  - Left 0GQ6
  - Right 0GQ7
- Carpal
  - Left 0PQN
  - Right 0PQM
- Cecum 0DQH
- Cerebellum 00QC
- Cerebral Hemisphere 00Q7
- Cerebral Meninges 00Q1
- Cerebral Ventricle 00Q6
- Cervix 0UQC
- Chest Wall 0WQ8
- Chordae Tendineae 02Q9
- Choroid
  - Left 08QB
  - Right 08QA
- Cisterna Chyli 07QL
- Clavicle
  - Left 0PQB
  - Right 0PQ9
- Clitoris 0UQJ
- Coccygeal Glomus 0GQB
- Coccyx 0QQS
- Colon
  - Ascending 0DQK
  - Descending 0DQM
  - Sigmoid 0DQN
  - Transverse 0DQL
- Conduction Mechanism 02Q8
- Conjunctiva
  - Left 08QTXZZ
  - Right 08QSXZZ
- Cord
  - Bilateral 0VQH
  - Left 0VQG
  - Right 0VQF
- Cornea
  - Left 08Q9XZZ
  - Right 08Q8XZZ
- Cul-de-sac 0UQF
- Diaphragm 0BQT

Repair — *continued*
- Disc
  - Cervical Vertebral 0RQ3
  - Cervicothoracic Vertebral 0RQ5
  - Lumbar Vertebral 0SQ2
  - Lumbosacral 0SQ4
  - Thoracic Vertebral 0RQ9
  - Thoracolumbar Vertebral 0RQB
- Duct
  - Common Bile 0FQ9
  - Cystic 0FQ8
  - Hepatic
    - Common 0FQ7
    - Left 0FQ6
    - Right 0FQ5
  - Lacrimal
    - Left 08QY
    - Right 08QX
  - Pancreatic 0FQD
    - Accessory 0FQF
  - Parotid
    - Left 0CQC
    - Right 0CQB
- Duodenum 0DQ9
- Dura Mater 00Q2
- Ear
  - External
    - Bilateral 09Q2
    - Left 09Q1
    - Right 09Q0
  - External Auditory Canal
    - Left 09Q4
    - Right 09Q3
  - Inner
    - Left 09QE
    - Right 09QD
  - Middle
    - Left 09Q6
    - Right 09Q5
- Elbow Region
  - Left 0XQC
  - Right 0XQB
- Epididymis
  - Bilateral 0VQL
  - Left 0VQK
  - Right 0VQJ
- Epiglottis 0CQR
- Esophagogastric Junction 0DQ4
- Esophagus 0DQ5
  - Lower 0DQ3
  - Middle 0DQ2
  - Upper 0DQ1
- Eustachian Tube
  - Left 09QG
  - Right 09QF
- Extremity
  - Lower
    - Left 0YQB
    - Right 0YQ9
  - Upper
    - Left 0XQ7
    - Right 0XQ6
- Eye
  - Left 08Q1XZZ
  - Right 08Q0XZZ
- Eyelid
  - Lower
    - Left 08QR
    - Right 08QQ
  - Upper
    - Left 08QP
    - Right 08QN
- Face 0WQ2
- Fallopian Tube
  - Left 0UQ6
  - Right 0UQ5
- Fallopian Tubes, Bilateral 0UQ7
- Femoral Region
  - Bilateral 0YQE
  - Left 0YQ8
  - Right 0YQ7
- Femoral Shaft
  - Left 0QQ9
  - Right 0QQ8
- Femur
  - Lower
    - Left 0QQC
    - Right 0QQB

Repair — continued
  Femur — continued
    Upper
      Left 0QQ7
      Right 0QQ6
  Fibula
    Left 0QQK
    Right 0QQJ
  Finger
    Index
      Left 0XQP
      Right 0XQN
    Little
      Left 0XQW
      Right 0XQV
    Middle
      Left 0XQR
      Right 0XQQ
    Ring
      Left 0XQT
      Right 0XQS
  Finger Nail 0HQQXZZ
  Floor of mouth *see* Repair, Oral Cavity and Throat 0WQ3
  Foot
    Left 0YQN
    Right 0YQM
  Gallbladder 0FQ4
  Gingiva
    Lower 0CQ6
    Upper 0CQ5
  Gland
    Adrenal
      Bilateral 0GQ4
      Left 0GQ2
      Right 0GQ3
    Lacrimal
      Left 08QW
      Right 08QV
    Minor Salivary 0CQJ
    Parotid
      Left 0CQ9
      Right 0CQ8
    Pituitary 0GQ0
    Sublingual
      Left 0CQF
      Right 0CQD
    Submaxillary
      Left 0CQH
      Right 0CQG
    Vestibular 0UQL
  Glenoid Cavity
    Left 0PQ8
    Right 0PQ7
  Glomus Jugulare 0GQC
  Hand
    Left 0XQK
    Right 0XQJ
  Head 0WQ0
  Heart 02QA
    Left 02QC
    Right 02QB
  Humeral Head
    Left 0PQD
    Right 0PQC
  Humeral Shaft
    Left 0PQG
    Right 0PQF
  Hymen 0UQK
  Hypothalamus 00QA
  Ileocecal Valve 0DQC
  Ileum 0DQB
  Inguinal Region
    Bilateral 0YQA
    Left 0YQ6
    Right 0YQ5
  Intestine
    Large 0DQE
      Left 0DQG
      Right 0DQF
    Small 0DQ8
  Iris
    Left 08QD3ZZ
    Right 08QC3ZZ
  Jaw
    Lower 0WQ5
    Upper 0WQ4
  Jejunum 0DQA

Repair — continued
  Joint
    Acromioclavicular
      Left 0RQH
      Right 0RQG
    Ankle
      Left 0SQG
      Right 0SQF
    Carpal
      Left 0RQR
      Right 0RQQ
    Carpometacarpal
      Left 0RQT
      Right 0RQS
    Cervical Vertebral 0RQ1
    Cervicothoracic Vertebral 0RQ4
    Coccygeal 0SQ6
    Elbow
      Left 0RQM
      Right 0RQL
    Finger Phalangeal
      Left 0RQX
      Right 0RQW
    Hip
      Left 0SQB
      Right 0SQ9
    Knee
      Left 0SQD
      Right 0SQC
    Lumbar Vertebral 0SQ0
    Lumbosacral 0SQ3
    Metacarpophalangeal
      Left 0RQV
      Right 0RQU
    Metatarsal-Phalangeal
      Left 0SQN
      Right 0SQM
    Occipital-cervical 0RQ0
    Sacrococcygeal 0SQ5
    Sacroiliac
      Left 0SQ8
      Right 0SQ7
    Shoulder
      Left 0RQK
      Right 0RQJ
    Sternoclavicular
      Left 0RQF
      Right 0RQE
    Tarsal
      Left 0SQJ
      Right 0SQH
    Tarsometatarsal
      Left 0SQL
      Right 0SQK
    Temporomandibular
      Left 0RQD
      Right 0RQC
    Thoracic Vertebral 0RQ6
    Thoracolumbar Vertebral 0RQA
    Toe Phalangeal
      Left 0SQQ
      Right 0SQP
    Wrist
      Left 0RQP
      Right 0RQN
  Kidney
    Left 0TQ1
    Right 0TQ0
  Kidney Pelvis
    Left 0TQ4
    Right 0TQ3
  Knee Region
    Left 0YQG
    Right 0YQF
  Larynx 0CQS
  Leg
    Lower
      Left 0YQJ
      Right 0YQH
    Upper
      Left 0YQD
      Right 0YQC
  Lens
    Left 08QK3ZZ
    Right 08QJ3ZZ
  Lip
    Lower 0CQ1
    Upper 0CQ0
  Liver 0FQ0

Repair — continued
  Liver — continued
    Left Lobe 0FQ2
    Right Lobe 0FQ1
  Lung
    Bilateral 0BQM
    Left 0BQL
    Lower Lobe
      Left 0BQJ
      Right 0BQF
    Middle Lobe, Right 0BQD
    Right 0BQK
    Upper Lobe
      Left 0BQG
      Right 0BQC
  Lung Lingula 0BQH
  Lymphatic
    Aortic 07QD
    Axillary
      Left 07Q6
      Right 07Q5
    Head 07Q0
    Inguinal
      Left 07QJ
      Right 07QH
    Internal Mammary
      Left 07Q9
      Right 07Q8
    Lower Extremity
      Left 07QG
      Right 07QF
    Mesenteric 07QB
    Neck
      Left 07Q2
      Right 07Q1
    Pelvis 07QC
    Thoracic Duct 07QK
    Thorax 07Q7
    Upper Extremity
      Left 07Q4
      Right 07Q3
  Mandible
    Left 0NQV
    Right 0NQT
  Maxilla 0NQR
  Mediastinum 0WQC
  Medulla Oblongata 00QD
  Mesentery 0DQV
  Metacarpal
    Left 0PQQ
    Right 0PQP
  Metatarsal
    Left 0QQP
    Right 0QQN
  Muscle
    Abdomen
      Left 0KQL
      Right 0KQK
    Extraocular
      Left 08QM
      Right 08QL
    Facial 0KQ1
    Foot
      Left 0KQW
      Right 0KQV
    Hand
      Left 0KQD
      Right 0KQC
    Head 0KQ0
    Hip
      Left 0KQP
      Right 0KQN
    Lower Arm and Wrist
      Left 0KQB
      Right 0KQ9
    Lower Leg
      Left 0KQT
      Right 0KQS
    Neck
      Left 0KQ3
      Right 0KQ2
    Papillary 02QD
    Perineum 0KQM
    Shoulder
      Left 0KQ6
      Right 0KQ5
    Thorax
      Left 0KQJ
      Right 0KQH

▽ **Subterms under main terms may continue to next column or page**

Repair — *continued*
  Muscle — *continued*
    Tongue, Palate, Pharynx 0KQ4
    Trunk
      Left 0KQG
      Right 0KQF
    Upper Arm
      Left 0KQ8
      Right 0KQ7
    Upper Leg
      Left 0KQR
      Right 0KQQ
  Nasal Mucosa and Soft Tissue 09QK
  Nasopharynx 09QN
  Neck 0WQ6
  Nerve
    Abdominal Sympathetic 01QM
    Abducens 00QL
    Accessory 00QR
    Acoustic 00QN
    Brachial Plexus 01Q3
    Cervical 01Q1
    Cervical Plexus 01Q0
    Facial 00QM
    Femoral 01QD
    Glossopharyngeal 00QP
    Head and Neck Sympathetic 01QK
    Hypoglossal 00QS
    Lumbar 01QB
    Lumbar Plexus 01Q9
    Lumbar Sympathetic 01QN
    Lumbosacral Plexus 01QA
    Median 01Q5
    Oculomotor 00QH
    Olfactory 00QF
    Optic 00QG
    Peroneal 01QH
    Phrenic 01Q2
    Pudendal 01QC
    Radial 01Q6
    Sacral 01QR
    Sacral Plexus 01QQ
    Sacral Sympathetic 01QP
    Sciatic 01QF
    Thoracic 01Q8
    Thoracic Sympathetic 01QL
    Tibial 01QG
    Trigeminal 00QK
    Trochlear 00QJ
    Ulnar 01Q4
    Vagus 00QQ
  Nipple
    Left 0HQX
    Right 0HQW
  Omentum 0DQU
  Oral Cavity and Throat 0WQ3
  Orbit
    Left 0NQQ
    Right 0NQP
  Ovary
    Bilateral 0UQ2
    Left 0UQ1
    Right 0UQ0
  Palate
    Hard 0CQ2
    Soft 0CQ3
  Pancreas 0FQG
  Para-aortic Body 0GQ9
  Paraganglion Extremity 0GQF
  Parathyroid Gland 0GQR
    Inferior
      Left 0GQP
      Right 0GQN
    Multiple 0GQQ
    Superior
      Left 0GQM
      Right 0GQL
  Patella
    Left 0QQF
    Right 0QQD
  Penis 0VQS
  Pericardium 02QN
  Perineum
    Female 0WQN
    Male 0WQM
  Peritoneum 0DQW
  Phalanx
    Finger
      Left 0PQV

Repair — *continued*
  Phalanx — *continued*
    Finger — *continued*
      Right 0PQT
    Thumb
      Left 0PQS
      Right 0PQR
    Toe
      Left 0QQR
      Right 0QQQ
  Pharynx 0CQM
  Pineal Body 0GQ1
  Pleura
    Left 0BQP
    Right 0BQN
  Pons 00QB
  Prepuce 0VQT
  Products of Conception 10Q0
  Prostate 0VQ0
  Radius
    Left 0PQJ
    Right 0PQH
  Rectum 0DQP
  Retina
    Left 08QF3ZZ
    Right 08QE3ZZ
  Retinal Vessel
    Left 08QH3ZZ
    Right 08QG3ZZ
  Ribs
    1 to 2 0PQ1
    3 or More 0PQ2
  Sacrum 0QQ1
  Scapula
    Left 0PQ6
    Right 0PQ5
  Sclera
    Left 08Q7XZZ
    Right 08Q6XZZ
  Scrotum 0VQ5
  Septum
    Atrial 02Q5
    Nasal 09QM
    Ventricular 02QM
  Shoulder Region
    Left 0XQ3
    Right 0XQ2
  Sinus
    Accessory 09QP
    Ethmoid
      Left 09QV
      Right 09QU
    Frontal
      Left 09QT
      Right 09QS
    Mastoid
      Left 09QC
      Right 09QB
    Maxillary
      Left 09QR
      Right 09QQ
    Sphenoid
      Left 09QX
      Right 09QW
  Skin
    Abdomen 0HQ7XZZ
    Back 0HQ6XZZ
    Buttock 0HQ8XZZ
    Chest 0HQ5XZZ
    Ear
      Left 0HQ3XZZ
      Right 0HQ2XZZ
    Face 0HQ1XZZ
    Foot
      Left 0HQNXZZ
      Right 0HQMXZZ
    Hand
      Left 0HQGXZZ
      Right 0HQFXZZ
    Inguinal 0HQAXZZ
    Lower Arm
      Left 0HQEXZZ
      Right 0HQDXZZ
    Lower Leg
      Left 0HQLXZZ
      Right 0HQKXZZ
    Neck 0HQ4XZZ
    Perineum 0HQ9XZZ
    Scalp 0HQ0XZZ

Repair — *continued*
  Skin — *continued*
    Upper Arm
      Left 0HQCXZZ
      Right 0HQBXZZ
    Upper Leg
      Left 0HQJXZZ
      Right 0HQHXZZ
  Skull 0NQ0
  Spinal Cord
    Cervical 00QW
    Lumbar 00QY
    Thoracic 00QX
  Spinal Meninges 00QT
  Spleen 07QP
  Sternum 0PQ0
  Stomach 0DQ6
    Pylorus 0DQ7
  Subcutaneous Tissue and Fascia
    Abdomen 0JQ8
    Back 0JQ7
    Buttock 0JQ9
    Chest 0JQ6
    Face 0JQ1
    Foot
      Left 0JQR
      Right 0JQQ
    Hand
      Left 0JQK
      Right 0JQJ
    Lower Arm
      Left 0JQH
      Right 0JQG
    Lower Leg
      Left 0JQP
      Right 0JQN
    Neck
      Left 0JQ5
      Right 0JQ4
    Pelvic Region 0JQC
    Perineum 0JQB
    Scalp 0JQ0
    Upper Arm
      Left 0JQF
      Right 0JQD
    Upper Leg
      Left 0JQM
      Right 0JQL
  Tarsal
    Left 0QQM
    Right 0QQL
  Tendon
    Abdomen
      Left 0LQG
      Right 0LQF
    Ankle
      Left 0LQT
      Right 0LQS
    Foot
      Left 0LQW
      Right 0LQV
    Hand
      Left 0LQ8
      Right 0LQ7
    Head and Neck 0LQ0
    Hip
      Left 0LQK
      Right 0LQJ
    Knee
      Left 0LQR
      Right 0LQQ
    Lower Arm and Wrist
      Left 0LQ6
      Right 0LQ5
    Lower Leg
      Left 0LQP
      Right 0LQN
    Perineum 0LQH
    Shoulder
      Left 0LQ2
      Right 0LQ1
    Thorax
      Left 0LQD
      Right 0LQC
    Trunk
      Left 0LQB
      Right 0LQ9
    Upper Arm
      Left 0LQ4

Repair — *continued*
  Tendon — *continued*
    Upper Arm — *continued*
      Right ØLQ3
    Upper Leg
      Left ØLQM
      Right ØLQL
  Testis
    Bilateral ØVQC
    Left ØVQB
    Right ØVQ9
  Thalamus ØØQ9
  Thumb
    Left ØXQM
    Right ØXQL
  Thymus Ø7QM
  Thyroid Gland ØGQK
    Left Lobe ØGQG
    Right Lobe ØGQH
  Thyroid Gland Isthmus ØGQJ
  Tibia
    Left ØQQH
    Right ØQQG
  Toe
    1st
      Left ØYQQ
      Right ØYQP
    2nd
      Left ØYQS
      Right ØYQR
    3rd
      Left ØYQU
      Right ØYQT
    4th
      Left ØYQW
      Right ØYQV
    5th
      Left ØYQY
      Right ØYQX
  Toe Nail ØHQRXZZ
  Tongue ØCQ7
  Tonsils ØCQP
  Tooth
    Lower ØCQX
    Upper ØCQW
  Trachea ØBQ1
  Tunica Vaginalis
    Left ØVQ7
    Right ØVQ6
  Turbinate, Nasal Ø9QL
  Tympanic Membrane
    Left Ø9Q8
    Right Ø9Q7
  Ulna
    Left ØPQL
    Right ØPQK
  Ureter
    Left ØTQ7
    Right ØTQ6
  Urethra ØTQD
  Uterine Supporting Structure ØUQ4
  Uterus ØUQ9
  Uvula ØCQN
  Vagina ØUQG
  Valve
    Aortic Ø2QF
    Mitral Ø2QG
    Pulmonary Ø2QH
    Tricuspid Ø2QJ
  Vas Deferens
    Bilateral ØVQQ
    Left ØVQP
    Right ØVQN
  Vein
    Axillary
      Left Ø5Q8
      Right Ø5Q7
    Azygos Ø5QØ
    Basilic
      Left Ø5QC
      Right Ø5QB
    Brachial
      Left Ø5QA
      Right Ø5Q9
    Cephalic
      Left Ø5QF
      Right Ø5QD
    Colic Ø6Q7

Repair — *continued*
  Vein — *continued*
    Common Iliac
      Left Ø6QD
      Right Ø6QC
    Coronary Ø2Q4
    Esophageal Ø6Q3
    External Iliac
      Left Ø6QG
      Right Ø6QF
    External Jugular
      Left Ø5QQ
      Right Ø5QP
    Face
      Left Ø5QV
      Right Ø5QT
    Femoral
      Left Ø6QN
      Right Ø6QM
    Foot
      Left Ø6QV
      Right Ø6QT
    Gastric Ø6Q2
    Hand
      Left Ø5QH
      Right Ø5QG
    Hemiazygos Ø5Q1
    Hepatic Ø6Q4
    Hypogastric
      Left Ø6QJ
      Right Ø6QH
    Inferior Mesenteric Ø6Q6
    Innominate
      Left Ø5Q4
      Right Ø5Q3
    Internal Jugular
      Left Ø5QN
      Right Ø5QM
    Intracranial Ø5QL
    Lower Ø6QY
    Portal Ø6Q8
    Pulmonary
      Left Ø2QT
      Right Ø2QS
    Renal
      Left Ø6QB
      Right Ø6Q9
    Saphenous
      Left Ø6QQ
      Right Ø6QP
    Splenic Ø6Q1
    Subclavian
      Left Ø5Q6
      Right Ø5Q5
    Superior Mesenteric Ø6Q5
    Upper Ø5QY
    Vertebral
      Left Ø5QS
      Right Ø5QR
  Vena Cava
    Inferior Ø6QØ
    Superior Ø2QV
  Ventricle
    Left Ø2QL
    Right Ø2QK
  Vertebra
    Cervical ØPQ3
    Lumbar ØQQØ
    Thoracic ØPQ4
  Vesicle
    Bilateral ØVQ3
    Left ØVQ2
    Right ØVQ1
  Vitreous
    Left Ø8Q53ZZ
    Right Ø8Q43ZZ
  Vocal Cord
    Left ØCQV
    Right ØCQT
  Vulva ØUQM
  Wrist Region
    Left ØXQH
    Right ØXQG
Repair, obstetric laceration, periurethral ØUQMXZZ
Replacement
  Acetabulum
    Left ØQR5
    Right ØQR4
  Ampulla of Vater ØFRC

Replacement — *continued*
  Anal Sphincter ØDRR
  Aorta
    Abdominal Ø4RØ
    Thoracic
      Ascending/Arch Ø2RX
      Descending Ø2RW
  Artery
    Anterior Tibial
      Left Ø4RQ
      Right Ø4RP
    Axillary
      Left Ø3R6
      Right Ø3R5
    Brachial
      Left Ø3R8
      Right Ø3R7
    Celiac Ø4R1
    Colic
      Left Ø4R7
      Middle Ø4R8
      Right Ø4R6
    Common Carotid
      Left Ø3RJ
      Right Ø3RH
    Common Iliac
      Left Ø4RD
      Right Ø4RC
    External Carotid
      Left Ø3RN
      Right Ø3RM
    External Iliac
      Left Ø4RJ
      Right Ø4RH
    Face Ø3RR
    Femoral
      Left Ø4RL
      Right Ø4RK
    Foot
      Left Ø4RW
      Right Ø4RV
    Gastric Ø4R2
    Hand
      Left Ø3RF
      Right Ø3RD
    Hepatic Ø4R3
    Inferior Mesenteric Ø4RB
    Innominate Ø3R2
    Internal Carotid
      Left Ø3RL
      Right Ø3RK
    Internal Iliac
      Left Ø4RF
      Right Ø4RE
    Internal Mammary
      Left Ø3R1
      Right Ø3RØ
    Intracranial Ø3RG
    Lower Ø4RY
    Peroneal
      Left Ø4RU
      Right Ø4RT
    Popliteal
      Left Ø4RN
      Right Ø4RM
    Posterior Tibial
      Left Ø4RS
      Right Ø4RR
    Pulmonary
      Left Ø2RR
      Right Ø2RQ
    Pulmonary Trunk Ø2RP
    Radial
      Left Ø3RC
      Right Ø3RB
    Renal
      Left Ø4RA
      Right Ø4R9
    Splenic Ø4R4
    Subclavian
      Left Ø3R4
      Right Ø3R3
    Superior Mesenteric Ø4R5
    Temporal
      Left Ø3RT
      Right Ø3RS
    Thyroid
      Left Ø3RV
      Right Ø3RU

Replacement

Replacement — continued
  Artery — continued
    Ulnar
      Left 03RA
      Right 03R9
    Upper 03RY
    Vertebral
      Left 03RQ
      Right 03RP
  Atrium
    Left 02R7
    Right 02R6
  Auditory Ossicle
    Left 09RA0
    Right 09R90
  Bladder 0TRB
  Bladder Neck 0TRC
  Bone
    Ethmoid
      Left 0NRG
      Right 0NRF
    Frontal 0NR1
    Hyoid 0NRX
    Lacrimal
      Left 0NRJ
      Right 0NRH
    Nasal 0NRB
    Occipital 0NR7
    Palatine
      Left 0NRL
      Right 0NRK
    Parietal
      Left 0NR4
      Right 0NR3
    Pelvic
      Left 0QR3
      Right 0QR2
    Sphenoid 0NRC
    Temporal
      Left 0NR6
      Right 0NR5
    Zygomatic
      Left 0NRN
      Right 0NRM
  Breast
    Bilateral 0HRV
    Left 0HRU
    Right 0HRT
  Bronchus
    Lingula 0BR9
    Lower Lobe
      Left 0BRB
      Right 0BR6
    Main
      Left 0BR7
      Right 0BR3
    Middle Lobe, Right 0BR5
    Upper Lobe
      Left 0BR8
      Right 0BR4
  Buccal Mucosa 0CR4
  Bursa and Ligament
    Abdomen
      Left 0MRJ
      Right 0MRH
    Ankle
      Left 0MRR
      Right 0MRQ
    Elbow
      Left 0MR4
      Right 0MR3
    Foot
      Left 0MRT
      Right 0MRS
    Hand
      Left 0MR8
      Right 0MR7
    Head and Neck 0MR0
    Hip
      Left 0MRM
      Right 0MRL
    Knee
      Left 0MRP
      Right 0MRN
    Lower Extremity
      Left 0MRW
      Right 0MRV
    Perineum 0MRK
    Rib(s) 0MRG

Replacement — continued
  Bursa and Ligament — continued
    Shoulder
      Left 0MR2
      Right 0MR1
    Spine
      Lower 0MRD
      Upper 0MRC
    Sternum 0MRF
    Upper Extremity
      Left 0MRB
      Right 0MR9
    Wrist
      Left 0MR6
      Right 0MR5
  Carina 0BR2
  Carpal
    Left 0PRN
    Right 0PRM
  Cerebral Meninges 00R1
  Cerebral Ventricle 00R6
  Chordae Tendineae 02R9
  Choroid
    Left 08RB
    Right 08RA
  Clavicle
    Left 0PRB
    Right 0PR9
  Coccyx 0QRS
  Conjunctiva
    Left 08RTX
    Right 08RSX
  Cornea
    Left 08R9
    Right 08R8
  Diaphragm 0BRT
  Disc
    Cervical Vertebral 0RR30
    Cervicothoracic Vertebral 0RR50
    Lumbar Vertebral 0SR20
    Lumbosacral 0SR40
    Thoracic Vertebral 0RR90
    Thoracolumbar Vertebral 0RRB0
  Duct
    Common Bile 0FR9
    Cystic 0FR8
    Hepatic
      Common 0FR7
      Left 0FR6
      Right 0FR5
    Lacrimal
      Left 08RY
      Right 08RX
    Pancreatic 0FRD
      Accessory 0FRF
    Parotid
      Left 0CRC
      Right 0CRB
  Dura Mater 00R2
  Ear
    External
      Bilateral 09R2
      Left 09R1
      Right 09R0
    Inner
      Left 09RE0
      Right 09RD0
    Middle
      Left 09R60
      Right 09R50
  Epiglottis 0CRR
  Esophagus 0DR5
  Eye
    Left 08R1
    Right 08R0
  Eyelid
    Lower
      Left 08RR
      Right 08RQ
    Upper
      Left 08RP
      Right 08RN
  Femoral Shaft
    Left 0QR9
    Right 0QR8
  Femur
    Lower
      Left 0QRC
      Right 0QRB

Replacement — continued
  Femur — continued
    Upper
      Left 0QR7
      Right 0QR6
  Fibula
    Left 0QRK
    Right 0QRJ
  Finger Nail 0HRQX
  Gingiva
    Lower 0CR6
    Upper 0CR5
  Glenoid Cavity
    Left 0PR8
    Right 0PR7
  Hair 0HRSX
  Heart 02RA0
  Humeral Head
    Left 0PRD
    Right 0PRC
  Humeral Shaft
    Left 0PRG
    Right 0PRF
  Iris
    Left 08RD3
    Right 08RC3
  Joint
    Acromioclavicular
      Left 0RRH0
      Right 0RRG0
    Ankle
      Left 0SRG
      Right 0SRF
    Carpal
      Left 0RRR0
      Right 0RRQ0
    Carpometacarpal
      Left 0RRT0
      Right 0RRS0
    Cervical Vertebral 0RR10
    Cervicothoracic Vertebral 0RR40
    Coccygeal 0SR60
    Elbow
      Left 0RRM0
      Right 0RRL0
    Finger Phalangeal
      Left 0RRX0
      Right 0RRW0
    Hip
      Left 0SRB
        Acetabular Surface 0SRE
        Femoral Surface 0SRS
      Right 0SR9
        Acetabular Surface 0SRA
        Femoral Surface 0SRR
    Knee
      Left 0SRD
        Femoral Surface 0SRU
        Tibial Surface 0SRW
      Right 0SRC
        Femoral Surface 0SRT
        Tibial Surface 0SRV
    Lumbar Vertebral 0SR00
    Lumbosacral 0SR30
    Metacarpophalangeal
      Left 0RRV0
      Right 0RRU0
    Metatarsal-Phalangeal
      Left 0SRN0
      Right 0SRM0
    Occipital-cervical 0RR00
    Sacrococcygeal 0SR50
    Sacroiliac
      Left 0SR80
      Right 0SR70
    Shoulder
      Left 0RRK
      Right 0RRJ
    Sternoclavicular
      Left 0RRF0
      Right 0RRE0
    Tarsal
      Left 0SRJ0
      Right 0SRH0
    Tarsometatarsal
      Left 0SRL0
      Right 0SRK0
    Temporomandibular
      Left 0RRD0

Replacement — *continued*
  Joint — *continued*
    Temporomandibular — *continued*
      Right 0RRC0
    Thoracic Vertebral 0RR60
    Thoracolumbar Vertebral 0RRA0
    Toe Phalangeal
      Left 0SRQ0
      Right 0SRP0
    Wrist
      Left 0RRP0
      Right 0RRN0
  Kidney Pelvis
    Left 0TR4
    Right 0TR3
  Larynx 0CRS
  Lens
    Left 08RK30Z
    Right 08RJ30Z
  Lip
    Lower 0CR1
    Upper 0CR0
  Mandible
    Left 0NRV
    Right 0NRT
  Maxilla 0NRR
  Mesentery 0DRV
  Metacarpal
    Left 0PRQ
    Right 0PRP
  Metatarsal
    Left 0QRP
    Right 0QRN
  Muscle
    Abdomen
      Left 0KRL
      Right 0KRK
    Facial 0KR1
    Foot
      Left 0KRW
      Right 0KRV
    Hand
      Left 0KRD
      Right 0KRC
    Head 0KR0
    Hip
      Left 0KRP
      Right 0KRN
    Lower Arm and Wrist
      Left 0KRB
      Right 0KR9
    Lower Leg
      Left 0KRT
      Right 0KRS
    Neck
      Left 0KR3
      Right 0KR2
    Papillary 02RD
    Perineum 0KRM
    Shoulder
      Left 0KR6
      Right 0KR5
    Thorax
      Left 0KRJ
      Right 0KRH
    Tongue, Palate, Pharynx 0KR4
    Trunk
      Left 0KRG
      Right 0KRF
    Upper Arm
      Left 0KR8
      Right 0KR7
    Upper Leg
      Left 0KRR
      Right 0KRQ
  Nasal Mucosa and Soft Tissue 09RK
  Nasopharynx 09RN
  Nerve
    Abducens 00RL
    Accessory 00RR
    Acoustic 00RN
    Cervical 01R1
    Facial 00RM
    Femoral 01RD
    Glossopharyngeal 00RP
    Hypoglossal 00RS
    Lumbar 01RB
    Median 01R5
    Oculomotor 00RH

Replacement — *continued*
  Nerve — *continued*
    Olfactory 00RF
    Optic 00RG
    Peroneal 01RH
    Phrenic 01R2
    Pudendal 01RC
    Radial 01R6
    Sacral 01RR
    Sciatic 01RF
    Thoracic 01R8
    Tibial 01RG
    Trigeminal 00RK
    Trochlear 00RJ
    Ulnar 01R4
    Vagus 00RQ
  Nipple
    Left 0HRX
    Right 0HRW
  Omentum 0DRU
  Orbit
    Left 0NRQ
    Right 0NRP
  Palate
    Hard 0CR2
    Soft 0CR3
  Patella
    Left 0QRF
    Right 0QRD
  Pericardium 02RN
  Peritoneum 0DRW
  Phalanx
    Finger
      Left 0PRV
      Right 0PRT
    Thumb
      Left 0PRS
      Right 0PRR
    Toe
      Left 0QRR
      Right 0QRQ
  Pharynx 0CRM
  Radius
    Left 0PRJ
    Right 0PRH
  Retinal Vessel
    Left 08RH3
    Right 08RG3
  Ribs
    1 to 2 0PR1
    3 or More 0PR2
  Sacrum 0QR1
  Scapula
    Left 0PR6
    Right 0PR5
  Sclera
    Left 08R7X
    Right 08R6X
  Septum
    Atrial 02R5
    Nasal 09RM
    Ventricular 02RM
  Skin
    Abdomen 0HR7
    Back 0HR6
    Buttock 0HR8
    Chest 0HR5
    Ear
      Left 0HR3
      Right 0HR2
    Face 0HR1
    Foot
      Left 0HRN
      Right 0HRM
    Hand
      Left 0HRG
      Right 0HRF
    Inguinal 0HRA
    Lower Arm
      Left 0HRE
      Right 0HRD
    Lower Leg
      Left 0HRL
      Right 0HRK
    Neck 0HR4
    Perineum 0HR9
    Scalp 0HR0
    Upper Arm
      Left 0HRC

Replacement — *continued*
  Skin — *continued*
    Upper Arm — *continued*
      Right 0HRB
    Upper Leg
      Left 0HRJ
      Right 0HRH
  Skull 0NR0
  Spinal Meninges 00RT
  Sternum 0PR0
  Subcutaneous Tissue and Fascia
    Abdomen 0JR8
    Back 0JR7
    Buttock 0JR9
    Chest 0JR6
    Face 0JR1
    Foot
      Left 0JRR
      Right 0JRQ
    Hand
      Left 0JRK
      Right 0JRJ
    Lower Arm
      Left 0JRH
      Right 0JRG
    Lower Leg
      Left 0JRP
      Right 0JRN
    Neck
      Left 0JR5
      Right 0JR4
    Pelvic Region 0JRC
    Perineum 0JRB
    Scalp 0JR0
    Upper Arm
      Left 0JRF
      Right 0JRD
    Upper Leg
      Left 0JRM
      Right 0JRL
  Tarsal
    Left 0QRM
    Right 0QRL
  Tendon
    Abdomen
      Left 0LRG
      Right 0LRF
    Ankle
      Left 0LRT
      Right 0LRS
    Foot
      Left 0LRW
      Right 0LRV
    Hand
      Left 0LR8
      Right 0LR7
    Head and Neck 0LR0
    Hip
      Left 0LRK
      Right 0LRJ
    Knee
      Left 0LRR
      Right 0LRQ
    Lower Arm and Wrist
      Left 0LR6
      Right 0LR5
    Lower Leg
      Left 0LRP
      Right 0LRN
    Perineum 0LRH
    Shoulder
      Left 0LR2
      Right 0LR1
    Thorax
      Left 0LRD
      Right 0LRC
    Trunk
      Left 0LRB
      Right 0LR9
    Upper Arm
      Left 0LR4
      Right 0LR3
    Upper Leg
      Left 0LRM
      Right 0LRL
  Testis
    Bilateral 0VRC0JZ
    Left 0VRB0JZ
    Right 0VR90JZ

Replacement

Replacement — continued
- Thumb
  - Left 0XRM
  - Right 0XRL
- Tibia
  - Left 0QRH
  - Right 0QRG
- Toe Nail 0HRRX
- Tongue 0CR7
- Tooth
  - Lower 0CRX
  - Upper 0CRW
- Trachea 0BR1
- Turbinate, Nasal 09RL
- Tympanic Membrane
  - Left 09R8
  - Right 09R7
- Ulna
  - Left 0PRL
  - Right 0PRK
- Ureter
  - Left 0TR7
  - Right 0TR6
- Urethra 0TRD
- Uvula 0CRN
- Valve
  - Aortic 02RF
  - Mitral 02RG
  - Pulmonary 02RH
  - Tricuspid 02RJ
- Vein
  - Axillary
    - Left 05R8
    - Right 05R7
  - Azygos 05R0
  - Basilic
    - Left 05RC
    - Right 05RB
  - Brachial
    - Left 05RA
    - Right 05R9
  - Cephalic
    - Left 05RF
    - Right 05RD
  - Colic 06R7
  - Common Iliac
    - Left 06RD
    - Right 06RC
  - Esophageal 06R3
  - External Iliac
    - Left 06RG
    - Right 06RF
  - External Jugular
    - Left 05RQ
    - Right 05RP
  - Face
    - Left 05RV
    - Right 05RT
  - Femoral
    - Left 06RN
    - Right 06RM
  - Foot
    - Left 06RV
    - Right 06RT
  - Gastric 06R2
  - Hand
    - Left 05RH
    - Right 05RG
  - Hemiazygos 05R1
  - Hepatic 06R4
  - Hypogastric
    - Left 06RJ
    - Right 06RH
  - Inferior Mesenteric 06R6
  - Innominate
    - Left 05R4
    - Right 05R3
  - Internal Jugular
    - Left 05RN
    - Right 05RM
  - Intracranial 05RL
  - Lower 06RY
  - Portal 06R8
  - Pulmonary
    - Left 02RT
    - Right 02RS
  - Renal
    - Left 06RB
    - Right 06R9

Replacement — continued
- Vein — continued
  - Saphenous
    - Left 06RQ
    - Right 06RP
  - Splenic 06R1
  - Subclavian
    - Left 05R6
    - Right 05R5
  - Superior Mesenteric 06R5
  - Upper 05RY
  - Vertebral
    - Left 05RS
    - Right 05RR
- Vena Cava
  - Inferior 06R0
  - Superior 02RV
- Ventricle
  - Left 02RL
  - Right 02RK
- Vertebra
  - Cervical 0PR3
  - Lumbar 0QR0
  - Thoracic 0PR4
- Vitreous
  - Left 08R53
  - Right 08R43
- Vocal Cord
  - Left 0CRV
  - Right 0CRT

Replacement, hip
- Partial or total see Replacement, Lower Joints 0SR
- Resurfacing only see Supplement, Lower Joints 0SU

Replacement, knee
- Meniscus implant only see New Technology, Joints XRR
- Partial or total see Replacement, Lower Joints 0SR

Replantation see Reposition

Replantation, scalp see Reattachment, Skin, Scalp 0HM0

Reposition
- Acetabulum
  - Left 0QS5
  - Right 0QS4
- Ampulla of Vater 0FSC
- Anus 0DSQ
- Aorta
  - Abdominal 04S0
  - Thoracic
    - Ascending/Arch 02SX0ZZ
    - Descending 02SW0ZZ
- Artery
  - Anterior Tibial
    - Left 04SQ
    - Right 04SP
  - Axillary
    - Left 03S6
    - Right 03S5
  - Brachial
    - Left 03S8
    - Right 03S7
  - Celiac 04S1
  - Colic
    - Left 04S7
    - Middle 04S8
    - Right 04S6
  - Common Carotid
    - Left 03SJ
    - Right 03SH
  - Common Iliac
    - Left 04SD
    - Right 04SC
  - Coronary
    - One Artery 02S00ZZ
    - Two Arteries 02S10ZZ
  - External Carotid
    - Left 03SN
    - Right 03SM
  - External Iliac
    - Left 04SJ
    - Right 04SH
  - Face 03SR
  - Femoral
    - Left 04SL
    - Right 04SK
  - Foot
    - Left 04SW

Reposition — continued
- Artery — continued
  - Foot — continued
    - Right 04SV
  - Gastric 04S2
  - Hand
    - Left 03SF
    - Right 03SD
  - Hepatic 04S3
  - Inferior Mesenteric 04SB
  - Innominate 03S2
  - Internal Carotid
    - Left 03SL
    - Right 03SK
  - Internal Iliac
    - Left 04SF
    - Right 04SE
  - Internal Mammary
    - Left 03S1
    - Right 03S0
  - Intracranial 03SG
  - Lower 04SY
  - Peroneal
    - Left 04SU
    - Right 04ST
  - Popliteal
    - Left 04SN
    - Right 04SM
  - Posterior Tibial
    - Left 04SS
    - Right 04SR
  - Pulmonary
    - Left 02SR0ZZ
    - Right 02SQ0ZZ
  - Pulmonary Trunk 02SP0ZZ
  - Radial
    - Left 03SC
    - Right 03SB
  - Renal
    - Left 04SA
    - Right 04S9
  - Splenic 04S4
  - Subclavian
    - Left 03S4
    - Right 03S3
  - Superior Mesenteric 04S5
  - Temporal
    - Left 03ST
    - Right 03SS
  - Thyroid
    - Left 03SV
    - Right 03SU
  - Ulnar
    - Left 03SA
    - Right 03S9
  - Upper 03SY
  - Vertebral
    - Left 03SQ
    - Right 03SP
- Auditory Ossicle
  - Left 09SA
  - Right 09S9
- Bladder 0TSB
- Bladder Neck 0TSC
- Bone
  - Ethmoid
    - Left 0NSG
    - Right 0NSF
  - Frontal 0NS1
  - Hyoid 0NSX
  - Lacrimal
    - Left 0NSJ
    - Right 0NSH
  - Nasal 0NSB
  - Occipital 0NS7
  - Palatine
    - Left 0NSL
    - Right 0NSK
  - Parietal
    - Left 0NS4
    - Right 0NS3
  - Pelvic
    - Left 0QS3
    - Right 0QS2
  - Sphenoid 0NSC
  - Temporal
    - Left 0NS6
    - Right 0NS5

Reposition — continued
  Bone — continued
    Zygomatic
      Left ØNSN
      Right ØNSM
  Breast
    Bilateral ØHSVØZZ
    Left ØHSUØZZ
    Right ØHSTØZZ
  Bronchus
    Lingula ØBS9ØZZ
    Lower Lobe
      Left ØBSBØZZ
      Right ØBS6ØZZ
    Main
      Left ØBS7ØZZ
      Right ØBS3ØZZ
    Middle Lobe, Right ØBS5ØZZ
    Upper Lobe
      Left ØBS8ØZZ
      Right ØBS4ØZZ
  Bursa and Ligament
    Abdomen
      Left ØMSJ
      Right ØMSH
    Ankle
      Left ØMSR
      Right ØMSQ
    Elbow
      Left ØMS4
      Right ØMS3
    Foot
      Left ØMST
      Right ØMSS
    Hand
      Left ØMS8
      Right ØMS7
    Head and Neck ØMSØ
    Hip
      Left ØMSM
      Right ØMSL
    Knee
      Left ØMSP
      Right ØMSN
    Lower Extremity
      Left ØMSW
      Right ØMSV
    Perineum ØMSK
    Rib(s) ØMSG
    Shoulder
      Left ØMS2
      Right ØMS1
    Spine
      Lower ØMSD
      Upper ØMSC
    Sternum ØMSF
    Upper Extremity
      Left ØMSB
      Right ØMS9
    Wrist
      Left ØMS6
      Right ØMS5
  Carina ØBS2ØZZ
  Carpal
    Left ØPSN
    Right ØPSM
  Cecum ØDSH
  Cervix ØUSC
  Clavicle
    Left ØPSB
    Right ØPS9
  Coccyx ØQSS
  Colon
    Ascending ØDSK
    Descending ØDSM
    Sigmoid ØDSN
    Transverse ØDSL
  Cord
    Bilateral ØVSH
    Left ØVSG
    Right ØVSF
  Cul-de-sac ØUSF
  Diaphragm ØBSTØZZ
  Duct
    Common Bile ØFS9
    Cystic ØFS8
    Hepatic
      Common ØFS7
      Left ØFS6

Reposition — continued
  Duct — continued
    Hepatic — continued
      Right ØFS5
    Lacrimal
      Left Ø8SY
      Right Ø8SX
    Pancreatic ØFSD
      Accessory ØFSF
    Parotid
      Left ØCSC
      Right ØCSB
  Duodenum ØDS9
  Ear
    Bilateral Ø9S2
    Left Ø9S1
    Right Ø9SØ
  Epiglottis ØCSR
  Esophagus ØDS5
  Eustachian Tube
    Left Ø9SG
    Right Ø9SF
  Eyelid
    Lower
      Left Ø8SR
      Right Ø8SQ
    Upper
      Left Ø8SP
      Right Ø8SN
  Fallopian Tube
    Left ØUS6
    Right ØUS5
  Fallopian Tubes, Bilateral ØUS7
  Femoral Shaft
    Left ØQS9
    Right ØQS8
  Femur
    Lower
      Left ØQSC
      Right ØQSB
    Upper
      Left ØQS7
      Right ØQS6
  Fibula
    Left ØQSK
    Right ØQSJ
  Gallbladder ØFS4
  Gland
    Adrenal
      Left ØGS2
      Right ØGS3
    Lacrimal
      Left Ø8SW
      Right Ø8SV
  Glenoid Cavity
    Left ØPS8
    Right ØPS7
  Hair ØHSSXZZ
  Humeral Head
    Left ØPSD
    Right ØPSC
  Humeral Shaft
    Left ØPSG
    Right ØPSF
  Ileum ØDSB
  Intestine
    Large ØDSE
    Small ØDS8
  Iris
    Left Ø8SD3ZZ
    Right Ø8SC3ZZ
  Jejunum ØDSA
  Joint
    Acromioclavicular
      Left ØRSH
      Right ØRSG
    Ankle
      Left ØSSG
      Right ØSSF
    Carpal
      Left ØRSR
      Right ØRSQ
    Carpometacarpal
      Left ØRST
      Right ØRSS
    Cervical Vertebral ØRS1
    Cervicothoracic Vertebral ØRS4
    Coccygeal ØSS6

Reposition — continued
  Joint — continued
    Elbow
      Left ØRSM
      Right ØRSL
    Finger Phalangeal
      Left ØRSX
      Right ØRSW
    Hip
      Left ØSSB
      Right ØSS9
    Knee
      Left ØSSD
      Right ØSSC
    Lumbar Vertebral ØSSØ
    Lumbosacral ØSS3
    Metacarpophalangeal
      Left ØRSV
      Right ØRSU
    Metatarsal-Phalangeal
      Left ØSSN
      Right ØSSM
    Occipital-cervical ØRSØ
    Sacrococcygeal ØSS5
    Sacroiliac
      Left ØSS8
      Right ØSS7
    Shoulder
      Left ØRSK
      Right ØRSJ
    Sternoclavicular
      Left ØRSF
      Right ØRSE
    Tarsal
      Left ØSSJ
      Right ØSSH
    Tarsometatarsal
      Left ØSSL
      Right ØSSK
    Temporomandibular
      Left ØRSD
      Right ØRSC
    Thoracic Vertebral ØRS6
    Thoracolumbar Vertebral ØRSA
    Toe Phalangeal
      Left ØSSQ
      Right ØSSP
    Wrist
      Left ØRSP
      Right ØRSN
  Kidney
    Left ØTS1
    Right ØTSØ
  Kidney Pelvis
    Left ØTS4
    Right ØTS3
  Kidneys, Bilateral ØTS2
  Larynx ØCSS
  Lens
    Left Ø8SK3ZZ
    Right Ø8SJ3ZZ
  Lip
    Lower ØCS1
    Upper ØCSØ
  Liver ØFSØ
  Lung
    Left ØBSLØZZ
    Lower Lobe
      Left ØBSJØZZ
      Right ØBSFØZZ
    Middle Lobe, Right ØBSDØZZ
    Right ØBSKØZZ
    Upper Lobe
      Left ØBSGØZZ
      Right ØBSCØZZ
  Lung Lingula ØBSHØZZ
  Mandible
    Left ØNSV
    Right ØNST
  Maxilla ØNSR
  Metacarpal
    Left ØPSQ
    Right ØPSP
  Metatarsal
    Left ØQSP
    Right ØQSN
  Muscle
    Abdomen
      Left ØKSL

▼ **Subterms under main terms may continue to next column or page**

Reposition

Reposition — *continued*
- Muscle — *continued*
  - Abdomen — *continued*
    - Right 0KSK
  - Extraocular
    - Left 08SM
    - Right 08SL
  - Facial 0KS1
  - Foot
    - Left 0KSW
    - Right 0KSV
  - Hand
    - Left 0KSD
    - Right 0KSC
  - Head 0KS0
  - Hip
    - Left 0KSP
    - Right 0KSN
  - Lower Arm and Wrist
    - Left 0KSB
    - Right 0KS9
  - Lower Leg
    - Left 0KST
    - Right 0KSS
  - Neck
    - Left 0KS3
    - Right 0KS2
  - Perineum 0KSM
  - Shoulder
    - Left 0KS6
    - Right 0KS5
  - Thorax
    - Left 0KSJ
    - Right 0KSH
  - Tongue, Palate, Pharynx 0KS4
  - Trunk
    - Left 0KSG
    - Right 0KSF
  - Upper Arm
    - Left 0KS8
    - Right 0KS7
  - Upper Leg
    - Left 0KSR
    - Right 0KSQ
- Nasal Mucosa and Soft Tissue 09SK
- Nerve
  - Abducens 00SL
  - Accessory 00SR
  - Acoustic 00SN
  - Brachial Plexus 01S3
  - Cervical 01S1
  - Cervical Plexus 01S0
  - Facial 00SM
  - Femoral 01SD
  - Glossopharyngeal 00SP
  - Hypoglossal 00SS
  - Lumbar 01SB
  - Lumbar Plexus 01S9
  - Lumbosacral Plexus 01SA
  - Median 01S5
  - Oculomotor 00SH
  - Olfactory 00SF
  - Optic 00SG
  - Peroneal 01SH
  - Phrenic 01S2
  - Pudendal 01SC
  - Radial 01S6
  - Sacral 01SR
  - Sacral Plexus 01SQ
  - Sciatic 01SF
  - Thoracic 01S8
  - Tibial 01SG
  - Trigeminal 00SK
  - Trochlear 00SJ
  - Ulnar 01S4
  - Vagus 00SQ
- Nipple
  - Left 0HSXXZZ
  - Right 0HSWXZZ
- Orbit
  - Left 0NSQ
  - Right 0NSP
- Ovary
  - Bilateral 0US2
  - Left 0US1
  - Right 0US0
- Palate
  - Hard 0CS2
  - Soft 0CS3

Reposition — *continued*
- Pancreas 0FSG
- Parathyroid Gland 0GSR
  - Inferior
    - Left 0GSP
    - Right 0GSN
  - Multiple 0GSQ
  - Superior
    - Left 0GSM
    - Right 0GSL
- Patella
  - Left 0QSF
  - Right 0QSD
- Phalanx
  - Finger
    - Left 0PSV
    - Right 0PST
  - Thumb
    - Left 0PSS
    - Right 0PSR
  - Toe
    - Left 0QSR
    - Right 0QSQ
- Products of Conception 10S0
  - Ectopic 10S2
- Radius
  - Left 0PSJ
  - Right 0PSH
- Rectum 0DSP
- Retinal Vessel
  - Left 08SH3ZZ
  - Right 08SG3ZZ
- Ribs
  - 1 to 2 0PS1
  - 3 or More 0PS2
- Sacrum 0QS1
- Scapula
  - Left 0PS6
  - Right 0PS5
- Septum, Nasal 09SM
- Sesamoid Bone(s) 1st Toe
  - *see* Reposition, Metatarsal, Left 0QSP
  - *see* Reposition, Metatarsal, Right 0QSN
- Skull 0NS0
- Spinal Cord
  - Cervical 00SW
  - Lumbar 00SY
  - Thoracic 00SX
- Spleen 07SP0ZZ
- Sternum 0PS0
- Stomach 0DS6
- Tarsal
  - Left 0QSM
  - Right 0QSL
- Tendon
  - Abdomen
    - Left 0LSG
    - Right 0LSF
  - Ankle
    - Left 0LST
    - Right 0LSS
  - Foot
    - Left 0LSW
    - Right 0LSV
  - Hand
    - Left 0LS8
    - Right 0LS7
  - Head and Neck 0LS0
  - Hip
    - Left 0LSK
    - Right 0LSJ
  - Knee
    - Left 0LSR
    - Right 0LSQ
  - Lower Arm and Wrist
    - Left 0LS6
    - Right 0LS5
  - Lower Leg
    - Left 0LSP
    - Right 0LSN
  - Perineum 0LSH
  - Shoulder
    - Left 0LS2
    - Right 0LS1
  - Thorax
    - Left 0LSD
    - Right 0LSC
  - Trunk
    - Left 0LSB

Reposition — *continued*
- Tendon — *continued*
  - Trunk — *continued*
    - Right 0LS9
  - Upper Arm
    - Left 0LS4
    - Right 0LS3
  - Upper Leg
    - Left 0LSM
    - Right 0LSL
- Testis
  - Bilateral 0VSC
  - Left 0VSB
  - Right 0VS9
- Thymus 07SM0ZZ
- Thyroid Gland
  - Left Lobe 0GSG
  - Right Lobe 0GSH
- Tibia
  - Left 0QSH
  - Right 0QSG
- Tongue 0CS7
- Tooth
  - Lower 0CSX
  - Upper 0CSW
- Trachea 0BS10ZZ
- Turbinate, Nasal 09SL
- Tympanic Membrane
  - Left 09S8
  - Right 09S7
- Ulna
  - Left 0PSL
  - Right 0PSK
- Ureter
  - Left 0TS7
  - Right 0TS6
- Ureters, Bilateral 0TS8
- Urethra 0TSD
- Uterine Supporting Structure 0US4
- Uterus 0US9
- Uvula 0CSN
- Vagina 0USG
- Vein
  - Axillary
    - Left 05S8
    - Right 05S7
  - Azygos 05S0
  - Basilic
    - Left 05SC
    - Right 05SB
  - Brachial
    - Left 05SA
    - Right 05S9
  - Cephalic
    - Left 05SF
    - Right 05SD
  - Colic 06S7
  - Common Iliac
    - Left 06SD
    - Right 06SC
  - Esophageal 06S3
  - External Iliac
    - Left 06SG
    - Right 06SF
  - External Jugular
    - Left 05SQ
    - Right 05SP
  - Face
    - Left 05SV
    - Right 05ST
  - Femoral
    - Left 06SN
    - Right 06SM
  - Foot
    - Left 06SV
    - Right 06ST
  - Gastric 06S2
  - Hand
    - Left 05SH
    - Right 05SG
  - Hemiazygos 05S1
  - Hepatic 06S4
  - Hypogastric
    - Left 06SJ
    - Right 06SH
  - Inferior Mesenteric 06S6
  - Innominate
    - Left 05S4
    - Right 05S3

Reposition — *continued*
  Vein — *continued*
    Internal Jugular
      Left 05SN
      Right 05SM
    Intracranial 05SL
    Lower 06SY
    Portal 06S8
    Pulmonary
      Left 02ST0ZZ
      Right 02SS0ZZ
    Renal
      Left 06SB
      Right 06S9
    Saphenous
      Left 06SQ
      Right 06SP
    Splenic 06S1
    Subclavian
      Left 05S6
      Right 05S5
    Superior Mesenteric 06S5
    Upper 05SY
    Vertebral
      Left 05SS
      Right 05SR
  Vena Cava
    Inferior 06S0
    Superior 02SV0ZZ
  Vertebra
    Cervical 0PS3
      Magnetically Controlled Growth Rod(s) XNS3
    Lumbar 0QS0
      Magnetically Controlled Growth Rod(s) XNS0
      Posterior (Dynamic) Distraction Device XNS0
    Thoracic 0PS4
      Magnetically Controlled Growth Rod(s) XNS4
      Posterior (Dynamic) Distraction Device XNS4
  Vocal Cord
    Left 0CSV
    Right 0CST

Resection
  Acetabulum
    Left 0QT50ZZ
    Right 0QT40ZZ
  Adenoids 0CTQ
  Ampulla of Vater 0FTC
  Anal Sphincter 0DTR
  Anus 0DTQ
  Aortic Body 0GTD
  Appendix 0DTJ
  Auditory Ossicle
    Left 09TA
    Right 09T9
  Bladder 0TTB
  Bladder Neck 0TTC
  Bone
    Ethmoid
      Left 0NTG0ZZ
      Right 0NTF0ZZ
    Frontal 0NT10ZZ
    Hyoid 0NTX0ZZ
    Lacrimal
      Left 0NTJ0ZZ
      Right 0NTH0ZZ
    Nasal 0NTB0ZZ
    Occipital 0NT70ZZ
    Palatine
      Left 0NTL0ZZ
      Right 0NTK0ZZ
    Parietal
      Left 0NT40ZZ
      Right 0NT30ZZ
    Pelvic
      Left 0QT30ZZ
      Right 0QT20ZZ
    Sphenoid 0NTC0ZZ
    Temporal
      Left 0NT60ZZ
      Right 0NT50ZZ
    Zygomatic
      Left 0NTN0ZZ
      Right 0NTM0ZZ

Resection — *continued*
  Breast
    Bilateral 0HTV0ZZ
    Left 0HTU0ZZ
    Right 0HTT0ZZ
    Supernumerary 0HTY0ZZ
  Bronchus
    Lingula 0BT9
    Lower Lobe
      Left 0BTB
      Right 0BT6
    Main
      Left 0BT7
      Right 0BT3
    Middle Lobe, Right 0BT5
    Upper Lobe
      Left 0BT8
      Right 0BT4
  Bursa and Ligament
    Abdomen
      Left 0MTJ
      Right 0MTH
    Ankle
      Left 0MTR
      Right 0MTQ
    Elbow
      Left 0MT4
      Right 0MT3
    Foot
      Left 0MTT
      Right 0MTS
    Hand
      Left 0MT8
      Right 0MT7
    Head and Neck 0MT0
    Hip
      Left 0MTM
      Right 0MTL
    Knee
      Left 0MTP
      Right 0MTN
    Lower Extremity
      Left 0MTW
      Right 0MTV
    Perineum 0MTK
    Rib(s) 0MTG
    Shoulder
      Left 0MT2
      Right 0MT1
    Spine
      Lower 0MTD
      Upper 0MTC
    Sternum 0MTF
    Upper Extremity
      Left 0MTB
      Right 0MT9
    Wrist
      Left 0MT6
      Right 0MT5
  Carina 0BT2
  Carotid Bodies, Bilateral 0GT8
  Carotid Body
    Left 0GT6
    Right 0GT7
  Carpal
    Left 0PTN0ZZ
    Right 0PTM0ZZ
  Cecum 0DTH
  Cerebral Hemisphere 00T7
  Cervix 0UTC
  Chordae Tendineae 02T9
  Cisterna Chyli 07TL
  Clavicle
    Left 0PTB0ZZ
    Right 0PT90ZZ
  Clitoris 0UTJ
  Coccygeal Glomus 0GTB
  Coccyx 0QTS0ZZ
  Colon
    Ascending 0DTK
    Descending 0DTM
    Sigmoid 0DTN
    Transverse 0DTL
  Conduction Mechanism 02T8
  Cord
    Bilateral 0VTH
    Left 0VTG
    Right 0VTF

Resection — *continued*
  Cornea
    Left 08T9XZZ
    Right 08T8XZZ
  Cul-de-sac 0UTF
  Diaphragm 0BTT
  Disc
    Cervical Vertebral 0RT30ZZ
    Cervicothoracic Vertebral 0RT50ZZ
    Lumbar Vertebral 0ST20ZZ
    Lumbosacral 0ST40ZZ
    Thoracic Vertebral 0RT90ZZ
    Thoracolumbar Vertebral 0RTB0ZZ
  Duct
    Common Bile 0FT9
    Cystic 0FT8
    Hepatic
      Common 0FT7
      Left 0FT6
      Right 0FT5
    Lacrimal
      Left 08TY
      Right 08TX
    Pancreatic 0FTD
      Accessory 0FTF
    Parotid
      Left 0CTC0ZZ
      Right 0CTB0ZZ
  Duodenum 0DT9
  Ear
    External
      Left 09T1
      Right 09T0
    Inner
      Left 09TE
      Right 09TD
    Middle
      Left 09T6
      Right 09T5
  Epididymis
    Bilateral 0VTL
    Left 0VTK
    Right 0VTJ
  Epiglottis 0CTR
  Esophagogastric Junction 0DT4
  Esophagus 0DT5
    Lower 0DT3
    Middle 0DT2
    Upper 0DT1
  Eustachian Tube
    Left 09TG
    Right 09TF
  Eye
    Left 08T1XZZ
    Right 08T0XZZ
  Eyelid
    Lower
      Left 08TR
      Right 08TQ
    Upper
      Left 08TP
      Right 08TN
  Fallopian Tube
    Left 0UT6
    Right 0UT5
  Fallopian Tubes, Bilateral 0UT7
  Femoral Shaft
    Left 0QT90ZZ
    Right 0QT80ZZ
  Femur
    Lower
      Left 0QTC0ZZ
      Right 0QTB0ZZ
    Upper
      Left 0QT70ZZ
      Right 0QT60ZZ
  Fibula
    Left 0QTK0ZZ
    Right 0QTJ0ZZ
  Finger Nail 0HTQXZZ
  Gallbladder 0FT4
  Gland
    Adrenal
      Bilateral 0GT4
      Left 0GT2
      Right 0GT3
    Lacrimal
      Left 08TW
      Right 08TV

▽ **Subterms under main terms may continue to next column or page**

Resection — *continued*
  Gland — *continued*
    Minor Salivary ØCTJØZZ
    Parotid
      Left ØCT9ØZZ
      Right ØCT8ØZZ
    Pituitary ØGTØ
    Sublingual
      Left ØCTFØZZ
      Right ØCTDØZZ
    Submaxillary
      Left ØCTHØZZ
      Right ØCTGØZZ
    Vestibular ØUTL
  Glenoid Cavity
    Left ØPT8ØZZ
    Right ØPT7ØZZ
  Glomus Jugulare ØGTC
  Humeral Head
    Left ØPTDØZZ
    Right ØPTCØZZ
  Humeral Shaft
    Left ØPTGØZZ
    Right ØPTFØZZ
  Hymen ØUTK
  Ileocecal Valve ØDTC
  Ileum ØDTB
  Intestine
    Large ØDTE
      Left ØDTG
      Right ØDTF
    Small ØDT8
  Iris
    Left Ø8TD3ZZ
    Right Ø8TC3ZZ
  Jejunum ØDTA
  Joint
    Acromioclavicular
      Left ØRTHØZZ
      Right ØRTGØZZ
    Ankle
      Left ØSTGØZZ
      Right ØSTFØZZ
    Carpal
      Left ØRTRØZZ
      Right ØRTQØZZ
    Carpometacarpal
      Left ØRTTØZZ
      Right ØRTSØZZ
    Cervicothoracic Vertebral ØRT4ØZZ
    Coccygeal ØST6ØZZ
    Elbow
      Left ØRTMØZZ
      Right ØRTLØZZ
    Finger Phalangeal
      Left ØRTXØZZ
      Right ØRTWØZZ
    Hip
      Left ØSTBØZZ
      Right ØST9ØZZ
    Knee
      Left ØSTDØZZ
      Right ØSTCØZZ
    Metacarpophalangeal
      Left ØRTVØZZ
      Right ØRTUØZZ
    Metatarsal-Phalangeal
      Left ØSTNØZZ
      Right ØSTMØZZ
    Sacrococcygeal ØST5ØZZ
    Sacroiliac
      Left ØST8ØZZ
      Right ØST7ØZZ
    Shoulder
      Left ØRTKØZZ
      Right ØRTJØZZ
    Sternoclavicular
      Left ØRTFØZZ
      Right ØRTEØZZ
    Tarsal
      Left ØSTJØZZ
      Right ØSTHØZZ
    Tarsometatarsal
      Left ØSTLØZZ
      Right ØSTKØZZ
    Temporomandibular
      Left ØRTDØZZ
      Right ØRTCØZZ

Resection — *continued*
  Joint — *continued*
    Toe Phalangeal
      Left ØSTQØZZ
      Right ØSTPØZZ
    Wrist
      Left ØRTPØZZ
      Right ØRTNØZZ
  Kidney
    Left ØTT1
    Right ØTTØ
  Kidney Pelvis
    Left ØTT4
    Right ØTT3
  Kidneys, Bilateral ØTT2
  Larynx ØCTS
  Lens
    Left Ø8TK3ZZ
    Right Ø8TJ3ZZ
  Lip
    Lower ØCT1
    Upper ØCTØ
  Liver ØFTØ
    Left Lobe ØFT2
    Right Lobe ØFT1
  Lung
    Bilateral ØBTM
    Left ØBTL
    Lower Lobe
      Left ØBTJ
      Right ØBTF
    Middle Lobe, Right ØBTD
    Right ØBTK
    Upper Lobe
      Left ØBTG
      Right ØBTC
  Lung Lingula ØBTH
  Lymphatic
    Aortic Ø7TD
    Axillary
      Left Ø7T6
      Right Ø7T5
    Head Ø7TØ
    Inguinal
      Left Ø7TJ
      Right Ø7TH
    Internal Mammary
      Left Ø7T9
      Right Ø7T8
    Lower Extremity
      Left Ø7TG
      Right Ø7TF
    Mesenteric Ø7TB
    Neck
      Left Ø7T2
      Right Ø7T1
    Pelvis Ø7TC
    Thoracic Duct Ø7TK
    Thorax Ø7T7
    Upper Extremity
      Left Ø7T4
      Right Ø7T3
  Mandible
    Left ØNTVØZZ
    Right ØNTTØZZ
  Maxilla ØNTRØZZ
  Metacarpal
    Left ØPTQØZZ
    Right ØPTPØZZ
  Metatarsal
    Left ØQTPØZZ
    Right ØQTNØZZ
  Muscle
    Abdomen
      Left ØKTL
      Right ØKTK
    Extraocular
      Left Ø8TM
      Right Ø8TL
    Facial ØKT1
    Foot
      Left ØKTW
      Right ØKTV
    Hand
      Left ØKTD
      Right ØKTC
    Head ØKTØ
    Hip
      Left ØKTP

Resection — *continued*
  Muscle — *continued*
    Hip — *continued*
      Right ØKTN
    Lower Arm and Wrist
      Left ØKTB
      Right ØKT9
    Lower Leg
      Left ØKTT
      Right ØKTS
    Neck
      Left ØKT3
      Right ØKT2
    Papillary Ø2TD
    Perineum ØKTM
    Shoulder
      Left ØKT6
      Right ØKT5
    Thorax
      Left ØKTJ
      Right ØKTH
    Tongue, Palate, Pharynx ØKT4
    Trunk
      Left ØKTG
      Right ØKTF
    Upper Arm
      Left ØKT8
      Right ØKT7
    Upper Leg
      Left ØKTR
      Right ØKTQ
  Nasal Mucosa and Soft Tissue Ø9TK
  Nasopharynx Ø9TN
  Nipple
    Left ØHTXXZZ
    Right ØHTWXZZ
  Omentum ØDTU
  Orbit
    Left ØNTQØZZ
    Right ØNTPØZZ
  Ovary
    Bilateral ØUT2
    Left ØUT1
    Right ØUTØ
  Palate
    Hard ØCT2
    Soft ØCT3
  Pancreas ØFTG
  Para-aortic Body ØGT9
  Paraganglion Extremity ØGTF
  Parathyroid Gland ØGTR
    Inferior
      Left ØGTP
      Right ØGTN
    Multiple ØGTQ
    Superior
      Left ØGTM
      Right ØGTL
  Patella
    Left ØQTFØZZ
    Right ØQTDØZZ
  Penis ØVTS
  Pericardium Ø2TN
  Phalanx
    Finger
      Left ØPTVØZZ
      Right ØPTTØZZ
    Thumb
      Left ØPTSØZZ
      Right ØPTRØZZ
    Toe
      Left ØQTRØZZ
      Right ØQTQØZZ
  Pharynx ØCTM
  Pineal Body ØGT1
  Prepuce ØVTT
  Products of Conception, Ectopic 1ØT2
  Prostate ØVTØ
  Radius
    Left ØPTJØZZ
    Right ØPTHØZZ
  Rectum ØDTP
  Ribs
    1 to 2 ØPT1ØZZ
    3 or More ØPT2ØZZ
  Scapula
    Left ØPT6ØZZ
    Right ØPT5ØZZ
  Scrotum ØVT5

Resection — *continued*
- Septum
  - Atrial 02T5
  - Nasal 09TM
  - Ventricular 02TM
- Sinus
  - Accessory 09TP
  - Ethmoid
    - Left 09TV
    - Right 09TU
  - Frontal
    - Left 09TT
    - Right 09TS
  - Mastoid
    - Left 09TC
    - Right 09TB
  - Maxillary
    - Left 09TR
    - Right 09TQ
  - Sphenoid
    - Left 09TX
    - Right 09TW
- Spleen 07TP
- Sternum 0PT00ZZ
- Stomach 0DT6
  - Pylorus 0DT7
- Tarsal
  - Left 0QTM0ZZ
  - Right 0QTL0ZZ
- Tendon
  - Abdomen
    - Left 0LTG
    - Right 0LTF
  - Ankle
    - Left 0LTT
    - Right 0LTS
  - Foot
    - Left 0LTW
    - Right 0LTV
  - Hand
    - Left 0LT8
    - Right 0LT7
  - Head and Neck 0LT0
  - Hip
    - Left 0LTK
    - Right 0LTJ
  - Knee
    - Left 0LTR
    - Right 0LTQ
  - Lower Arm and Wrist
    - Left 0LT6
    - Right 0LT5
  - Lower Leg
    - Left 0LTP
    - Right 0LTN
  - Perineum 0LTH
  - Shoulder
    - Left 0LT2
    - Right 0LT1
  - Thorax
    - Left 0LTD
    - Right 0LTC
  - Trunk
    - Left 0LTB
    - Right 0LT9
  - Upper Arm
    - Left 0LT4
    - Right 0LT3
  - Upper Leg
    - Left 0LTM
    - Right 0LTL
- Testis
  - Bilateral 0VTC
  - Left 0VTB
  - Right 0VT9
- Thymus 07TM
- Thyroid Gland 0GTK
  - Left Lobe 0GTG
  - Right Lobe 0GTH
- Thyroid Gland Isthmus 0GTJ
- Tibia
  - Left 0QTH0ZZ
  - Right 0QTG0ZZ
- Toe Nail 0HTRXZZ
- Tongue 0CT7
- Tonsils 0CTP
- Tooth
  - Lower 0CTX0Z
  - Upper 0CTW0Z

Resection — *continued*
- Trachea 0BT1
- Tunica Vaginalis
  - Left 0VT7
  - Right 0VT6
- Turbinate, Nasal 09TL
- Tympanic Membrane
  - Left 09T8
  - Right 09T7
- Ulna
  - Left 0PTL0ZZ
  - Right 0PTK0ZZ
- Ureter
  - Left 0TT7
  - Right 0TT6
- Urethra 0TTD
- Uterine Supporting Structure 0UT4
- Uterus 0UT9
- Uvula 0CTN
- Vagina 0UTG
- Valve, Pulmonary 02TH
- Vas Deferens
  - Bilateral 0VTQ
  - Left 0VTP
  - Right 0VTN
- Vesicle
  - Bilateral 0VT3
  - Left 0VT2
  - Right 0VT1
- Vitreous
  - Left 08T53ZZ
  - Right 08T43ZZ
- Vocal Cord
  - Left 0CTV
  - Right 0CTT
- Vulva 0UTM

Resection, Left ventricular outflow tract obstruction (LVOT) *see* Dilation, Ventricle, Left 027L

Resection, Subaortic membrane (Left ventricular outflow tract obstruction) *see* Dilation, Ventricle, Left 027L

restor3d TIDAL™ Fusion Cage *use* Internal Fixation Device, Gyroid-Sheet Lattice Design in New Technology

Restoration, Cardiac, Single, Rhythm 5A2204Z

RestoreAdvanced neurostimulator (SureScan) (MRI Safe) *use* Stimulator Generator, Multiple Array Rechargeable in 0JH

RestoreSensor neurostimulator (SureScan) (MRI Safe) *use* Stimulator Generator, Multiple Array Rechargeable in 0JH

RestoreUltra neurostimulator (SureScan) (MRI Safe) *use* Stimulator Generator, Multiple Array Rechargeable in 0JH

Restriction
- Ampulla of Vater 0FVC
- Anus 0DVQ
- Aorta
  - Abdominal 04V0
    - Intraluminal Device, Branched or Fenestrated 04V0
  - Thoracic
    - Ascending/Arch, Intraluminal Device, Branched or Fenestrated 02VX
    - Descending, Intraluminal Device, Branched or Fenestrated 02VW
- Artery
  - Anterior Tibial
    - Left 04VQ
    - Right 04VP
  - Axillary
    - Left 03V6
    - Right 03V5
  - Brachial
    - Left 03V8
    - Right 03V7
  - Celiac 04V1
  - Colic
    - Left 04V7
    - Middle 04V8
    - Right 04V6
  - Common Carotid
    - Left 03VJ
    - Right 03VH
  - Common Iliac
    - Left 04VD
    - Right 04VC

Restriction — *continued*
- Artery — *continued*
  - External Carotid
    - Left 03VN
    - Right 03VM
  - External Iliac
    - Left 04VJ
    - Right 04VH
  - Face 03VR
  - Femoral
    - Left 04VL
    - Right 04VK
  - Foot
    - Left 04VW
    - Right 04VV
  - Gastric 04V2
  - Hand
    - Left 03VF
    - Right 03VD
  - Hepatic 04V3
  - Inferior Mesenteric 04VB
  - Innominate 03V2
  - Internal Carotid
    - Left 03VL
    - Right 03VK
  - Internal Iliac
    - Left 04VF
    - Right 04VE
  - Internal Mammary
    - Left 03V1
    - Right 03V0
  - Intracranial 03VG
  - Lower 04VY
  - Peroneal
    - Left 04VU
    - Right 04VT
  - Popliteal
    - Left 04VN
    - Right 04VM
  - Posterior Tibial
    - Left 04VS
    - Right 04VR
  - Pulmonary
    - Left 02VR
    - Right 02VQ
  - Pulmonary Trunk 02VP
  - Radial
    - Left 03VC
    - Right 03VB
  - Renal
    - Left 04VA
    - Right 04V9
  - Splenic 04V4
  - Subclavian
    - Left 03V4
    - Right 03V3
  - Superior Mesenteric 04V5
  - Temporal
    - Left 03VT
    - Right 03VS
  - Thyroid
    - Left 03VV
    - Right 03VU
  - Ulnar
    - Left 03VA
    - Right 03V9
  - Upper 03VY
  - Vertebral
    - Left 03VQ
    - Right 03VP
- Bladder 0TVB
- Bladder Neck 0TVC
- Bronchus
  - Lingula 0BV9
  - Lower Lobe
    - Left 0BVB
    - Right 0BV6
  - Main
    - Left 0BV7
    - Right 0BV3
  - Middle Lobe, Right 0BV5
  - Upper Lobe
    - Left 0BV8
    - Right 0BV4
- Carina 0BV2
- Cecum 0DVH
- Cervix 0UVC
- Cisterna Chyli 07VL

Restriction — continued
  Colon
    Ascending 0DVK
    Descending 0DVM
    Sigmoid 0DVN
    Transverse 0DVL
  Duct
    Common Bile 0FV9
    Cystic 0FV8
    Hepatic
      Common 0FV7
      Left 0FV6
      Right 0FV5
    Lacrimal
      Left 08VY
      Right 08VX
    Pancreatic 0FVD
      Accessory 0FVF
    Parotid
      Left 0CVC
      Right 0CVB
  Duodenum 0DV9
  Esophagogastric Junction 0DV4
  Esophagus 0DV5
    Lower 0DV3
    Middle 0DV2
    Upper 0DV1
  Heart 02VA
  Ileocecal Valve 0DVC
  Ileum 0DVB
  Intestine
    Large 0DVE
      Left 0DVG
      Right 0DVF
    Small 0DV8
  Jejunum 0DVA
  Kidney Pelvis
    Left 0TV4
    Right 0TV3
  Lymphatic
    Aortic 07VD
    Axillary
      Left 07V6
      Right 07V5
    Head 07V0
    Inguinal
      Left 07VJ
      Right 07VH
    Internal Mammary
      Left 07V9
      Right 07V8
    Lower Extremity
      Left 07VG
      Right 07VF
    Mesenteric 07VB
    Neck
      Left 07V2
      Right 07V1
    Pelvis 07VC
    Thoracic Duct 07VK
    Thorax 07V7
    Upper Extremity
      Left 07V4
      Right 07V3
  Rectum 0DVP
  Stomach 0DV6
    Pylorus 0DV7
  Trachea 0BV1
  Ureter
    Left 0TV7
    Right 0TV6
  Urethra 0TVD
  Valve, Mitral 02VG
  Vein
    Axillary
      Left 05V8
      Right 05V7
    Azygos 05V0
    Basilic
      Left 05VC
      Right 05VB
    Brachial
      Left 05VA
      Right 05V9
    Cephalic
      Left 05VF
      Right 05VD
    Colic 06V7

Restriction — continued
  Vein — continued
    Common Iliac
      Left 06VD
      Right 06VC
    Esophageal 06V3
    External Iliac
      Left 06VG
      Right 06VF
    External Jugular
      Left 05VQ
      Right 05VP
    Face
      Left 05VV
      Right 05VT
    Femoral
      Left 06VN
      Right 06VM
    Foot
      Left 06VV
      Right 06VT
    Gastric 06V2
    Hand
      Left 05VH
      Right 05VG
    Hemiazygos 05V1
    Hepatic 06V4
    Hypogastric
      Left 06VJ
      Right 06VH
    Inferior Mesenteric 06V6
    Innominate
      Left 05V4
      Right 05V3
    Internal Jugular
      Left 05VN
      Right 05VM
    Intracranial 05VL
    Lower 06VY
    Portal 06V8
    Pulmonary
      Left 02VT
      Right 02VS
    Renal
      Left 06VB
      Right 06V9
    Saphenous
      Left 06VQ
      Right 06VP
    Splenic 06V1
    Subclavian
      Left 05V6
      Right 05V5
    Superior Mesenteric 06V5
    Upper 05VY
    Vertebral
      Left 05VS
      Right 05VR
    Vena Cava
      Inferior 06V0
      Superior 02VV
  Ventricle, Left 02VL
Resurfacing Device
  Removal of device from
    Left 0SPB0BZ
    Right 0SP90BZ
  Revision of device in
    Left 0SWB0BZ
    Right 0SW90BZ
  Supplement
    Left 0SUB0BZ
      Acetabular Surface 0SUE0BZ
      Femoral Surface 0SUS0BZ
    Right 0SU90BZ
      Acetabular Surface 0SUA0BZ
      Femoral Surface 0SUR0BZ
Resuscitation
  Cardiopulmonary see Assistance, Cardiac 5A02
  Cardioversion 5A2204Z
  Defibrillation 5A2204Z
  Endotracheal intubation see Insertion of device in, Trachea 0BH1
  External chest compression, manual 5A12012
  External chest compression, mechanical 5A1221J
  Pulmonary 5A19054

Resuscitative endovascular balloon occlusion of the aorta (REBOA)
  02LW3DJ
  04L03DJ
Resuscitative thoracotomy
  see Control bleeding in, Mediastinum 0W3C
  see Control bleeding in, Pericardial Cavity 0W3D
Resuture, Heart valve prosthesis see Revision of device in, Heart and Great Vessels 02W
Retained placenta, manual removal see Extraction, Products of Conception, Retained 10D1
RETHYMIC® use Engineered Allogeneic Thymus Tissue
Retraining
  Cardiac see Motor Treatment, Rehabilitation F07
  Vocational see Activities of Daily Living Treatment, Rehabilitation F08
Retrogasserian rhizotomy see Division, Nerve, Trigeminal 008K
Retroperitoneal cavity use Retroperitoneum
Retroperitoneal lymph node use Lymphatic, Aortic
Retroperitoneal space use Retroperitoneum
Retropharyngeal lymph node
  use Lymphatic, Left Neck
  use Lymphatic, Right Neck
Retropharyngeal space use Neck
Retropubic space use Pelvic Cavity
Reveal (LINQ) (DX) (XT) use Monitoring Device
Reverse total shoulder replacement see Replacement, Upper Joints 0RR
Reverse® Shoulder Prosthesis use Synthetic Substitute, Reverse Ball and Socket in 0RR
Revision
  Correcting a portion of existing device see Revision of device in
  Removal of device without replacement see Removal of device from
  Replacement of existing device
    see Removal of device from
    see Root operation to place new device, e.g., Insertion, Replacement, Supplement
Revision of device in
  Abdominal Wall 0WWF
  Acetabulum
    Left 0QW5
    Right 0QW4
  Anal Sphincter 0DWR
  Anus 0DWQ
  Aorta, Thoracic, Descending 02WW3RZ
  Artery
    Lower 04WY
    Upper 03WY
  Auditory Ossicle
    Left 09WA
    Right 09W9
  Back
    Lower 0WWL
    Upper 0WWK
  Bladder 0TWB
  Bone
    Facial 0NWW
    Lower 0QWY
    Nasal 0NWB
    Pelvic
      Left 0QW3
      Right 0QW2
    Upper 0PWY
  Bone Marrow 07WT
  Brain 00W0
  Breast
    Left 0HWU
    Right 0HWT
  Bursa and Ligament
    Lower 0MWY
    Upper 0MWX
  Carpal
    Left 0PWN
    Right 0PWM
  Cavity, Cranial 0WW1
  Cerebral Ventricle 00W6
  Chest Wall 0WW8
  Cisterna Chyli 07WL
  Clavicle
    Left 0PWB
    Right 0PW9
  Coccyx 0QWS
  Diaphragm 0BWT
  Disc
    Cervical Vertebral 0RW3

Revision of device in — *continued*
  Disc — *continued*
    Cervicothoracic Vertebral ØRW5
    Lumbar Vertebral ØSW2
    Lumbosacral ØSW4
    Thoracic Vertebral ØRW9
    Thoracolumbar Vertebral ØRWB
  Duct
    Hepatobiliary ØFWB
    Pancreatic ØFWD
  Ear
    Inner
      Left Ø9WE
      Right Ø9WD
    Left Ø9WJ
    Right Ø9WH
  Epididymis and Spermatic Cord ØVWM
  Esophagus ØDW5
  Extremity
    Lower
      Left ØYWB
      Right ØYW9
    Upper
      Left ØXW7
      Right ØXW6
  Eye
    Left Ø8W1
    Right Ø8WØ
  Face ØWW2
  Fallopian Tube ØUW8
  Femoral Shaft
    Left ØQW9
    Right ØQW8
  Femur
    Lower
      Left ØQWC
      Right ØQWB
    Upper
      Left ØQW7
      Right ØQW6
  Fibula
    Left ØQWK
    Right ØQWJ
  Finger Nail ØHWQX
  Gallbladder ØFW4
  Gastrointestinal Tract ØWWP
  Genitourinary Tract ØWWR
  Gland
    Adrenal ØGW5
    Endocrine ØGWS
    Pituitary ØGWØ
    Salivary ØCWA
  Glenoid Cavity
    Left ØPW8
    Right ØPW7
  Great Vessel Ø2WY
  Hair ØHWSX
  Head ØWWØ
  Heart Ø2WA
  Humeral Head
    Left ØPWD
    Right ØPWC
  Humeral Shaft
    Left ØPWG
    Right ØPWF
  Intestinal Tract
    Lower Intestinal Tract ØDWD
    Upper Intestinal Tract ØDWØ
  Intestine
    Large ØDWE
    Small ØDW8
  Jaw
    Lower ØWW5
    Upper ØWW4
  Joint
    Acromioclavicular
      Left ØRWH
      Right ØRWG
    Ankle
      Left ØSWG
      Right ØSWF
    Carpal
      Left ØRWR
      Right ØRWQ
    Carpometacarpal
      Left ØRWT
      Right ØRWS
    Cervical Vertebral ØRW1
    Cervicothoracic Vertebral ØRW4

Revision of device in — *continued*
  Joint — *continued*
    Coccygeal ØSW6
    Elbow
      Left ØRWM
      Right ØRWL
    Finger Phalangeal
      Left ØRWX
      Right ØRWW
    Hip
      Left ØSWB
        Acetabular Surface ØSWE
        Femoral Surface ØSWS
      Right ØSW9
        Acetabular Surface ØSWA
        Femoral Surface ØSWR
    Knee
      Left ØSWD
        Femoral Surface ØSWU
        Tibial Surface ØSWW
      Right ØSWC
        Femoral Surface ØSWT
        Tibial Surface ØSWV
    Lumbar Vertebral ØSWØ
    Lumbosacral ØSW3
    Metacarpophalangeal
      Left ØRWV
      Right ØRWU
    Metatarsal-Phalangeal
      Left ØSWN
      Right ØSWM
    Occipital-cervical ØRWØ
    Sacrococcygeal ØSW5
    Sacroiliac
      Left ØSW8
      Right ØSW7
    Shoulder
      Left ØRWK
      Right ØRWJ
    Sternoclavicular
      Left ØRWF
      Right ØRWE
    Tarsal
      Left ØSWJ
      Right ØSWH
    Tarsometatarsal
      Left ØSWL
      Right ØSWK
    Temporomandibular
      Left ØRWD
      Right ØRWC
    Thoracic Vertebral ØRW6
    Thoracolumbar Vertebral ØRWA
    Toe Phalangeal
      Left ØSWQ
      Right ØSWP
    Wrist
      Left ØRWP
      Right ØRWN
  Kidney ØTW5
  Larynx ØCWS
  Lens
    Left Ø8WK
    Right Ø8WJ
  Liver ØFWØ
  Lung
    Left ØBWL
    Right ØBWK
  Lymphatic Ø7WN
    Thoracic Duct Ø7WK
  Mediastinum ØWWC
  Mesentery ØDWV
  Metacarpal
    Left ØPWQ
    Right ØPWP
  Metatarsal
    Left ØQWP
    Right ØQWN
  Mouth and Throat ØCWY
  Muscle
    Extraocular
      Left Ø8WM
      Right Ø8WL
    Lower ØKWY
    Upper ØKWX
  Nasal Mucosa and Soft Tissue Ø9WK
  Neck ØWW6
  Nerve
    Cranial ØØWE

Revision of device in — *continued*
  Nerve — *continued*
    Peripheral Ø1WY
  Omentum ØDWU
  Ovary ØUW3
  Pancreas ØFWG
  Parathyroid Gland ØGWR
  Patella
    Left ØQWF
    Right ØQWD
  Pelvic Cavity ØWWJ
  Penis ØVWS
  Pericardial Cavity ØWWD
  Perineum
    Female ØWWN
    Male ØWWM
  Peritoneal Cavity ØWWG
  Peritoneum ØDWW
  Phalanx
    Finger
      Left ØPWV
      Right ØPWT
    Thumb
      Left ØPWS
      Right ØPWR
    Toe
      Left ØQWR
      Right ØQWQ
  Pineal Body ØGW1
  Pleura ØBWQ
  Pleural Cavity
    Left ØWWB
    Right ØWW9
  Prostate and Seminal Vesicles ØVW4
  Radius
    Left ØPWJ
    Right ØPWH
  Respiratory Tract ØWWQ
  Retroperitoneum ØWWH
  Ribs
    1 to 2 ØPW1
    3 or More ØPW2
  Sacrum ØQW1
  Scapula
    Left ØPW6
    Right ØPW5
  Scrotum and Tunica Vaginalis ØVW8
  Septum
    Atrial Ø2W5
    Ventricular Ø2WM
  Sinus Ø9WY
  Skin ØHWPX
  Skull ØNWØ
  Spinal Canal ØØWU
  Spinal Cord ØØWV
  Spleen Ø7WP
  Sternum ØPWØ
  Stomach ØDW6
  Subcutaneous Tissue and Fascia
    Head and Neck ØJWS
    Lower Extremity ØJWW
    Trunk ØJWT
    Upper Extremity ØJWV
  Tarsal
    Left ØQWM
    Right ØQWL
  Tendon
    Lower ØLWY
    Upper ØLWX
  Testis ØVWD
  Thymus Ø7WM
  Thyroid Gland ØGWK
  Tibia
    Left ØQWH
    Right ØQWG
  Toe Nail ØHWRX
  Trachea ØBW1
  Tracheobronchial Tree ØBWØ
  Tympanic Membrane
    Left Ø9W8
    Right Ø9W7
  Ulna
    Left ØPWL
    Right ØPWK
  Ureter ØTW9
  Urethra ØTWD
  Uterus and Cervix ØUWD
  Vagina and Cul-de-sac ØUWH

Revision of device in — *continued*
- Valve
  - Aortic 02WF
  - Mitral 02WG
  - Pulmonary 02WH
  - Tricuspid 02WJ
- Vas Deferens 0VWR
- Vein
  - Azygos 05W0
  - Innominate
    - Left 05W4
    - Right 05W3
  - Lower 06WY
  - Upper 05WY
- Vertebra
  - Cervical 0PW3
  - Lumbar 0QW0
  - Thoracic 0PW4
- Vulva 0UWM

Revo MRI™ SureScan® pacemaker *use* Pacemaker, Dual Chamber in 0JH
Rezafungin XW0
rhBMP-2 *use* Recombinant Bone Morphogenetic Protein
Rheos® System device *use* Stimulator Generator in Subcutaneous Tissue and Fascia
Rheos® System lead *use* Stimulator Lead in Upper Arteries
Rhinopharynx *use* Nasopharynx
Rhinoplasty
  see Alteration, Nasal Mucosa and Soft Tissue 090K
  see Repair, Nasal Mucosa and Soft Tissue 09QK
  see Replacement, Nasal Mucosa and Soft Tissue 09RK
  see Supplement, Nasal Mucosa and Soft Tissue 09UK
Rhinorrhaphy *see* Repair, Nasal Mucosa and Soft Tissue 09QK
Rhinoscopy 09JKXZZ
Rhizotomy
  see Division, Central Nervous System and Cranial Nerves 008
  see Division, Peripheral Nervous System 018
Rhomboid major muscle
  use Trunk Muscle, Left
  use Trunk Muscle, Right
Rhomboid minor muscle
  use Trunk Muscle, Left
  use Trunk Muscle, Right
Rhythm electrocardiogram *see* Measurement, Cardiac 4A02
Rhytidectomy *see* Alteration, Face 0W02
Right ascending lumbar vein *use* Azygos Vein
Right atrioventricular valve *use* Tricuspid Valve
Right auricular appendix *use* Atrium, Right
Right colic vein *use* Colic Vein
Right coronary sulcus *use* Heart, Right
Right gastric artery *use* Gastric Artery
Right gastroepiploic vein *use* Superior Mesenteric Vein
Right inferior phrenic vein *use* Inferior Vena Cava
Right inferior pulmonary vein *use* Pulmonary Vein, Right
Right jugular trunk *use* Lymphatic, Right Neck
Right lateral ventricle *use* Cerebral Ventricle
Right lymphatic duct *use* Lymphatic, Right Neck
Right ovarian vein *use* Inferior Vena Cava
Right second lumbar vein *use* Inferior Vena Cava
Right subclavian trunk *use* Lymphatic, Right Neck
Right subcostal vein *use* Azygos Vein
Right superior pulmonary vein *use* Pulmonary Vein, Right
Right suprarenal vein *use* Inferior Vena Cava
Right testicular vein *use* Inferior Vena Cava
Rima glottidis *use* Larynx
Risorius muscle *use* Facial Muscle
RNS System lead *use* Neurostimulator Lead in Central Nervous System and Cranial Nerves
RNS system neurostimulator generator *use* Neurostimulator Generator in Head and Facial Bones
Robotic Assisted Procedure
- Extremity
  - Lower 8E0Y
  - Upper 8E0X
- Head and Neck Region 8E09
- Trunk Region 8E0W

Rotation of fetal head
  Forceps 10S07ZZ
  Manual 10S0XZZ
Round ligament of uterus *use* Uterine Supporting Structure
Round window
  use Inner Ear, Left
  use Inner Ear, Right
Roux-en-Y operation
  see Bypass, Gastrointestinal System 0D1
  see Bypass, Hepatobiliary System and Pancreas 0F1
RP-L201 *use* Marnetegragene Autotemcel
Rupture
  Adhesions *see* Release
  Fluid collection *see* Drainage
Ruxolitinib *use* Other Substance
RYBREVANT™ *use* Amivantamab Monoclonal Antibody

S

Sabizabulin XW0
Sacral ganglion *use* Sacral Sympathetic Nerve
Sacral lymph node *use* Lymphatic, Pelvis
Sacral nerve modulation (SNM) lead *use* Stimulator Lead in Urinary System
Sacral neuromodulation lead *use* Stimulator Lead in Urinary System
Sacral splanchnic nerve *use* Sacral Sympathetic Nerve
Sacrectomy *see* Excision, Lower Bones 0QB
Sacrococcygeal ligament *use* Lower Spine Bursa and Ligament
Sacrococcygeal symphysis *use* Sacrococcygeal Joint
Sacroiliac ligament *use* Lower Spine Bursa and Ligament
Sacrospinous ligament *use* Lower Spine Bursa and Ligament
Sacrotuberous ligament *use* Lower Spine Bursa and Ligament
Salpingectomy
  see Excision, Female Reproductive System 0UB
  see Resection, Female Reproductive System 0UT
Salpingolysis *see* Release, Female Reproductive System 0UN
Salpingopexy
  see Repair, Female Reproductive System 0UQ
  see Reposition, Female Reproductive System 0US
Salpingopharyngeus muscle *use* Tongue, Palate, Pharynx Muscle
Salpingoplasty
  see Repair, Female Reproductive System 0UQ
  see Supplement, Female Reproductive System 0UU
Salpingorrhaphy *see* Repair, Female Reproductive System 0UQ
Salpingoscopy 0UJ88ZZ
Salpingostomy *see* Drainage, Female Reproductive System 0U9
Salpingotomy *see* Drainage, Female Reproductive System 0U9
Salpinx
  use Fallopian Tube, Left
  use Fallopian Tube, Right
Saphenous nerve *use* Femoral Nerve
SAPIEN transcatheter aortic valve *use* Zooplastic Tissue in Heart and Great Vessels
Sarilumab XW0
SARS-CoV-2 Antibody Detection, Serum/Plasma Nanoparticle Fluorescence XXE5XV7
SARS-CoV-2 Polymerase Chain Reaction, Nasopharyngeal Fluid XXE97U7
Sartorius muscle
  use Upper Leg Muscle, Left
  use Upper Leg Muscle, Right
Satralizumab-mwge XW01397
SAVAL below-the-knee (BTK) drug-eluting stent system
  use Intraluminal Device, Drug-eluting in Lower Arteries
  use Intraluminal Device, Drug-eluting, Two in Lower Arteries
  use Intraluminal Device, Drug-eluting, Three in Lower Arteries
  use Intraluminal Device, Drug-eluting, Four or More in Lower Arteries
Scalene muscle
  use Neck Muscle, Left

Scalene muscle — *continued*
  use Neck Muscle, Right
Scan
  Computerized Tomography (CT) *see* Computerized Tomography (CT Scan)
  Radioisotope *see* Planar Nuclear Medicine Imaging
Scaphoid bone
  use Carpal, Left
  use Carpal, Right
Scapholunate ligament
  use Wrist Bursa and Ligament, Left
  use Wrist Bursa and Ligament, Right
Scaphotrapezium ligament
  use Hand Bursa and Ligament, Left
  use Hand Bursa and Ligament, Right
Scapulectomy
  see Excision, Upper Bones 0PB
  see Resection, Upper Bones 0PT
Scapulopexy
  see Repair, Upper Bones 0PQ
  see Reposition, Upper Bones 0PS
Scarpa's (vestibular) ganglion *use* Acoustic Nerve
Sclerectomy *see* Excision, Eye 08B
Sclerotherapy, mechanical *see* Destruction
Sclerotherapy, via injection of sclerosing agent
  see Introduction, Destructive Agent
Sclerotomy *see* Drainage, Eye 089
Scrotectomy
  see Excision, Male Reproductive System 0VB
  see Resection, Male Reproductive System 0VT
Scrotoplasty
  see Repair, Male Reproductive System 0VQ
  see Supplement, Male Reproductive System 0VU
Scrotorrhaphy *see* Repair, Male Reproductive System 0VQ
Scrototomy *see* Drainage, Male Reproductive System 0V9
Sebaceous gland *use* Skin
Second cranial nerve *use* Optic Nerve
Section, cesarean *see* Extraction, Pregnancy 10D
Secura (DR) (VR) *use* Defibrillator Generator in 0JH
sEEG radiofrequency ablation (RFA) 00503Z4
Sella turcica *use* Sphenoid Bone
Selux Rapid AST Platform XXE5XY9
Semicircular canal
  use Inner Ear, Left
  use Inner Ear, Right
Semimembranosus muscle
  use Upper Leg Muscle, Left
  use Upper Leg Muscle, Right
Semitendinosus muscle
  use Upper Leg Muscle, Left
  use Upper Leg Muscle, Right
Sentinel™ Cerebral Protection System (CPS) X2A5312
Seprafilm *use* Adhesion Barrier
Septal cartilage *use* Nasal Septum
Septectomy
  see Excision, Ear, Nose, Sinus 09B
  see Excision, Heart and Great Vessels 02B
  see Resection, Ear, Nose, Sinus 09T
  see Resection, Heart and Great Vessels 02T
SeptiCyte® RAPID XXE5X38
Septoplasty
  see Repair, Ear, Nose, Sinus 09Q
  see Repair, Heart and Great Vessels 02Q
  see Replacement, Ear, Nose, Sinus 09R
  see Replacement, Heart and Great Vessels 02R
  see Reposition, Ear, Nose, Sinus 09S
  see Supplement, Ear, Nose, Sinus 09U
  see Supplement, Heart and Great Vessels 02U
Septostomy, balloon atrial 02163Z7
Septotomy *see* Drainage, Ear, Nose, Sinus 099
Sequestrectomy, bone *see* Extirpation
SER-109 XW0DXN9
Seraph® 100 Microbind® Affinity Blood Filter XXA536A
Serratus anterior muscle
  use Thorax Muscle, Left
  use Thorax Muscle, Right
Serratus posterior muscle
  use Trunk Muscle, Left
  use Trunk Muscle, Right
Seventh cranial nerve *use* Facial Nerve
Shapshot_NIR 8E02XDZ

Sheffield hybrid external fixator
 use External Fixation Device, Hybrid in 0PH
 use External Fixation Device, Hybrid in 0PS
 use External Fixation Device, Hybrid in 0QH
 use External Fixation Device, Hybrid in 0QS
Sheffield ring external fixator
 use External Fixation Device, Ring in 0PH
 use External Fixation Device, Ring in 0PS
 use External Fixation Device, Ring in 0QH
 use External Fixation Device, Ring in 0QS
Shirodkar cervical cerclage 0UVC7ZZ
Shock Wave Therapy, Musculoskeletal 6A93
Shockwave Intravascular Lithotripsy (Shockwave IVL) see Fragmentation
Short gastric artery use Splenic Artery
ShortCut™, used during transcatheter aortic valve replacement (TAVR) procedure X28F3VA
Shortening
 see Excision
 see Repair
 see Reposition
Shunt creation see Bypass
Sialoadenectomy
 Complete see Resection, Mouth and Throat 0CT
 Partial see Excision, Mouth and Throat 0CB
Sialodochoplasty
 see Repair, Mouth and Throat 0CQ
 see Replacement, Mouth and Throat 0CR
 see Supplement, Mouth and Throat 0CU
Sialoectomy
 see Excision, Mouth and Throat 0CB
 see Resection, Mouth and Throat 0CT
Sialography see Plain Radiography, Ear, Nose, Mouth and Throat B90
Sialolithotomy see Extirpation, Mouth and Throat 0CC
S-ICD™ lead use Subcutaneous Defibrillator Lead in Subcutaneous Tissue and Fascia
Sigmoid artery use Inferior Mesenteric Artery
Sigmoid flexure use Sigmoid Colon
Sigmoid vein use Inferior Mesenteric Vein
Sigmoidectomy
 see Excision, Gastrointestinal System 0DB
 see Resection, Gastrointestinal System 0DT
Sigmoidorrhaphy see Repair, Gastrointestinal System 0DQ
Sigmoidoscopy 0DJD8ZZ
Sigmoidotomy see Drainage, Gastrointestinal System 0D9
Single lead pacemaker (atrium) (ventricle) use Pacemaker, Single Chamber in 0JH
Single lead rate responsive pacemaker (atrium) (ventricle) use Pacemaker, Single Chamber Rate Responsive in 0JH
Single-use Duodenoscope XFJ
Single-use Oversleeve with Intraoperative Colonic Irrigation XDPH8K7
Sinoatrial node use Conduction Mechanism
Sinogram
 Abdominal Wall see Fluoroscopy, Abdomen and Pelvis BW11
 Chest Wall see Plain Radiography, Chest BW03
 Retroperitoneum see Fluoroscopy, Abdomen and Pelvis BW11
Sinus venosus use Atrium, Right
Sinusectomy
 see Excision, Ear, Nose, Sinus 09B
 see Resection, Ear, Nose, Sinus 09T
Sinusoscopy 09JY4ZZ
Sinusotomy see Drainage, Ear, Nose, Sinus 099
Sirolimus-eluting coronary stent use Intraluminal Device, Drug-eluting in Heart and Great Vessels
Sixth cranial nerve use Abducens Nerve
Size reduction, breast see Excision, Skin and Breast 0HB
SJM Biocor® Stented Valve System use Zooplastic Tissue in Heart and Great Vessels
Skene's (paraurethral) gland use Vestibular Gland
Sling
 Fascial, orbicularis muscle (mouth) see Supplement, Muscle, Facial 0KU1
 Levator muscle, for urethral suspension see Reposition, Bladder Neck 0TSC
 Pubococcygeal, for urethral suspension see Reposition, Bladder Neck 0TSC
 Rectum see Reposition, Rectum 0DSP
Small bowel series see Fluoroscopy, Bowel, Small BD13

Small saphenous vein
 use Saphenous Vein, Left
 use Saphenous Vein, Right
Snapshot_NIR 8E02XDZ
Snaring, polyp, colon see Excision, Gastrointestinal System 0DB
Solar (celiac) plexus use Abdominal Sympathetic Nerve
Soleus muscle
 use Lower Leg Muscle, Left
 use Lower Leg Muscle, Right
Soliris® use Eculizumab
Space of Retzius use Pelvic Cavity
Spacer
 Insertion of device in
  Disc
   Lumbar Vertebral 0SH2
   Lumbosacral 0SH4
  Joint
   Acromioclavicular
    Left 0RHH
    Right 0RHG
   Ankle
    Left 0SHG
    Right 0SHF
   Carpal
    Left 0RHR
    Right 0RHQ
   Carpometacarpal
    Left 0RHT
    Right 0RHS
   Cervical Vertebral 0RH1
   Cervicothoracic Vertebral 0RH4
   Coccygeal 0SH6
   Elbow
    Left 0RHM
    Right 0RHL
   Finger Phalangeal
    Left 0RHX
    Right 0RHW
   Hip
    Left 0SHB
    Right 0SH9
   Knee
    Left 0SHD
    Right 0SHC
   Lumbar Vertebral 0SH0
   Lumbosacral 0SH3
   Metacarpophalangeal
    Left 0RHV
    Right 0RHU
   Metatarsal-Phalangeal
    Left 0SHN
    Right 0SHM
   Occipital-cervical 0RH0
   Sacrococcygeal 0SH5
   Sacroiliac
    Left 0SH8
    Right 0SH7
   Shoulder
    Left 0RHK
    Right 0RHJ
   Sternoclavicular
    Left 0RHF
    Right 0RHE
   Tarsal
    Left 0SHJ
    Right 0SHH
   Tarsometatarsal
    Left 0SHL
    Right 0SHK
   Temporomandibular
    Left 0RHD
    Right 0RHC
   Thoracic Vertebral 0RH6
   Thoracolumbar Vertebral 0RHA
   Toe Phalangeal
    Left 0SHQ
    Right 0SHP
   Wrist
    Left 0RHP
    Right 0RHN
 Removal of device from
  Acromioclavicular
   Left 0RPH
   Right 0RPG
  Ankle
   Left 0SPG

Spacer — continued
 Removal of device from — continued
  Ankle — continued
   Right 0SPF
  Carpal
   Left 0RPR
   Right 0RPQ
  Carpometacarpal
   Left 0RPT
   Right 0RPS
  Cervical Vertebral 0RP1
  Cervicothoracic Vertebral 0RP4
  Coccygeal 0SP6
  Elbow
   Left 0RPM
   Right 0RPL
  Finger Phalangeal
   Left 0RPX
   Right 0RPW
  Hip
   Left 0SPB
   Right 0SP9
  Knee
   Left 0SPD
   Right 0SPC
  Lumbar Vertebral 0SP0
  Lumbosacral 0SP3
  Metacarpophalangeal
   Left 0RPV
   Right 0RPU
  Metatarsal-Phalangeal
   Left 0SPN
   Right 0SPM
  Occipital-cervical 0RP0
  Sacrococcygeal 0SP5
  Sacroiliac
   Left 0SP8
   Right 0SP7
  Shoulder
   Left 0RPK
   Right 0RPJ
  Sternoclavicular
   Left 0RPF
   Right 0RPE
  Tarsal
   Left 0SPJ
   Right 0SPH
  Tarsometatarsal
   Left 0SPL
   Right 0SPK
  Temporomandibular
   Left 0RPD
   Right 0RPC
  Thoracic Vertebral 0RP6
  Thoracolumbar Vertebral 0RPA
  Toe Phalangeal
   Left 0SPQ
   Right 0SPP
  Wrist
   Left 0RPP
   Right 0RPN
 Revision of device in
  Acromioclavicular
   Left 0RWH
   Right 0RWG
  Ankle
   Left 0SWG
   Right 0SWF
  Carpal
   Left 0RWR
   Right 0RWQ
  Carpometacarpal
   Left 0RWT
   Right 0RWS
  Cervical Vertebral 0RW1
  Cervicothoracic Vertebral 0RW4
  Coccygeal 0SW6
  Elbow
   Left 0RWM
   Right 0RWL
  Finger Phalangeal
   Left 0RWX
   Right 0RWW
  Hip
   Left 0SWB
   Right 0SW9
  Knee
   Left 0SWD
   Right 0SWC

Spacer — *continued*
  Revision of device in — *continued*
    Lumbar Vertebral 0SW0
    Lumbosacral 0SW3
    Metacarpophalangeal
      Left 0RWV
      Right 0RWU
    Metatarsal-Phalangeal
      Left 0SWN
      Right 0SWM
    Occipital-cervical 0RW0
    Sacrococcygeal 0SW5
    Sacroiliac
      Left 0SW8
      Right 0SW7
    Shoulder
      Left 0RWK
      Right 0RWJ
    Sternoclavicular
      Left 0RWF
      Right 0RWE
    Tarsal
      Left 0SWJ
      Right 0SWH
    Tarsometatarsal
      Left 0SWL
      Right 0SWK
    Temporomandibular
      Left 0RWD
      Right 0RWC
    Thoracic Vertebral 0RW6
    Thoracolumbar Vertebral 0RWA
    Toe Phalangeal
      Left 0SWQ
      Right 0SWP
    Wrist
      Left 0RWP
      Right 0RWN
Spacer, Articulating (Antibiotic) *use* Articulating Spacer in Lower Joints
Spacer, Static (Antibiotic) *use* Spacer in Lower Joints
Spectroscopy
  Intravascular Near Infrared 8E023DZ
  Near Infrared *see* Physiological Systems and Anatomical Regions 8E0
Speech Assessment F00
Speech therapy *see* Speech Treatment, Rehabilitation F06
Speech Treatment F06
Spesolimab Monoclonal Antibody XW0
SPEVIGO® *use* Spesolimab Monoclonal Antibody
Sphenoidectomy
  see Excision, Ear, Nose, Sinus 09B
  see Excision, Head and Facial Bones 0NB
  see Resection, Ear, Nose, Sinus 09T
  see Resection, Head and Facial Bones 0NT
Sphenoidotomy *see* Drainage, Ear, Nose, Sinus 099
Sphenomandibular ligament *use* Head and Neck Bursa and Ligament
Sphenopalatine (pterygopalatine) ganglion *use* Head and Neck Sympathetic Nerve
Sphincterorrhaphy, anal *see* Repair, Anal Sphincter 0DQR
Sphincterotomy, anal
  see Division, Anal Sphincter 0D8R
  see Drainage, Anal Sphincter 0D9R
SPIKEVAX™
  use COVID-19 Vaccine
  use COVID-19 Vaccine Booster
  use COVID-19 Vaccine Dose 1
  use COVID-19 Vaccine Dose 2
  use COVID-19 Vaccine Dose 3
Spinal cord neurostimulator lead *use* Neurostimulator Lead in Central Nervous System and Cranial Nerves
Spinal growth rods, magnetically controlled *use* Magnetically Controlled Growth Rod(s) in New Technology
Spinal nerve, cervical *use* Cervical Nerve
Spinal nerve, lumbar *use* Lumbar Nerve
Spinal nerve, sacral *use* Sacral Nerve
Spinal nerve, thoracic *use* Thoracic Nerve
Spinal Stabilization Device
  Facet Replacement
    Cervical Vertebral 0RH1
    Cervicothoracic Vertebral 0RH4
    Lumbar Vertebral 0SH0
    Lumbosacral 0SH3

Spinal Stabilization Device — *continued*
  Facet Replacement — *continued*
    Occipital-cervical 0RH0
    Thoracic Vertebral 0RH6
    Thoracolumbar Vertebral 0RHA
  Interspinous Process
    Cervical Vertebral 0RH1
    Cervicothoracic Vertebral 0RH4
    Lumbar Vertebral 0SH0
    Lumbosacral 0SH3
    Occipital-cervical 0RH0
    Thoracic Vertebral 0RH6
    Thoracolumbar Vertebral 0RHA
  Pedicle-Based
    Cervical Vertebral 0RH1
    Cervicothoracic Vertebral 0RH4
    Lumbar Vertebral 0SH0
    Lumbosacral 0SH3
    Occipital-cervical 0RH0
    Thoracic Vertebral 0RH6
    Thoracolumbar Vertebral 0RHA
SpineJack® system *use* Synthetic Substitute, Mechanically Expandable (Paired) in New Technology
Spinous process
  use Cervical Vertebra
  use Lumbar Vertebra
  use Thoracic Vertebra
Spiral ganglion *use* Acoustic Nerve
Spiration IBV™ Valve System *use* Intraluminal Device, Endobronchial Valve in Respiratory System
Splenectomy
  see Excision, Lymphatic and Hemic Systems 07B
  see Resection, Lymphatic and Hemic Systems 07T
Splenic flexure *use* Transverse Colon
Splenic plexus *use* Abdominal Sympathetic Nerve
Splenius capitis muscle *use* Head Muscle
Splenius cervicis muscle
  use Neck Muscle, Left
  use Neck Muscle, Right
Splenolysis *see* Release, Lymphatic and Hemic Systems 07N
Splenopexy
  see Repair, Lymphatic and Hemic Systems 07Q
  see Reposition, Lymphatic and Hemic Systems 07S
Splenoplasty *see* Repair, Lymphatic and Hemic Systems 07Q
Splenorrhaphy *see* Repair, Lymphatic and Hemic Systems 07Q
Splenotomy *see* Drainage, Lymphatic and Hemic Systems 079
Splinting, musculoskeletal *see* Immobilization, Anatomical Regions 2W3
SPRAVATO™ (Esketamine Hydrochloride) *use* Other Substance
SPY PINPOINT fluorescence imaging system
  see Monitoring, Physiological Systems 4A1
  see Other Imaging, Hepatobiliary System and Pancreas BF5
SPY system intraoperative fluorescence cholangiography *see* Other Imaging, Hepatobiliary System and Pancreas BF5
SPY system intravascular fluorescence angiography *see* Monitoring, Physiological Systems 4A1
SSO2 (Supersaturated Oxygen) therapy, cardiac intra-arterial 5A0222C
Staged hepatectomy
  see Division, Hepatobiliary System and Pancreas 0F8
  see Resection, Hepatobiliary System and Pancreas 0FT
Stapedectomy
  see Excision, Ear, Nose, Sinus 09B
  see Resection, Ear, Nose, Sinus 09T
Stapediolysis *see* Release, Ear, Nose, Sinus 09N
Stapedioplasty
  see Repair, Ear, Nose, Sinus 09Q
  see Replacement, Ear, Nose, Sinus 09R
  see Supplement, Ear, Nose, Sinus 09U
Stapedotomy *see* Drainage, Ear, Nose, Sinus 099
Stapes
  use Auditory Ossicle, Left
  use Auditory Ossicle, Right
Static Spacer (Antibiotic) *use* Spacer in Lower Joints
STELARA® *use* Other New Technology Therapeutic Substance
Stellate ganglion *use* Head and Neck Sympathetic Nerve

Stem cell transplant *see* Transfusion, Circulatory 302
Stensen's duct
  use Parotid Duct, Left
  use Parotid Duct, Right
Stent, intraluminal (cardiovascular) (gastrointestinal) (hepatobiliary) (urinary) *use* Intraluminal Device
Stent retriever thrombectomy *see* Extirpation, Upper Arteries 03C
Stented tissue valve *use* Zooplastic Tissue in Heart and Great Vessels
Stereoelectroencephalographic Radiofrequency (sEEG) Ablation 00503Z4
Stereotactic Radiosurgery
  Abdomen DW23
  Adrenal Gland DG22
  Bile Ducts DF22
  Bladder DT22
  Bone Marrow D720
  Brain D020
  Brain Stem D021
  Breast
    Left DM20
    Right DM21
  Bronchus DB21
  Cervix DU21
  Chest DW22
  Chest Wall DB27
  Colon DD25
  Diaphragm DB28
  Duodenum DD22
  Ear D920
  Esophagus DD20
  Eye D820
  Gallbladder DF21
  Gamma Beam
    Abdomen DW23JZZ
    Adrenal Gland DG22JZZ
    Bile Ducts DF22JZZ
    Bladder DT22JZZ
    Bone Marrow D720JZZ
    Brain D020JZZ
    Brain Stem D021JZZ
    Breast
      Left DM20JZZ
      Right DM21JZZ
    Bronchus DB21JZZ
    Cervix DU21JZZ
    Chest DW22JZZ
    Chest Wall DB27JZZ
    Colon DD25JZZ
    Diaphragm DB28JZZ
    Duodenum DD22JZZ
    Ear D920JZZ
    Esophagus DD20JZZ
    Eye D820JZZ
    Gallbladder DF21JZZ
    Gland
      Adrenal DG22JZZ
      Parathyroid DG24JZZ
      Pituitary DG20JZZ
      Thyroid DG25JZZ
    Glands, Salivary D926JZZ
    Head and Neck DW21JZZ
    Ileum DD24JZZ
    Jejunum DD23JZZ
    Kidney DT20JZZ
    Larynx D92BJZZ
    Liver DF20JZZ
    Lung DB22JZZ
    Lymphatics
      Abdomen D726JZZ
      Axillary D724JZZ
      Inguinal D728JZZ
      Neck D723JZZ
      Pelvis D727JZZ
      Thorax D725JZZ
    Mediastinum DB26JZZ
    Mouth D924JZZ
    Nasopharynx D92DJZZ
    Neck and Head DW21JZZ
    Nerve, Peripheral D027JZZ
    Nose D921JZZ
    Ovary DU20JZZ
    Palate
      Hard D928JZZ
      Soft D929JZZ
    Pancreas DF23JZZ

Stereotactic Radiosurgery — continued
  Gamma Beam — continued
    Parathyroid Gland DG24JZZ
    Pelvic Region DW26JZZ
    Pharynx D92CJZZ
    Pineal Body DG21JZZ
    Pituitary Gland DG20JZZ
    Pleura DB25JZZ
    Prostate DV20JZZ
    Rectum DD27JZZ
    Sinuses D927JZZ
    Spinal Cord D026JZZ
    Spleen D722JZZ
    Stomach DD21JZZ
    Testis DV21JZZ
    Thymus D721JZZ
    Thyroid Gland DG25JZZ
    Tongue D925JZZ
    Trachea DB20JZZ
    Ureter DT21JZZ
    Urethra DT23JZZ
    Uterus DU22JZZ
  Gland
    Adrenal DG22
    Parathyroid DG24
    Pituitary DG20
    Thyroid DG25
  Glands, Salivary D926
  Head and Neck DW21
  Ileum DD24
  Jejunum DD23
  Kidney DT20
  Larynx D92B
  Liver DF20
  Lung DB22
  Lymphatics
    Abdomen D726
    Axillary D724
    Inguinal D728
    Neck D723
    Pelvis D727
    Thorax D725
  Mediastinum DB26
  Mouth D924
  Nasopharynx D92D
  Neck and Head DW21
  Nerve, Peripheral D027
  Nose D921
  Other Photon
    Abdomen DW23DZZ
    Adrenal Gland DG22DZZ
    Bile Ducts DF22DZZ
    Bladder DT22DZZ
    Bone Marrow D720DZZ
    Brain D020DZZ
    Brain Stem D021DZZ
    Breast
      Left DM20DZZ
      Right DM21DZZ
    Bronchus DB21DZZ
    Cervix DU21DZZ
    Chest DW22DZZ
    Chest Wall DB27DZZ
    Colon DD25DZZ
    Diaphragm DB28DZZ
    Duodenum DD22DZZ
    Ear D920DZZ
    Esophagus DD20DZZ
    Eye D820DZZ
    Gallbladder DF21DZZ
    Gland
      Adrenal DG22DZZ
      Parathyroid DG24DZZ
      Pituitary DG20DZZ
      Thyroid DG25DZZ
    Glands, Salivary D926DZZ
    Head and Neck DW21DZZ
    Ileum DD24DZZ
    Jejunum DD23DZZ
    Kidney DT20DZZ
    Larynx D92BDZZ
    Liver DF20DZZ
    Lung DB22DZZ
    Lymphatics
      Abdomen D726DZZ
      Axillary D724DZZ
      Inguinal D728DZZ
      Neck D723DZZ
      Pelvis D727DZZ

Stereotactic Radiosurgery — continued
  Other Photon — continued
    Lymphatics — continued
      Thorax D725DZZ
    Mediastinum DB26DZZ
    Mouth D924DZZ
    Nasopharynx D92DDZZ
    Neck and Head DW21DZZ
    Nerve, Peripheral D027DZZ
    Nose D921DZZ
    Ovary DU20DZZ
    Palate
      Hard D928DZZ
      Soft D929DZZ
    Pancreas DF23DZZ
    Parathyroid Gland DG24DZZ
    Pelvic Region DW26DZZ
    Pharynx D92CDZZ
    Pineal Body DG21DZZ
    Pituitary Gland DG20DZZ
    Pleura DB25DZZ
    Prostate DV20DZZ
    Rectum DD27DZZ
    Sinuses D927DZZ
    Spinal Cord D026DZZ
    Spleen D722DZZ
    Stomach DD21DZZ
    Testis DV21DZZ
    Thymus D721DZZ
    Thyroid Gland DG25DZZ
    Tongue D925DZZ
    Trachea DB20DZZ
    Ureter DT21DZZ
    Urethra DT23DZZ
    Uterus DU22DZZ
  Ovary DU20
  Palate
    Hard D928
    Soft D929
  Pancreas DF23
  Parathyroid Gland DG24
  Particulate
    Abdomen DW23HZZ
    Adrenal Gland DG22HZZ
    Bile Ducts DF22HZZ
    Bladder DT22HZZ
    Bone Marrow D720HZZ
    Brain D020HZZ
    Brain Stem D021HZZ
    Breast
      Left DM20HZZ
      Right DM21HZZ
    Bronchus DB21HZZ
    Cervix DU21HZZ
    Chest DW22HZZ
    Chest Wall DB27HZZ
    Colon DD25HZZ
    Diaphragm DB28HZZ
    Duodenum DD22HZZ
    Ear D920HZZ
    Esophagus DD20HZZ
    Eye D820HZZ
    Gallbladder DF21HZZ
    Gland
      Adrenal DG22HZZ
      Parathyroid DG24HZZ
      Pituitary DG20HZZ
      Thyroid DG25HZZ
    Glands, Salivary D926HZZ
    Head and Neck DW21HZZ
    Ileum DD24HZZ
    Jejunum DD23HZZ
    Kidney DT20HZZ
    Larynx D92BHZZ
    Liver DF20HZZ
    Lung DB22HZZ
    Lymphatics
      Abdomen D726HZZ
      Axillary D724HZZ
      Inguinal D728HZZ
      Neck D723HZZ
      Pelvis D727HZZ
      Thorax D725HZZ
    Mediastinum DB26HZZ
    Mouth D924HZZ
    Nasopharynx D92DHZZ
    Neck and Head DW21HZZ
    Nerve, Peripheral D027HZZ
    Nose D921HZZ

Stereotactic Radiosurgery — continued
  Particulate — continued
    Ovary DU20HZZ
    Palate
      Hard D928HZZ
      Soft D929HZZ
    Pancreas DF23HZZ
    Parathyroid Gland DG24HZZ
    Pelvic Region DW26HZZ
    Pharynx D92CHZZ
    Pineal Body DG21HZZ
    Pituitary Gland DG20HZZ
    Pleura DB25HZZ
    Prostate DV20HZZ
    Rectum DD27HZZ
    Sinuses D927HZZ
    Spinal Cord D026HZZ
    Spleen D722HZZ
    Stomach DD21HZZ
    Testis DV21HZZ
    Thymus D721HZZ
    Thyroid Gland DG25HZZ
    Tongue D925HZZ
    Trachea DB20HZZ
    Ureter DT21HZZ
    Urethra DT23HZZ
    Uterus DU22HZZ
  Pelvic Region DW26
  Pharynx D92C
  Pineal Body DG21
  Pituitary Gland DG20
  Pleura DB25
  Prostate DV20
  Rectum DD27
  Sinuses D927
  Spinal Cord D026
  Spleen D722
  Stomach DD21
  Testis DV21
  Thymus D721
  Thyroid Gland DG25
  Tongue D925
  Trachea DB20
  Ureter DT21
  Urethra DT23
  Uterus DU22
Steripath® Micro™ Blood Collection System
  XXE5XR7
Sternoclavicular ligament
  use Shoulder Bursa and Ligament, Left
  use Shoulder Bursa and Ligament, Right
Sternocleidomastoid artery
  use Thyroid Artery, Left
  use Thyroid Artery, Right
Sternocleidomastoid muscle
  use Neck Muscle, Left
  use Neck Muscle, Right
Sternocostal ligament *use* Sternum Bursa and Ligament
Sternotomy
  see Division, Sternum 0P80
  see Drainage, Sternum 0P90
Stimulation, cardiac
  Cardioversion 5A2204Z
  Electrophysiologic testing *see* Measurement, Cardiac 4A02
Stimulator Generator
  Insertion of device in
    Abdomen 0JH8
    Back 0JH7
    Chest 0JH6
  Multiple Array
    Abdomen 0JH8
    Back 0JH7
    Chest 0JH6
  Multiple Array Rechargeable
    Abdomen 0JH8
    Back 0JH7
    Chest 0JH6
  Removal of device from, Subcutaneous Tissue and Fascia, Trunk 0JPT
  Revision of device in, Subcutaneous Tissue and Fascia, Trunk 0JWT
  Single Array
    Abdomen 0JH8
    Back 0JH7
    Chest 0JH6

Stimulator Generator — continued
  Single Array Rechargeable
    Abdomen 0JH8
    Back 0JH7
    Chest 0JH6
Stimulator Lead
  Insertion of device in
    Anal Sphincter 0DHR
    Artery
      Left 03HL
      Right 03HK
    Bladder 0THB
    Muscle
      Lower 0KHY
      Upper 0KHX
    Stomach 0DH6
    Ureter 0TH9
  Removal of device from
    Anal Sphincter 0DPR
    Artery, Upper 03PY
    Bladder 0TPB
    Muscle
      Lower 0KPY
      Upper 0KPX
    Stomach 0DP6
    Ureter 0TP9
  Revision of device in
    Anal Sphincter 0DWR
    Artery, Upper 03WY
    Bladder 0TWB
    Muscle
      Lower 0KWY
      Upper 0KWX
    Stomach 0DW6
    Ureter 0TW9
Stoma
  Excision
    Abdominal Wall 0WBFXZ2
    Neck 0WB6XZ2
  Repair
    Abdominal Wall 0WQFXZ2
    Neck 0WQ6XZ2
Stomatoplasty
  see Repair, Mouth and Throat 0CQ
  see Replacement, Mouth and Throat 0CR
  see Supplement, Mouth and Throat 0CU
Stomatorrhaphy see Repair, Mouth and Throat 0CQ
StrataGraft® use Bioengineered Allogeneic Construct
Stratos LV use Cardiac Resynchronization Pacemaker Pulse Generator in 0JH
Stress test 4A02XM4, 4A12XM4
Stripping see Extraction
Study
  Electrophysiologic stimulation, cardiac see Measurement, Cardiac 4A02
  Ocular motility 4A07X7Z
  Pulmonary airway flow measurement see Measurement, Respiratory 4A09
  Visual acuity 4A07X0Z
Styloglossus muscle use Tongue, Palate, Pharynx Muscle
Stylomandibular ligament use Head and Neck Bursa and Ligament
Stylopharyngeus muscle use Tongue, Palate, Pharynx Muscle
Subacromial bursa
  use Shoulder Bursa and Ligament, Left
  use Shoulder Bursa and Ligament, Right
Subaortic (common iliac) lymph node use Lymphatic, Pelvis
Subarachnoid space, spinal use Spinal Canal
Subclavicular (apical) lymph node
  use Lymphatic, Left Axillary
  use Lymphatic, Right Axillary
Subclavius muscle
  use Thorax Muscle, Left
  use Thorax Muscle, Right
Subclavius nerve use Brachial Plexus
Subcostal artery use Upper Artery
Subcostal muscle
  use Thorax Muscle, Left
  use Thorax Muscle, Right
Subcostal nerve use Thoracic Nerve
Subcutaneous Defibrillator Lead
  Insertion of device in, Subcutaneous Tissue and Fascia, Chest 0JH6
  Removal of device from, Subcutaneous Tissue and Fascia, Trunk 0JPT

Subcutaneous Defibrillator Lead — continued
  Revision of device in, Subcutaneous Tissue and Fascia, Trunk 0JWT
Subcutaneous injection reservoir, port use Vascular Access Device, Totally Implantable in Subcutaneous Tissue and Fascia
Subcutaneous injection reservoir, pump use Infusion Device, Pump in Subcutaneous Tissue and Fascia
Subdermal progesterone implant use Contraceptive Device in Subcutaneous Tissue and Fascia
Subdural space, spinal use Spinal Canal
Submandibular ganglion
  use Facial Nerve
  use Head and Neck Sympathetic Nerve
Submandibular gland
  use Submaxillary Gland, Left
  use Submaxillary Gland, Right
Submandibular lymph node use Lymphatic, Head
Submandibular space use Subcutaneous Tissue and Fascia, Face
Submaxillary ganglion use Head and Neck Sympathetic Nerve
Submaxillary lymph node use Lymphatic, Head
Submental artery use Face Artery
Submental lymph node use Lymphatic, Head
Submucous (Meissner's) plexus use Abdominal Sympathetic Nerve
Suboccipital nerve use Cervical Nerve
Suboccipital venous plexus
  use Vertebral Vein, Left
  use Vertebral Vein, Right
Subparotid lymph node use Lymphatic, Head
Subscapular aponeurosis
  use Subcutaneous Tissue and Fascia, Left Upper Arm
  use Subcutaneous Tissue and Fascia, Right Upper Arm
Subscapular artery
  use Axillary Artery, Left
  use Axillary Artery, Right
Subscapular (posterior) lymph node
  use Lymphatic, Axillary, Left
  use Lymphatic, Axillary, Right
Subscapularis muscle
  use Shoulder Muscle, Left
  use Shoulder Muscle, Right
Substance Abuse Treatment
  Counseling
    Family, for substance abuse, Other Family Counseling HZ63ZZZ
    Group
      12-Step HZ43ZZZ
      Behavioral HZ41ZZZ
      Cognitive HZ40ZZZ
      Cognitive-Behavioral HZ42ZZZ
      Confrontational HZ48ZZZ
      Continuing Care HZ49ZZZ
      Infectious Disease
        Post-Test HZ4CZZZ
        Pre-Test HZ4CZZZ
      Interpersonal HZ44ZZZ
      Motivational Enhancement HZ47ZZZ
      Psychoeducation HZ46ZZZ
      Spiritual HZ4BZZZ
      Vocational HZ45ZZZ
    Individual
      12-Step HZ33ZZZ
      Behavioral HZ31ZZZ
      Cognitive HZ30ZZZ
      Cognitive-Behavioral HZ32ZZZ
      Confrontational HZ38ZZZ
      Continuing Care HZ39ZZZ
      Infectious Disease
        Post-Test HZ3CZZZ
        Pre-Test HZ3CZZZ
      Interpersonal HZ34ZZZ
      Motivational Enhancement HZ37ZZZ
      Psychoeducation HZ36ZZZ
      Spiritual HZ3BZZZ
      Vocational HZ35ZZZ
    Detoxification Services, for substance abuse HZ2ZZZZ
  Medication Management
    Antabuse HZ83ZZZ
    Bupropion HZ87ZZZ
    Clonidine HZ86ZZZ

Substance Abuse Treatment — continued
  Medication Management — continued
    Levo-alpha-acetyl-methadol (LAAM) HZ82ZZZ
    Methadone Maintenance HZ81ZZZ
    Naloxone HZ85ZZZ
    Naltrexone HZ84ZZZ
    Nicotine Replacement HZ80ZZZ
    Other Replacement Medication HZ89ZZZ
    Psychiatric Medication HZ88ZZZ
  Pharmacotherapy
    Antabuse HZ93ZZZ
    Bupropion HZ97ZZZ
    Clonidine HZ96ZZZ
    Levo-alpha-acetyl-methadol (LAAM) HZ92ZZZ
    Methadone Maintenance HZ91ZZZ
    Naloxone HZ95ZZZ
    Naltrexone HZ94ZZZ
    Nicotine Replacement HZ90ZZZ
    Psychiatric Medication HZ98ZZZ
    Replacement Medication, Other HZ99ZZZ
  Psychotherapy
    12-Step HZ53ZZZ
    Behavioral HZ51ZZZ
    Cognitive HZ50ZZZ
    Cognitive-Behavioral HZ52ZZZ
    Confrontational HZ58ZZZ
    Interactive HZ55ZZZ
    Interpersonal HZ54ZZZ
    Motivational Enhancement HZ57ZZZ
    Psychoanalysis HZ5BZZZ
    Psychodynamic HZ5CZZZ
    Psychoeducation HZ56ZZZ
    Psychophysiological HZ5DZZZ
    Supportive HZ59ZZZ
Substantia nigra use Basal Ganglia
Subtalar (talocalcaneal) joint
  use Tarsal Joint, Left
  use Tarsal Joint, Right
Subtalar ligament
  use Foot Bursa and Ligament, Left
  use Foot Bursa and Ligament, Right
Subthalamic nucleus use Basal Ganglia
Suction curettage (D&C), nonobstetric see Extraction, Endometrium 0UDB
Suction curettage, obstetric post-delivery see Extraction, Products of Conception, Retained 10D1
Sulbactam-Durlobactam XW0
SUL-DUR use Sulbactam-Durlobactam
Superficial circumflex iliac vein
  use Saphenous Vein, Left
  use Saphenous Vein, Right
Superficial epigastric artery
  use Femoral Artery, Left
  use Femoral Artery, Right
Superficial epigastric vein
  use Saphenous Vein, Left
  use Saphenous Vein, Right
Superficial Inferior Epigastric Artery Flap
  Replacement
    Bilateral 0HRV078
    Left 0HRU078
    Right 0HRT078
  Transfer
    Left 0KXG
    Right 0KXF
Superficial palmar arch
  use Hand Artery, Left
  use Hand Artery, Right
Superficial palmar venous arch
  use Hand Vein, Left
  use Hand Vein, Right
Superficial temporal artery
  use Temporal Artery, Left
  use Temporal Artery, Right
Superficial transverse perineal muscle use Perineum Muscle
Superior cardiac nerve use Thoracic Sympathetic Nerve
Superior cerebellar vein use Intracranial Vein
Superior cerebral vein use Intracranial Vein
Superior clunic (cluneal) nerve use Lumbar Nerve
Superior epigastric artery
  use Internal Mammary Artery, Left
  use Internal Mammary Artery, Right

Superior genicular artery
  use Popliteal Artery, Left
  use Popliteal Artery, Right
Superior gluteal artery
  use Internal Iliac Artery, Left
  use Internal Iliac Artery, Right
Superior gluteal nerve use Lumbar Plexus
Superior hypogastric plexus use Abdominal Sympathetic Nerve
Superior labial artery use Face Artery
Superior laryngeal artery
  use Thyroid Artery, Left
  use Thyroid Artery, Right
Superior laryngeal nerve use Vagus Nerve
Superior longitudinal muscle use Tongue, Palate, Pharynx Muscle
Superior mesenteric ganglion use Abdominal Sympathetic Nerve
Superior mesenteric lymph node use Lymphatic, Mesenteric
Superior mesenteric plexus use Abdominal Sympathetic Nerve
Superior oblique muscle
  use Extraocular Muscle, Left
  use Extraocular Muscle, Right
Superior olivary nucleus use Pons
Superior rectal artery use Inferior Mesenteric Artery
Superior rectal vein use Inferior Mesenteric Vein
Superior rectus muscle
  use Extraocular Muscle, Left
  use Extraocular Muscle, Right
Superior tarsal plate
  use Upper Eyelid, Left
  use Upper Eyelid, Right
Superior thoracic artery
  use Axillary Artery, Left
  use Axillary Artery, Right
Superior thyroid artery
  use External Carotid Artery, Left
  use External Carotid Artery, Right
  use Thyroid Artery, Left
  use Thyroid Artery, Right
Superior turbinate use Nasal Turbinate
Superior ulnar collateral artery
  use Brachial Artery, Left
  use Brachial Artery, Right
Superior vesical artery
  use Internal Iliac Artery, Left
  use Internal Iliac Artery, Right
Supersaturated Oxygen (SSO2) therapy, cardiac intra-arterial 5A0222C
Supplement
  Abdominal Wall 0WUF
  Acetabulum
    Left 0QU5
    Right 0QU4
  Ampulla of Vater 0FUC
  Anal Sphincter 0DUR
  Ankle Region
    Left 0YUL
    Right 0YUK
  Anus 0DUQ
  Aorta
    Abdominal 04U0
    Thoracic
      Ascending/Arch 02UX
      Descending 02UW
  Arm
    Lower
      Left 0XUF
      Right 0XUD
    Upper
      Left 0XU9
      Right 0XU8
  Arteriovenous Fistula, Extraluminal Support Device X2U
  Artery
    Anterior Tibial
      Left 04UQ
      Right 04UP
    Axillary
      Left 03U6
      Right 03U5
    Brachial
      Left 03U8
      Right 03U7
    Celiac 04U1

Supplement — continued
  Artery — continued
    Colic
      Left 04U7
      Middle 04U8
      Right 04U6
    Common Carotid
      Left 03UJ
      Right 03UH
    Common Iliac
      Left 04UD
      Right 04UC
    Coronary
      Four or More Arteries 02U3
      One Artery 02U0
      Three Arteries 02U2
      Two Arteries 02U1
    External Carotid
      Left 03UN
      Right 03UM
    External Iliac
      Left 04UJ
      Right 04UH
    Face 03UR
    Femoral
      Left 04UL
      Right 04UK
    Foot
      Left 04UW
      Right 04UV
    Gastric 04U2
    Hand
      Left 03UF
      Right 03UD
    Hepatic 04U3
    Inferior Mesenteric 04UB
    Innominate 03U2
    Internal Carotid
      Left 03UL
      Right 03UK
    Internal Iliac
      Left 04UF
      Right 04UE
    Internal Mammary
      Left 03U1
      Right 03U0
    Intracranial 03UG
    Lower 04UY
    Peroneal
      Left 04UU
      Right 04UT
    Popliteal
      Left 04UN
      Right 04UM
    Posterior Tibial
      Left 04US
      Right 04UR
    Pulmonary
      Left 02UR
      Right 02UQ
    Pulmonary Trunk 02UP
    Radial
      Left 03UC
      Right 03UB
    Renal
      Left 04UA
      Right 04U9
    Splenic 04U4
    Subclavian
      Left 03U4
      Right 03U3
    Superior Mesenteric 04U5
    Temporal
      Left 03UT
      Right 03US
    Thyroid
      Left 03UV
      Right 03UU
    Ulnar
      Left 03UA
      Right 03U9
    Upper 03UY
    Vertebral
      Left 03UQ
      Right 03UP
  Atrium
    Left 02U7
    Right 02U6

Supplement — continued
  Auditory Ossicle
    Left 09UA
    Right 09U9
  Axilla
    Left 0XU5
    Right 0XU4
  Back
    Lower 0WUL
    Upper 0WUK
  Bladder 0TUB
  Bladder Neck 0TUC
  Bone
    Ethmoid
      Left 0NUG
      Right 0NUF
    Frontal 0NU1
    Hyoid 0NUX
    Lacrimal
      Left 0NUJ
      Right 0NUH
    Nasal 0NUB
    Occipital 0NU7
    Palatine
      Left 0NUL
      Right 0NUK
    Parietal
      Left 0NU4
      Right 0NU3
    Pelvic
      Left 0QU3
      Right 0QU2
    Sphenoid 0NUC
    Temporal
      Left 0NU6
      Right 0NU5
    Zygomatic
      Left 0NUN
      Right 0NUM
  Breast
    Bilateral 0HUV
    Left 0HUU
    Right 0HUT
  Bronchus
    Lingula 0BU9
    Lower Lobe
      Left 0BUB
      Right 0BU6
    Main
      Left 0BU7
      Right 0BU3
    Middle Lobe, Right 0BU5
    Upper Lobe
      Left 0BU8
      Right 0BU4
  Buccal Mucosa 0CU4
  Bursa and Ligament
    Abdomen
      Left 0MUJ
      Right 0MUH
    Ankle
      Left 0MUR
      Right 0MUQ
    Elbow
      Left 0MU4
      Right 0MU3
    Foot
      Left 0MUT
      Right 0MUS
    Hand
      Left 0MU8
      Right 0MU7
    Head and Neck 0MU0
    Hip
      Left 0MUM
      Right 0MUL
    Knee
      Left 0MUP
      Right 0MUN
    Lower Extremity
      Left 0MUW
      Right 0MUV
    Perineum 0MUK
    Rib(s) 0MUG
    Shoulder
      Left 0MU2
      Right 0MU1
    Spine
      Lower 0MUD

Supplement — continued
  Bursa and Ligament — continued
    Spine — continued
      Posterior Vertebral Tether XKU
      Upper ØMUC
    Sternum ØMUF
    Upper Extremity
      Left ØMUB
      Right ØMU9
    Wrist
      Left ØMU6
      Right ØMU5
  Buttock
    Left ØYU1
    Right ØYUØ
  Carina ØBU2
  Carpal
    Left ØPUN
    Right ØPUM
  Cecum ØDUH
  Cerebral Meninges ØØU1
  Cerebral Ventricle ØØU6
  Chest Wall ØWU8
  Chordae Tendineae Ø2U9
  Cisterna Chyli Ø7UL
  Clavicle
    Left ØPUB
    Right ØPU9
  Clitoris ØUUJ
  Coccyx ØQUS
  Colon
    Ascending ØDUK
    Descending ØDUM
    Sigmoid ØDUN
    Transverse ØDUL
  Cord
    Bilateral ØVUH
    Left ØVUG
    Right ØVUF
  Cornea
    Left Ø8U9
    Right Ø8U8
  Coronary Artery/Arteries, Vein Graft Extraluminal Support Device(s) X2U4Ø79
  Cul-de-sac ØUUF
  Diaphragm ØBUT
  Disc
    Cervical Vertebral ØRU3
    Cervicothoracic Vertebral ØRU5
    Lumbar Vertebral ØSU2
    Lumbosacral ØSU4
    Thoracic Vertebral ØRU9
    Thoracolumbar Vertebral ØRUB
  Duct
    Common Bile ØFU9
    Cystic ØFU8
    Hepatic
      Common ØFU7
      Left ØFU6
      Right ØFU5
    Lacrimal
      Left Ø8UY
      Right Ø8UX
    Pancreatic ØFUD
      Accessory ØFUF
  Duodenum ØDU9
  Dura Mater ØØU2
  Ear
    External
      Bilateral Ø9U2
      Left Ø9U1
      Right Ø9UØ
    Inner
      Left Ø9UE
      Right Ø9UD
    Middle
      Left Ø9U6
      Right Ø9U5
  Elbow Region
    Left ØXUC
    Right ØXUB
  Epididymis
    Bilateral ØVUL
    Left ØVUK
    Right ØVUJ
  Epiglottis ØCUR
  Esophagogastric Junction ØDU4
  Esophagus ØDU5
    Lower ØDU3

Supplement — continued
  Esophagus — continued
    Middle ØDU2
    Upper ØDU1
  Extremity
    Lower
      Left ØYUB
      Right ØYU9
    Upper
      Left ØXU7
      Right ØXU6
  Eye
    Left Ø8U1
    Right Ø8UØ
  Eyelid
    Lower
      Left Ø8UR
      Right Ø8UQ
    Upper
      Left Ø8UP
      Right Ø8UN
  Face ØWU2
  Fallopian Tube
    Left ØUU6
    Right ØUU5
  Fallopian Tubes, Bilateral ØUU7
  Femoral Region
    Bilateral ØYUE
    Left ØYU8
    Right ØYU7
  Femoral Shaft
    Left ØQU9
    Right ØQU8
  Femur
    Lower
      Left ØQUC
      Right ØQUB
    Upper
      Left ØQU7
      Right ØQU6
  Fibula
    Left ØQUK
    Right ØQUJ
  Finger
    Index
      Left ØXUP
      Right ØXUN
    Little
      Left ØXUW
      Right ØXUV
    Middle
      Left ØXUR
      Right ØXUQ
    Ring
      Left ØXUT
      Right ØXUS
  Foot
    Left ØYUN
    Right ØYUM
  Gingiva
    Lower ØCU6
    Upper ØCU5
  Glenoid Cavity
    Left ØPU8
    Right ØPU7
  Hand
    Left ØXUK
    Right ØXUJ
  Head ØWUØ
  Heart Ø2UA
  Humeral Head
    Left ØPUD
    Right ØPUC
  Humeral Shaft
    Left ØPUG
    Right ØPUF
  Hymen ØUUK
  Ileocecal Valve ØDUC
  Ileum ØDUB
  Inguinal Region
    Bilateral ØYUA
    Left ØYU6
    Right ØYU5
  Intestine
    Large ØDUE
      Left ØDUG
      Right ØDUF
    Small ØDU8

Supplement — continued
  Iris
    Left Ø8UD
    Right Ø8UC
  Jaw
    Lower ØWU5
    Upper ØWU4
  Jejunum ØDUA
  Joint
    Acromioclavicular
      Left ØRUH
      Right ØRUG
    Ankle
      Left ØSUG
      Right ØSUF
    Carpal
      Left ØRUR
      Right ØRUQ
    Carpometacarpal
      Left ØRUT
      Right ØRUS
    Cervical Vertebral ØRU1
    Cervicothoracic Vertebral ØRU4
    Coccygeal ØSU6
    Elbow
      Left ØRUM
      Right ØRUL
    Finger Phalangeal
      Left ØRUX
      Right ØRUW
    Hip
      Left ØSUB
        Acetabular Surface ØSUE
        Femoral Surface ØSUS
      Right ØSU9
        Acetabular Surface ØSUA
        Femoral Surface ØSUR
    Knee
      Left ØSUD
        Femoral Surface ØSUUØ9Z
        Tibial Surface ØSUWØ9Z
      Right ØSUC
        Femoral Surface ØSUTØ9Z
        Tibial Surface ØSUVØ9Z
    Lumbar Vertebral ØSUØ
    Lumbosacral ØSU3
    Metacarpophalangeal
      Left ØRUV
      Right ØRUU
    Metatarsal-Phalangeal
      Left ØSUN
      Right ØSUM
    Occipital-cervical ØRUØ
    Sacrococcygeal ØSU5
    Sacroiliac
      Left ØSU8
      Right ØSU7
    Shoulder
      Left ØRUK
      Right ØRUJ
    Sternoclavicular
      Left ØRUF
      Right ØRUE
    Tarsal
      Left ØSUJ
      Right ØSUH
    Tarsometatarsal
      Left ØSUL
      Right ØSUK
    Temporomandibular
      Left ØRUD
      Right ØRUC
    Thoracic Vertebral ØRU6
    Thoracolumbar Vertebral ØRUA
    Toe Phalangeal
      Left ØSUQ
      Right ØSUP
    Wrist
      Left ØRUP
      Right ØRUN
  Kidney Pelvis
    Left ØTU4
    Right ØTU3
  Knee Region
    Left ØYUG
    Right ØYUF
  Larynx ØCUS

Supplement — *continued*
- Leg
  - Lower
    - Left ØYUJ
    - Right ØYUH
  - Upper
    - Left ØYUD
    - Right ØYUC
- Lip
  - Lower ØCU1
  - Upper ØCUØ
- Lymphatic
  - Aortic Ø7UD
  - Axillary
    - Left Ø7U6
    - Right Ø7U5
  - Head Ø7UØ
  - Inguinal
    - Left Ø7UJ
    - Right Ø7UH
  - Internal Mammary
    - Left Ø7U9
    - Right Ø7U8
  - Lower Extremity
    - Left Ø7UG
    - Right Ø7UF
  - Mesenteric Ø7UB
  - Neck
    - Left Ø7U2
    - Right Ø7U1
  - Pelvis Ø7UC
  - Thoracic Duct Ø7UK
  - Thorax Ø7U7
  - Upper Extremity
    - Left Ø7U4
    - Right Ø7U3
- Mandible
  - Left ØNUV
  - Right ØNUT
- Maxilla ØNUR
- Mediastinum ØWUC
- Mesentery ØDUV
- Metacarpal
  - Left ØPUQ
  - Right ØPUP
- Metatarsal
  - Left ØQUP
  - Right ØQUN
- Muscle
  - Abdomen
    - Left ØKUL
    - Right ØKUK
  - Extraocular
    - Left Ø8UM
    - Right Ø8UL
  - Facial ØKU1
  - Foot
    - Left ØKUW
    - Right ØKUV
  - Hand
    - Left ØKUD
    - Right ØKUC
  - Head ØKUØ
  - Hip
    - Left ØKUP
    - Right ØKUN
  - Lower Arm and Wrist
    - Left ØKUB
    - Right ØKU9
  - Lower Leg
    - Left ØKUT
    - Right ØKUS
  - Neck
    - Left ØKU3
    - Right ØKU2
  - Papillary Ø2UD
  - Perineum ØKUM
  - Shoulder
    - Left ØKU6
    - Right ØKU5
  - Thorax
    - Left ØKUJ
    - Right ØKUH
  - Tongue, Palate, Pharynx ØKU4
  - Trunk
    - Left ØKUG
    - Right ØKUF
  - Upper Arm
    - Left ØKU8

Supplement — *continued*
- Muscle — *continued*
  - Upper Arm — *continued*
    - Right ØKU7
  - Upper Leg
    - Left ØKUR
    - Right ØKUQ
- Nasal Mucosa and Soft Tissue Ø9UK
- Nasopharynx Ø9UN
- Neck ØWU6
- Nerve
  - Abducens ØØUL
  - Accessory ØØUR
  - Acoustic ØØUN
  - Cervical Ø1U1
  - Facial ØØUM
  - Femoral Ø1UD
  - Glossopharyngeal ØØUP
  - Hypoglossal ØØUS
  - Lumbar Ø1UB
  - Median Ø1U5
  - Oculomotor ØØUH
  - Olfactory ØØUF
  - Optic ØØUG
  - Peroneal Ø1UH
  - Phrenic Ø1U2
  - Pudendal Ø1UC
  - Radial Ø1U6
  - Sacral Ø1UR
  - Sciatic Ø1UF
  - Thoracic Ø1U8
  - Tibial Ø1UG
  - Trigeminal ØØUK
  - Trochlear ØØUJ
  - Ulnar Ø1U4
  - Vagus ØØUQ
- Nipple
  - Left ØHUX
  - Right ØHUW
- Omentum ØDUU
- Orbit
  - Left ØNUQ
  - Right ØNUP
- Palate
  - Hard ØCU2
  - Soft ØCU3
- Patella
  - Left ØQUF
  - Right ØQUD
- Penis ØVUS
- Pericardium Ø2UN
- Perineum
  - Female ØWUN
  - Male ØWUM
- Peritoneum ØDUW
- Phalanx
  - Finger
    - Left ØPUV
    - Right ØPUT
  - Thumb
    - Left ØPUS
    - Right ØPUR
  - Toe
    - Left ØQUR
    - Right ØQUQ
- Pharynx ØCUM
- Prepuce ØVUT
- Radius
  - Left ØPUJ
  - Right ØPUH
- Rectum ØDUP
- Retina
  - Left Ø8UF
  - Right Ø8UE
- Retinal Vessel
  - Left Ø8UH
  - Right Ø8UG
- Ribs
  - 1 to 2 ØPU1
  - 3 or More ØPU2
- Sacrum ØQU1
- Scapula
  - Left ØPU6
  - Right ØPU5
- Scrotum ØVU5
- Septum
  - Atrial Ø2U5
  - Nasal Ø9UM
  - Ventricular Ø2UM

Supplement — *continued*
- Shoulder Region
  - Left ØXU3
  - Right ØXU2
- Sinus
  - Accessory Ø9UP
  - Ethmoid
    - Left Ø9UV
    - Right Ø9UU
  - Frontal
    - Left Ø9UT
    - Right Ø9US
  - Mastoid
    - Left Ø9UC
    - Right Ø9UB
  - Maxillary
    - Left Ø9UR
    - Right Ø9UQ
  - Sphenoid
    - Left Ø9UX
    - Right Ø9UW
- Skull ØNUØ
- Spinal Meninges ØØUT
- Sternum ØPUØ
- Stomach ØDU6
  - Pylorus ØDU7
- Subcutaneous Tissue and Fascia
  - Abdomen ØJU8
  - Back ØJU7
  - Buttock ØJU9
  - Chest ØJU6
  - Face ØJU1
  - Foot
    - Left ØJUR
    - Right ØJUQ
  - Hand
    - Left ØJUK
    - Right ØJUJ
  - Lower Arm
    - Left ØJUH
    - Right ØJUG
  - Lower Leg
    - Left ØJUP
    - Right ØJUN
  - Neck
    - Left ØJU5
    - Right ØJU4
  - Pelvic Region ØJUC
  - Perineum ØJUB
  - Scalp ØJUØ
  - Upper Arm
    - Left ØJUF
    - Right ØJUD
  - Upper Leg
    - Left ØJUM
    - Right ØJUL
- Tarsal
  - Left ØQUM
  - Right ØQUL
- Tendon
  - Abdomen
    - Left ØLUG
    - Right ØLUF
  - Ankle
    - Left ØLUT
    - Right ØLUS
  - Foot
    - Left ØLUW
    - Right ØLUV
  - Hand
    - Left ØLU8
    - Right ØLU7
  - Head and Neck ØLUØ
  - Hip
    - Left ØLUK
    - Right ØLUJ
  - Knee
    - Left ØLUR
    - Right ØLUQ
  - Lower Arm and Wrist
    - Left ØLU6
    - Right ØLU5
  - Lower Leg
    - Left ØLUP
    - Right ØLUN
  - Perineum ØLUH
  - Shoulder
    - Left ØLU2
    - Right ØLU1

Supplement — *continued*
  Tendon — *continued*
    Thorax
      Left 0LUD
      Right 0LUC
    Trunk
      Left 0LUB
      Right 0LU9
    Upper Arm
      Left 0LU4
      Right 0LU3
    Upper Leg
      Left 0LUM
      Right 0LUL
  Testis
    Bilateral 0VUC0
    Left 0VUB0
    Right 0VU90
  Thumb
    Left 0XUM
    Right 0XUL
  Tibia
    Left 0QUH
    Right 0QUG
  Toe
    1st
      Left 0YUQ
      Right 0YUP
    2nd
      Left 0YUS
      Right 0YUR
    3rd
      Left 0YUU
      Right 0YUT
    4th
      Left 0YUW
      Right 0YUV
    5th
      Left 0YUY
      Right 0YUX
  Tongue 0CU7
  Trachea 0BU1
  Tunica Vaginalis
    Left 0VU7
    Right 0VU6
  Turbinate, Nasal 09UL
  Tympanic Membrane
    Left 09U8
    Right 09U7
  Ulna
    Left 0PUL
    Right 0PUK
  Ureter
    Left 0TU7
    Right 0TU6
  Urethra 0TUD
  Uterine Supporting Structure 0UU4
  Uvula 0CUN
  Vagina 0UUG
  Valve
    Aortic 02UF
    Mitral 02UG
    Pulmonary 02UH
    Tricuspid 02UJ
  Vas Deferens
    Bilateral 0VUQ
    Left 0VUP
    Right 0VUN
  Vein
    Axillary
      Left 05U8
      Right 05U7
    Azygos 05U0
    Basilic
      Left 05UC
      Right 05UB
    Brachial
      Left 05UA
      Right 05U9
    Cephalic
      Left 05UF
      Right 05UD
    Colic 06U7
    Common Iliac
      Left 06UD
      Right 06UC
    Esophageal 06U3
    External Iliac
      Left 06UG

Supplement — *continued*
  Vein — *continued*
    External Iliac — *continued*
      Right 06UF
    External Jugular
      Left 05UQ
      Right 05UP
    Face
      Left 05UV
      Right 05UT
    Femoral
      Left 06UN
      Right 06UM
    Foot
      Left 06UV
      Right 06UT
    Gastric 06U2
    Hand
      Left 05UH
      Right 05UG
    Hemiazygos 05U1
    Hepatic 06U4
    Hypogastric
      Left 06UJ
      Right 06UH
    Inferior Mesenteric 06U6
    Innominate
      Left 05U4
      Right 05U3
    Internal Jugular
      Left 05UN
      Right 05UM
    Intracranial 05UL
    Lower 06UY
    Portal 06U8
    Pulmonary
      Left 02UT
      Right 02US
    Renal
      Left 06UB
      Right 06U9
    Saphenous
      Left 06UQ
      Right 06UP
    Splenic 06U1
    Subclavian
      Left 05U6
      Right 05U5
    Superior Mesenteric 06U5
    Upper 05UY
    Vertebral
      Left 05US
      Right 05UR
  Vena Cava
    Inferior 06U0
    Superior 02UV
  Ventricle
    Left 02UL
    Right 02UK
  Vertebra
    Cervical 0PU3
    Lumbar 0QU0
      Mechanically Expandable (Paired) Synthetic Substitute XNU0356
    Thoracic 0PU4
      Mechanically Expandable (Paired) Synthetic Substitute XNU4356
  Vesicle
    Bilateral 0VU3
    Left 0VU2
    Right 0VU1
  Vocal Cord
    Left 0CUV
    Right 0CUT
  Vulva 0UUM
  Wrist Region
    Left 0XUH
    Right 0XUG
Supraclavicular (Virchow's) lymph node
  use Lymphatic, Left Neck
  use Lymphatic, Right Neck
Supraclavicular nerve *use* Cervical Plexus
Suprahyoid lymph node *use* Lymphatic, Head
Suprahyoid muscle
  use Neck Muscle, Left
  use Neck Muscle, Right
Suprainguinal lymph node *use* Lymphatic, Pelvis

Supraorbital vein
  use Face Vein, Left
  use Face Vein, Right
Suprarenal gland
  use Adrenal Gland
  use Adrenal Gland, Bilateral
  use Adrenal Gland, Left
  use Adrenal Gland, Right
Suprarenal plexus *use* Abdominal Sympathetic Nerve
Suprascapular nerve *use* Brachial Plexus
Supraspinatus fascia
  use Subcutaneous Tissue and Fascia, Left Upper Arm
  use Subcutaneous Tissue and Fascia, Right Upper Arm
Supraspinatus muscle
  use Shoulder Muscle, Left
  use Shoulder Muscle, Right
Supraspinous ligament
  use Lower Spine Bursa and Ligament
  use Upper Spine Bursa and Ligament
Suprasternal notch *use* Sternum
Supratrochlear lymph node
  use Lymphatic, Left Upper Extremity
  use Lymphatic, Right Upper Extremity
Sural artery
  use Popliteal Artery, Left
  use Popliteal Artery, Right
Surpass Streamline™ Flow Diverter *use* Intraluminal Device, Flow Diverter in 03V
Suspension
  Bladder Neck *see* Reposition, Bladder Neck 0TSC
  Kidney *see* Reposition, Urinary System 0TS
  Urethra *see* Reposition, Urinary System 0TS
  Urethrovesical *see* Reposition, Bladder Neck 0TSC
  Uterus *see* Reposition, Uterus 0US9
  Vagina *see* Reposition, Vagina 0USG
Suture
  Laceration repair *see* Repair
  Ligation *see* Occlusion
Suture Removal
  Extremity
    Lower 8E0YXY8
    Upper 8E0XXY8
  Head and Neck Region 8E09XY8
  Trunk Region 8E0WXY8
Sutureless valve, Perceval (rapid deployment technique) *see* Replacement, Valve, Aortic 02RF
Sweat gland *use* Skin
Sympathectomy *see* Excision, Peripheral Nervous System 01B
Symplicity Spyral™ Renal Denervation System X05133A
SynCardia (temporary) total artificial heart (TAH)
  use Synthetic Substitute, Pneumatic in 02R
SynCardia Total Artificial Heart *use* Synthetic Substitute
SynchroMed pump *use* Infusion Device, Pump in Subcutaneous Tissue and Fascia
Syncra CRT-P *use* Cardiac Resynchronization Pacemaker Pulse Generator in 0JH
Synechiotomy, iris *see* Release, Eye 08N
Synovectomy
  Lower joint *see* Excision, Lower Joints 0SB
  Upper joint *see* Excision, Upper Joints 0RB
Systemic Nuclear Medicine Therapy
  Abdomen CW70
  Anatomical Regions, Multiple CW7YYZZ
  Chest CW73
  Thyroid CW7G
  Whole Body CW7N

T

tab-cel® *use* Tabelecleucel Immunotherapy
Tabelecleucel Immunotherapy XW0
Tagraxofusp-erzs Antineoplastic XW0
Takedown
  Arteriovenous shunt *see* Removal of device from, Upper Arteries 03P
  Arteriovenous shunt, with creation of new shunt *see* Bypass, Upper Arteries 031
  Stoma
    see Excision
    see Reposition
Talent® Converter *use* Intraluminal Device

Talent® Occluder use Intraluminal Device
Talent® Stent Graft (abdominal) (thoracic) use Intraluminal Device
Talocalcaneal (subtalar) joint
  use Tarsal Joint, Left
  use Tarsal Joint, Right
Talocalcaneal ligament
  use Foot Bursa and Ligament, Left
  use Foot Bursa and Ligament, Right
Talocalcaneonavicular joint
  use Tarsal Joint, Left
  use Tarsal Joint, Right
Talocalcaneonavicular ligament
  use Foot Bursa and Ligament, Left
  use Foot Bursa and Ligament, Right
Talocrural joint
  use Ankle Joint, Left
  use Joint, Ankle, Right
Talofibular ligament
  use Ankle Bursa and Ligament, Left
  use Ankle Bursa and Ligament, Right
Talquetamab Antineoplastic XW01329
Talus bone
  use Tarsal, Left
  use Tarsal, Right
TALVEY™ use Talquetamab Antineoplastic
TAMBE Device (Thoracoabdominal Branch Endoprosthesis), GORE® EXCLUDER® use Branched Intraluminal Device, Manufactured Integrated System, Four or More Arteries in New Technology
TandemHeart® System use Short-term External Heart Assist System in Heart and Great Vessels
Tarsectomy
  see Excision, Lower Bones 0QB
  see Resection, Lower Bones 0QT
Tarsometatarsal ligament
  use Foot Bursa and Ligament, Left
  use Foot Bursa and Ligament, Right
Tarsorrhaphy see Repair, Eye 08Q
Tattooing
  Cornea 3E0CXMZ
  Skin see Introduction of substance in or on, Skin 3E00
Taurolidine Anti-infective and Heparin Anticoagulant XY0YX28
TAXUS® Liberte® Paclitaxel-eluting Coronary Stent System use Intraluminal Device, Drug-eluting in Heart and Great Vessels
TBNA (transbronchial needle aspiration)
  Fluid or gas see Drainage, Respiratory System 0B9
  Tissue biopsy see Extraction, Respiratory System 0BD
T-cell Antigen Coupler T-cell (TAC-T) Therapy use Non-Chimeric Antigen Receptor T-cell Immune Effector Cell Therapy
T-cell Receptor-Engineered T-cell (TCR-T) Therapy use Non-Chimeric Antigen Receptor T-cell Immune Effector Cell Therapy
Tecartus™ use Brexucabtagene Autoleucel Immunotherapy
TECENTRIQ® use Atezolizumab Antineoplastic
Teclistamab Antineoplastic XW01348
TECVAYLI™ use Teclistamab Antineoplastic
Telemetry 4A12X4Z
  Ambulatory 4A12X45
Temperature gradient study 4A0ZXKZ
Temperature-controlled sEEG radiofrequency ablation 00503Z4
Temporal lobe use Cerebral Hemisphere
Temporalis muscle use Head Muscle
Temporoparietalis muscle use Head Muscle
Tendolysis see Release, Tendons 0LN
Tendonectomy
  see Excision, Tendons 0LB
  see Resection, Tendons 0LT
Tendonoplasty, tenoplasty
  see Repair, Tendons 0LQ
  see Replacement, Tendons 0LR
  see Supplement, Tendons 0LU
Tendorrhaphy see Repair, Tendons 0LQ
Tendototomy
  see Division, Tendons 0L8
  see Drainage, Tendons 0L9
Tenectomy, tenonectomy
  see Excision, Tendons 0LB
  see Resection, Tendons 0LT

Tenolysis see Release, Tendons 0LN
Tenontorrhaphy see Repair, Tendons 0LQ
Tenontotomy
  see Division, Tendons 0L8
  see Drainage, Tendons 0L9
Tenorrhaphy see Repair, Tendons 0LQ
Tenosynovectomy
  see Excision, Tendons 0LB
  see Resection, Tendons 0LT
Tenotomy
  see Division, Tendons 0L8
  see Drainage, Tendons 0L9
Tensor fasciae latae muscle
  use Hip Muscle, Left
  use Hip Muscle, Right
Tensor veli palatini muscle use Tongue, Palate, Pharynx Muscle
Tenth cranial nerve use Vagus Nerve
Tentorium cerebelli use Dura Mater
Teres major muscle
  use Shoulder Muscle, Left
  use Shoulder Muscle, Right
Teres minor muscle
  use Shoulder Muscle, Left
  use Shoulder Muscle, Right
Terlipressin XW0
TERLIVAZ® use Terlipressin
Termination of pregnancy
  Aspiration curettage 10A07ZZ
  Dilation and curettage 10A07ZZ
  Hysterotomy 10A00ZZ
  Intra-amniotic injection 10A03ZZ
  Laminaria 10A07ZW
  Vacuum 10A07Z6
Testectomy
  see Excision, Male Reproductive System 0VB
  see Resection, Male Reproductive System 0VT
Testicular artery use Abdominal Aorta
Testing
  Glaucoma 4A07XBZ
  Hearing see Hearing Assessment, Diagnostic Audiology F13
  Mental health see Psychological Tests
  Muscle function, electromyography (EMG) see Measurement, Musculoskeletal 4A0F
  Muscle function, manual see Motor Function Assessment, Rehabilitation F01
  Neurophysiologic monitoring, intra-operative see Monitoring, Physiological Systems 4A1
  Range of motion see Motor Function Assessment, Rehabilitation F01
  Vestibular function see Vestibular Assessment, Diagnostic Audiology F15
Thalamectomy see Excision, Thalamus 00B9
Thalamotomy see Drainage, Thalamus 0099
Thenar muscle
  use Hand Muscle, Left
  use Hand Muscle, Right
Therapeutic Massage
  Musculoskeletal System 8E0KX1Z
  Reproductive System
    Prostate 8E0VX1C
    Rectum 8E0VX1D
Therapeutic occlusion coil(s) use Intraluminal Device
Thermography 4A0ZXKZ
Thermotherapy, prostate see Destruction, Prostate 0V50
Third cranial nerve use Oculomotor Nerve
Third occipital nerve use Cervical Nerve
Third ventricle use Cerebral Ventricle
Thoracectomy see Excision, Anatomical Regions, General 0WB
Thoracentesis see Drainage, Anatomical Regions, General 0W9
Thoracic aortic plexus use Thoracic Sympathetic Nerve
Thoracic esophagus use Esophagus, Middle
Thoracic facet joint use Thoracic Vertebral Joint
Thoracic ganglion use Thoracic Sympathetic Nerve
Thoracoacromial artery
  use Axillary Artery, Left
  use Axillary Artery, Right
Thoracocentesis see Drainage, Anatomical Regions, General 0W9
Thoracolumbar facet joint use Thoracolumbar Vertebral Joint
Thoracoplasty
  see Repair, Anatomical Regions, General 0WQ

Thoracoplasty — continued
  see Supplement, Anatomical Regions, General 0WU
Thoracostomy, for lung collapse see Drainage, Respiratory System 0B9
Thoracostomy tube use Drainage Device
Thoracotomy
  see Control bleeding in, Mediastinum 0W3C
  see Control bleeding in, Pericardial Cavity 0W3D
  see Drainage, Anatomical Regions, General 0W9
  Exploratory see Inspection, Anatomical Regions, General 0WJ
Thoraflex™ Hybrid device use Branched Synthetic Substitute with Intraluminal Device in New Technology
Thoratec IVAD (Implantable Ventricular Assist Device) use Implantable Heart Assist System in Heart and Great Vessels
Thoratec Paracorporeal Ventricular Assist Device use Short-term External Heart Assist System in Heart and Great Vessels
Thrombectomy see Extirpation
Thrombolysis
  Catheter-directed see Fragmentation
  Systemic see Introduction of substance in or on, Physiological Systems and Anatomical Regions 3E0
  Ultrasound assisted
    see Fragmentation, Artery
    see Fragmentation, Vein
Thymectomy
  see Excision, Lymphatic and Hemic Systems 07B
  see Resection, Lymphatic and Hemic Systems 07T
Thymopexy
  see Repair, Lymphatic and Hemic Systems 07Q
  see Reposition, Lymphatic and Hemic Systems 07S
Thymus gland use Thymus
Thyroarytenoid muscle
  use Neck Muscle, Left
  use Neck Muscle, Right
Thyrocervical trunk
  use Thyroid Artery, Left
  use Thyroid Artery, Right
Thyroid cartilage use Larynx
Thyroidectomy
  see Excision, Endocrine System 0GB
  see Resection, Endocrine System 0GT
Thyroidorrhaphy see Repair, Endocrine System 0GQ
Thyroidoscopy 0GJK4ZZ
Thyroidotomy see Drainage, Endocrine System 0G9
Tibial Extension with Motion Sensors, Insertion XNH
Tibial insert use Liner in Lower Joints
Tibial sesamoid
  use Metatarsal, Left
  use Metatarsal, Right
Tibialis anterior muscle
  use Lower Leg Muscle, Left
  use Lower Leg Muscle, Right
Tibialis posterior muscle
  use Lower Leg Muscle, Left
  use Lower Leg Muscle, Right
Tibiofemoral joint
  use Knee Joint, Left
  use Knee Joint, Right
  use Knee Joint, Tibial Surface, Left
  use Knee Joint, Tibial Surface, Right
Tibioperoneal trunk
  use Popliteal Artery, Left
  use Popliteal Artery, Right
Tisagenlecleucel use Tisagenlecleucel Immunotherapy
Tisagenlecleucel Immunotherapy XW0
Tissue bank graft use Nonautologous Tissue Substitute
Tissue expander (inflatable) (injectable)
  use Tissue Expander in Skin and Breast
  use Tissue Expander in Subcutaneous Tissue and Fascia
Tissue Expander
  Insertion of device in
    Breast
      Bilateral 0HHV
      Left 0HHU
      Right 0HHT
    Nipple
      Left 0HHX
      Right 0HHW
    Subcutaneous Tissue and Fascia
      Abdomen 0JH8

Tissue Expander — *continued*
  Insertion of device in — *continued*
    Subcutaneous Tissue and Fascia — *continued*
      Back 0JH7
      Buttock 0JH9
      Chest 0JH6
      Face 0JH1
      Foot
        Left 0JHR
        Right 0JHQ
      Hand
        Left 0JHK
        Right 0JHJ
      Lower Arm
        Left 0JHH
        Right 0JHG
      Lower Leg
        Left 0JHP
        Right 0JHN
      Neck
        Left 0JH5
        Right 0JH4
      Pelvic Region 0JHC
      Perineum 0JHB
      Scalp 0JH0
      Upper Arm
        Left 0JHF
        Right 0JHD
      Upper Leg
        Left 0JHM
        Right 0JHL
  Removal of device from
    Breast
      Left 0HPU
      Right 0HPT
    Subcutaneous Tissue and Fascia
      Head and Neck 0JPS
      Lower Extremity 0JPW
      Trunk 0JPT
      Upper Extremity 0JPV
  Revision of device in
    Breast
      Left 0HWU
      Right 0HWT
    Subcutaneous Tissue and Fascia
      Head and Neck 0JWS
      Lower Extremity 0JWW
      Trunk 0JWT
      Upper Extremity 0JWV
Tissue Plasminogen Activator (tPA) (r-tPA) *use* Other Thrombolytic
Titan Endoskeleton™
  use Interbody Fusion Device in Lower Joints
  use Interbody Fusion Device in Upper Joints
Titanium Sternal Fixation System (TSFS)
  use Internal Fixation Device, Rigid Plate in 0PS
  use Internal Fixation Device, Rigid Plate in 0PH
Tixagevimab and Cilgavimab Monoclonal Antibody XW023X7
Tocilizumab XW0
Tomographic (Tomo) Nuclear Medicine Imaging
  Abdomen CW20
  Abdomen and Chest CW24
  Abdomen and Pelvis CW21
  Anatomical Regions, Multiple CW2YYZZ
  Bladder, Kidneys and Ureters CT23
  Brain C020
  Breast CH2YYZZ
    Bilateral CH22
    Left CH21
    Right CH20
  Bronchi and Lungs CB22
  Central Nervous System C02YYZZ
  Cerebrospinal Fluid C025
  Chest CW23
  Chest and Abdomen CW24
  Chest and Neck CW26
  Digestive System CD2YYZZ
  Endocrine System CG2YYZZ
  Extremity
    Lower CW2D
      Bilateral CP2F
      Left CP2D
      Right CP2C
    Upper CW2M
      Bilateral CP2B
      Left CP29

Tomographic (Tomo) Nuclear Medicine Imaging — *continued*
  Extremity — *continued*
    Upper — *continued*
      Right CP28
  Gallbladder CF24
  Gastrointestinal Tract CD27
  Gland, Parathyroid CG21
  Head and Neck CW2B
  Heart C22YYZZ
    Right and Left C226
  Hepatobiliary System and Pancreas CF2YYZZ
  Kidneys, Ureters and Bladder CT23
  Liver CF25
  Liver and Spleen CF26
  Lungs and Bronchi CB22
  Lymphatics and Hematologic System C72YYZZ
  Musculoskeletal System, Other CP2YYZZ
  Myocardium C22G
  Neck and Chest CW26
  Neck and Head CW2B
  Pancreas and Hepatobiliary System CF2YYZZ
  Pelvic Region CW2J
  Pelvis CP26
  Pelvis and Abdomen CW21
  Pelvis and Spine CP27
  Respiratory System CB2YYZZ
  Skin CH2YYZZ
  Skull CP21
  Skull and Cervical Spine CP23
  Spine
    Cervical CP22
    Cervical and Skull CP23
    Lumbar CP2H
    Thoracic CP2G
    Thoracolumbar CP2J
  Spine and Pelvis CP27
  Spleen C722
  Spleen and Liver CF26
  Subcutaneous Tissue CH2YYZZ
  Thorax CP24
  Ureters, Kidneys and Bladder CT23
  Urinary System CT2YYZZ
Tomography, computerized *see* Computerized Tomography (CT Scan)
Tongue, base of *use* Pharynx
Tonometry 4A07XBZ
Tonsillectomy
  see Excision, Mouth and Throat 0CB
  see Resection, Mouth and Throat 0CT
Tonsillotomy *see* Drainage, Mouth and Throat 0C9
TOPS™ System *use* Posterior Spinal Motion Preservation Device in New Technology
Total Ankle Talar Replacement™ (TATR) *use* Synthetic Substitute, Talar Prosthesis in New Technology
Total Anomalous Pulmonary Venous Return (TAPVR) repair
  see Bypass, Atrium, Left 0217
  see Bypass, Vena Cava, Superior 021V
Total artificial (replacement) heart *use* Synthetic Substitute
Total parenteral nutrition (TPN) *see* Introduction of Nutritional Substance
Tourniquet, External *see* Compression, Anatomical Regions 2W1
Trachectomy
  see Excision, Trachea 0BB1
  see Resection, Trachea 0BT1
Trachelectomy
  see Excision, Cervix 0UBC
  see Resection, Cervix 0UTC
Trachelopexy
  see Repair, Cervix 0UQC
  see Reposition, Cervix 0USC
Tracheloplasty *see* Repair, Cervix 0UQC
Trachelorrhaphy *see* Repair, Cervix 0UQC
Trachelotomy *see* Drainage, Cervix 0U9C
Tracheobronchial lymph node *use* Lymphatic, Thorax
Tracheoesophageal fistulization 0B110D6
Tracheoesophageal Puncture (TEP) 0B110D6
Tracheolysis *see* Release, Respiratory System 0BN
Tracheoplasty
  see Repair, Respiratory System 0BQ
  see Supplement, Respiratory System 0BU
Tracheorrhaphy *see* Repair, Respiratory System 0BQ
Tracheoscopy 0BJ18ZZ
Tracheostomy *see* Bypass, Respiratory System 0B1

Tracheostomy Device
  Bypass, Trachea 0B11
  Change device in, Trachea 0B21XFZ
  Removal of device from, Trachea 0BP1
  Revision of device in, Trachea 0BW1
Tracheostomy tube *use* Tracheostomy Device in Respiratory System
Tracheotomy *see* Drainage, Respiratory System 0B9
Traction
  Abdominal Wall 2W63X
  Arm
    Lower
      Left 2W6DX
      Right 2W6CX
    Upper
      Left 2W6BX
      Right 2W6AX
  Back 2W65X
  Chest Wall 2W64X
  Extremity
    Lower
      Left 2W6MX
      Right 2W6LX
    Upper
      Left 2W69X
      Right 2W68X
  Face 2W61X
  Finger
    Left 2W6KX
    Right 2W6JX
  Foot
    Left 2W6TX
    Right 2W6SX
  Hand
    Left 2W6FX
    Right 2W6EX
  Head 2W60X
  Inguinal Region
    Left 2W67X
    Right 2W66X
  Leg
    Lower
      Left 2W6RX
      Right 2W6QX
    Upper
      Left 2W6PX
      Right 2W6NX
  Neck 2W62X
  Thumb
    Left 2W6HX
    Right 2W6GX
  Toe
    Left 2W6VX
    Right 2W6UX
Tractotomy *see* Division, Central Nervous System and Cranial Nerves 008
Tragus
  use External Ear, Bilateral
  use External Ear, Left
  use External Ear, Right
Training, caregiver *see* Caregiver Training
TRAM (transverse rectus abdominis myocutaneous) flap reconstruction
  Free *see* Replacement, Skin and Breast 0HR
  Pedicled *see* Transfer, Muscles 0KX
Transcatheter Pulmonary Valve (TPV) placement
  In conduit 02RH38L
  Native site 02RH38M
Transcatheter tricuspid valve replacement
  EVOQUE valve/system (Edwards) X2RJ3RA
  Other valve/system 02RJ38Z
Transdermal Glomerular Filtration Rate (GFR) Measurement System XT25XE5
Transection *see* Division
Transfer
  Buccal Mucosa 0CX4
  Bursa and Ligament
    Abdomen
      Left 0MXJ
      Right 0MXH
    Ankle
      Left 0MXR
      Right 0MXQ
    Elbow
      Left 0MX4
      Right 0MX3
    Foot
      Left 0MXT

Transfer — continued
  Bursa and Ligament — continued
    Foot — continued
      Right 0MXS
    Hand
      Left 0MX8
      Right 0MX7
    Head and Neck 0MX0
    Hip
      Left 0MXM
      Right 0MXL
    Knee
      Left 0MXP
      Right 0MXN
    Lower Extremity
      Left 0MXW
      Right 0MXV
    Perineum 0MXK
    Rib(s) 0MXG
    Shoulder
      Left 0MX2
      Right 0MX1
    Spine
      Lower 0MXD
      Upper 0MXC
    Sternum 0MXF
    Upper Extremity
      Left 0MXB
      Right 0MX9
    Wrist
      Left 0MX6
      Right 0MX5
  Finger
    Left 0XXP0ZM
    Right 0XXN0ZL
  Gingiva
    Lower 0CX6
    Upper 0CX5
  Intestine
    Large 0DXE
    Small 0DX8
  Lip
    Lower 0CX1
    Upper 0CX0
  Muscle
    Abdomen
      Left 0KXL
      Right 0KXK
    Extraocular
      Left 08XM
      Right 08XL
    Facial 0KX1
    Foot
      Left 0KXW
      Right 0KXV
    Hand
      Left 0KXD
      Right 0KXC
    Head 0KX0
    Hip
      Left 0KXP
      Right 0KXN
    Lower Arm and Wrist
      Left 0KXB
      Right 0KX9
    Lower Leg
      Left 0KXT
      Right 0KXS
    Neck
      Left 0KX3
      Right 0KX2
    Perineum 0KXM
    Shoulder
      Left 0KX6
      Right 0KX5
    Thorax
      Left 0KXJ
      Right 0KXH
    Tongue, Palate, Pharynx 0KX4
    Trunk
      Left 0KXG
      Right 0KXF
    Upper Arm
      Left 0KX8
      Right 0KX7
    Upper Leg
      Left 0KXR
      Right 0KXQ

Transfer — continued
  Nerve
    Abducens 00XL
    Accessory 00XR
    Acoustic 00XN
    Cervical 01X1
    Facial 00XM
    Femoral 01XD
    Glossopharyngeal 00XP
    Hypoglossal 00XS
    Lumbar 01XB
    Median 01X5
    Oculomotor 00XH
    Olfactory 00XF
    Optic 00XG
    Peroneal 01XH
    Phrenic 01X2
    Pudendal 01XC
    Radial 01X6
    Sciatic 01XF
    Thoracic 01X8
    Tibial 01XG
    Trigeminal 00XK
    Trochlear 00XJ
    Ulnar 01X4
    Vagus 00XQ
  Omentum 0DXU
  Palate, Soft 0CX3
  Prepuce 0VXT
  Skin
    Abdomen 0HX7XZZ
    Back 0HX6XZZ
    Buttock 0HX8XZZ
    Chest 0HX5XZZ
    Ear
      Left 0HX3XZZ
      Right 0HX2XZZ
    Face 0HX1XZZ
    Foot
      Left 0HXNXZZ
      Right 0HXMXZZ
    Hand
      Left 0HXGXZZ
      Right 0HXFXZZ
    Inguinal 0HXAXZZ
    Lower Arm
      Left 0HXEXZZ
      Right 0HXDXZZ
    Lower Leg
      Left 0HXLXZZ
      Right 0HXKXZZ
    Neck 0HX4XZZ
    Perineum 0HX9XZZ
    Scalp 0HX0XZZ
    Upper Arm
      Left 0HXCXZZ
      Right 0HXBXZZ
    Upper Leg
      Left 0HXJXZZ
      Right 0HXHXZZ
  Stomach 0DX6
  Subcutaneous Tissue and Fascia
    Abdomen 0JX8
    Back 0JX7
    Buttock 0JX9
    Chest 0JX6
    Face 0JX1
    Foot
      Left 0JXR
      Right 0JXQ
    Hand
      Left 0JXK
      Right 0JXJ
    Lower Arm
      Left 0JXH
      Right 0JXG
    Lower Leg
      Left 0JXP
      Right 0JXN
    Neck
      Left 0JX5
      Right 0JX4
    Pelvic Region 0JXC
    Perineum 0JXB
    Scalp 0JX0
    Upper Arm
      Left 0JXF
      Right 0JXD

Transfer — continued
  Subcutaneous Tissue and Fascia — continued
    Upper Leg
      Left 0JXM
      Right 0JXL
  Tendon
    Abdomen
      Left 0LXG
      Right 0LXF
    Ankle
      Left 0LXT
      Right 0LXS
    Foot
      Left 0LXW
      Right 0LXV
    Hand
      Left 0LX8
      Right 0LX7
    Head and Neck 0LX0
    Hip
      Left 0LXK
      Right 0LXJ
    Knee
      Left 0LXR
      Right 0LXQ
    Lower Arm and Wrist
      Left 0LX6
      Right 0LX5
    Lower Leg
      Left 0LXP
      Right 0LXN
    Perineum 0LXH
    Shoulder
      Left 0LX2
      Right 0LX1
    Thorax
      Left 0LXD
      Right 0LXC
    Trunk
      Left 0LXB
      Right 0LX9
    Upper Arm
      Left 0LX4
      Right 0LX3
    Upper Leg
      Left 0LXM
      Right 0LXL
  Tongue 0CX7
Transfusion
  Bone Marrow
    Blood
      Platelets 302A3R
      Red Cells 302A3N
        Frozen 302A3P
      Whole 302A3H
    Plasma
      Fresh 302A3L
      Frozen 302A3K
    Serum Albumin 302A3J
  New Technology see New Technology, Anatomical Regions XW1
  Products of Conception
    Antihemophilic Factors 3027
    Blood
      Platelets 3027
      Red Cells 3027
        Frozen 3027
      White Cells 3027
      Whole 3027
    Factor IX 3027
    Fibrinogen 3027
    Globulin 3027
    Plasma
      Fresh 3027
      Frozen 3027
    Plasma Cryoprecipitate 3027
    Serum Albumin 3027
  Vein
    4-Factor Prothrombin Complex Concentrate 30283B1
    Central
      Antihemophilic Factors 30243V
      Blood
        Platelets 30243R
        Red Cells 30243N
          Frozen 30243P
        White Cells 30243Q
        Whole 30243H
      Bone Marrow 30243G

Transfusion — continued
　Vein — continued
　　Central — continued
　　　Factor IX 30243W
　　　Fibrinogen 30243T
　　　Globulin 30243S
　　　Hematopoietic Stem/Progenitor Cells (HSPC), Genetically Modified 30243C0
　　　Pathogen Reduced Cryoprecipitated Fibrinogen Complex 30243D1
　　　Plasma
　　　　Fresh 30243L
　　　　Frozen 30243K
　　　Plasma Cryoprecipitate 30243M
　　　Serum Albumin 30243J
　　　Stem Cells
　　　　Cord Blood 30243X
　　　　Embryonic 30243AZ
　　　　Hematopoietic 30243Y
　　　　T-cell Depleted Hematopoietic 30243U
　　Peripheral
　　　Antihemophilic Factors 30233V
　　　Blood
　　　　Platelets 30233R
　　　　Red Cells 30233N
　　　　　Frozen 30233P
　　　　White Cells 30233Q
　　　　Whole 30233H
　　　Bone Marrow 30233G
　　　Factor IX 30233W
　　　Fibrinogen 30233T
　　　Globulin 30233S
　　　Hematopoietic Stem/Progenitor Cells (HSPC), Genetically Modified 30233C0
　　　Pathogen Reduced Cryoprecipitated Fibrinogen Complex 30233D1
　　　Plasma
　　　　Fresh 30233L
　　　　Frozen 30233K
　　　Plasma Cryoprecipitate 30233M
　　　Serum Albumin 30233J
　　　Stem Cells
　　　　Cord Blood 30233X
　　　　Embryonic 30233AZ
　　　　Hematopoietic 30233Y
　　　　T-cell Depleted Hematopoietic 30233U
Transplant *see* Transplantation
Transplantation
　Bone marrow
　　see Transfusion, Vein, Central 30243G
　　see Transfusion, Vein, Peripheral 30233G
　Esophagus 0DY50Z
　Face 0WY20Z
　Hand
　　Left 0XYK0Z
　　Right 0XYJ0Z
　Heart 02YA0Z
　Hematopoietic cell *see* Transfusion, Circulatory 302
　Intestine
　　Large 0DYE0Z
　　Small 0DY80Z
　Kidney
　　Left 0TY10Z
　　Right 0TY00Z
　Liver 0FY00Z
　Lung
　　Bilateral 0BYM0Z
　　Left 0BYL0Z
　　Lower Lobe
　　　Left 0BYJ0Z
　　　Right 0BYF0Z
　　Middle Lobe, Right 0BYD0Z
　　Right 0BYK0Z
　　Upper Lobe
　　　Left 0BYG0Z
　　　Right 0BYC0Z
　Lung Lingula 0BYH0Z
　Ovary
　　Left 0UY10Z
　　Right 0UY00Z
　Pancreas 0FYG0Z
　Penis 0VYS0Z
　Products of Conception 10Y0
　Scrotum 0VY50Z

Transplantation — continued
　Spleen 07YP0Z
　Stem cell *see* Transfusion, Circulatory 302
　Stomach 0DY60Z
　Thymus 07YM0Z
　Uterus 0UY90Z
Transposition
　see Bypass
　see Reposition
　see Transfer
Transversalis fascia *use* Subcutaneous Tissue and Fascia, Trunk
Transverse acetabular ligament
　use Hip Bursa and Ligament, Left
　use Hip Bursa and Ligament, Right
Transverse (cutaneous) cervical nerve *use* Cervical Plexus
Transverse facial artery
　use Temporal Artery, Left
　use Temporal Artery, Right
Transverse foramen *use* Cervical Vertebra
Transverse humeral ligament
　use Shoulder Bursa and Ligament, Left
　use Shoulder Bursa and Ligament, Right
Transverse ligament of atlas *use* Head and Neck Bursa and Ligament
Transverse process
　use Cervical Vertebra
　use Lumbar Vertebra
　use Thoracic Vertebra
Transverse Rectus Abdominis Myocutaneous Flap
　Replacement
　　Bilateral 0HRV076
　　Left 0HRU076
　　Right 0HRT076
　Transfer
　　Left 0KXL
　　Right 0KXK
Transverse scapular ligament
　use Shoulder Bursa and Ligament, Left
　use Shoulder Bursa and Ligament, Right
Transverse thoracis muscle
　use Thorax Muscle, Left
　use Thorax Muscle, Right
Transversospinalis muscle
　use Trunk Muscle, Left
　use Trunk Muscle, Right
Transversus abdominis muscle
　use Abdomen Muscle, Left
　use Abdomen Muscle, Right
Trapezium bone
　use Carpal, Left
　use Carpal, Right
Trapezius muscle
　use Trunk Muscle, Left
　use Trunk Muscle, Right
Trapezoid bone
　use Carpal, Left
　use Carpal, Right
Treosulfan XW0
Triceps brachii muscle
　use Upper Arm Muscle, Left
　use Upper Arm Muscle, Right
Tricuspid annulus *use* Tricuspid Valve
TricValve® Transcatheter Bicaval Valve System *use* Intraluminal Device, Bioprosthetic Valve in New Technology
Trifacial nerve *use* Trigeminal Nerve
Trifecta™ Valve (aortic) *use* Zooplastic Tissue in Heart and Great Vessels
Trigone of bladder *use* Bladder
TriGuard 3™ CEPD (cerebral embolic protection device) X2A6325
Trilaciclib XW0
Trimming, excisional *see* Excision
Triquetral bone
　use Carpal, Left
　use Carpal, Right
Trochanteric bursa
　use Hip Bursa and Ligament, Left
　use Hip Bursa and Ligament, Right
TTVR *see* Transcatheter tricuspid valve replacement
Tumor-Infiltrating Lymphocyte (TIL) Therapy *use* Non-Chimeric Antigen Receptor T-cell Immune Effector Cell Therapy
TUMT (transurethral microwave thermotherapy of prostate) 0V507ZZ

TUNA (transurethral needle ablation of prostate) 0V507ZZ
Tunneled central venous catheter *use* Vascular Access Device, Tunneled in Subcutaneous Tissue and Fascia
Tunneled spinal (intrathecal) catheter *use* Infusion Device
Turbinectomy
　see Excision, Ear, Nose, Sinus 09B
　see Resection, Ear, Nose, Sinus 09T
Turbinoplasty
　see Repair, Ear, Nose, Sinus 09Q
　see Replacement, Ear, Nose, Sinus 09R
　see Supplement, Ear, Nose, Sinus 09U
Turbinotomy
　see Division, Ear, Nose, Sinus 098
　see Drainage, Ear, Nose, Sinus 099
TURP (transurethral resection of prostate) 0VB07ZZ
　see Excision, Prostate 0VB0
　see Resection, Prostate 0VT0
Twelfth cranial nerve *use* Hypoglossal Nerve
Two lead pacemaker *use* Pacemaker, Dual Chamber in 0JH
Tympanic cavity
　use Middle Ear, Left
　use Middle Ear, Right
Tympanic nerve *use* Glossopharyngeal Nerve
Tympanic part of temporal bone
　use Temporal Bone, Left
　use Temporal Bone, Right
Tympanogram *see* Hearing Assessment, Diagnostic Audiology F13
Tympanoplasty
　see Repair, Ear, Nose, Sinus 09Q
　see Replacement, Ear, Nose, Sinus 09R
　see Supplement, Ear, Nose, Sinus 09U
Tympanosympathectomy *see* Excision, Nerve, Head and Neck Sympathetic 01BK
Tympanotomy *see* Drainage, Ear, Nose, Sinus 099
TYRX Antibacterial Envelope *use* Anti-Infective Envelope

U

Ulnar collateral carpal ligament
　use Wrist Bursa and Ligament, Left
　use Wrist Bursa and Ligament, Right
Ulnar collateral ligament
　use Elbow Bursa and Ligament, Left
　use Elbow Bursa and Ligament, Right
Ulnar notch
　use Radius, Left
　use Radius, Right
Ulnar vein
　use Brachial Vein, Left
　use Brachial Vein, Right
Ultrafiltration
　Hemodialysis *see* Performance, Urinary 5A1D
　Therapeutic plasmapheresis *see* Pheresis, Circulatory 6A55
Ultraflex™ Precision Colonic Stent System *use* Intraluminal Device
ULTRAPRO Hernia System (UHS) *use* Synthetic Substitute
ULTRAPRO Partially Absorbable Lightweight Mesh *use* Synthetic Substitute
ULTRAPRO Plug *use* Synthetic Substitute
Ultrasonic osteogenic stimulator
　use Bone Growth Stimulator in Head and Facial Bones
　use Bone Growth Stimulator in Lower Bones
　use Bone Growth Stimulator in Upper Bones
Ultrasonography
　Abdomen BW40ZZZ
　Abdomen and Pelvis BW41ZZZ
　Abdominal Wall BH49ZZZ
　Aorta
　　Abdominal, Intravascular B440ZZ3
　　Thoracic, Intravascular B340ZZ3
　Appendix BD48ZZZ
　Artery
　　Brachiocephalic-Subclavian, Right, Intravascular B341ZZ3
　　Celiac and Mesenteric, Intravascular B44KZZ3
　　Common Carotid
　　　Bilateral, Intravascular B345ZZ3

Ultrasonography — continued
  Artery — continued
    Common Carotid — continued
      Left, Intravascular B344ZZ3
      Right, Intravascular B343ZZ3
    Coronary
      Multiple B241YZZ
        Intravascular B241ZZ3
        Transesophageal B241ZZ4
      Single B240YZZ
        Intravascular B240ZZ3
        Transesophageal B240ZZ4
    Femoral, Intravascular B44LZZ3
    Inferior Mesenteric, Intravascular B445ZZ3
    Internal Carotid
      Bilateral, Intravascular B348ZZ3
      Left, Intravascular B347ZZ3
      Right, Intravascular B346ZZ3
    Intra-Abdominal, Other, Intravascular B44BZZ3
    Intracranial, Intravascular B34RZZ3
    Lower Extremity
      Bilateral, Intravascular B44HZZ3
      Left, Intravascular B44GZZ3
      Right, Intravascular B44FZZ3
    Mesenteric and Celiac, Intravascular B44KZZ3
    Ophthalmic, Intravascular B34VZZ3
    Penile, Intravascular B44NZZ3
    Pulmonary
      Left, Intravascular B34TZZ3
      Right, Intravascular B34SZZ3
    Renal
      Bilateral, Intravascular B448ZZ3
      Left, Intravascular B447ZZ3
      Right, Intravascular B446ZZ3
    Subclavian, Left, Intravascular B342ZZ3
    Superior Mesenteric, Intravascular B444ZZ3
    Upper Extremity
      Bilateral, Intravascular B34KZZ3
      Left, Intravascular B34JZZ3
      Right, Intravascular B34HZZ3
  Bile Duct BF40ZZZ
  Bile Duct and Gallbladder BF43ZZZ
  Bladder BT40ZZZ
    and Kidney BT4JZZZ
  Brain B040ZZZ
  Breast
    Bilateral BH42ZZZ
    Left BH41ZZZ
    Right BH40ZZZ
  Chest Wall BH4BZZZ
  Coccyx BR4FZZZ
  Connective Tissue
    Lower Extremity BL41ZZZ
    Upper Extremity BL40ZZZ
  Duodenum BD49ZZZ
  Elbow
    Left, Densitometry BP4HZZ1
    Right, Densitometry BP4GZZ1
  Esophagus BD41ZZZ
  Extremity
    Lower BH48ZZZ
    Upper BH47ZZZ
  Eye
    Bilateral B847ZZZ
    Left B846ZZZ
    Right B845ZZZ
  Fallopian Tube
    Bilateral BU42
    Left BU41
    Right BU40
  Fetal Umbilical Cord BY47ZZZ
  Fetus
    First Trimester, Multiple Gestation BY4BZZZ
    Second Trimester, Multiple Gestation BY4DZZZ
    Single
      First Trimester BY49ZZZ
      Second Trimester BY4CZZZ
      Third Trimester BY4FZZZ
    Third Trimester, Multiple Gestation BY4GZZZ
  Gallbladder BF42ZZZ
  Gallbladder and Bile Duct BF43ZZZ
  Gastrointestinal Tract BD47ZZZ
  Gland
    Adrenal
      Bilateral BG42ZZZ
      Left BG41ZZZ
      Right BG40ZZZ

Ultrasonography — continued
  Gland — continued
    Parathyroid BG43ZZZ
    Thyroid BG44ZZZ
  Hand
    Left, Densitometry BP4PZZ1
    Right, Densitometry BP4NZZ1
  Head and Neck BH4CZZZ
  Heart
    Left B245YZZ
      Intravascular B245ZZ3
      Transesophageal B245ZZ4
    Pediatric B24DYZZ
      Intravascular B24DZZ3
      Transesophageal B24DZZ4
    Right B244YZZ
      Intravascular B244ZZ3
      Transesophageal B244ZZ4
    Right and Left B246YZZ
      Intravascular B246ZZ3
      Transesophageal B246ZZ4
  Heart with Aorta B24BYZZ
    Intravascular B24BZZ3
    Transesophageal B24BZZ4
  Hepatobiliary System, All BF4CZZZ
  Hip
    Bilateral BQ42ZZZ
    Left BQ41ZZZ
    Right BQ40ZZZ
  Kidney
    and Bladder BT4JZZZ
    Bilateral BT43ZZZ
    Left BT42ZZZ
    Right BT41ZZZ
    Transplant BT49ZZZ
  Knee
    Bilateral BQ49ZZZ
    Left BQ48ZZZ
    Right BQ47ZZZ
  Liver BF45ZZZ
  Liver and Spleen BF46ZZZ
  Mediastinum BB4CZZZ
  Neck BW4FZZZ
  Ovary
    Bilateral BU45
    Left BU44
    Right BU43
  Ovary and Uterus BU4C
  Pancreas BF47ZZZ
  Pelvic Region BW4GZZZ
  Pelvis and Abdomen BW41ZZZ
  Penis BV4BZZZ
  Pericardium B24CYZZ
    Intravascular B24CZZ3
    Transesophageal B24CZZ4
  Placenta BY48ZZZ
  Pleura BB4BZZZ
  Prostate and Seminal Vesicle BV49ZZZ
  Rectum BD4CZZZ
  Sacrum BR4FZZZ
  Scrotum BV44ZZZ
  Seminal Vesicle and Prostate BV49ZZZ
  Shoulder
    Left, Densitometry BP49ZZ1
    Right, Densitometry BP48ZZ1
  Spinal Cord B04BZZZ
  Spine
    Cervical BR40ZZZ
    Lumbar BR49ZZZ
    Thoracic BR47ZZZ
  Spleen and Liver BF46ZZZ
  Stomach BD42ZZZ
  Tendon
    Lower Extremity BL43ZZZ
    Upper Extremity BL42ZZZ
  Ureter
    Bilateral BT48ZZZ
    Left BT47ZZZ
    Right BT46ZZZ
  Urethra BT45ZZZ
  Uterus BU46
  Uterus and Ovary BU4C
  Vein
    Jugular
      Left, Intravascular B544ZZ3
      Right, Intravascular B543ZZ3
    Lower Extremity
      Bilateral, Intravascular B54DZZ3
      Left, Intravascular B54CZZ3

Ultrasonography — continued
  Vein — continued
    Lower Extremity — continued
      Right, Intravascular B54BZZ3
    Portal, Intravascular B54TZZ3
    Renal
      Bilateral, Intravascular B54LZZ3
      Left, Intravascular B54KZZ3
      Right, Intravascular B54JZZ3
    Splanchnic, Intravascular B54TZZ3
    Subclavian
      Left, Intravascular B547ZZ3
      Right, Intravascular B546ZZ3
    Upper Extremity
      Bilateral, Intravascular B54PZZ3
      Left, Intravascular B54NZZ3
      Right, Intravascular B54MZZ3
    Vena Cava
      Inferior, Intravascular B549ZZ3
      Superior, Intravascular B548ZZ3
  Wrist
    Left, Densitometry BP4MZZ1
    Right, Densitometry BP4LZZ1

Ultrasound Ablation, Destruction, Renal Sympathetic Nerve(s) X051329

Ultrasound bone healing system
  use Bone Growth Stimulator in Head and Facial Bones
  use Bone Growth Stimulator in Lower Bones
  use Bone Growth Stimulator in Upper Bones

Ultrasound Penetrable Synthetic Substitute, Skull XNR80D9

Ultrasound Therapy
  Heart 6A75
  No Qualifier 6A75
  Vessels
    Head and Neck 6A75
    Other 6A75
    Peripheral 6A75

Ultraviolet Light Therapy, Skin 6A80

Umbilical artery
  use Internal Iliac Artery, Left
  use Internal Iliac Artery, Right
  use Lower Artery

Uniplanar external fixator
  use External Fixation Device, Monoplanar in 0PH
  use External Fixation Device, Monoplanar in 0PS
  use External Fixation Device, Monoplanar in 0QH
  use External Fixation Device, Monoplanar in 0QS

UPLIZNA® *use* Inebilizumab-cdon

Upper GI series *see* Fluoroscopy, Gastrointestinal, Upper BD15

Ureteral orifice
  use Ureter
  use Ureter, Left
  use Ureter, Right
  use Ureters, Bilateral

Ureterectomy
  see Excision, Urinary System 0TB
  see Resection, Urinary System 0TT

Ureterocolostomy *see* Bypass, Urinary System 0T1
Ureterocystostomy *see* Bypass, Urinary System 0T1
Ureteroenterostomy *see* Bypass, Urinary System 0T1
Ureteroileostomy *see* Bypass, Urinary System 0T1
Ureterolithotomy *see* Extirpation, Urinary System 0TC
Ureterolysis *see* Release, Urinary System 0TN

Ureteroneocystostomy
  see Bypass, Urinary System 0T1
  see Reposition, Urinary System 0TS

Ureteropelvic junction (UPJ)
  use Kidney Pelvis, Left
  use Kidney Pelvis, Right

Ureteropexy
  see Repair, Urinary System 0TQ
  see Reposition, Urinary System 0TS

Ureteroplasty
  see Repair, Urinary System 0TQ
  see Replacement, Urinary System 0TR
  see Supplement, Urinary System 0TU

Ureteroplication *see* Restriction, Urinary System 0TV
Ureteropyelography *see* Fluoroscopy, Urinary System BT1
Ureterorrhaphy *see* Repair, Urinary System 0TQ
Ureteroscopy 0TJ98ZZ

Ureterostomy
  see Bypass, Urinary System 0T1
  see Drainage, Urinary System 0T9

Ureterotomy see Drainage, Urinary System 0T9
Ureteroureterostomy see Bypass, Urinary System 0T1
Ureterovesical orifice
  use Ureter
  use Ureter, Left
  use Ureter, Right
  use Ureters, Bilateral
Urethral catheterization, indwelling 0T9B70Z
Urethrectomy
  see Excision, Urethra 0TBD
  see Resection, Urethra 0TTD
Urethrolithotomy see Extirpation, Urethra 0TCD
Urethrolysis see Release, Urethra 0TND
Urethropexy
  see Repair, Urethra 0TQD
  see Reposition, Urethra 0TSD
Urethroplasty
  see Repair, Urethra 0TQD
  see Replacement, Urethra 0TRD
  see Supplement, Urethra 0TUD
Urethrorrhaphy see Repair, Urethra 0TQD
Urethroscopy 0TJD8ZZ
Urethrotomy see Drainage, Urethra 0T9D
Uridine Triacetate XW0DX82
Urinary incontinence stimulator lead use Stimulator Lead in Urinary System
Urography see Fluoroscopy, Urinary System BT1
Ustekinumab use Other New Technology Therapeutic Substance
Uterine Artery
  use Internal Iliac Artery, Left
  use Internal Iliac Artery, Right
Uterine artery embolization (UAE) see Occlusion, Lower Arteries 04L
Uterine cornu use Uterus
Uterine tube
  use Fallopian Tube, Left
  use Fallopian Tube, Right
Uterine vein
  use Hypogastric Vein, Left
  use Hypogastric Vein, Right
Uvulectomy
  see Excision, Uvula 0CBN
  see Resection, Uvula 0CTN
Uvulorrhaphy see Repair, Uvula 0CQN
Uvulotomy see Drainage, Uvula 0C9N

V

VABOMERE™ (Meropenem-vaborbactam Anti-infective) use Other Anti-infective
Vaccination see Introduction of Serum, Toxoid, and Vaccine
Vacuum extraction, obstetric 10D07Z6
VADER® Pedicle System use Carbon/PEEK Spinal Stabilization Device, Pedicle Based in New Technology
Vaginal artery
  use Internal Iliac Artery, Left
  use Internal Iliac Artery, Right
Vaginal pessary use Intraluminal Device, Pessary in Female Reproductive System
Vaginal vein
  use Hypogastric Vein, Left
  use Hypogastric Vein, Right
Vaginectomy
  see Excision, Vagina 0UBG
  see Resection, Vagina 0UTG
Vaginofixation
  see Repair, Vagina 0UQG
  see Reposition, Vagina 0USG
Vaginoplasty
  see Repair, Vagina 0UQG
  see Supplement, Vagina 0UUG
Vaginorrhaphy see Repair, Vagina 0UQG
Vaginoscopy 0UJH8ZZ
Vaginotomy see Drainage, Female Reproductive System 0U9
Vagotomy see Division, Nerve, Vagus 008Q
Valiant Thoracic Stent Graft use Intraluminal Device
Valvotomy, valvulotomy
  see Division, Heart and Great Vessels 028
  see Release, Heart and Great Vessels 02N
Valvuloplasty
  see Repair, Heart and Great Vessels 02Q
  see Replacement, Heart and Great Vessels 02R

Valvuloplasty — continued
  see Supplement, Heart and Great Vessels 02U
Valvuloplasty, Alfieri Stitch see Restriction, Valve, Mitral 02VG
Vancomycin Hydrochloride and Tobramycin Sulfate Anti-infective, Temporary Irrigation Spacer System XW0U0GA
Vanta™ PC neurostimulator use Stimulator Generator, Multiple Array in 0JH
Vascular Access Device
  Totally Implantable
    Insertion of device in
      Abdomen 0JH8
      Chest 0JH6
      Lower Arm
        Left 0JHH
        Right 0JHG
      Lower Leg
        Left 0JHP
        Right 0JHN
      Upper Arm
        Left 0JHF
        Right 0JHD
      Upper Leg
        Left 0JHM
        Right 0JHL
    Removal of device from
      Lower Extremity 0JPW
      Trunk 0JPT
      Upper Extremity 0JPV
    Revision of device in
      Lower Extremity 0JWW
      Trunk 0JWT
      Upper Extremity 0JWV
  Tunneled
    Insertion of device in
      Abdomen 0JH8
      Chest 0JH6
      Lower Arm
        Left 0JHH
        Right 0JHG
      Lower Leg
        Left 0JHP
        Right 0JHN
      Upper Arm
        Left 0JHF
        Right 0JHD
      Upper Leg
        Left 0JHM
        Right 0JHL
    Removal of device from
      Lower Extremity 0JPW
      Trunk 0JPT
      Upper Extremity 0JPV
    Revision of device in
      Lower Extremity 0JWW
      Trunk 0JWT
      Upper Extremity 0JWV
Vasectomy see Excision, Male Reproductive System 0VB
Vasography
  see Fluoroscopy, Male Reproductive System BV1
  see Plain Radiography, Male Reproductive System BV0
Vasoligation see Occlusion, Male Reproductive System 0VL
Vasorrhaphy see Repair, Male Reproductive System 0VQ
Vasostomy see Bypass, Male Reproductive System 0V1
Vasotomy
  Drainage see Drainage, Male Reproductive System 0V9
  With ligation see Occlusion, Male Reproductive System 0VL
Vasovasostomy see Repair, Male Reproductive System 0VQ
VasQ™ External Support device use Synthetic Substitute, Extraluminal Support Device in New Technology
Vastus intermedius muscle
  use Upper Leg Muscle, Left
  use Upper Leg Muscle, Right
Vastus lateralis muscle
  use Upper Leg Muscle, Left
  use Upper Leg Muscle, Right
Vastus medialis muscle
  use Upper Leg Muscle, Left
  use Upper Leg Muscle, Right

VCG (vectorcardiogram) see Measurement, Cardiac 4A02
Vectra® Vascular Access Graft use Vascular Access Device, Tunneled in Subcutaneous Tissue and Fascia
Vein Graft Extraluminal Support Device(s), Supplement, Coronary Artery/Arteries X2U4079
Veklury use Remdesivir Anti-infective
Venclexta® (Venetoclax Antineoplastic tablets) use Other Antineoplastic
Venectomy
  see Excision, Lower Veins 06B
  see Excision, Upper Veins 05B
Venetoclax Antineoplastic (tablets) use Other Antineoplastic
Venography
  see Fluoroscopy, Veins B51
  see Plain Radiography, Veins B50
Venorrhaphy
  see Repair, Lower Veins 06Q
  see Repair, Upper Veins 05Q
Venotripsy
  see Occlusion, Lower Veins 06L
  see Occlusion, Upper Veins 05L
VenoValve® use Intraluminal Device, Bioprosthetic Valve in New Technology
Veno-venous bypass, during percutaneous thrombectomy 5A05A0L
Veno-venous circuit, during percutaneous thrombectomy 5A05A0L
Ventricular fold use Larynx
Ventriculoatriostomy see Bypass, Central Nervous System and Cranial Nerves 001
Ventriculocisternostomy see Bypass, Central Nervous System and Cranial Nerves 001
Ventriculogram, cardiac
  Combined left and right heart see Fluoroscopy, Heart, Right and Left B216
  Left ventricle see Fluoroscopy, Heart, Left B215
  Right ventricle see Fluoroscopy, Heart, Right B214
Ventriculopuncture, through previously implanted catheter 8C01X6J
Ventriculoscopy 00J04ZZ
Ventriculostomy
  External drainage see Drainage, Cerebral Ventricle 0096
  Internal shunt see Bypass, Cerebral Ventricle 0016
Ventriculovenostomy see Bypass, Cerebral Ventricle 0016
Ventrio™ Hernia Patch use Synthetic Substitute
VEP (visual evoked potential) 4A07X0Z
Vermiform appendix use Appendix
Vermilion border
  use Lower Lip
  use Upper Lip
Versa use Pacemaker, Dual Chamber in 0JH
Version, obstetric
  External 10S0XZZ
  Internal 10S07ZZ
Vertebral arch
  use Cervical Vertebra
  use Lumbar Vertebra
  use Thoracic Vertebra
Vertebral artery, intracranial portion use Intracranial Artery
Vertebral body
  use Cervical Vertebra
  use Lumbar Vertebra
  use Thoracic Vertebra
Vertebral canal use Spinal Canal
Vertebral foramen
  use Cervical Vertebra
  use Lumbar Vertebra
  use Thoracic Vertebra
Vertebral lamina
  use Cervical Vertebra
  use Lumbar Vertebra
  use Thoracic Vertebra
Vertebral pedicle
  use Cervical Vertebra
  use Lumbar Vertebra
  use Thoracic Vertebra
Vesical vein
  use Hypogastric Vein, Left
  use Hypogastric Vein, Right
Vesicotomy see Drainage, Urinary System 0T9

Vesiculectomy
  see Excision, Male Reproductive System ØVB
  see Resection, Male Reproductive System ØVT
Vesiculogram, seminal *see* Plain Radiography, Male Reproductive System BVØ
Vesiculotomy *see* Drainage, Male Reproductive System ØV9
Vestibular Assessment F15Z
Vestibular (Scarpa's) ganglion *use* Acoustic Nerve
Vestibular nerve *use* Acoustic Nerve
Vestibular Treatment FØC
Vestibulocochlear nerve *use* Acoustic Nerve
VEST™ Venous External Support device *use* Vein Graft Extraluminal Support Device(s) in New Technology
VH-IVUS (virtual histology intravascular ultrasound) *see* Ultrasonography, Heart B24
Virchow's (supraclavicular) lymph node
  use Lymphatic, Left Neck
  use Lymphatic, Right Neck
Virtuoso (II) (DR) (VR) *use* Defibrillator Generator in ØJH
Vistogard® *use* Uridine Triacetate
Visualase™ MRI-Guided Laser Ablation System *see* Destruction
VITEK® REVEAL™ Rapid AST System XXE5X4A
Vitrectomy
  see Excision, Eye Ø8B
  see Resection, Eye Ø8T
Vitreous body
  use Vitreous, Left
  use Vitreous, Right
Viva (XT) (S) *use* Cardiac Resynchronization Defibrillator Pulse Generator in ØJH
Vivistim® Paired VNS System Lead *use* Neurostimulator Lead with Paired Stimulation System in New Technology
Vocal fold
  use Vocal Cord, Left
  use Vocal Cord, Right
Vocational
  Assessment *see* Activities of Daily Living Assessment, Rehabilitation FØ2
  Retraining *see* Activities of Daily Living Treatment, Rehabilitation FØ8
Volar (palmar) digital vein
  use Hand Vein, Left
  use Hand Vein, Right
Volar (palmar) metacarpal vein
  use Hand Vein, Left
  use Hand Vein, Right
Vomer bone *use* Nasal Septum
Vomer of nasal septum *use* Nasal Bone
Voraxaze *use* Glucarpidase
VOWST™ *use* SER-109

VT-X7 (Irrigation System) (Spacer) *use* Vancomycin Hydrochloride and Tobramycin Sulfate Anti-infective, Temporary Irrigation Spacer System
Vulvectomy
  see Excision, Female Reproductive System ØUB
  see Resection, Female Reproductive System ØUT
V-Wave Interatrial Shunt System *use* Synthetic Substitute
VYXEOS™ *use* Cytarabine and Daunorubicin Liposome Antineoplastic

W

WALLSTENT® Endoprosthesis *use* Intraluminal Device
Washing *see* Irrigation
WavelinQ EndoAVF system
  Radial Artery, Left Ø31C3ZF
  Radial Artery, Right Ø31B3ZF
  Ulnar Artery, Left Ø31A3ZF
  Ulnar Artery, Right Ø3193ZF
Wedge resection, pulmonary *see* Excision, Respiratory System ØBB
Whole Blood Reverse Transcription and Quantitative Real-time Polymerase Chain Reaction XXE5X38
Window *see* Drainage
Wiring, dental 2W31X9Z

X

Xacduro® *use* Sulbactam-Durlobactam
Xact Carotid Stent System *use* Intraluminal Device
XENLETA™ *use* Lefamulin Anti-infective
Xenograft *use* Zooplastic Tissue in Heart and Great Vessels
XENOVIEW™ BB34Z3Z
XIENCE Everolimus Eluting Coronary Stent System *use* Intraluminal Device, Drug-eluting in Heart and Great Vessels
Xiphoid process *use* Sternum
XLIF® System *use* Interbody Fusion Device in Lower Joints
XOSPATA® (Gilteritinib) *use* Other Antineoplastic
X-ray *see* Plain Radiography
X-Spine Axle Cage
  use Spinal Stabilization Device, Interspinous Process in ØRH
  use Spinal Stabilization Device, Interspinous Process in ØSH
X-STOP® Spacer
  use Spinal Stabilization Device, Interspinous Process in ØRH
  use Spinal Stabilization Device, Interspinous Process in ØSH

Y

Yescarta® *use* Axicabtagene Ciloleucel Immunotherapy
Yoga Therapy 8EØZXY4

Z

Zanidatamab Antineoplastic XWØ
Zenith AAA Endovascular Graft *use* Intraluminal Device
Zenith Flex® AAA Endovascular Graft *use* Intraluminal Device
Zenith TX2® TAA Endovascular Graft *use* Intraluminal Device
Zenith® Fenestrated AAA Endovascular Graft
  use Intraluminal Device, Branched or Fenestrated, One or Two Arteries in Ø4V
  use Intraluminal Device, Branched or Fenestrated, Three or More Arteries in Ø4V
Zenith® Renu™ AAA Ancillary Graft *use* Intraluminal Device
ZEPZELCA™ *use* Lurbinectedin
ZERBAXA® *use* Ceftolozane/Tazobactam Anti-infective
Zilver® PTX® (paclitaxel) Drug-Eluting Peripheral Stent
  use Intraluminal Device, Drug-eluting in Lower Arteries
  use Intraluminal Device, Drug-eluting in Upper Arteries
Zimmer® NexGen® LPS Mobile Bearing Knee *use* Synthetic Substitute
Zimmer® NexGen® LPS-Flex Mobile Knee *use* Synthetic Substitute
ZINPLAVA™ Infusion *see* Introduction with qualifier Other Therapeutic Monoclonal Antibody
Zonule of Zinn
  use Lens, Left
  use Lens, Right
Zotarolimus-eluting Coronary Stent *use* Intraluminal Device, Drug-eluting in Heart and Great Vessels
Z-plasty, skin for scar contracture *see* Release, Skin and Breast ØHN
ZULRESSO™ *use* Brexanolone
Zygomatic process of frontal bone *use* Frontal Bone
Zygomatic process of temporal bone
  use Temporal Bone, Left
  use Temporal Bone, Right
Zygomaticus muscle *use* Facial Muscle
ZYNTEGLO® *use* Betibeglogene Autotemcel
Zyvox *use* Oxazolidinones

ICD-10-PCS Tables

Central Nervous System and Cranial Nerves Ø01–ØØX

Character Meanings

This Character Meaning table is provided as a guide to assist the user in the identification of character members that may be found in this section of code tables. It **SHOULD NOT** be used to build a PCS code.

Operation–Character 3	Body Part–Character 4	Approach–Character 5	Device–Character 6	Qualifier–Character 7
1 Bypass	Ø Brain	Ø Open	Ø Drainage Device	Ø Nasopharynx
2 Change	1 Cerebral Meninges	3 Percutaneous	1 Radioactive Element	1 Mastoid Sinus OR Connectomic Analysis
5 Destruction	2 Dura Mater	4 Percutaneous Endoscopic	2 Monitoring Device	2 Atrium
7 Dilation	3 Epidural Space, Intracranial	X External	3 Infusion Device	3 Blood Vessel OR Laser Interstitial Thermal Therapy
8 Division	4 Subdural Space, Intracranial		4 Radioactive Element, Cesium-131 Collagen Implant	4 Pleural Cavity OR Stereoelectroencephalographic Radiofrequency Ablation
9 Drainage	5 Subarachnoid Space, Intracranial		5 Radioactive Element, Palladium-103 Collagen Implant	5 Intestine
B Excision	6 Cerebral Ventricle		7 Autologous Tissue Substitute	6 Peritoneal Cavity
C Extirpation	7 Cerebral Hemisphere		J Synthetic Substitute	7 Urinary Tract
D Extraction	8 Basal Ganglia		K Nonautologous Tissue Substitute	8 Bone Marrow
F Fragmentation	9 Thalamus		M Neurostimulator Lead	9 Fallopian Tube
H Insertion	A Hypothalamus		Y Other Device	A Subgaleal Space
J Inspection	B Pons		Z No Device	B Cerebral Cisterns
K Map	C Cerebellum			F Olfactory Nerve
N Release	D Medulla Oblongata			G Optic Nerve
P Removal	E Cranial Nerve			H Oculomotor Nerve
Q Repair	F Olfactory Nerve			J Trochlear Nerve
R Replacement	G Optic Nerve			K Trigeminal Nerve
S Reposition	H Oculomotor Nerve			L Abducens Nerve
T Resection	J Trochlear Nerve			M Facial Nerve
U Supplement	K Trigeminal Nerve			N Acoustic Nerve
W Revision	L Abducens Nerve			P Glossopharyngeal Nerve
X Transfer	M Facial Nerve			Q Vagus Nerve
	N Acoustic Nerve			R Accessory Nerve
	P Glossopharyngeal Nerve			S Hypoglossal Nerve
	Q Vagus Nerve			X Diagnostic
	R Accessory Nerve			Z No Qualifier
	S Hypoglossal Nerve			
	T Spinal Meninges			
	U Spinal Canal			
	V Spinal Cord			
	W Cervical Spinal Cord			
	X Thoracic Spinal Cord			
	Y Lumbar Spinal Cord			

Central Nervous System and Cranial Nerves

AHA Coding Clinic for table 001
2021, 2Q, 19	Electromagnetic stealth guided ventriculoperitoneal shunt insertion with endoscopy
2019, 4Q, 21-22	Cerebral ventricle bypass Qualifier
2018, 4Q, 86	Placement of lumboatrial shunt
2017, 4Q, 39-41	Dilation and bypass of cerebral ventricle
2015, 2Q, 9	Revision of ventriculoperitoneal (VP) shunt
2013, 2Q, 36	Insertion of ventriculoperitoneal shunt with laparoscopic assistance

AHA Coding Clinic for table 005
2022, 4Q, 53-54	Laser interstitial thermal therapy
2022, 1Q, 50	Percutaneous ganglion balloon compression
2021, 3Q, 16	Decompression of Chiari malformation by excision
2021, 2Q, 17	Dorsal root entry zone procedure

AHA Coding Clinic for table 007
2017, 4Q, 39-41	Dilation and bypass of cerebral ventricle

AHA Coding Clinic for table 009
2018, 4Q, 85	Externalization of lumboatrial shunt
2017, 1Q, 50	Failed lumbar puncture
2015, 3Q, 10	Open evacuation of subdural hematoma
2015, 3Q, 11	Percutaneous drainage of subdural hematoma
2015, 3Q, 12	Subdural evacuation portal system (SEPS) placement
2015, 3Q, 12	Placement of ventriculostomy catheter via burr hole
2015, 2Q, 30	Drainage of syrinx
2015, 1Q, 31	Intrathecal chemotherapy
2014, 1Q, 8	Diagnostic lumbar tap
2014, 1Q, 8	Lumbar drainage port aspiration

AHA Coding Clinic for table 00B
2021, 3Q, 16	Decompression of Chiari malformation by excision
2017, 3Q, 17	Resection of schwannoma and placement of DuraGen and Lorenz cranial plating system
2016, 2Q, 12	Resection of malignant neoplasm of infratemporal fossa
2016, 2Q, 18	Amygdalohippocampectomy
2014, 4Q, 34	Resection of brain malignancy with implantation of chemotherapeutic wafer
2014, 3Q, 24	Repair of lipomyelomeningocele and tethered cord

AHA Coding Clinic for table 00C
2019, 3Q, 4	Evacuation of subdural hematoma and control of bleeding artery
2019, 2Q, 36	Evacuation of hematoma using NICO Brainpath® technology
2017, 4Q, 48	New and revised body part values - Extirpation spinal canal
2016, 2Q, 29	Decompressive craniectomy with cryopreservation and storage of bone flap
2015, 3Q, 10	Open evacuation of subdural hematoma
2015, 3Q, 11	Percutaneous drainage of subdural hematoma
2015, 3Q, 13	Evacuation of intracerebral hematoma

AHA Coding Clinic for table 00D
2022, 4Q, 54	Ultrasonic surgical aspiration of brain
2021, 4Q, 38-40	Ultrasonic surgical aspiration of brain
2015, 3Q, 13	Nonexcisional debridement of cranial wound with removal and replacement of hardware

AHA Coding Clinic for table 00H
2024, 1Q, 5-6	Insertion of Palladium-103 radioactive implant
2020, 4Q, 43-44	Insertion of radioactive element
2020, 2Q, 15	Ommaya reservoir with ventricular catheter placement
2020, 2Q, 16	Ommaya reservoir placement for cerebrospinal fluid infusion therapy
2017, 4Q, 30-31	Radiotherapeutic brain implant
2017, 3Q, 13	Implantation of bilateral neurostimulator electrodes
2014, 3Q, 19	End of life replacement of Baclofen pump

AHA Coding Clinic for table 00J
2021, 2Q, 19	Electromagnetic stealth guided ventriculoperitoneal shunt insertion with endoscopy
2019, 2Q, 36	Evacuation of hematoma using NICO Brainpath® technology
2017, 1Q, 50	Failed lumbar puncture

AHA Coding Clinic for table 00N
2019, 2Q, 19	Cervical spinal fusion, decompression and placement of interfacet stabilization device
2019, 1Q, 28	Decompressive laminectomy of both spinal cord and nerve roots
2018, 3Q, 30	Decompressive laminectomy (release of spinal cord versus release of spinal meninges)
2017, 3Q, 10	Repair of Chiari malformation
2017, 2Q, 23	Decompression of spinal cord and placement of instrumentation
2016, 2Q, 29	Decompressive craniectomy with cryopreservation and storage of bone flap
2015, 2Q, 20	Cervical laminoplasty
2015, 2Q, 21	Multiple decompressive cervical laminectomies
2015, 2Q, 34	Decompressive laminectomy
2014, 3Q, 24	Repair of lipomyelomeningocele and tethered cord

AHA Coding Clinic for table 00P
2014, 3Q, 19	End of life replacement of Baclofen pump

AHA Coding Clinic for table 00Q
2014, 3Q, 7	Hemi-cranioplasty for repair of cranial defect
2013, 3Q, 25	Fracture of frontal bone with repair and coagulation for hemostasis

AHA Coding Clinic for table 00S
2014, 4Q, 35	Reimplantation of buccal nerve

AHA Coding Clinic for table 00U
2021, 3Q, 16	Decompression of Chiari malformation by excision
2018, 1Q, 9	Craniectomy with DuraGaurd placement
2017, 4Q, 62	Added and revised device values - Nerve substitutes
2017, 3Q, 10	Repair of Chiari malformation
2017, 3Q, 17	Resection of schwannoma and placement of DuraGen and Lorenz cranial plating system
2015, 4Q, 39	Dural patch graft
2014, 3Q, 24	Repair of lipomyelomeningocele and tethered cord

AHA Coding Clinic for table 00W
2018, 4Q, 86	Placement of lumboatrial shunt

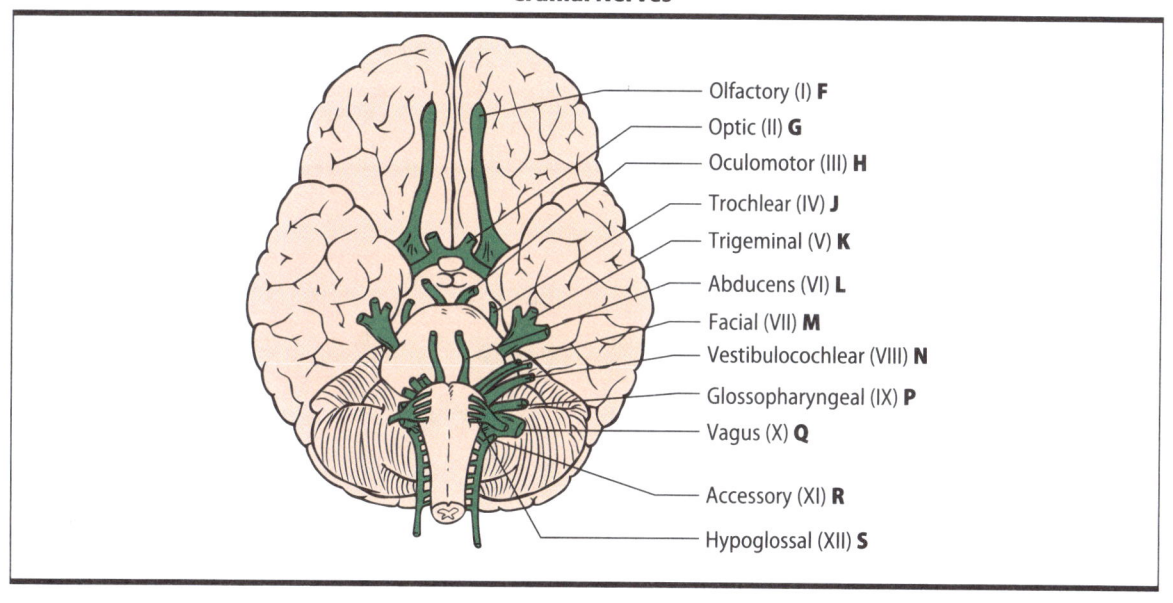

Central Nervous System and Cranial Nerves

Brain

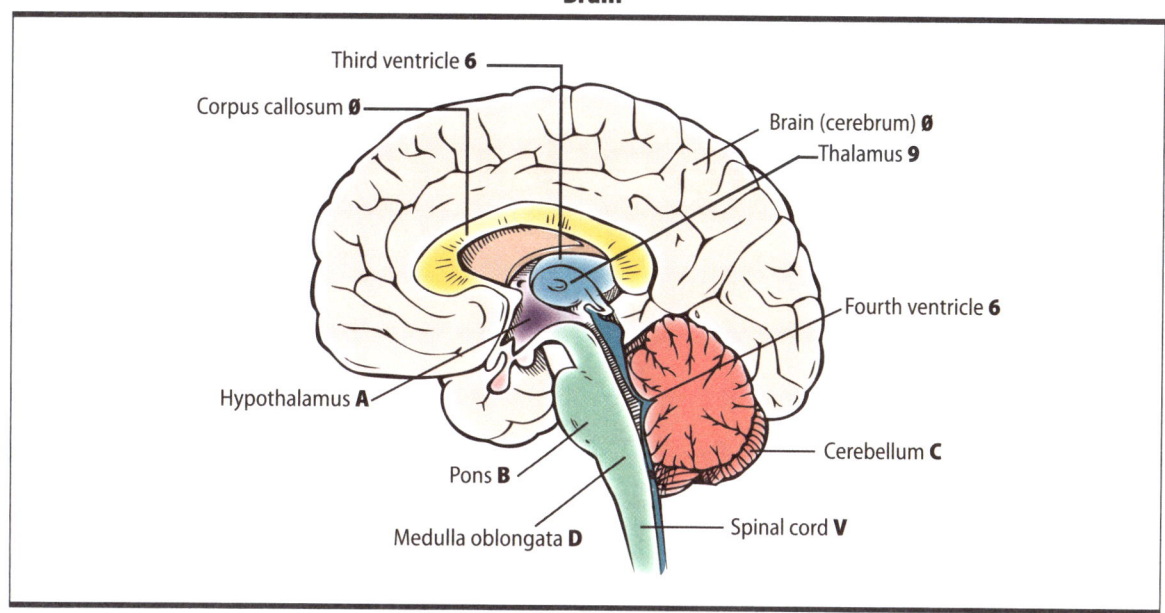

- Third ventricle **6**
- Corpus callosum **0**
- Brain (cerebrum) **0**
- Thalamus **9**
- Fourth ventricle **6**
- Hypothalamus **A**
- Cerebellum **C**
- Pons **B**
- Spinal cord **V**
- Medulla oblongata **D**

Cranial Nerves

- Olfactory (I) **F**
- Optic (II) **G**
- Oculomotor (III) **H**
- Trochlear (IV) **J**
- Trigeminal (V) **K**
- Abducens (VI) **L**
- Facial (VII) **M**
- Vestibulocochlear (VIII) **N**
- Glossopharyngeal (IX) **P**
- Vagus (X) **Q**
- Accessory (XI) **R**
- Hypoglossal (XII) **S**

Central Nervous System and Cranial Nerves

0 Medical and Surgical
0 Central Nervous System and Cranial Nerves
1 Bypass   Definition: Altering the route of passage of the contents of a tubular body part
Explanation: Rerouting contents of a body part to a downstream area of the normal route, to a similar route and body part, or to an abnormal route and dissimilar body part. Includes one or more anastomoses, with or without the use of a device.

Body Part Character 4	Approach Character 5	Device Character 6	Qualifier Character 7
6 Cerebral Ventricle Aqueduct of Sylvius Cerebral aqueduct (Sylvius) Choroid plexus Ependyma Foramen of Monro (intraventricular) Fourth ventricle Interventricular foramen (Monro) Left lateral ventricle Right lateral ventricle Third ventricle	**0** Open **3** Percutaneous **4** Percutaneous Endoscopic	**7** Autologous Tissue Substitute **J** Synthetic Substitute **K** Nonautologous Tissue Substitute	**0** Nasopharynx **1** Mastoid Sinus **2** Atrium **3** Blood Vessel **4** Pleural Cavity **5** Intestine **6** Peritoneal Cavity **7** Urinary Tract **8** Bone Marrow **A** Subgaleal Space **B** Cerebral Cisterns
6 Cerebral Ventricle Aqueduct of Sylvius Cerebral aqueduct (Sylvius) Choroid plexus Ependyma Foramen of Monro (intraventricular) Fourth ventricle Interventricular foramen (Monro) Left lateral ventricle Right lateral ventricle Third ventricle	**0** Open **3** Percutaneous **4** Percutaneous Endoscopic	**Z** No Device	**B** Cerebral Cisterns
U Spinal Canal Epidural space, spinal Extradural space, spinal Subarachnoid space, spinal Subdural space, spinal Vertebral canal	**0** Open **3** Percutaneous **4** Percutaneous Endoscopic	**7** Autologous Tissue Substitute **J** Synthetic Substitute **K** Nonautologous Tissue Substitute	**2** Atrium **4** Pleural Cavity **6** Peritoneal Cavity **7** Urinary Tract **9** Fallopian Tube

0 Medical and Surgical
0 Central Nervous System and Cranial Nerves
2 Change   Definition: Taking out or off a device from a body part and putting back an identical or similar device in or on the same body part without cutting or puncturing the skin or a mucous membrane
Explanation: All CHANGE procedures are coded using the approach EXTERNAL

Body Part Character 4	Approach Character 5	Device Character 6	Qualifier Character 7
0 Brain Cerebrum Corpus callosum Encephalon **E** Cranial Nerve **U** Spinal Canal Epidural space, spinal Extradural space, spinal Subarachnoid space, spinal Subdural space, spinal Vertebral canal	**X** External	**0** Drainage Device **Y** Other Device	**Z** No Qualifier

Non-OR   All body part, approach, device, and qualifier values

ICD-10-PCS 2025 — Central Nervous System and Cranial Nerves — 005-005

- **0** Medical and Surgical
- **0** Central Nervous System and Cranial Nerves
- **5** Destruction

Definition: Physical eradication of all or a portion of a body part by the direct use of energy, force, or a destructive agent
Explanation: None of the body part is physically taken out

Body Part Character 4	Approach Character 5	Device Character 6	Qualifier Character 7

0 Brain
  Cerebrum
  Corpus callosum
  Encephalon
	0 Open
	4 Percutaneous Endoscopic
		Z No Device	**3** Laser Interstitial Thermal Therapy
			Z No Qualifier

0 Brain
  Cerebrum
  Corpus callosum
  Encephalon
	3 Percutaneous	**Z** No Device	**3** Laser Interstitial Thermal Therapy
			4 Stereoelectroencephalographic Radiofrequency Ablation
			Z No Qualifier

1 Cerebral Meninges
  Arachnoid mater, intracranial
  Leptomeninges, intracranial
  Pia mater, intracranial
2 Dura Mater
  Diaphragma sellae
  Dura mater, intracranial
  Falx cerebri
  Tentorium cerebelli
6 Cerebral Ventricle
  Aqueduct of Sylvius
  Cerebral aqueduct (Sylvius)
  Choroid plexus
  Ependyma
  Foramen of Monro (intraventricular)
  Fourth ventricle
  Interventricular foramen (Monro)
  Left lateral ventricle
  Right lateral ventricle
  Third ventricle
7 Cerebral Hemisphere
  Frontal lobe
  Occipital lobe
  Parietal lobe
  Temporal lobe
8 Basal Ganglia
  Basal nuclei
  Claustrum
  Corpus striatum
  Globus pallidus
  Substantia nigra
  Subthalamic nucleus
9 Thalamus
  Epithalamus
  Geniculate nucleus
  Metathalamus
  Pulvinar
A Hypothalamus
  Mammillary body
B Pons
  Apneustic center
  Basis pontis
  Locus ceruleus
  Pneumotaxic center
  Pontine tegmentum
  Superior olivary nucleus
C Cerebellum
  Culmen
D Medulla Oblongata
  Myelencephalon
F Olfactory Nerve
  First cranial nerve
  Olfactory bulb
G Optic Nerve
  Optic chiasma
  Second cranial nerve
	H Oculomotor Nerve
	  Third cranial nerve
	J Trochlear Nerve
	  Fourth cranial nerve
	K Trigeminal Nerve
	  Fifth cranial nerve
	  Gasserian ganglion
	  Mandibular nerve
	  Maxillary nerve
	  Ophthalmic nerve
	  Trifacial nerve
	L Abducens Nerve
	  Sixth cranial nerve
	M Facial Nerve
	  Chorda tympani
	  Geniculate ganglion
	  Greater superficial petrosal nerve
	  Nerve to the stapedius
	  Parotid plexus
	  Posterior auricular nerve
	  Seventh cranial nerve
	  Submandibular ganglion
	N Acoustic Nerve
	  Cochlear nerve
	  Eighth cranial nerve
	  Scarpa's (vestibular) ganglion
	  Spiral ganglion
	  Vestibular (Scarpa's) ganglion
	  Vestibular nerve
	  Vestibulocochlear nerve
	P Glossopharyngeal Nerve
	  Carotid sinus nerve
	  Ninth cranial nerve
	  Tympanic nerve
	Q Vagus Nerve
	  Anterior vagal trunk
	  Pharyngeal plexus
	  Pneumogastric nerve
	  Posterior vagal trunk
	  Pulmonary plexus
	  Recurrent laryngeal nerve
	  Superior laryngeal nerve
	  Tenth cranial nerve
	R Accessory Nerve
	  Eleventh cranial nerve
	S Hypoglossal Nerve
	  Twelfth cranial nerve
	T Spinal Meninges
	  Arachnoid mater, spinal
	  Denticulate (dentate) ligament
	  Dura mater, spinal
	  Filum terminale
	  Leptomeninges, spinal
	  Pia mater, spinal
		0 Open
		3 Percutaneous
		4 Percutaneous Endoscopic
			Z No Device	**Z** No Qualifier

W Cervical Spinal Cord **X** Thoracic Spinal Cord **Y** Lumbar Spinal Cord	**0** Open **3** Percutaneous **4** Percutaneous Endoscopic	**Z** No Device	**3** Laser Interstitial Thermal Therapy **Z** No Qualifier

Non-OR 005[F,G,H,J,K,L,M,N,P,Q,R,S][0,3,4]ZZ

0 Medical and Surgical
0 Central Nervous System and Cranial Nerves
7 Dilation

Definition: Expanding an orifice or the lumen of a tubular body part

Explanation: The orifice can be a natural orifice or an artificially created orifice. Accomplished by stretching a tubular body part using intraluminal pressure or by cutting part of the orifice or wall of the tubular body part.

Body Part Character 4	Approach Character 5	Device Character 6	Qualifier Character 7

6 Cerebral Ventricle
  Aqueduct of Sylvius
  Cerebral aqueduct (Sylvius)
  Choroid plexus
  Ependyma
  Foramen of Monro (intraventricular)
  Fourth ventricle
  Interventricular foramen (Monro)
  Left lateral ventricle
  Right lateral ventricle
  Third ventricle
	0 Open
	3 Percutaneous
	4 Percutaneous Endoscopic
		Z No Device	Z No Qualifier

0 Medical and Surgical
0 Central Nervous System and Cranial Nerves
8 Division

Definition: Cutting into a body part, without draining fluids and/or gases from the body part, in order to separate or transect a body part

Explanation: All or a portion of the body part is separated into two or more portions

Body Part Character 4	Approach Character 5	Device Character 6	Qualifier Character 7

0 Brain
  Cerebrum
  Corpus callosum
  Encephalon
7 Cerebral Hemisphere
  Frontal lobe
  Occipital lobe
  Parietal lobe
  Temporal lobe
8 Basal Ganglia
  Basal nuclei
  Claustrum
  Corpus striatum
  Globus pallidus
  Substantia nigra
  Subthalamic nucleus
F Olfactory Nerve
  First cranial nerve
  Olfactory bulb
G Optic Nerve
  Optic chiasma
  Second cranial nerve
H Oculomotor Nerve
  Third cranial nerve
J Trochlear Nerve
  Fourth cranial nerve
K Trigeminal Nerve
  Fifth cranial nerve
  Gasserian ganglion
  Mandibular nerve
  Maxillary nerve
  Ophthalmic nerve
  Trifacial nerve
L Abducens Nerve
  Sixth cranial nerve
M Facial Nerve
  Chorda tympani
  Geniculate ganglion
  Greater superficial petrosal nerve
  Nerve to the stapedius
  Parotid plexus
  Posterior auricular nerve
  Seventh cranial nerve
  Submandibular ganglion
	N Acoustic Nerve
	  Cochlear nerve
	  Eighth cranial nerve
	  Scarpa's (vestibular) ganglion
	  Spiral ganglion
	  Vestibular (Scarpa's) ganglion
	  Vestibular nerve
	  Vestibulocochlear nerve
	P Glossopharyngeal Nerve
	  Carotid sinus nerve
	  Ninth cranial nerve
	  Tympanic nerve
	Q Vagus Nerve
	  Anterior vagal trunk
	  Pharyngeal plexus
	  Pneumogastric nerve
	  Posterior vagal trunk
	  Pulmonary plexus
	  Recurrent laryngeal nerve
	  Superior laryngeal nerve
	  Tenth cranial nerve
	R Accessory Nerve
	  Eleventh cranial nerve
	S Hypoglossal Nerve
	  Twelfth cranial nerve
	W Cervical Spinal Cord
	  Dorsal root ganglion
	X Thoracic Spinal Cord
	  Dorsal root ganglion
	Y Lumbar Spinal Cord
	  Cauda equina
	  Conus medullaris
	  Dorsal root ganglion
		0 Open
		3 Percutaneous
		4 Percutaneous Endoscopic
			Z No Device	Z No Qualifier

Non-OR Procedure   DRG Non-OR Procedure   Valid OR Procedure   HAC Associated Procedure   Combination Only   New/Revised April   New/Revised October

0 Medical and Surgical
0 Central Nervous System and Cranial Nerves
9 Drainage Definition: Taking or letting out fluids and/or gases from a body part
  Explanation: The qualifier DIAGNOSTIC is used to identify drainage procedures that are biopsies

Body Part Character 4	Approach Character 5	Device Character 6	Qualifier Character 7
0 Brain
Cerebrum
Corpus callosum
Encephalon
1 Cerebral Meninges
Arachnoid mater, intracranial
Leptomeninges, intracranial
Pia mater, intracranial
2 Dura Mater
Diaphragma sellae
Dura mater, intracranial
Falx cerebri
Tentorium cerebelli
3 Epidural Space, Intracranial
Extradural space, intracranial
4 Subdural Space, Intracranial
5 Subarachnoid Space, Intracranial
6 Cerebral Ventricle
Aqueduct of Sylvius
Cerebral aqueduct (Sylvius)
Choroid plexus
Ependyma
Foramen of Monro (intraventricular)
Fourth ventricle
Interventricular foramen (Monro)
Left lateral ventricle
Right lateral ventricle
Third ventricle
7 Cerebral Hemisphere
Frontal lobe
Occipital lobe
Parietal lobe
Temporal lobe
8 Basal Ganglia
Basal nuclei
Claustrum
Corpus striatum
Globus pallidus
Substantia nigra
Subthalamic nucleus
9 Thalamus
Epithalamus
Geniculate nucleus
Metathalamus
Pulvinar
A Hypothalamus
Mammillary body
B Pons
Apneustic center
Basis pontis
Locus ceruleus
Pneumotaxic center
Pontine tegmentum
Superior olivary nucleus
C Cerebellum
Culmen
D Medulla Oblongata
Myelencephalon
F Olfactory Nerve
First cranial nerve
Olfactory bulb
G Optic Nerve
Optic chiasma
Second cranial nerve
H Oculomotor Nerve
Third cranial nerve
J Trochlear Nerve
Fourth cranial nerve
K Trigeminal Nerve
Fifth cranial nerve
Gasserian ganglion
Mandibular nerve
Maxillary nerve
Ophthalmic nerve
Trifacial nerve
L Abducens Nerve
Sixth cranial nerve
M Facial Nerve
Chorda tympani
Geniculate ganglion
Greater superficial petrosal nerve
Nerve to the stapedius
Parotid plexus
Posterior auricular nerve
Seventh cranial nerve
Submandibular ganglion
N Acoustic Nerve
Cochlear nerve
Eighth cranial nerve
Scarpa's (vestibular) ganglion
Spiral ganglion
Vestibular (Scarpa's) ganglion
Vestibular nerve
Vestibulocochlear nerve
P Glossopharyngeal Nerve
Carotid sinus nerve
Ninth cranial nerve
Tympanic nerve
Q Vagus Nerve
Anterior vagal trunk
Pharyngeal plexus
Pneumogastric nerve
Posterior vagal trunk
Pulmonary plexus
Recurrent laryngeal nerve
Superior laryngeal nerve
Tenth cranial nerve
R Accessory Nerve
Eleventh cranial nerve
S Hypoglossal Nerve
Twelfth cranial nerve
T Spinal Meninges
Arachnoid mater, spinal
Denticulate (dentate) ligament
Dura mater, spinal
Filum terminale
Leptomeninges, spinal
Pia mater, spinal
U Spinal Canal
Epidural space, spinal
Extradural space, spinal
Subarachnoid space, spinal
Subdural space, spinal
Vertebral canal
W Cervical Spinal Cord
Dorsal root ganglion
X Thoracic Spinal Cord
Dorsal root ganglion
Y Lumbar Spinal Cord
Cauda equina
Conus medullaris
Dorsal root ganglion	**0** Open
3 Percutaneous
4 Percutaneous Endoscopic	**0** Drainage Device	**Z** No Qualifier

Non-OR 009[T,W,X,Y]30Z
Non-OR 009U[3,4]0Z

009 Continued on next page

009–009   **Central Nervous System and Cranial Nerves**   ICD-10-PCS 2025

009 Continued

0 Medical and Surgical
0 Central Nervous System and Cranial Nerves
9 Drainage   Definition: Taking or letting out fluids and/or gases from a body part
Explanation: The qualifier DIAGNOSTIC is used to identify drainage procedures that are biopsies

Body Part Character 4	Approach Character 5	Device Character 6	Qualifier Character 7
0 Brain Cerebrum Corpus callosum Encephalon **1 Cerebral Meninges** Arachnoid mater, intracranial Leptomeninges, intracranial Pia mater, intracranial **2 Dura Mater** Diaphragma sellae Dura mater, intracranial Falx cerebri Tentorium cerebelli **3 Epidural Space, Intracranial** Extradural space, intracranial **4 Subdural Space, Intracranial** **5 Subarachnoid Space, Intracranial** **6 Cerebral Ventricle** Aqueduct of Sylvius Cerebral aqueduct (Sylvius) Choroid plexus Ependyma Foramen of Monro (intraventricular) Fourth ventricle Interventricular foramen (Monro) Left lateral ventricle Right lateral ventricle Third ventricle **7 Cerebral Hemisphere** Frontal lobe Occipital lobe Parietal lobe Temporal lobe **8 Basal Ganglia** Basal nuclei Claustrum Corpus striatum Globus pallidus Substantia nigra Subthalamic nucleus **9 Thalamus** Epithalamus Geniculate nucleus Metathalamus Pulvinar **A Hypothalamus** Mammillary body **B Pons** Apneustic center Basis pontis Locus ceruleus Pneumotaxic center Pontine tegmentum Superior olivary nucleus **C Cerebellum** Culmen **D Medulla Oblongata** Myelencephalon **F Olfactory Nerve** First cranial nerve Olfactory bulb **G Optic Nerve** Optic chiasma Second cranial nerve **H Oculomotor Nerve** Third cranial nerve **J Trochlear Nerve** Fourth cranial nerve **K Trigeminal Nerve** Fifth cranial nerve Gasserian ganglion Mandibular nerve Maxillary nerve Ophthalmic nerve Trifacial nerve **L Abducens Nerve** Sixth cranial nerve **M Facial Nerve** Chorda tympani Geniculate ganglion Greater superficial petrosal nerve Nerve to the stapedius Parotid plexus Posterior auricular nerve Seventh cranial nerve Submandibular ganglion **N Acoustic Nerve** Cochlear nerve Eighth cranial nerve Scarpa's (vestibular) ganglion Spiral ganglion Vestibular (Scarpa's) ganglion Vestibular nerve Vestibulocochlear nerve **P Glossopharyngeal Nerve** Carotid sinus nerve Ninth cranial nerve Tympanic nerve **Q Vagus Nerve** Anterior vagal trunk Pharyngeal plexus Pneumogastric nerve Posterior vagal trunk Pulmonary plexus Recurrent laryngeal nerve Superior laryngeal nerve Tenth cranial nerve **R Accessory Nerve** Eleventh cranial nerve **S Hypoglossal Nerve** Twelfth cranial nerve **T Spinal Meninges** Arachnoid mater, spinal Denticulate (dentate) ligament Dura mater, spinal Filum terminale Leptomeninges, spinal Pia mater, spinal **U Spinal Canal** Epidural space, spinal Extradural space, spinal Subarachnoid space, spinal Subdural space, spinal Vertebral canal **W Cervical Spinal Cord** Dorsal root ganglion **X Thoracic Spinal Cord** Dorsal root ganglion **Y Lumbar Spinal Cord** Cauda equina Conus medullaris Dorsal root ganglion	**0** Open **3** Percutaneous **4** Percutaneous Endoscopic	**Z** No Device	**X** Diagnostic **Z** No Qualifier

Non-OR   009[0,1,2,3,4,5,6,7,8,9,A,B,C,D,F,G,H,J,K,L,M,N,P,Q,R,S][3,4]ZX
Non-OR   009[T,W,X,Y]3Z[X,Z]
Non-OR   009U[3,4]Z[X,Z]

Non-OR Procedure   DRG Non-OR Procedure   Valid OR Procedure   HAC Associated Procedure   Combination Only   New/Revised April   New/Revised October

ICD-10-PCS 2025 — Central Nervous System and Cranial Nerves — 00B–00B

- 0 Medical and Surgical
- 0 Central Nervous System and Cranial Nerves
- B Excision   Definition: Cutting out or off, without replacement, a portion of a body part
  Explanation: The qualifier DIAGNOSTIC is used to identify excision procedures that are biopsies

Body Part Character 4	Approach Character 5	Device Character 6	Qualifier Character 7
0 Brain Cerebrum Corpus callosum Encephalon **1 Cerebral Meninges** Arachnoid mater, intracranial Leptomeninges, intracranial Pia mater, intracranial **2 Dura Mater** Diaphragma sellae Dura mater, intracranial Falx cerebri Tentorium cerebelli **6 Cerebral Ventricle** Aqueduct of Sylvius Cerebral aqueduct (Sylvius) Choroid plexus Ependyma Foramen of Monro (intraventricular) Fourth ventricle Interventricular foramen (Monro) Left lateral ventricle Right lateral ventricle Third ventricle **7 Cerebral Hemisphere** Frontal lobe Occipital lobe Parietal lobe Temporal lobe **8 Basal Ganglia** Basal nuclei Claustrum Corpus striatum Globus pallidus Substantia nigra Subthalamic nucleus **9 Thalamus** Epithalamus Geniculate nucleus Metathalamus Pulvinar **A Hypothalamus** Mammillary body **B Pons** Apneustic center Basis pontis Locus ceruleus Pneumotaxic center Pontine tegmentum Superior olivary nucleus **C Cerebellum** Culmen **D Medulla Oblongata** Myelencephalon **F Olfactory Nerve** First cranial nerve Olfactory bulb **G Optic Nerve** Optic chiasma Second cranial nerve **H Oculomotor Nerve** Third cranial nerve **J Trochlear Nerve** Fourth cranial nerve **K Trigeminal Nerve** Fifth cranial nerve Gasserian ganglion Mandibular nerve Maxillary nerve Ophthalmic nerve Trifacial nerve **L Abducens Nerve** Sixth cranial nerve **M Facial Nerve** Chorda tympani Geniculate ganglion Greater superficial petrosal nerve Nerve to the stapedius Parotid plexus Posterior auricular nerve Seventh cranial nerve Submandibular ganglion **N Acoustic Nerve** Cochlear nerve Eighth cranial nerve Scarpa's (vestibular) ganglion Spiral ganglion Vestibular (Scarpa's) ganglion Vestibular nerve Vestibulocochlear nerve **P Glossopharyngeal Nerve** Carotid sinus nerve Ninth cranial nerve Tympanic nerve **Q Vagus Nerve** Anterior vagal trunk Pharyngeal plexus Pneumogastric nerve Posterior vagal trunk Pulmonary plexus Recurrent laryngeal nerve Superior laryngeal nerve Tenth cranial nerve **R Accessory Nerve** Eleventh cranial nerve **S Hypoglossal Nerve** Twelfth cranial nerve **T Spinal Meninges** Arachnoid mater, spinal Denticulate (dentate) ligament Dura mater, spinal Filum terminale Leptomeninges, spinal Pia mater, spinal **W Cervical Spinal Cord** Dorsal root ganglion **X Thoracic Spinal Cord** Dorsal root ganglion **Y Lumbar Spinal Cord** Cauda equina Conus medullaris Dorsal root ganglion	0 Open 3 Percutaneous 4 Percutaneous Endoscopic	Z No Device	X Diagnostic Z No Qualifier

Non-OR   00B[F,G,H,J,K,L,M,N,P,Q,R,S][3,4]ZX

0 Medical and Surgical
0 Central Nervous System and Cranial Nerves
C Extirpation Definition: Taking or cutting out solid matter from a body part
Explanation: The solid matter may be an abnormal byproduct of a biological function or a foreign body; it may be imbedded in a body part or in the lumen of a tubular body part. The solid matter may or may not have been previously broken into pieces.

Body Part Character 4	Approach Character 5	Device Character 6	Qualifier Character 7
0 Brain 　Cerebrum 　Corpus callosum 　Encephalon **1** Cerebral Meninges 　Arachnoid mater, intracranial 　Leptomeninges, intracranial 　Pia mater, intracranial **2** Dura Mater 　Diaphragma sellae 　Dura mater, intracranial 　Falx cerebri 　Tentorium cerebelli **3** Epidural Space, Intracranial 　Extradural space, intracranial **4** Subdural Space, Intracranial **5** Subarachnoid Space, Intracranial **6** Cerebral Ventricle 　Aqueduct of Sylvius 　Cerebral aqueduct (Sylvius) 　Choroid plexus 　Ependyma 　Foramen of Monro (intraventricular) 　Fourth ventricle 　Interventricular foramen (Monro) 　Left lateral ventricle 　Right lateral ventricle 　Third ventricle **7** Cerebral Hemisphere 　Frontal lobe 　Occipital lobe 　Parietal lobe 　Temporal lobe **8** Basal Ganglia 　Basal nuclei 　Claustrum 　Corpus striatum 　Globus pallidus 　Substantia nigra 　Subthalamic nucleus **9** Thalamus 　Epithalamus 　Geniculate nucleus 　Metathalamus 　Pulvinar **A** Hypothalamus 　Mammillary body **B** Pons 　Apneustic center 　Basis pontis 　Locus ceruleus 　Pneumotaxic center 　Pontine tegmentum 　Superior olivary nucleus **C** Cerebellum 　Culmen **D** Medulla Oblongata 　Myelencephalon **F** Olfactory Nerve 　First cranial nerve 　Olfactory bulb	**G** Optic Nerve 　Optic chiasma 　Second cranial nerve **H** Oculomotor Nerve 　Third cranial nerve **J** Trochlear Nerve 　Fourth cranial nerve **K** Trigeminal Nerve 　Fifth cranial nerve 　Gasserian ganglion 　Mandibular nerve 　Maxillary nerve 　Ophthalmic nerve 　Trifacial nerve **L** Abducens Nerve 　Sixth cranial nerve **M** Facial Nerve 　Chorda tympani 　Geniculate ganglion 　Greater superficial petrosal nerve 　Nerve to the stapedius 　Parotid plexus 　Posterior auricular nerve 　Seventh cranial nerve 　Submandibular ganglion **N** Acoustic Nerve 　Cochlear nerve 　Eighth cranial nerve 　Scarpa's (vestibular) ganglion 　Spiral ganglion 　Vestibular (Scarpa's) ganglion 　Vestibular nerve 　Vestibulocochlear nerve **P** Glossopharyngeal Nerve 　Carotid sinus nerve 　Ninth cranial nerve 　Tympanic nerve **Q** Vagus Nerve 　Anterior vagal trunk 　Pharyngeal plexus 　Pneumogastric nerve 　Posterior vagal trunk 　Pulmonary plexus 　Recurrent laryngeal nerve 　Superior laryngeal nerve 　Tenth cranial nerve **R** Accessory Nerve 　Eleventh cranial nerve **S** Hypoglossal Nerve 　Twelfth cranial nerve **T** Spinal Meninges 　Arachnoid mater, spinal 　Denticulate (dentate) ligament 　Dura mater, spinal 　Filum terminale 　Leptomeninges, spinal 　Pia mater, spinal **U** Spinal Canal **W** Cervical Spinal Cord 　Dorsal root ganglion **X** Thoracic Spinal Cord 　Dorsal root ganglion **Y** Lumbar Spinal Cord 　Cauda equina 　Conus medullaris 　Dorsal root ganglion	**0** Open **3** Percutaneous **4** Percutaneous Endoscopic	**Z** No Device	**Z** No Qualifier

ICD-10-PCS 2025 — Central Nervous System and Cranial Nerves — 00D-00D

- **0** Medical and Surgical
- **0** Central Nervous System and Cranial Nerves
- **D** Extraction Definition: Pulling or stripping out or off all or a portion of a body part by the use of force
  Explanation: The qualifier DIAGNOSTIC is used to identify extraction procedures that are biopsies

Body Part Character 4	Approach Character 5	Device Character 6	Qualifier Character 7
0 Brain 　Cerebrum 　Corpus callosum 　Encephalon **1 Cerebral Meninges** 　Arachnoid mater, intracranial 　Leptomeninges, intracranial 　Pia mater, intracranial **2 Dura Mater** 　Diaphragma sellae 　Dura mater, intracranial 　Falx cerebri 　Tentorium cerebelli **7 Cerebral Hemisphere** 　Frontal lobe 　Occipital lobe 　Parietal lobe 　Temporal lobe **C Cerebellum** 　Culmen **F Olfactory Nerve** 　First cranial nerve 　Olfactory bulb **G Optic Nerve** 　Optic chiasma 　Second cranial nerve **H Oculomotor Nerve** 　Third cranial nerve **J Trochlear Nerve** 　Fourth cranial nerve **K Trigeminal Nerve** 　Fifth cranial nerve 　Gasserian ganglion 　Mandibular nerve 　Maxillary nerve 　Ophthalmic nerve 　Trifacial nerve **L Abducens Nerve** 　Sixth cranial nerve **M Facial Nerve** 　Chorda tympani 　Geniculate ganglion 　Greater superficial petrosal nerve 　Nerve to the stapedius 　Parotid plexus 　Posterior auricular nerve 　Seventh cranial nerve 　Submandibular ganglion **N Acoustic Nerve** 　Cochlear nerve 　Eighth cranial nerve 　Scarpa's (vestibular) ganglion 　Spiral ganglion 　Vestibular (Scarpa's) ganglion 　Vestibular nerve 　Vestibulocochlear nerve **P Glossopharyngeal Nerve** 　Carotid sinus nerve 　Ninth cranial nerve 　Tympanic nerve **Q Vagus Nerve** 　Anterior vagal trunk 　Pharyngeal plexus 　Pneumogastric nerve 　Posterior vagal trunk 　Pulmonary plexus 　Recurrent laryngeal nerve 　Superior laryngeal nerve 　Tenth cranial nerve **R Accessory Nerve** 　Eleventh cranial nerve **S Hypoglossal Nerve** 　Twelfth cranial nerve **T Spinal Meninges** 　Arachnoid mater, spinal 　Denticulate (dentate) ligament 　Dura mater, spinal 　Filum terminale 　Leptomeninges, spinal 　Pia mater, spinal	**0** Open **3** Percutaneous **4** Percutaneous Endoscopic	**Z** No Device	**Z** No Qualifier

0 Medical and Surgical
0 Central Nervous System and Cranial Nerves
F Fragmentation Definition: Breaking solid matter in a body part into pieces
Explanation: Physical force (e.g., manual, ultrasonic) applied directly or indirectly is used to break the solid matter into pieces. The solid matter may be an abnormal byproduct of a biological function or a foreign body. The pieces of solid matter are not taken out.

Body Part Character 4	Approach Character 5	Device Character 6	Qualifier Character 7

3 Epidural Space, Intracranial NC
  Extradural space, intracranial
4 Subdural Space, Intracranial NC
5 Subarachnoid Space, Intracranial NC
6 Cerebral Ventricle
  Aqueduct of Sylvius
  Cerebral aqueduct (Sylvius)
  Choroid plexus
  Ependyma
  Foramen of Monro (intraventricular)
  Fourth ventricle
  Interventricular foramen (Monro)
  Left lateral ventricle
  Right lateral ventricle
  Third ventricle
U Spinal Canal
  Epidural space, spinal
  Extradural space, spinal
  Subarachnoid space, spinal
  Subdural space, spinal
  Vertebral canal
	0 Open
	3 Percutaneous
	4 Percutaneous Endoscopic
	X External
		Z No Device	Z No Qualifier

Non-OR   00F[3,4,5,6]XZZ
NC   00F[3,4,5,6]XZZ

0 Medical and Surgical
0 Central Nervous System and Cranial Nerves
H Insertion Definition: Putting in a nonbiological appliance that monitors, assists, performs, or prevents a physiological function but does not physically take the place of a body part
Explanation: None

Body Part Character 4	Approach Character 5	Device Character 6	Qualifier Character 7

0 Brain
  Cerebrum
  Corpus callosum
  Encephalon
	0 Open	1 Radioactive Element
		2 Monitoring Device
		3 Infusion Device
		4 Radioactive Element, Cesium-131 Collagen Implant
		5 Radioactive Element, Palladium-103 Collagen Implant
		M Neurostimulator Lead
		Y Other Device
			Z No Qualifier

0 Brain
  Cerebrum
  Corpus callosum
  Encephalon
	3 Percutaneous
	4 Percutaneous Endoscopic
		1 Radioactive Element
		2 Monitoring Device
		3 Infusion Device
		M Neurostimulator Lead
		Y Other Device
			Z No Qualifier

6 Cerebral Ventricle
  Aqueduct of Sylvius
  Cerebral aqueduct (Sylvius)
  Choroid plexus
  Ependyma
  Foramen of Monro (intraventricular)
  Fourth ventricle Interventricular foramen (Monro)
  Left lateral ventricle
  Right lateral ventricle
  Third ventricle
E Cranial Nerve
U Spinal Canal
  Epidural space, spinal
  Extradural space, spinal
  Subarachnoid space, spinal
  Subdural space, spinal
  Vertebral canal
V Spinal Cord
  Dorsal root ganglion
	0 Open
	3 Percutaneous
	4 Percutaneous Endoscopic
		1 Radioactive Element
		2 Monitoring Device
		3 Infusion Device
		M Neurostimulator Lead
		Y Other Device
			Z No Qualifier

DRG Non-OR 00H004Z
Non-OR   00H[E,U,V]32Z
Non-OR   00H[E,U][3,4]YZ
Non-OR   00H[U,V][0,3,4]3Z

See Appendix L for Procedure Combinations
  00H00MZ
  00H0[3,4]MZ
  00H[6,E,U,V][0,3,4]MZ

ICD-10-PCS 2025 — Central Nervous System and Cranial Nerves — 00J–00K

0 Medical and Surgical
0 Central Nervous System and Cranial Nerves
J Inspection Definition: Visually and/or manually exploring a body part
Explanation: Visual exploration may be performed with or without optical instrumentation. Manual exploration may be performed directly or through intervening body layers.

Body Part Character 4	Approach Character 5	Device Character 6	Qualifier Character 7
0 Brain Cerebrum Corpus callosum Encephalon **E Cranial Nerve** **U Spinal Canal** Epidural space, spinal Extradural space, spinal Subarachnoid space, spinal Subdural space, spinal Vertebral canal **V Spinal Cord** Dorsal root ganglion	**0** Open **3** Percutaneous **4** Percutaneous Endoscopic	**Z** No Device	**Z** No Qualifier

Non-OR 00J[0,E,U,V]3ZZ

0 Medical and Surgical
0 Central Nervous System and Cranial Nerves
K Map Definition: Locating the route of passage of electrical impulses and/or locating functional areas in a body part
Explanation: Applicable only to the cardiac conduction mechanism and the central nervous system

Body Part Character 4	Approach Character 5	Device Character 6	Qualifier Character 7
0 Brain Cerebrum Corpus callosum Encephalon	**0** Open **3** Percutaneous **4** Percutaneous Endoscopic	**Z** No Device	**Z** No Qualifier
0 Brain Cerebrum Corpus callosum Encephalon	**X** External	**Z** No Device	**1** Connectomic Analysis
7 Cerebral Hemisphere Frontal lobe Occipital lobe Parietal lobe Temporal lobe **8 Basal Ganglia** Basal nuclei Claustrum Corpus striatum Globus pallidus Substantia nigra Subthalamic nucleus **9 Thalamus** Epithalamus Geniculate nucleus Metathalamus Pulvinar **A Hypothalamus** Mammillary body **B Pons** Apneustic center Basis pontis Locus ceruleus Pneumotaxic center Pontine tegmentum Superior olivary nucleus **C Cerebellum** Culmen **D Medulla Oblongata** Myelencephalon	**0** Open **3** Percutaneous **4** Percutaneous Endoscopic	**Z** No Device	**Z** No Qualifier

Central Nervous System and Cranial Nerves

0 Medical and Surgical
0 Central Nervous System and Cranial Nerves
N Release
 Definition: Freeing a body part from an abnormal physical constraint by cutting or by the use of force
 Explanation: Some of the restraining tissue may be taken out but none of the body part is taken out

Body Part — Character 4	Approach — Character 5	Device — Character 6	Qualifier — Character 7

0 Brain
  Cerebrum
  Corpus callosum
  Encephalon
1 Cerebral Meninges
  Arachnoid mater, intracranial
  Leptomeninges, intracranial
  Pia mater, intracranial
2 Dura Mater
  Diaphragma sellae
  Dura mater, intracranial
  Falx cerebri
  Tentorium cerebelli
6 Cerebral Ventricle
  Aqueduct of Sylvius
  Cerebral aqueduct (Sylvius)
  Choroid plexus
  Ependyma
  Foramen of Monro (intraventricular)
  Fourth ventricle
  Interventricular foramen (Monro)
  Left lateral ventricle
  Right lateral ventricle
  Third ventricle
7 Cerebral Hemisphere
  Frontal lobe
  Occipital lobe
  Parietal lobe
  Temporal lobe
8 Basal Ganglia
  Basal nuclei
  Claustrum
  Corpus striatum
  Globus pallidus
  Substantia nigra
  Subthalamic nucleus
9 Thalamus
  Epithalamus
  Geniculate nucleus
  Metathalamus
  Pulvinar
A Hypothalamus
  Mammillary body
B Pons
  Apneustic center
  Basis pontis
  Locus ceruleus
  Pneumotaxic center
  Pontine tegmentum
  Superior olivary nucleus
C Cerebellum
  Culmen
D Medulla Oblongata
  Myelencephalon
F Olfactory Nerve
  First cranial nerve
  Olfactory bulb
G Optic Nerve
  Optic chiasma
  Second cranial nerve
H Oculomotor Nerve
  Third cranial nerve
J Trochlear Nerve
  Fourth cranial nerve
K Trigeminal Nerve
  Fifth cranial nerve
  Gasserian ganglion
  Mandibular nerve
  Maxillary nerve
  Ophthalmic nerve
  Trifacial nerve
L Abducens Nerve
  Sixth cranial nerve
M Facial Nerve
  Chorda tympani
  Geniculate ganglion
  Greater superficial petrosal nerve
  Nerve to the stapedius
  Parotid plexus
  Posterior auricular nerve
  Seventh cranial nerve
  Submandibular ganglion
N Acoustic Nerve
  Cochlear nerve
  Eighth cranial nerve
  Scarpa's (vestibular) ganglion
  Spiral ganglion
  Vestibular (Scarpa's) ganglion
  Vestibular nerve
  Vestibulocochlear nerve
P Glossopharyngeal Nerve
  Carotid sinus nerve
  Ninth cranial nerve
  Tympanic nerve
Q Vagus Nerve
  Anterior vagal trunk
  Pharyngeal plexus
  Pneumogastric nerve
  Posterior vagal trunk
  Pulmonary plexus
  Recurrent laryngeal nerve
  Superior laryngeal nerve
  Tenth cranial nerve
R Accessory Nerve
  Eleventh cranial nerve
S Hypoglossal Nerve
  Twelfth cranial nerve
T Spinal Meninges
  Arachnoid mater, spinal
  Denticulate (dentate) ligament
  Dura mater, spinal
  Filum terminale
  Leptomeninges, spinal
  Pia mater, spinal
W Cervical Spinal Cord
  Dorsal root ganglion
X Thoracic Spinal Cord
  Dorsal root ganglion
Y Lumbar Spinal Cord
  Cauda equina
  Conus medullaris
  Dorsal root ganglion
	0 Open
	3 Percutaneous
	4 Percutaneous Endoscopic
		Z No Device	**Z** No Qualifier

ICD-10-PCS 2025   Central Nervous System and Cranial Nerves   00P–00P

- **0** Medical and Surgical
- **0** Central Nervous System and Cranial Nerves
- **P** Removal   Definition: Taking out or off a device from a body part

Explanation: If a device is taken out and a similar device put in without cutting or puncturing the skin or mucous membrane, the procedure is coded to the root operation CHANGE. Otherwise, the procedure for taking out a device is coded to the root operation REMOVAL.

Body Part Character 4	Approach Character 5	Device Character 6	Qualifier Character 7

0 Brain
    Cerebrum
    Corpus callosum
    Encephalon
V Spinal Cord
    Dorsal root ganglion
	0 Open
	3 Percutaneous
	4 Percutaneous Endoscopic
		0 Drainage Device
		2 Monitoring Device
		3 Infusion Device
		7 Autologous Tissue Substitute
		J Synthetic Substitute
		K Nonautologous Tissue Substitute
		M Neurostimulator Lead
		Y Other Device
			Z No Qualifier

0 Brain
    Cerebrum
    Corpus callosum
    Encephalon
V Spinal Cord
    Dorsal root ganglion
	X External	**0** Drainage Device
		2 Monitoring Device
		3 Infusion Device
		M Neurostimulator Lead
			Z No Qualifier

6 Cerebral Ventricle
    Aqueduct of Sylvius
    Cerebral aqueduct (Sylvius)
    Choroid plexus
    Ependyma
    Foramen of Monro (intraventricular)
    Fourth ventricle
    Interventricular foramen (Monro)
    Left lateral ventricle
    Right lateral ventricle
    Third ventricle
U Spinal Canal
    Epidural space, spinal
    Extradural space, spinal
    Subarachnoid space, spinal
    Subdural space, spinal
    Vertebral canal
	0 Open
	3 Percutaneous
	4 Percutaneous Endoscopic
		0 Drainage Device
		2 Monitoring Device
		3 Infusion Device
		J Synthetic Substitute
		M Neurostimulator Lead
		Y Other Device
			Z No Qualifier

6 Cerebral Ventricle
    Aqueduct of Sylvius
    Cerebral aqueduct (Sylvius)
    Choroid plexus
    Ependyma
    Foramen of Monro (intraventricular)
    Fourth ventricle
    Interventricular foramen (Monro)
    Left lateral ventricle
    Right lateral ventricle
    Third ventricle
U Spinal Canal
    Epidural space, spinal
    Extradural space, spinal
    Subarachnoid space, spinal
    Subdural space, spinal
    Vertebral canal
	X External	**0** Drainage Device
		2 Monitoring Device
		3 Infusion Device
		M Neurostimulator Lead
			Z No Qualifier

E Cranial Nerve	**0** Open **3** Percutaneous **4** Percutaneous Endoscopic	**0** Drainage Device **2** Monitoring Device **3** Infusion Device **7** Autologous Tissue Substitute **M** Neurostimulator Lead **Y** Other Device	**Z** No Qualifier
E Cranial Nerve	**X** External	**0** Drainage Device **2** Monitoring Device **3** Infusion Device **M** Neurostimulator Lead	**Z** No Qualifier

Non-OR   00P[0,V]3[0,2,3]Z
Non-OR   00P[0,V][3,4]YZ
Non-OR   00P[0,V]X[0,2,3,M]Z
Non-OR   00P[6,U]3[0,2,3]Z
Non-OR   00P[6,U][3,4]YZ
Non-OR   00P[6,U]X[0,2,3,M]Z
Non-OR   00PE3[0,2,3]Z
Non-OR   00PE[3,4]YZ
Non-OR   00PEX[0,2,3,M]Z

NC Noncovered Procedure   **LC** Limited Coverage   **QA** Questionable OB Admit   **NT** New Tech Add-on   ✚ Combination Member   ♂ Male   ♀ Female

Central Nervous System and Cranial Nerves

0 Medical and Surgical
0 Central Nervous System and Cranial Nerves
Q Repair Definition: Restoring, to the extent possible, a body part to its normal anatomic structure and function
Explanation: Used only when the method to accomplish the repair is not one of the other root operations

Body Part Character 4	Approach Character 5	Device Character 6	Qualifier Character 7
0 Brain Cerebrum Corpus callosum Encephalon **1 Cerebral Meninges** Arachnoid mater, intracranial Leptomeninges, intracranial Pia mater, intracranial **2 Dura Mater** Diaphragma sellae Dura mater, intracranial Falx cerebri Tentorium cerebelli **6 Cerebral Ventricle** Aqueduct of Sylvius Cerebral aqueduct (Sylvius) Choroid plexus Ependyma Foramen of Monro (intraventricular) Fourth ventricle Interventricular foramen (Monro) Left lateral ventricle Right lateral ventricle Third ventricle **7 Cerebral Hemisphere** Frontal lobe Occipital lobe Parietal lobe Temporal lobe **8 Basal Ganglia** Basal nuclei Claustrum Corpus striatum Globus pallidus Substantia nigra Subthalamic nucleus **9 Thalamus** Epithalamus Geniculate nucleus Metathalamus Pulvinar **A Hypothalamus** Mammillary body **B Pons** Apneustic center Basis pontis Locus ceruleus Pneumotaxic center Pontine tegmentum Superior olivary nucleus **C Cerebellum** Culmen **D Medulla Oblongata** Myelencephalon **F Olfactory Nerve** First cranial nerve Olfactory bulb **G Optic Nerve** Optic chiasma Second cranial nerve	**H Oculomotor Nerve** Third cranial nerve **J Trochlear Nerve** Fourth cranial nerve **K Trigeminal Nerve** Fifth cranial nerve Gasserian ganglion Mandibular nerve Maxillary nerve Ophthalmic nerve Trifacial nerve **L Abducens Nerve** Sixth cranial nerve **M Facial Nerve** Chorda tympani Geniculate ganglion Greater superficial petrosal nerve Nerve to the stapedius Parotid plexus Posterior auricular nerve Seventh cranial nerve Submandibular ganglion **N Acoustic Nerve** Cochlear nerve Eighth cranial nerve Scarpa's (vestibular) ganglion Spiral ganglion Vestibular (Scarpa's) ganglion Vestibular nerve Vestibulocochlear nerve **P Glossopharyngeal Nerve** Carotid sinus nerve Ninth cranial nerve Tympanic nerve **Q Vagus Nerve** Anterior vagal trunk Pharyngeal plexus Pneumogastric nerve Posterior vagal trunk Pulmonary plexus Recurrent laryngeal nerve Superior laryngeal nerve Tenth cranial nerve **R Accessory Nerve** Eleventh cranial nerve **S Hypoglossal Nerve** Twelfth cranial nerve **T Spinal Meninges** Arachnoid mater, spinal Denticulate (dentate) ligament Dura mater, spinal Filum terminale Leptomeninges, spinal Pia mater, spinal **W Cervical Spinal Cord** Dorsal root ganglion **X Thoracic Spinal Cord** Dorsal root ganglion **Y Lumbar Spinal Cord** Cauda equina Conus medullaris Dorsal root ganglion	**0** Open **3** Percutaneous **4** Percutaneous Endoscopic	**Z** No Device	**Z** No Qualifier

0 Medical and Surgical
0 Central Nervous System and Cranial Nerves
R Replacement Definition: Putting in or on biological or synthetic material that physically takes the place and/or function of all or a portion of a body part
Explanation: The body part may have been taken out or replaced, or may be taken out, physically eradicated, or rendered nonfunctional during the REPLACEMENT procedure. A REMOVAL procedure is coded for taking out the device used in a previous replacement procedure.

Body Part Character 4	Approach Character 5	Device Character 6	Qualifier Character 7

1 Cerebral Meninges
  Arachnoid mater, intracranial
  Leptomeninges, intracranial
  Pia mater, intracranial
2 Dura Mater
  Diaphragma sellae
  Dura mater, intracranial
  Falx cerebri
  Tentorium cerebelli
6 Cerebral Ventricle
  Aqueduct of Sylvius
  Cerebral aqueduct (Sylvius)
  Choroid plexus
  Ependyma
  Foramen of Monro (intraventricular)
  Fourth ventricle
  Interventricular foramen (Monro)
  Left lateral ventricle
  Right lateral ventricle
  Third ventricle
F Olfactory Nerve
  First cranial nerve
  Olfactory bulb
G Optic Nerve
  Optic chiasma
  Second cranial nerve
H Oculomotor Nerve
  Third cranial nerve
J Trochlear Nerve
  Fourth cranial nerve
K Trigeminal Nerve
  Fifth cranial nerve
  Gasserian ganglion
  Mandibular nerve
  Maxillary nerve
  Ophthalmic nerve
  Trifacial nerve
L Abducens Nerve
  Sixth cranial nerve
M Facial Nerve
  Chorda tympani
  Geniculate ganglion
  Greater superficial petrosal nerve
  Nerve to the stapedius
  Parotid plexus
  Posterior auricular nerve
  Seventh cranial nerve
  Submandibular ganglion
N Acoustic Nerve
  Cochlear nerve
  Eighth cranial nerve
  Scarpa's (vestibular) ganglion
  Spiral ganglion
  Vestibular (Scarpa's) ganglion
  Vestibular nerve
  Vestibulocochlear nerve
P Glossopharyngeal Nerve
  Carotid sinus nerve
  Ninth cranial nerve
  Tympanic nerve
Q Vagus Nerve
  Anterior vagal trunk
  Pharyngeal plexus
  Pneumogastric nerve
  Posterior vagal trunk
  Pulmonary plexus
  Recurrent laryngeal nerve
  Superior laryngeal nerve
  Tenth cranial nerve
R Accessory Nerve
  Eleventh cranial nerve
S Hypoglossal Nerve
  Twelfth cranial nerve
T Spinal Meninges
  Arachnoid mater, spinal
  Denticulate (dentate) ligament
  Dura mater, spinal
  Filum terminale
  Leptomeninges, spinal
  Pia mater, spinal
	0 Open
	4 Percutaneous Endoscopic
		7 Autologous Tissue Substitute
		J Synthetic Substitute
		K Nonautologous Tissue Substitute
			Z No Qualifier

0 Medical and Surgical
0 Central Nervous System and Cranial Nerves
S Reposition

Definition: Moving to its normal location, or other suitable location, all or a portion of a body part

Explanation: The body part is moved to a new location from an abnormal location, or from a normal location where it is not functioning correctly. The body part may or may not be cut out or off to be moved to the new location.

Body Part Character 4	Approach Character 5	Device Character 6	Qualifier Character 7

F Olfactory Nerve
  First cranial nerve
  Olfactory bulb
G Optic Nerve
  Optic chiasma
  Second cranial nerve
H Oculomotor Nerve
  Third cranial nerve
J Trochlear Nerve
  Fourth cranial nerve
K Trigeminal Nerve
  Fifth cranial nerve
  Gasserian ganglion
  Mandibular nerve
  Maxillary nerve
  Ophthalmic nerve
  Trifacial nerve
L Abducens Nerve
  Sixth cranial nerve
M Facial Nerve
  Chorda tympani
  Geniculate ganglion
  Greater superficial petrosal nerve
  Nerve to the stapedius
  Parotid plexus
  Posterior auricular nerve
  Seventh cranial nerve
  Submandibular ganglion
N Acoustic Nerve
  Cochlear nerve
  Eighth cranial nerve
  Scarpa's (vestibular) ganglion
  Spiral ganglion
  Vestibular (Scarpa's) ganglion
  Vestibular nerve
  Vestibulocochlear nerve
P Glossopharyngeal Nerve
  Carotid sinus nerve
  Ninth cranial nerve
  Tympanic nerve
Q Vagus Nerve
  Anterior vagal trunk
  Pharyngeal plexus
  Pneumogastric nerve
  Posterior vagal trunk
  Pulmonary plexus
  Recurrent laryngeal nerve
  Superior laryngeal nerve
  Tenth cranial nerve
R Accessory Nerve
  Eleventh cranial nerve
S Hypoglossal Nerve
  Twelfth cranial nerve
W Cervical Spinal Cord
  Dorsal root ganglion
X Thoracic Spinal Cord
  Dorsal root ganglion
Y Lumbar Spinal Cord
  Cauda equina
  Conus medullaris
  Dorsal root ganglion
	0 Open
	3 Percutaneous
	4 Percutaneous Endoscopic
		Z No Device	**Z** No Qualifier

0 Medical and Surgical
0 Central Nervous System and Cranial Nerves
T Resection

Definition: Cutting out or off, without replacement, all of a body part

Explanation: None

Body Part Character 4	Approach Character 5	Device Character 6	Qualifier Character 7

7 Cerebral Hemisphere
  Frontal lobe
  Occipital lobe
  Parietal lobe
  Temporal lobe
	0 Open
	3 Percutaneous
	4 Percutaneous Endoscopic
		Z No Device	**Z** No Qualifier

Non-OR Procedure   DRG Non-OR Procedure   Valid OR Procedure   HAC Associated Procedure   Combination Only   New/Revised April   New/Revised October

0 Medical and Surgical
0 Central Nervous System and Cranial Nerves
U Supplement   Definition: Putting in or on biological or synthetic material that physically reinforces and/or augments the function of a portion of a body part
Explanation: The biological material is non-living, or is living and from the same individual. The body part may have been previously replaced, and the SUPPLEMENT procedure is performed to physically reinforce and/or augment the function of the replaced body part.

Body Part Character 4	Approach Character 5	Device Character 6	Qualifier Character 7

1 Cerebral Meninges
   Arachnoid mater, intracranial
   Leptomeninges, intracranial
   Pia mater, intracranial
2 Dura Mater
   Diaphragma sellae
   Dura mater, intracranial
   Falx cerebri
   Tentorium cerebelli
6 Cerebral Ventricle
   Aqueduct of Sylvius
   Cerebral aqueduct (Sylvius)
   Choroid plexus
   Ependyma
   Foramen of Monro (intraventricular)
   Fourth ventricle
   Interventricular foramen (Monro)
   Left lateral ventricle
   Right lateral ventricle
   Third ventricle
F Olfactory Nerve
   First cranial nerve
   Olfactory bulb
G Optic Nerve
   Optic chiasma
   Second cranial nerve
H Oculomotor Nerve
   Third cranial nerve
J Trochlear Nerve
   Fourth cranial nerve
K Trigeminal Nerve
   Fifth cranial nerve
   Gasserian ganglion
   Mandibular nerve
   Maxillary nerve
   Ophthalmic nerve
   Trifacial nerve
L Abducens Nerve
   Sixth cranial nerve
M Facial Nerve
   Chorda tympani
   Geniculate ganglion
   Greater superficial petrosal nerve
   Nerve to the stapedius
   Parotid plexus
   Posterior auricular nerve
   Seventh cranial nerve
   Submandibular ganglion
N Acoustic Nerve
   Cochlear nerve
   Eighth cranial nerve
   Scarpa's (vestibular) ganglion
   Spiral ganglion
   Vestibular (Scarpa's) ganglion
   Vestibular nerve
   Vestibulocochlear nerve
P Glossopharyngeal Nerve
   Carotid sinus nerve
   Ninth cranial nerve
   Tympanic nerve
Q Vagus Nerve
   Anterior vagal trunk
   Pharyngeal plexus
   Pneumogastric nerve
   Posterior vagal trunk
   Pulmonary plexus
   Recurrent laryngeal nerve
   Superior laryngeal nerve
   Tenth cranial nerve
R Accessory Nerve
   Eleventh cranial nerve
S Hypoglossal Nerve
   Twelfth cranial nerve
T Spinal Meninges
   Arachnoid mater, spinal
   Denticulate (dentate) ligament
   Dura mater, spinal
   Filum terminale
   Leptomeninges, spinal
   Pia mater, spinal
	0 Open
	3 Percutaneous
	4 Percutaneous Endoscopic
		7 Autologous Tissue Substitute
		J Synthetic Substitute
		K Nonautologous Tissue Substitute
			Z No Qualifier

Central Nervous System and Cranial Nerves

0 Medical and Surgical
0 Central Nervous System and Cranial Nerves
W Revision — Definition: Correcting, to the extent possible, a portion of a malfunctioning device or the position of a displaced device
Explanation: Revision can include correcting a malfunctioning or displaced device by taking out or putting in components of the device such as a screw or pin

Body Part Character 4	Approach Character 5	Device Character 6	Qualifier Character 7

0 Brain
   Cerebrum
   Corpus callosum
   Encephalon
V Spinal Cord
   Dorsal root ganglion
	0 Open
	3 Percutaneous
	4 Percutaneous Endoscopic
		0 Drainage Device
		2 Monitoring Device
		3 Infusion Device
		7 Autologous Tissue Substitute
		J Synthetic Substitute
		K Nonautologous Tissue Substitute
		M Neurostimulator Lead
		Y Other Device
			Z No Qualifier

0 Brain
   Cerebrum
   Corpus callosum
   Encephalon
V Spinal Cord
   Dorsal root ganglion
	X External	**0** Drainage Device
		2 Monitoring Device
		3 Infusion Device
		7 Autologous Tissue Substitute
		J Synthetic Substitute
		K Nonautologous Tissue Substitute
		M Neurostimulator Lead
			Z No Qualifier

6 Cerebral Ventricle
   Aqueduct of Sylvius
   Cerebral aqueduct (Sylvius)
   Choroid plexus
   Ependyma
   Foramen of Monro (intraventricular)
   Fourth ventricle
   Interventricular foramen (Monro)
   Left lateral ventricle
   Right lateral ventricle
   Third ventricle
U Spinal Canal
   Epidural space, spinal
   Extradural space, spinal
   Subarachnoid space, spinal
   Subdural space, spinal
   Vertebral canal
	0 Open
	3 Percutaneous
	4 Percutaneous Endoscopic
		0 Drainage Device
		2 Monitoring Device
		3 Infusion Device
		J Synthetic Substitute
		M Neurostimulator Lead
		Y Other Device
			Z No Qualifier

6 Cerebral Ventricle
   Aqueduct of Sylvius
   Cerebral aqueduct (Sylvius)
   Choroid plexus
   Ependyma
   Foramen of Monro (intraventricular)
   Fourth ventricle
   Interventricular foramen (Monro)
   Left lateral ventricle
   Right lateral ventricle
   Third ventricle
U Spinal Canal
   Epidural space, spinal
   Extradural space, spinal
   Subarachnoid space, spinal
   Subdural space, spinal
   Vertebral canal
	X External	**0** Drainage Device
		2 Monitoring Device
		3 Infusion Device
		J Synthetic Substitute
		M Neurostimulator Lead
			Z No Qualifier

E Cranial Nerve	**0** Open **3** Percutaneous **4** Percutaneous Endoscopic	**0** Drainage Device **2** Monitoring Device **3** Infusion Device **7** Autologous Tissue Substitute **M** Neurostimulator Lead **Y** Other Device	**Z** No Qualifier
E Cranial Nerve	**X** External	**0** Drainage Device **2** Monitoring Device **3** Infusion Device **7** Autologous Tissue Substitute **M** Neurostimulator Lead	**Z** No Qualifier

Non-OR   00W[0,V][3,4]YZ
Non-OR   00W[0,V]X[0,2,3,7,J,K,M]Z
Non-OR   00W[6,U][3,4]YZ
Non-OR   00W[6,U]X[0,2,3,J,M]Z
Non-OR   00WE[3,4]YZ
Non-OR   00WEX[0,2,3,7,M]Z

0 Medical and Surgical
0 Central Nervous System and Cranial Nerves
X Transfer Definition: Moving, without taking out, all or a portion of a body part to another location to take over the function of all or a portion of a body part
Explanation: The body part transferred remains connected to its vascular and nervous supply

Body Part Character 4	Approach Character 5	Device Character 6	Qualifier Character 7

F Olfactory Nerve
  First cranial nerve
  Olfactory bulb
G Optic Nerve
  Optic chiasma
  Second cranial nerve
H Oculomotor Nerve
  Third cranial nerve
J Trochlear Nerve
  Fourth cranial nerve
K Trigeminal Nerve
  Fifth cranial nerve
  Gasserian ganglion
  Mandibular nerve
  Maxillary nerve
  Ophthalmic nerve
  Trifacial nerve
L Abducens Nerve
  Sixth cranial nerve
M Facial Nerve
  Chorda tympani
  Geniculate ganglion
  Greater superficial petrosal nerve
  Nerve to the stapedius
  Parotid plexus
  Posterior auricular nerve
  Seventh cranial nerve
  Submandibular ganglion
N Acoustic Nerve
  Cochlear nerve
  Eighth cranial nerve
  Scarpa's (vestibular) ganglion
  Spiral ganglion
  Vestibular (Scarpa's) ganglion
  Vestibular nerve
  Vestibulocochlear nerve
P Glossopharyngeal Nerve
  Carotid sinus nerve
  Ninth cranial nerve
  Tympanic nerve
Q Vagus Nerve
  Anterior vagal trunk
  Pharyngeal plexus
  Pneumogastric nerve
  Posterior vagal trunk
  Pulmonary plexus
  Recurrent laryngeal nerve
  Superior laryngeal nerve
  Tenth cranial nerve
R Accessory Nerve
  Eleventh cranial nerve
S Hypoglossal Nerve
  Twelfth cranial nerve
	0 Open
	4 Percutaneous Endoscopic
		Z No Device	**F** Olfactory Nerve
			G Optic Nerve
			H Oculomotor Nerve
			J Trochlear Nerve
			K Trigeminal Nerve
			L Abducens Nerve
			M Facial Nerve
			N Acoustic Nerve
			P Glossopharyngeal Nerve
			Q Vagus Nerve
			R Accessory Nerve
			S Hypoglossal Nerve

Peripheral Nervous System Ø12–Ø1X

Character Meanings

This Character Meaning table is provided as a guide to assist the user in the identification of character members that may be found in this section of code tables. It **SHOULD NOT** be used to build a PCS code.

Operation–Character 3	Body Part–Character 4	Approach–Character 5	Device–Character 6	Qualifier–Character 7
2 Change	Ø Cervical Plexus	Ø Open	Ø Drainage Device	1 Cervical Nerve
5 Destruction	1 Cervical Nerve	3 Percutaneous	1 Radioactive Element	2 Phrenic Nerve
8 Division	2 Phrenic Nerve	4 Percutaneous Endoscopic	2 Monitoring Device	4 Ulnar Nerve
9 Drainage	3 Brachial Plexus	X External	7 Autologous Tissue Substitute	5 Median Nerve
B Excision	4 Ulnar Nerve		J Synthetic Substitute	6 Radial Nerve
C Extirpation	5 Median Nerve		K Nonautologous Tissue Substitute	8 Thoracic Nerve
D Extraction	6 Radial Nerve		M Neurostimulator Lead	B Lumbar Nerve
H Insertion	8 Thoracic Nerve		Y Other Device	C Perineal Nerve
J Inspection	9 Lumbar Plexus		Z No Device	D Femoral Nerve
N Release	A Lumbosacral Plexus			F Sciatic Nerve
P Removal	B Lumbar Nerve			G Tibial Nerve
Q Repair	C Pudendal Nerve			H Peroneal Nerve
R Replacement	D Femoral Nerve			X Diagnostic
S Reposition	F Sciatic Nerve			Z No Qualifier
U Supplement	G Tibial Nerve			
W Revision	H Peroneal Nerve			
X Transfer	K Head and Neck Sympathetic Nerve			
	L Thoracic Sympathetic Nerve			
	M Abdominal Sympathetic Nerve			
	N Lumbar Sympathetic Nerve			
	P Sacral Sympathetic Nerve			
	Q Sacral Plexus			
	R Sacral Nerve			
	Y Peripheral Nerve			

AHA Coding Clinic for table Ø1B
2018, 2Q, 22 — Excision of synovial cyst
2017, 2Q, 19 — Thoracic outlet decompression with sympathectomy

AHA Coding Clinic for table Ø1H
2020, 4Q, 43-44 — Insertion of radioactive element

AHA Coding Clinic for table Ø1N
2019, 1Q, 28 — Decompressive laminectomy of both spinal cord and nerve roots
2018, 2Q, 22 — Excision of synovial cyst
2017, 2Q, 19 — Thoracic outlet decompression with sympathectomy
2016, 2Q, 16 — Decompressive laminectomy/foraminotomy and lumbar discectomy
2016, 2Q, 17 — Removal of longitudinal ligament to decompress cervical nerve root
2016, 2Q, 23 — Thoracic outlet syndrome and release of brachial plexus
2015, 2Q, 34 — Decompressive laminectomy
2014, 3Q, 33 — Radial fracture treatment with open reduction internal fixation, and release of carpal ligament

AHA Coding Clinic for table Ø1Q
2019, 3Q, 32 — Breast reconstruction with neurotization

AHA Coding Clinic for table Ø1S
2021, 3Q, 19 — Elbow amputation and targeted muscle reinnervation

AHA Coding Clinic for table Ø1U
2019, 3Q, 32 — Breast reconstruction with neurotization
2017, 4Q, 62 — Added and revised device values - Nerve substitutes

Median and Ulnar Nerves

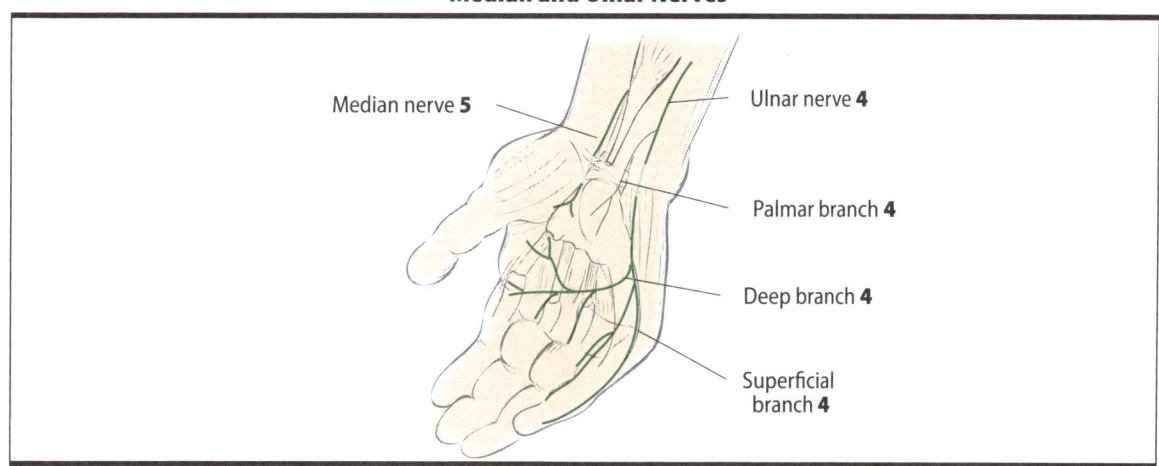

Median nerve **5**
Ulnar nerve **4**
Palmar branch **4**
Deep branch **4**
Superficial branch **4**

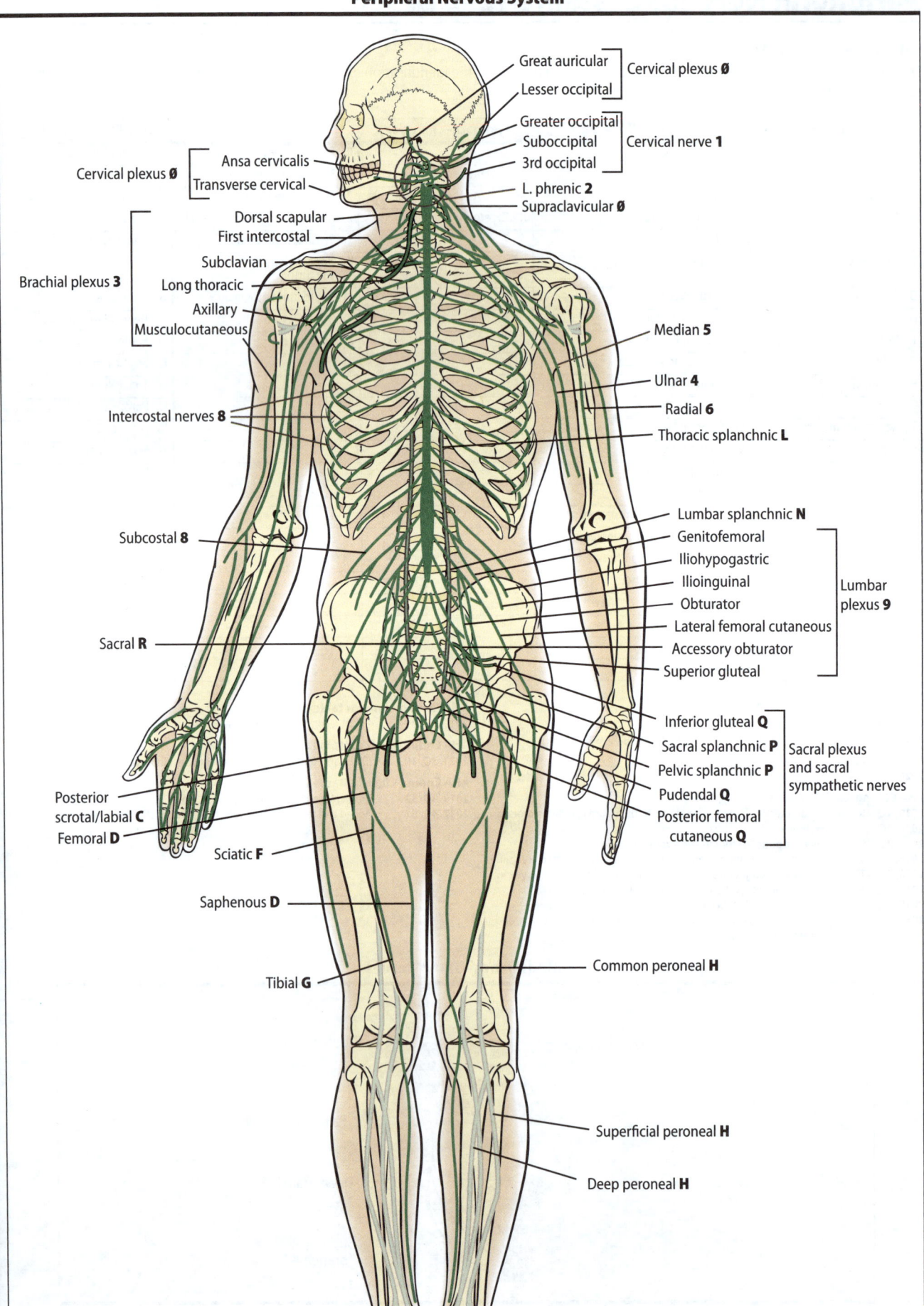

Peripheral Nervous System

Peripheral Nervous System

- Great auricular — Cervical plexus 0
- Lesser occipital
- Greater occipital
- Suboccipital — Cervical nerve 1
- 3rd occipital
- L. phrenic 2
- Supraclavicular 0

Cervical plexus 0:
- Ansa cervicalis
- Transverse cervical

Brachial plexus 3:
- Dorsal scapular
- First intercostal
- Subclavian
- Long thoracic
- Axillary
- Musculocutaneous

- Median 5
- Ulnar 4
- Radial 6
- Thoracic splanchnic L
- Intercostal nerves 8
- Subcostal 8

Lumbar plexus 9:
- Lumbar splanchnic N
- Genitofemoral
- Iliohypogastric
- Ilioinguinal
- Obturator
- Lateral femoral cutaneous
- Accessory obturator
- Superior gluteal

Sacral plexus and sacral sympathetic nerves:
- Inferior gluteal Q
- Sacral splanchnic P
- Pelvic splanchnic P
- Pudendal Q
- Posterior femoral cutaneous Q

- Sacral R
- Posterior scrotal/labial C
- Femoral D
- Sciatic F
- Saphenous D
- Tibial G
- Common peroneal H
- Superficial peroneal H
- Deep peroneal H

ICD-10-PCS 2025 — Peripheral Nervous System — 012–015

0 Medical and Surgical
1 Peripheral Nervous System
2 Change — Definition: Taking out or off a device from a body part and putting back an identical or similar device in or on the same body part without cutting or puncturing the skin or a mucous membrane
Explanation: All CHANGE procedures are coded using the approach EXTERNAL

Body Part Character 4	Approach Character 5	Device Character 6	Qualifier Character 7
Y Peripheral Nerve	X External	0 Drainage Device Y Other Device	Z No Qualifier

Non-OR All body part, approach, device, and qualifier values

---

0 Medical and Surgical
1 Peripheral Nervous System
5 Destruction — Definition: Physical eradication of all or a portion of a body part by the direct use of energy, force, or a destructive agent
Explanation: None of the body part is physically taken out

Body Part Character 4	Approach Character 5	Device Character 6	Qualifier Character 7
0 Cervical Plexus Ansa cervicalis Cutaneous (transverse) cervical nerve Great auricular nerve Lesser occipital nerve Supraclavicular nerve Transverse (cutaneous) cervical nerve **1 Cervical Nerve** Greater occipital nerve Spinal nerve, cervical Suboccipital nerve Third occipital nerve **2 Phrenic Nerve** Accessory phrenic nerve **3 Brachial Plexus** Axillary nerve Dorsal scapular nerve First intercostal nerve Long thoracic nerve Musculocutaneous nerve Subclavius nerve Suprascapular nerve **4 Ulnar Nerve** Cubital nerve **5 Median Nerve** Anterior interosseous nerve Palmar cutaneous nerve **6 Radial Nerve** Dorsal digital nerve Musculospiral nerve Palmar cutaneous nerve Posterior interosseous nerve **8 Thoracic Nerve** Intercostal nerve Intercostobrachial nerve Spinal nerve, thoracic Subcostal nerve **9 Lumbar Plexus** Accessory obturator nerve Genitofemoral nerve Iliohypogastric nerve Ilioinguinal nerve Lateral femoral cutaneous nerve Obturator nerve Superior gluteal nerve **A Lumbosacral Plexus** **B Lumbar Nerve** Lumbosacral trunk Spinal nerve, lumbar Superior clunic (cluneal) nerve **C Pudendal Nerve** Posterior labial nerve Posterior scrotal nerve **D Femoral Nerve** Anterior crural nerve Saphenous nerve **F Sciatic Nerve** Ischiatic nerve **G Tibial Nerve** Lateral plantar nerve Medial plantar nerve Medial popliteal nerve Medial sural cutaneous nerve **H Peroneal Nerve** Common fibular nerve Common peroneal nerve External popliteal nerve Lateral sural cutaneous nerve **K Head and Neck Sympathetic Nerve** Cavernous plexus Cervical ganglion Ciliary ganglion Internal carotid plexus Otic ganglion Pterygopalatine (sphenopalatine) ganglion Sphenopalatine (pterygopalatine) ganglion Stellate ganglion Submandibular ganglion Submaxillary ganglion **L Thoracic Sympathetic Nerve** Cardiac plexus Esophageal plexus Greater splanchnic nerve Inferior cardiac nerve Least splanchnic nerve Lesser splanchnic nerve Middle cardiac nerve Pulmonary plexus Superior cardiac nerve Thoracic aortic plexus Thoracic ganglion **M Abdominal Sympathetic Nerve** Abdominal aortic plexus Auerbach's (myenteric) plexus Celiac (solar) plexus Celiac ganglion Gastric plexus Hepatic plexus Inferior hypogastric plexus Inferior mesenteric ganglion Inferior mesenteric plexus Meissner's (submucous) plexus Myenteric (Auerbach's) plexus Pancreatic plexus Pelvic splanchnic nerve Renal nerve Renal plexus Solar (celiac) plexus Splenic plexus Submucous (Meissner's) plexus Superior hypogastric plexus Superior mesenteric ganglion Superior mesenteric plexus Suprarenal plexus **N Lumbar Sympathetic Nerve** Lumbar ganglion Lumbar splanchnic nerve **P Sacral Sympathetic Nerve** Ganglion impar (ganglion of Walther) Pelvic splanchnic nerve Sacral ganglion Sacral splanchnic nerve **Q Sacral Plexus** Inferior gluteal nerve Posterior femoral cutaneous nerve Pudendal nerve **R Sacral Nerve** Spinal nerve, sacral	0 Open 3 Percutaneous 4 Percutaneous Endoscopic	Z No Device	Z No Qualifier

Non-OR 015[0,2,3,4,5,6,9,A,C,D,F,G,H,Q][0,3,4]ZZ
Non-OR 015[1,8,B,R]3ZZ

018–018   Peripheral Nervous System   ICD-10-PCS 2025

0 Medical and Surgical
1 Peripheral Nervous System
8 Division   Definition: Cutting into a body part, without draining fluids and/or gases from the body part, in order to separate or transect a body part
Explanation: All or a portion of the body part is separated into two or more portions

Body Part Character 4	Approach Character 5	Device Character 6	Qualifier Character 7
0 Cervical Plexus Ansa cervicalis Cutaneous (transverse) cervical nerve Great auricular nerve Lesser occipital nerve Supraclavicular nerve Transverse (cutaneous) cervical nervef **1 Cervical Nerve** Greater occipital nerve Spinal nerve, cervical Suboccipital nerve Third occipital nerve **2 Phrenic Nerve** Accessory phrenic nerve **3 Brachial Plexus** Axillary nerve Dorsal scapular nerve First intercostal nerve Long thoracic nerve Musculocutaneous nerve Subclavius nerve Suprascapular nerve **4 Ulnar Nerve** Cubital nerve **5 Median Nerve** Anterior interosseous nerve Palmar cutaneous nerve **6 Radial Nerve** Dorsal digital nerve Musculospiral nerve Palmar cutaneous nerve Posterior interosseous nerve **8 Thoracic Nerve** Intercostal nerve Intercostobrachial nerve Spinal nerve, thoracic Subcostal nerve **9 Lumbar Plexus** Accessory obturator nerve Genitofemoral nerve Iliohypogastric nerve Ilioinguinal nerve Lateral femoral cutaneous nerve Obturator nerve Superior gluteal nerve **A Lumbosacral Plexus** **B Lumbar Nerve** Lumbosacral trunk Spinal nerve, lumbar Superior clunic (cluneal) nerve **C Pudendal Nerve** Posterior labial nerve Posterior scrotal nerve **D Femoral Nerve** Anterior crural nerve Saphenous nerve **F Sciatic Nerve** Ischiatic nerve **G Tibial Nerve** Lateral plantar nerve Medial plantar nerve Medial popliteal nerve Medial sural cutaneous nerve	**H Peroneal Nerve** Common fibular nerve Common peroneal nerve External popliteal nerve Lateral sural cutaneous nerve **K Head and Neck Sympathetic Nerve** Cavernous plexus Cervical ganglion Ciliary ganglion Internal carotid plexus Otic ganglion Pterygopalatine (sphenopalatine) ganglion Sphenopalatine (pterygopalatine) ganglion Stellate ganglion Submandibular ganglion Submaxillary ganglion **L Thoracic Sympathetic Nerve** Cardiac plexus Esophageal plexus Greater splanchnic nerve Inferior cardiac nerve Least splanchnic nerve Lesser splanchnic nerve Middle cardiac nerve Pulmonary plexus Superior cardiac nerve Thoracic aortic plexus Thoracic ganglion **M Abdominal Sympathetic Nerve** Abdominal aortic plexus Auerbach's (myenteric) plexus Celiac (solar) plexus Celiac ganglion Gastric plexus Hepatic plexus Inferior hypogastric plexus Inferior mesenteric ganglion Inferior mesenteric plexus Meissner's (submucous) plexus Myenteric (Auerbach's) plexus Pancreatic plexus Pelvic splanchnic nerve Renal nerve Renal plexus Solar (celiac) plexus Splenic plexus Submucous (Meissner's) plexus Superior hypogastric plexus Superior mesenteric ganglion Superior mesenteric plexus Suprarenal plexus **N Lumbar Sympathetic Nerve** Lumbar ganglion Lumbar splanchnic nerve **P Sacral Sympathetic Nerve** Ganglion impar (ganglion of Walther) Pelvic splanchnic nerve Sacral ganglion Sacral splanchnic nerve **Q Sacral Plexus** Inferior gluteal nerve Posterior femoral cutaneous nerve Pudendal nerve **R Sacral Nerve** Spinal nerve, sacral	**0** Open **3** Percutaneous **4** Percutaneous Endoscopic	**Z** No Device	**Z** No Qualifier

Non-OR Procedure   DRG Non-OR Procedure   Valid OR Procedure   HAC Associated Procedure   Combination Only   New/Revised April   New/Revised October

ICD-10-PCS 2025   Peripheral Nervous System   019–019

0 Medical and Surgical
1 Peripheral Nervous System
9 Drainage   Definition: Taking or letting out fluids and/or gases from a body part
                 Explanation: The qualifier DIAGNOSTIC is used to identify drainage procedures that are biopsies

Body Part Character 4	Approach Character 5	Device Character 6	Qualifier Character 7

0 Cervical Plexus
    Ansa cervicalis
    Cutaneous (transverse) cervical nerve
    Great auricular nerve
    Lesser occipital nerve
    Supraclavicular nerve
    Transverse (cutaneous) cervical nerve
1 Cervical Nerve
    Greater occipital nerve
    Spinal nerve, cervical
    Suboccipital nerve
    Third occipital nerve
2 Phrenic Nerve
    Accessory phrenic nerve
3 Brachial Plexus
    Axillary nerve
    Dorsal scapular nerve
    First intercostal nerve
    Long thoracic nerve
    Musculocutaneous nerve
    Subclavius nerve
    Suprascapular nerve
4 Ulnar Nerve
    Cubital nerve
5 Median Nerve
    Anterior interosseous nerve
    Palmar cutaneous nerve
6 Radial Nerve
    Dorsal digital nerve
    Musculospiral nerve
    Palmar cutaneous nerve
    Posterior interosseous nerve
8 Thoracic Nerve
    Intercostal nerve
    Intercostobrachial nerve
    Spinal nerve, thoracic
    Subcostal nerve
9 Lumbar Plexus
    Accessory obturator nerve
    Genitofemoral nerve
    Iliohypogastric nerve
    Ilioinguinal nerve
    Lateral femoral cutaneous nerve
    Obturator nerve
    Superior gluteal nerve
A Lumbosacral Plexus
B Lumbar Nerve
    Lumbosacral trunk
    Spinal nerve, lumbar
    Superior clunic (cluneal) nerve
C Pudendal Nerve
    Posterior labial nerve
    Posterior scrotal nerve
D Femoral Nerve
    Anterior crural nerve
    Saphenous nerve
F Sciatic Nerve
    Ischiatic nerve
G Tibial Nerve
    Lateral plantar nerve
    Medial plantar nerve
    Medial popliteal nerve
    Medial sural cutaneous nerve
	H Peroneal Nerve
	    Common fibular nerve
	    Common peroneal nerve
	    External popliteal nerve
	    Lateral sural cutaneous nerve
	K Head and Neck Sympathetic Nerve
	    Cavernous plexus
	    Cervical ganglion
	    Ciliary ganglion
	    Internal carotid plexus
	    Otic ganglion
	    Pterygopalatine (sphenopalatine) ganglion
	    Sphenopalatine (pterygopalatine) ganglion
	    Stellate ganglion
	    Submandibular ganglion
	    Submaxillary ganglion
	L Thoracic Sympathetic Nerve
	    Cardiac plexus
	    Esophageal plexus
	    Greater splanchnic nerve
	    Inferior cardiac nerve
	    Least splanchnic nerve
	    Lesser splanchnic nerve
	    Middle cardiac nerve
	    Pulmonary plexus
	    Superior cardiac nerve
	    Thoracic aortic plexus
	    Thoracic ganglion
	M Abdominal Sympathetic Nerve
	    Abdominal aortic plexus
	    Auerbach's (myenteric) plexus
	    Celiac (solar) plexus
	    Celiac ganglion
	    Gastric plexus
	    Hepatic plexus
	    Inferior hypogastric plexus
	    Inferior mesenteric ganglion
	    Inferior mesenteric plexus
	    Meissner's (submucous) plexus
	    Myenteric (Auerbach's) plexus
	    Pancreatic plexus
	    Pelvic splanchnic nerve
	    Renal nerve
	    Renal plexus
	    Solar (celiac) plexus
	    Splenic plexus
	    Submucous (Meissner's) plexus
	    Superior hypogastric plexus
	    Superior mesenteric ganglion
	    Superior mesenteric plexus
	    Suprarenal plexus
	N Lumbar Sympathetic Nerve
	    Lumbar ganglion
	    Lumbar splanchnic nerve
	P Sacral Sympathetic Nerve
	    Ganglion impar (ganglion of Walther)
	    Pelvic splanchnic nerve
	    Sacral ganglion
	    Sacral splanchnic nerve
	Q Sacral Plexus
	    Inferior gluteal nerve
	    Posterior femoral cutaneous nerve
	    Pudendal nerve
	R Sacral Nerve
	    Spinal nerve, sacral
		0 Open
		3 Percutaneous
		4 Percutaneous Endoscopic
			0 Drainage Device	**Z** No Qualifier

Non-OR   019[0,1,2,3,4,5,6,8,9,A,B,C,D,F,G,H,K,L,M,N,P,Q,R]30Z

019 Continued on next page

019 Continued

0 Medical and Surgical
1 Peripheral Nervous System
9 Drainage — Definition: Taking or letting out fluids and/or gases from a body part
Explanation: The qualifier DIAGNOSTIC is used to identify drainage procedures that are biopsies

Body Part — Character 4	Approach — Character 5	Device — Character 6	Qualifier — Character 7
0 Cervical Plexus Ansa cervicalis Cutaneous (transverse) cervical nerve Great auricular nerve Lesser occipital nerve Supraclavicular nerve Transverse (cutaneous) cervical nerve **1 Cervical Nerve** Greater occipital nerve Spinal nerve, cervical Suboccipital nerve Third occipital nerve **2 Phrenic Nerve** Accessory phrenic nerve **3 Brachial Plexus** Axillary nerve Dorsal scapular nerve First intercostal nerve Long thoracic nerve Musculocutaneous nerve Subclavius nerve Suprascapular nerve **4 Ulnar Nerve** Cubital nerve **5 Median Nerve** Anterior interosseous nerve Palmar cutaneous nerve **6 Radial Nerve** Dorsal digital nerve Musculospiral nerve Palmar cutaneous nerve Posterior interosseous nerve **8 Thoracic Nerve** Intercostal nerve Intercostobrachial nerve Spinal nerve, thoracic Subcostal nerve **9 Lumbar Plexus** Accessory obturator nerve Genitofemoral nerve Iliohypogastric nerve Ilioinguinal nerve Lateral femoral cutaneous nerve Obturator nerve Superior gluteal nerve **A Lumbosacral Plexus** **B Lumbar Nerve** Lumbosacral trunk Spinal nerve, lumbar Superior clunic (cluneal) nerve **C Pudendal Nerve** Posterior labial nerve Posterior scrotal nerve **D Femoral Nerve** Anterior crural nerve Saphenous nerve **F Sciatic Nerve** Ischiatic nerve **G Tibial Nerve** Lateral plantar nerve Medial plantar nerve Medial popliteal nerve Medial sural cutaneous nerve	**H Peroneal Nerve** Common fibular nerve Common peroneal nerve External popliteal nerve Lateral sural cutaneous nerve **K Head and Neck Sympathetic Nerve** Cavernous plexus Cervical ganglion Ciliary ganglion Internal carotid plexus Otic ganglion Pterygopalatine (sphenopalatine) ganglion Sphenopalatine (pterygopalatine) ganglion Stellate ganglion Submandibular ganglion Submaxillary ganglion **L Thoracic Sympathetic Nerve** Cardiac plexus Esophageal plexus Greater splanchnic nerve Inferior cardiac nerve Least splanchnic nerve Lesser splanchnic nerve Middle cardiac nerve Pulmonary plexus Superior cardiac nerve Thoracic aortic plexus Thoracic ganglion **M Abdominal Sympathetic Nerve** Abdominal aortic plexus Auerbach's (myenteric) plexus Celiac (solar) plexus Celiac ganglion Gastric plexus Hepatic plexus Inferior hypogastric plexus Inferior mesenteric ganglion Inferior mesenteric plexus Meissner's (submucous) plexus Myenteric (Auerbach's) plexus Pancreatic plexus Pelvic splanchnic nerve Renal nerve Renal plexus Solar (celiac) plexus Splenic plexus Submucous (Meissner's) plexus Superior hypogastric plexus Superior mesenteric ganglion Superior mesenteric plexus Suprarenal plexus **N Lumbar Sympathetic Nerve** Lumbar ganglion Lumbar splanchnic nerve **P Sacral Sympathetic Nerve** Ganglion impar (ganglion of Walther) Pelvic splanchnic nerve Sacral ganglion Sacral splanchnic nerve **Q Sacral Plexus** Inferior gluteal nerve Posterior femoral cutaneous nerve Pudendal nerve **R Sacral Nerve** Spinal nerve, sacral	**0** Open **3** Percutaneous **4** Percutaneous Endoscopic	**Z** No Device	**X** Diagnostic **Z** No Qualifier

Non-OR 019[0,1,2,3,4,5,6,8,9,A,B,C,D,F,G,H,Q,R][3,4]ZX
Non-OR 019[0,1,2,3,4,5,6,8,9,A,B,C,D,F,G,H,K,L,M,N,P,Q,R]3ZZ

0 Medical and Surgical
1 Peripheral Nervous System
B Excision Definition: Cutting out or off, without replacement, a portion of a body part
Explanation: The qualifier DIAGNOSTIC is used to identify excision procedures that are biopsies

Body Part Character 4	Approach Character 5	Device Character 6	Qualifier Character 7

0 Cervical Plexus
  Ansa cervicalis
  Cutaneous (transverse) cervical nerve
  Great auricular nerve
  Lesser occipital nerve
  Supraclavicular nerve
  Transverse (cutaneous) cervical nerve
1 Cervical Nerve
  Greater occipital nerve
  Spinal nerve, cervical
  Suboccipital nerve
  Third occipital nerve
2 Phrenic Nerve
  Accessory phrenic nerve
3 Brachial Plexus
  Axillary nerve
  Dorsal scapular nerve
  First intercostal nerve
  Long thoracic nerve
  Musculocutaneous nerve
  Subclavius nerve
  Suprascapular nerve
4 Ulnar Nerve
  Cubital nerve
5 Median Nerve
  Anterior interosseous nerve
  Palmar cutaneous nerve
6 Radial Nerve
  Dorsal digital nerve
  Musculospiral nerve
  Palmar cutaneous nerve
  Posterior interosseous nerve
8 Thoracic Nerve
  Intercostal nerve
  Intercostobrachial nerve
  Spinal nerve, thoracic
  Subcostal nerve
9 Lumbar Plexus
  Accessory obturator nerve
  Genitofemoral nerve
  Iliohypogastric nerve
  Ilioinguinal nerve
  Lateral femoral cutaneous nerve
  Obturator nerve
  Superior gluteal nerve
A Lumbosacral Plexus
B Lumbar Nerve
  Lumbosacral trunk
  Spinal nerve, lumbar
  Superior clunic (cluneal) nerve
C Pudendal Nerve
  Posterior labial nerve
  Posterior scrotal nerve
D Femoral Nerve
  Anterior crural nerve
  Saphenous nerve
F Sciatic Nerve
  Ischiatic nerve
G Tibial Nerve
  Lateral plantar nerve
  Medial plantar nerve
  Medial popliteal nerve
  Medial sural cutaneous nerve
	H Peroneal Nerve
	  Common fibular nerve
	  Common peroneal nerve
	  External popliteal nerve
	  Lateral sural cutaneous nerve
	K Head and Neck Sympathetic Nerve
	  Cavernous plexus
	  Cervical ganglion
	  Ciliary ganglion
	  Internal carotid plexus
	  Otic ganglion
	  Pterygopalatine (sphenopalatine) ganglion
	  Sphenopalatine (pterygopalatine) ganglion
	  Stellate ganglion
	  Submandibular ganglion
	  Submaxillary ganglion
	L Thoracic Sympathetic Nerve
	  Cardiac plexus
	  Esophageal plexus
	  Greater splanchnic nerve
	  Inferior cardiac nerve
	  Least splanchnic nerve
	  Lesser splanchnic nerve
	  Middle cardiac nerve
	  Pulmonary plexus
	  Superior cardiac nerve
	  Thoracic aortic plexus
	  Thoracic ganglion
	M Abdominal Sympathetic Nerve
	  Abdominal aortic plexus
	  Auerbach's (myenteric) plexus
	  Celiac (solar) plexus
	  Celiac ganglion
	  Gastric plexus
	  Hepatic plexus
	  Inferior hypogastric plexus
	  Inferior mesenteric ganglion
	  Inferior mesenteric plexus
	  Meissner's (submucous) plexus
	  Myenteric (Auerbach's) plexus
	  Pancreatic plexus
	  Pelvic splanchnic nerve
	  Renal nerve
	  Renal plexus
	  Solar (celiac) plexus
	  Splenic plexus
	  Submucous (Meissner's) plexus
	  Superior hypogastric plexus
	  Superior mesenteric ganglion
	  Superior mesenteric plexus
	  Suprarenal plexus
	N Lumbar Sympathetic Nerve
	  Lumbar ganglion
	  Lumbar splanchnic nerve
	P Sacral Sympathetic Nerve
	  Ganglion impar (ganglion of Walther)
	  Pelvic splanchnic nerve
	  Sacral ganglion
	  Sacral splanchnic nerve
	Q Sacral Plexus
	  Inferior gluteal nerve
	  Posterior femoral cutaneous nerve
	  Pudendal nerve
	R Sacral Nerve
	  Spinal nerve, sacral
		0 Open
		3 Percutaneous
		4 Percutaneous Endoscopic
			Z No Device	**X** Diagnostic
				Z No Qualifier

Non-OR 01B[0,1,2,3,4,5,6,8,9,A,B,C,D,F,G,H,Q,R][3,4]ZX

0 Medical and Surgical
1 Peripheral Nervous System
C Extirpation   Definition: Taking or cutting out solid matter from a body part

Explanation: The solid matter may be an abnormal byproduct of a biological function or a foreign body; it may be imbedded in a body part or in the lumen of a tubular body part. The solid matter may or may not have been previously broken into pieces.

Body Part — Character 4	Approach — Character 5	Device — Character 6	Qualifier — Character 7

0 Cervical Plexus
  Ansa cervicalis
  Cutaneous (transverse) cervical nerve
  Great auricular nerve
  Lesser occipital nerve
  Supraclavicular nerve
  Transverse (cutaneous) cervical nerve
1 Cervical Nerve
  Greater occipital nerve
  Spinal nerve, cervical
  Suboccipital nerve
  Third occipital nerve
2 Phrenic Nerve
  Accessory phrenic nerve
3 Brachial Plexus
  Axillary nerve
  Dorsal scapular nerve
  First intercostal nerve
  Long thoracic nerve
  Musculocutaneous nerve
  Subclavius nerve
  Suprascapular nerve
4 Ulnar Nerve
  Cubital nerve
5 Median Nerve
  Anterior interosseous nerve
  Palmar cutaneous nerve
6 Radial Nerve
  Dorsal digital nerve
  Musculospiral nerve
  Palmar cutaneous nerve
  Posterior interosseous nerve
8 Thoracic Nerve
  Intercostal nerve
  Intercostobrachial nerve
  Spinal nerve, thoracic
  Subcostal nerve
9 Lumbar Plexus
  Accessory obturator nerve
  Genitofemoral nerve
  Iliohypogastric nerve
  Ilioinguinal nerve
  Lateral femoral cutaneous nerve
  Obturator nerve
  Superior gluteal nerve
A Lumbosacral Plexus
B Lumbar Nerve
  Lumbosacral trunk
  Spinal nerve, lumbar
  Superior clunic (cluneal) nerve
C Pudendal Nerve
  Posterior labial nerve
  Posterior scrotal nerve
D Femoral Nerve
  Anterior crural nerve
  Saphenous nerve
F Sciatic Nerve
  Ischiatic nerve
G Tibial Nerve
  Lateral plantar nerve
  Medial plantar nerve
  Medial popliteal nerve
  Medial sural cutaneous nerve
	0 Open
	3 Percutaneous
	4 Percutaneous Endoscopic
		Z No Device	**Z No Qualifier**

H Peroneal Nerve
  Common fibular nerve
  Common peroneal nerve
  External popliteal nerve
  Lateral sural cutaneous nerve
K Head and Neck Sympathetic Nerve
  Cavernous plexus
  Cervical ganglion
  Ciliary ganglion
  Internal carotid plexus
  Otic ganglion
  Pterygopalatine (sphenopalatine) ganglion
  Sphenopalatine (pterygopalatine) ganglion
  Stellate ganglion
  Submandibular ganglion
  Submaxillary ganglion
L Thoracic Sympathetic Nerve
  Cardiac plexus
  Esophageal plexus
  Greater splanchnic nerve
  Inferior cardiac nerve
  Least splanchnic nerve
  Lesser splanchnic nerve
  Middle cardiac nerve
  Pulmonary plexus
  Superior cardiac nerve
  Thoracic aortic plexus
  Thoracic ganglion
M Abdominal Sympathetic Nerve
  Abdominal aortic plexus
  Auerbach's (myenteric) plexus
  Celiac (solar) plexus
  Celiac ganglion
  Gastric plexus
  Hepatic plexus
  Inferior hypogastric plexus
  Inferior mesenteric ganglion
  Inferior mesenteric plexus
  Meissner's (submucous) plexus
  Myenteric (Auerbach's) plexus
  Pancreatic plexus
  Pelvic splanchnic nerve
  Renal nerve
  Renal plexus
  Solar (celiac) plexus
  Splenic plexus
  Submucous (Meissner's) plexus
  Superior hypogastric plexus
  Superior mesenteric ganglion
  Superior mesenteric plexus
  Suprarenal plexus
N Lumbar Sympathetic Nerve
  Lumbar ganglion
  Lumbar splanchnic nerve
P Sacral Sympathetic Nerve
  Ganglion impar (ganglion of Walther)
  Pelvic splanchnic nerve
  Sacral ganglion
  Sacral splanchnic nerve
Q Sacral Plexus
  Inferior gluteal nerve
  Posterior femoral cutaneous nerve
  Pudendal nerve
R Sacral Nerve
  Spinal nerve, sacral			

Non-OR Procedure   DRG Non-OR Procedure   Valid OR Procedure   HAC Associated Procedure   Combination Only   New/Revised April   New/Revised October

0 Medical and Surgical
1 Peripheral Nervous System
D Extraction Definition: Pulling or stripping out or off all or a portion of a body part by the use of force
Explanation: The qualifier DIAGNOSTIC is used to identify extraction procedures that are biopsies

Body Part Character 4	Approach Character 5	Device Character 6	Qualifier Character 7
0 Cervical Plexus 　Ansa cervicalis 　Cutaneous (transverse) cervical nerve 　Great auricular nerve 　Lesser occipital nerve 　Supraclavicular nerve 　Transverse (cutaneous) cervical nerve **1 Cervical Nerve** 　Greater occipital nerve 　Spinal nerve, cervical 　Suboccipital nerve 　Third occipital nerve **2 Phrenic Nerve** 　Accessory phrenic nerve **3 Brachial Plexus** 　Axillary nerve 　Dorsal scapular nerve 　First intercostal nerve 　Long thoracic nerve 　Musculocutaneous nerve 　Subclavius nerve 　Suprascapular nerve **4 Ulnar Nerve** 　Cubital nerve **5 Median Nerve** 　Anterior interosseous nerve 　Palmar cutaneous nerve **6 Radial Nerve** 　Dorsal digital nerve 　Musculospiral nerve 　Palmar cutaneous nerve 　Posterior interosseous nerve **8 Thoracic Nerve** 　Intercostal nerve 　Intercostobrachial nerve 　Spinal nerve, thoracic 　Subcostal nerve **9 Lumbar Plexus** 　Accessory obturator nerve 　Genitofemoral nerve 　Iliohypogastric nerve 　Ilioinguinal nerve 　Lateral femoral cutaneous nerve 　Obturator nerve 　Superior gluteal nerve **A Lumbosacral Plexus** **B Lumbar Nerve** 　Lumbosacral trunk 　Spinal nerve, lumbar 　Superior clunic (cluneal) nerve **C Pudendal Nerve]** 　Posterior labial nerve 　Posterior scrotal nerve **D Femoral Nerve** 　Anterior crural nerve 　Saphenous nerve **F Sciatic Nerve** 　Ischiatic nerve **G Tibial Nerve** 　Lateral plantar nerve 　Medial plantar nerve 　Medial popliteal nerve 　Medial sural cutaneous nerve	**H Peroneal Nerve** 　Common fibular nerve 　Common peroneal nerve 　External popliteal nerve 　Lateral sural cutaneous nerve **K Head and Neck Sympathetic Nerve** 　Cavernous plexus 　Cervical ganglion 　Ciliary ganglion 　Internal carotid plexus 　Otic ganglion 　Pterygopalatine (sphenopalatine) ganglion 　Sphenopalatine (pterygopalatine) ganglion 　Stellate ganglion 　Submandibular ganglion 　Submaxillary ganglion **L Thoracic Sympathetic Nerve** 　Cardiac plexus 　Esophageal plexus 　Greater splanchnic nerve 　Inferior cardiac nerve 　Least splanchnic nerve 　Lesser splanchnic nerve 　Middle cardiac nerve 　Pulmonary plexus 　Superior cardiac nerve 　Thoracic aortic plexus 　Thoracic ganglion **M Abdominal Sympathetic Nerve** 　Abdominal aortic plexus 　Auerbach's (myenteric) plexus 　Celiac (solar) plexus 　Celiac ganglion 　Gastric plexus 　Hepatic plexus 　Inferior hypogastric plexus 　Inferior mesenteric ganglion 　Inferior mesenteric plexus 　Meissner's (submucous) plexus 　Myenteric (Auerbach's) plexus 　Pancreatic plexus 　Pelvic splanchnic nerve 　Renal nerve 　Renal plexus 　Solar (celiac) plexus 　Splenic plexus 　Submucous (Meissner's) plexus 　Superior hypogastric plexus 　Superior mesenteric ganglion 　Superior mesenteric plexus 　Suprarenal plexus **N Lumbar Sympathetic Nerve** 　Lumbar ganglion 　Lumbar splanchnic nerve **P Sacral Sympathetic Nerve** 　Ganglion impar (ganglion of Walther) 　Pelvic splanchnic nerve 　Sacral ganglion 　Sacral splanchnic nerve **Q Sacral Plexus** 　Inferior gluteal nerve 　Posterior femoral cutaneous nerve 　Pudendal nerve **R Sacral Nerve** 　Spinal nerve, sacral	**0** Open **3** Percutaneous **4** Percutaneous Endoscopic	**Z** No Device	**Z** No Qualifier

0 Medical and Surgical
1 Peripheral Nervous System
H Insertion Definition: Putting in a nonbiological appliance that monitors, assists, performs, or prevents a physiological function but does not physically take the place of a body part
Explanation: None

Body Part Character 4	Approach Character 5	Device Character 6	Qualifier Character 7
Y Peripheral Nerve	0 Open 3 Percutaneous 4 Percutaneous Endoscopic	1 Radioactive Element 2 Monitoring Device M Neurostimulator Lead Y Other Device	Z No Qualifier

Non-OR 01HY31Z
Non-OR 01HY[3,4]YZ

See Appendix L for Procedure Combinations
01HY[0,3,4]MZ

0 Medical and Surgical
1 Peripheral Nervous System
J Inspection Definition: Visually and/or manually exploring a body part
Explanation: Visual exploration may be performed with or without optical instrumentation. Manual exploration may be performed directly or through intervening body layers.

Body Part Character 4	Approach Character 5	Device Character 6	Qualifier Character 7
Y Peripheral Nerve	0 Open 3 Percutaneous 4 Percutaneous Endoscopic	Z No Device	Z No Qualifier

Non-OR 01JY3ZZ

0 Medical and Surgical
1 Peripheral Nervous System
N Release   Definition: Freeing a body part from an abnormal physical constraint by cutting or by the use of force
               Explanation: Some of the restraining tissue may be taken out but none of the body part is taken out

Body Part Character 4	Approach Character 5	Device Character 6	Qualifier Character 7

0 Cervical Plexus
   Ansa cervicalis
   Cutaneous (transverse) cervical nerve
   Great auricular nerve
   Lesser occipital nerve
   Supraclavicular nerve
   Transverse (cutaneous) cervical nerve
1 Cervical Nerve
   Greater occipital nerve
   Spinal nerve, cervical
   Suboccipital nerve
   Third occipital nerve
2 Phrenic Nerve
   Accessory phrenic nerve
3 Brachial Plexus
   Axillary nerve
   Dorsal scapular nerve
   First intercostal nerve
   Long thoracic nerve
   Musculocutaneous nerve
   Subclavius nerve
   Suprascapular nerve
4 Ulnar Nerve
   Cubital nerve
5 Median Nerve
   Anterior interosseous nerve
   Palmar cutaneous nerve
6 Radial Nerve
   Dorsal digital nerve
   Musculospiral nerve
   Palmar cutaneous nerve
   Posterior interosseous nerve
8 Thoracic Nerve
   Intercostal nerve
   Intercostobrachial nerve
   Spinal nerve, thoracic
   Subcostal nerve
9 Lumbar Plexus
   Accessory obturator nerve
   Genitofemoral nerve
   Iliohypogastric nerve
   Ilioinguinal nerve
   Lateral femoral cutaneous nerve
   Obturator nerve
   Superior gluteal nerve
A Lumbosacral Plexus
B Lumbar Nerve
   Lumbosacral trunk
   Spinal nerve, lumbar
   Superior clunic (cluneal) nerve
C Pudendal Nerve
   Posterior labial nerve
   Posterior scrotal nerve
D Femoral Nerve
   Anterior crural nerve
   Saphenous nerve
F Sciatic Nerve
   Ischiatic nerve
G Tibial Nerve
   Lateral plantar nerve
   Medial plantar nerve
   Medial popliteal nerve
   Medial sural cutaneous nerve
H Peroneal Nerve
   Common fibular nerve
   Common peroneal nerve
   External popliteal nerve
   Lateral sural cutaneous nerve
K Head and Neck Sympathetic Nerve
   Cavernous plexus
   Cervical ganglion
   Ciliary ganglion
   Internal carotid plexus
   Otic ganglion
   Pterygopalatine (sphenopalatine) ganglion
   Sphenopalatine (pterygopalatine) ganglion
   Stellate ganglion
   Submandibular ganglion
   Submaxillary ganglion
L Thoracic Sympathetic Nerve
   Cardiac plexus
   Esophageal plexus
   Greater splanchnic nerve
   Inferior cardiac nerve
   Least splanchnic nerve
   Lesser splanchnic nerve
   Middle cardiac nerve
   Pulmonary plexus
   Superior cardiac nerve
   Thoracic aortic plexus
   Thoracic ganglion
M Abdominal Sympathetic Nerve
   Abdominal aortic plexus
   Auerbach's (myenteric) plexus
   Celiac (solar) plexus
   Celiac ganglion
   Gastric plexus
   Hepatic plexus
   Inferior hypogastric plexus
   Inferior mesenteric ganglion
   Inferior mesenteric plexus
   Meissner's (submucous) plexus
   Myenteric (Auerbach's) plexus
   Pancreatic plexus
   Pelvic splanchnic nerve
   Renal nerve
   Renal plexus
   Solar (celiac) plexus
   Splenic plexus
   Submucous (Meissner's) plexus
   Superior hypogastric plexus
   Superior mesenteric ganglion
   Superior mesenteric plexus
   Suprarenal plexus
N Lumbar Sympathetic Nerve
   Lumbar ganglion
   Lumbar splanchnic nerve
P Sacral Sympathetic Nerve
   Ganglion impar (ganglion of Walther)
   Pelvic splanchnic nerve
   Sacral ganglion
   Sacral splanchnic nerve
Q Sacral Plexus
   Inferior gluteal nerve
   Posterior femoral cutaneous nerve
   Pudendal nerve
R Sacral Nerve
   Spinal nerve, sacral
	0 Open
	3 Percutaneous
	4 Percutaneous Endoscopic
		Z No Device	**Z** No Qualifier

0 Medical and Surgical
1 Peripheral Nervous System
P Removal

Definition: Taking out or off a device from a body part

Explanation: If a device is taken out and a similar device put in without cutting or puncturing the skin or mucous membrane, the procedure is coded to the root operation CHANGE. Otherwise, the procedure for taking out a device is coded to the root operation REMOVAL.

Body Part Character 4	Approach Character 5	Device Character 6	Qualifier Character 7
Y Peripheral Nerve	0 Open 3 Percutaneous 4 Percutaneous Endoscopic	0 Drainage Device 2 Monitoring Device 7 Autologous Tissue Substitute M Neurostimulator Lead Y Other Device	Z No Qualifier
Y Peripheral Nerve	X External	0 Drainage Device 2 Monitoring Device M Neurostimulator Lead	Z No Qualifier

Non-OR 01PY3[0,2]Z
Non-OR 01PY[3,4]YZ
Non-OR 01PYX[0,2,M]Z

0 Medical and Surgical
1 Peripheral Nervous System
Q Repair Definition: Restoring, to the extent possible, a body part to its normal anatomic structure and function
Explanation: Used only when the method to accomplish the repair is not one of the other root operations

Body Part Character 4	Approach Character 5	Device Character 6	Qualifier Character 7
0 Cervical Plexus Ansa cervicalis Cutaneous (transverse) cervical nerve Great auricular nerve Lesser occipital nerve Supraclavicular nerve Transverse (cutaneous) cervical nerve **1 Cervical Nerve** Greater occipital nerve Spinal nerve, cervical Suboccipital nerve Third occipital nerve **2 Phrenic Nerve** Accessory phrenic nerve **3 Brachial Plexus** Axillary nerve Dorsal scapular nerve First intercostal nerve Long thoracic nerve Musculocutaneous nerve Subclavius nerve Suprascapular nerve **4 Ulnar Nerve** Cubital nerve **5 Median Nerve** Anterior interosseous nerve Palmar cutaneous nerve **6 Radial Nerve** Dorsal digital nerve Musculospiral nerve Palmar cutaneous nerve Posterior interosseous nerve **8 Thoracic Nerve** Intercostal nerve Intercostobrachial nerve Spinal nerve, thoracic Subcostal nerve **9 Lumbar Plexus** Accessory obturator nerve Genitofemoral nerve Iliohypogastric nerve Ilioinguinal nerve Lateral femoral cutaneous nerve Obturator nerve Superior gluteal nerve **A Lumbosacral Plexus** **B Lumbar Nerve** Lumbosacral trunk Spinal nerve, lumbar Superior clunic (cluneal) nerve **C Pudendal Nerve** Posterior labial nerve Posterior scrotal nerve **D Femoral Nerve** Anterior crural nerve Saphenous nerve **F Sciatic Nerve** Ischiatic nerve **G Tibial Nerve** Lateral plantar nerve Medial plantar nerve Medial popliteal nerve Medial sural cutaneous nerve	**H Peroneal Nerve** Common fibular nerve Common peroneal nerve External popliteal nerve Lateral sural cutaneous nerve **K Head and Neck Sympathetic Nerve** Cavernous plexus Cervical ganglion Ciliary ganglion Internal carotid plexus Otic ganglion Pterygopalatine (sphenopalatine) ganglion Sphenopalatine (pterygopalatine) ganglion Stellate ganglion Submandibular ganglion Submaxillary ganglion **L Thoracic Sympathetic Nerve** Cardiac plexus Esophageal plexus Greater splanchnic nerve Inferior cardiac nerve Least splanchnic nerve Lesser splanchnic nerve Middle cardiac nerve Pulmonary plexus Superior cardiac nerve Thoracic aortic plexus Thoracic ganglion **M Abdominal Sympathetic Nerve** Abdominal aortic plexus Auerbach's (myenteric) plexus Celiac (solar) plexus Celiac ganglion Gastric plexus Hepatic plexus Inferior hypogastric plexus Inferior mesenteric ganglion Inferior mesenteric plexus Meissner's (submucous) plexus Myenteric (Auerbach's) plexus Pancreatic plexus Pelvic splanchnic nerve Renal nerve Renal plexus Solar (celiac) plexus Splenic plexus Submucous (Meissner's) plexus Superior hypogastric plexus Superior mesenteric ganglion Superior mesenteric plexus Suprarenal plexus **N Lumbar Sympathetic Nerve** Lumbar ganglion Lumbar splanchnic nerve **P Sacral Sympathetic Nerve** Ganglion impar (ganglion of Walther) Pelvic splanchnic nerve Sacral ganglion Sacral splanchnic nerve **Q Sacral Plexus** Inferior gluteal nerve Posterior femoral cutaneous nerve Pudendal nerve **R Sacral Nerve** Spinal nerve, sacral	**0** Open **3** Percutaneous **4** Percutaneous Endoscopic	**Z** No Device	**Z** No Qualifier

0 Medical and Surgical
1 Peripheral Nervous System
R Replacement   Definition: Putting in or on biological or synthetic material that physically takes the place and/or function of all or a portion of a body part
Explanation: The body part may have been taken out or replaced, or may be taken out, physically eradicated, or rendered nonfunctional during the REPLACEMENT procedure. A REMOVAL procedure is coded for taking out the device used in a previous replacement procedure.

Body Part Character 4	Approach Character 5	Device Character 6	Qualifier Character 7

1 Cervical Nerve
  Greater occipital nerve
  Spinal nerve, cervical
  Suboccipital nerve
  Third occipital nerve
2 Phrenic Nerve
  Accessory phrenic nerve
4 Ulnar Nerve
  Cubital nerve
5 Median Nerve
  Anterior interosseous nerve
  Palmar cutaneous nerve
6 Radial Nerve
  Dorsal digital nerve
  Musculospiral nerve
  Palmar cutaneous nerve
  Posterior interosseous nerve
8 Thoracic Nerve
  Intercostal nerve
  Intercostobrachial nerve
  Spinal nerve, thoracic
  Subcostal nerve
B Lumbar Nerve
  Lumbosacral trunk
  Spinal nerve, lumbar
  Superior clunic (cluneal) nerve
C Pudendal Nerve
  Posterior labial nerve
  Posterior scrotal nerve
D Femoral Nerve
  Anterior crural nerve
  Saphenous nerve
F Sciatic Nerve
  Ischiatic nerve
G Tibial Nerve
  Lateral plantar nerve
  Medial plantar nerve
  Medial popliteal nerve
  Medial sural cutaneous nerve
H Peroneal Nerve
  Common fibular nerve
  Common peroneal nerve
  External popliteal nerve
  Lateral sural cutaneous nerve
R Sacral Nerve
  Spinal nerve, sacral
	0 Open
	4 Percutaneous Endoscopic
		7 Autologous Tissue Substitute
		J Synthetic Substitute
		K Nonautologous Tissue Substitute
			Z No Qualifier

ICD-10-PCS 2025 — Peripheral Nervous System — 01S–01S

- **0** Medical and Surgical
- **1** Peripheral Nervous System
- **S** Reposition

Definition: Moving to its normal location, or other suitable location, all or a portion of a body part

Explanation: The body part is moved to a new location from an abnormal location, or from a normal location where it is not functioning correctly. The body part may or may not be cut out or off to be moved to the new location.

Body Part Character 4	Approach Character 5	Device Character 6	Qualifier Character 7
0 Cervical Plexus Ansa cervicalis; Cutaneous (transverse) cervical nerve; Great auricular nerve; Lesser occipital nerve; Supraclavicular nerve; Transverse (cutaneous) cervical nerve **1 Cervical Nerve** Greater occipital nerve; Spinal nerve, cervical; Suboccipital nerve; Third occipital nerve **2 Phrenic Nerve** Accessory phrenic nerve **3 Brachial Plexus** Axillary nerve; Dorsal scapular nerve; First intercostal nerve; Long thoracic nerve; Musculocutaneous nerve; Subclavius nerve; Suprascapular nerve **4 Ulnar Nerve** Cubital nerve **5 Median Nerve** Anterior interosseous nerve; Palmar cutaneous nerve **6 Radial Nerve** Dorsal digital nerve; Musculospiral nerve; Palmar cutaneous nerve; Posterior interosseous nerve **8 Thoracic Nerve** Intercostal nerve; Intercostobrachial nerve; Spinal nerve, thoracic; Subcostal nerve **9 Lumbar Plexus** Accessory obturator nerve; Genitofemoral nerve; Iliohypogastric nerve; Ilioinguinal nerve; Lateral femoral cutaneous nerve; Obturator nerve; Superior gluteal nerve **A Lumbosacral Plexus** **B Lumbar Nerve** Lumbosacral trunk; Spinal nerve, lumbar; Superior clunic (cluneal) nerve **C Pudendal Nerve** Posterior labial nerve; Posterior scrotal nerve **D Femoral Nerve** Anterior crural nerve; Saphenous nerve **F Sciatic Nerve** Ischiatic nerve **G Tibial Nerve** Lateral plantar nerve; Medial plantar nerve; Medial popliteal nerve; Medial sural cutaneous nerve **H Peroneal Nerve** Common fibular nerve; Common peroneal nerve; External popliteal nerve; Lateral sural cutaneous nerve **Q Sacral Plexus** Inferior gluteal nerve; Posterior femoral cutaneous nerve; Pudendal nerve **R Sacral Nerve** Spinal nerve, sacral	**0** Open **3** Percutaneous **4** Percutaneous Endoscopic	**Z** No Device	**Z** No Qualifier

NC Noncovered Procedure · LC Limited Coverage · QA Questionable OB Admit · NT New Tech Add-on · ➕ Combination Member · ♂ Male · ♀ Female

0 Medical and Surgical
1 Peripheral Nervous System
U Supplement Definition: Putting in or on biological or synthetic material that physically reinforces and/or augments the function of a portion of a body part
Explanation: The biological material is non-living, or is living and from the same individual. The body part may have been previously replaced, and the SUPPLEMENT procedure is performed to physically reinforce and/or augment the function of the replaced body part.

Body Part Character 4	Approach Character 5	Device Character 6	Qualifier Character 7

1 Cervical Nerve
  Greater occipital nerve
  Spinal nerve, cervical
  Suboccipital nerve
  Third occipital nerve
2 Phrenic Nerve
  Accessory phrenic nerve
4 Ulnar Nerve
  Cubital nerve
5 Median Nerve
  Anterior interosseous nerve
  Palmar cutaneous nerve
6 Radial Nerve
  Dorsal digital nerve
  Musculospiral nerve
  Palmar cutaneous nerve
  Posterior interosseous nerve
8 Thoracic Nerve
  Intercostal nerve
  Intercostobrachial nerve
  Spinal nerve, thoracic
  Subcostal nerve
B Lumbar Nerve
  Lumbosacral trunk
  Spinal nerve, lumbar
  Superior clunic (cluneal) nerve
C Pudendal Nerve
  Posterior labial nerve
  Posterior scrotal nerve
D Femoral Nerve
  Anterior crural nerve
  Saphenous nerve
F Sciatic Nerve
  Ischiatic nerve
G Tibial Nerve
  Lateral plantar nerve
  Medial plantar nerve
  Medial popliteal nerve
  Medial sural cutaneous nerve
H Peroneal Nerve
  Common fibular nerve
  Common peroneal nerve
  External popliteal nerve
  Lateral sural cutaneous nerve
R Sacral Nerve
  Spinal nerve, sacral
	0 Open
	3 Percutaneous
	4 Percutaneous Endoscopic
		7 Autologous Tissue Substitute
		J Synthetic Substitute
		K Nonautologous Tissue Substitute
			Z No Qualifier

0 Medical and Surgical
1 Peripheral Nervous System
W Revision Definition: Correcting, to the extent possible, a portion of a malfunctioning device or the position of a displaced device
Explanation: Revision can include correcting a malfunctioning or displaced device by taking out or putting in components of the device such as a screw or pin

Body Part Character 4	Approach Character 5	Device Character 6	Qualifier Character 7
Y Peripheral Nerve	**0** Open **3** Percutaneous **4** Percutaneous Endoscopic	**0** Drainage Device **2** Monitoring Device **7** Autologous Tissue Substitute **M** Neurostimulator Lead **Y** Other Device	**Z** No Qualifier
Y Peripheral Nerve	**X** External	**0** Drainage Device **2** Monitoring Device **7** Autologous Tissue Substitute **M** Neurostimulator Lead	**Z** No Qualifier

Non-OR 01WY[3,4]YZ
Non-OR 01WYX[0,2,7,M]Z

0 Medical and Surgical
1 Peripheral Nervous System
X Transfer   Definition: Moving, without taking out, all or a portion of a body part to another location to take over the function of all or a portion of a body part
Explanation: The body part transferred remains connected to its vascular and nervous supply

Body Part Character 4	Approach Character 5	Device Character 6	Qualifier Character 7

1 Cervical Nerve
  Greater occipital nerve
  Spinal nerve, cervical
  Suboccipital nerve
  Third occipital nerve
2 Phrenic Nerve
  Accessory phrenic nerve
	0 Open
	4 Percutaneous Endoscopic
		Z No Device	1 Cervical Nerve
			2 Phrenic Nerve

4 Ulnar Nerve
  Cubital nerve
5 Median Nerve
  Anterior interosseous nerve
  Palmar cutaneous nerve
6 Radial Nerve
  Dorsal digital nerve
  Musculospiral nerve
  Palmar cutaneous nerve
  Posterior interosseous nerve
	0 Open
	4 Percutaneous Endoscopic
		Z No Device	4 Ulnar Nerve
			5 Median Nerve
			6 Radial Nerve

8 Thoracic Nerve
  Intercostal nerve
  Intercostobrachial nerve
  Spinal nerve, thoracic
  Subcostal nerve
	0 Open
	4 Percutaneous Endoscopic
		Z No Device	8 Thoracic Nerve

B Lumbar Nerve
  Lumbosacral trunk
  Spinal nerve, lumbar
  Superior clunic (cluneal) nerve
C Pudendal Nerve
  Posterior labial nerve
  Posterior scrotal nerve
	0 Open
	4 Percutaneous Endoscopic
		Z No Device	B Lumbar Nerve
			C Perineal Nerve

D Femoral Nerve
  Anterior crural nerve
  Saphenous nerve
F Sciatic Nerve
  Ischiatic nerve
G Tibial Nerve
  Lateral plantar nerve
  Medial plantar nerve
  Medial popliteal nerve
  Medial sural cutaneous nerve
H Peroneal Nerve
  Common fibular nerve
  Common peroneal nerve
  External popliteal nerve
  Lateral sural cutaneous nerve
	0 Open
	4 Percutaneous Endoscopic
		Z No Device	D Femoral Nerve
			F Sciatic Nerve
			G Tibial Nerve
			H Peroneal Nerve

Heart and Great Vessels Ø21–Ø2Y

Character Meanings

This Character Meaning table is provided as a guide to assist the user in the identification of character members that may be found in this section of code tables. It **SHOULD NOT** be used to build a PCS code.

Operation–Character 3	Body Part–Character 4	Approach–Character 5	Device–Character 6	Qualifier–Character 7
1 Bypass	Ø Coronary Artery, One Artery	Ø Open	Ø Monitoring Device, Pressure Sensor	Ø Allogeneic OR Ultrasonic
4 Creation	1 Coronary Artery, Two Arteries	3 Percutaneous	2 Monitoring Device	1 Syngeneic
5 Destruction	2 Coronary Artery, Three Arteries	4 Percutaneous Endoscopic	3 Infusion Device	2 Zooplastic OR Common Atrioventricular Valve
7 Dilation	3 Coronary Artery, Four or More Arteries	X External	4 Intraluminal Device, Drug-eluting	3 Coronary Artery
8 Division	4 Coronary Vein		5 Intraluminal Device, Drug-eluting, Two	4 Coronary Vein
B Excision	5 Atrial Septum		6 Intraluminal Device, Drug-eluting, Three	5 Coronary Circulation
C Extirpation	6 Atrium, Right		7 Intraluminal Device, Drug-eluting, Four or More OR Autologous Tissue Substitute	6 Bifurcation OR Atrium, Right
F Fragmentation	7 Atrium, Left		8 Zooplastic Tissue	7 Atrium, Left OR Orbital Atherectomy Technique
H Insertion	8 Conduction Mechanism		9 Autologous Venous Tissue	8 Internal Mammary, Right
J Inspection	9 Chordae Tendineae		A Autologous Arterial Tissue	9 Internal Mammary, Left
K Map	A Heart		C Extraluminal Device	A Innominate Artery
L Occlusion	B Heart, Right		D Intraluminal Device	B Subclavian
N Release	C Heart, Left		E Intraluminal Device, Two OR Intraluminal Device, Branched or Fenestrated, One or Two Arteries	C Thoracic Artery
P Removal	D Papillary Muscle		F Intraluminal Device, Three OR Intraluminal Device, Branched or Fenestrated, Three or More Arteries	D Carotid
Q Repair	F Aortic Valve		G Intraluminal Device, Four or More	E Atrioventricular Valve, Left
R Replacement	G Mitral Valve		J Synthetic Substitute OR Cardiac Lead, Pacemaker	F Abdominal Artery OR Irreversible Electroporation
S Reposition	H Pulmonary Valve		K Nonautologous Tissue Substitute OR Cardiac Lead, Defibrillator	G Atrioventricular Valve, Right OR Axillary Artery
T Resection	J Tricuspid Valve		L Biologic with Synthetic Substitute, Autoregulated Electrohydraulic	H Transapical OR Brachial Artery
U Supplement	K Ventricle, Right		M Cardiac Lead OR Synthetic Substitute, Pneumatic	J Truncal Valve OR Temporary OR Intraoperative
V Restriction	L Ventricle, Left		N Intracardiac Pacemaker	K Left Atrial Appendage
W Revision	M Ventricular Septum		Q Implantable Heart Assist System	L In Existing Conduit
Y Transplantation	N Pericardium		R Short-term External Heart Assist System	M Native Site
	P Pulmonary Trunk		T Intraluminal Device, Radioactive	N Rapid Deployment Technique
	Q Pulmonary Artery, Right		Y Other Device	P Pulmonary Trunk
	R Pulmonary Artery, Left		Z No Device	Q Pulmonary Artery, Right
	S Pulmonary Vein, Right			R Pulmonary Artery, Left
	T Pulmonary Vein, Left			S Pulmonary Vein, Right OR Biventricular
	V Superior Vena Cava			T Pulmonary Vein, Left OR Ductus Arteriosus
	W Thoracic Aorta, Descending			U Pulmonary Vein, Confluence
	X Thoracic Aorta, Ascending/Arch			V Lower Extremity Artery
	Y Great Vessel			W Aorta
				X Diagnostic
				Z No Qualifier

Heart and Great Vessels

AHA Coding Clinic for Heart and Great Vessels
2022, 1Q, 10-13	Procedures performed on a continuous vessel, ICD-10-PCS Guideline B4.1c

AHA Coding Clinic for table 021
2023, 2Q, 22	Norwood procedure with excision of thymus
2022, 1Q, 54	Coronary artery bypass graft surgery
2021, 3Q, 22	Left internal mammary artery free graft between obtuse marginal saphenous vein graft and left anterior descending artery
2020, 4Q, 44-45	Atrium bypass qualifier
2020, 1Q, 24	Pulmonary artery unifocalization
2020, 1Q, 37	Bypass of ascending aorta to brachiocephalic artery
2019, 4Q, 23	Bypass thoracic aorta to innominate artery
2019, 3Q, 30	Aortic aneurysm repair with debranching of common carotid and brachiocephalic arteries
2018, 4Q, 45-46	Descending thoracic aorta bypass
2018, 3Q, 8	Coronary artery bypass graft surgery (revision versus total redo)
2018, 3Q, 26	Coronary artery bypass graft surgery with endarterectomy
2017, 4Q, 56	Added approach values - Percutaneous heart valve procedures
2017, 1Q, 19	Norwood Sano procedure
2016, 4Q, 80-81	Thoracic aorta, ascending/arch and descending
2016, 4Q, 82-83	Coronary artery, number of arteries
2016, 4Q, 102-109	Correction of congenital heart defects
2016, 4Q, 144	Repair of atrial septal defect and anomalous pulmonary venous return
2016, 4Q, 145	Modified Warden procedure for repair of septal defect and right partial anomalous pulmonary venous return
2016, 1Q, 27	Aortocoronary bypass graft utilizing Y-graft
2015, 4Q, 22, 24	Congenital heart corrective procedures
2015, 3Q, 16	Revision of previous truncus arteriosus surgery with ventricle to pulmonary artery conduit
2014, 3Q, 3	Blalock-Taussig shunt procedure
2014, 3Q, 8	Coronary artery bypass graft utilizing internal mammary as pedicle graft
2014, 3Q, 20	MAZE procedure performed with coronary artery bypass graft
2014, 3Q, 29	Fontan completion procedure stage II
2014, 3Q, 30	Creation of conduit from right ventricle to pulmonary artery
2014, 1Q, 10	Repair of thoracic aortic aneurysm & coronary artery bypass graft
2013, 2Q, 37	Coronary artery release performed during coronary artery bypass graft

AHA Coding Clinic for table 024
2016, 4Q, 101	Root operation Creation
2016, 4Q, 102-109	Correction of congenital heart defects

AHA Coding Clinic for table 025
2024, 1Q, 6	Irreversible electroporation for cardiac ablation
2020, 1Q, 32	Ablation convergent procedure (catheter-based and thoracoscopic ablations)
2018, 3Q, 27	Alcohol septal ablation
2016, 4Q, 80-81	Thoracic aorta, ascending/arch and descending
2016, 3Q, 43-44	Peri-pulmonary catheter ablation
2016, 3Q, 44-45	Maze procedure
2016, 2Q, 17	Photodynamic therapy for treatment of malignant mesothelioma
2014, 4Q, 47	Catheter ablation of peripulmonary veins
2014, 3Q, 19	Ablation of ventricular tachycardia with Impella® support
2014, 3Q, 20	MAZE procedure performed with coronary artery bypass graft
2013, 2Q, 38	Catheter ablation to treat atrial fibrillation

AHA Coding Clinic for table 027
2018, 3Q, 7	Coronary brachytherapy with angioplasty
2018, 3Q, 10	Disruption of perma-catheter fibrin sheath via angioplasty of superior vena cava
2018, 2Q, 24	Coronary artery bifurcation
2017, 4Q, 32-33	Corrective surgery of left ventricular outflow tract obstruction
2016, 4Q, 80-81	Thoracic aorta, ascending/arch and descending
2016, 4Q, 82-83	Coronary artery, number of arteries
2016, 4Q, 84-85	Coronary artery, number of stents
2016, 4Q, 86-88	Coronary and peripheral artery bifurcation
2016, 1Q, 16	Pulmonary valvotomy and dilation of annulus
2015, 4Q, 13	New Section X codes—New Technology procedures
2015, 3Q, 9	Failed attempt to treat coronary artery occlusion
2015, 3Q, 10	Coronary angioplasty with unsuccessful stent insertion
2015, 3Q, 16	Revision of previous truncus arteriosus surgery with ventricle to pulmonary artery conduit
2015, 2Q, 3-5	Coronary artery intervention site
2014, 2Q, 4	Coronary angioplasty of bypassed vessel

AHA Coding Clinic for table 02B
2019, 3Q, 32	Endomyocardial biopsy and right heart catheterization
2019, 2Q, 20	Pericardiectomy for constrictive pericarditis
2017, 1Q, 38	Mitral valve repair and chordae tendineae transfer
2016, 4Q, 80-81	Thoracic aorta, ascending/arch and descending
2015, 2Q, 23	Annuloplasty ring

AHA Coding Clinic for table 02C
2021, 4Q, 41	Coronary orbital atherectomy
2019, 4Q, 25	Coronary artery to root operation Supplement
2018, 3Q, 26	Coronary artery bypass graft surgery with endarterectomy
2018, 2Q, 24	Coronary artery bifurcation
2017, 2Q, 23	Thrombectomy via Fogarty catheter
2016, 4Q, 80-81	Thoracic aorta, ascending/arch and descending
2016, 4Q, 82-83	Coronary artery, number of arteries
2016, 4Q, 86-87	Coronary and peripheral artery bifurcation
2016, 2Q, 24	Repair/decalcification of mitral valve
2016, 2Q, 25	Aortic valve surgery with excision of calcium deposits

AHA Coding Clinic for table 02F
2021, 4Q, 41-42	Coronary intravascular lithotripsy
2020, 4Q, 45-49	New fragmentation tables
2020, 4Q, 49-50	Intravascular ultrasound assisted thrombolysis
2020, 4Q, 50	Intravascular lithotripsy

AHA Coding Clinic for table 02H
2024, 2Q, 29	Wireless stimulation endocardially for cardiac resynchronization (WiSE®-CRT) system
2024, 1Q, 30	PROTEKDuo® cannula insertion with CentriMag®
2023, 4Q, 51-52	Short-term external heart assist system in descending thoracic aorta
2022, 3Q, 19	Placement of stent into aorta to secure debris
2022, 2Q, 25	Temporary-permanent pacemaker placement
2021, 2Q, 23	Clarification of lead placement in bundle of HIS
2019, 4Q, 23-24	Coronary artery Body Part to root operation Insertion
2019, 3Q, 19	Insertion of left ventricular catheter
2019, 3Q, 23	Placement of pacemaker lead in Bundle of HIS
2019, 1Q, 24	Replacement of left ventricular assist device with retention of outflow graft
2018, 4Q, 94	Insertion and removal of failed Watchman™ device
2018, 2Q, 3-5	Intra-aortic balloon pump
2018, 2Q, 19	Pacing lead attached to automatic implantable cardioverter defibrillator
2017, 4Q, 42-45	Insertion of external heart assist devices
2017, 4Q, 63-64	Added and revised device values - Vascular access reservoir
2017, 4Q, 104	Placement of Watchman™ left atrial appendage device
2017, 3Q, 11	Placement of peripherally inserted central catheter using 3CG ECG technology
2017, 2Q, 24	Tunneled catheter versus totally implantable catheter
2017, 2Q, 26	Exchange of tunneled catheter
2017, 1Q, 10-11	External heart assist device
2016, 4Q, 80-81	Thoracic aorta, ascending/arch and descending
2016, 4Q, 95	Intracardiac pacemaker
2016, 4Q, 137-138	Heart assist device systems
2016, 2Q, 15	Removal and replacement of tunneled internal jugular catheter
2015, 4Q, 14	New Section X codes—New Technology procedures
2015, 4Q, 26-31	Vascular access devices
2015, 3Q, 35	Swan Ganz catheterization
2015, 2Q, 31	Leadless pacemaker insertion
2015, 2Q, 33	Totally implantable central venous access device (Port-a-Cath)
2013, 3Q, 18	Placement of peripherally inserted central catheter (PICC)

AHA Coding Clinic for table 02J
2015, 3Q, 9	Failed attempt to treat coronary artery occlusion

AHA Coding Clinic for table 02K
2020, 1Q, 32	Ablation convergent procedure (catheter-based and thoracoscopic ablations)

AHA Coding Clinic for table 02L
2023, 1Q, 9	Temporary balloon occlusion of aorta
2018, 4Q, 94	Insertion and removal of failed Watchman™ device
2017, 4Q, 31	Resuscitative endovascular balloon occlusion of the aorta
2017, 4Q, 33-34	Occlusion/ligation of pulmonary trunk & right pulmonary artery
2016, 4Q, 102-109	Correction of congenital heart defects
2016, 2Q, 26	Embolization of pulmonary arteriovenous fistula
2015, 4Q, 23	Congenital heart corrective procedures
2014, 3Q, 20	MAZE procedure performed with coronary artery bypass graft

AHA Coding Clinic for table 02N
2021, 3Q, 26	Cavoatrial junction tear with repair and relief of cardiac tamponade
2019, 2Q, 13	Unroofing of anomalous coronary artery
2019, 2Q, 20	Pericardiectomy for constrictive pericarditis
2017, 4Q, 35	Release of myocardial bridge
2016, 4Q, 80-81	Thoracic aorta, ascending/arch and descending
2014, 3Q, 16	Repair of Tetralogy of Fallot

AHA Coding Clinic for table 02P

2023, 4Q, 51-52	Short-term external heart assist system in descending thoracic aorta
2022, 2Q, 25	Temporary-permanent pacemaker placement
2019, 1Q, 24	Replacement of left ventricular assist device with retention of outflow graft
2018, 4Q, 52-54	Percutaneous extracorporeal membrane oxygenation
2018, 4Q, 85	Externalization of lumboatrial shunt
2018, 4Q, 94	Insertion and removal of failed Watchman™ device
2018, 2Q, 3-5	Intra-aortic balloon pump
2017, 4Q, 42-45	Insertion of external heart assist devices
2017, 4Q, 104	Placement of Watchman™ left atrial appendage device
2017, 3Q, 18	Intra-aortic balloon pump removal
2017, 2Q, 24	Tunneled catheter versus totally implantable catheter
2017, 2Q, 26	Exchange of tunneled catheter
2017, 1Q, 11	External heart assist device
2017, 1Q, 13	SynCardia total artificial heart
2016, 4Q, 95-96	Intracardiac pacemaker

AHA Coding Clinic for table 02P (Continued)

2016, 4Q, 137-139	Heart assist device systems
2016, 3Q, 19	Nonoperative removal of peripherally inserted central catheter
2016, 2Q, 15	Removal and replacement of tunneled internal jugular catheter
2015, 4Q, 31	Vascular access devices
2015, 3Q, 33	Approach values for repositioning and removal of cardiac lead

AHA Coding Clinic for table 02Q

2023, 3Q, 27	Fenestration of aortic dissection flap
2022, 1Q, 40	Repair of common atrioventricular valve using Alfieri stitch
2022, 1Q, 41	Common atrioventricular valve repair with commissuroplasty sutures
2021, 3Q, 26	Cavoatrial junction tear with repair and relief of cardiac tamponade
2018, 1Q, 12	Percutaneous balloon valvuloplasty & cardiac catheterization with ventriculogram
2017, 1Q, 18	Sutureless repair of pulmonary vein stenosis
2016, 4Q, 80-81	Thoracic aorta, ascending/arch and descending
2016, 4Q, 82-83	Coronary artery, number of arteries
2016, 4Q, 101	Root operation Creation
2016, 4Q, 102-109	Correction of congenital heart defects
2015, 4Q, 23	Congenital heart corrective procedures
2015, 3Q, 16	Vascular ring surgery and double aortic arch
2015, 2Q, 23	Annuloplasty ring
2013, 3Q, 26	Transcatheter replacement of heart valve (TAVR) with measurements

AHA Coding Clinic for table 02R

2024, 2Q, 18	Ascending aorta and total aortic arch repair with extension frozen elephant trunk
2024, 2Q, 30	Aortic valve and aortic root replacement with aortic valve conduit
2022, 4Q, 54-55	Rapid deployment technique for replacement of aortic valve using zooplastic tissue
2021, 4Q, 42-43	Total artificial heart systems
2021, 4Q, 43	Transcatheter replacement of pulmonary valve
2020, 1Q, 25	Elephant trunk repair of aortic dissection
2019, 4Q, 24	Coronary artery Body Part to root operation Insertion
2019, 4Q, 46	Cerebral embolic filtration
2019, 3Q, 23	Replacement of atrioventricular valve
2019, 3Q, 24	Valve sparing aortic root replacement with modified Gleason Vascutek® graft to ascending aorta
2019, 1Q, 31	Transcatheter aortic valve in valve replacement
2018, 3Q, 11	Transcatheter aortic valve replacement via transaortic approach
2018, 1Q, 12	Percutaneous balloon valvuloplasty & cardiac catheterization with ventriculogram
2017, 4Q, 55-56	Added approach values - Percutaneous heart valve procedures
2017, 1Q, 13	SynCardia total artificial heart
2016, 4Q, 80-81	Thoracic aorta, ascending/arch and descending
2016, 3Q, 32	Transcatheter tricuspid valve replacement
2014, 1Q, 10	Repair of thoracic aortic aneurysm & coronary artery bypass graft

AHA Coding Clinic for table 02S

2016, 4Q, 80-81	Thoracic aorta, ascending/arch and descending
2016, 4Q, 82-83	Coronary artery, number of arteries
2016, 4Q, 102-109	Correction of congenital heart defects
2015, 4Q, 23	Congenital heart corrective procedures

AHA Coding Clinic for table 02U

2023, 2Q, 21	Placement of Carillon Mitral Contour System®
2023, 2Q, 22	Norwood procedure with excision of thymus
2022, 1Q, 37	Insertion of amplatzer occluder device into atrium
2022, 1Q, 38	Reconstruction of aorto-mitral curtain using bovine pericardium
2021, 3Q, 28	Repair mitral valve with Pascal® system
2020, 4Q, 52	Transapical mitral valve repair with device
2020, 1Q, 24	Pulmonary artery unifocalization
2019, 4Q, 25	Coronary artery to root operation Supplement
2018, 1Q, 12	Percutaneous balloon valvuloplasty & cardiac catheterization with ventriculogram
2017, 4Q, 36	Alfieri stitch procedure
2017, 3Q, 7	Senning procedure (arterial switch)
2017, 1Q, 19	Norwood Sano procedure
2016, 4Q, 80-81	Thoracic aorta, ascending/arch and descending
2016, 4Q, 101	Root operation Creation
2016, 4Q, 102-109	Correction of congenital heart defects
2016, 2Q, 23	Repair of tetralogy of Fallot with autologous pericardial patch graft
2016, 2Q, 26	Aortic valve replacement with aortic root enlargement
2015, 4Q, 22-24	Congenital heart corrective procedures
2015, 3Q, 16	Revision of previous truncus arteriosus surgery with ventricle to pulmonary artery conduit
2015, 2Q, 23	Annuloplasty ring
2014, 3Q, 16	Repair of tetralogy of Fallot

AHA Coding Clinic for table 02V

2022, 1Q, 40	Repair of common atrioventricular valve using Alfieri stitch
2021, 4Q, 44	Restriction of left ventricle
2020, 1Q, 25	Elephant trunk repair of aortic dissection
2017, 4Q, 35-36	Alfieri stitch procedure
2016, 4Q, 80-81	Thoracic aorta, ascending/arch and descending
2016, 4Q, 89-92	Branched and fenestrated endograft repair of aneurysms

AHA Coding Clinic for table 02W

2023, 4Q, 51-52	Short-term external heart assist system in descending thoracic aorta
2019, 1Q, 24	Replacement of left ventricular assist device with retention of outflow graft
2018, 3Q, 8	Coronary artery bypass graft surgery (revision versus total redo)
2018, 3Q, 9	Fibrin sheath stripping of malfunctioning port-a-cath
2018, 1Q, 17	Repositioning of Impella short-term external heart assist device
2017, 4Q, 42-45	Insertion of external heart assist devices
2017, 4Q, 55-56	Added approach values - Percutaneous heart valve procedures
2016, 4Q, 85	Coronary artery, number of stents
2016, 4Q, 95-96	Intracardiac pacemaker
2015, 3Q, 32	Approach values for repositioning and removal of cardiac lead
2014, 3Q, 31	Closure of paravalvular leak using Amplatzer® vascular plug

AHA Coding Clinic for table 02Y

2023, 2Q, 32	Preparation of donor organ before transplantation
2013, 3Q, 18	Heart transplant surgery

Heart and Great Vessels

Coronary Arteries

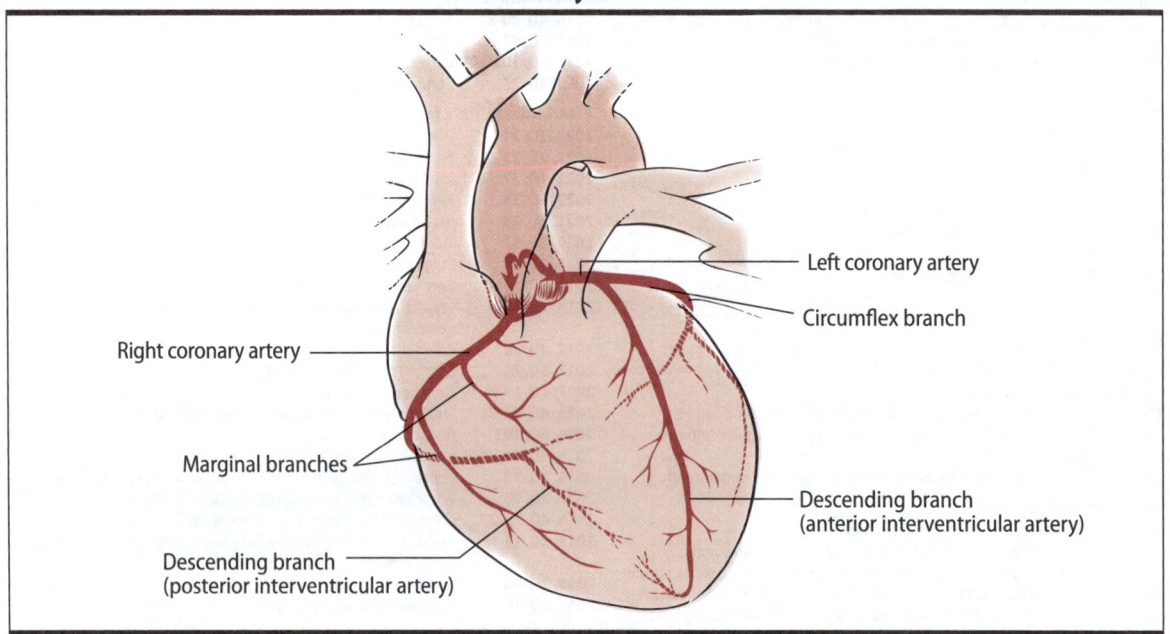

- Right coronary artery
- Marginal branches
- Descending branch (posterior interventricular artery)
- Left coronary artery
- Circumflex branch
- Descending branch (anterior interventricular artery)

Heart Anatomy

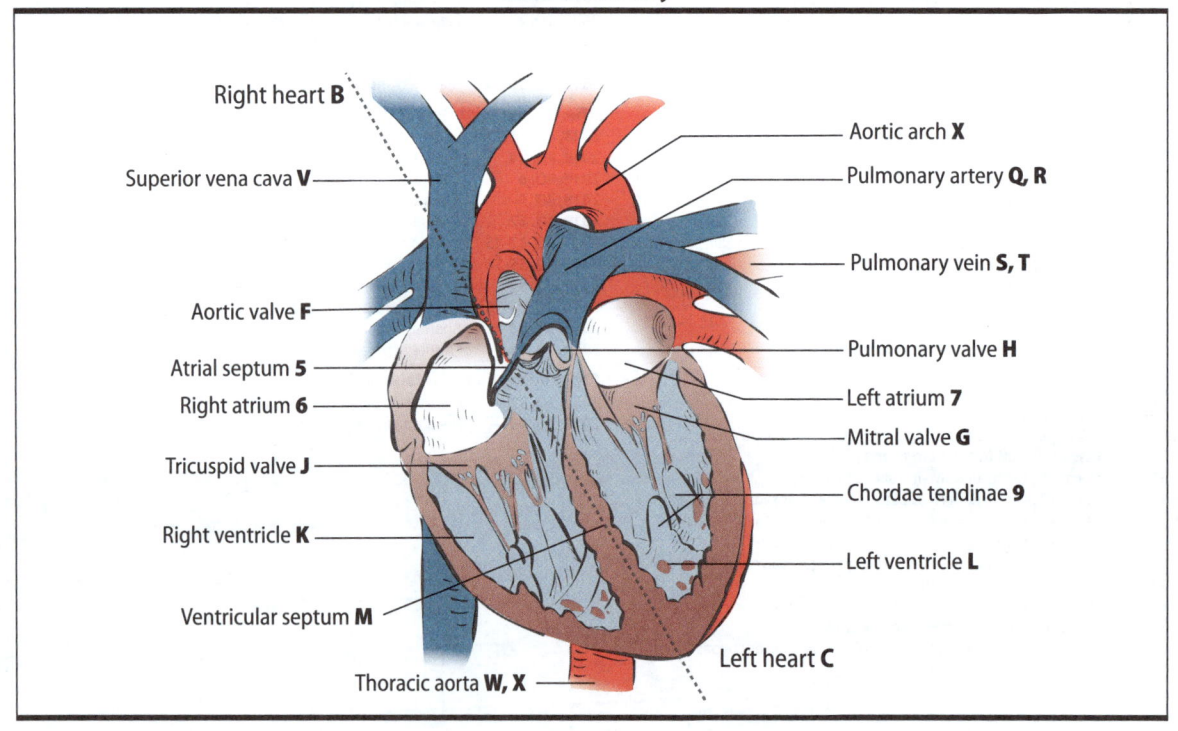

- Right heart **B**
- Superior vena cava **V**
- Aortic valve **F**
- Atrial septum **5**
- Right atrium **6**
- Tricuspid valve **J**
- Right ventricle **K**
- Ventricular septum **M**
- Thoracic aorta **W, X**
- Aortic arch **X**
- Pulmonary artery **Q, R**
- Pulmonary vein **S, T**
- Pulmonary valve **H**
- Left atrium **7**
- Mitral valve **G**
- Chordae tendinae **9**
- Left ventricle **L**
- Left heart **C**

ICD-10-PCS 2025 — Heart and Great Vessels — 021-021

- 0 Medical and Surgical
- 2 Heart and Great Vessels
- 1 Bypass Definition: Altering the route of passage of the contents of a tubular body part
  Explanation: Rerouting contents of a body part to a downstream area of the normal route, to a similar route and body part, or to an abnormal route and dissimilar body part. Includes one or more anastomoses, with or without the use of a device.

Body Part Character 4	Approach Character 5	Device Character 6	Qualifier Character 7
0 Coronary Artery, One Artery 1 Coronary Artery, Two Arteries 2 Coronary Artery, Three Arteries 3 Coronary Artery, Four or More Arteries	0 Open	8 Zooplastic Tissue 9 Autologous Venous Tissue A Autologous Arterial Tissue J Synthetic Substitute K Nonautologous Tissue Substitute	3 Coronary Artery 8 Internal Mammary, Right 9 Internal Mammary, Left C Thoracic Artery F Abdominal Artery W Aorta
0 Coronary Artery, One Artery 1 Coronary Artery, Two Arteries 2 Coronary Artery, Three Arteries 3 Coronary Artery, Four or More Arteries	0 Open	Z No Device	3 Coronary Artery 8 Internal Mammary, Right 9 Internal Mammary, Left C Thoracic Artery F Abdominal Artery
0 Coronary Artery, One Artery 1 Coronary Artery, Two Arteries 2 Coronary Artery, Three Arteries 3 Coronary Artery, Four or More Arteries	3 Percutaneous	4 Intraluminal Device, Drug-eluting D Intraluminal Device	4 Coronary Vein
0 Coronary Artery, One Artery 1 Coronary Artery, Two Arteries 2 Coronary Artery, Three Arteries 3 Coronary Artery, Four or More Arteries	4 Percutaneous Endoscopic	4 Intraluminal Device, Drug-eluting D Intraluminal Device	4 Coronary Vein
0 Coronary Artery, One Artery 1 Coronary Artery, Two Arteries 2 Coronary Artery, Three Arteries 3 Coronary Artery, Four or More Arteries	4 Percutaneous Endoscopic	8 Zooplastic Tissue 9 Autologous Venous Tissue A Autologous Arterial Tissue J Synthetic Substitute K Nonautologous Tissue Substitute	3 Coronary Artery 8 Internal Mammary, Right 9 Internal Mammary, Left C Thoracic Artery F Abdominal Artery W Aorta
0 Coronary Artery, One Artery 1 Coronary Artery, Two Arteries 2 Coronary Artery, Three Arteries 3 Coronary Artery, Four or More Arteries	4 Percutaneous Endoscopic	Z No Device	3 Coronary Artery 8 Internal Mammary, Right 9 Internal Mammary, Left C Thoracic Artery F Abdominal Artery

6 Atrium, Right
  Atrium dextrum cordis
  Right auricular appendix
  Sinus venosus
	0 Open
	4 Percutaneous Endoscopic
		8 Zooplastic Tissue
		9 Autologous Venous Tissue
		A Autologous Arterial Tissue
		J Synthetic Substitute
		K Nonautologous Tissue Substitute
			P Pulmonary Trunk
			Q Pulmonary Artery, Right
			R Pulmonary Artery, Left

6 Atrium, Right
  Atrium dextrum cordis
  Right auricular appendix
  Sinus venosus
	0 Open
	4 Percutaneous Endoscopic
		Z No Device	7 Atrium, Left
			P Pulmonary Trunk
			Q Pulmonary Artery, Right
			R Pulmonary Artery, Left

6 Atrium, Right
  Atrium dextrum cordis
  Right auricular appendix
  Sinus venosus
	3 Percutaneous	Z No Device	7 Atrium, Left

7 Atrium, Left
  Atrium pulmonale
  Left auricular appendix
	0 Open
	4 Percutaneous Endoscopic
		8 Zooplastic Tissue
		9 Autologous Venous Tissue
		A Autologous Arterial Tissue
		J Synthetic Substitute
		K Nonautologous Tissue Substitute
		Z No Device
			P Pulmonary Trunk
			Q Pulmonary Artery, Right
			R Pulmonary Artery, Left
			S Pulmonary Vein, Right
			T Pulmonary Vein, Left
			U Pulmonary Vein, Confluence

7 Atrium, Left
  Atrium pulmonale
  Left auricular appendix
	3 Percutaneous	J Synthetic Substitute	6 Atrium, Right

K Ventricle, Right Conus arteriosus L Ventricle, Left	0 Open 4 Percutaneous Endoscopic	8 Zooplastic Tissue 9 Autologous Venous Tissue A Autologous Arterial Tissue J Synthetic Substitute K Nonautologous Tissue Substitute	P Pulmonary Trunk Q Pulmonary Artery, Right R Pulmonary Artery, Left

HAC 021[0,1,2,3]0[8,9,A,J,K][3,8,9,C,F,W] when reported with SDx J98.51 or J98.59
HAC 021[0,1,2,3]0Z[3,8,9,C,F] when reported with SDx J98.51 or J98.59
HAC 021[0,1,2,3]4[8,9,A,J,K][3,8,9,C,F,W] when reported with SDx J98.51 or J98.59
HAC 021[0,1,2,3]4Z[3,8,9,C,F] when reported with SDx J98.51 or J98.59

021 Continued on next page

NC Noncovered Procedure LC Limited Coverage QA Questionable OB Admit NT New Tech Add-on ✚ Combination Member ♂ Male ♀ Female

0 Medical and Surgical
2 Heart and Great Vessels
1 Bypass Definition: Altering the route of passage of the contents of a tubular body part
Explanation: Rerouting contents of a body part to a downstream area of the normal route, to a similar route and body part, or to an abnormal route and dissimilar body part. Includes one or more anastomoses, with or without the use of a device.

Ø21 Continued

Body Part Character 4	Approach Character 5	Device Character 6	Qualifier Character 7
K Ventricle, Right Conus arteriosus L Ventricle, Left	Ø Open 4 Percutaneous Endoscopic	Z No Device	5 Coronary Circulation 8 Internal Mammary, Right 9 Internal Mammary, Left C Thoracic Artery F Abdominal Artery P Pulmonary Trunk Q Pulmonary Artery, Right R Pulmonary Artery, Left W Aorta

P Pulmonary Trunk
Q Pulmonary Artery, Right
R Pulmonary Artery, Left
   Arterial canal (duct)
   Botallo's duct
   Pulmoaortic canal
	Ø Open
	4 Percutaneous Endoscopic
		8 Zooplastic Tissue
		9 Autologous Venous Tissue
		A Autologous Arterial Tissue
		J Synthetic Substitute
		K Nonautologous Tissue Substitute
		Z No Device
			A Innominate Artery
			B Subclavian
			D Carotid

V Superior Vena Cava
   Cavoatrial junction
   Precava
	Ø Open
	4 Percutaneous Endoscopic
		8 Zooplastic Tissue
		9 Autologous Venous Tissue
		A Autologous Arterial Tissue
		J Synthetic Substitute
		K Nonautologous Tissue Substitute
		Z No Device
			P Pulmonary Trunk
			Q Pulmonary Artery, Right
			R Pulmonary Artery, Left
			S Pulmonary Vein, Right
			T Pulmonary Vein, Left
			U Pulmonary Vein, Confluence

W Thoracic Aorta, Descending	Ø Open	8 Zooplastic Tissue 9 Autologous Venous Tissue A Autologous Arterial Tissue J Synthetic Substitute K Nonautologous Tissue Substitute	A Innominate Artery B Subclavian D Carotid F Abdominal Artery G Axillary Artery H Brachial Artery P Pulmonary Trunk Q Pulmonary Artery, Right R Pulmonary Artery, Left V Lower Extremity Artery
W Thoracic Aorta, Descending	Ø Open	Z No Device	A Innominate Artery B Subclavian D Carotid P Pulmonary Trunk Q Pulmonary Artery, Right R Pulmonary Artery, Left
W Thoracic Aorta, Descending	4 Percutaneous Endoscopic	8 Zooplastic Tissue 9 Autologous Venous Tissue A Autologous Arterial Tissue J Synthetic Substitute K Nonautologous Tissue Substitute Z No Device	A Innominate Artery B Subclavian D Carotid P Pulmonary Trunk Q Pulmonary Artery, Right R Pulmonary Artery, Left

X Thoracic Aorta, Ascending/Arch
   Aortic arch
   Aortic isthmus
   Ascending aorta
   Juxtaductal aorta
	Ø Open
	4 Percutaneous Endoscopic
		8 Zooplastic Tissue
		9 Autologous Venous Tissue
		A Autologous Arterial Tissue
		J Synthetic Substitute
		K Nonautologous Tissue Substitute
		Z No Device
			A Innominate Artery
			B Subclavian
			D Carotid
			P Pulmonary Trunk
			Q Pulmonary Artery, Right
			R Pulmonary Artery, Left

0 Medical and Surgical
2 Heart and Great Vessels
4 Creation Definition: Putting in or on biological or synthetic material to form a new body part that to the extent possible replicates the anatomic structure or function of an absent body part
Explanation: Used for gender reassignment surgery and corrective procedures in individuals with congenital anomalies

Body Part Character 4	Approach Character 5	Device Character 6	Qualifier Character 7
F Aortic Valve Aortic annulus	Ø Open	7 Autologous Tissue 8 Zooplastic Tissue J Synthetic Substitute K Nonautologous Tissue Substitute	J Truncal Valve

G Mitral Valve
   Bicuspid valve
   Left atrioventricular valve
   Mitral annulus
J Tricuspid Valve
   Right atrioventricular valve
   Tricuspid annulus
	Ø Open	7 Autologous Tissue
		8 Zooplastic Tissue
		J Synthetic Substitute
		K Nonautologous Tissue Substitute
			2 Common Atrioventricular Valve

Non-OR Procedure DRG Non-OR Procedure Valid OR Procedure HAC Associated Procedure Combination Only New/Revised April New/Revised October

0 Medical and Surgical
2 Heart and Great Vessels
5 Destruction — Definition: Physical eradication of all or a portion of a body part by the direct use of energy, force, or a destructive agent
Explanation: None of the body part is physically taken out

Body Part Character 4	Approach Character 5	Device Character 6	Qualifier Character 7

4 Coronary Vein
5 Atrial Septum
    Interatrial septum
6 Atrium, Right
    Atrium dextrum cordis
    Right auricular appendix
    Sinus venosus
9 Chordae Tendineae
D Papillary Muscle
F Aortic Valve
    Aortic annulus
G Mitral Valve
    Bicuspid valve
    Left atrioventricular valve
    Mitral annulus
H Pulmonary Valve
    Pulmonary annulus
    Pulmonic valve
J Tricuspid Valve
    Right atrioventricular valve
    Tricuspid annulus
K Ventricle, Right
    Conus arteriosus
L Ventricle, Left
M Ventricular Septum
    Interventricular septum
N Pericardium
P Pulmonary Trunk
Q Pulmonary Artery, Right
R Pulmonary Artery, Left
    Arterial canal (duct)
    Botallo's duct
    Pulmoaortic canal
S Pulmonary Vein, Right
    Right inferior pulmonary vein
    Right superior pulmonary vein
T Pulmonary Vein, Left
    Left inferior pulmonary vein
    Left superior pulmonary vein
V Superior Vena Cava
    Cavoatrial junction
    Precava
W Thoracic Aorta, Descending
X Thoracic Aorta, Ascending/Arch
    Aortic arch
    Aortic isthmus
    Ascending aorta
    Juxtaductal aorta
	0 Open
	3 Percutaneous
	4 Percutaneous Endoscopic
		Z No Device	**Z** No Qualifier

7 Atrium, Left
    Atrium pulmonale
    Left auricular appendix
	0 Open
	3 Percutaneous
	4 Percutaneous Endoscopic
		Z No Device	**K** Left Atrial Appendage
			Z No Qualifier

8 Conduction Mechanism
    Atrioventricular node
    Bundle of His
    Bundle of Kent
    Sinoatrial node
	0 Open
	4 Percutaneous Endoscopic
		Z No Device	**Z** No Qualifier

8 Conduction Mechanism
    Atrioventricular node
    Bundle of His
    Bundle of Kent
    Sinoatrial node
	3 Percutaneous	**Z** No Device	**F** Irreversible Electroporation
			Z No Qualifier

DRG Non-OR 0257[0,3,4]ZK

027-028   Heart and Great Vessels   ICD-10-PCS 2025

0 Medical and Surgical
2 Heart and Great Vessels
7 Dilation Definition: Expanding an orifice or the lumen of a tubular body part
Explanation: The orifice can be a natural orifice or an artificially created orifice. Accomplished by stretching a tubular body part using intraluminal pressure or by cutting part of the orifice or wall of the tubular body part.

Body Part Character 4	Approach Character 5	Device Character 6	Qualifier Character 7
0 Coronary Artery, One Artery 1 Coronary Artery, Two Arteries 2 Coronary Artery, Three Arteries 3 Coronary Artery, Four or More Arteries	0 Open 3 Percutaneous 4 Percutaneous Endoscopic	4 Intraluminal Device, Drug-eluting 5 Intraluminal Device, Drug-eluting, Two 6 Intraluminal Device, Drug-eluting, Three 7 Intraluminal Device, Drug-eluting, Four or More D Intraluminal Device E Intraluminal Device, Two F Intraluminal Device, Three G Intraluminal Device, Four or More T Intraluminal Device, Radioactive Z No Device	6 Bifurcation Z No Qualifier

F Aortic Valve
   Aortic annulus
G Mitral Valve
   Bicuspid valve
   Left atrioventricular valve
   Mitral annulus
H Pulmonary Valve
   Pulmonary annulus
   Pulmonic valve
J Tricuspid Valve
   Right atrioventricular valve
   Tricuspid annulus
K Ventricle, Right
   Conus arteriosus
L Ventricle, Left
P Pulmonary Trunk
Q Pulmonary Artery, Right
S Pulmonary Vein, Right
   Right inferior pulmonary vein
   Right superior pulmonary vein
T Pulmonary Vein, Left
   Left inferior pulmonary vein
   Left superior pulmonary vein
V Superior Vena Cava
   Cavoatrial junction
   Precava
W Thoracic Aorta, Descending
X Thoracic Aorta, Ascending/Arch
   Aortic arch
   Aortic isthmus
   Ascending aorta
   Juxtaductal aorta
	0 Open
	3 Percutaneous
	4 Percutaneous Endoscopic
		4 Intraluminal Device, Drug-eluting
		D Intraluminal Device
		Z No Device
			Z No Qualifier

R Pulmonary Artery, Left
   Arterial canal (duct)
   Botallo's duct
   Pulmoaortic canal
	0 Open
	3 Percutaneous
	4 Percutaneous Endoscopic
		4 Intraluminal Device, Drug-eluting
		D Intraluminal Device
		Z No Device
			T Ductus Arteriosus
			Z No Qualifier

0 Medical and Surgical
2 Heart and Great Vessels
8 Division Definition: Cutting into a body part, without draining fluids and/or gases from the body part, in order to separate or transect a body part
Explanation: All or a portion of the body part is separated into two or more portions

Body Part Character 4	Approach Character 5	Device Character 6	Qualifier Character 7

8 Conduction Mechanism
   Atrioventricular node
   Bundle of His
   Bundle of Kent
   Sinoatrial node
9 Chordae Tendineae
D Papillary Muscle
	0 Open
	3 Percutaneous
	4 Percutaneous Endoscopic
		Z No Device	Z No Qualifier

Non-OR Procedure   DRG Non-OR Procedure   Valid OR Procedure   HAC Associated Procedure   Combination Only   New/Revised April   New/Revised October

ICD-10-PCS 2025 — Heart and Great Vessels — 02B–02B

- **0** Medical and Surgical
- **2** Heart and Great Vessels
- **B** Excision Definition: Cutting out or off, without replacement, a portion of a body part
  Explanation: The qualifier DIAGNOSTIC is used to identify excision procedures that are biopsies

Body Part Character 4	Approach Character 5	Device Character 6	Qualifier Character 7

4 Coronary Vein
5 Atrial Septum
   Interatrial septum
6 Atrium, Right
   Atrium dextrum cordis
   Right auricular appendix
   Sinus venosus
8 Conduction Mechanism
   Atrioventricular node
   Bundle of His
   Bundle of Kent
   Sinoatrial node
9 Chordae Tendineae
D Papillary Muscle
F Aortic Valve
   Aortic annulus
G Mitral Valve
   Bicuspid valve
   Left atrioventricular valve
   Mitral annulus
H Pulmonary Valve
   Pulmonary annulus
   Pulmonic valve
J Tricuspid Valve
   Right atrioventricular valve
   Tricuspid annulus
K Ventricle, Right [NC]
   Conus arteriosus
L Ventricle, Left [NC]
M Ventricular Septum
   Interventricular septum
N Pericardium
P Pulmonary Trunk
Q Pulmonary Artery, Right
R Pulmonary Artery, Left
   Arterial canal (duct)
   Botallo's duct
   Pulmoaortic canal
S Pulmonary Vein, Right
   Right inferior pulmonary vein
   Right superior pulmonary vein
T Pulmonary Vein, Left
   Left inferior pulmonary vein
   Left superior pulmonary vein
V Superior Vena Cava
   Cavoatrial junction
   Precava
W Thoracic Aorta, Descending
X Thoracic Aorta, Ascending/Arch
   Aortic arch
   Aortic isthmus
   Ascending aorta
   Juxtaductal aorta
	0 Open
	3 Percutaneous
	4 Percutaneous Endoscopic
		Z No Device	**X** Diagnostic
			Z No Qualifier

7 Atrium, Left
   Atrium pulmonale
   Left auricular appendix
	0 Open
	3 Percutaneous
	4 Percutaneous Endoscopic
		Z No Device	**K** Left Atrial Appendage
			X Diagnostic
			Z No Qualifier

DRG Non-OR 02B7[0,3,4]ZK
Non-OR 02B[4,5,6,8,9,D,F,G,H,J,K,L,M][0,3,4]ZX
NC 02B[K,L][0,3,4]ZZ

[NC] Noncovered Procedure [LC] Limited Coverage [QA] Questionable OB Admit [NT] New Tech Add-on ✚ Combination Member ♂ Male ♀ Female

0 Medical and Surgical
2 Heart and Great Vessels
C Extirpation Definition: Taking or cutting out solid matter from a body part
Explanation: The solid matter may be an abnormal byproduct of a biological function or a foreign body; it may be imbedded in a body part or in the lumen of a tubular body part. The solid matter may or may not have been previously broken into pieces.

Body Part Character 4	Approach Character 5	Device Character 6	Qualifier Character 7
0 Coronary Artery, One Artery **1** Coronary Artery, Two Arteries **2** Coronary Artery, Three Arteries **3** Coronary Artery, Four or More Arteries	**0** Open **4** Percutaneous Endoscopic	**Z** No Device	**6** Bifurcation **Z** No Qualifier
0 Coronary Artery, One Artery **1** Coronary Artery, Two Arteries **2** Coronary Artery, Three Arteries **3** Coronary Artery, Four or More Arteries	**3** Percutaneous	**Z** No Device	**6** Bifurcation **7** Orbital Atherectomy Technique **Z** No Qualifier

4 Coronary Vein
5 Atrial Septum
  Interatrial septum
6 Atrium, Right
  Atrium dextrum cordis
  Right auricular appendix
  Sinus venosus
7 Atrium, Left
  Atrium pulmonale
  Left auricular appendix
8 Conduction Mechanism
  Atrioventricular node
  Bundle of His
  Bundle of Kent
  Sinoatrial node
9 Chordae Tendineae
D Papillary Muscle
F Aortic Valve
  Aortic annulus
G Mitral Valve
  Bicuspid valve
  Left atrioventricular valve
  Mitral annulus
H Pulmonary Valve
  Pulmonary annulus
  Pulmonic valve
J Tricuspid Valve
  Right atrioventricular valve
  Tricuspid annulus
K Ventricle, Right
  Conus arteriosus
L Ventricle, Left
M Ventricular Septum
  Interventricular septum
N Pericardium
P Pulmonary Trunk
Q Pulmonary Artery, Right
R Pulmonary Artery, Left
  Arterial canal (duct)
  Botallo's duct
  Pulmoaortic canal
S Pulmonary Vein, Right
  Right inferior pulmonary vein
  Right superior pulmonary vein
T Pulmonary Vein, Left
  Left inferior pulmonary vein
  Left superior pulmonary vein
V Superior Vena Cava
  Cavoatrial junction
  Precava
W Thoracic Aorta, Descending
X Thoracic Aorta, Ascending/Arch
  Aortic arch
  Aortic isthmus
  Ascending aorta
  Juxtaductal aorta
	0 Open
	3 Percutaneous
	4 Percutaneous Endoscopic
		Z No Device	**Z** No Qualifier

ICD-10-PCS 2025 — Heart and Great Vessels — 02F–02F

- **0** Medical and Surgical
- **2** Heart and Great Vessels
- **F** Fragmentation Definition: Breaking solid matter in a body part into pieces
  Explanation: Physical force (e.g., manual, ultrasonic) applied directly or indirectly is used to break the solid matter into pieces. The solid matter may be an abnormal byproduct of a biological function or a foreign body. The pieces of solid matter are not taken out.

Body Part Character 4	Approach Character 5	Device Character 6	Qualifier Character 7
0 Coronary Artery, One Artery **1** Coronary Artery, Two Arteries **2** Coronary Artery, Three Arteries **3** Coronary Artery, Four or More Arteries	**3** Percutaneous	**Z** No Device	**Z** No Qualifier
N Pericardium NC	**0** Open **3** Percutaneous **4** Percutaneous Endoscopic **X** External	**Z** No Device	**Z** No Qualifier

P Pulmonary Trunk
Q Pulmonary Artery, Right
R Pulmonary Artery, Left
  Arterial canal (duct)
  Botallo's duct
  Pulmoaortic canal
S Pulmonary Vein, Right
  Right inferior pulmonary vein
  Right superior pulmonary vein
T Pulmonary Vein, Left
  Left inferior pulmonary vein
  Left superior pulmonary vein
	3 Percutaneous	**Z** No Device	**0** Ultrasonic
			Z No Qualifier

Non-OR 02FNXZZ
NC 02FNXZZ

Heart and Great Vessels

0 Medical and Surgical
2 Heart and Great Vessels
H Insertion Definition: Putting in a nonbiological appliance that monitors, assists, performs, or prevents a physiological function but does not physically take the place of a body part
Explanation: None

Body Part — Character 4	Approach — Character 5	Device — Character 6	Qualifier — Character 7
0 Coronary Artery, One Artery 1 Coronary Artery, Two Arteries 2 Coronary Artery, Three Arteries 3 Coronary Artery, Four or More Arteries	0 Open 3 Percutaneous 4 Percutaneous Endoscopic	D Intraluminal Device Y Other Device	Z No Qualifier

4 Coronary Vein
6 Atrium, Right
  Atrium dextrum cordis
  Right auricular appendix
  Sinus venosus
7 Atrium, Left
  Atrium pulmonale
  Left auricular appendix
K Ventricle, Right
  Conus arteriosus
L Ventricle, Left
	0 Open
	3 Percutaneous
	4 Percutaneous Endoscopic
		0 Monitoring Device, Pressure Sensor
		2 Monitoring Device
		3 Infusion Device
		D Intraluminal Device
		J Cardiac Lead, Pacemaker
		K Cardiac Lead, Defibrillator
		M Cardiac Lead
		N Intracardiac Pacemaker
		Y Other Device
			Z No Qualifier

A Heart	0 Open 3 Percutaneous 4 Percutaneous Endoscopic	Q Implantable Heart Assist System Y Other Device	Z No Qualifier
A Heart	0 Open 3 Percutaneous 4 Percutaneous Endoscopic	R Short-term External Heart Assist System	J Intraoperative S Biventricular Z No Qualifier
N Pericardium	0 Open 3 Percutaneous 4 Percutaneous Endoscopic	0 Monitoring Device, Pressure Sensor 2 Monitoring Device J Cardiac Lead, Pacemaker K Cardiac Lead, Defibrillator M Cardiac Lead Y Other Device	Z No Qualifier

P Pulmonary Trunk
Q Pulmonary Artery, Right
R Pulmonary Artery, Left
  Arterial canal (duct)
  Botallo's duct
  Pulmoaortic canal
S Pulmonary Vein, Right
  Right inferior pulmonary vein
  Right superior pulmonary vein
T Pulmonary Vein, Left
  Left inferior pulmonary vein
  Left superior pulmonary vein
V Superior Vena Cava
  Cavoatrial junction
  Precava
	0 Open
	3 Percutaneous
	4 Percutaneous Endoscopic
		0 Monitoring Device, Pressure Sensor
		2 Monitoring Device
		3 Infusion Device
		D Intraluminal Device
		Y Other Device
			Z No Qualifier

W Thoracic Aorta, Descending	0 Open 4 Percutaneous Endoscopic	0 Monitoring Device, Pressure Sensor 2 Monitoring Device 3 Infusion Device D Intraluminal Device Y Other Device	Z No Qualifier
W Thoracic Aorta, Descending	3 Percutaneous	0 Monitoring Device, Pressure Sensor 2 Monitoring Device 3 Infusion Device D Intraluminal Device R Short-term External Heart Assist System Y Other Device	Z No Qualifier

DRG Non-OR 02H[4,6,7,K,L][0,3,4][J,M]Z
DRG Non-OR 02HK32Z
DRG Non-OR 02HN[0,3,4][J,M]Z
Non-OR 02H[4,6,7,L]3[2,3]Z
Non-OR 02H[6,7]3MZ
Non-OR 02HK3[0,3]Z
Non-OR 02HN32Z
Non-OR 02HP[0,3,4][0,2,3]Z
Non-OR 02H[Q,R][0,3,4][2,3]Z
Non-OR 02H[S,T,V][0,3,4]3Z
Non-OR 02H[S,T,V]32Z
Non-OR 02HW0[0,3]Z
Non-OR 02HW43Z
Non-OR 02HW3[0,2,3]Z
02HA[3,4]QZ

HAC 02H[4,6,7,K,L][0,3,4][J,K,N]Z when reported with SDx K68.11, or T81.40-T81.49, T82.7 with 7th character A
HAC 02H[4,6,7]3MZ when reported with SDx K68.11, or T81.40-T81.49, T82.7 with 7th character A
HAC 02H[6,K]33Z when reported with SDx J95.811
HAC 02HN[0,3,4][J,K,M]Z when reported with SDx K68.11, or T81.40-T81.49, T82.7 with 7th character A
HAC 02H[S,T,V][3,4]3Z when reported with SDx J95.811

See Appendix L for Procedure Combinations
  02H[4,6,7,K,L][0,3,4][J,K,M]Z
  02HA[0,3,4]R[S,Z]
  02HN[0,3,4][J,K,M]Z

02H Continued on next page

0 Medical and Surgical
2 Heart and Great Vessels
H Insertion — Definition: Putting in a nonbiological appliance that monitors, assists, performs, or prevents a physiological function but does not physically take the place of a body part
Explanation: None

Body Part Character 4	Approach Character 5	Device Character 6	Qualifier Character 7

X Thoracic Aorta, Ascending/Arch
  Aortic arch
  Aortic isthmus
  Ascending aorta
  Juxtaductal aorta
	0 Open
	3 Percutaneous
	4 Percutaneous Endoscopic
		0 Monitoring Device, Pressure Sensor
		2 Monitoring Device
		3 Infusion Device
		D Intraluminal Device
			Z No Qualifier

Non-OR 02HX[0,3,4][0,3]Z

0 Medical and Surgical
2 Heart and Great Vessels
J Inspection — Definition: Visually and/or manually exploring a body part
Explanation: Visual exploration may be performed with or without optical instrumentation. Manual exploration may be performed directly or through intervening body layers.

Body Part Character 4	Approach Character 5	Device Character 6	Qualifier Character 7
A Heart Y Great Vessel	0 Open 3 Percutaneous 4 Percutaneous Endoscopic	Z No Device	Z No Qualifier

Non-OR 02J[A,Y]3ZZ

0 Medical and Surgical
2 Heart and Great Vessels
K Map — Definition: Locating the route of passage of electrical impulses and/or locating functional areas in a body part
Explanation: Applicable only to the cardiac conduction mechanism and the central nervous system

Body Part Character 4	Approach Character 5	Device Character 6	Qualifier Character 7

8 Conduction Mechanism
  Atrioventricular node
  Bundle of His
  Bundle of Kent
  Sinoatrial node
	0 Open
	3 Percutaneous
	4 Percutaneous Endoscopic
		Z No Device	Z No Qualifier

DRG Non-OR 02K8[0,3,4]ZZ

0 Medical and Surgical
2 Heart and Great Vessels
L Occlusion — Definition: Completely closing an orifice or the lumen of a tubular body part
Explanation: The orifice can be a natural orifice or an artificially created orifice

Body Part Character 4	Approach Character 5	Device Character 6	Qualifier Character 7

7 Atrium, Left
  Atrium pulmonale
  Left auricular appendix
	0 Open
	3 Percutaneous
	4 Percutaneous Endoscopic
		C Extraluminal Device
		D Intraluminal Device
		Z No Device
			K Left Atrial Appendage

H Pulmonary Valve
  Pulmonary annulus
  Pulmonic valve
P Pulmonary Trunk
Q Pulmonary Artery, Right
S Pulmonary Vein, Right
  Right inferior pulmonary vein
  Right superior pulmonary vein
T Pulmonary Vein, Left
  Left inferior pulmonary vein
  Left superior pulmonary vein
V Superior Vena Cava
  Cavoatrial junction
  Precava
	0 Open
	3 Percutaneous
	4 Percutaneous Endoscopic
		C Extraluminal Device
		D Intraluminal Device
		Z No Device
			Z No Qualifier

R Pulmonary Artery, Left
  Arterial canal (duct)
  Botallo's duct
  Pulmoaortic canal
	0 Open
	3 Percutaneous
	4 Percutaneous Endoscopic
		C Extraluminal Device
		D Intraluminal Device
		Z No Device
			T Ductus Arteriosus
			Z No Qualifier

W Thoracic Aorta, Descending	0 Open 3 Percutaneous	D Intraluminal Device	J Temporary

DRG Non-OR 02L7[0,3,4][C,D,Z]K

0 Medical and Surgical
2 Heart and Great Vessels
N Release Definition: Freeing a body part from an abnormal physical constraint by cutting or by the use of force
Explanation: Some of the restraining tissue may be taken out but none of the body part is taken out

Body Part Character 4	Approach Character 5	Device Character 6	Qualifier Character 7

0 Coronary Artery, One Artery
1 Coronary Artery, Two Arteries
2 Coronary Artery, Three Arteries
3 Coronary Artery, Four or More Arteries
4 Coronary Vein
5 Atrial Septum
   Interatrial septum
6 Atrium, Right
   Atrium dextrum cordis
   Right auricular appendix
   Sinus venosus
7 Atrium, Left
   Atrium pulmonale
   Left auricular appendix
8 Conduction Mechanism
   Atrioventricular node
   Bundle of His
   Bundle of Kent
   Sinoatrial node
9 Chordae Tendineae
D Papillary Muscle
F Aortic Valve
   Aortic annulus
G Mitral Valve
   Bicuspid valve
   Left atrioventricular valve
   Mitral annulus
H Pulmonary Valve
   Pulmonary annulus
   Pulmonic valve
J Tricuspid Valve
   Right atrioventricular valve
   Tricuspid annulus
K Ventricle, Right
   Conus arteriosus
L Ventricle, Left
M Ventricular Septum
   Interventricular septum
N Pericardium
P Pulmonary Trunk
Q Pulmonary Artery, Right
R Pulmonary Artery, Left
   Arterial canal (duct)
   Botallo's duct
   Pulmoaortic canal
S Pulmonary Vein, Right
   Right inferior pulmonary vein
   Right superior pulmonary vein
T Pulmonary Vein, Left
   Left inferior pulmonary vein
   Left superior pulmonary vein
V Superior Vena Cava
   Cavoatrial junction
   Precava
W Thoracic Aorta, Descending
X Thoracic Aorta, Ascending/Arch
   Aortic arch
   Aortic isthmus
   Ascending aorta
   Juxtaductal aorta
	0 Open
	3 Percutaneous
	4 Percutaneous Endoscopic
		Z No Device	Z No Qualifier

ICD-10-PCS 2025 — Heart and Great Vessels — 02P–02P

- 0 Medical and Surgical
- 2 Heart and Great Vessels
- P Removal

Definition: Taking out or off a device from a body part

Explanation: If a device is taken out and a similar device put in without cutting or puncturing the skin or mucous membrane, the procedure is coded to the root operation CHANGE. Otherwise, the procedure for taking out a device is coded to the root operation REMOVAL.

Body Part Character 4	Approach Character 5	Device Character 6	Qualifier Character 7
A Heart	0 Open 3 Percutaneous 4 Percutaneous Endoscopic	2 Monitoring Device 3 Infusion Device 7 Autologous Tissue Substitute 8 Zooplastic Tissue C Extraluminal Device D Intraluminal Device J Synthetic Substitute K Nonautologous Tissue Substitute M Cardiac Lead N Intracardiac Pacemaker Q Implantable Heart Assist System Y Other Device	Z No Qualifier
A Heart ✚	0 Open 3 Percutaneous 4 Percutaneous Endoscopic	R Short-term External Heart Assist System	S Biventricular Z No Qualifier
A Heart	X External	2 Monitoring Device 3 Infusion Device D Intraluminal Device M Cardiac Lead	Z No Qualifier
W Thoracic Aorta, Descending ✚	3 Percutaneous	R Short-term External Heart Assist System	Z No Qualifier
Y Great Vessel	0 Open 3 Percutaneous 4 Percutaneous Endoscopic	2 Monitoring Device 3 Infusion Device 7 Autologous Tissue Substitute 8 Zooplastic Tissue C Extraluminal Device D Intraluminal Device J Synthetic Substitute K Nonautologous Tissue Substitute Y Other Device	Z No Qualifier
Y Great Vessel	X External	2 Monitoring Device 3 Infusion Device D Intraluminal Device	Z No Qualifier

Non-OR 02PA3[2,3,D]Z
Non-OR 02PA[3,4]YZ
Non-OR 02PAX[2,3,D,M]Z
Non-OR 02PY3[2,3,D]Z
Non-OR 02PY[3,4]YZ
Non-OR 02PYX[2,3,D]Z
HAC 02PA[0,3,4][M,N]Z when reported with SDx K68.11 or T81.40-T81.49, T82.7 with 7th character A
HAC 02PAXMZ when reported with SDx K68.11 or T81.40-T81.49, T82.7 with 7th character A

See Appendix L for Procedure Combinations
✚ 02PA[0,3,4]RZ
✚ 02PW3RZ

0 Medical and Surgical
2 Heart and Great Vessels
Q Repair   Definition: Restoring, to the extent possible, a body part to its normal anatomic structure and function
           Explanation: Used only when the method to accomplish the repair is not one of the other root operations

Body Part Character 4	Approach Character 5	Device Character 6	Qualifier Character 7

0 Coronary Artery, One Artery
1 Coronary Artery, Two Arteries
2 Coronary Artery, Three Arteries
3 Coronary Artery, Four or More Arteries
4 Coronary Vein
5 Atrial Septum
   Interatrial septum
6 Atrium, Right
   Atrium dextrum cordis
   Right auricular appendix
   Sinus venosus
7 Atrium, Left
   Atrium pulmonale
   Left auricular appendix
8 Conduction Mechanism
   Atrioventricular node
   Bundle of His
   Bundle of Kent
   Sinoatrial node
9 Chordae Tendineae
A Heart
B Heart, Right
   Right coronary sulcus
C Heart, Left
   Left coronary sulcus
   Obtuse margin
D Papillary Muscle
H Pulmonary Valve
   Pulmonary annulus
   Pulmonic valve
K Ventricle, Right
   Conus arteriosus
L Ventricle, Left
M Ventricular Septum
   Interventricular septum
N Pericardium
P Pulmonary Trunk
Q Pulmonary Artery, Right
R Pulmonary Artery, Left
   Arterial canal (duct)
   Botallo's duct
   Pulmoaortic canal
S Pulmonary Vein, Right
   Right inferior pulmonary vein
   Right superior pulmonary vein
T Pulmonary Vein, Left
   Left inferior pulmonary vein
   Left superior pulmonary vein
V Superior Vena Cava
   Cavoatrial junction
   Precava
W Thoracic Aorta, Descending
X Thoracic Aorta, Ascending/Arch
   Aortic arch
   Aortic isthmus
   Ascending aorta
   Juxtaductal aorta
	0 Open
	3 Percutaneous
	4 Percutaneous Endoscopic
		Z No Device	Z No Qualifier

F Aortic Valve Aortic annulus	0 Open 3 Percutaneous 4 Percutaneous Endoscopic	Z No Device	J Truncal Valve Z No Qualifier

G Mitral Valve
   Bicuspid valve
   Left atrioventricular valve
   Mitral annulus
	0 Open
	3 Percutaneous
	4 Percutaneous Endoscopic
		Z No Device	E Atrioventricular Valve, Left
			Z No Qualifier

J Tricuspid Valve
   Right atrioventricular valve
   Tricuspid annulus
	0 Open
	3 Percutaneous
	4 Percutaneous Endoscopic
		Z No Device	G Atrioventricular Valve, Right
			Z No Qualifier

ICD-10-PCS 2025 — Heart and Great Vessels — 02R–02R

- **0** Medical and Surgical
- **2** Heart and Great Vessels
- **R** Replacement **Definition:** Putting in or on biological or synthetic material that physically takes the place and/or function of all or a portion of a body part
  Explanation: The body part may have been taken out or replaced, or may be taken out, physically eradicated, or rendered nonfunctional during the REPLACEMENT procedure. A REMOVAL procedure is coded for taking out the device used in a previous replacement procedure.

Body Part – Character 4	Approach – Character 5	Device – Character 6	Qualifier – Character 7

5 Atrial Septum
  Interatrial septum
6 Atrium, Right
  Atrium dextrum cordis
  Right auricular appendix
  Sinus venosus
7 Atrium, Left
  Atrium pulmonale
  Left auricular appendix
9 Chordae Tendineae
D Papillary Muscle
K Ventricle, Right ✚
  Conus arteriosus
L Ventricle, Left ✚
M Ventricular Septum
  Interventricular septum
N Pericardium
P Pulmonary Trunk
Q Pulmonary Artery, Right
R Pulmonary Artery, Left
  Arterial canal (duct)
  Botallo's duct
  Pulmoaortic canal
S Pulmonary Vein, Right
  Right inferior pulmonary vein
  Right superior pulmonary vein
T Pulmonary Vein, Left
  Left inferior pulmonary vein
  Left superior pulmonary vein
V Superior Vena Cava
  Cavoatrial junction
  Precava
W Thoracic Aorta, Descending
X Thoracic Aorta, Ascending/Arch
  Aortic arch
  Aortic isthmus
  Ascending aorta
  Juxtaductal aorta
	0 Open
	4 Percutaneous Endoscopic
		7 Autologous Tissue Substitute
		8 Zooplastic Tissue
		J Synthetic Substitute
		K Nonautologous Tissue Substitute
			Z No Qualifier

A Heart	**0** Open	**L** Biologic with Synthetic Substitute, Autoregulated Electrohydraulic **M** Synthetic Substitute, Pneumatic	**Z** No Qualifier
F Aortic Valve Aortic annulus	**0** Open **4** Percutaneous Endoscopic	**7** Autologous Tissue Substitute **J** Synthetic Substitute **K** Nonautologous Tissue Substitute	**Z** No Qualifier
F Aortic Valve Aortic annulus	**0** Open **4** Percutaneous Endoscopic	**8** Zooplastic Tissue	**N** Rapid Deployment Technique **Z** No Qualifier
F Aortic Valve Aortic annulus	**3** Percutaneous	**7** Autologous Tissue Substitute **J** Synthetic Substitute **K** Nonautologous Tissue Substitute	**H** Transapical **Z** No Qualifier
F Aortic Valve Aortic annulus	**3** Percutaneous	**8** Zooplastic Tissue	**H** Transapical **N** Rapid Deployment Technique **Z** No Qualifier

G Mitral Valve
  Bicuspid valve
  Left atrioventricular valve
  Mitral annulus
J Tricuspid Valve
  Right atrioventricular valve
  Tricuspid annulus
	0 Open
	4 Percutaneous Endoscopic
		7 Autologous Tissue Substitute
		8 Zooplastic Tissue
		J Synthetic Substitute
		K Nonautologous Tissue Substitute
			Z No Qualifier

G Mitral Valve
  Bicuspid valve
  Left atrioventricular valve
  Mitral annulus
J Tricuspid Valve
  Right atrioventricular valve
  Tricuspid annulus
	3 Percutaneous	**7** Autologous Tissue Substitute
		8 Zooplastic Tissue
		J Synthetic Substitute
		K Nonautologous Tissue Substitute
			H Transapical
			Z No Qualifier

H Pulmonary Valve
  Pulmonary annulus
  Pulmonic valve
	0 Open
	4 Percutaneous Endoscopic
		7 Autologous Tissue Substitute
		8 Zooplastic Tissue
		J Synthetic Substitute
		K Nonautologous Tissue Substitute
			Z No Qualifier

H Pulmonary Valve
  Pulmonary annulus
  Pulmonic valve
	3 Percutaneous	**7** Autologous Tissue Substitute
		J Synthetic Substitute
		K Nonautologous Tissue Substitute
			H Transapical
			Z No Qualifier

H Pulmonary Valve
  Pulmonary annulus
  Pulmonic valve
	3 Percutaneous	**8** Zooplastic Tissue	**H** Transapical
			L In Existing Conduit
			M Native Site
			Z No Qualifier

See Appendix L for Procedure Combinations
  ✚ 02R[K,L]0JZ

NC Noncovered Procedure   **LC** Limited Coverage   **QA** Questionable OB Admit   **NT** New Tech Add-on   ✚ Combination Member   ♂ Male   ♀ Female

0	Medical and Surgical
2	Heart and Great Vessels
S	Reposition

Definition: Moving to its normal location, or other suitable location, all or a portion of a body part

Explanation: The body part is moved to a new location from an abnormal location, or from a normal location where it is not functioning correctly. The body part may or may not be cut out or off to be moved to the new location.

Body Part Character 4	Approach Character 5	Device Character 6	Qualifier Character 7

0 Coronary Artery, One Artery
1 Coronary Artery, Two Arteries
P Pulmonary Trunk
Q Pulmonary Artery, Right
R Pulmonary Artery, Left
   Arterial canal (duct)
   Botallo's duct
   Pulmoaortic canal
S Pulmonary Vein, Right
   Right inferior pulmonary vein
   Right superior pulmonary vein
T Pulmonary Vein, Left
   Left inferior pulmonary vein
   Left superior pulmonary vein
V Superior Vena Cava
   Cavoatrial junction
   Precava
W Thoracic Aorta, Descending
X Thoracic Aorta, Ascending/Arch
   Aortic arch
   Aortic isthmus
   Ascending aorta
   Juxtaductal aorta
	0 Open	Z No Device	Z No Qualifier

0	Medical and Surgical
2	Heart and Great Vessels
T	Resection

Definition: Cutting out or off, without replacement, all of a body part

Explanation: None

Body Part Character 4	Approach Character 5	Device Character 6	Qualifier Character 7

5 Atrial Septum
   Interatrial septum
8 Conduction Mechanism
   Atrioventricular node
   Bundle of His
   Bundle of Kent
   Sinoatrial node
9 Chordae Tendineae
D Papillary Muscle
H Pulmonary Valve
   Pulmonary annulus
   Pulmonic valve
M Ventricular Septum
   Interventricular septum
N Pericardium
	0 Open
	3 Percutaneous
	4 Percutaneous Endoscopic
		Z No Device	Z No Qualifier

Heart and Great Vessels

0 Medical and Surgical
2 Heart and Great Vessels
U Supplement   Definition: Putting in or on biological or synthetic material that physically reinforces and/or augments the function of a portion of a body part
Explanation: The biological material is non-living, or is living and from the same individual. The body part may have been previously replaced, and the SUPPLEMENT procedure is performed to physically reinforce and/or augment the function of the replaced body part.

Body Part Character 4	Approach Character 5	Device Character 6	Qualifier Character 7

0 Coronary Artery, One Artery
1 Coronary Artery, Two Arteries
2 Coronary Artery, Three Arteries
3 Coronary Artery, Four or More Arteries
5 Atrial Septum
   Interatrial septum
6 Atrium, Right
   Atrium dextrum cordis
   Right auricular appendix
   Sinus venosus
7 Atrium, Left
   Atrium pulmonale
   Left auricular appendix
9 Chordae Tendineae
A Heart
D Papillary Muscle
H Pulmonary Valve
   Pulmonary annulus
   Pulmonic valve
K Ventricle, Right
   Conus arteriosus
L Ventricle, Left
M Ventricular Septum
   Interventricular septum
N Pericardium
P Pulmonary Trunk
Q Pulmonary Artery, Right
R Pulmonary Artery, Left
   Arterial canal (duct)
   Botallo's duct
   Pulmoaortic canal
S Pulmonary Vein, Right
   Right inferior pulmonary vein
   Right superior pulmonary vein
T Pulmonary Vein, Left
   Left inferior pulmonary vein
   Left superior pulmonary vein
V Superior Vena Cava
   Cavoatrial junction
   Precava
W Thoracic Aorta, Descending
X Thoracic Aorta, Ascending/Arch
   Aortic arch
   Aortic isthmus
   Ascending aorta
   Juxtaductal aorta
	0 Open
	3 Percutaneous
	4 Percutaneous Endoscopic
		7 Autologous Tissue Substitute
		8 Zooplastic Tissue
		J Synthetic Substitute
		K Nonautologous Tissue Substitute
			Z No Qualifier

F Aortic Valve Aortic annulus	**0** Open **3** Percutaneous **4** Percutaneous Endoscopic	**7** Autologous Tissue Substitute **8** Zooplastic Tissue **J** Synthetic Substitute **K** Nonautologous Tissue Substitute	**J** Truncal Valve **Z** No Qualifier

G Mitral Valve
   Bicuspid valve
   Left atrioventricular valve
   Mitral annulus
	0 Open
	4 Percutaneous Endoscopic
		7 Autologous Tissue Substitute
		8 Zooplastic Tissue
		J Synthetic Substitute
		K Nonautologous Tissue Substitute
			E Atrioventricular Valve, Left
			Z No Qualifier

G Mitral Valve
   Bicuspid valve
   Left atrioventricular valve
   Mitral annulus
	3 Percutaneous	**7** Autologous Tissue Substitute
		8 Zooplastic Tissue
		K Nonautologous Tissue Substitute
			E Atrioventricular Valve, Left
			Z No Qualifier

G Mitral Valve
   Bicuspid valve
   Left atrioventricular valve
   Mitral annulus
	3 Percutaneous	**J** Synthetic Substitute	**E** Atrioventricular Valve, Left
			H Transapical
			Z No Qualifier

J Tricuspid Valve
   Right atrioventricular valve
   Tricuspid annulus
	0 Open
	3 Percutaneous
	4 Percutaneous Endoscopic
		7 Autologous Tissue Substitute
		8 Zooplastic Tissue
		J Synthetic Substitute
		K Nonautologous Tissue Substitute
			G Atrioventricular Valve, Right
			Z No Qualifier

DRG Non-OR   02U7[3,4]JZ

0 Medical and Surgical
2 Heart and Great Vessels
V Restriction   Definition: Partially closing an orifice or the lumen of a tubular body part
Explanation: The orifice can be a natural orifice or an artificially created orifice

Body Part Character 4	Approach Character 5	Device Character 6	Qualifier Character 7
A Heart	0 Open 3 Percutaneous 4 Percutaneous Endoscopic	C Extraluminal Device Z No Device	Z No Qualifier

G Mitral Valve
  Bicuspid valve
  Left atrioventricular valve
  Mitral annulus
	0 Open
	3 Percutaneous
	4 Percutaneous Endoscopic
		Z No Device	Z No Qualifier

L Ventricle, Left
P Pulmonary Trunk
Q Pulmonary Artery, Right
S Pulmonary Vein, Right
  Right inferior pulmonary vein
  Right superior pulmonary vein
T Pulmonary Vein, Left
  Left inferior pulmonary vein
  Left superior pulmonary vein
V Superior Vena Cava
  Cavoatrial junction
  Precava
	0 Open
	3 Percutaneous
	4 Percutaneous Endoscopic
		C Extraluminal Device
		D Intraluminal Device
		Z No Device
			Z No Qualifier

R Pulmonary Artery, Left
  Arterial canal (duct)
  Botallo's duct
  Pulmoaortic canal
	0 Open
	3 Percutaneous
	4 Percutaneous Endoscopic
		C Extraluminal Device
		D Intraluminal Device
		Z No Device
			T Ductus Arteriosus
			Z No Qualifier

W Thoracic Aorta, Descending
X Thoracic Aorta, Ascending/Arch
  Aortic arch
  Aortic isthmus
  Ascending aorta
  Juxtaductal aorta
	0 Open
	3 Percutaneous
	4 Percutaneous Endoscopic
		C Extraluminal Device
		D Intraluminal Device [NT]
		E Intraluminal Device, Branched [NT]
		  or Fenestrated, One or Two Arteries
		F Intraluminal Device, Branched or
		  Fenestrated, Three or More Arteries
		Z No Device
			Z No Qualifier

[NT] 02VW3DZ with 02VX3EZ for GORE® TAG® Thoracic Branch Endoprosthesis

ICD-10-PCS 2025 — Heart and Great Vessels — 02W–02W

0 Medical and Surgical
2 Heart and Great Vessels
W Revision — Definition: Correcting, to the extent possible, a portion of a malfunctioning device or the position of a displaced device
Explanation: Revision can include correcting a malfunctioning or displaced device by taking out or putting in components of the device such as a screw or pin

Body Part Character 4	Approach Character 5	Device Character 6	Qualifier Character 7

5 Atrial Septum
  Interatrial septum
 	
M Ventricular Septum
  Interventricular septum
	0 Open
	4 Percutaneous Endoscopic
		J Synthetic Substitute	Z No Qualifier

A Heart LC ✚	0 Open 3 Percutaneous 4 Percutaneous Endoscopic	2 Monitoring Device 3 Infusion Device 7 Autologous Tissue Substitute 8 Zooplastic Tissue C Extraluminal Device D Intraluminal Device J Synthetic Substitute K Nonautologous Tissue Substitute M Cardiac Lead N Intracardiac Pacemaker Q Implantable Heart Assist System Y Other Device	Z No Qualifier
A Heart ✚	0 Open 3 Percutaneous 4 Percutaneous Endoscopic	R Short-term External Heart Assist System	S Biventricular Z No Qualifier
A Heart	X External	2 Monitoring Device 3 Infusion Device 7 Autologous Tissue Substitute 8 Zooplastic Tissue C Extraluminal Device D Intraluminal Device J Synthetic Substitute K Nonautologous Tissue Substitute M Cardiac Lead N Intracardiac Pacemaker Q Implantable Heart Assist System	Z No Qualifier
A Heart	X External	R Short-term External Heart Assist System	S Biventricular Z No Qualifier

F Aortic Valve
  Aortic annulus
G Mitral Valve
  Bicuspid valve
  Left atrioventricular valve
  Mitral annulus
H Pulmonary Valve
  Pulmonary annulus
  Pulmonic valve
J Tricuspid Valve
  Right atrioventricular valve
  Tricuspid annulus
	0 Open
	3 Percutaneous
	4 Percutaneous Endoscopic
		7 Autologous Tissue Substitute
		8 Zooplastic Tissue
		J Synthetic Substitute
		K Nonautologous Tissue Substitute
			Z No Qualifier

W Thoracic Aorta, Descending ✚	3 Percutaneous	R Short-term External Heart Assist System	Z No Qualifier
Y Great Vessel	0 Open 3 Percutaneous 4 Percutaneous Endoscopic	2 Monitoring Device 3 Infusion Device 7 Autologous Tissue Substitute 8 Zooplastic Tissue C Extraluminal Device D Intraluminal Device J Synthetic Substitute K Nonautologous Tissue Substitute Y Other Device	Z No Qualifier

Non-OR 02WA3[2,3,D]Z
Non-OR 02WA[3,4]YZ
Non-OR 02WAX[2,3,7,8,C,D,J,K,M,N,Q]Z
Non-OR 02WAXRZ
Non-OR 02WY3[2,3]Z
Non-OR 02WY[3,4]YZ
LC 02WA[3,4]QZ

HAC 02WA[0,3,4][M,N]Z when reported with SDx K68.11, or T81.40-T81.49, T82.7 with 7th character A
HAC 02WAXNZ when reported with SDx K68.11, or T81.40-T81.49, T82.7 with 7th character A

See Appendix L for Procedure Combinations
✚ 02WA[0,3,4]QZ
✚ 02WA[0,3,4]RZ
✚ 02WW3RZ

02W Continued on next page

02W–02Y   Heart and Great Vessels   ICD-10-PCS 2025

02W Continued

0 Medical and Surgical
2 Heart and Great Vessels
W Revision   Definition: Correcting, to the extent possible, a portion of a malfunctioning device or the position of a displaced device
               Explanation: Revision can include correcting a malfunctioning or displaced device by taking out or putting in components of the device such as a screw or pin

Body Part Character 4	Approach Character 5	Device Character 6	Qualifier Character 7
Y Great Vessel	X External	2 Monitoring Device 3 Infusion Device 7 Autologous Tissue Substitute 8 Zooplastic Tissue C Extraluminal Device D Intraluminal Device J Synthetic Substitute K Nonautologous Tissue Substitute	Z No Qualifier

Non-OR   02WYX[2,3,7,8,C,D,J,K]Z

0 Medical and Surgical
2 Heart and Great Vessels
Y Transplantation   Definition: Putting in or on all or a portion of a living body part taken from another individual or animal to physically take the place and/or function of all or a portion of a similar body part
               Explanation: The native body part may or may not be taken out, and the transplanted body part may take over all or a portion of its function

Body Part Character 4	Approach Character 5	Device Character 6	Qualifier Character 7
A Heart LC	0 Open	Z No Device	0 Allogeneic 1 Syngeneic 2 Zooplastic

LC   02YA0Z[0,1,2]

Upper Arteries Ø31–Ø3W

Character Meanings

This Character Meaning table is provided as a guide to assist the user in the identification of character members that may be found in this section of code tables. It **SHOULD NOT** be used to build a PCS code.

Operation–Character 3	Body Part–Character 4	Approach–Character 5	Device–Character 6	Qualifier–Character 7
1 Bypass	Ø Internal Mammary Artery, Right	Ø Open	Ø Drainage Device	Ø Upper Arm Artery, Right OR Ultrasonic
5 Destruction	1 Internal Mammary Artery, Left	3 Percutaneous	2 Monitoring Device	1 Upper Arm Artery, Left OR Drug-Coated Balloon
7 Dilation	2 Innominate Artery	4 Percutaneous Endoscopic	3 Infusion Device	2 Upper Arm Artery, Bilateral
9 Drainage	3 Subclavian Artery, Right	X External	4 Intraluminal Device, Drug-eluting	3 Lower Arm Artery, Right
B Excision	4 Subclavian Artery, Left		5 Intraluminal Device, Drug-eluting, Two	4 Lower Arm Artery, Left
C Extirpation	5 Axillary Artery, Right		6 Intraluminal Device, Drug-eluting, Three	5 Lower Arm Artery, Bilateral
F Fragmentation	6 Axillary Artery, Left		7 Intraluminal Device, Drug-eluting, Four or More OR Autologous Tissue Substitute	6 Upper Leg Artery, Right
H Insertion	7 Brachial Artery, Right		9 Autologous Venous Tissue	7 Upper Leg Artery, Left OR Stent Retriever
J Inspection	8 Brachial Artery, Left		A Autologous Arterial Tissue	8 Upper Leg Artery, Bilateral
L Occlusion	9 Ulnar Artery, Right		B Intraluminal Device, Bioactive	9 Lower Leg Artery, Right
N Release	A Ulnar Artery, Left		C Extraluminal Device	B Lower Leg Artery, Left
P Removal	B Radial Artery, Right		D Intraluminal Device	C Lower Leg Artery, Bilateral
Q Repair	C Radial Artery, Left		E Intraluminal Device, Two	D Upper Arm Vein
R Replacement	D Hand Artery, Right		F Intraluminal Device, Three	F Lower Arm Vein
S Reposition	F Hand Artery, Left		G Intraluminal Device, Four or More	G Intracranial Artery
U Supplement	G Intracranial Artery		H Intraluminal Device, Flow Diverter	J Extracranial Artery, Right
V Restriction	H Common Carotid Artery, Right		J Synthetic Substitute	K Extracranial Artery, Left
W Revision	J Common Carotid Artery, Left		K Nonautologous Tissue Substitute	M Pulmonary Artery, Right
	K Internal Carotid Artery, Right		M Stimulator Lead	N Pulmonary Artery, Left
	L Internal Carotid Artery, Left		Y Other Device	T Abdominal Artery
	M External Carotid Artery, Right		Z No Device	V Superior Vena Cava
	N External Carotid Artery, Left			W Lower Extremity Vein
	P Vertebral Artery, Right			X Diagnostic
	Q Vertebral Artery, Left			Y Upper Artery
	R Face Artery			Z No Qualifier
	S Temporal Artery, Right			
	T Temporal Artery, Left			
	U Thyroid Artery, Right			
	V Thyroid Artery, Left			
	Y Upper Artery			

Upper Arteries

AHA Coding Clinic for Upper Arteries
2022, 1Q, 10-13	Procedures performed on a continuous vessel, ICD-10-PCS Guideline B4.1c

AHA Coding Clinic for table 031
2024, 1Q, 32	Percutaneous creation of arteriovenous fistula with Ellipsys® Vascular Access System
2021, 4Q, 45-46	Percutaneous bypass of brachial artery for arteriovenous fistula creation
2021, 4Q, 60	Percutaneous creation of arteriovenous fistula using thermal resistance energy
2021, 3Q, 14	Arteriovenous fistula revision with graft to cephalic vein stump
2019, 4Q, 26	Upper artery bypass Qualifier
2019, 4Q, 26	Percutaneous approach upper artery bypass
2017, 4Q, 64-65	New qualifier values - Left to right carotid bypass
2017, 2Q, 22	Carotid artery to subclavian artery transposition
2017, 1Q, 31	Left to right common carotid artery bypass
2016, 3Q, 37	Insertion of arteriovenous graft using HeRO device
2016, 3Q, 39	Revision of arteriovenous graft
2013, 4Q, 125	Stage II cephalic vein transposition (superficialization) of arteriovenous fistula
2013, 1Q, 27	Creation of radial artery fistula

AHA Coding Clinic for table 037
2020, 4Q, 70-71	Cerebral embolic filtration extracorporeal flow reversal circuit
2019, 4Q, 27	Bifurcation Qualifier
2019, 3Q, 29	Transcarotid arterial catheterization
2018, 2Q, 24	Coronary artery bifurcation
2016, 4Q, 86	Peripheral artery, number of stents
2016, 4Q, 86-87	Coronary and peripheral artery bifurcation
2015, 1Q, 32	Deployment of stent for herniated/migrated coil in basilar artery

AHA Coding Clinic for table 03B
2016, 2Q, 12	Resection of malignant neoplasm of infratemporal fossa

AHA Coding Clinic for table 03C
2023, 3Q, 24	Thrombectomy of HeRO® graft
2022, 1Q, 43	Cerebral thrombectomy with failed stent retriever deployment and aspiration of thrombus
2021, 2Q, 13	Thromboendarterectomy with deconstruction of internal carotid artery
2020, 3Q, 38	Thrombectomy of arteriovenous fistula with angioplasty and stent placement
2019, 4Q, 27	Bifurcation Qualifier
2018, 4Q, 47-48	Endovascular thrombectomy with stent retriever
2018, 2Q, 24	Coronary artery bifurcation
2017, 4Q, 64-65	New qualifier values - Left to right carotid bypass
2017, 2Q, 23	Thrombectomy via Fogarty catheter
2016, 4Q, 86-87	Coronary and peripheral artery bifurcation
2016, 2Q, 11	Carotid endarterectomy with patch angioplasty
2015, 1Q, 29	Discontinued carotid endarterectomy

AHA Coding Clinic for table 03F
2021, 4Q, 46	Fragmentation of intracranial artery
2020, 4Q, 45-49	New fragmentation tables
2020, 4Q, 49-50	Intravascular ultrasound assisted thrombolysis
2020, 4Q, 50	Intravascular lithotripsy

AHA Coding Clinic for table 03H
2024, 2Q, 18	Ascending aorta and total aortic arch repair with extension frozen elephant trunk
2019, 1Q, 23	Endovascular repair of shaggy aorta and deployment of chimney stent grafts
2020, 1Q, 25	Elephant trunk repair of aortic dissection
2016, 2Q, 32	Arterial catheter placement

AHA Coding Clinic for table 03J
2021, 1Q, 16	Placement of Sentinel™ embolic protection device with deployment of single filter
2015, 1Q, 29	Discontinued carotid endarterectomy

AHA Coding Clinic for table 03L
2021, 2Q, 13	Thromboendarterectomy with deconstruction of internal carotid artery
2016, 2Q, 30	Clipping (occlusion) of cerebral artery, decompressive craniectomy and storage of bone flap in abdominal wall
2014, 4Q, 20	Control of epistaxis
2014, 4Q, 37	Endovascular embolization of arteriovenous malformation using Onyx-18 liquid

AHA Coding Clinic for table 03Q
2017, 1Q, 31	Left to right common carotid artery bypass

AHA Coding Clinic for table 03S
2017, 2Q, 22	Carotid artery to subclavian artery transposition
2015, 3Q, 27	Moyamoya disease and hemispheric pial synangiosis with craniotomy

AHA Coding Clinic for table 03U
2023, 1Q, 35	Carotid artery endarterectomy with imbrication
2019, 1Q, 22	Cerebral artery fusiform aneurysm repair via wrapping
2016, 2Q, 11	Carotid endarterectomy with patch angioplasty

AHA Coding Clinic for table 03V
2023, 3Q, 26	Body part value for posterior inferior cerebellar artery branch of vertebral artery
2023, 1Q, 34	Carotid artery pseudoaneurysm embolization using flow diverter stent and coils
2019, 4Q, 27-28	Aneurysm treatment using flow diverter stent
2019, 1Q, 22	Cerebral artery fusiform aneurysm repair via wrapping
2016, 1Q, 19	Embolization of superior hypophyseal aneurysm using stent-assisted coil

AHA Coding Clinic for table 03W
2023, 3Q, 24	Thrombectomy of HeRO® graft
2016, 3Q, 39	Revision of arteriovenous graft
2015, 1Q, 32	Deployment of stent for herniated/migrated coil in basilar artery

Upper Arteries

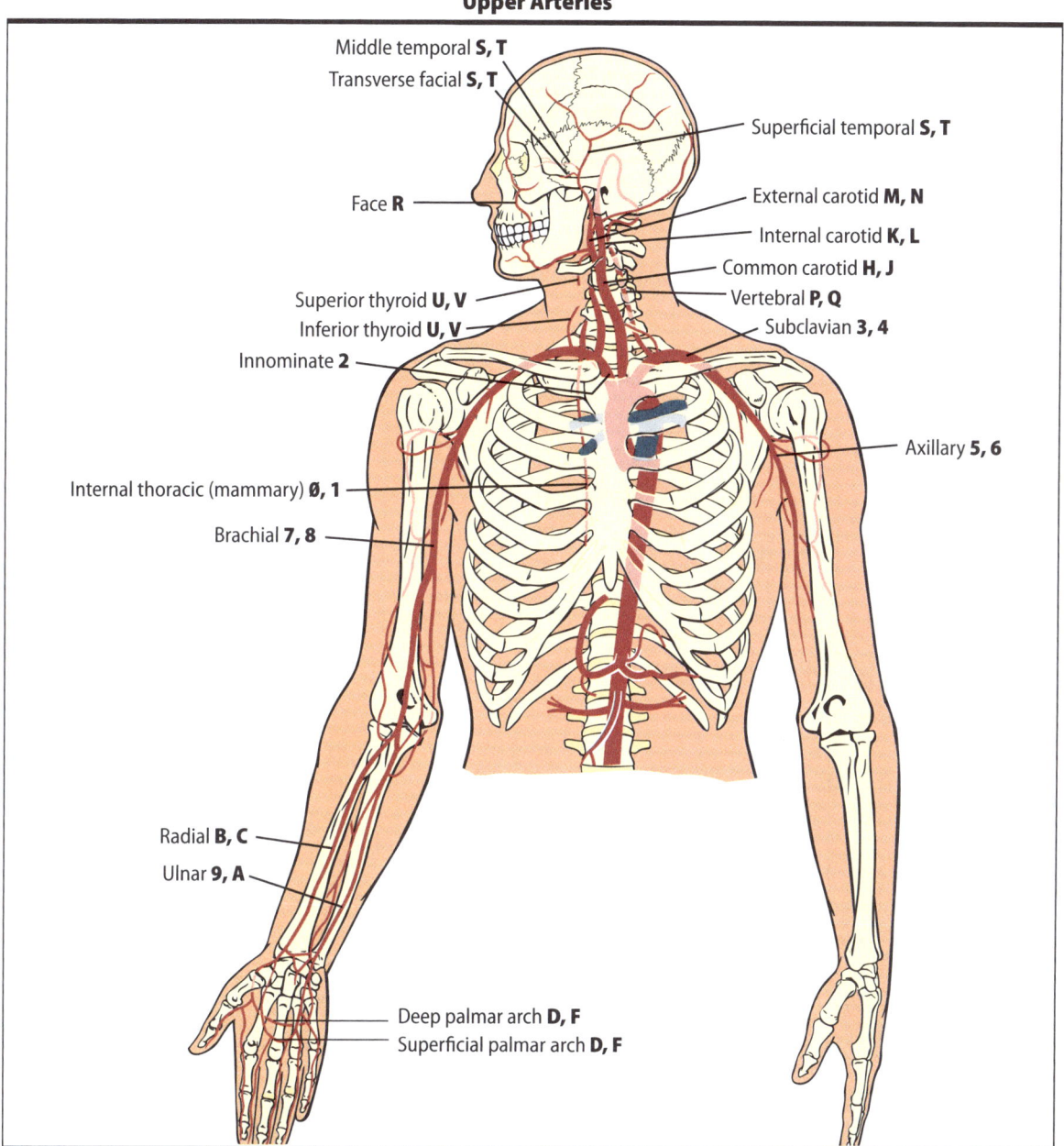

- Middle temporal **S, T**
- Transverse facial **S, T**
- Superficial temporal **S, T**
- Face **R**
- External carotid **M, N**
- Internal carotid **K, L**
- Common carotid **H, J**
- Superior thyroid **U, V**
- Vertebral **P, Q**
- Inferior thyroid **U, V**
- Subclavian **3, 4**
- Innominate **2**
- Axillary **5, 6**
- Internal thoracic (mammary) **Ø, 1**
- Brachial **7, 8**
- Radial **B, C**
- Ulnar **9, A**
- Deep palmar arch **D, F**
- Superficial palmar arch **D, F**

Head and Neck Arteries

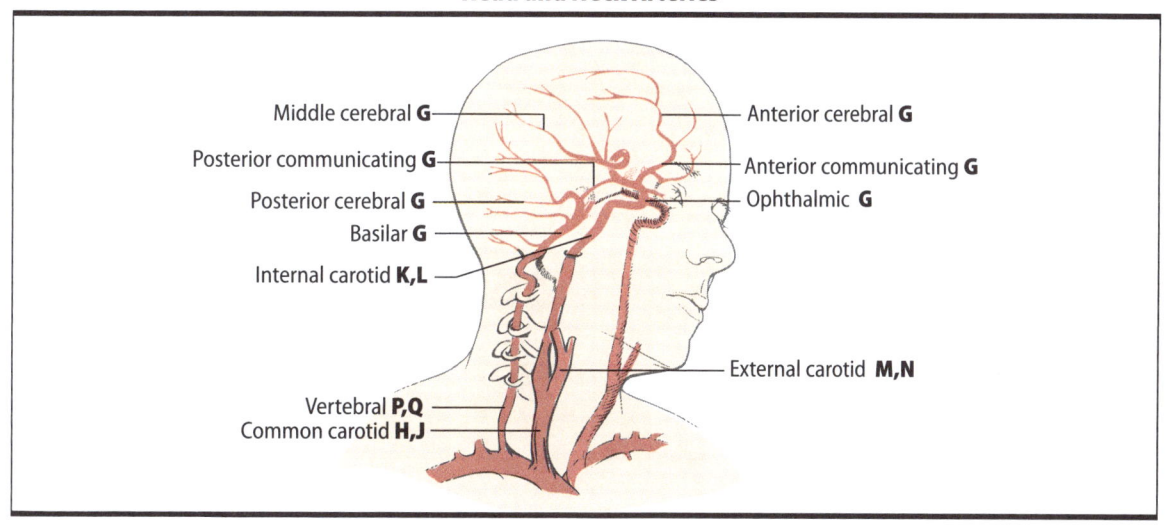

- Middle cerebral **G**
- Anterior cerebral **G**
- Posterior communicating **G**
- Anterior communicating **G**
- Posterior cerebral **G**
- Ophthalmic **G**
- Basilar **G**
- Internal carotid **K, L**
- External carotid **M, N**
- Vertebral **P, Q**
- Common carotid **H, J**

Upper Arteries

0 Medical and Surgical
3 Upper Arteries
1 Bypass Definition: Altering the route of passage of the contents of a tubular body part
Explanation: Rerouting contents of a body part to a downstream area of the normal route, to a similar route and body part, or to an abnormal route and dissimilar body part. Includes one or more anastomoses, with or without the use of a device.

Body Part Character 4	Approach Character 5	Device Character 6	Qualifier Character 7
2 Innominate Artery Brachiocephalic artery Brachiocephalic trunk	**0** Open	**9** Autologous Venous Tissue **A** Autologous Arterial Tissue **J** Synthetic Substitute **K** Nonautologous Tissue Substitute **Z** No Device	**0** Upper Arm Artery, Right **1** Upper Arm Artery, Left **2** Upper Arm Artery, Bilateral **3** Lower Arm Artery, Right **4** Lower Arm Artery, Left **5** Lower Arm Artery, Bilateral **6** Upper Leg Artery, Right **7** Upper Leg Artery, Left **8** Upper Leg Artery, Bilateral **9** Lower Leg Artery, Right **B** Lower Leg Artery, Left **C** Lower Leg Artery, Bilateral **D** Upper Arm Vein **F** Lower Arm Vein **J** Extracranial Artery, Right **K** Extracranial Artery, Left **W** Lower Extremity Vein
3 Subclavian Artery, Right Costocervical trunk Dorsal scapular artery Internal thoracic artery **4 Subclavian Artery, Left** See 3 Subclavian Artery, Right	**0** Open	**9** Autologous Venous Tissue **A** Autologous Arterial Tissue **J** Synthetic Substitute **K** Nonautologous Tissue Substitute **Z** No Device	**0** Upper Arm Artery, Right **1** Upper Arm Artery, Left **2** Upper Arm Artery, Bilateral **3** Lower Arm Artery, Right **4** Lower Arm Artery, Left **5** Lower Arm Artery, Bilateral **6** Upper Leg Artery, Right **7** Upper Leg Artery, Left **8** Upper Leg Artery, Bilateral **9** Lower Leg Artery, Right **B** Lower Leg Artery, Left **C** Lower Leg Artery, Bilateral **D** Upper Arm Vein **F** Lower Arm Vein **J** Extracranial Artery, Right **K** Extracranial Artery, Left **M** Pulmonary Artery, Right **N** Pulmonary Artery, Left **W** Lower Extremity Vein
5 Axillary Artery, Right Anterior circumflex humeral artery Lateral thoracic artery Posterior circumflex humeral artery Subscapular artery Superior thoracic artery Thoracoacromial artery **6 Axillary Artery, Left** See 5 Axillary Artery, Right	**0** Open	**9** Autologous Venous Tissue **A** Autologous Arterial Tissue **J** Synthetic Substitute **K** Nonautologous Tissue Substitute **Z** No Device	**0** Upper Arm Artery, Right **1** Upper Arm Artery, Left **2** Upper Arm Artery, Bilateral **3** Lower Arm Artery, Right **4** Lower Arm Artery, Left **5** Lower Arm Artery, Bilateral **6** Upper Leg Artery, Right **7** Upper Leg Artery, Left **8** Upper Leg Artery, Bilateral **9** Lower Leg Artery, Right **B** Lower Leg Artery, Left **C** Lower Leg Artery, Bilateral **D** Upper Arm Vein **F** Lower Arm Vein **J** Extracranial Artery, Right **K** Extracranial Artery, Left **T** Abdominal Artery **V** Superior Vena Cava **W** Lower Extremity Vein
7 Brachial Artery, Right Inferior ulnar collateral artery Profunda brachii Superior ulnar collateral artery	**0** Open	**9** Autologous Venous Tissue **A** Autologous Arterial Tissue **J** Synthetic Substitute **K** Nonautologous Tissue Substitute **Z** No Device	**0** Upper Arm Artery, Right **3** Lower Arm Artery, Right **D** Upper Arm Vein **F** Lower Arm Vein **V** Superior Vena Cava **W** Lower Extremity Vein
7 Brachial Artery, Right Inferior ulnar collateral artery Profunda brachii Superior ulnar collateral artery	**3** Percutaneous	**Z** No Device	**F** Lower Arm Vein

031 Continued on next page

ICD-10-PCS 2025 — Upper Arteries — 031–031

031 Continued

- **0** Medical and Surgical
- **3** Upper Arteries
- **1** Bypass

Definition: Altering the route of passage of the contents of a tubular body part

Explanation: Rerouting contents of a body part to a downstream area of the normal route, to a similar route and body part, or to an abnormal route and dissimilar body part. Includes one or more anastomoses, with or without the use of a device.

Body Part Character 4	Approach Character 5	Device Character 6	Qualifier Character 7
8 Brachial Artery, Left Inferior ulnar collateral artery Profunda brachii Superior ulnar collateral artery	**0** Open	**9** Autologous Venous Tissue **A** Autologous Arterial Tissue **J** Synthetic Substitute **K** Nonautologous Tissue Substitute **Z** No Device	**1** Upper Arm Artery, Left **4** Lower Arm Artery, Left **D** Upper Arm Vein **F** Lower Arm Vein **V** Superior Vena Cava **W** Lower Extremity Vein
8 Brachial Artery, Left Inferior ulnar collateral artery Profunda brachii Superior ulnar collateral artery	**3** Percutaneous	**Z** No Device	**F** Lower Arm Vein
9 Ulnar Artery, Right Anterior ulnar recurrent artery Common interosseous artery Posterior ulnar recurrent artery **B** Radial Artery, Right Radial recurrent artery	**0** Open	**9** Autologous Venous Tissue **A** Autologous Arterial Tissue **J** Synthetic Substitute **K** Nonautologous Tissue Substitute **Z** No Device	**3** Lower Arm Artery, Right **F** Lower Arm Vein
9 Ulnar Artery, Right Anterior ulnar recurrent artery Common interosseous artery Posterior ulnar recurrent artery **B** Radial Artery, Right Radial recurrent artery	**3** Percutaneous	**Z** No Device	**F** Lower Arm Vein
A Ulnar Artery, Left Anterior ulnar recurrent artery Common interosseous artery Posterior ulnar recurrent artery **C** Radial Artery, Left Radial recurrent artery	**0** Open	**9** Autologous Venous Tissue **A** Autologous Arterial Tissue **J** Synthetic Substitute **K** Nonautologous Tissue Substitute **Z** No Device	**4** Lower Arm Artery, Left **F** Lower Arm Vein
A Ulnar Artery, Left Anterior ulnar recurrent artery Common interosseous artery Posterior ulnar recurrent artery **C** Radial Artery, Left Radial recurrent artery	**3** Percutaneous	**Z** No Device	**F** Lower Arm Vein
G Intracranial Artery Anterior cerebral artery Anterior choroidal artery Anterior communicating artery Basilar artery Circle of Willis Internal carotid artery, intracranial portion Middle cerebral artery Middle meningeal artery, intracranial portion Ophthalmic artery Posterior cerebral artery Posterior communicating artery Posterior inferior cerebellar artery (PICA) Vertebral artery, intracranial portion **S** Temporal Artery, Right Middle temporal artery Superficial temporal artery Transverse facial artery **T** Temporal Artery, Left *See S Temporal Artery, Right*	**0** Open	**9** Autologous Venous Tissue **A** Autologous Arterial Tissue **J** Synthetic Substitute **K** Nonautologous Tissue Substitute **Z** No Device	**G** Intracranial Artery
H Common Carotid Artery, Right **J** Common Carotid Artery, Left	**0** Open	**9** Autologous Venous Tissue **A** Autologous Arterial Tissue **J** Synthetic Substitute **K** Nonautologous Tissue Substitute **Z** No Device	**G** Intracranial Artery **J** Extracranial Artery, Right **K** Extracranial Artery, Left **Y** Upper Artery

031 Continued on next page

0 Medical and Surgical
3 Upper Arteries
1 Bypass — Definition: Altering the route of passage of the contents of a tubular body part
Explanation: Rerouting contents of a body part to a downstream area of the normal route, to a similar route and body part, or to an abnormal route and dissimilar body part. Includes one or more anastomoses, with or without the use of a device.

Body Part Character 4	Approach Character 5	Device Character 6	Qualifier Character 7
K Internal Carotid Artery, Right Caroticotympanic artery Carotid sinus **L Internal Carotid Artery, Left** Caroticotympanic artery Carotid sinus **M External Carotid Artery, Right** Ascending pharyngeal artery Internal maxillary artery Lingual artery Maxillary artery Occipital artery Posterior auricular artery Superior thyroid artery **N External Carotid Artery, Left** Ascending pharyngeal artery Internal maxillary artery Lingual artery Maxillary artery Occipital artery Posterior auricular artery Superior thyroid artery	**0** Open	**9** Autologous Venous Tissue **A** Autologous Arterial Tissue **J** Synthetic Substitute **K** Nonautologous Tissue Substitute **Z** No Device	**J** Extracranial Artery, Right **K** Extracranial Artery, Left

ICD-10-PCS 2025 — Upper Arteries — 035–035

- **0** Medical and Surgical
- **3** Upper Arteries
- **5** Destruction **Definition:** Physical eradication of all or a portion of a body part by the direct use of energy, force, or a destructive agent
  Explanation: None of the body part is physically taken out

Body Part – Character 4	Approach – Character 5	Device – Character 6	Qualifier – Character 7

0 Internal Mammary Artery, Right
  Anterior intercostal artery
  Internal thoracic artery
  Musculophrenic artery
  Pericardiophrenic artery
  Superior epigastric artery
1 Internal Mammary Artery, Left
  See 0 Internal Mammary Artery, Right
2 Innominate Artery
  Brachiocephalic artery
  Brachiocephalic trunk
3 Subclavian Artery, Right
  Costocervical trunk
  Dorsal scapular artery
  Internal thoracic artery
4 Subclavian Artery, Left
  See 3 Subclavian Artery, Right
5 Axillary Artery, Right
  Anterior circumflex humeral artery
  Lateral thoracic artery
  Posterior circumflex humeral artery
  Subscapular artery
  Superior thoracic artery
  Thoracoacromial artery
6 Axillary Artery, Left
  See 5 Axillary Artery, Right
7 Brachial Artery, Right
  Inferior ulnar collateral artery
  Profunda brachii
  Superior ulnar collateral artery
8 Brachial Artery, Left
  See 7 Brachial Artery, Right
9 Ulnar Artery, Right
  Anterior ulnar recurrent artery
  Common interosseous artery
  Posterior ulnar recurrent artery
A Ulnar Artery, Left
  See 9 Ulnar Artery, Right
B Radial Artery, Right
  Radial recurrent artery
C Radial Artery, Left
  See B Radial Artery, Right
D Hand Artery, Right
  Deep palmar arch
  Princeps pollicis artery
  Radialis indicis
  Superficial palmar arch
F Hand Artery, Left
  See D Hand Artery, Right
G Intracranial Artery
  Anterior cerebral artery
  Anterior choroidal artery
  Anterior communicating artery
  Basilar artery
  Circle of Willis
  Internal carotid artery, intracranial portion
  Middle cerebral artery
  Middle meningeal artery, intracranial portion
  Ophthalmic artery
  Posterior cerebral artery
  Posterior communicating artery
  Posterior inferior cerebellar artery (PICA)
  Vertebral artery, intracranial portion
H Common Carotid Artery, Right
J Common Carotid Artery, Left
K Internal Carotid Artery, Right
  Caroticotympanic artery
  Carotid sinus
L Internal Carotid Artery, Left
  See K Internal Carotid Artery, Right
M External Carotid Artery, Right
  Ascending pharyngeal artery
  Internal maxillary artery
  Lingual artery
  Maxillary artery
  Occipital artery
  Posterior auricular artery
  Superior thyroid artery
N External Carotid Artery, Left
  See M External Carotid Artery, Right
P Vertebral Artery, Right
  Anterior spinal artery
  Posterior spinal artery
Q Vertebral Artery, Left
  See P Vertebral Artery, Right
R Face Artery
  Angular artery
  Ascending palatine artery
  External maxillary artery
  Facial artery
  Inferior labial artery
  Submental artery
  Superior labial artery
S Temporal Artery, Right
  Middle temporal artery
  Superficial temporal artery
  Transverse facial artery
T Temporal Artery, Left
  See S Temporal Artery, Right
U Thyroid Artery, Right
  Cricothyroid artery
  Hyoid artery
  Sternocleidomastoid artery
  Superior laryngeal artery
  Superior thyroid artery
  Thyrocervical trunk
V Thyroid Artery, Left
  See U Thyroid Artery, Right
Y Upper Artery
  Aortic intercostal artery
  Bronchial artery
  Esophageal artery
  Subcostal artery
	0 Open
	3 Percutaneous
	4 Percutaneous Endoscopic
		Z No Device	**Z** No Qualifier

NC Noncovered Procedure **LC** Limited Coverage **QA** Questionable OB Admit **NT** New Tech Add-on ✚ Combination Member ♂ Male ♀ Female

0 Medical and Surgical
3 Upper Arteries
7 Dilation Definition: Expanding an orifice or the lumen of a tubular body part
Explanation: The orifice can be a natural orifice or an artificially created orifice. Accomplished by stretching a tubular body part using intraluminal pressure or by cutting part of the orifice or wall of the tubular body part.

Body Part Character 4	Approach Character 5	Device Character 6	Qualifier Character 7

0 Internal Mammary Artery, Right
  Anterior intercostal artery
  Internal thoracic artery
  Musculophrenic artery
  Pericardiophrenic artery
  Superior epigastric artery
1 Internal Mammary Artery, Left
  See 0 Internal Mammary Artery, Right
2 Innominate Artery
  Brachiocephalic artery
  Brachiocephalic trunk
3 Subclavian Artery, Right
  Costocervical trunk
  Dorsal scapular artery
  Internal thoracic artery
4 Subclavian Artery, Left
  See 3 Subclavian Artery, Right
5 Axillary Artery, Right
  Anterior circumflex humeral artery
  Lateral thoracic artery
  Posterior circumflex humeral artery
  Subscapular artery
  Superior thoracic artery
  Thoracoacromial artery
6 Axillary Artery, Left
  See 5 Axillary Artery, Right
7 Brachial Artery, Right
  Inferior ulnar collateral artery
  Profunda brachii
  Superior ulnar collateral artery
8 Brachial Artery, Left
  See 7 Brachial Artery, Right
9 Ulnar Artery, Right
  Anterior ulnar recurrent artery
  Common interosseous artery
  Posterior ulnar recurrent artery
A Ulnar Artery, Left
  See 9 Ulnar Artery, Right
B Radial Artery, Right
  Radial recurrent artery
C Radial Artery, Left
  See B Radial Artery, Right
	0 Open
	3 Percutaneous
	4 Percutaneous Endoscopic
		4 Intraluminal Device, Drug-eluting
		5 Intraluminal Device, Drug-eluting, Two
		6 Intraluminal Device, Drug-eluting, Three
		7 Intraluminal Device, Drug-eluting, Four or More
		E Intraluminal Device, Two
		F Intraluminal Device, Three
		G Intraluminal Device, Four or More
			Z No Qualifier

0 Internal Mammary Artery, Right
  Anterior intercostal artery
  Internal thoracic artery
  Musculophrenic artery
  Pericardiophrenic artery
  Superior epigastric artery
1 Internal Mammary Artery, Left
  See 0 Internal Mammary Artery, Right
2 Innominate Artery
  Brachiocephalic artery
  Brachiocephalic trunk
3 Subclavian Artery, Right
  Costocervical trunk
  Dorsal scapular artery
  Internal thoracic artery
4 Subclavian Artery, Left
  See 3 Subclavian Artery, Right
5 Axillary Artery, Right
  Anterior circumflex humeral artery
  Lateral thoracic artery
  Posterior circumflex humeral artery
  Subscapular artery
  Superior thoracic artery
  Thoracoacromial artery
6 Axillary Artery, Left
  See 5 Axillary Artery, Right
7 Brachial Artery, Right
  Inferior ulnar collateral artery
  Profunda brachii
  Superior ulnar collateral artery
8 Brachial Artery, Left
  See 7 Brachial Artery, Right
9 Ulnar Artery, Right
  Anterior ulnar recurrent artery
  Common interosseous artery
  Posterior ulnar recurrent artery
A Ulnar Artery, Left
  See 9 Ulnar Artery, Right
B Radial Artery, Right
  Radial recurrent artery
C Radial Artery, Left
  See B Radial Artery, Right
	0 Open
	3 Percutaneous
	4 Percutaneous Endoscopic
		D Intraluminal Device
		Z No Device
			1 Drug-Coated Balloon
			Z No Qualifier

037 Continued on next page

ICD-10-PCS 2025 — Upper Arteries — 037 Continued

0 Medical and Surgical
3 Upper Arteries
7 Dilation

Definition: Expanding an orifice or the lumen of a tubular body part
Explanation: The orifice can be a natural orifice or an artificially created orifice. Accomplished by stretching a tubular body part using intraluminal pressure or by cutting part of the orifice or wall of the tubular body part.

Body Part — Character 4	Approach — Character 5	Device — Character 6	Qualifier — Character 7
D Hand Artery, Right Deep palmar arch Princeps pollicis artery Radialis indicis Superficial palmar arch **F Hand Artery, Left** *See D Hand Artery, Right* **G Intracranial Artery** Anterior cerebral artery Anterior choroidal artery Anterior communicating artery Basilar artery Circle of Willis Internal carotid artery, intracranial portion Middle cerebral artery Middle meningeal artery, intracranial portion Ophthalmic artery Posterior cerebral artery Posterior communicating artery Posterior inferior cerebellar artery (PICA) Vertebral artery, intracranial portion **H Common Carotid Artery, Right** **J Common Carotid Artery, Left** **K Internal Carotid Artery, Right** Caroticotympanic artery Carotid sinus **L Internal Carotid Artery, Left** *See K Internal Carotid Artery, Right* **M External Carotid Artery, Right** Ascending pharyngeal artery Internal maxillary artery Lingual artery Maxillary artery Occipital artery Posterior auricular artery Superior thyroid artery **N External Carotid Artery, Left** *See M External Carotid Artery, Right* **P Vertebral Artery, Right** Anterior spinal artery Posterior spinal artery **Q Vertebral Artery, Left** *See P Vertebral Artery, Right* **R Face Artery** Angular artery Ascending palatine artery External maxillary artery Facial artery Inferior labial artery Submental artery Superior labial artery **S Temporal Artery, Right** Middle temporal artery Superficial temporal artery Transverse facial artery **T Temporal Artery, Left** *See S Temporal Artery, Right* **U Thyroid Artery, Right** Cricothyroid artery Hyoid artery Sternocleidomastoid artery Superior laryngeal artery Superior thyroid artery Thyrocervical trunk **V Thyroid Artery, Left** *See U Thyroid Artery, Right* **Y Upper Artery** Aortic intercostal artery Bronchial artery Esophageal artery Subcostal artery	0 Open 3 Percutaneous 4 Percutaneous Endoscopic	4 Intraluminal Device, Drug-eluting 5 Intraluminal Device, Drug-eluting, Two 6 Intraluminal Device, Drug-eluting, Three 7 Intraluminal Device, Drug-eluting, Four or More D Intraluminal Device E Intraluminal Device, Two F Intraluminal Device, Three G Intraluminal Device, Four or More Z No Device	Z No Qualifier

NC 037G[3,4]ZZ

0 Medical and Surgical
3 Upper Arteries
9 Drainage Definition: Taking or letting out fluids and/or gases from a body part
Explanation: The qualifier DIAGNOSTIC is used to identify drainage procedures that are biopsies

Body Part Character 4		Approach Character 5	Device Character 6	Qualifier Character 7
0 Internal Mammary Artery, Right Anterior intercostal artery Internal thoracic artery Musculophrenic artery Pericardiophrenic artery Superior epigastric artery **1 Internal Mammary Artery, Left** See 0 Internal Mammary Artery, Right above **2 Innominate Artery** Brachiocephalic artery Brachiocephalic trunk **3 Subclavian Artery, Right** Costocervical trunk Dorsal scapular artery Internal thoracic artery **4 Subclavian Artery, Left** See 3 Subclavian Artery, Right **5 Axillary Artery, Right** Anterior circumflex humeral artery Lateral thoracic artery Posterior circumflex humeral artery Subscapular artery Superior thoracic artery Thoracoacromial artery **6 Axillary Artery, Left** See 5 Axillary Artery, Right **7 Brachial Artery, Right** Inferior ulnar collateral artery Profunda brachii Superior ulnar collateral artery **8 Brachial Artery, Left** See 7 Brachial Artery, Right **9 Ulnar Artery, Right** Anterior ulnar recurrent artery Common interosseous artery Posterior ulnar recurrent artery **A Ulnar Artery, Left** See 9 Ulnar Artery, Right **B Radial Artery, Right** Radial recurrent artery **C Radial Artery, Left** See B Radial Artery, Right **D Hand Artery, Right** Deep palmar arch Princeps pollicis artery Radialis indicis Superficial palmar arch **F Hand Artery, Left** See D Hand Artery, Right **G Intracranial Artery** Anterior cerebral artery Anterior choroidal artery Anterior communicating artery Basilar artery Circle of Willis Internal carotid artery, intracranial portion Middle cerebral artery Middle meningeal artery, intracranial portion Ophthalmic artery Posterior cerebral artery Posterior communicating artery Posterior inferior cerebellar artery (PICA) Vertebral artery, intracranial portion	**H Common Carotid Artery, Right** **J Common Carotid Artery, Left** **K Internal Carotid Artery, Right** Caroticotympanic artery Carotid sinus **L Internal Carotid Artery, Left** See K Internal Carotid Artery, Right **M External Carotid Artery, Right** Ascending pharyngeal artery Internal maxillary artery Lingual artery Maxillary artery Occipital artery Posterior auricular artery Superior thyroid artery **N External Carotid Artery, Left** See M External Carotid Artery, Right **P Vertebral Artery, Right** Anterior spinal artery Posterior spinal artery **Q Vertebral Artery, Left** See P Vertebral Artery, Right **R Face Artery** Angular artery Ascending palatine artery External maxillary artery Facial artery Inferior labial artery Submental artery Superior labial artery **S Temporal Artery, Right** Middle temporal artery Superficial temporal artery Transverse facial artery **T Temporal Artery, Left** See S Temporal Artery, Right **U Thyroid Artery, Right** Cricothyroid artery Hyoid artery Sternocleidomastoid artery Superior laryngeal artery Superior thyroid artery Thyrocervical trunk **V Thyroid Artery, Left** See U Thyroid Artery, Right **Y Upper Artery** Aortic intercostal artery Bronchial artery Esophageal artery Subcostal artery	0 Open 3 Percutaneous 4 Percutaneous Endoscopic	0 Drainage Device	Z No Qualifier

Non-OR 039[0,1,2,3,4,5,6,7,8,9,A,B,C,D,F,G,H,J,K,L,M,N,P,Q,R,S,T,U,V,Y][0,3,4]0Z

039 Continued on next page

ICD-10-PCS 2025 — Upper Arteries — 039–039

0 Medical and Surgical
3 Upper Arteries
9 Drainage

039 Continued

Definition: Taking or letting out fluids and/or gases from a body part
Explanation: The qualifier DIAGNOSTIC is used to identify drainage procedures that are biopsies

Body Part Character 4	Approach Character 5	Device Character 6	Qualifier Character 7
0 Internal Mammary Artery, Right Anterior intercostal artery Internal thoracic artery Musculophrenic artery Pericardiophrenic artery Superior epigastric artery **1 Internal Mammary Artery, Left** See 0 Internal Mammary Artery, Right **2 Innominate Artery** Brachiocephalic artery Brachiocephalic trunk **3 Subclavian Artery, Right** Costocervical trunk Dorsal scapular artery Internal thoracic artery **4 Subclavian Artery, Left** See 3 Subclavian Artery, Right **5 Axillary Artery, Right** Anterior circumflex humeral artery Lateral thoracic artery Posterior circumflex humeral artery Subscapular artery Superior thoracic artery Thoracoacromial artery **6 Axillary Artery, Left** See 5 Axillary Artery, Right **7 Brachial Artery, Right** Inferior ulnar collateral artery Profunda brachii Superior ulnar collateral artery **8 Brachial Artery, Left** See 7 Brachial Artery, Right **9 Ulnar Artery, Right** Anterior ulnar recurrent artery Common interosseous artery Posterior ulnar recurrent artery **A Ulnar Artery, Left** See 9 Ulnar Artery, Right **B Radial Artery, Right** Radial recurrent artery **C Radial Artery, Left** See B Radial Artery, Right **D Hand Artery, Right** Deep palmar arch Princeps pollicis artery Radialis indicis Superficial palmar arch **F Hand Artery, Left** See D Hand Artery, Right **G Intracranial Artery** Anterior cerebral artery Anterior choroidal artery Anterior communicating artery Basilar artery Circle of Willis Internal carotid artery, intracranial portion Middle cerebral artery Middle meningeal artery, intracranial portion Ophthalmic artery Posterior cerebral artery Posterior communicating artery Posterior inferior cerebellar artery (PICA) Vertebral artery, intracranial portion **H Common Carotid Artery, Right** **J Common Carotid Artery, Left** **K Internal Carotid Artery, Right** Caroticotympanic artery Carotid sinus **L Internal Carotid Artery, Left** See K Internal Carotid Artery, Right **M External Carotid Artery, Right** Ascending pharyngeal artery Internal maxillary artery Lingual artery Maxillary artery Occipital artery Posterior auricular artery Superior thyroid artery **N External Carotid Artery, Left** See M External Carotid Artery, Right **P Vertebral Artery, Right** Anterior spinal artery Posterior spinal artery **Q Vertebral Artery, Left** See P Vertebral Artery, Right **R Face Artery** Angular artery Ascending palatine artery External maxillary artery Facial artery Inferior labial artery Submental artery Superior labial artery **S Temporal Artery, Right** Middle temporal artery Superficial temporal artery Transverse facial artery **T Temporal Artery, Left** See S Temporal Artery, Right **U Thyroid Artery, Right** Cricothyroid artery Hyoid artery Sternocleidomastoid artery Superior laryngeal artery Superior thyroid artery Thyrocervical trunk **V Thyroid Artery, Left** See U Thyroid Artery, Right **Y Upper Artery** Aortic intercostal artery Bronchial artery Esophageal artery Subcostal artery	**0** Open **3** Percutaneous **4** Percutaneous Endoscopic	**Z** No Device	**X** Diagnostic **Z** No Qualifier

Non-OR 039[0,1,2,3,4,5,6,7,8,9,A,B,C,D,F,G,H,J,K,L,M,N,P,Q,R,S,T,U,V,Y]3ZX
Non-OR 039[0,1,2,3,4,5,6,7,8,9,A,B,C,D,F,G,H,J,K,L,M,N,P,Q,R,S,T,U,V,Y][0,3,4]ZZ

Upper Arteries

0 Medical and Surgical
3 Upper Arteries
B Excision — Definition: Cutting out or off, without replacement, a portion of a body part
Explanation: The qualifier DIAGNOSTIC is used to identify excision procedures that are biopsies

Body Part — Character 4	Approach — Character 5	Device — Character 6	Qualifier — Character 7

0 Internal Mammary Artery, Right
  Anterior intercostal artery
  Internal thoracic artery
  Musculophrenic artery
  Pericardiophrenic artery
  Superior epigastric artery
1 Internal Mammary Artery, Left
  See 0 Internal Mammary Artery, Right
2 Innominate Artery
  Brachiocephalic artery
  Brachiocephalic trunk
3 Subclavian Artery, Right
  Costocervical trunk
  Dorsal scapular artery
  Internal thoracic artery
4 Subclavian Artery, Left
  See 3 Subclavian Artery, Right
5 Axillary Artery, Right
  Anterior circumflex humeral artery
  Lateral thoracic artery
  Posterior circumflex humeral artery
  Subscapular artery
  Superior thoracic artery
  Thoracoacromial artery
6 Axillary Artery, Left
  See 5 Axillary Artery, Right
7 Brachial Artery, Right
  Inferior ulnar collateral artery
  Profunda brachii
  Superior ulnar collateral artery
8 Brachial Artery, Left
  See 7 Brachial Artery, Right
9 Ulnar Artery, Right
  Anterior ulnar recurrent artery
  Common interosseous artery
  Posterior ulnar recurrent artery
A Ulnar Artery, Left
  See 9 Ulnar Artery, Right
B Radial Artery, Right
  Radial recurrent artery
C Radial Artery, Left
  See B Radial Artery, Right
D Hand Artery, Right
  Deep palmar arch
  Princeps pollicis artery
  Radialis indicis
  Superficial palmar arch
F Hand Artery, Left
  See D Hand Artery, Right
G Intracranial Artery
  Anterior cerebral artery
  Anterior choroidal artery
  Anterior communicating artery
  Basilar artery
  Circle of Willis
  Internal carotid artery, intracranial portion
  Middle cerebral artery
  Middle meningeal artery, intracranial portion
  Ophthalmic artery
  Posterior cerebral artery
  Posterior communicating artery
  Posterior inferior cerebellar artery (PICA)
  Vertebral artery, intracranial portion
	0 Open
	3 Percutaneous
	4 Percutaneous Endoscopic
		Z No Device	**X** Diagnostic
			Z No Qualifier

H Common Carotid Artery, Right
J Common Carotid Artery, Left
K Internal Carotid Artery, Right
  Caroticotympanic artery
  Carotid sinus
L Internal Carotid Artery, Left
  See K Internal Carotid Artery, Right
M External Carotid Artery, Right
  Ascending pharyngeal artery
  Internal maxillary artery
  Lingual artery
  Maxillary artery
  Occipital artery
  Posterior auricular artery
  Superior thyroid artery
N External Carotid Artery, Left
  See M External Carotid Artery, Right
P Vertebral Artery, Right
  Anterior spinal artery
  Posterior spinal artery
Q Vertebral Artery, Left
  See P Vertebral Artery, Right
R Face Artery
  Angular artery
  Ascending palatine artery
  External maxillary artery
  Facial artery
  Inferior labial artery
  Submental artery
  Superior labial artery
S Temporal Artery, Right
  Middle temporal artery
  Superficial temporal artery
  Transverse facial artery
T Temporal Artery, Left
  See S Temporal Artery, Right
U Thyroid Artery, Right
  Cricothyroid artery
  Hyoid artery
  Sternocleidomastoid artery
  Superior laryngeal artery
  Superior thyroid artery
  Thyrocervical trunk
V Thyroid Artery, Left
  See U Thyroid Artery, Right
Y Upper Artery
  Aortic intercostal artery
  Bronchial artery
  Esophageal artery
  Subcostal artery			

Non-OR Procedure | DRG Non-OR Procedure | Valid OR Procedure | HAC Associated Procedure | Combination Only | New/Revised April | New/Revised October

Upper Arteries

0 Medical and Surgical
3 Upper Arteries
C Extirpation Definition: Taking or cutting out solid matter from a body part
Explanation: The solid matter may be an abnormal byproduct of a biological function or a foreign body; it may be imbedded in a body part or in the lumen of a tubular body part. The solid matter may or may not have been previously broken into pieces.

Body Part Character 4	Approach Character 5	Device Character 6	Qualifier Character 7
0 Internal Mammary Artery, Right 　Anterior intercostal artery 　Internal thoracic artery 　Musculophrenic artery 　Pericardiophrenic artery 　Superior epigastric artery **1** Internal Mammary Artery, Left 　*See 0 Internal Mammary Artery, Right* **2** Innominate Artery 　Brachiocephalic artery 　Brachiocephalic trunk **3** Subclavian Artery, Right 　Costocervical trunk 　Dorsal scapular artery 　Internal thoracic artery **4** Subclavian Artery, Left 　*See 3 Subclavian Artery, Right* **5** Axillary Artery, Right 　Anterior circumflex humeral artery 　Lateral thoracic artery 　Posterior circumflex humeral artery 　Subscapular artery 　Superior thoracic artery 　Thoracoacromial artery **6** Axillary Artery, Left 　*See 5 Axillary Artery, Right* **7** Brachial Artery, Right 　Inferior ulnar collateral artery 　Profunda brachii 　Superior ulnar collateral artery **8** Brachial Artery, Left 　*See 7 Brachial Artery, Right* **9** Ulnar Artery, Right 　Anterior ulnar recurrent artery 　Common interosseous artery 　Posterior ulnar recurrent artery **A** Ulnar Artery, Left 　*See 9 Ulnar Artery, Right* **B** Radial Artery, Right 　Radial recurrent artery **C** Radial Artery, Left 　*See B Radial Artery, Right* **D** Hand Artery, Right 　Deep palmar arch 　Princeps pollicis artery 　Radialis indicis 　Superficial palmar arch **F** Hand Artery, Left 　*See D Hand Artery, Right* **R** Face Artery 　Angular artery 　Ascending palatine artery 　External maxillary artery 　Facial artery 　Inferior labial artery 　Submental artery 　Superior labial artery **S** Temporal Artery, Right 　Middle temporal artery 　Superficial temporal artery 　Transverse facial artery **T** Temporal Artery, Left 　*See S Temporal Artery, Right* **U** Thyroid Artery, Right 　Cricothyroid artery 　Hyoid artery 　Sternocleidomastoid artery 　Superior laryngeal artery 　Superior thyroid artery 　Thyrocervical trunk **V** Thyroid Artery, Left 　*See U Thyroid Artery, Right* **Y** Upper Artery 　Aortic intercostal artery 　Bronchial artery 　Esophageal artery 　Subcostal artery	**0** Open **3** Percutaneous **4** Percutaneous Endoscopic	**Z** No Device	**Z** No Qualifier
G Intracranial Artery 　Anterior cerebral artery 　Anterior choroidal artery 　Anterior communicating artery 　Basilar artery 　Circle of Willis 　Internal carotid artery, intracranial portion 　Middle cerebral artery 　Middle meningeal artery, intracranial portion 　Ophthalmic artery 　Posterior cerebral artery 　Posterior communicating artery 　Posterior inferior cerebellar artery (PICA) 　Vertebral artery, intracranial portion **H** Common Carotid Artery, Right **J** Common Carotid Artery, Left **K** Internal Carotid Artery, Right 　Caroticotympanic artery 　Carotid sinus	**L** Internal Carotid Artery, Left 　*See K Internal Carotid Artery, Right* **M** External Carotid Artery, Right 　Ascending pharyngeal artery 　Internal maxillary artery 　Lingual artery 　Maxillary artery 　Occipital artery 　Posterior auricular artery 　Superior thyroid artery **N** External Carotid Artery, Left 　*See M External Carotid Artery, Right* **P** Vertebral Artery, Right 　Anterior spinal artery 　Posterior spinal artery **Q** Vertebral Artery, Left 　*See P Vertebral Artery, Right*	**0** Open **4** Percutaneous Endoscopic	**Z** No Device	**Z** No Qualifier

03C Continued on next page

03C–03F Upper Arteries — ICD-10-PCS 2025

0 Medical and Surgical
3 Upper Arteries
C Extirpation

03C Continued

Definition: Taking or cutting out solid matter from a body part
Explanation: The solid matter may be an abnormal byproduct of a biological function or a foreign body; it may be imbedded in a body part or in the lumen of a tubular body part. The solid matter may or may not have been previously broken into pieces.

Body Part Character 4	Approach Character 5	Device Character 6	Qualifier Character 7

G Intracranial Artery
  Anterior cerebral artery
  Anterior choroidal artery
  Anterior communicating artery
  Basilar artery
  Circle of Willis
  Internal carotid artery, intracranial portion
  Middle cerebral artery
  Middle meningeal artery, intracranial portion
  Ophthalmic artery
  Posterior cerebral artery
  Posterior communicating artery
  Posterior inferior cerebellar artery (PICA)
  Vertebral artery, intracranial portion
H Common Carotid Artery, Right
J Common Carotid Artery, Left
K Internal Carotid Artery, Right
  Caroticotympanic artery
  Carotid sinus
L Internal Carotid Artery, Left
  See K Internal Carotid Artery, Right
M External Carotid Artery, Right
  Ascending pharyngeal artery
  Internal maxillary artery
  Lingual artery
  Maxillary artery
  Occipital artery
  Posterior auricular artery
  Superior thyroid artery
N External Carotid Artery, Left
  See M External Carotid Artery, Right
P Vertebral Artery, Right
  Anterior spinal artery
  Posterior spinal artery
Q Vertebral Artery, Left
  See P Vertebral Artery, Right
	3 Percutaneous	**Z** No Device	**7** Stent Retriever
			Z No Qualifier

---

0 Medical and Surgical
3 Upper Arteries
F Fragmentation

Definition: Breaking solid matter in a body part into pieces
Explanation: Physical force (e.g., manual, ultrasonic) applied directly or indirectly is used to break the solid matter into pieces. The solid matter may be an abnormal byproduct of a biological function or a foreign body. The pieces of solid matter are not taken out.

Body Part Character 4	Approach Character 5	Device Character 6	Qualifier Character 7

2 Innominate Artery
  Brachiocephalic artery
  Brachiocephalic trunk
3 Subclavian Artery, Right
  Costocervical trunk
  Dorsal scapular artery
  Internal thoracic artery
4 Subclavian Artery, Left
  See 3 Subclavian Artery, Right
5 Axillary Artery, Right
  Anterior circumflex humeral artery
  Lateral thoracic artery
  Posterior circumflex humeral artery
  Subscapular artery
  Superior thoracic artery
  Thoracoacromial artery
6 Axillary Artery, Left
  See 5 Axillary Artery, Right
7 Brachial Artery, Right
  Inferior ulnar collateral artery
  Profunda brachii
  Superior ulnar collateral artery
8 Brachial Artery, Left
  See 7 Brachial Artery, Right
9 Ulnar Artery, Right
  Anterior ulnar recurrent artery
  Common interosseous artery
  Posterior ulnar recurrent artery
A Ulnar Artery, Left
  See 9 Ulnar Artery, Right
B Radial Artery, Right
  Radial recurrent artery
C Radial Artery, Left
  See B Radial Artery, Right
G Intracranial Artery
  Anterior cerebral artery
  Anterior choroidal artery
  Anterior communicating artery
  Basilar artery
  Circle of Willis
  Internal carotid artery, intracranial portion
  Middle cerebral artery
  Middle meningeal artery, intracranial portion
  Ophthalmic artery
  Posterior cerebral artery
  Posterior communicating artery
  Posterior inferior cerebellar artery (PICA)
  Vertebral artery, intracranial portion
Y Upper Artery
  Aortic intercostal artery
  Bronchial artery
  Esophageal artery
  Subcostal artery
	3 Percutaneous	**Z** No Device	**0** Ultrasonic
			Z No Qualifier

Non-OR Procedure | DRG Non-OR Procedure | Valid OR Procedure | HAC Associated Procedure | Combination Only | New/Revised April | New/Revised October

ICD-10-PCS 2025 — Upper Arteries — 03H–03H

0 Medical and Surgical
3 Upper Arteries
H Insertion

Definition: Putting in a nonbiological appliance that monitors, assists, performs, or prevents a physiological function but does not physically take the place of a body part
Explanation: None

Body Part Character 4	Approach Character 5	Device Character 6	Qualifier Character 7
0 Internal Mammary Artery, Right Anterior intercostal artery Internal thoracic artery Musculophrenic artery Pericardiophrenic artery Superior epigastric artery **1 Internal Mammary Artery, Left** *See 0 Internal Mammary Artery, Right* **2 Innominate Artery** Brachiocephalic artery Brachiocephalic trunk **3 Subclavian Artery, Right** Costocervical trunk Dorsal scapular artery Internal thoracic artery **4 Subclavian Artery, Left** *See 3 Subclavian Artery, Right* **5 Axillary Artery, Right** Anterior circumflex humeral artery Lateral thoracic artery Posterior circumflex humeral artery Subscapular artery Superior thoracic artery Thoracoacromial artery **6 Axillary Artery, Left** *See 5 Axillary Artery, Right* **7 Brachial Artery, Right** Inferior ulnar collateral artery Profunda brachii Superior ulnar collateral artery **8 Brachial Artery, Left** *See 7 Brachial Artery, Right* **9 Ulnar Artery, Right** Anterior ulnar recurrent artery Common interosseous artery Posterior ulnar recurrent artery **A Ulnar Artery, Left** *See 9 Ulnar Artery, Right* **B Radial Artery, Right** Radial recurrent artery **C Radial Artery, Left** *See B Radial Artery, Right* **D Hand Artery, Right** Deep palmar arch Princeps pollicis artery Radialis indicis Superficial palmar arch **F Hand Artery, Left** *See D Hand Artery, Right* **G Intracranial Artery** Anterior cerebral artery Anterior choroidal artery Anterior communicating artery Basilar artery Circle of Willis Internal carotid artery, intracranial portion Middle cerebral artery Middle meningeal artery, intracranial portion Ophthalmic artery Posterior cerebral artery Posterior communicating artery Posterior inferior cerebellar artery (PICA) Vertebral artery, intracranial portion **H Common Carotid Artery, Right** **J Common Carotid Artery, Left** **M External Carotid Artery, Right** Ascending pharyngeal artery Internal maxillary artery Lingual artery Maxillary artery Occipital artery Posterior auricular artery Superior thyroid artery **N External Carotid Artery, Left** *See M External Carotid Artery, Right* **P Vertebral Artery, Right** Anterior spinal artery Posterior spinal artery **Q Vertebral Artery, Left** *See P Vertebral Artery, Right* **R Face Artery** Angular artery Ascending palatine artery External maxillary artery Facial artery Inferior labial artery Submental artery Superior labial artery **S Temporal Artery, Right** Middle temporal artery Superficial temporal artery Transverse facial artery **T Temporal Artery, Left** *See S Temporal Artery, Right* **U Thyroid Artery, Right** Cricothyroid artery Hyoid artery Sternocleidomastoid artery Superior laryngeal artery Superior thyroid artery Thyrocervical trunk **V Thyroid Artery, Left** *See U Thyroid Artery, Right*	0 Open 3 Percutaneous 4 Percutaneous Endoscopic	3 Infusion Device D Intraluminal Device	Z No Qualifier

Non-OR 03H[0,1,2,3,4,5,6,7,8,9,A,B,C,D,F,G,H,J,M,N,P,Q,R,S,T,U,V][0,3,4]3Z

03H Continued on next page

Ø3H–Ø3J Upper Arteries ICD-10-PCS 2025

Ø3H Continued

Ø Medical and Surgical
3 Upper Arteries
H Insertion Definition: Putting in a nonbiological appliance that monitors, assists, performs, or prevents a physiological function but does not physically take the place of a body part
Explanation: None

Body Part Character 4	Approach Character 5	Device Character 6	Qualifier Character 7

K Internal Carotid Artery, Right ✚
  Caroticotympanic artery
  Carotid sinus
L Internal Carotid Artery, Left ✚
  See K Internal Carotid Artery, Right
	Ø Open
	3 Percutaneous
	4 Percutaneous Endoscope
		3 Infusion Device
		D Intraluminal Device
		M Stimulator Lead
			Z No Qualifier

Y Upper Artery
  Aortic intercostal artery
  Bronchial artery
  Esophageal artery
  Subcostal artery
	Ø Open
	3 Percutaneous
	4 Percutaneous Endoscopic
		2 Monitoring Device
		3 Infusion Device
		D Intraluminal Device
		Y Other Device
			Z No Qualifier

Non-OR   Ø3H[K,L][Ø,3,4]3Z
Non-OR   Ø3HY[Ø,3,4]3Z
Non-OR   Ø3HY32Z
Non-OR   Ø3HY[3,4]YZ

See Appendix L for Procedure Combinations
✚ Ø3H[K,L]3MZ

Ø Medical and Surgical
3 Upper Arteries
J Inspection Definition: Visually and/or manually exploring a body part
Explanation: Visual exploration may be performed with or without optical instrumentation. Manual exploration may be performed directly or through intervening body layers.

Body Part Character 4	Approach Character 5	Device Character 6	Qualifier Character 7

Y Upper Artery
  Aortic intercostal artery
  Bronchial artery
  Esophageal artery
  Subcostal artery
	Ø Open
	3 Percutaneous
	4 Percutaneous Endoscopic
	X External
		Z No Device	**Z** No Qualifier

Non-OR   Ø3JY[3,4,X]ZZ

ICD-10-PCS 2025 — Upper Arteries — 03L–03L

- **0** Medical and Surgical
- **3** Upper Arteries
- **L** Occlusion

Definition: Completely closing an orifice or the lumen of a tubular body part
Explanation: The orifice can be a natural orifice or an artificially created orifice

Body Part (Character 4)	Approach (Character 5)	Device (Character 6)	Qualifier (Character 7)

0 Internal Mammary Artery, Right
  Anterior intercostal artery
  Internal thoracic artery
  Musculophrenic artery
  Pericardiophrenic artery
  Superior epigastric artery
1 Internal Mammary Artery, Left
  See 0 Internal Mammary Artery, Left
2 Innominate Artery
  Brachiocephalic artery
  Brachiocephalic trunk
3 Subclavian Artery, Right
  Costocervical trunk
  Dorsal scapular artery
  Internal thoracic artery
4 Subclavian Artery, Left
  See 3 Subclavian Artery, Right
5 Axillary Artery, Right
  Anterior circumflex humeral artery
  Lateral thoracic artery
  Posterior circumflex humeral artery
  Subscapular artery
  Superior thoracic artery
  Thoracoacromial artery
6 Axillary Artery, Left
  See 5 Axillary Artery, Right
7 Brachial Artery, Right
  Inferior ulnar collateral artery
  Profunda brachii
  Superior ulnar collateral artery
8 Brachial Artery, Left
  See 7 Brachial Artery, Right
9 Ulnar Artery, Right
  Anterior ulnar recurrent artery
  Common interosseous artery
  Posterior ulnar recurrent artery
A Ulnar Artery, Left
  See 9 Ulnar Artery, Right
B Radial Artery, Right
  Radial recurrent artery
C Radial Artery, Left
  See B Radial Artery, Right
D Hand Artery, Right
  Deep palmar arch
  Princeps pollicis artery
  Radialis indicis
  Superficial palmar arch
F Hand Artery, Left
  See D Hand Artery, Right
R Face Artery
  Angular artery
  Ascending palatine artery
  External maxillary artery
  Facial artery
  Inferior labial artery
  Submental artery
  Superior labial artery
S Temporal Artery, Right
  Middle temporal artery
  Superficial temporal artery
  Transverse facial artery
T Temporal Artery, Left
  See S Temporal Artery, Right
U Thyroid Artery, Right
  Cricothyroid artery
  Hyoid artery
  Sternocleidomastoid artery
  Superior laryngeal artery
  Superior thyroid artery
  Thyrocervical trunk
V Thyroid Artery, Left
  See U Thyroid Artery, Right
Y Upper Artery
  Aortic intercostal artery
  Bronchial artery
  Esophageal artery
  Subcostal artery
	0 Open
	3 Percutaneous
	4 Percutaneous Endoscopic
		C Extraluminal Device
		D Intraluminal Device
		Z No Device
			Z No Qualifier

G Intracranial Artery
  Anterior cerebral artery
  Anterior choroidal artery
  Anterior communicating artery
  Basilar artery
  Circle of Willis
  Internal carotid artery, intracranial portion
  Middle cerebral artery
  Middle meningeal artery, intracranial portion
  Ophthalmic artery
  Posterior cerebral artery
  Posterior communicating artery
  Posterior inferior cerebellar artery (PICA)
  Vertebral artery, intracranial portion
H Common Carotid Artery, Right
J Common Carotid Artery, Left
K Internal Carotid Artery, Right
  Caroticotympanic artery
  Carotid sinus
L Internal Carotid Artery, Left
  See K Internal Carotid Artery, Right
M External Carotid Artery, Right
  Ascending pharyngeal artery
  Internal maxillary artery
  Lingual artery
  Maxillary artery
  Occipital artery
  Posterior auricular artery
  Superior thyroid artery
N External Carotid Artery, Left
  See M External Carotid Artery, Right
P Vertebral Artery, Right
  Anterior spinal artery
  Posterior spinal artery
Q Vertebral Artery, Left
  See P Vertebral Artery, Right
	0 Open
	3 Percutaneous
	4 Percutaneous Endoscopic
		B Intraluminal Device, Bioactive
		C Extraluminal Device
		D Intraluminal Device
		Z No Device
			Z No Qualifier

0 Medical and Surgical
3 Upper Arteries
N Release Definition: Freeing a body part from an abnormal physical constraint by cutting or by the use of force
Explanation: Some of the restraining tissue may be taken out but none of the body part is taken out

Body Part Character 4	Approach Character 5	Device Character 6	Qualifier Character 7
0 Internal Mammary Artery, Right Anterior intercostal artery Internal thoracic artery Musculophrenic artery Pericardiophrenic artery Superior epigastric artery **1 Internal Mammary Artery, Left** See 0 Internal Mammary Artery, Right **2 Innominate Artery** Brachiocephalic artery Brachiocephalic trunk **3 Subclavian Artery, Right** Costocervical trunk Dorsal scapular artery Internal thoracic artery **4 Subclavian Artery, Left** See 3 Subclavian Artery, Right **5 Axillary Artery, Right** Anterior circumflex humeral artery Lateral thoracic artery Posterior circumflex humeral artery Subscapular artery Superior thoracic artery Thoracoacromial artery **6 Axillary Artery, Left** See 5 Axillary Artery, Right **7 Brachial Artery, Right** Inferior ulnar collateral artery Profunda brachii Superior ulnar collateral artery **8 Brachial Artery, Left** See 7 Brachial Artery, Right **9 Ulnar Artery, Right** Anterior ulnar recurrent artery Common interosseous artery Posterior ulnar recurrent artery **A Ulnar Artery, Left** See 9 Ulnar Artery, Right **B Radial Artery, Right** Radial recurrent artery **C Radial Artery, Left** See B Radial Artery, Right **D Hand Artery, Right** Deep palmar arch Princeps pollicis artery Radialis indicis Superficial palmar arch **F Hand Artery, Left** See D Hand Artery, Right **G Intracranial Artery** Anterior cerebral artery Anterior choroidal artery Anterior communicating artery Basilar artery Circle of Willis Internal carotid artery, intracranial portion Middle cerebral artery Middle meningeal artery, intracranial portion Ophthalmic artery Posterior cerebral artery Posterior communicating artery Posterior inferior cerebellar artery (PICA) Vertebral artery, intracranial portion	**H Common Carotid Artery, Right** **J Common Carotid Artery, Left** **K Internal Carotid Artery, Right** Caroticotympanic artery Carotid sinus **L Internal Carotid Artery, Left** See K Internal Carotid Artery, Right **M External Carotid Artery, Right** Ascending pharyngeal artery Internal maxillary artery Lingual artery Maxillary artery Occipital artery Posterior auricular artery Superior thyroid artery **N External Carotid Artery, Left** See M External Carotid Artery, Right **P Vertebral Artery, Right** Anterior spinal artery Posterior spinal artery **Q Vertebral Artery, Left** See P Vertebral Artery, Right **R Face Artery** Angular artery Ascending palatine artery External maxillary artery Facial artery Inferior labial artery Submental artery Superior labial artery **S Temporal Artery, Right** Middle temporal artery Superficial temporal artery Transverse facial artery **T Temporal Artery, Left** See S Temporal Artery, Right **U Thyroid Artery, Right** Cricothyroid artery Hyoid artery Sternocleidomastoid artery Superior laryngeal artery Superior thyroid artery Thyrocervical trunk **V Thyroid Artery, Left** See U Thyroid Artery, Right **Y Upper Artery** Aortic intercostal artery Bronchial artery Esophageal artery Subcostal artery	**0 Open** **3 Percutaneous** **4 Percutaneous Endoscopic**	**Z No Device**	**Z No Qualifier**

Non-OR Procedure   DRG Non-OR Procedure   Valid OR Procedure   HAC Associated Procedure   Combination Only   New/Revised April   New/Revised October

0 Medical and Surgical
3 Upper Arteries
P Removal

Definition: Taking out or off a device from a body part
Explanation: If a device is taken out and a similar device put in without cutting or puncturing the skin or mucous membrane, the procedure is coded to the root operation CHANGE. Otherwise, the procedure for taking out a device is coded to the root operation REMOVAL.

Body Part Character 4	Approach Character 5	Device Character 6	Qualifier Character 7
Y Upper Artery Aortic intercostal artery Bronchial artery Esophageal artery Subcostal artery	**0** Open **3** Percutaneous **4** Percutaneous Endoscopic	**0** Drainage Device **2** Monitoring Device **3** Infusion Device **7** Autologous Tissue Substitute **C** Extraluminal Device **D** Intraluminal Device **J** Synthetic Substitute **K** Nonautologous Tissue Substitute **M** Stimulator Lead **Y** Other Device	**Z** No Qualifier
Y Upper Artery Aortic intercostal artery Bronchial artery Esophageal artery Subcostal artery	**X** External	**0** Drainage Device **2** Monitoring Device **3** Infusion Device **D** Intraluminal Device **M** Stimulator Lead	**Z** No Qualifier

Non-OR 03PY3[0,2,3,D]Z
Non-OR 03PY[3,4]YZ
Non-OR 03PYX[0,2,3,D,M]Z

0 Medical and Surgical
3 Upper Arteries
Q Repair   Definition: Restoring, to the extent possible, a body part to its normal anatomic structure and function
          Explanation: Used only when the method to accomplish the repair is not one of the other root operations

Body Part Character 4	Approach Character 5	Device Character 6	Qualifier Character 7
0 Internal Mammary Artery, Right Anterior intercostal artery Internal thoracic artery Musculophrenic artery Pericardiophrenic artery Superior epigastric artery **1 Internal Mammary Artery, Left** See 0 Internal Mammary Artery, Right **2 Innominate Artery** Brachiocephalic artery Brachiocephalic trunk **3 Subclavian Artery, Right** Costocervical trunk Dorsal scapular artery Internal thoracic artery **4 Subclavian Artery, Left** See 3 Subclavian Artery, Right **5 Axillary Artery, Right** Anterior circumflex humeral artery Lateral thoracic artery Posterior circumflex humeral artery Subscapular artery Superior thoracic artery Thoracoacromial artery **6 Axillary Artery, Left** See 5 Axillary Artery, Right **7 Brachial Artery, Right** Inferior ulnar collateral artery Profunda brachii Superior ulnar collateral artery **8 Brachial Artery, Left** See 7 Brachial Artery, Right **9 Ulnar Artery, Right** Anterior ulnar recurrent artery Common interosseous artery Posterior ulnar recurrent artery **A Ulnar Artery, Left** See 9 Ulnar Artery, Right **B Radial Artery, Right** Radial recurrent artery **C Radial Artery, Left** See B Radial Artery, Right **D Hand Artery, Right** Deep palmar arch Princeps pollicis artery Radialis indicis Superficial palmar arch **F Hand Artery, Left** See D Hand Artery, Right **G Intracranial Artery** Anterior cerebral artery Anterior choroidal artery Anterior communicating artery Basilar artery Circle of Willis Internal carotid artery, intracranial portion Middle cerebral artery Middle meningeal artery, intracranial portion Ophthalmic artery Posterior cerebral artery Posterior communicating artery Posterior inferior cerebellar artery (PICA) Vertebral artery, intracranial portion	**H Common Carotid Artery, Right** **J Common Carotid Artery, Left** **K Internal Carotid Artery, Right** Caroticotympanic artery Carotid sinus **L Internal Carotid Artery, Left** See K Internal Carotid Artery, Right **M External Carotid Artery, Right** Ascending pharyngeal artery Internal maxillary artery Lingual artery Maxillary artery Occipital artery Posterior auricular artery Superior thyroid artery **N External Carotid Artery, Left** See M External Carotid Artery, Right **P Vertebral Artery, Right** Anterior spinal artery Posterior spinal artery **Q Vertebral Artery, Left** See P Vertebral Artery, Right **R Face Artery** Angular artery Ascending palatine artery External maxillary artery Facial artery Inferior labial artery Submental artery Superior labial artery **S Temporal Artery, Right** Middle temporal artery Superficial temporal artery Transverse facial artery **T Temporal Artery, Left** See S Temporal Artery, Right **U Thyroid Artery, Right** Cricothyroid artery Hyoid artery Sternocleidomastoid artery Superior laryngeal artery Superior thyroid artery Thyrocervical trunk **V Thyroid Artery, Left** See U Thyroid Artery, Right **Y Upper Artery** Aortic intercostal artery Bronchial artery Esophageal artery Subcostal artery	**0** Open **3** Percutaneous **4** Percutaneous Endoscopic	**Z** No Device	**Z** No Qualifier

ICD-10-PCS 2025 — Upper Arteries — 03R–03R

0 Medical and Surgical
3 Upper Arteries
R Replacement — Definition: Putting in or on biological or synthetic material that physically takes the place and/or function of all or a portion of a body part
Explanation: The body part may have been taken out or replaced, or may be taken out, physically eradicated, or rendered nonfunctional during the REPLACEMENT procedure. A REMOVAL procedure is coded for taking out the device used in a previous replacement procedure.

Body Part Character 4	Approach Character 5	Device Character 6	Qualifier Character 7

0 Internal Mammary Artery, Right
  Anterior intercostal artery
  Internal thoracic artery
  Musculophrenic artery
  Pericardiophrenic artery
  Superior epigastric artery
1 Internal Mammary Artery, Left
  See 0 Internal Mammary Artery, Right
2 Innominate Artery
  Brachiocephalic artery
  Brachiocephalic trunk
3 Subclavian Artery, Right
  Costocervical trunk
  Dorsal scapular artery
  Internal thoracic artery
4 Subclavian Artery, Left
  See 3 Subclavian Artery, Right
5 Axillary Artery, Right
  Anterior circumflex humeral artery
  Lateral thoracic artery
  Posterior circumflex humeral artery
  Subscapular artery
  Superior thoracic artery
  Thoracoacromial artery
6 Axillary Artery, Left
  See 5 Axillary Artery, Right
7 Brachial Artery, Right
  Inferior ulnar collateral artery
  Profunda brachii
  Superior ulnar collateral artery
8 Brachial Artery, Left
  See 7 Brachial Artery, Right
9 Ulnar Artery, Right
  Anterior ulnar recurrent artery
  Common interosseous artery
  Posterior ulnar recurrent artery
A Ulnar Artery, Left
  See 9 Ulnar Artery, Right
B Radial Artery, Right
  Radial recurrent artery
C Radial Artery, Left
  See B Radial Artery, Right
D Hand Artery, Right
  Deep palmar arch
  Princeps pollicis artery
  Radialis indicis
  Superficial palmar arch
F Hand Artery, Left
  See D Hand Artery, Right
G Intracranial Artery
  Anterior cerebral artery
  Anterior choroidal artery
  Anterior communicating artery
  Basilar artery
  Circle of Willis
  Internal carotid artery, intracranial portion
  Middle cerebral artery
  Middle meningeal artery, intracranial portion
  Ophthalmic artery
  Posterior cerebral artery
  Posterior communicating artery
  Posterior inferior cerebellar artery (PICA)
  Vertebral artery, intracranial portion
H Common Carotid Artery, Right
J Common Carotid Artery, Left
K Internal Carotid Artery, Right
  Caroticotympanic artery
  Carotid sinus
L Internal Carotid Artery, Left
  See K Internal Carotid Artery, Right
M External Carotid Artery, Right
  Ascending pharyngeal artery
  Internal maxillary artery
  Lingual artery
  Maxillary artery
  Occipital artery
  Posterior auricular artery
  Superior thyroid artery
N External Carotid Artery, Left
  See M External Carotid Artery, Right
P Vertebral Artery, Right
  Anterior spinal artery
  Posterior spinal artery
Q Vertebral Artery, Left
  See P Vertebral Artery, Right
R Face Artery
  Angular artery
  Ascending palatine artery
  External maxillary artery
  Facial artery
  Inferior labial artery
  Submental artery
  Superior labial artery
S Temporal Artery, Right
  Middle temporal artery
  Superficial temporal artery
  Transverse facial artery
T Temporal Artery, Left
  See S Temporal Artery, Right
U Thyroid Artery, Right
  Cricothyroid artery
  Hyoid artery
  Sternocleidomastoid artery
  Superior laryngeal artery
  Superior thyroid artery
  Thyrocervical trunk
V Thyroid Artery, Left
  See U Thyroid Artery, Right
Y Upper Artery
  Aortic intercostal artery
  Bronchial artery
  Esophageal artery
  Subcostal artery
	0 Open
	4 Percutaneous Endoscopic
		7 Autologous Tissue Substitute
		J Synthetic Substitute
		K Nonautologous Tissue Substitute
			Z No Qualifier

0 Medical and Surgical
3 Upper Arteries
S Reposition

Definition: Moving to its normal location, or other suitable location, all or a portion of a body part
Explanation: The body part is moved to a new location from an abnormal location, or from a normal location where it is not functioning correctly. The body part may or may not be cut out or off to be moved to the new location.

Body Part Character 4	Approach Character 5	Device Character 6	Qualifier Character 7
0 Internal Mammary Artery, Right Anterior intercostal artery Internal thoracic artery Musculophrenic artery Pericardiophrenic artery Superior epigastric artery **1 Internal Mammary Artery, Left** See 0 Internal Mammary Artery, Right **2 Innominate Artery** Brachiocephalic artery Brachiocephalic trunk **3 Subclavian Artery, Right** Costocervical trunk Dorsal scapular artery Internal thoracic artery **4 Subclavian Artery, Left** See 3 Subclavian Artery, Right **5 Axillary Artery, Right** Anterior circumflex humeral artery Lateral thoracic artery Posterior circumflex humeral artery Subscapular artery Superior thoracic artery Thoracoacromial artery **6 Axillary Artery, Left** See 5 Axillary Artery, Right **7 Brachial Artery, Right** Inferior ulnar collateral artery Profunda brachii Superior ulnar collateral artery **8 Brachial Artery, Left** See 7 Brachial Artery, Right **9 Ulnar Artery, Right** Anterior ulnar recurrent artery Common interosseous artery Posterior ulnar recurrent artery **A Ulnar Artery, Left** See 9 Ulnar Artery, Right **B Radial Artery, Right** Radial recurrent artery **C Radial Artery, Left** See B Radial Artery, Right **D Hand Artery, Right** Deep palmar arch Princeps pollicis artery Radialis indicis Superficial palmar arch **F Hand Artery, Left** See D Hand Artery, Right **G Intracranial Artery** Anterior cerebral artery Anterior choroidal artery Anterior communicating artery Basilar artery Circle of Willis Internal carotid artery, intracranial portion Middle cerebral artery Middle meningeal artery, intracranial portion Ophthalmic artery Posterior cerebral artery Posterior communicating artery Posterior inferior cerebellar artery (PICA) Vertebral artery, intracranial portion	**H Common Carotid Artery, Right** **J Common Carotid Artery, Left** **K Internal Carotid Artery, Right** Caroticotympanic artery Carotid sinus **L Internal Carotid Artery, Left** See K Internal Carotid Artery, Right **M External Carotid Artery, Right** Ascending pharyngeal artery Internal maxillary artery Lingual artery Maxillary artery Occipital artery Posterior auricular artery Superior thyroid artery **N External Carotid Artery, Left** See M External Carotid Artery, Right **P Vertebral Artery, Right** Anterior spinal artery Posterior spinal artery **Q Vertebral Artery, Left** See P Vertebral Artery, Right **R Face Artery** Angular artery Ascending palatine artery External maxillary artery Facial artery Inferior labial artery Submental artery Superior labial artery **S Temporal Artery, Right** Middle temporal artery Superficial temporal artery Transverse facial artery **T Temporal Artery, Left** See S Temporal Artery, Right **U Thyroid Artery, Right** Cricothyroid artery Hyoid artery Sternocleidomastoid artery Superior laryngeal artery Superior thyroid artery Thyrocervical trunk **V Thyroid Artery, Left** See U Thyroid Artery, Right **Y Upper Artery** Aortic intercostal artery Bronchial artery Esophageal artery Subcostal artery	**0 Open** **3 Percutaneous** **4 Percutaneous Endoscopic**	**Z No Device**	**Z No Qualifier**

ICD-10-PCS 2025 — Upper Arteries — 03U–03U

- **0** Medical and Surgical
- **3** Upper Arteries
- **U** Supplement

Definition: Putting in or on biological or synthetic material that physically reinforces and/or augments the function of a portion of a body part

Explanation: The biological material is non-living, or is living and from the same individual. The body part may have been previously replaced, and the SUPPLEMENT procedure is performed to physically reinforce and/or augment the function of the replaced body part.

Body Part — Character 4	Approach — Character 5	Device — Character 6	Qualifier — Character 7

0 Internal Mammary Artery, Right
  Anterior intercostal artery
  Internal thoracic artery
  Musculophrenic artery
  Pericardiophrenic artery
  Superior epigastric artery
1 Internal Mammary Artery, Left
  See 0 Internal Mammary Artery, Right
2 Innominate Artery
  Brachiocephalic artery
  Brachiocephalic trunk
3 Subclavian Artery, Right
  Costocervical trunk
  Dorsal scapular artery
  Internal thoracic artery
4 Subclavian Artery, Left
  See 3 Subclavian Artery, Right
5 Axillary Artery, Right
  Anterior circumflex humeral artery
  Lateral thoracic artery
  Posterior circumflex humeral artery
  Subscapular artery
  Superior thoracic artery
  Thoracoacromial artery
6 Axillary Artery, Left
  See 5 Axillary Artery, Right
7 Brachial Artery, Right
  Inferior ulnar collateral artery
  Profunda brachii
  Superior ulnar collateral artery
8 Brachial Artery, Left
  See 7 Brachial Artery, Right
9 Ulnar Artery, Right
  Anterior ulnar recurrent artery
  Common interosseous artery
  Posterior ulnar recurrent artery
A Ulnar Artery, Left
  See 9 Ulnar Artery, Right
B Radial Artery, Right
  Radial recurrent artery
C Radial Artery, Left
  See B Radial Artery, Right
D Hand Artery, Right
  Deep palmar arch
  Princeps pollicis artery
  Radialis indicis
  Superficial palmar arch
F Hand Artery, Left
  See D Hand Artery, Right
G Intracranial Artery
  Anterior cerebral artery
  Anterior choroidal artery
  Anterior communicating artery
  Basilar artery
  Circle of Willis
  Internal carotid artery, intracranial portion
  Middle cerebral artery
  Middle meningeal artery, intracranial portion
  Ophthalmic artery
  Posterior cerebral artery
  Posterior communicating artery
  Posterior inferior cerebellar artery (PICA)
  Vertebral artery, intracranial portion
H Common Carotid Artery, Right
J Common Carotid Artery, Left
K Internal Carotid Artery, Right
  Caroticotympanic artery
  Carotid sinus
L Internal Carotid Artery, Left
  See K Internal Carotid Artery, Right
M External Carotid Artery, Right
  Ascending pharyngeal artery
  Internal maxillary artery
  Lingual artery
  Maxillary artery
  Occipital artery
  Posterior auricular artery
  Superior thyroid artery
N External Carotid Artery, Left
  See M External Carotid Artery, Right
P Vertebral Artery, Right
  Anterior spinal artery
  Posterior spinal artery
Q Vertebral Artery, Left
  See P Vertebral Artery, Right
R Face Artery
  Angular artery
  Ascending palatine artery
  External maxillary artery
  Facial artery
  Inferior labial artery
  Submental artery
  Superior labial artery
S Temporal Artery, Right
  Middle temporal artery
  Superficial temporal artery
  Transverse facial artery
T Temporal Artery, Left
  See S Temporal Artery, Right
U Thyroid Artery, Right
  Cricothyroid artery
  Hyoid artery
  Sternocleidomastoid artery
  Superior laryngeal artery
  Superior thyroid artery
  Thyrocervical trunk
V Thyroid Artery, Left
  See U Thyroid Artery, Right
Y Upper Artery
  Aortic intercostal artery
  Bronchial artery
  Esophageal artery
  Subcostal artery
	0 Open
	3 Percutaneous
	4 Percutaneous Endoscopic
		7 Autologous Tissue Substitute
		J Synthetic Substitute
		K Nonautologous Tissue Substitute
			Z No Qualifier

NC Noncovered Procedure   **LC** Limited Coverage   **QA** Questionable OB Admit   **NT** New Tech Add-on   ✚ Combination Member   ♂ Male   ♀ Female

0 Medical and Surgical
3 Upper Arteries
V Restriction Definition: Partially closing an orifice or the lumen of a tubular body part
Explanation: The orifice can be a natural orifice or an artificially created orifice

Body Part Character 4	Approach Character 5	Device Character 6	Qualifier Character 7

0 Internal Mammary Artery, Right
  Anterior intercostal artery
  Internal thoracic artery
  Musculophrenic artery
  Pericardiophrenic artery
  Superior epigastric artery
1 Internal Mammary Artery, Left
  See 0 Internal Mammary Artery, Right
2 Innominate Artery
  Brachiocephalic artery
  Brachiocephalic trunk
3 Subclavian Artery, Right
  Costocervical trunk
  Dorsal scapular artery
  Internal thoracic artery
4 Subclavian Artery, Left
  See 3 Subclavian Artery, Right
5 Axillary Artery, Right
  Anterior circumflex humeral artery
  Lateral thoracic artery
  Posterior circumflex humeral artery
  Subscapular artery
  Superior thoracic artery
  Thoracoacromial artery
6 Axillary Artery, Left
  See 5 Axillary Artery, Right
7 Brachial Artery, Right
  Inferior ulnar collateral artery
  Profunda brachii
  Superior ulnar collateral artery
8 Brachial Artery, Left
  See 7 Brachial Artery, Right
9 Ulnar Artery, Right
  Anterior ulnar recurrent artery
  Common interosseous artery
  Posterior ulnar recurrent artery
A Ulnar Artery, Left
  See 9 Ulnar Artery, Right
B Radial Artery, Right
  Radial recurrent artery
C Radial Artery, Left
  See B Radial Artery, Right
D Hand Artery, Right
  Deep palmar arch
  Princeps pollicis artery
  Radialis indicis
  Superficial palmar arch
F Hand Artery, Left
  See D Hand Artery, Right
R Face Artery
  Angular artery
  Ascending palatine artery
  External maxillary artery
  Facial artery
  Inferior labial artery
  Submental artery
  Superior labial artery
S Temporal Artery, Right
  Middle temporal artery
  Superficial temporal artery
  Transverse facial artery
T Temporal Artery, Left
  See S Temporal Artery, Right
U Thyroid Artery, Right
  Cricothyroid artery
  Hyoid artery
  Sternocleidomastoid artery
  Superior laryngeal artery
  Superior thyroid artery
  Thyrocervical trunk
V Thyroid Artery, Left
  See U Thyroid Artery, Right
Y Upper Artery
  Aortic intercostal artery
  Bronchial artery
  Esophageal artery
  Subcostal artery
	0 Open
	3 Percutaneous
	4 Percutaneous Endoscopic
		C Extraluminal Device
		D Intraluminal Device
		Z No Device
			Z No Qualifier

G Intracranial Artery
  Anterior cerebral artery
  Anterior choroidal artery
  Anterior communicating artery
  Basilar artery
  Circle of Willis
  Internal carotid artery, intracranial portion
  Middle cerebral artery
  Middle meningeal artery, intracranial portion
  Ophthalmic artery
  Posterior cerebral artery
  Posterior communicating artery
  Posterior inferior cerebellar artery (PICA)
  Vertebral artery, intracranial portion
H Common Carotid Artery, Right
J Common Carotid Artery, Left
K Internal Carotid Artery, Right
  Caroticotympanic artery
  Carotid sinus
L Internal Carotid Artery, Left
  See K Internal Carotid Artery, Right
M External Carotid Artery, Right
  Ascending pharyngeal artery
  Internal maxillary artery
  Lingual artery
  Maxillary artery
  Occipital artery
  Posterior auricular artery
  Superior thyroid artery
N External Carotid Artery, Left
  See M External Carotid Artery, Right
P Vertebral Artery, Right
  Anterior spinal artery
  Posterior spinal artery
Q Vertebral Artery, Left
  See P Vertebral Artery, Right
	0 Open
	3 Percutaneous
	4 Percutaneous Endoscopic
		B Intraluminal Device, Bioactive
		C Extraluminal Device
		D Intraluminal Device
		H Intraluminal Device, Flow Diverter
		Z No Device
			Z No Qualifier

0 Medical and Surgical
3 Upper Arteries
W Revision

Definition: Correcting, to the extent possible, a portion of a malfunctioning device or the position of a displaced device

Explanation: Revision can include correcting a malfunctioning or displaced device by taking out or putting in components of the device such as a screw or pin

Body Part Character 4	Approach Character 5	Device Character 6	Qualifier Character 7

Y Upper Artery
   Aortic intercostal artery
   Bronchial artery
   Esophageal artery
   Subcostal artery
	0 Open
	3 Percutaneous
	4 Percutaneous Endoscopic
		0 Drainage Device
		2 Monitoring Device
		3 Infusion Device
		7 Autologous Tissue Substitute
		C Extraluminal Device
		D Intraluminal Device
		J Synthetic Substitute
		K Nonautologous Tissue Substitute
		M Stimulator Lead
		Y Other Device
			Z No Qualifier

Y Upper Artery
   Aortic intercostal artery
   Bronchial artery
   Esophageal artery
   Subcostal artery
	X External	0 Drainage Device
		2 Monitoring Device
		3 Infusion Device
		7 Autologous Tissue Substitute
		C Extraluminal Device
		D Intraluminal Device
		J Synthetic Substitute
		K Nonautologous Tissue Substitute
		M Stimulator Lead
			Z No Qualifier

Non-OR 03WY3[0,2,3]Z
Non-OR 03WY[3,4]YZ
Non-OR 03WYX[0,2,3,7,C,D,J,K,M]Z

Lower Arteries 041–04W

Character Meanings

This Character Meaning table is provided as a guide to assist the user in the identification of character members that may be found in this section of code tables. It **SHOULD NOT** be used to build a PCS code.

Operation–Character 3	Body Part–Character 4	Approach–Character 5	Device–Character 6	Qualifier–Character 7
1 Bypass	0 Abdominal Aorta	0 Open	0 Drainage Device	0 Abdominal Aorta OR Ultrasonic
5 Destruction	1 Celiac Artery	3 Percutaneous	1 Radioactive Element	1 Celiac Artery OR Drug-Coated Balloon
7 Dilation	2 Gastric Artery	4 Percutaneous Endoscopic	2 Monitoring Device	2 Mesenteric Artery OR Sustained Release
9 Drainage	3 Hepatic Artery	X External	3 Infusion Device	3 Renal Artery, Right
B Excision	4 Splenic Artery		4 Intraluminal Device, Drug-eluting	4 Renal Artery, Left
C Extirpation	5 Superior Mesenteric Artery		5 Intraluminal Device, Drug-eluting, Two	5 Renal Artery, Bilateral
F Fragmentation	6 Colic Artery, Right		6 Intraluminal Device, Drug-eluting, Three	6 Common Iliac Artery, Right
H Insertion	7 Colic Artery, Left		7 Intraluminal Device, Drug-eluting, Four or More OR Autologous Tissue Substitute	7 Common Iliac Artery, Left
J Inspection	8 Colic Artery, Middle		9 Autologous Venous Tissue	8 Common Iliac Arteries, Bilateral
L Occlusion	9 Renal Artery, Right		A Autologous Arterial Tissue	9 Internal Iliac Artery, Right
N Release	A Renal Artery, Left		C Extraluminal Device	B Internal Iliac Artery, Left
P Removal	B Inferior Mesenteric Artery		D Intraluminal Device	C Internal Iliac Arteries, Bilateral
Q Repair	C Common Iliac Artery, Right		E Intraluminal Device, Two OR Intraluminal Device, Branched or Fenestrated, One or Two Arteries	D External Iliac Artery, Right
R Replacement	D Common Iliac Artery, Left		F Intraluminal Device, Three OR Intraluminal Device, Branched or Fenestrated, Three or More Arteries	F External Iliac Artery, Left
S Reposition	E Internal Iliac Artery, Right		G Intraluminal Device, Four or More	G External Iliac Arteries, Bilateral
U Supplement	F Internal Iliac Artery, Left		J Synthetic Substitute	H Femoral Artery, Right
V Restriction	H External Iliac Artery, Right		K Nonautologous Tissue Substitute	J Femoral Artery, Left OR Temporary
W Revision	J External Iliac Artery, Left		Y Other Device	K Femoral Arteries, Bilateral
	K Femoral Artery, Right		Z No Device	L Popliteal Artery
	L Femoral Artery, Left			M Peroneal Artery
	M Popliteal Artery, Right			N Posterior Tibial Artery
	N Popliteal Artery, Left			P Foot Artery
	P Anterior Tibial Artery, Right			Q Lower Extremity Artery
	Q Anterior Tibial Artery, Left			R Lower Artery
	R Posterior Tibial Artery, Right			S Lower Extremity Vein
	S Posterior Tibial Artery, Left			T Uterine Artery, Right
	T Peroneal Artery, Right			U Uterine Artery, Left
	U Peroneal Artery, Left			V Prostatic Artery, Right
	V Foot Artery, Right			W Prostatic Artery, Left
	W Foot Artery, Left			X Diagnostic
	Y Lower Artery			Z No Qualifier

Lower Arteries

AHA Coding Clinic for Lower Arteries
2022, 1Q, 10-13	Procedures performed on a continuous vessel, ICD-10-PCS Guideline B4.1c

AHA Coding Clinic for table 041
2022, 3Q, 5	Aortoiliac aneurysm repair
2019, 1Q, 23	Endovascular repair of shaggy aorta and deployment of chimney stent grafts
2018, 3Q, 25	Femoral artery to tibioperoneal trunk bypass
2017, 4Q, 46-47	New and revised body part values - Bypass hepatic artery to renal artery
2017, 3Q, 5	Femoral artery to posterior tibial artery bypass using autologous and synthetic grafts
2017, 3Q, 16	Abdominal aortic debranching with bypass of external iliac artery to bilateral renal arteries and superior mesenteric artery
2017, 1Q, 32	Peroneal artery to dorsalis pedis artery bypass using saphenous vein graft
2016, 2Q, 18	Femoral-tibial artery bypass and saphenous vein graft
2015, 3Q, 28	Bilateral renal artery bypass

AHA Coding Clinic for table 047
2020, 4Q, 50	Intravascular lithotripsy
2019, 4Q, 27	Bifurcation Qualifier
2019, 2Q, 14	Revision of occluded femoral-popliteal bypass graft
2018, 2Q, 24	Coronary artery bifurcation
2016, 4Q, 86	Peripheral artery, number of stents
2016, 4Q, 86-88	Coronary and peripheral artery bifurcation
2016, 3Q, 39	Infrarenal abdominal aortic aneurysm repair with iliac graft extension
2015, 4Q, 4-7, 15	Drug-coated balloon angioplasty in peripheral vessels
2015, 3Q, 9	Aborted endovascular stenting of superficial femoral artery

AHA Coding Clinic for table 04C
2021, 1Q, 15	Iliofemoral endarterectomy and furthest point of entry
2019, 4Q, 27	Bifurcation Qualifier
2019, 1Q, 23	Endovascular repair of shaggy aorta and deployment of chimney stent grafts
2018, 2Q, 24	Coronary artery bifurcation
2017, 2Q, 23	Thrombectomy via Fogarty catheter
2016, 4Q, 86-88	Coronary and peripheral artery bifurcation
2016, 1Q, 31	Iliofemoral endarterectomy with patch repair
2015, 1Q, 29	Discontinued carotid endarterectomy
2015, 1Q, 36	Percutaneous mechanical thrombectomy of femoropopliteal bypass graft

AHA Coding Clinic for table 04F
2020, 4Q, 45-49	New fragmentation tables
2020, 4Q, 49-50	Intravascular ultrasound assisted thrombolysis
2020, 4Q, 50-51	Intravascular lithotripsy

AHA Coding Clinic for table 04H
2022, 3Q, 19	Placement of stent into aorta to secure debris
2019, 3Q, 20	Removal and revision of ECMO component
2019, 1Q, 23	Endovascular repair of shaggy aorta and deployment of chimney stent grafts
2017, 1Q, 30	Insertion of umbilical artery catheter

AHA Coding Clinic for table 04J
2022, 4Q, 56	Embolization of prostatic artery

AHA Coding Clinic for table 04L
2023, 1Q, 9	Temporary balloon occlusion of aorta
2022, 4Q, 55-56	Embolization of prostatic artery
2020, 3Q, 43	Staged laparoscopic gastric conduit and placement of feeding tube
2018, 2Q, 18	Transverse rectus abdominis myocutaneous (TRAM) delay
2017, 4Q, 31	Resuscitative endovascular balloon occlusion of the aorta
2015, 2Q, 27	Uterine artery embolization using Gelfoam
2014, 3Q, 26	Coil embolization of gastroduodenal artery with chemoembolization of hepatic artery
2014, 1Q, 24	Endovascular embolization for gastrointestinal bleeding

AHA Coding Clinic for table 04N
2015, 2Q, 28	Release and replacement of celiac artery

AHA Coding Clinic for table 04P
2019, 3Q, 20	Removal and revision of ECMO component

AHA Coding Clinic for table 04Q
2023, 3Q, 27	Fenestration of aortic dissection flap
2014, 1Q, 21	Repair of femoral artery pseudoaneurysm

AHA Coding Clinic for table 04R
2022, 3Q, 5	Aortoiliac aneurysm repair
2019, 1Q, 22	Abdominal aortic aneurysm repair using tube graft
2015, 2Q, 28	Release and replacement of celiac artery

AHA Coding Clinic for table 04U
2023, 3Q, 25	Deployment of Tack Endovascular System® for vessel dissection
2019, 1Q, 22	Abdominal aortic aneurysm repair using tube graft
2016, 2Q, 18	Femoral-tibial artery bypass and saphenous vein graft
2016, 1Q, 31	Iliofemoral endarterectomy with patch repair
2014, 4Q, 37	Bovine patch arterioplasty
2014, 1Q, 22	Repair of pseudoaneurysm of femoral-popliteal bypass graft

AHA Coding Clinic for table 04V
2024, 2Q, 18	Ascending aorta and total aortic arch repair with extension frozen elephant trunk
2021, 3Q, 23	Transcatheter embolization of splenic artery
2019, 4Q, 27	Bifurcation Qualifier
2019, 1Q, 22	Abdominal aortic aneurysm repair using tube graft
2018, 2Q, 24	Coronary artery bifurcation
2016, 4Q, 86-87	Coronary and peripheral artery bifurcation
2016, 4Q, 89-93	Branched and fenestrated endograft repair of aneurysms
2016, 3Q, 39	Infrarenal abdominal aortic aneurysm repair with iliac graft extension
2014, 1Q, 9	Endovascular repair of abdominal aortic aneurysm

AHA Coding Clinic for table 04W
2020, 3Q, 5	Types of endoleaks following endovascular aneurysm repair
2019, 2Q, 14	Revision of occluded femoral-popliteal bypass graft
2015, 1Q, 36	Revision of femoropopliteal bypass graft
2014, 1Q, 9	Endovascular repair of endoleak
2014, 1Q, 22	Repair of pseudoaneurysm of femoral-popliteal bypass graft

Lower Arteries

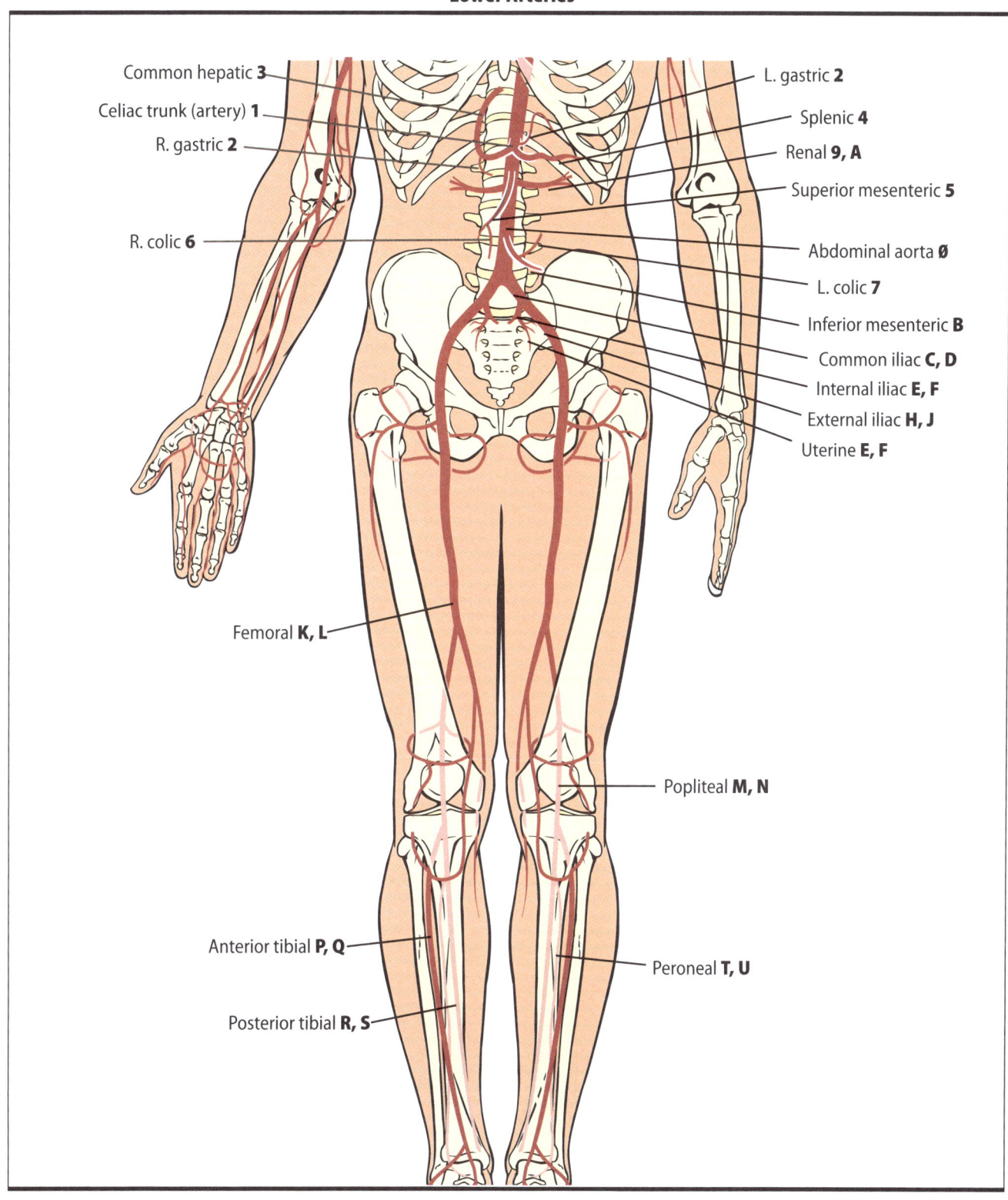

- Common hepatic **3**
- Celiac trunk (artery) **1**
- R. gastric **2**
- R. colic **6**
- L. gastric **2**
- Splenic **4**
- Renal **9, A**
- Superior mesenteric **5**
- Abdominal aorta **Ø**
- L. colic **7**
- Inferior mesenteric **B**
- Common iliac **C, D**
- Internal iliac **E, F**
- External iliac **H, J**
- Uterine **E, F**
- Femoral **K, L**
- Popliteal **M, N**
- Anterior tibial **P, Q**
- Peroneal **T, U**
- Posterior tibial **R, S**

041–041 Lower Arteries — ICD-10-PCS 2025

0 Medical and Surgical
4 Lower Arteries
1 Bypass

Definition: Altering the route of passage of the contents of a tubular body part
Explanation: Rerouting contents of a body part to a downstream area of the normal route, to a similar route and body part, or to an abnormal route and dissimilar body part. Includes one or more anastomoses, with or without the use of a device.

Body Part — Character 4	Approach — Character 5	Device — Character 6	Qualifier — Character 7

0 Abdominal Aorta
  Inferior phrenic artery
  Lumbar artery
  Median sacral artery
  Middle suprarenal artery
  Ovarian artery
  Testicular artery
C Common Iliac Artery, Right
D Common Iliac Artery, Left
	0 Open
	4 Percutaneous Endoscopic
		9 Autologous Venous Tissue
		A Autologous Arterial Tissue
		J Synthetic Substitute
		K Nonautologous Tissue Substitute
		Z No Device
			0 Abdominal Aorta
			1 Celiac Artery
			2 Mesenteric Artery
			3 Renal Artery, Right
			4 Renal Artery, Left
			5 Renal Artery, Bilateral
			6 Common Iliac Artery, Right
			7 Common Iliac Artery, Left
			8 Common Iliac Arteries, Bilateral
			9 Internal Iliac Artery, Right
			B Internal Iliac Artery, Left
			C Internal Iliac Arteries, Bilateral
			D External Iliac Artery, Right
			F External Iliac Artery, Left
			G External Iliac Arteries, Bilateral
			H Femoral Artery, Right
			J Femoral Artery, Left
			K Femoral Arteries, Bilateral
			Q Lower Extremity Artery
			R Lower Artery

3 Hepatic Artery
  Common hepatic artery
  Gastroduodenal artery
  Hepatic artery proper
4 Splenic Artery
  Left gastroepiploic artery
  Pancreatic artery
  Short gastric artery
	0 Open
	4 Percutaneous Endoscopic
		9 Autologous Venous Tissue
		A Autologous Arterial Tissue
		J Synthetic Substitute
		K Nonautologous Tissue Substitute
		Z No Device
			3 Renal Artery, Right
			4 Renal Artery, Left
			5 Renal Artery, Bilateral
			R Lower Artery

E Internal Iliac Artery, Right
  Deferential artery
  Hypogastric artery
  Iliolumbar artery
  Inferior gluteal artery
  Inferior vesical artery
  Internal pudendal artery
  Lateral sacral artery
  Middle rectal artery
  Obturator artery
  Prostatic artery
  Superior gluteal artery
  Superior vesical artery
  Umbilical artery
  Uterine artery
  Vaginal artery
F Internal Iliac Artery, Left
  See E Internal Iliac Artery, Right
H External Iliac Artery, Right
  Deep circumflex iliac artery
  Inferior epigastric artery
J External Iliac Artery, Left
  See H External Iliac Artery, Right
	0 Open
	4 Percutaneous Endoscopic
		9 Autologous Venous Tissue
		A Autologous Arterial Tissue
		J Synthetic Substitute
		K Nonautologous Tissue Substitute
		Z No Device
			9 Internal Iliac Artery, Right
			B Internal Iliac Artery, Left
			C Internal Iliac Arteries, Bilateral
			D External Iliac Artery, Right
			F External Iliac Artery, Left
			G External Iliac Arteries, Bilateral
			H Femoral Artery, Right
			J Femoral Artery, Left
			K Femoral Arteries, Bilateral
			P Foot Artery
			Q Lower Extremity Artery

K Femoral Artery, Right
  Circumflex iliac artery
  Deep femoral artery
  Descending genicular artery
  External pudendal artery
  Superficial epigastric artery
L Femoral Artery, Left
  See K Femoral Artery, Right
	0 Open
	4 Percutaneous Endoscopic
		9 Autologous Venous Tissue
		A Autologous Arterial Tissue
		J Synthetic Substitute
		K Nonautologous Tissue Substitute
		Z No Device
			H Femoral Artery, Right
			J Femoral Artery, Left
			K Femoral Arteries, Bilateral
			L Popliteal Artery
			M Peroneal Artery
			N Posterior Tibial Artery
			P Foot Artery
			Q Lower Extremity Artery
			S Lower Extremity Vein

K Femoral Artery, Right
  Circumflex iliac artery
  Deep femoral artery
  Descending genicular artery
  External pudendal artery
  Superficial epigastric artery
L Femoral Artery, Left
  See K Femoral Artery, Right
	3 Percutaneous	**J** Synthetic Substitute	**Q** Lower Extremity Artery
			S Lower Extremity Vein

M Popliteal Artery, Right
  Inferior genicular artery
  Middle genicular artery
  Superior genicular artery
  Sural artery
  Tibioperoneal trunk
N Popliteal Artery, Left
  See M Popliteal Artery, Right
	0 Open
	4 Percutaneous Endoscopic
		9 Autologous Venous Tissue
		A Autologous Arterial Tissue
		J Synthetic Substitute
		K Nonautologous Tissue Substitute
		Z No Device
			L Popliteal Artery
			M Peroneal Artery
			P Foot Artery
			Q Lower Extremity Artery
			S Lower Extremity Vein

041 Continued on next page

Non-OR Procedure | DRG Non-OR Procedure | Valid OR Procedure | HAC Associated Procedure | Combination Only | New/Revised April | New/Revised October

ICD-10-PCS 2025 — Lower Arteries — 041–041

041 Continued

- 0 Medical and Surgical
- 4 Lower Arteries
- 1 Bypass Definition: Altering the route of passage of the contents of a tubular body part
  Explanation: Rerouting contents of a body part to a downstream area of the normal route, to a similar route and body part, or to an abnormal route and dissimilar body part. Includes one or more anastomoses, with or without the use of a device.

Body Part — Character 4	Approach — Character 5	Device — Character 6	Qualifier — Character 7

M Popliteal Artery, Right
  Inferior genicular artery
  Middle genicular artery
  Superior genicular artery
  Sural artery
  Tibioperoneal trunk
N Popliteal Artery, Left
  See M Popliteal Artery, Right
	3 Percutaneous	**J** Synthetic Substitute	**Q** Lower Extremity Artery
			S Lower Extremity Vein

P Anterior Tibial Artery, Right
  Anterior lateral malleolar artery
  Anterior medial malleolar artery
  Anterior tibial recurrent artery
  Dorsalis pedis artery
  Posterior tibial recurrent artery
Q Anterior Tibial Artery, Left
  See P Anterior Tibial Artery, Right
R Posterior Tibial Artery, Right
S Posterior Tibial Artery, Left
	0 Open
	3 Percutaneous
	4 Percutaneous Endoscopic
		J Synthetic Substitute	**Q** Lower Extremity Artery
			S Lower Extremity Vein

T Peroneal Artery, Right
  Fibular artery
U Peroneal Artery, Left
  See T Peroneal Artery, Right
V Foot Artery, Right
  Arcuate artery
  Dorsal metatarsal artery
  Lateral plantar artery
  Lateral tarsal artery
  Medial plantar artery
W Foot Artery, Left
  See V Foot Artery, Right
	0 Open
	4 Percutaneous Endoscopic
		9 Autologous Venous Tissue
		A Autologous Arterial Tissue
		J Synthetic Substitute
		K Nonautologous Tissue Substitute
		Z No Device
			P Foot Artery
			Q Lower Extremity Artery
			S Lower Extremity Vein

T Peroneal Artery, Right
  Fibular artery
U Peroneal Artery, Left
  See T Peroneal Artery, Right
V Foot Artery, Right
  Arcuate artery
  Dorsal metatarsal artery
  Lateral plantar artery
  Lateral tarsal artery
  Medial plantar artery
W Foot Artery, Left
  See V Foot Artery, Right
	3 Percutaneous	**J** Synthetic Substitute	**Q** Lower Extremity Artery
			S Lower Extremity Vein

NC Noncovered Procedure   **LC** Limited Coverage   **QA** Questionable OB Admit   **NT** New Tech Add-on   ✚ Combination Member   ♂ Male   ♀ Female

0 Medical and Surgical
4 Lower Arteries
5 Destruction Definition: Physical eradication of all or a portion of a body part by the direct use of energy, force, or a destructive agent
Explanation: None of the body part is physically taken out

Body Part Character 4	Approach Character 5	Device Character 6	Qualifier Character 7

0 Abdominal Aorta
  Inferior phrenic artery
  Lumbar artery
  Median sacral artery
  Middle suprarenal artery
  Ovarian artery
  Testicular artery
1 Celiac Artery
  Celiac trunk
2 Gastric Artery
  Left gastric artery
  Right gastric artery
3 Hepatic Artery
  Common hepatic artery
  Gastroduodenal artery
  Hepatic artery proper
4 Splenic Artery
  Left gastroepiploic artery
  Pancreatic artery
  Short gastric artery
5 Superior Mesenteric Artery
  Ileal artery
  Ileocolic artery
  Inferior pancreaticoduodenal artery
  Jejunal artery
6 Colic Artery, Right
7 Colic Artery, Left
8 Colic Artery, Middle
9 Renal Artery, Right
  Inferior suprarenal artery
  Renal segmental artery
A Renal Artery, Left
  See 9 Renal Artery, Right
B Inferior Mesenteric Artery
  Sigmoid artery
  Superior rectal artery
C Common Iliac Artery, Right
D Common Iliac Artery, Left
E Internal Iliac Artery, Right
  Deferential artery
  Hypogastric artery
  Iliolumbar artery
  Inferior gluteal artery
  Inferior vesical artery
  Internal pudendal artery
  Lateral sacral artery
  Middle rectal artery
  Obturator artery
  Prostatic artery
  Superior gluteal artery
  Superior vesical artery
  Umbilical artery
  Uterine artery
  Vaginal artery
	F Internal Iliac Artery, Left
	  See E Internal Iliac Artery, Right
	H External Iliac Artery, Right
	  Deep circumflex iliac artery
	  Inferior epigastric artery
	J External Iliac Artery, Left
	  See H External Iliac Artery, Right
	K Femoral Artery, Right
	  Circumflex iliac artery
	  Deep femoral artery
	  Descending genicular artery
	  External pudendal artery
	  Superficial epigastric artery
	L Femoral Artery, Left
	  See K Femoral Artery, Right
	M Popliteal Artery, Right
	  Inferior genicular artery
	  Middle genicular artery
	  Superior genicular artery
	  Sural artery
	  Tibioperoneal trunk
	N Popliteal Artery, Left
	  See M Popliteal Artery, Right
	P Anterior Tibial Artery, Right
	  Anterior lateral malleolar artery
	  Anterior medial malleolar artery
	  Anterior tibial recurrent artery
	  Dorsalis pedis artery
	  Posterior tibial recurrent artery
	Q Anterior Tibial Artery, Left
	  See P Anterior Tibial Artery, Right
	R Posterior Tibial Artery, Right
	S Posterior Tibial Artery, Left
	T Peroneal Artery, Right
	  Fibular artery
	U Peroneal Artery, Left
	  See T Peroneal Artery, Right
	V Foot Artery, Right
	  Arcuate artery
	  Dorsal metatarsal artery
	  Lateral plantar artery
	  Lateral tarsal artery
	  Medial plantar artery
	W Foot Artery, Left
	  See V Foot Artery, Right
	Y Lower Artery
	  Umbilical artery
		0 Open
		3 Percutaneous
		4 Percutaneous Endoscopic
			Z No Device	**Z** No Qualifier

0 Medical and Surgical
4 Lower Arteries
7 Dilation Definition: Expanding an orifice or the lumen of a tubular body part
Explanation: The orifice can be a natural orifice or an artificially created orifice. Accomplished by stretching a tubular body part using intraluminal pressure or by cutting part of the orifice or wall of the tubular body part.

Body Part Character 4	Approach Character 5	Device Character 6	Qualifier Character 7
0 Abdominal Aorta Inferior phrenic artery Lumbar artery Median sacral artery Middle suprarenal artery Ovarian artery Testicular artery **1 Celiac Artery** Celiac trunk **2 Gastric Artery** Left gastric artery Right gastric artery **3 Hepatic Artery** Common hepatic artery Gastroduodenal artery Hepatic artery proper **4 Splenic Artery** Left gastroepiploic artery Pancreatic artery Short gastric artery **5 Superior Mesenteric Artery** Ileal artery Ileocolic artery Inferior pancreaticoduodenal artery Jejunal artery **6 Colic Artery, Right** **7 Colic Artery, Left** **8 Colic Artery, Middle** **9 Renal Artery, Right** Inferior suprarenal artery Renal segmental artery **A Renal Artery, Left** *See 9 Renal Artery, Right* **B Inferior Mesenteric Artery** Sigmoid artery Superior rectal artery	**C Common Iliac Artery, Right** **D Common Iliac Artery, Left** **E Internal Iliac Artery, Right** Deferential artery Hypogastric artery Iliolumbar artery Inferior gluteal artery Inferior vesical artery Internal pudendal artery Lateral sacral artery Middle rectal artery Obturator artery Prostatic artery Superior gluteal artery Superior vesical artery Umbilical artery Uterine artery Vaginal artery **F Internal Iliac Artery, Left** *See E Internal Iliac Artery, Right* **H External Iliac Artery, Right** Deep circumflex iliac artery Inferior epigastric artery **J External Iliac Artery, Left** *See H External Iliac Artery, Right* **V Foot Artery, Right** Arcuate artery Dorsal metatarsal artery Lateral plantar artery Lateral tarsal artery Medial plantar artery **W Foot Artery, Left** *See V Foot Artery, Right* **Y Lower Artery** Umbilical artery	**0 Open** **3 Percutaneous** **4 Percutaneous Endoscopic**	**4 Intraluminal Device, Drug-eluting** **D Intraluminal Device** **Z No Device**	**1 Drug-Coated Balloon** **Z No Qualifier**
0 Abdominal Aorta Inferior phrenic artery Lumbar artery Median sacral artery Middle suprarenal artery Ovarian artery Testicular artery **1 Celiac Artery** Celiac trunk **2 Gastric Artery** Left gastric artery Right gastric artery **3 Hepatic Artery** Common hepatic artery Gastroduodenal artery Hepatic artery proper **4 Splenic Artery** Left gastroepiploic artery Pancreatic artery Short gastric artery **5 Superior Mesenteric Artery** Ileal artery Ileocolic artery Inferior pancreaticoduodenal artery Jejunal artery **6 Colic Artery, Right** **7 Colic Artery, Left** **8 Colic Artery, Middle** **9 Renal Artery, Right** Inferior suprarenal artery Renal segmental artery **A Renal Artery, Left** *See 9 Renal Artery, Right* **B Inferior Mesenteric Artery** Sigmoid artery Superior rectal artery	**C Common Iliac Artery, Right** **D Common Iliac Artery, Left** **E Internal Iliac Artery, Right** Deferential artery Hypogastric artery Iliolumbar artery Inferior gluteal artery Inferior vesical artery Internal pudendal artery Lateral sacral artery Middle rectal artery Obturator artery Prostatic artery Superior gluteal artery Superior vesical artery Umbilical artery Uterine artery Vaginal artery **F Internal Iliac Artery, Left** *See E Internal Iliac Artery, Right* **H External Iliac Artery, Right** Deep circumflex iliac artery Inferior epigastric artery **J External Iliac Artery, Left** *See H External Iliac Artery, Right* **V Foot Artery, Right** Arcuate artery Dorsal metatarsal artery Lateral plantar artery Lateral tarsal artery Medial plantar artery **W Foot Artery, Left** *See V Foot Artery, Right* **Y Lower Artery** Umbilical artery	**0 Open** **3 Percutaneous** **4 Percutaneous Endoscopic**	**5 Intraluminal Device, Drug-eluting, Two** **6 Intraluminal Device, Drug-eluting, Three** **7 Intraluminal Device, Drug-eluting, Four or More** **E Intraluminal Device, Two** **F Intraluminal Device, Three** **G Intraluminal Device, Four or More**	**Z No Qualifier**

047 Continued on next page

0 Medical and Surgical
4 Lower Arteries
7 Dilation   Definition: Expanding an orifice or the lumen of a tubular body part
Explanation: The orifice can be a natural orifice or an artificially created orifice. Accomplished by stretching a tubular body part using intraluminal pressure or by cutting part of the orifice or wall of the tubular body part.

047 Continued

Body Part — Character 4	Approach — Character 5	Device — Character 6	Qualifier — Character 7
K Femoral Artery, Right 　Circumflex iliac artery 　Deep femoral artery 　Descending genicular artery 　External pudendal artery 　Superficial epigastric artery **L** Femoral Artery, Left 　See K Femoral Artery, Right **M** Popliteal Artery, Right 　Inferior genicular artery 　Middle genicular artery 　Superior genicular artery 　Sural artery 　Tibioperoneal trunk **N** Popliteal Artery, Left 　See M Popliteal Artery, Right **P** Anterior Tibial Artery, Right 　Anterior lateral malleolar artery 　Anterior medial malleolar artery 　Anterior tibial recurrent artery 　Dorsalis pedis artery 　Posterior tibial recurrent artery **Q** Anterior Tibial Artery, Left 　See P Anterior Tibial Artery, Right **R** Posterior Tibial Artery, Right **S** Posterior Tibial Artery, Left **T** Peroneal Artery, Right 　Fibular artery **U** Peroneal Artery, Left 　See T Peroneal Artery, Right	**0** Open **4** Percutaneous Endoscopic	**4** Intraluminal Device, Drug-eluting **D** Intraluminal Device **Z** No Device	**1** Drug-Coated Balloon **Z** No Qualifier
K Femoral Artery, Right 　Circumflex iliac artery 　Deep femoral artery 　Descending genicular artery 　External pudendal artery 　Superficial epigastric artery **L** Femoral Artery, Left 　See K Femoral Artery, Right **M** Popliteal Artery, Right 　Inferior genicular artery 　Middle genicular artery 　Superior genicular artery 　Sural artery 　Tibioperoneal trunk **N** Popliteal Artery, Left 　See M Popliteal Artery, Right **P** Anterior Tibial Artery, Right 　Anterior lateral malleolar artery 　Anterior medial malleolar artery 　Anterior tibial recurrent artery 　Dorsalis pedis artery 　Posterior tibial recurrent artery **Q** Anterior Tibial Artery, Left 　See P Anterior Tibial Artery, Right **R** Posterior Tibial Artery, Right **S** Posterior Tibial Artery, Left **T** Peroneal Artery, Right 　Fibular artery **U** Peroneal Artery, Left 　See T Peroneal Artery, Right	**0** Open **4** Percutaneous Endoscopic	**5** Intraluminal Device, Drug-eluting, Two **6** Intraluminal Device, Drug-eluting, Three **7** Intraluminal Device, Drug-eluting, Four or More **E** Intraluminal Device, Two **F** Intraluminal Device, Three **G** Intraluminal Device, Four or More	**Z** No Qualifier
K Femoral Artery, Right 　Circumflex iliac artery 　Deep femoral artery 　Descending genicular artery 　External pudendal artery 　Superficial epigastric artery **L** Femoral Artery, Left 　See K Femoral Artery, Right **M** Popliteal Artery, Right 　Inferior genicular artery 　Middle genicular artery 　Superior genicular artery 　Sural artery 　Tibioperoneal trunk **N** Popliteal Artery, Left 　See M Popliteal Artery, Right **P** Anterior Tibial Artery, Right 　Anterior lateral malleolar artery 　Anterior medial malleolar artery 　Anterior tibial recurrent artery 　Dorsalis pedis artery 　Posterior tibial recurrent artery **Q** Anterior Tibial Artery, Left 　See P Anterior Tibial Artery, Right **R** Posterior Tibial Artery, Right **S** Posterior Tibial Artery, Left **T** Peroneal Artery, Right 　Fibular artery **U** Peroneal Artery, Left 　See T Peroneal Artery, Right	**3** Percutaneous	**4** Intraluminal Device, Drug-eluting	**1** Drug-Coated Balloon **2** Sustained Release **Z** No Qualifier
K Femoral Artery, Right 　Circumflex iliac artery 　Deep femoral artery 　Descending genicular artery 　External pudendal artery 　Superficial epigastric artery **L** Femoral Artery, Left 　See K Femoral Artery, Right **M** Popliteal Artery, Right 　Inferior genicular artery 　Middle genicular artery 　Superior genicular artery 　Sural artery 　Tibioperoneal trunk **N** Popliteal Artery, Left 　See M Popliteal Artery, Right **P** Anterior Tibial Artery, Right 　Anterior lateral malleolar artery 　Anterior medial malleolar artery 　Anterior tibial recurrent artery 　Dorsalis pedis artery 　Posterior tibial recurrent artery **Q** Anterior Tibial Artery, Left 　See P Anterior Tibial Artery, Right **R** Posterior Tibial Artery, Right **S** Posterior Tibial Artery, Left **T** Peroneal Artery, Right 　Fibular artery **U** Peroneal Artery, Left 　See T Peroneal Artery, Right	**3** Percutaneous	**5** Intraluminal Device, Drug-eluting, Two **6** Intraluminal Device, Drug-eluting, Three **7** Intraluminal Device, Drug-eluting, Four or More	**2** Sustained Release **Z** No Qualifier

047 Continued on next page

Non-OR Procedure　DRG Non-OR Procedure　Valid OR Procedure　HAC Associated Procedure　Combination Only　New/Revised April　New/Revised October

ICD-10-PCS 2025 — Lower Arteries — 047–047

047 Continued

- **0** Medical and Surgical
- **4** Lower Arteries
- **7** Dilation

Definition: Expanding an orifice or the lumen of a tubular body part

Explanation: The orifice can be a natural orifice or an artificially created orifice. Accomplished by stretching a tubular body part using intraluminal pressure or by cutting part of the orifice or wall of the tubular body part.

Body Part Character 4	Approach Character 5	Device Character 6	Qualifier Character 7
K Femoral Artery, Right 　Circumflex iliac artery 　Deep femoral artery 　Descending genicular artery 　External pudendal artery 　Superficial epigastric artery **L** Femoral Artery, Left 　See K Femoral Artery, Right **M** Popliteal Artery, Right 　Inferior genicular artery 　Middle genicular artery 　Superior genicular artery 　Sural artery 　Tibioperoneal trunk **N** Popliteal Artery, Left 　See M Popliteal Artery, Right **P** Anterior Tibial Artery, Right 　Anterior lateral malleolar artery 　Anterior medial malleolar artery 　Anterior tibial recurrent artery 　Dorsalis pedis artery 　Posterior tibial recurrent artery **Q** Anterior Tibial Artery, Left 　See P Anterior Tibial Artery, Right **R** Posterior Tibial Artery, Right **S** Posterior Tibial Artery, Left **T** Peroneal Artery, Right 　Fibular artery **U** Peroneal Artery, Left 　See T Peroneal Artery, Right	**3** Percutaneous	**D** Intraluminal Device **Z** No Device	**1** Drug-Coated Balloon **Z** No Qualifier
K Femoral Artery, Right 　Circumflex iliac artery 　Deep femoral artery 　Descending genicular artery 　External pudendal artery 　Superficial epigastric artery **L** Femoral Artery, Left 　See K Femoral Artery, Right **M** Popliteal Artery, Right 　Inferior genicular artery 　Middle genicular artery 　Superior genicular artery 　Sural artery 　Tibioperoneal trunk **N** Popliteal Artery, Left 　See M Popliteal Artery, Right **P** Anterior Tibial Artery, Right 　Anterior lateral malleolar artery 　Anterior medial malleolar artery 　Anterior tibial recurrent artery 　Dorsalis pedis artery 　Posterior tibial recurrent artery **Q** Anterior Tibial Artery, Left 　See P Anterior Tibial Artery, Right **R** Posterior Tibial Artery, Right **S** Posterior Tibial Artery, Left **T** Peroneal Artery, Right 　Fibular artery **U** Peroneal Artery, Left 　See T Peroneal Artery, Right	**3** Percutaneous	**E** Intraluminal Device, Two **F** Intraluminal Device, Three **G** Intraluminal Device, Four or More	**Z** No Qualifier

NC Noncovered Procedure　　LC Limited Coverage　　QA Questionable OB Admit　　NT New Tech Add-on　　✚ Combination Member　　♂ Male　　♀ Female

Lower Arteries

0 Medical and Surgical
4 Lower Arteries
9 Drainage   Definition: Taking or letting out fluids and/or gases from a body part
Explanation: The qualifier DIAGNOSTIC is used to identify drainage procedures that are biopsies

Body Part Character 4	Approach Character 5	Device Character 6	Qualifier Character 7
0 Abdominal Aorta Inferior phrenic artery Lumbar artery Median sacral artery Middle suprarenal artery Ovarian artery Testicular artery **1 Celiac Artery** Celiac trunk **2 Gastric Artery** Left gastric artery Right gastric artery **3 Hepatic Artery** Common hepatic artery Gastroduodenal artery Hepatic artery proper **4 Splenic Artery** Left gastroepiploic artery Pancreatic artery Short gastric artery **5 Superior Mesenteric Artery** Ileal artery Ileocolic artery Inferior pancreaticoduodenal artery Jejunal artery **6 Colic Artery, Right** **7 Colic Artery, Left** **8 Colic Artery, Middle** **9 Renal Artery, Right** Inferior suprarenal artery Renal segmental artery **A Renal Artery, Left** See 9 Renal Artery, Right **B Inferior Mesenteric Artery** Sigmoid artery Superior rectal artery **C Common Iliac Artery, Right** **D Common Iliac Artery, Left** **E Internal Iliac Artery, Right** Deferential artery Hypogastric artery Iliolumbar artery Inferior gluteal artery Inferior vesical artery Internal pudendal artery Lateral sacral artery Middle rectal artery Obturator artery Prostatic artery Superior gluteal artery Superior vesical artery Umbilical artery Uterine artery Vaginal artery	**F Internal Iliac Artery, Left** See E Internal Iliac Artery, Right **H External Iliac Artery, Right** Deep circumflex iliac artery Inferior epigastric artery **J External Iliac Artery, Left** See H External Iliac Artery, Right **K Femoral Artery, Right** Circumflex iliac artery Deep femoral artery Descending genicular artery External pudendal artery Superficial epigastric artery **L Femoral Artery, Left** See K Femoral Artery, Right **M Popliteal Artery, Right** Inferior genicular artery Middle genicular artery Superior genicular artery Sural artery Tibioperoneal trunk **N Popliteal Artery, Left** See M Popliteal Artery, Right **P Anterior Tibial Artery, Right** Anterior lateral malleolar artery Anterior medial malleolar artery Anterior tibial recurrent artery Dorsalis pedis artery Posterior tibial recurrent artery **Q Anterior Tibial Artery, Left** See P Anterior Tibial Artery, Right **R Posterior Tibial Artery, Right** **S Posterior Tibial Artery, Left** **T Peroneal Artery, Right** Fibular artery **U Peroneal Artery, Left** See T Peroneal Artery, Right **V Foot Artery, Right** Arcuate artery Dorsal metatarsal artery Lateral plantar artery Lateral tarsal artery Medial plantar artery **W Foot Artery, Left** See V Foot Artery, Right **Y Lower Artery** Umbilical artery	**0** Open **3** Percutaneous **4** Percutaneous Endoscopic	**0** Drainage Device	**Z** No Qualifier

Non-OR 049[0,1,2,3,4,5,6,7,8,9,A,B,C,D,E,F,H,J,K,L,M,N,P,Q,R,S,T,U,V,W,Y][0,3,4]0Z

049 Continued on next page

ICD-10-PCS 2025 — Lower Arteries — 049–049

0 Medical and Surgical
4 Lower Arteries
9 Drainage Definition: Taking or letting out fluids and/or gases from a body part
Explanation: The qualifier DIAGNOSTIC is used to identify drainage procedures that are biopsies

049 Continued

Body Part Character 4	Approach Character 5	Device Character 6	Qualifier Character 7

0 **Abdominal Aorta**
  Inferior phrenic artery
  Lumbar artery
  Median sacral artery
  Middle suprarenal artery
  Ovarian artery
  Testicular artery
1 **Celiac Artery**
  Celiac trunk
2 **Gastric Artery**
  Left gastric artery
  Right gastric artery
3 **Hepatic Artery**
  Common hepatic artery
  Gastroduodenal artery
  Hepatic artery proper
4 **Splenic Artery**
  Left gastroepiploic artery
  Pancreatic artery
  Short gastric artery
5 **Superior Mesenteric Artery**
  Ileal artery
  Ileocolic artery
  Inferior pancreaticoduodenal artery
  Jejunal artery
6 **Colic Artery, Right**
7 **Colic Artery, Left**
8 **Colic Artery, Middle**
9 **Renal Artery, Right**
  Inferior suprarenal artery
  Renal segmental artery
A **Renal Artery, Left**
  See 9 Renal Artery, Right
B **Inferior Mesenteric Artery**
  Sigmoid artery
  Superior rectal artery
C **Common Iliac Artery, Right**
D **Common Iliac Artery, Left**
E **Internal Iliac Artery, Right**
  Deferential artery
  Hypogastric artery
  Iliolumbar artery
  Inferior gluteal artery
  Inferior vesical artery
  Internal pudendal artery
  Lateral sacral artery
  Middle rectal artery
  Obturator artery
  Prostatic artery
  Superior gluteal artery
  Superior vesical artery
  Umbilical artery
  Uterine artery
  Vaginal artery
	F **Internal Iliac Artery, Left**
	  See E Internal Iliac Artery, Right
	H **External Iliac Artery, Right**
	  Deep circumflex iliac artery
	  Inferior epigastric artery
	J **External Iliac Artery, Left**
	  See H External Iliac Artery, Right
	K **Femoral Artery, Right**
	  Circumflex iliac artery
	  Deep femoral artery
	  Descending genicular artery
	  External pudendal artery
	  Superficial epigastric artery
	L **Femoral Artery, Left**
	  See K Femoral Artery, Right
	M **Popliteal Artery, Right**
	  Inferior genicular artery
	  Middle genicular artery
	  Superior genicular artery
	  Sural artery
	  Tibioperoneal trunk
	N **Popliteal Artery, Left**
	  See M Popliteal Artery, Right
	P **Anterior Tibial Artery, Right**
	  Anterior lateral malleolar artery
	  Anterior medial malleolar artery
	  Anterior tibial recurrent artery
	  Dorsalis pedis artery
	  Posterior tibial recurrent artery
	Q **Anterior Tibial Artery, Left**
	  See P Anterior Tibial Artery, Right
	R **Posterior Tibial Artery, Right**
	S **Posterior Tibial Artery, Left**
	T **Peroneal Artery, Right**
	  Fibular artery
	U **Peroneal Artery, Left**
	  See T Peroneal Artery, Right
	V **Foot Artery, Right**
	  Arcuate artery
	  Dorsal metatarsal artery
	  Lateral plantar artery
	  Lateral tarsal artery
	  Medial plantar artery
	W **Foot Artery, Left**
	  See V Foot Artery, Right
	Y **Lower Artery**
	  Umbilical artery
		0 Open
		3 Percutaneous
		4 Percutaneous Endoscopic
			Z No Device	**X** Diagnostic
				Z No Qualifier

Non-OR 049[0,1,2,3,4,5,6,7,8,9,A,B,C,D,E,F,H,J,K,L,M,N,P,Q,R,S,T,U,V,W,Y]3ZX
Non-OR 049[0,1,2,3,4,5,6,7,8,9,A,B,C,D,E,F,H,J,K,L,M,N,P,Q,R,S,T,U,V,W,Y][0,3,4]ZZ

0 Medical and Surgical
4 Lower Arteries
B Excision   Definition: Cutting out or off, without replacement, a portion of a body part
Explanation: The qualifier DIAGNOSTIC is used to identify excision procedures that are biopsies

Body Part Character 4	Approach Character 5	Device Character 6	Qualifier Character 7
0 Abdominal Aorta Inferior phrenic artery Lumbar artery Median sacral artery Middle suprarenal artery Ovarian artery Testicular artery **1 Celiac Artery** Celiac trunk **2 Gastric Artery** Left gastric artery Right gastric artery **3 Hepatic Artery** Common hepatic artery Gastroduodenal artery Hepatic artery proper **4 Splenic Artery** Left gastroepiploic artery Pancreatic artery Short gastric artery **5 Superior Mesenteric Artery** Ileal artery Ileocolic artery Inferior pancreaticoduodenal artery Jejunal artery **6 Colic Artery, Right** **7 Colic Artery, Left** **8 Colic Artery, Middle** **9 Renal Artery, Right** Inferior suprarenal artery Renal segmental artery **A Renal Artery, Left** See 9 Renal Artery, Right **B Inferior Mesenteric Artery** Sigmoid artery Superior rectal artery **C Common Iliac Artery, Right** **D Common Iliac Artery, Left** **E Internal Iliac Artery, Right** Deferential artery Hypogastric artery Iliolumbar artery Inferior gluteal artery Inferior vesical artery Internal pudendal artery Lateral sacral artery Middle rectal artery Obturator artery Prostatic artery Superior gluteal artery Superior vesical artery Umbilical artery Uterine artery Vaginal artery **F Internal Iliac Artery, Left** See E Internal Iliac Artery, Right **H External Iliac Artery, Right** Deep circumflex iliac artery Inferior epigastric artery **J External Iliac Artery, Left** See H External Iliac Artery, Right **K Femoral Artery, Right** Circumflex iliac artery Deep femoral artery Descending genicular artery External pudendal artery Superficial epigastric artery **L Femoral Artery, Left** See K Femoral Artery, Right **M Popliteal Artery, Right** Inferior genicular artery Middle genicular artery Superior genicular artery Sural artery Tibioperoneal trunk **N Popliteal Artery, Left** See M Popliteal Artery, Right **P Anterior Tibial Artery, Right** Anterior lateral malleolar artery Anterior medial malleolar artery Anterior tibial recurrent artery Dorsalis pedis artery Posterior tibial recurrent artery **Q Anterior Tibial Artery, Left** See P Anterior Tibial Artery, Right **R Posterior Tibial Artery, Right** **S Posterior Tibial Artery, Left** **T Peroneal Artery, Right** Fibular artery **U Peroneal Artery, Left** See T Peroneal Artery, Right **V Foot Artery, Right** Arcuate artery Dorsal metatarsal artery Lateral plantar artery Lateral tarsal artery Medial plantar artery **W Foot Artery, Left** See V Foot Artery, Right **Y Lower Artery** Umbilical artery	**0** Open **3** Percutaneous **4** Percutaneous Endoscopic	**Z** No Device	**X** Diagnostic **Z** No Qualifier

0　Medical and Surgical
4　Lower Arteries
C　Extirpation　Definition: Taking or cutting out solid matter from a body part
Explanation: The solid matter may be an abnormal byproduct of a biological function or a foreign body; it may be imbedded in a body part or in the lumen of a tubular body part. The solid matter may or may not have been previously broken into pieces.

Body Part — Character 4	Approach — Character 5	Device — Character 6	Qualifier — Character 7
0　Abdominal Aorta 　Inferior phrenic artery 　Lumbar artery 　Median sacral artery 　Middle suprarenal artery 　Ovarian artery 　Testicular artery **1　Celiac Artery** 　Celiac trunk **2　Gastric Artery** 　Left gastric artery 　Right gastric artery **3　Hepatic Artery** 　Common hepatic artery 　Gastroduodenal artery 　Hepatic artery proper **4　Splenic Artery** 　Left gastroepiploic artery 　Pancreatic artery 　Short gastric artery **5　Superior Mesenteric Artery** 　Ileal artery 　Ileocolic artery 　Inferior pancreaticoduodenal artery 　Jejunal artery **6　Colic Artery, Right** **7　Colic Artery, Left** **8　Colic Artery, Middle** **9　Renal Artery, Right** 　Inferior suprarenal artery 　Renal segmental artery **A　Renal Artery, Left** 　See 9 Renal Artery, Right **B　Inferior Mesenteric Artery** 　Sigmoid artery 　Superior rectal artery **C　Common Iliac Artery, Right** **D　Common Iliac Artery, Left** **E　Internal Iliac Artery, Right** 　Deferential artery 　Hypogastric artery 　Iliolumbar artery 　Inferior gluteal artery 　Inferior vesical artery 　Internal pudendal artery 　Lateral sacral artery 　Middle rectal artery 　Obturator artery 　Prostatic artery 　Superior gluteal artery 　Superior vesical artery 　Umbilical artery 　Uterine artery 　Vaginal artery	**F　Internal Iliac Artery, Left** 　See E Internal Iliac Artery, Right **H　External Iliac Artery, Right** 　Deep circumflex iliac artery 　Inferior epigastric artery **J　External Iliac Artery, Left** 　See H External Iliac Artery, Right **K　Femoral Artery, Right** 　Circumflex iliac artery 　Deep femoral artery 　Descending genicular artery 　External pudendal artery 　Superficial epigastric artery **L　Femoral Artery, Left** 　See K Femoral Artery, Right **M　Popliteal Artery, Right** 　Inferior genicular artery 　Middle genicular artery 　Superior genicular artery 　Sural artery 　Tibioperoneal trunk **N　Popliteal Artery, Left** 　See M Popliteal Artery, Right **P　Anterior Tibial Artery, Right** 　Anterior lateral malleolar artery 　Anterior medial malleolar artery 　Anterior tibial recurrent artery 　Dorsalis pedis artery 　Posterior tibial recurrent artery **Q　Anterior Tibial Artery, Left** 　See P Anterior Tibial Artery, Right **R　Posterior Tibial Artery, Right** **S　Posterior Tibial Artery, Left** **T　Peroneal Artery, Right** 　Fibular artery **U　Peroneal Artery, Left** 　See T Peroneal Artery, Right **V　Foot Artery, Right** 　Arcuate artery 　Dorsal metatarsal artery 　Lateral plantar artery 　Lateral tarsal artery 　Medial plantar artery **W　Foot Artery, Left** 　See V Foot Artery, Right **Y　Lower Artery** 　Umbilical artery	**0**　Open **3**　Percutaneous **4**　Percutaneous Endoscopic	**Z**　No Device	**Z**　No Qualifier

0 Medical and Surgical
4 Lower Arteries
F Fragmentation Definition: Breaking solid matter in a body part into pieces
Explanation: Physical force (e.g., manual, ultrasonic) applied directly or indirectly is used to break the solid matter into pieces. The solid matter may be an abnormal byproduct of a biological function or a foreign body. The pieces of solid matter are not taken out.

Body Part Character 4	Approach Character 5	Device Character 6	Qualifier Character 7

C Common Iliac Artery, Right
D Common Iliac Artery, Left
E Internal Iliac Artery, Right
   Deferential artery
   Hypogastric artery
   Iliolumbar artery
   Inferior gluteal artery
   Inferior vesical artery
   Internal pudendal artery
   Lateral sacral artery
   Middle rectal artery
   Obturator artery
   Prostatic artery
   Superior gluteal artery
   Superior vesical artery
   Umbilical artery
   Uterine artery
   Vaginal artery
F Internal Iliac Artery, Left
   See E Internal Iliac Artery, Right
H External Iliac Artery, Right
   Deep circumflex iliac artery
   Inferior epigastric artery
J External Iliac Artery, Left
   See H External Iliac Artery, Right
K Femoral Artery, Right
   Circumflex iliac artery
   Deep femoral artery
   Descending genicular artery
   External pudendal artery
   Superficial epigastric artery
L Femoral Artery, Left
   See K Femoral Artery, Right
M Popliteal Artery, Right
   Inferior genicular artery
   Middle genicular artery
   Superior genicular artery
   Sural artery
   Tibioperoneal trunk
N Popliteal Artery, Left
   See M Popliteal Artery, Right
P Anterior Tibial Artery, Right
   Anterior lateral malleolar artery
   Anterior medial malleolar artery
   Anterior tibial recurrent artery
   Dorsalis pedis artery
   Posterior tibial recurrent artery
Q Anterior Tibial Artery, Left
   See P Anterior Tibial Artery, Right
R Posterior Tibial Artery, Right
S Posterior Tibial Artery, Left
T Peroneal Artery, Right
   Fibular artery
U Peroneal Artery, Left
   See T Peroneal Artery, Right
Y Lower Artery
   Umbilical artery
	3 Percutaneous	Z No Device	0 Ultrasonic
			Z No Qualifier

0 Medical and Surgical
4 Lower Arteries
H Insertion   Definition: Putting in a nonbiological appliance that monitors, assists, performs, or prevents a physiological function but does not physically take the place of a body part
Explanation: None

Body Part Character 4	Approach Character 5	Device Character 6	Qualifier Character 7
0 Abdominal Aorta Inferior phrenic artery Lumbar artery Median sacral artery Middle suprarenal artery Ovarian artery Testicular artery	**0** Open **3** Percutaneous **4** Percutaneous Endoscopic	**2** Monitoring Device **3** Infusion Device **D** Intraluminal Device	**Z** No Qualifier
1 Celiac Artery Celiac trunk **2 Gastric Artery** Left gastric artery Right gastric artery **3 Hepatic Artery** Common hepatic artery Gastroduodenal artery Hepatic artery proper **4 Splenic Artery** Left gastroepiploic artery Pancreatic artery Short gastric artery **5 Superior Mesenteric Artery** Ileal artery Ileocolic artery Inferior pancreaticoduodenal artery Jejunal artery **6 Colic Artery, Right** **7 Colic Artery, Left** **8 Colic Artery, Middle** **9 Renal Artery, Right** Inferior suprarenal artery Renal segmental artery **A Renal Artery, Left** See 9 Renal Artery, Right **B Inferior Mesenteric Artery** Sigmoid artery Superior rectal artery **C Common Iliac Artery, Right** **D Common Iliac Artery, Left** **E Internal Iliac Artery, Right** Deferential artery Hypogastric artery Iliolumbar artery Inferior gluteal artery Inferior vesical artery Internal pudendal artery Lateral sacral artery Middle rectal artery Obturator artery Prostatic artery Superior gluteal artery Superior vesical artery Umbilical artery Uterine artery Vaginal artery	**F Internal Iliac Artery, Left** See E Internal Iliac Artery, Right **H External Iliac Artery, Right** Deep circumflex iliac artery Inferior epigastric artery **J External Iliac Artery, Left** See H External Iliac Artery, Right **K Femoral Artery, Right** Circumflex iliac artery Deep femoral artery Descending genicular artery External pudendal artery Superficial epigastric artery **L Femoral Artery, Left** See K Femoral Artery, Right **M Popliteal Artery, Right** Inferior genicular artery Middle genicular artery Superior genicular artery Sural artery Tibioperoneal trunk **N Popliteal Artery, Left** See M Popliteal Artery, Right **P Anterior Tibial Artery, Right** Anterior lateral malleolar artery Anterior medial malleolar artery Anterior tibial recurrent artery Dorsalis pedis artery Posterior tibial recurrent artery **Q Anterior Tibial Artery, Left** See P Anterior Tibial Artery, Right **R Posterior Tibial Artery, Right** **S Posterior Tibial Artery, Left** **T Peroneal Artery, Right** Fibular artery **U Peroneal Artery, Left** See T Peroneal Artery, Right **V Foot Artery, Right** Arcuate artery Dorsal metatarsal artery Lateral plantar artery Lateral tarsal artery Medial plantar artery **W Foot Artery, Left** See V Foot Artery, Right	**0** Open **3** Percutaneous **4** Percutaneous Endoscopic	**3** Infusion Device **D** Intraluminal Device	**Z** No Qualifier
Y Lower Artery Umbilical artery		**0** Open **3** Percutaneous **4** Percutaneous Endoscopic	**2** Monitoring Device **3** Infusion Device **D** Intraluminal Device **Y** Other Device	**Z** No Qualifier

Non-OR   04H0[0,3,4][2,3]Z
Non-OR   04H[1,2,3,4,5,6,7,8,9,A,B,C,D,E,F,H,J,K,L,M,N,P,Q,R,S,T,U,V,W][0,3,4]3Z
Non-OR   04HY32Z
Non-OR   04HY[0,3,4]3Z
Non-OR   04HY[3,4]YZ

0 Medical and Surgical
4 Lower Arteries
J Inspection

Definition: Visually and/or manually exploring a body part

Explanation: Visual exploration may be performed with or without optical instrumentation. Manual exploration may be performed directly or through intervening body layers.

Body Part Character 4	Approach Character 5	Device Character 6	Qualifier Character 7
Y Lower Artery Umbilical artery	0 Open 3 Percutaneous 4 Percutaneous Endoscopic X External	Z No Device	Z No Qualifier

Non-OR   04JY[3,4,X]ZZ

---

0 Medical and Surgical
4 Lower Arteries
L Occlusion

Definition: Completely closing an orifice or the lumen of a tubular body part

Explanation: The orifice can be a natural orifice or an artificially created orifice

Body Part Character 4	Approach Character 5	Device Character 6	Qualifier Character 7

0 Abdominal Aorta
   Inferior phrenic artery
   Lumbar artery
   Median sacral artery
   Middle suprarenal artery
   Ovarian artery
   Testicular artery
	0 Open
	3 Percutaneous
		C Extraluminal Device
		Z No Device
			Z No Qualifier

0 Abdominal Aorta
   Inferior phrenic artery
   Lumbar artery
   Median sacral artery
   Middle suprarenal artery
   Ovarian artery
   Testicular artery
	0 Open
	3 Percutaneous
		D Intraluminal Device	J Temporary
			Z No Qualifier

0 Abdominal Aorta
   Inferior phrenic artery
   Lumbar artery
   Median sacral artery
   Middle suprarenal artery
   Ovarian artery
   Testicular artery
	4 Percutaneous Endoscopic	C Extraluminal Device
		D Intraluminal Device
		Z No Device
			Z No Qualifier

04L Continued on next page

Lower Arteries

0 Medical and Surgical
4 Lower Arteries
L Occlusion

04L Continued

Definition: Completely closing an orifice or the lumen of a tubular body part
Explanation: The orifice can be a natural orifice or an artificially created orifice

Body Part Character 4	Approach Character 5	Device Character 6	Qualifier Character 7

1 Celiac Artery
   Celiac trunk
2 Gastric Artery
   Left gastric artery
   Right gastric artery
3 Hepatic Artery
   Common hepatic artery
   Gastroduodenal artery
   Hepatic artery proper
4 Splenic Artery
   Left gastroepiploic artery
   Pancreatic artery
   Short gastric artery
5 Superior Mesenteric Artery
   Ileal artery
   Ileocolic artery
   Inferior pancreaticoduodenal artery
   Jejunal artery
6 Colic Artery, Right
7 Colic Artery, Left
8 Colic Artery, Middle
9 Renal Artery, Right
   Inferior suprarenal artery
   Renal segmental artery
A Renal Artery, Left
   See 9 Renal Artery, Right
B Inferior Mesenteric Artery
   Sigmoid artery
   Superior rectal artery
C Common Iliac Artery, Right
D Common Iliac Artery, Left
H External Iliac Artery, Right
   Deep circumflex iliac artery
   Inferior epigastric artery
J External Iliac Artery, Left
   See H External Iliac Artery, Right
K Femoral Artery, Right
   Circumflex iliac artery
   Deep femoral artery
   Descending genicular artery
   External pudendal artery
   Superficial epigastric artery
L Femoral Artery, Left
   See K Femoral Artery, Right
M Popliteal Artery, Right
   Inferior genicular artery
   Middle genicular artery
   Superior genicular artery
   Sural artery
   Tibioperoneal trunk
N Popliteal Artery, Left
   See M Popliteal Artery, Right
P Anterior Tibial Artery, Right
   Anterior lateral malleolar artery
   Anterior medial malleolar artery
   Anterior tibial recurrent artery
   Dorsalis pedis artery
   Posterior tibial recurrent artery
Q Anterior Tibial Artery, Left
   See P Anterior Tibial Artery, Right
R Posterior Tibial Artery, Right
S Posterior Tibial Artery, Left
T Peroneal Artery, Right
   Fibular artery
U Peroneal Artery, Left
   See T Peroneal Artery, Right
V Foot Artery, Right
   Arcuate artery
   Dorsal metatarsal artery
   Lateral plantar artery
   Lateral tarsal artery
   Medial plantar artery
W Foot Artery, Left
   See V Foot Artery, Right
Y Lower Artery
   Umbilical artery
	0 Open
	3 Percutaneous
	4 Percutaneous Endoscopic
		C Extraluminal Device
		D Intraluminal Device
		Z No Device
			Z No Qualifier

E Internal Iliac Artery, Right
   Deferential artery
   Hypogastric artery
   Iliolumbar artery
   Inferior gluteal artery
   Inferior vesical artery
   Internal pudendal artery
   Lateral sacral artery
   Middle rectal artery
   Obturator artery
   Prostatic artery
   Superior gluteal artery
   Superior vesical artery
   Umbilical artery
   Uterine artery
   Vaginal artery
	0 Open
	3 Percutaneous
	4 Percutaneous Endoscopic
		C Extraluminal Device
		D Intraluminal Device
		Z No Device
			T Uterine Artery, Right
			V Prostatic Artery, Right
			Z No Qualifier

F Internal Iliac Artery, Left
   Deferential artery
   Hypogastric artery
   Iliolumbar artery
   Inferior gluteal artery
   Inferior vesical artery
   Internal pudendal artery
   Lateral sacral artery
   Middle rectal artery
   Obturator artery
   Prostatic artery
   Superior gluteal artery
   Superior vesical artery
   Umbilical artery
   Uterine artery
   Vaginal artery
	0 Open
	3 Percutaneous
	4 Percutaneous Endoscopic
		C Extraluminal Device
		D Intraluminal Device
		Z No Device
			U Uterine Artery, Left
			W Prostatic Artery, Left
			Z No Qualifier

NC Noncovered Procedure   **LC** Limited Coverage   **QA** Questionable OB Admit   **NT** New Tech Add-on   ✚ Combination Member   ♂ Male   ♀ Female

0 Medical and Surgical
4 Lower Arteries
N Release Definition: Freeing a body part from an abnormal physical constraint by cutting or by the use of force
Explanation: Some of the restraining tissue may be taken out but none of the body part is taken out

Body Part Character 4	Approach Character 5	Device Character 6	Qualifier Character 7

0 Abdominal Aorta
  Inferior phrenic artery
  Lumbar artery
  Median sacral artery
  Middle suprarenal artery
  Ovarian artery
  Testicular artery
1 Celiac Artery
  Celiac trunk
2 Gastric Artery
  Left gastric artery
  Right gastric artery
3 Hepatic Artery
  Common hepatic artery
  Gastroduodenal artery
  Hepatic artery proper
4 Splenic Artery
  Left gastroepiploic artery
  Pancreatic artery
  Short gastric artery
5 Superior Mesenteric Artery
  Ileal artery
  Ileocolic artery
  Inferior pancreaticoduodenal artery
  Jejunal artery
6 Colic Artery, Right
7 Colic Artery, Left
8 Colic Artery, Middle
9 Renal Artery, Right
  Inferior suprarenal artery
  Renal segmental artery
A Renal Artery, Left
  See 9 Renal Artery, Right
B Inferior Mesenteric Artery
  Sigmoid artery
  Superior rectal artery
C Common Iliac Artery, Right
D Common Iliac Artery, Left
E Internal Iliac Artery, Right
  Deferential artery
  Hypogastric artery
  Iliolumbar artery
  Inferior gluteal artery
  Inferior vesical artery
  Internal pudendal artery
  Lateral sacral artery
  Middle rectal artery
  Obturator artery
  Prostatic artery
  Superior gluteal artery
  Superior vesical artery
  Umbilical artery
  Uterine artery
  Vaginal artery
F Internal Iliac Artery, Left
  See E Internal Iliac Artery, Right
H External Iliac Artery, Right
  Deep circumflex iliac artery
  Inferior epigastric artery
J External Iliac Artery, Left
  See H External Iliac Artery, Right
K Femoral Artery, Right
  Circumflex iliac artery
  Deep femoral artery
  Descending genicular artery
  External pudendal artery
  Superficial epigastric artery
L Femoral Artery, Left
  See K Femoral Artery, Right
M Popliteal Artery, Right
  Inferior genicular artery
  Middle genicular artery
  Superior genicular artery
  Sural artery
  Tibioperoneal trunk
N Popliteal Artery, Left
  See M Popliteal Artery, Right
P Anterior Tibial Artery, Right
  Anterior lateral malleolar artery
  Anterior medial malleolar artery
  Anterior tibial recurrent artery
  Dorsalis pedis artery
  Posterior tibial recurrent artery
Q Anterior Tibial Artery, Left
  See P Anterior Tibial Artery, Right
R Posterior Tibial Artery, Right
S Posterior Tibial Artery, Left
T Peroneal Artery, Right
  Fibular artery
U Peroneal Artery, Left
  See T Peroneal Artery, Right
V Foot Artery, Right
  Arcuate artery
  Dorsal metatarsal artery
  Lateral plantar artery
  Lateral tarsal artery
  Medial plantar artery
W Foot Artery, Left
  See V Foot Artery, Right
Y Lower Artery
  Umbilical artery
	0 Open
	3 Percutaneous
	4 Percutaneous Endoscopic
		Z No Device	**Z** No Qualifier

0 Medical and Surgical
4 Lower Arteries
P Removal Definition: Taking out or off a device from a body part

Explanation: If a device is taken out and a similar device put in without cutting or puncturing the skin or mucous membrane, the procedure is coded to the root operation CHANGE. Otherwise, the procedure for taking out a device is coded to the root operation REMOVAL.

Body Part Character 4	Approach Character 5	Device Character 6	Qualifier Character 7
Y Lower Artery Umbilical artery	0 Open 3 Percutaneous 4 Percutaneous Endoscopic	0 Drainage Device 2 Monitoring Device 3 Infusion Device 7 Autologous Tissue Substitute C Extraluminal Device D Intraluminal Device J Synthetic Substitute K Nonautologous Tissue Substitute Y Other Device	Z No Qualifier
Y Lower Artery Umbilical artery	X External	0 Drainage Device 1 Radioactive Element 2 Monitoring Device 3 Infusion Device D Intraluminal Device	Z No Qualifier

Non-OR 04PY3[0,2,3,D]Z
Non-OR 04PY[3,4]YZ
Non-OR 04PYX[0,1,2,3,D]Z

0 Medical and Surgical
4 Lower Arteries
Q Repair Definition: Restoring, to the extent possible, a body part to its normal anatomic structure and function
Explanation: Used only when the method to accomplish the repair is not one of the other root operations

Body Part Character 4	Approach Character 5	Device Character 6	Qualifier Character 7
0 Abdominal Aorta Inferior phrenic artery Lumbar artery Median sacral artery Middle suprarenal artery Ovarian artery Testicular artery **1 Celiac Artery** Celiac trunk **2 Gastric Artery** Left gastric artery Right gastric artery **3 Hepatic Artery** Common hepatic artery Gastroduodenal artery Hepatic artery proper **4 Splenic Artery** Left gastroepiploic artery Pancreatic artery Short gastric artery **5 Superior Mesenteric Artery** Ileal artery Ileocolic artery Inferior pancreaticoduodenal artery Jejunal artery **6 Colic Artery, Right** **7 Colic Artery, Left** **8 Colic Artery, Middle** **9 Renal Artery, Right** Inferior suprarenal artery Renal segmental artery **A Renal Artery, Left** See 9 Renal Artery, Right **B Inferior Mesenteric Artery** Sigmoid artery Superior rectal artery **C Common Iliac Artery, Right** **D Common Iliac Artery, Left** **E Internal Iliac Artery, Right** Deferential artery Hypogastric artery Iliolumbar artery Inferior gluteal artery Inferior vesical artery Internal pudendal artery Lateral sacral artery Middle rectal artery Obturator artery Prostatic artery Superior gluteal artery Superior vesical artery Umbilical artery Uterine artery Vaginal artery	**F Internal Iliac Artery, Left** See E Internal Iliac Artery, Right **H External Iliac Artery, Right** Deep circumflex iliac artery Inferior epigastric artery **J External Iliac Artery, Left** See H External Iliac Artery, Right **K Femoral Artery, Right** Circumflex iliac artery Deep femoral artery Descending genicular artery External pudendal artery Superficial epigastric artery **L Femoral Artery, Left** See K Femoral Artery, Right **M Popliteal Artery, Right** Inferior genicular artery Middle genicular artery Superior genicular artery Sural artery Tibioperoneal trunk **N Popliteal Artery, Left** See M Popliteal Artery, Right **P Anterior Tibial Artery, Right** Anterior lateral malleolar artery Anterior medial malleolar artery Anterior tibial recurrent artery Dorsalis pedis artery Posterior tibial recurrent artery **Q Anterior Tibial Artery, Left** See P Anterior Tibial Artery, Right **R Posterior Tibial Artery, Right** **S Posterior Tibial Artery, Left** **T Peroneal Artery, Right** Fibular artery **U Peroneal Artery, Left** See T Peroneal Artery, Right **V Foot Artery, Right** Arcuate artery Dorsal metatarsal artery Lateral plantar artery Lateral tarsal artery Medial plantar artery **W Foot Artery, Left** See V Foot Artery, Right **Y Lower Artery** Umbilical artery	**0 Open** **3 Percutaneous** **4 Percutaneous Endoscopic**	**Z No Device**	**Z No Qualifier**

0   Medical and Surgical
4   Lower Arteries
R   Replacement Definition: Putting in or on biological or synthetic material that physically takes the place and/or function of all or a portion of a body part
Explanation: The body part may have been taken out or replaced, or may be taken out, physically eradicated, or rendered nonfunctional during the REPLACEMENT procedure. A REMOVAL procedure is coded for taking out the device used in a previous replacement procedure.

Body Part Character 4	Approach Character 5	Device Character 6	Qualifier Character 7

0 Abdominal Aorta
  Inferior phrenic artery
  Lumbar artery
  Median sacral artery
  Middle suprarenal artery
  Ovarian artery
  Testicular artery
1 Celiac Artery
  Celiac trunk
2 Gastric Artery
  Left gastric artery
  Right gastric artery
3 Hepatic Artery
  Common hepatic artery
  Gastroduodenal artery
  Hepatic artery proper
4 Splenic Artery
  Left gastroepiploic artery
  Pancreatic artery
  Short gastric artery
5 Superior Mesenteric Artery
  Ileal artery
  Ileocolic artery
  Inferior pancreaticoduodenal artery
  Jejunal artery
6 Colic Artery, Right
7 Colic Artery, Left
8 Colic Artery, Middle
9 Renal Artery, Right
  Inferior suprarenal artery
  Renal segmental artery
A Renal Artery, Left
  See 9 Renal Artery, Right
B Inferior Mesenteric Artery
  Sigmoid artery
  Superior rectal artery
C Common Iliac Artery, Right
D Common Iliac Artery, Left
E Internal Iliac Artery, Right
  Deferential artery
  Hypogastric artery
  Iliolumbar artery
  Inferior gluteal artery
  Inferior vesical artery
  Internal pudendal artery
  Lateral sacral artery
  Middle rectal artery
  Obturator artery
  Prostatic artery
  Superior gluteal artery
  Superior vesical artery
  Umbilical artery
  Uterine artery
  Vaginal artery
F Internal Iliac Artery, Left
  See E Internal Iliac Artery, Right
H External Iliac Artery, Right
  Deep circumflex iliac artery
  Inferior epigastric artery
J External Iliac Artery, Left
  See H External Iliac Artery, Right
K Femoral Artery, Right
  Circumflex iliac artery
  Deep femoral artery
  Descending genicular artery
  External pudendal artery
  Superficial epigastric artery
L Femoral Artery, Left
  See K Femoral Artery, Right
M Popliteal Artery, Right
  Inferior genicular artery
  Middle genicular artery
  Superior genicular artery
  Sural artery
  Tibioperoneal trunk
N Popliteal Artery, Left
  See M Popliteal Artery, Right
P Anterior Tibial Artery, Right
  Anterior lateral malleolar artery
  Anterior medial malleolar artery
  Anterior tibial recurrent artery
  Dorsalis pedis artery
  Posterior tibial recurrent artery
Q Anterior Tibial Artery, Left
  See P Anterior Tibial Artery, Right
R Posterior Tibial Artery, Right
S Posterior Tibial Artery, Left
T Peroneal Artery, Right
  Fibular artery
U Peroneal Artery, Left
  See T Peroneal Artery, Right
V Foot Artery, Right
  Arcuate artery
  Dorsal metatarsal artery
  Lateral plantar artery
  Lateral tarsal artery
  Medial plantar artery
W Foot Artery, Left
  See V Foot Artery, Right
Y Lower Artery
  Umbilical artery
	0 Open
	4 Percutaneous Endoscopic
		7 Autologous Tissue Substitute
		J Synthetic Substitute
		K Nonautologous Tissue Substitute
			Z No Qualifier

0 Medical and Surgical
4 Lower Arteries
S Reposition

Definition: Moving to its normal location, or other suitable location, all or a portion of a body part
Explanation: The body part is moved to a new location from an abnormal location, or from a normal location where it is not functioning correctly. The body part may or may not be cut out or off to be moved to the new location.

Body Part Character 4	Approach Character 5	Device Character 6	Qualifier Character 7
0 Abdominal Aorta Inferior phrenic artery Lumbar artery Median sacral artery Middle suprarenal artery Ovarian artery Testicular artery **1 Celiac Artery** Celiac trunk **2 Gastric Artery** Left gastric artery Right gastric artery **3 Hepatic Artery** Common hepatic artery Gastroduodenal artery Hepatic artery proper **4 Splenic Artery** Left gastroepiploic artery Pancreatic artery Short gastric artery **5 Superior Mesenteric Artery** Ileal artery Ileocolic artery Inferior pancreaticoduodenal artery Jejunal artery **6 Colic Artery, Right** **7 Colic Artery, Left** **8 Colic Artery, Middle** **9 Renal Artery, Right** Inferior suprarenal artery Renal segmental artery **A Renal Artery, Left** See 9 Renal Artery, Right **B Inferior Mesenteric Artery** Sigmoid artery Superior rectal artery **C Common Iliac Artery, Right** **D Common Iliac Artery, Left** **E Internal Iliac Artery, Right** Deferential artery Hypogastric artery Iliolumbar artery Inferior gluteal artery Inferior vesical artery Internal pudendal artery Lateral sacral artery Middle rectal artery Obturator artery Prostatic artery Superior gluteal artery Superior vesical artery Umbilical artery Uterine artery Vaginal artery	**F Internal Iliac Artery, Left** See E Internal Iliac Artery, Right **H External Iliac Artery, Right** Deep circumflex iliac artery Inferior epigastric artery **J External Iliac Artery, Left** See H External Iliac Artery, Right **K Femoral Artery, Right** Circumflex iliac artery Deep femoral artery Descending genicular artery External pudendal artery Superficial epigastric artery **L Femoral Artery, Left** See K Femoral Artery, Right **M Popliteal Artery, Right** Inferior genicular artery Middle genicular artery Superior genicular artery Sural artery Tibioperoneal trunk **N Popliteal Artery, Left** See M Popliteal Artery, Right **P Anterior Tibial Artery, Right** Anterior lateral malleolar artery Anterior medial malleolar artery Anterior tibial recurrent artery Dorsalis pedis artery Posterior tibial recurrent artery **Q Anterior Tibial Artery, Left** See P Anterior Tibial Artery, Right **R Posterior Tibial Artery, Right** **S Posterior Tibial Artery, Left** **T Peroneal Artery, Right** Fibular artery **U Peroneal Artery, Left** See T Peroneal Artery, Right **V Foot Artery, Right** Arcuate artery Dorsal metatarsal artery Lateral plantar artery Lateral tarsal artery Medial plantar artery **W Foot Artery, Left** See V Foot Artery, Right **Y Lower Artery** Umbilical artery	**0** Open **3** Percutaneous **4** Percutaneous Endoscopic	**Z** No Device	**Z** No Qualifier

ICD-10-PCS 2025 — Lower Arteries — 04U–04U

- **0** Medical and Surgical
- **4** Lower Arteries
- **U** Supplement

Definition: Putting in or on biological or synthetic material that physically reinforces and/or augments the function of a portion of a body part

Explanation: The biological material is non-living, or is living and from the same individual. The body part may have been previously replaced, and the SUPPLEMENT procedure is performed to physically reinforce and/or augment the function of the replaced body part.

Body Part — Character 4	Approach — Character 5	Device — Character 6	Qualifier — Character 7

0 Abdominal Aorta
  Inferior phrenic artery
  Lumbar artery
  Median sacral artery
  Middle suprarenal artery
  Ovarian artery
  Testicular artery
1 Celiac Artery
  Celiac trunk
2 Gastric Artery
  Left gastric artery
  Right gastric artery
3 Hepatic Artery
  Common hepatic artery
  Gastroduodenal artery
  Hepatic artery proper
4 Splenic Artery
  Left gastroepiploic artery
  Pancreatic artery
  Short gastric artery
5 Superior Mesenteric Artery
  Ileal artery
  Ileocolic artery
  Inferior pancreaticoduodenal artery
  Jejunal artery
6 Colic Artery, Right
7 Colic Artery, Left
8 Colic Artery, Middle
9 Renal Artery, Right
  Inferior suprarenal artery
  Renal segmental artery
A Renal Artery, Left
  See 9 Renal Artery, Right
B Inferior Mesenteric Artery
  Sigmoid artery
  Superior rectal artery
C Common Iliac Artery, Right
D Common Iliac Artery, Left
E Internal Iliac Artery, Right
  Deferential artery
  Hypogastric artery
  Iliolumbar artery
  Inferior gluteal artery
  Inferior vesical artery
  Internal pudendal artery
  Lateral sacral artery
  Middle rectal artery
  Obturator artery
  Prostatic artery
  Superior gluteal artery
  Superior vesical artery
  Umbilical artery
  Uterine artery
  Vaginal artery
F Internal Iliac Artery, Left
  See E Internal Iliac Artery, Right
H External Iliac Artery, Right
  Deep circumflex iliac artery
  Inferior epigastric artery
J External Iliac Artery, Left
  See H External Iliac Artery, Right
K Femoral Artery, Right
  Circumflex iliac artery
  Deep femoral artery
  Descending genicular artery
  External pudendal artery
  Superficial epigastric artery
L Femoral Artery, Left
  See K Femoral Artery, Right
M Popliteal Artery, Right
  Inferior genicular artery
  Middle genicular artery
  Superior genicular artery
  Sural artery
  Tibioperoneal trunk
N Popliteal Artery, Left
  See M Popliteal Artery, Right
P Anterior Tibial Artery, Right
  Anterior lateral malleolar artery
  Anterior medial malleolar artery
  Anterior tibial recurrent artery
  Dorsalis pedis artery
  Posterior tibial recurrent artery
Q Anterior Tibial Artery, Left
  See P Anterior Tibial Artery, Right
R Posterior Tibial Artery, Right
S Posterior Tibial Artery, Left
T Peroneal Artery, Right
  Fibular artery
U Peroneal Artery, Left
  See T Peroneal Artery, Right
V Foot Artery, Right
  Arcuate artery
  Dorsal metatarsal artery
  Lateral plantar artery
  Lateral tarsal artery
  Medial plantar artery
W Foot Artery, Left
  See V Foot Artery, Right
Y Lower Artery
  Umbilical artery
	0 Open
	3 Percutaneous
	4 Percutaneous Endoscopic
		7 Autologous Tissue Substitute
		J Synthetic Substitute
		K Nonautologous Tissue Substitute
			Z No Qualifier

Ø Medical and Surgical
4 Lower Arteries
V Restriction

Definition: Partially closing an orifice or the lumen of a tubular body part
Explanation: The orifice can be a natural orifice or an artificially created orifice

Body Part Character 4	Approach Character 5	Device Character 6	Qualifier Character 7
Ø Abdominal Aorta Inferior phrenic artery Lumbar artery Median sacral artery Middle suprarenal artery Ovarian artery Testicular artery	**Ø** Open **3** Percutaneous **4** Percutaneous Endoscopic	**C** Extraluminal Device **E** Intraluminal Device, Branched or Fenestrated, One or Two Arteries **F** Intraluminal Device, Branched or Fenestrated, Three or More Arteries **Z** No Device	**Z** No Qualifier
Ø Abdominal Aorta Inferior phrenic artery Lumbar artery Median sacral artery Middle suprarenal artery Ovarian artery Testicular artery	**Ø** Open **3** Percutaneous **4** Percutaneous Endoscopic	**D** Intraluminal Device	**J** Temporary **Z** No Qualifier
1 Celiac Artery Celiac trunk **2 Gastric Artery** Left gastric artery Right gastric artery **3 Hepatic Artery** Common hepatic artery Gastroduodenal artery Hepatic artery proper **4 Splenic Artery** Left gastroepiploic artery Pancreatic artery Short gastric artery **5 Superior Mesenteric Artery** Ileal artery Ileocolic artery Inferior pancreaticoduodenal artery Jejunal artery **6 Colic Artery, Right** **7 Colic Artery, Left** **8 Colic Artery, Middle** **9 Renal Artery, Right** Inferior suprarenal artery Renal segmental artery **A Renal Artery, Left** See 9 Renal Artery, Right **B Inferior Mesenteric Artery** Sigmoid artery Superior rectal artery **E Internal Iliac Artery, Right** Deferential artery Hypogastric artery Iliolumbar artery Inferior gluteal artery Inferior vesical artery Internal pudendal artery Lateral sacral artery Middle rectal artery Obturator artery Prostatic artery Superior gluteal artery Superior vesical artery Umbilical artery Uterine artery Vaginal artery **F Internal Iliac Artery, Left** See E Internal Iliac Artery, Right **H External Iliac Artery, Right** Deep circumflex iliac artery Inferior epigastric artery **J External Iliac Artery, Left** See H External Iliac Artery, Right **K Femoral Artery, Right** Circumflex iliac artery Deep femoral artery Descending genicular artery External pudendal artery Superficial epigastric artery **L Femoral Artery, Left** See K Femoral Artery, Right **M Popliteal Artery, Right** Inferior genicular artery Middle genicular artery Superior genicular artery Sural artery Tibioperoneal trunk **N Popliteal Artery, Left** See M Popliteal Artery, Right **P Anterior Tibial Artery, Right** Anterior lateral malleolar artery Anterior medial malleolar artery Anterior tibial recurrent artery Dorsalis pedis artery Posterior tibial recurrent artery **Q Anterior Tibial Artery, Left** See P Anterior Tibial Artery, Right **R Posterior Tibial Artery, Right** **S Posterior Tibial Artery, Left** **T Peroneal Artery, Right** Fibular artery **U Peroneal Artery, Left** See T Peroneal Artery, Right **V Foot Artery, Right** Arcuate artery Dorsal metatarsal artery Lateral plantar artery Lateral tarsal artery Medial plantar artery **W Foot Artery, Left** See V Foot Artery, Right **Y Lower Artery** Umbilical artery	**Ø** Open **3** Percutaneous **4** Percutaneous Endoscopic	**C** Extraluminal Device **D** Intraluminal Device **Z** No Device	**Z** No Qualifier
C Common Iliac Artery, Right **D Common Iliac Artery, Left**	**Ø** Open **3** Percutaneous **4** Percutaneous Endoscopic	**C** Extraluminal Device **D** Intraluminal Device **E** Intraluminal Device, Branched or Fenestrated, One or Two Arteries **Z** No Device	**Z** No Qualifier

0 Medical and Surgical
4 Lower Arteries
W Revision

Definition: Correcting, to the extent possible, a portion of a malfunctioning device or the position of a displaced device

Explanation: Revision can include correcting a malfunctioning or displaced device by taking out or putting in components of the device such as a screw or pin

Body Part Character 4	Approach Character 5	Device Character 6	Qualifier Character 7
Y Lower Artery Umbilical artery	0 Open 3 Percutaneous 4 Percutaneous Endoscopic	0 Drainage Device 2 Monitoring Device 3 Infusion Device 7 Autologous Tissue Substitute C Extraluminal Device D Intraluminal Device J Synthetic Substitute K Nonautologous Tissue Substitute Y Other Device	Z No Qualifier
Y Lower Artery Umbilical artery	X External	0 Drainage Device 2 Monitoring Device 3 Infusion Device 7 Autologous Tissue Substitute C Extraluminal Device D Intraluminal Device J Synthetic Substitute K Nonautologous Tissue Substitute	Z No Qualifier

Non-OR 04WY3[0,2,3]Z
Non-OR 04WY[3,4]YZ
Non-OR 04WYX[0,2,3,7,C,D,J,K]Z

Upper Veins Ø51–Ø5W

Character Meanings

This Character Meaning table is provided as a guide to assist the user in the identification of character members that may be found in this section of code tables. It **SHOULD NOT** be used to build a PCS code.

Operation–Character 3		Body Part–Character 4		Approach–Character 5		Device–Character 6		Qualifier–Character 7	
1	Bypass	Ø	Azygos Vein	Ø	Open	Ø	Drainage Device	Ø	Ultrasonic
5	Destruction	1	Hemiazygos Vein	3	Percutaneous	2	Monitoring Device	1	Drug-Coated Balloon
7	Dilation	3	Innominate Vein, Right	4	Percutaneous Endoscopic	3	Infusion Device	X	Diagnostic
9	Drainage	4	Innominate Vein, Left	X	External	7	Autologous Tissue Substitute	Y	Upper Vein
B	Excision	5	Subclavian Vein, Right			9	Autologous Venous Tissue	Z	No Qualifier
C	Extirpation	6	Subclavian Vein, Left			A	Autologous Arterial Tissue		
D	Extraction	7	Axillary Vein, Right			C	Extraluminal Device		
F	Fragmentation	8	Axillary Vein, Left			D	Intraluminal Device		
H	Insertion	9	Brachial Vein, Right			J	Synthetic Substitute		
J	Inspection	A	Brachial Vein, Left			K	Nonautologous Tissue Substitute		
L	Occlusion	B	Basilic Vein, Right			M	Neurostimulator Lead		
N	Release	C	Basilic Vein, Left			Y	Other Device		
P	Removal	D	Cephalic Vein, Right			Z	No Device		
Q	Repair	F	Cephalic Vein, Left						
R	Replacement	G	Hand Vein, Right						
S	Reposition	H	Hand Vein, Left						
U	Supplement	L	Intracranial Vein						
V	Restriction	M	Internal Jugular Vein, Right						
W	Revision	N	Internal Jugular Vein, Left						
		P	External Jugular Vein, Right						
		Q	External Jugular Vein, Left						
		R	Vertebral Vein, Right						
		S	Vertebral Vein, Left						
		T	Face Vein, Right						
		V	Face Vein, Left						
		Y	Upper Vein						

AHA Coding Clinic for Upper Veins
2022, 1Q, 10-13 Procedures performed on a continuous vessel, ICD-10-PCS Guideline B4.1c

AHA Coding Clinic for table Ø51
2020, 1Q, 28 Free flap microvascular breast reconstruction
2017, 3Q, 15 Bypass of innominate vein to atrial appendage

AHA Coding Clinic for table Ø57
2020, 3Q, 38 Thrombectomy of arteriovenous fistula with angioplasty and stent placement

AHA Coding Clinic for table Ø59
2018, 3Q, 7 Catheter placement for treatment of congestive heart failure

AHA Coding Clinic for table Ø5B
2021, 2Q, 15 Excision of pituitary macroadenoma within cavernous sinus
2020, 3Q, 40 Excision of ulceration of arteriovenous fistula
2020, 1Q, 24 Resection of vascular malformation, likely cavernoma
2016, 2Q, 12 Resection of malignant neoplasm of infratemporal fossa

AHA Coding Clinic for table Ø5C
2023, 3Q, 24 Thrombectomy of HeRO® graft
2020, 3Q, 37 Repair of aneurysm of arteriovenous fistula with endovenectomy
2020, 3Q, 38 Thrombectomy of arteriovenous fistula with angioplasty and stent placement

AHA Coding Clinic for table Ø5F
2020, 4Q, 45-49 New fragmentation tables
2020, 4Q, 49-50 Intravascular ultrasound assisted thrombolysis
2020, 4Q, 50 Intravascular lithotripsy

AHA Coding Clinic for table Ø5H
2016, 4Q, 97-98 Phrenic neurostimulator

AHA Coding Clinic for table Ø5P
2016, 4Q, 97-98 Phrenic neurostimulator

AHA Coding Clinic for table Ø5Q
2017, 3Q, 15 Bypass of innominate vein to atrial appendage

AHA Coding Clinic for table Ø5S
2013, 4Q, 125 Stage II cephalic vein transposition (superficialization) of arteriovenous fistula

AHA Coding Clinic for table Ø5V
2020, 3Q, 37 Repair of aneurysm of arteriovenous fistula with endovenectomy

AHA Coding Clinic for table Ø5W
2023, 3Q, 24 Thrombectomy of HeRO® graft
2016, 4Q, 97-98 Phrenic neurostimulator

Upper Veins

Head and Neck Veins

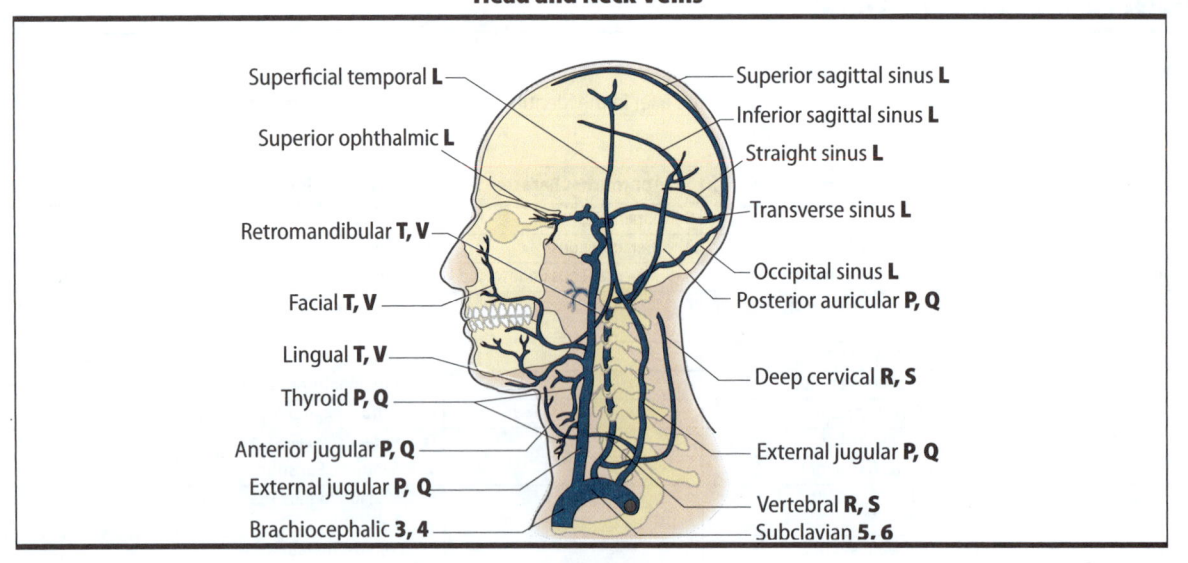

- Superficial temporal **L**
- Superior ophthalmic **L**
- Retromandibular **T, V**
- Facial **T, V**
- Lingual **T, V**
- Thyroid **P, Q**
- Anterior jugular **P, Q**
- External jugular **P, Q**
- Brachiocephalic **3, 4**
- Superior sagittal sinus **L**
- Inferior sagittal sinus **L**
- Straight sinus **L**
- Transverse sinus **L**
- Occipital sinus **L**
- Posterior auricular **P, Q**
- Deep cervical **R, S**
- External jugular **P, Q**
- Vertebral **R, S**
- Subclavian **5, 6**

Upper Veins

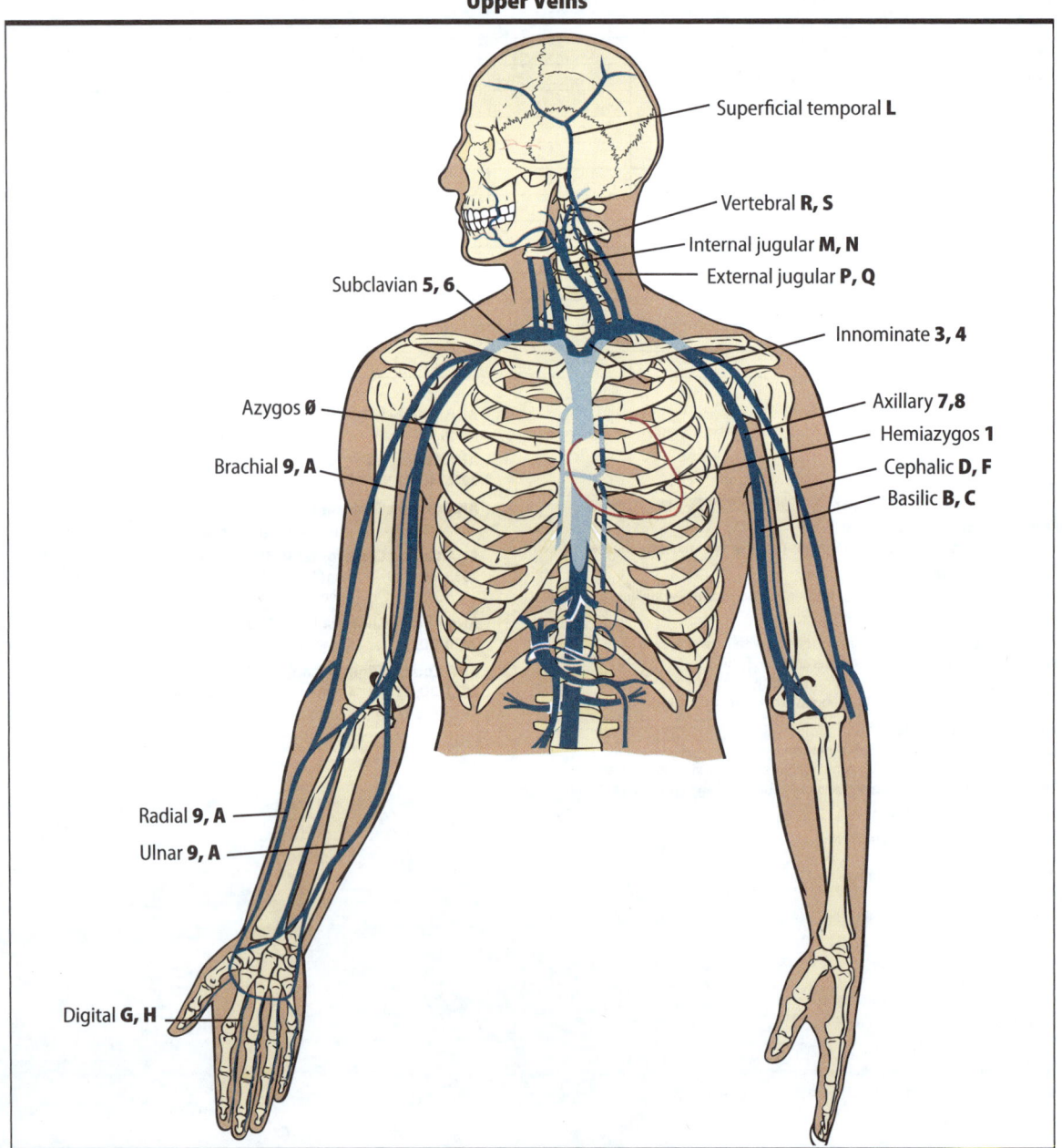

- Superficial temporal **L**
- Vertebral **R, S**
- Internal jugular **M, N**
- External jugular **P, Q**
- Subclavian **5, 6**
- Innominate **3, 4**
- Azygos **Ø**
- Axillary **7, 8**
- Brachial **9, A**
- Hemiazygos **1**
- Cephalic **D, F**
- Basilic **B, C**
- Radial **9, A**
- Ulnar **9, A**
- Digital **G, H**

ICD-10-PCS 2025 — Upper Veins — 051–051

0 Medical and Surgical
5 Upper Veins
1 Bypass — Definition: Altering the route of passage of the contents of a tubular body part
Explanation: Rerouting contents of a body part to a downstream area of the normal route, to a similar route and body part, or to an abnormal route and dissimilar body part. Includes one or more anastomoses, with or without the use of a device.

Body Part Character 4	Approach Character 5	Device Character 6	Qualifier Character 7
0 Azygos Vein Right ascending lumbar vein Right subcostal vein **1 Hemiazygos Vein** Left ascending lumbar vein Left subcostal vein **3 Innominate Vein, Right** Brachiocephalic vein Inferior thyroid vein **4 Innominate Vein, Left** See 3 Innominate Vein, Right **5 Subclavian Vein, Right** **6 Subclavian Vein, Left** **7 Axillary Vein, Right** **8 Axillary Vein, Left** **9 Brachial Vein, Right** Radial vein Ulnar vein **A Brachial Vein, Left** See 9 Brachial Vein, Right **B Basilic Vein, Right** Median antebrachial vein Median cubital vein **C Basilic Vein, Left** See B Basilic Vein, Right **D Cephalic Vein, Right** Accessory cephalic vein **F Cephalic Vein, Left** See D Cephalic Vein, Right **G Hand Vein, Right** Dorsal metacarpal vein Palmar (volar) digital vein Palmar (volar) metacarpal vein Superficial palmar venous arch Volar (palmar) digital vein Volar (palmar) metacarpal vein **H Hand Vein, Left** See G Hand Vein, Right **L Intracranial Vein** Anterior cerebral vein Basal (internal) cerebral vein Dural venous sinus Great cerebral vein Inferior cerebellar vein Inferior cerebral vein Internal (basal) cerebral vein Middle cerebral vein Ophthalmic vein Superior cerebellar vein Superior cerebral vein **M Internal Jugular Vein, Right** **N Internal Jugular Vein, Left** **P External Jugular Vein, Right** Posterior auricular vein **Q External Jugular Vein, Left** See P External Jugular Vein, Right **R Vertebral Vein, Right** Deep cervical vein Suboccipital venous plexus **S Vertebral Vein, Left** See R Vertebral Vein, Right **T Face Vein, Right** Angular vein Anterior facial vein Common facial vein Deep facial vein Frontal vein Posterior facial (retromandibular) vein Supraorbital vein **V Face Vein, Left** See T Face Vein, Right	**0** Open **4** Percutaneous Endoscopic	**7** Autologous Tissue Substitute **9** Autologous Venous Tissue **A** Autologous Arterial Tissue **J** Synthetic Substitute **K** Nonautologous Tissue Substitute **Z** No Device	**Y** Upper Vein

0 Medical and Surgical
5 Upper Veins
5 Destruction Definition: Physical eradication of all or a portion of a body part by the direct use of energy, force, or a destructive agent
Explanation: None of the body part is physically taken out

Body Part Character 4	Approach Character 5	Device Character 6	Qualifier Character 7

0 Azygos Vein
   Right ascending lumbar vein
   Right subcostal vein
1 Hemiazygos Vein
   Left ascending lumbar vein
   Left subcostal vein
3 Innominate Vein, Right
   Brachiocephalic vein
   Inferior thyroid vein
4 Innominate Vein, Left
   See *3 Innominate Vein, Right*
5 Subclavian Vein, Right
6 Subclavian Vein, Left
7 Axillary Vein, Right
8 Axillary Vein, Left
9 Brachial Vein, Right
   Radial vein
   Ulnar vein
A Brachial Vein, Left
   See *9 Brachial Vein, Right*
B Basilic Vein, Right
   Median antebrachial vein
   Median cubital vein
C Basilic Vein, Left
   See *B Basilic Vein, Right*
D Cephalic Vein, Right
   Accessory cephalic vein
F Cephalic Vein, Left
   See *D Cephalic Vein, Right*
G Hand Vein, Right
   Dorsal metacarpal vein
   Palmar (volar) digital vein
   Palmar (volar) metacarpal vein
   Superficial palmar venous arch
   Volar (palmar) digital vein
   Volar (palmar) metacarpal vein
H Hand Vein, Left
   See *G Hand Vein, Right*
L Intracranial Vein
   Anterior cerebral vein
   Basal (internal) cerebral vein
   Dural venous sinus
   Great cerebral vein
   Inferior cerebellar vein
   Inferior cerebral vein
   Internal (basal) cerebral vein
   Middle cerebral vein
   Ophthalmic vein
   Superior cerebellar vein
   Superior cerebral vein
M Internal Jugular Vein, Right
N Internal Jugular Vein, Left
P External Jugular Vein, Right
   Posterior auricular vein
Q External Jugular Vein, Left
   See *P External Jugular Vein, Right*
R Vertebral Vein, Right
   Deep cervical vein
   Suboccipital venous plexus
S Vertebral Vein, Left
   See *R Vertebral Vein, Right*
T Face Vein, Right
   Angular vein
   Anterior facial vein
   Common facial vein
   Deep facial vein
   Frontal vein
   Posterior facial (retromandibular) vein
   Supraorbital vein
V Face Vein, Left
   See *T Face Vein, Right*
Y Upper Vein
	0 Open
	3 Percutaneous
	4 Percutaneous Endoscopic
		Z No Device	**Z** No Qualifier

ICD-10-PCS 2025 — Upper Veins — 057–057

- 0 Medical and Surgical
- 5 Upper Veins
- 7 Dilation Definition: Expanding an orifice or the lumen of a tubular body part
  Explanation: The orifice can be a natural orifice or an artificially created orifice. Accomplished by stretching a tubular body part using intraluminal pressure or by cutting part of the orifice or wall of the tubular body part.

Body Part Character 4	Approach Character 5	Device Character 6	Qualifier Character 7

0 Azygos Vein
  Right ascending lumbar vein
  Right subcostal vein
1 Hemiazygos Vein
  Left ascending lumbar vein
  Left subcostal vein
G Hand Vein, Right
  Dorsal metacarpal vein
  Palmar (volar) digital vein
  Palmar (volar) metacarpal vein
  Superficial palmar venous arch
  Volar (palmar) digital vein
  Volar (palmar) metacarpal vein
H Hand Vein, Left
  See G Hand Vein, Right
L Intracranial Vein [NC]
  Anterior cerebral vein
  Basal (internal) cerebral vein
  Dural venous sinus
  Great cerebral vein
  Inferior cerebellar vein
  Inferior cerebral vein
  Internal (basal) cerebral vein
  Middle cerebral vein
  Ophthalmic vein
  Superior cerebellar vein
  Superior cerebral vein
M Internal Jugular Vein, Right
N Internal Jugular Vein, Left
P External Jugular Vein, Right
  Posterior auricular vein
Q External Jugular Vein, Left
  See P External Jugular Vein, Right
R Vertebral Vein, Right
  Deep cervical vein
  Suboccipital venous plexus
S Vertebral Vein, Left
  See R Vertebral Vein, Right
T Face Vein, Right
  Angular vein
  Anterior facial vein
  Common facial vein
  Deep facial vein
  Frontal vein
  Posterior facial (retromandibular) vein
  Supraorbital vein
V Face Vein, Left
  See T Face Vein, Right
Y Upper Vein
	0 Open
	3 Percutaneous
	4 Percutaneous Endoscopic
		D Intraluminal Device
		Z No Device
			Z No Qualifier

3 Innominate Vein, Right
  Brachiocephalic vein
  Inferior thyroid vein
4 Innominate Vein, Left
  See 3 Innominate Vein, Right
5 Subclavian Vein, Right
6 Subclavian Vein, Left
7 Axillary Vein, Right
8 Axillary Vein, Left
9 Brachial Vein, Right
  Radial vein
  Ulnar vein
A Brachial Vein, Left
  See 9 Brachial Vein, Right
B Basilic Vein, Right
  Median antebrachial vein
  Median cubital vein
C Basilic Vein, Left
  See B Basilic Vein, Right
D Cephalic Vein, Right
  Accessory cephalic vein
F Cephalic Vein, Left
  See D Cephalic Vein, Right
	0 Open
	3 Percutaneous
	4 Percutaneous Endoscopic
		D Intraluminal Device
		Z No Device
			1 Drug-Coated Balloon
			Z No Qualifier

[NC] 057L[3,4]ZZ

[NC] Noncovered Procedure [LC] Limited Coverage [QA] Questionable OB Admit [NT] New Tech Add-on ✚ Combination Member ♂ Male ♀ Female

Upper Veins

0 Medical and Surgical
5 Upper Veins
9 Drainage Definition: Taking or letting out fluids and/or gases from a body part
Explanation: The qualifier DIAGNOSTIC is used to identify drainage procedures that are biopsies

Body Part Character 4	Approach Character 5	Device Character 6	Qualifier Character 7

0 Azygos Vein
    Right ascending lumbar vein
    Right subcostal vein
1 Hemiazygos Vein
    Left ascending lumbar vein
    Left subcostal vein
3 Innominate Vein, Right
    Brachiocephalic vein
    Inferior thyroid vein
4 Innominate Vein, Left
    See 3 Innominate Vein, Right
5 Subclavian Vein, Right
6 Subclavian Vein, Left
7 Axillary Vein, Right
8 Axillary Vein, Left
9 Brachial Vein, Right
    Radial vein
    Ulnar vein
A Brachial Vein, Left
    See 9 Brachial Vein, Right
B Basilic Vein, Right
    Median antebrachial vein
    Median cubital vein
C Basilic Vein, Left
    See B Basilic Vein, Right
D Cephalic Vein, Right
    Accessory cephalic vein
F Cephalic Vein, Left
    See D Cephalic Vein, Right
G Hand Vein, Right
    Dorsal metacarpal vein
    Palmar (volar) digital vein
    Palmar (volar) metacarpal vein
    Superficial palmar venous arch
    Volar (palmar) digital vein
    Volar (palmar) metacarpal vein
H Hand Vein, Left
    See G Hand Vein, Right
L Intracranial Vein
    Anterior cerebral vein
    Basal (internal) cerebral vein
    Dural venous sinus
    Great cerebral vein
    Inferior cerebellar vein
    Inferior cerebral vein
    Internal (basal) cerebral vein
    Middle cerebral vein
    Ophthalmic vein
    Superior cerebellar vein
    Superior cerebral vein
M Internal Jugular Vein, Right
N Internal Jugular Vein, Left
P External Jugular Vein, Right
    Posterior auricular vein
Q External Jugular Vein, Left
    See P External Jugular Vein, Right
R Vertebral Vein, Right
    Deep cervical vein
    Suboccipital venous plexus
S Vertebral Vein, Left
    See R Vertebral Vein, Right
T Face Vein, Right
    Angular vein
    Anterior facial vein
    Common facial vein
    Deep facial vein
    Frontal vein
    Posterior facial (retromandibular) vein
    Supraorbital vein
V Face Vein, Left
    See T Face Vein, Right
Y Upper Vein
	0 Open
	3 Percutaneous
	4 Percutaneous Endoscopic
		0 Drainage Device	**Z** No Qualifier

0 Azygos Vein
    Right ascending lumbar vein
    Right subcostal vein
1 Hemiazygos Vein
    Left ascending lumbar vein
    Left subcostal vein
3 Innominate Vein, Right
    Brachiocephalic vein
    Inferior thyroid vein
4 Innominate Vein, Left
    See 3 Innominate Vein, Right
5 Subclavian Vein, Right
6 Subclavian Vein, Left
7 Axillary Vein, Right
8 Axillary Vein, Left
9 Brachial Vein, Right
    Radial vein
    Ulnar vein
A Brachial Vein, Left
    See 9 Brachial Vein, Right
B Basilic Vein, Right
    Median antebrachial vein
    Median cubital vein
C Basilic Vein, Left
    See B Basilic Vein, Right
D Cephalic Vein, Right
    Accessory cephalic vein
F Cephalic Vein, Left
    See D Cephalic Vein, Right
G Hand Vein, Right
    Dorsal metacarpal vein
    Palmar (volar) digital vein
    Palmar (volar) metacarpal vein
    Superficial palmar venous arch
    Volar (palmar) digital vein
    Volar (palmar) metacarpal vein
H Hand Vein, Left
    See G Hand Vein, Right
L Intracranial Vein
    Anterior cerebral vein
    Basal (internal) cerebral vein
    Dural venous sinus
    Great cerebral vein
    Inferior cerebellar vein
    Inferior cerebral vein
    Internal (basal) cerebral vein
    Middle cerebral vein
    Ophthalmic vein
    Superior cerebellar vein
    Superior cerebral vein
M Internal Jugular Vein, Right
N Internal Jugular Vein, Left
P External Jugular Vein, Right
    Posterior auricular vein
Q External Jugular Vein, Left
    See P External Jugular Vein, Right
R Vertebral Vein, Right
    Deep cervical vein
    Suboccipital venous plexus
S Vertebral Vein, Left
    See R Vertebral Vein, Right
T Face Vein, Right
    Angular vein
    Anterior facial vein
    Common facial vein
    Deep facial vein
    Frontal vein
    Posterior facial (retromandibular) vein
    Supraorbital vein
V Face Vein, Left
    See T Face Vein, Right
Y Upper Vein
	0 Open
	3 Percutaneous
	4 Percutaneous Endoscopic
		Z No Device	**X** Diagnostic
			Z No Qualifier

Non-OR 059[0,1,3,4,5,6,7,8,9,A,B,C,D,F,G,H,L,M,N,P,Q,R,S,T,V,Y][0,3,4]0Z
Non-OR 059[0,1,3,4,5,6,7,8,9,A,B,C,D,F,G,H,L,M,N,P,Q,R,S,T,V,Y]3ZX
Non-OR 059[0,1,3,4,5,6,7,8,9,A,B,C,D,F,G,H,L,M,N,P,Q,R,S,T,V,Y][0,3,4]ZZ

Non-OR Procedure   DRG Non-OR Procedure   Valid OR Procedure   HAC Associated Procedure   Combination Only   New/Revised April   New/Revised October

Upper Veins

05B–05B

- **0** Medical and Surgical
- **5** Upper Veins
- **B** Excision   Definition: Cutting out or off, without replacement, a portion of a body part
  Explanation: The qualifier DIAGNOSTIC is used to identify excision procedures that are biopsies

Body Part Character 4	Approach Character 5	Device Character 6	Qualifier Character 7

0 **Azygos Vein**
   Right ascending lumbar vein
   Right subcostal vein
1 **Hemiazygos Vein**
   Left ascending lumbar vein
   Left subcostal vein
3 **Innominate Vein, Right**
   Brachiocephalic vein
   Inferior thyroid vein
4 **Innominate Vein, Left**
   See 3 Innominate Vein, Right
5 **Subclavian Vein, Right**
6 **Subclavian Vein, Left**
7 **Axillary Vein, Right**
8 **Axillary Vein, Left**
9 **Brachial Vein, Right**
   Radial vein
   Ulnar vein
A **Brachial Vein, Left**
   See 9 Brachial Vein, Right
B **Basilic Vein, Right**
   Median antebrachial vein
   Median cubital vein
C **Basilic Vein, Left**
   See B Basilic Vein, Right
D **Cephalic Vein, Right**
   Accessory cephalic vein
F **Cephalic Vein, Left**
   See D Cephalic Vein, Right
G **Hand Vein, Right**
   Dorsal metacarpal vein
   Palmar (volar) digital vein
   Palmar (volar) metacarpal vein
   Superficial palmar venous arch
   Volar (palmar) digital vein
   Volar (palmar) metacarpal vein
H **Hand Vein, Left**
   See G Hand Vein, Right
L **Intracranial Vein**
   Anterior cerebral vein
   Basal (internal) cerebral vein
   Dural venous sinus
   Great cerebral vein
   Inferior cerebellar vein
   Inferior cerebral vein
   Internal (basal) cerebral vein
   Middle cerebral vein
   Ophthalmic vein
   Superior cerebellar vein
   Superior cerebral vein
M **Internal Jugular Vein, Right**
N **Internal Jugular Vein, Left**
P **External Jugular Vein, Right**
   Posterior auricular vein
Q **External Jugular Vein, Left**
   See P External Jugular Vein, Right
R **Vertebral Vein, Right**
   Deep cervical vein
   Suboccipital venous plexus
S **Vertebral Vein, Left**
   See R Vertebral Vein, Right
T **Face Vein, Right**
   Angular vein
   Anterior facial vein
   Common facial vein
   Deep facial vein
   Frontal vein
   Posterior facial (retromandibular) vein
   Supraorbital vein
V **Face Vein, Left**
   See T Face Vein, Right
Y **Upper Vein**
	0 Open
	3 Percutaneous
	4 Percutaneous Endoscopic
		Z No Device	**X** Diagnostic
			Z No Qualifier

0 Medical and Surgical
5 Upper Veins
C Extirpation Definition: Taking or cutting out solid matter from a body part
Explanation: The solid matter may be an abnormal byproduct of a biological function or a foreign body; it may be imbedded in a body part or in the lumen of a tubular body part. The solid matter may or may not have been previously broken into pieces.

Body Part Character 4	Approach Character 5	Device Character 6	Qualifier Character 7
0 Azygos Vein Right ascending lumbar vein Right subcostal vein **1 Hemiazygos Vein** Left ascending lumbar vein Left subcostal vein **3 Innominate Vein, Right** Brachiocephalic vein Inferior thyroid vein **4 Innominate Vein, Left** See 3 Innominate Vein, Right **5 Subclavian Vein, Right** **6 Subclavian Vein, Left** **7 Axillary Vein, Right** **8 Axillary Vein, Left** **9 Brachial Vein, Right** Radial vein Ulnar vein **A Brachial Vein, Left** See 9 Brachial Vein, Right **B Basilic Vein, Right** Median antebrachial vein Median cubital vein **C Basilic Vein, Left** See B Basilic Vein, Right **D Cephalic Vein, Right** Accessory cephalic vein **F Cephalic Vein, Left** See D Cephalic Vein, Right **G Hand Vein, Right** Dorsal metacarpal vein Palmar (volar) digital vein Palmar (volar) metacarpal vein Superficial palmar venous arch Volar (palmar) digital vein Volar (palmar) metacarpal vein **H Hand Vein, Left** See G Hand Vein, Right **L Intracranial Vein** Anterior cerebral vein Basal (internal) cerebral vein Dural venous sinus Great cerebral vein Inferior cerebellar vein Inferior cerebral vein Internal (basal) cerebral vein Middle cerebral vein Ophthalmic vein Superior cerebellar vein Superior cerebral vein **M Internal Jugular Vein, Right** **N Internal Jugular Vein, Left** **P External Jugular Vein, Right** Posterior auricular vein **Q External Jugular Vein, Left** See P External Jugular Vein, Right **R Vertebral Vein, Right** Deep cervical vein Suboccipital venous plexus **S Vertebral Vein, Left** See R Vertebral Vein, Right **T Face Vein, Right** Angular vein Anterior facial vein Common facial vein Deep facial vein Frontal vein Posterior facial (retromandibular) vein Supraorbital vein **V Face Vein, Left** See T Face Vein, Right **Y Upper Vein**	**0** Open **3** Percutaneous **4** Percutaneous Endoscopic	**Z** No Device	**Z** No Qualifier

0 Medical and Surgical
5 Upper Veins
D Extraction Definition: Pulling or stripping out or off all or a portion of a body part by the use of force
Explanation: The qualifier DIAGNOSTIC is used to identify extraction procedures that are biopsies

Body Part Character 4	Approach Character 5	Device Character 6	Qualifier Character 7

9 Brachial Vein, Right
  Radial vein
  Ulnar vein
A Brachial Vein, Left
  See 9 Brachial Vein, Right
B Basilic Vein, Right
  Median antebrachial vein
  Median cubital vein
C Basilic Vein, Left
  See B Basilic Vein, Right
D Cephalic Vein, Right
  Accessory cephalic vein
F Cephalic Vein, Left
  See D Cephalic Vein, Right
G Hand Vein, Right
  Dorsal metacarpal vein
  Palmar (volar) digital vein
  Palmar (volar) metacarpal vein
  Superficial palmar venous arch
  Volar (palmar) digital vein
  Volar (palmar) metacarpal vein
H Hand Vein, Left
  See G Hand Vein, Right
Y Upper Vein
	0 Open
	3 Percutaneous
		Z No Device	Z No Qualifier

0 Medical and Surgical
5 Upper Veins
F Fragmentation Definition: Breaking solid matter in a body part into pieces
Explanation: Physical force (e.g., manual, ultrasonic) applied directly or indirectly is used to break the solid matter into pieces. The solid matter may be an abnormal byproduct of a biological function or a foreign body. The pieces of solid matter are not taken out.

Body Part Character 4	Approach Character 5	Device Character 6	Qualifier Character 7

3 Innominate Vein, Right
  Brachiocephalic vein
  Inferior thyroid vein
4 Innominate Vein, Left
  See 3 Innominate Vein, Right
5 Subclavian Vein, Right
6 Subclavian Vein, Left
7 Axillary Vein, Right
8 Axillary Vein, Left
9 Brachial Vein, Right
  Radial vein
  Ulnar vein
A Brachial Vein, Left
  See 9 Brachial Vein, Right
B Basilic Vein, Right
  Median antebrachial vein
  Median cubital vein
C Basilic Vein, Left
  See B Basilic Vein, Right
D Cephalic Vein, Right
  Accessory cephalic vein
F Cephalic Vein, Left
  See D Cephalic Vein, Right
Y Upper Vein
	3 Percutaneous	Z No Device	0 Ultrasonic
			Z No Qualifier

Ø5H–Ø5J   **Upper Veins**   ICD-10-PCS 2025

Ø Medical and Surgical
5 Upper Veins
H Insertion

Definition: Putting in a nonbiological appliance that monitors, assists, performs, or prevents a physiological function but does not physically take the place of a body part
Explanation: None

Body Part Character 4	Approach Character 5	Device Character 6	Qualifier Character 7

Ø Azygos Vein ⊕
   Right ascending lumbar vein
   Right subcostal vein
	Ø Open
	3 Percutaneous
	4 Percutaneous Endoscopic
		2 Monitoring Device
		3 Infusion Device
		D Intraluminal Device
		M Neurostimulator Lead
			Z No Qualifier

1 Hemiazygos Vein
   Left ascending lumbar vein
   Left subcostal vein
5 Subclavian Vein, Right
6 Subclavian Vein, Left
7 Axillary Vein, Right
8 Axillary Vein, Left
9 Brachial Vein, Right
   Radial vein
   Ulnar vein
A Brachial Vein, Left
   See 9 Brachial Vein, Right
B Basilic Vein, Right
   Median antebrachial vein
   Median cubital vein
C Basilic Vein, Left
   See B Basilic Vein, Right
D Cephalic Vein, Right
   Accessory cephalic vein
F Cephalic Vein, Left
   See D Cephalic Vein, Right
G Hand Vein, Right
   Dorsal metacarpal vein
   Palmar (volar) digital vein
   Palmar (volar) metacarpal vein
   Superficial palmar venous arch
   Volar (palmar) digital vein
   Volar (palmar) metacarpal vein
H Hand Vein, Left
   See G Hand Vein, Right
	L Intracranial Vein
	   Anterior cerebral vein
	   Basal (internal) cerebral vein
	   Dural venous sinus
	   Great cerebral vein
	   Inferior cerebellar vein
	   Inferior cerebral vein
	   Internal (basal) cerebral vein
	   Middle cerebral vein
	   Ophthalmic vein
	   Superior cerebellar vein
	   Superior cerebral vein
	M Internal Jugular Vein, Right
	N Internal Jugular Vein, Left
	P External Jugular Vein, Right
	   Posterior auricular vein
	Q External Jugular Vein, Left
	   See P External Jugular Vein, Right
	R Vertebral Vein, Right
	   Deep cervical vein
	   Suboccipital venous plexus
	S Vertebral Vein, Left
	   See R Vertebral Vein, Right
	T Face Vein, Right
	   Angular vein
	   Anterior facial vein
	   Common facial vein
	   Deep facial vein
	   Frontal vein
	   Posterior facial (retromandibular) vein
	   Supraorbital vein
	V Face Vein, Left
	   See T Face Vein, Right
		Ø Open
		3 Percutaneous
		4 Percutaneous Endoscopic
			3 Infusion Device
			D Intraluminal Device
				Z No Qualifier

3 Innominate Vein, Right ⊕
   Brachiocephalic vein
   Inferior thyroid vein
4 Innominate Vein, Left ⊕
   See 3 Innominate Vein, Right
	Ø Open
	3 Percutaneous
	4 Percutaneous Endoscopic
		3 Infusion Device
		D Intraluminal Device
		M Neurostimulator Lead
			Z No Qualifier

Y Upper Vein	**Ø** Open **3** Percutaneous **4** Percutaneous Endoscopic	**2** Monitoring Device **3** Infusion Device **D** Intraluminal Device **Y** Other Device	**Z** No Qualifier

Non-OR   Ø5HØ[Ø,3,4]3Z
Non-OR   Ø5H[1,5,6,7,8,9,A,B,C,D,F,G,H,L,M,N,P,Q,R,S,T,V][Ø,3,4]3Z
Non-OR   Ø5H[3,4][Ø,3,4]3Z
Non-OR   Ø5HY[Ø,3,4]3Z
Non-OR   Ø5HY32Z
Non-OR   Ø5HY[3,4]YZ
HAC   Ø5HØ[3,4]3Z when reported with SDx J95.811
HAC   Ø5H[1,5,6][3,4]3Z when reported with SDx J95.811
HAC   Ø5H[M,N,P,Q]33Z when reported with SDx J95.811
HAC   Ø5H[3,4][3,4]3Z when reported with SDx J95.811

See Appendix L for Procedure Combinations
⊕   Ø5HØ[Ø,3,4]MZ
⊕   Ø5H[3,4][Ø,3,4]MZ

Ø Medical and Surgical
5 Upper Veins
J Inspection

Definition: Visually and/or manually exploring a body part
Explanation: Visual exploration may be performed with or without optical instrumentation. Manual exploration may be performed directly or through intervening body layers.

Body Part Character 4	Approach Character 5	Device Character 6	Qualifier Character 7
Y Upper Vein	**Ø** Open **3** Percutaneous **4** Percutaneous Endoscopic **X** External	**Z** No Device	**Z** No Qualifier

Non-OR   Ø5JY[3,X]ZZ

Non-OR Procedure   DRG Non-OR Procedure   Valid OR Procedure   HAC Associated Procedure   Combination Only   New/Revised April   New/Revised October

Upper Veins

0 Medical and Surgical
5 Upper Veins
L Occlusion

Definition: Completely closing an orifice or the lumen of a tubular body part
Explanation: The orifice can be a natural orifice or an artificially created orifice

Body Part Character 4	Approach Character 5	Device Character 6	Qualifier Character 7
0 Azygos Vein 　Right ascending lumbar vein 　Right subcostal vein **1** Hemiazygos Vein 　Left ascending lumbar vein 　Left subcostal vein **3** Innominate Vein, Right 　Brachiocephalic vein 　Inferior thyroid vein **4** Innominate Vein, Left 　*See* 3 Innominate Vein, Right **5** Subclavian Vein, Right **6** Subclavian Vein, Left **7** Axillary Vein, Right **8** Axillary Vein, Left **9** Brachial Vein, Right 　Radial vein 　Ulnar vein **A** Brachial Vein, Left 　*See* 9 Brachial Vein, Right **B** Basilic Vein, Right 　Median antebrachial vein 　Median cubital vein **C** Basilic Vein, Left 　*See* B Basilic Vein, Right **D** Cephalic Vein, Right 　Accessory cephalic vein **F** Cephalic Vein, Left 　*See* D Cephalic Vein, Right **G** Hand Vein, Right 　Dorsal metacarpal vein 　Palmar (volar) digital vein 　Palmar (volar) metacarpal vein 　Superficial palmar venous arch 　Volar (palmar) digital vein 　Volar (palmar) metacarpal vein **H** Hand Vein, Left 　*See* G Hand Vein, Right **L** Intracranial Vein 　Anterior cerebral vein 　Basal (internal) cerebral vein 　Dural venous sinus 　Great cerebral vein 　Inferior cerebellar vein 　Inferior cerebral vein 　Internal (basal) cerebral vein 　Middle cerebral vein 　Ophthalmic vein 　Superior cerebellar vein 　Superior cerebral vein **M** Internal Jugular Vein, Right **N** Internal Jugular Vein, Left **P** External Jugular Vein, Right 　Posterior auricular vein **Q** External Jugular Vein, Left 　*See* P External Jugular Vein, Right **R** Vertebral Vein, Right 　Deep cervical vein 　Suboccipital venous plexus **S** Vertebral Vein, Left 　*See* R Vertebral Vein, Right **T** Face Vein, Right 　Angular vein 　Anterior facial vein 　Common facial vein 　Deep facial vein 　Frontal vein 　Posterior facial (retromandibular) vein 　Supraorbital vein **V** Face Vein, Left 　*See* T Face Vein, Right **Y** Upper Vein	**0** Open **3** Percutaneous **4** Percutaneous Endoscopic	**C** Extraluminal Device **D** Intraluminal Device **Z** No Device	**Z** No Qualifier

Upper Veins

0 Medical and Surgical
5 Upper Veins
N Release

Definition: Freeing a body part from an abnormal physical constraint by cutting or by the use of force
Explanation: Some of the restraining tissue may be taken out but none of the body part is taken out

Body Part Character 4	Approach Character 5	Device Character 6	Qualifier Character 7
0 Azygos Vein Right ascending lumbar vein Right subcostal vein **1** Hemiazygos Vein Left ascending lumbar vein Left subcostal vein **3** Innominate Vein, Right Brachiocephalic vein Inferior thyroid vein **4** Innominate Vein, Left See 3 Innominate Vein, Right **5** Subclavian Vein, Right **6** Subclavian Vein, Left **7** Axillary Vein, Right **8** Axillary Vein, Left **9** Brachial Vein, Right Radial vein Ulnar vein **A** Brachial Vein, Left See 9 Brachial Vein, Right **B** Basilic Vein, Right Median antebrachial vein Median cubital vein **C** Basilic Vein, Left See B Basilic Vein, Right **D** Cephalic Vein, Right Accessory cephalic vein **F** Cephalic Vein, Left See D Cephalic Vein, Right **G** Hand Vein, Right Dorsal metacarpal vein Palmar (volar) digital vein Palmar (volar) metacarpal vein Superficial palmar venous arch Volar (palmar) digital vein Volar (palmar) metacarpal vein **H** Hand Vein, Left See G Hand Vein, Right **L** Intracranial Vein Anterior cerebral vein Basal (internal) cerebral vein Dural venous sinus Great cerebral vein Inferior cerebellar vein Inferior cerebral vein Internal (basal) cerebral vein Middle cerebral vein Ophthalmic vein Superior cerebellar vein Superior cerebral vein **M** Internal Jugular Vein, Right **N** Internal Jugular Vein, Left **P** External Jugular Vein, Right Posterior auricular vein **Q** External Jugular Vein, Left See P External Jugular Vein, Right **R** Vertebral Vein, Right Deep cervical vein Suboccipital venous plexus **S** Vertebral Vein, Left See R Vertebral Vein, Right **T** Face Vein, Right Angular vein Anterior facial vein Common facial vein Deep facial vein Frontal vein Posterior facial (retromandibular) vein Supraorbital vein **V** Face Vein, Left See T Face Vein, Right **Y** Upper Vein	**0** Open **3** Percutaneous **4** Percutaneous Endoscopic	**Z** No Device	**Z** No Qualifier

ICD-10-PCS 2025 — Upper Veins — 05P–05P

0 Medical and Surgical
5 Upper Veins
P Removal

Definition: Taking out or off a device from a body part

Explanation: If a device is taken out and a similar device put in without cutting or puncturing the skin or mucous membrane, the procedure is coded to the root operation CHANGE. Otherwise, the procedure for taking out a device is coded to the root operation REMOVAL.

Body Part Character 4	Approach Character 5	Device Character 6	Qualifier Character 7
0 Azygos Vein Right ascending lumbar vein Right subcostal vein	**0** Open **3** Percutaneous **4** Percutaneous Endoscopic **X** External	**2** Monitoring Device **M** Neurostimulator Lead	**Z** No Qualifier
3 Innominate Vein, Right Brachiocephalic vein Inferior thyroid vein **4** Innominate Vein, Left See 3 Innominate Vein, Right	**0** Open **3** Percutaneous **4** Percutaneous Endoscopic **X** External	**M** Neurostimulator Lead	**Z** No Qualifier
Y Upper Vein	**0** Open **3** Percutaneous **4** Percutaneous Endoscopic	**0** Drainage Device **2** Monitoring Device **3** Infusion Device **7** Autologous Tissue Substitute **C** Extraluminal Device **D** Intraluminal Device **J** Synthetic Substitute **K** Nonautologous Tissue Substitute **Y** Other Device	**Z** No Qualifier
Y Upper Vein	**X** External	**0** Drainage Device **2** Monitoring Device **3** Infusion Device **D** Intraluminal Device	**Z** No Qualifier

Non-OR 05P0[0,3,4,X]2Z
Non-OR 05PY3[0,2,3]Z
Non-OR 05PY[3,4]YZ
Non-OR 05PYX[0,2,3,D]Z

- **0** Medical and Surgical
- **5** Upper Veins
- **Q** Repair Definition: Restoring, to the extent possible, a body part to its normal anatomic structure and function
  Explanation: Used only when the method to accomplish the repair is not one of the other root operations

Body Part Character 4	Approach Character 5	Device Character 6	Qualifier Character 7

0 Azygos Vein
  Right ascending lumbar vein
  Right subcostal vein
1 Hemiazygos Vein
  Left ascending lumbar vein
  Left subcostal vein
3 Innominate Vein, Right
  Brachiocephalic vein
  Inferior thyroid vein
4 Innominate Vein, Left
  See 3 Innominate Vein, Right
5 Subclavian Vein, Right
6 Subclavian Vein, Left
7 Axillary Vein, Right
8 Axillary Vein, Left
9 Brachial Vein, Right
  Radial vein
  Ulnar vein
A Brachial Vein, Left
  See 9 Brachial Vein, Right
B Basilic Vein, Right
  Median antebrachial vein
  Median cubital vein
C Basilic Vein, Left
  See B Basilic Vein, Right
D Cephalic Vein, Right
  Accessory cephalic vein
F Cephalic Vein, Left
  See D Cephalic Vein, Right
G Hand Vein, Right
  Dorsal metacarpal vein
  Palmar (volar) digital vein
  Palmar (volar) metacarpal vein
  Superficial palmar venous arch
  Volar (palmar) digital vein
  Volar (palmar) metacarpal vein
H Hand Vein, Left
  See G Hand Vein, Right
L Intracranial Vein
  Anterior cerebral vein
  Basal (internal) cerebral vein
  Dural venous sinus
  Great cerebral vein
  Inferior cerebellar vein
  Inferior cerebral vein
  Internal (basal) cerebral vein
  Middle cerebral vein
  Ophthalmic vein
  Superior cerebellar vein
  Superior cerebral vein
M Internal Jugular Vein, Right
N Internal Jugular Vein, Left
P External Jugular Vein, Right
  Posterior auricular vein
Q External Jugular Vein, Left
  See P External Jugular Vein, Right
R Vertebral Vein, Right
  Deep cervical vein
  Suboccipital venous plexus
S Vertebral Vein, Left
  See R Vertebral Vein, Right
T Face Vein, Right
  Angular vein
  Anterior facial vein
  Common facial vein
  Deep facial vein
  Frontal vein
  Posterior facial (retromandibular) vein
  Supraorbital vein
V Face Vein, Left
  See T Face Vein, Right
Y Upper Vein
	0 Open
	3 Percutaneous
	4 Percutaneous Endoscopic
		Z No Device	**Z** No Qualifier

ICD-10-PCS 2025 — Upper Veins — 05R–05R

- **0** Medical and Surgical
- **5** Upper Veins
- **R** Replacement

Definition: Putting in or on biological or synthetic material that physically takes the place and/or function of all or a portion of a body part

Explanation: The body part may have been taken out or replaced, or may be taken out, physically eradicated, or rendered nonfunctional during the REPLACEMENT procedure. A REMOVAL procedure is coded for taking out the device used in a previous replacement procedure.

Body Part Character 4	Approach Character 5	Device Character 6	Qualifier Character 7

0 Azygos Vein
   Right ascending lumbar vein
   Right subcostal vein
1 Hemiazygos Vein
   Left ascending lumbar vein
   Left subcostal vein
3 Innominate Vein, Right
   Brachiocephalic vein
   Inferior thyroid vein
4 Innominate Vein, Left
   See 3 Innominate Vein, Right
5 Subclavian Vein, Right
6 Subclavian Vein, Left
7 Axillary Vein, Right
8 Axillary Vein, Left
9 Brachial Vein, Right
   Radial vein
   Ulnar vein
A Brachial Vein, Left
   See 9 Brachial Vein, Right
B Basilic Vein, Right
   Median antebrachial vein
   Median cubital vein
C Basilic Vein, Left
   See B Basilic Vein, Right
D Cephalic Vein, Right
   Accessory cephalic vein
F Cephalic Vein, Left
   See D Cephalic Vein, Right
G Hand Vein, Right
   Dorsal metacarpal vein
   Palmar (volar) digital vein
   Palmar (volar) metacarpal vein
   Superficial palmar venous arch
   Volar (palmar) digital vein
   Volar (palmar) metacarpal vein
H Hand Vein, Left
   See G Hand Vein, Right
L Intracranial Vein
   Anterior cerebral vein
   Basal (internal) cerebral vein
   Dural venous sinus
   Great cerebral vein
   Inferior cerebellar vein
   Inferior cerebral vein
   Internal (basal) cerebral vein
   Middle cerebral vein
   Ophthalmic vein
   Superior cerebellar vein
   Superior cerebral vein
M Internal Jugular Vein, Right
N Internal Jugular Vein, Left
P External Jugular Vein, Right
   Posterior auricular vein
Q External Jugular Vein, Left
   See P External Jugular Vein, Right
R Vertebral Vein, Right
   Deep cervical vein
   Suboccipital venous plexus
S Vertebral Vein, Left
   See R Vertebral Vein, Right
T Face Vein, Right
   Angular vein
   Anterior facial vein
   Common facial vein
   Deep facial vein
   Frontal vein
   Posterior facial (retromandibular) vein
   Supraorbital vein
V Face Vein, Left
   See T Face Vein, Right
Y Upper Vein
	0 Open
	4 Percutaneous Endoscopic
		7 Autologous Tissue Substitute
		J Synthetic Substitute
		K Nonautologous Tissue Substitute
			Z No Qualifier

NC Noncovered Procedure   **LC** Limited Coverage   **QA** Questionable OB Admit   **NT** New Tech Add-on   ✚ Combination Member   ♂ Male   ♀ Female

0 Medical and Surgical
5 Upper Veins
S Reposition Definition: Moving to its normal location, or other suitable location, all or a portion of a body part
Explanation: The body part is moved to a new location from an abnormal location, or from a normal location where it is not functioning correctly. The body part may or may not be cut out or off to be moved to the new location.

Body Part Character 4	Approach Character 5	Device Character 6	Qualifier Character 7
0 Azygos Vein Right ascending lumbar vein Right subcostal vein **1 Hemiazygos Vein** Left ascending lumbar vein Left subcostal vein **3 Innominate Vein, Right** Brachiocephalic vein Inferior thyroid vein **4 Innominate Vein, Left** See 3 Innominate Vein, Right **5 Subclavian Vein, Right** **6 Subclavian Vein, Left** **7 Axillary Vein, Right** **8 Axillary Vein, Left** **9 Brachial Vein, Right** Radial vein Ulnar vein **A Brachial Vein, Left** See 9 Brachial Vein, Right **B Basilic Vein, Right** Median antebrachial vein Median cubital vein **C Basilic Vein, Left** See B Basilic Vein, Right **D Cephalic Vein, Right** Accessory cephalic vein **F Cephalic Vein, Left** See D Cephalic Vein, Right **G Hand Vein, Right** Dorsal metacarpal vein Palmar (volar) digital vein Palmar (volar) metacarpal vein Superficial palmar venous arch Volar (palmar) digital vein Volar (palmar) metacarpal vein **H Hand Vein, Left** See G Hand Vein, Right **L Intracranial Vein** Anterior cerebral vein Basal (internal) cerebral vein Dural venous sinus Great cerebral vein Inferior cerebellar vein Inferior cerebral vein Internal (basal) cerebral vein Middle cerebral vein Ophthalmic vein Superior cerebellar vein Superior cerebral vein **M Internal Jugular Vein, Right** **N Internal Jugular Vein, Left** **P External Jugular Vein, Right** Posterior auricular vein **Q External Jugular Vein, Left** See P External Jugular Vein, Right **R Vertebral Vein, Right** Deep cervical vein Suboccipital venous plexus **S Vertebral Vein, Left** See R Vertebral Vein, Right **T Face Vein, Right** Angular vein Anterior facial vein Common facial vein Deep facial vein Frontal vein Posterior facial (retromandibular) vein Supraorbital vein **V Face Vein, Left** See T Face Vein, Right **Y Upper Vein**	**0** Open **3** Percutaneous **4** Percutaneous Endoscopic	**Z** No Device	**Z** No Qualifier

ICD-10-PCS 2025 — Upper Veins — 05U–05U

- **0** Medical and Surgical
- **5** Upper Veins
- **U** Supplement

Definition: Putting in or on biological or synthetic material that physically reinforces and/or augments the function of a portion of a body part
Explanation: The biological material is non-living, or is living and from the same individual. The body part may have been previously replaced, and the SUPPLEMENT procedure is performed to physically reinforce and/or augment the function of the replaced body part.

Body Part Character 4	Approach Character 5	Device Character 6	Qualifier Character 7
0 Azygos Vein 　Right ascending lumbar vein 　Right subcostal vein **1** Hemiazygos Vein 　Left ascending lumbar vein 　Left subcostal vein **3** Innominate Vein, Right 　Brachiocephalic vein 　Inferior thyroid vein **4** Innominate Vein, Left 　See 3 Innominate Vein, Right **5** Subclavian Vein, Right **6** Subclavian Vein, Left **7** Axillary Vein, Right **8** Axillary Vein, Left **9** Brachial Vein, Right 　Radial vein 　Ulnar vein **A** Brachial Vein, Left 　See 9 Brachial Vein, Right **B** Basilic Vein, Right 　Median antebrachial vein 　Median cubital vein **C** Basilic Vein, Left 　See B Basilic Vein, Right **D** Cephalic Vein, Right 　Accessory cephalic vein **F** Cephalic Vein, Left 　See D Cephalic Vein, Right **G** Hand Vein, Right 　Dorsal metacarpal vein 　Palmar (volar) digital vein 　Palmar (volar) metacarpal vein 　Superficial palmar venous arch 　Volar (palmar) digital vein 　Volar (palmar) metacarpal vein **H** Hand Vein, Left 　See G Hand Vein, Right **L** Intracranial Vein 　Anterior cerebral vein 　Basal (internal) cerebral vein 　Dural venous sinus 　Great cerebral vein 　Inferior cerebellar vein 　Inferior cerebral vein 　Internal (basal) cerebral vein 　Middle cerebral vein 　Ophthalmic vein 　Superior cerebellar vein 　Superior cerebral vein **M** Internal Jugular Vein, Right **N** Internal Jugular Vein, Left **P** External Jugular Vein, Right 　Posterior auricular vein **Q** External Jugular Vein, Left 　See P External Jugular Vein, Right **R** Vertebral Vein, Right 　Deep cervical vein 　Suboccipital venous plexus **S** Vertebral Vein, Left 　See R Vertebral Vein, Right **T** Face Vein, Right 　Angular vein 　Anterior facial vein 　Common facial vein 　Deep facial vein 　Frontal vein 　Posterior facial (retromandibular) vein 　Supraorbital vein **V** Face Vein, Left 　See T Face Vein, Right **Y** Upper Vein	**0** Open **3** Percutaneous **4** Percutaneous Endoscopic	**7** Autologous Tissue Substitute **J** Synthetic Substitute **K** Nonautologous Tissue Substitute	**Z** No Qualifier

0 Medical and Surgical
5 Upper Veins
V Restriction

Definition: Partially closing an orifice or the lumen of a tubular body part
Explanation: The orifice can be a natural orifice or an artificially created orifice

Body Part — Character 4	Approach — Character 5	Device — Character 6	Qualifier — Character 7

0 Azygos Vein
   Right ascending lumbar vein
   Right subcostal vein
1 Hemiazygos Vein
   Left ascending lumbar vein
   Left subcostal vein
3 Innominate Vein, Right
   Brachiocephalic vein
   Inferior thyroid vein
4 Innominate Vein, Left
   See 3 Innominate Vein, Right
5 Subclavian Vein, Right
6 Subclavian Vein, Left
7 Axillary Vein, Right
8 Axillary Vein, Left
9 Brachial Vein, Right
   Radial vein
   Ulnar vein
A Brachial Vein, Left
   See 9 Brachial Vein, Right
B Basilic Vein, Right
   Median antebrachial vein
   Median cubital vein
C Basilic Vein, Left
   See B Basilic Vein, Right
D Cephalic Vein, Right
   Accessory cephalic vein
F Cephalic Vein, Left
   See D Cephalic Vein, Right
G Hand Vein, Right
   Dorsal metacarpal vein
   Palmar (volar) digital vein
   Palmar (volar) metacarpal vein
   Superficial palmar venous arch
   Volar (palmar) digital vein
   Volar (palmar) metacarpal vein
H Hand Vein, Left
   See G Hand Vein, Right
L Intracranial Vein
   Anterior cerebral vein
   Basal (internal) cerebral vein
   Dural venous sinus
   Great cerebral vein
   Inferior cerebellar vein
   Inferior cerebral vein
   Internal (basal) cerebral vein
   Middle cerebral vein
   Ophthalmic vein
   Superior cerebellar vein
   Superior cerebral vein
M Internal Jugular Vein, Right
N Internal Jugular Vein, Left
P External Jugular Vein, Right
   Posterior auricular vein
Q External Jugular Vein, Left
   See P External Jugular Vein, Right
R Vertebral Vein, Right
   Deep cervical vein
   Suboccipital venous plexus
S Vertebral Vein, Left
   See R Vertebral Vein, Right
T Face Vein, Right
   Angular vein
   Anterior facial vein
   Common facial vein
   Deep facial vein
   Frontal vein
   Posterior facial (retromandibular) vein
   Supraorbital vein
V Face Vein, Left
   See T Face Vein, Right
Y Upper Vein
	0 Open
	3 Percutaneous
	4 Percutaneous Endoscopic
		C Extraluminal Device
		D Intraluminal Device
		Z No Device
			Z No Qualifier

ICD-10-PCS 2025 — Upper Veins — 05W–05W

0 Medical and Surgical
5 Upper Veins
W Revision Definition: Correcting, to the extent possible, a portion of a malfunctioning device or the position of a displaced device
Explanation: Revision can include correcting a malfunctioning or displaced device by taking out or putting in components of the device such as a screw or pin

Body Part Character 4	Approach Character 5	Device Character 6	Qualifier Character 7
0 Azygos Vein Right ascending lumbar vein Right subcostal vein	0 Open 3 Percutaneous 4 Percutaneous Endoscopic X External	2 Monitoring Device M Neurostimulator Lead	Z No Qualifier
3 Innominate Vein, Right Brachiocephalic vein Inferior thyroid vein **4 Innominate Vein, Left** See 3 Innominate Vein, Right	0 Open 3 Percutaneous 4 Percutaneous Endoscopic X External	M Neurostimulator Lead	Z No Qualifier
Y Upper Vein	0 Open 3 Percutaneous 4 Percutaneous Endoscopic	0 Drainage Device 2 Monitoring Device 3 Infusion Device 7 Autologous Tissue Substitute C Extraluminal Device D Intraluminal Device J Synthetic Substitute K Nonautologous Tissue Substitute Y Other Device	Z No Qualifier
Y Upper Vein	X External	0 Drainage Device 2 Monitoring Device 3 Infusion Device 7 Autologous Tissue Substitute C Extraluminal Device D Intraluminal Device J Synthetic Substitute K Nonautologous Tissue Substitute	Z No Qualifier

Non-OR 05W0XMZ
Non-OR 05W[3,4]XMZ
Non-OR 05WY3[0,2,3]Z
Non-OR 05WY[3,4]YZ
Non-OR 05WYX[0,2,3,7,C,D,J,K]Z

Lower Veins Ø61–Ø6W

Character Meanings
This Character Meaning table is provided as a guide to assist the user in the identification of character members that may be found in this section of code tables. It **SHOULD NOT** be used to build a PCS code.

Operation–Character 3		Body Part–Character 4		Approach–Character 5		Device–Character 6		Qualifier–Character 7	
1	Bypass	Ø	Inferior Vena Cava	Ø	Open	Ø	Drainage Device	Ø	Ultrasonic
5	Destruction	1	Splenic Vein	3	Percutaneous	2	Monitoring Device	4	Hepatic Vein
7	Dilation	2	Gastric Vein	4	Percutaneous Endoscopic	3	Infusion Device	5	Superior Mesenteric Vein
9	Drainage	3	Esophageal Vein	7	Via Natural or Artificial Opening	7	Autologous Tissue Substitute	6	Inferior Mesenteric Vein
B	Excision	4	Hepatic Vein	8	Via Natural or Artificial Opening Endoscopic	9	Autologous Venous Tissue	9	Renal Vein, Right
C	Extirpation	5	Superior Mesenteric Vein	X	External	A	Autologous Arterial Tissue	B	Renal Vein, Left
D	Extraction	6	Inferior Mesenteric Vein			C	Extraluminal Device	C	Hemorrhoidal Plexus
F	Fragmentation	7	Colic Vein			D	Intraluminal Device	P	Pulmonary Trunk
H	Insertion	8	Portal Vein			J	Synthetic Substitute	Q	Pulmonary Artery, Right
J	Inspection	9	Renal Vein, Right			K	Nonautologous Tissue Substitute	R	Pulmonary Artery, Left
L	Occlusion	B	Renal Vein, Left			Y	Other Device	T	Via Umbilical Vein
N	Release	C	Common Iliac Vein, Right			Z	No Device	X	Diagnostic
P	Removal	D	Common Iliac Vein, Left					Y	Lower Vein
Q	Repair	F	External Iliac Vein, Right					Z	No Qualifier
R	Replacement	G	External Iliac Vein, Left						
S	Reposition	H	Hypogastric Vein, Right						
U	Supplement	J	Hypogastric Vein, Left						
V	Restriction	M	Femoral Vein, Right						
W	Revision	N	Femoral Vein, Left						
		P	Saphenous Vein, Right						
		Q	Saphenous Vein, Left						
		T	Foot Vein, Right						
		V	Foot Vein, Left						
		Y	Lower Vein						

AHA Coding Clinic for Lower Veins
2022, 1Q, 10-13   Procedures performed on a continuous vessel, ICD-10-PCS Guideline B4.1c

AHA Coding Clinic for table Ø61
2017, 4Q, 36-38   Fontan completion procedure
2017, 4Q, 66-67   New qualifier values - Portal to hepatic shunt

AHA Coding Clinic for table Ø6B
2020, 1Q, 28   Free flap microvascular breast reconstruction
2017, 3Q, 5   Femoral artery to posterior tibial artery bypass using autologous and synthetic grafts
2017, 1Q, 31   Left to right common carotid artery bypass
2017, 1Q, 32   Peroneal artery to dorsalis pedis artery bypass using saphenous vein graft
2016, 3Q, 31   Femoral to peroneal artery bypass with in-situ saphenous vein graft and lysis of valves
2016, 2Q, 18   Femoral-tibial artery bypass and saphenous vein graft
2016, 1Q, 27   Aortocoronary bypass graft utilizing Y-graft
2014, 3Q, 8   Excision of saphenous vein for coronary artery bypass graft
2014, 3Q, 20   MAZE procedure performed with coronary artery bypass graft
2014, 1Q, 10   Repair of thoracic aortic aneurysm & coronary artery bypass graft

AHA Coding Clinic for table Ø6F
2020, 4Q, 45-49   New fragmentation tables
2020, 4Q, 49-50   Intravascular ultrasound assisted thrombolysis
2020, 4Q, 50   Intravascular lithotripsy

AHA Coding Clinic for table Ø6H
2021, 3Q, 18   Placement and removal of cannulas for extracorporeal membrane oxygenation
2017, 3Q, 11   Placement of peripherally inserted central catheter using 3CG ECG technology
2017, 1Q, 31   Umbilical vein catheterization
2017, 1Q, 31   Central catheter placement in femoral vein
2013, 3Q, 18   Heart transplant surgery

AHA Coding Clinic for table Ø6L
2021, 4Q, 47   Endoscopic banding of hemorrhoidal plexus
2021, 4Q, 49   Division of liver for staged hepatectomy
2020, 3Q, 44   Cardiophrenic vein embolization
2019, 4Q, 28   Transorifice occlusion of gastric varices
2018, 2Q, 18   Transverse rectus abdominis myocutaneous (TRAM) delay
2017, 4Q, 57-58   Added approach values - Transorifice esophageal vein banding
2013, 4Q, 112   Endoscopic banding of esophageal varices

AHA Coding Clinic for table Ø6P
2021, 3Q, 18   Placement and removal of cannulas for extracorporeal membrane oxygenation

AHA Coding Clinic for table Ø6V
2018, 3Q, 11   Transvenous transcatheter placement of valve in inferior vena cava
2018, 1Q, 10   Revision of transjugular intrahepatic portosystemic shunt

AHA Coding Clinic for table Ø6W
2019, 2Q, 39   Transjugular intrahepatic portosystemic shunt revision
2018, 1Q, 10   Revision of transjugular intrahepatic portosystemic shunt
2014, 3Q, 25   Revision of transjugular intrahepatic portosystemic shunt (TIPS)

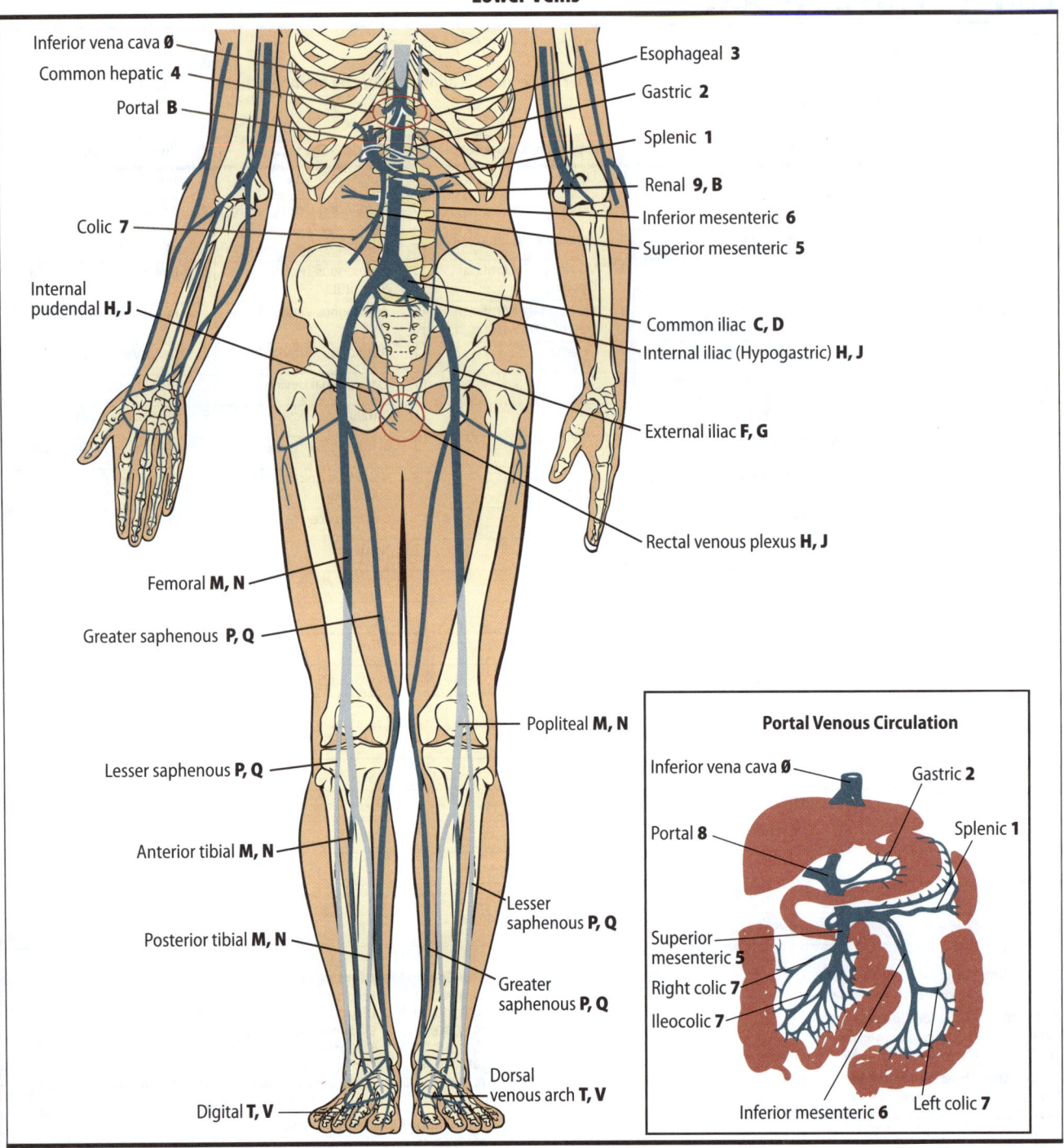

Lower Veins

Lower Veins

- Inferior vena cava **0**
- Common hepatic **4**
- Portal **B**
- Colic **7**
- Internal pudendal **H, J**
- Esophageal **3**
- Gastric **2**
- Splenic **1**
- Renal **9, B**
- Inferior mesenteric **6**
- Superior mesenteric **5**
- Common iliac **C, D**
- Internal iliac (Hypogastric) **H, J**
- External iliac **F, G**
- Rectal venous plexus **H, J**
- Femoral **M, N**
- Greater saphenous **P, Q**
- Popliteal **M, N**
- Lesser saphenous **P, Q**
- Anterior tibial **M, N**
- Lesser saphenous **P, Q**
- Posterior tibial **M, N**
- Greater saphenous **P, Q**
- Dorsal venous arch **T, V**
- Digital **T, V**

Portal Venous Circulation

- Inferior vena cava **0**
- Portal **8**
- Gastric **2**
- Splenic **1**
- Superior mesenteric **5**
- Right colic **7**
- Ileocolic **7**
- Inferior mesenteric **6**
- Left colic **7**

ICD-10-PCS 2025 — Lower Veins — 061–061

- 0 Medical and Surgical
- 6 Lower Veins
- 1 Bypass

Definition: Altering the route of passage of the contents of a tubular body part

Explanation: Rerouting contents of a body part to a downstream area of the normal route, to a similar route and body part, or to an abnormal route and dissimilar body part. Includes one or more anastomoses, with or without the use of a device.

Body Part Character 4	Approach Character 5	Device Character 6	Qualifier Character 7
0 Inferior Vena Cava Postcava Right inferior phrenic vein Right ovarian vein Right second lumbar vein Right suprarenal vein Right testicular vein	0 Open 4 Percutaneous Endoscopic	7 Autologous Tissue Substitute 9 Autologous Venous Tissue A Autologous Arterial Tissue J Synthetic Substitute K Nonautologous Tissue Substitute Z No Device	5 Superior Mesenteric Vein 6 Inferior Mesenteric Vein P Pulmonary Trunk Q Pulmonary Artery, Right R Pulmonary Artery, Left Y Lower Vein
1 Splenic Vein Left gastroepiploic vein Pancreatic vein	0 Open 4 Percutaneous Endoscopic	7 Autologous Tissue Substitute 9 Autologous Venous Tissue A Autologous Arterial Tissue J Synthetic Substitute K Nonautologous Tissue Substitute Z No Device	9 Renal Vein, Right B Renal Vein, Left Y Lower Vein

2 Gastric Vein
3 Esophageal Vein
4 Hepatic Vein
5 Superior Mesenteric Vein
   Right gastroepiploic vein
6 Inferior Mesenteric Vein
   Sigmoid vein
   Superior rectal vein
7 Colic Vein
   Ileocolic vein
   Left colic vein
   Middle colic vein
   Right colic vein
9 Renal Vein, Right
B Renal Vein, Left
   Left inferior phrenic vein
   Left ovarian vein
   Left second lumbar vein
   Left suprarenal vein
   Left testicular vein
C Common Iliac Vein, Right
D Common Iliac Vein, Left
F External Iliac Vein, Right
G External Iliac Vein, Left
H Hypogastric Vein, Right
   Gluteal vein
   Internal iliac vein
   Internal pudendal vein
   Lateral sacral vein
   Middle hemorrhoidal vein
   Obturator vein
   Uterine vein
   Vaginal vein
   Vesical vein
J Hypogastric Vein, Left
   See H Hypogastric Vein, Right
M Femoral Vein, Right
   Deep femoral (profunda femoris) vein
   Popliteal vein
   Profunda femoris (deep femoral) vein
N Femoral Vein, Left
   See M Femoral Vein, Right
P Saphenous Vein, Right
   External pudendal vein
   Great(er) saphenous vein
   Lesser saphenous vein
   Small saphenous vein
   Superficial circumflex iliac vein
   Superficial epigastric vein
Q Saphenous Vein, Left
   See P Saphenous Vein, Right
T Foot Vein, Right
   Common digital vein
   Dorsal metatarsal vein
   Dorsal venous arch
   Plantar digital vein
   Plantar metatarsal vein
   Plantar venous arch
V Foot Vein, Left
   See T Foot Vein, Right
	0 Open
	4 Percutaneous Endoscopic
		7 Autologous Tissue Substitute
		9 Autologous Venous Tissue
		A Autologous Arterial Tissue
		J Synthetic Substitute
		K Nonautologous Tissue Substitute
		Z No Device
			Y Lower Vein

8 Portal Vein Hepatic portal vein	0 Open	7 Autologous Tissue Substitute 9 Autologous Venous Tissue A Autologous Arterial Tissue J Synthetic Substitute K Nonautologous Tissue Substitute Z No Device	9 Renal Vein, Right B Renal Vein, Left Y Lower Vein
8 Portal Vein Hepatic portal vein	3 Percutaneous	J Synthetic Substitute	4 Hepatic Vein Y Lower Vein
8 Portal Vein Hepatic portal vein	4 Percutaneous Endoscopic	7 Autologous Tissue Substitute 9 Autologous Venous Tissue A Autologous Arterial Tissue K Nonautologous Tissue Substitute Z No Device	9 Renal Vein, Right B Renal Vein, Left Y Lower Vein
8 Portal Vein Hepatic portal vein	4 Percutaneous Endoscopic	J Synthetic Substitute	4 Hepatic Vein 9 Renal Vein, Right B Renal Vein, Left Y Lower Vein

NC Noncovered Procedure   LC Limited Coverage   QA Questionable OB Admit   NT New Tech Add-on   ✚ Combination Member   ♂ Male   ♀ Female

0 Medical and Surgical
6 Lower Veins
5 Destruction

Definition: Physical eradication of all or a portion of a body part by the direct use of energy, force, or a destructive agent
Explanation: None of the body part is physically taken out

Body Part Character 4	Approach Character 5	Device Character 6	Qualifier Character 7
0 Inferior Vena Cava Postcava Right inferior phrenic vein Right ovarian vein Right second lumbar vein Right suprarenal vein Right testicular vein **1 Splenic Vein** Left gastroepiploic vein Pancreatic vein **2 Gastric Vein** **3 Esophageal Vein** **4 Hepatic Vein** **5 Superior Mesenteric Vein** Right gastroepiploic vein **6 Inferior Mesenteric Vein** Sigmoid vein Superior rectal vein **7 Colic Vein** Ileocolic vein Left colic vein Middle colic vein Right colic vein **8 Portal Vein** Hepatic portal vein **9 Renal Vein, Right** **B Renal Vein, Left** Left inferior phrenic vein Left ovarian vein Left second lumbar vein Left suprarenal vein Left testicular vein **C Common Iliac Vein, Right** **D Common Iliac Vein, Left** **F External Iliac Vein, Right** **G External Iliac Vein, Left** **H Hypogastric Vein, Right** Gluteal vein Internal iliac vein Internal pudendal vein Lateral sacral vein Middle hemorrhoidal vein Obturator vein Uterine vein Vaginal vein Vesical vein **J Hypogastric Vein, Left** See H Hypogastric Vein, Right **M Femoral Vein, Right** Deep femoral (profunda femoris) vein Popliteal vein Profunda femoris (deep femoral) vein **N Femoral Vein, Left** See M Femoral Vein, Right **P Saphenous Vein, Right** External pudendal vein Great(er) saphenous vein Lesser saphenous vein Small saphenous vein Superficial circumflex iliac vein Superficial epigastric vein **Q Saphenous Vein, Left** See P Saphenous Vein, Right **T Foot Vein, Right** Common digital vein Dorsal metatarsal vein Dorsal venous arch Plantar digital vein Plantar metatarsal vein Plantar venous arch **V Foot Vein, Left** See T Foot Vein, Right	**0** Open **3** Percutaneous **4** Percutaneous Endoscopic	**Z** No Device	**Z** No Qualifier
Y Lower Vein	**0** Open **3** Percutaneous **4** Percutaneous Endoscopic	**Z** No Device	**C** Hemorrhoidal Plexus **Z** No Qualifier

Non-OR Procedure   DRG Non-OR Procedure   Valid OR Procedure   HAC Associated Procedure   Combination Only   New/Revised April   New/Revised October

0 Medical and Surgical
6 Lower Veins
7 Dilation

Definition: Expanding an orifice or the lumen of a tubular body part

Explanation: The orifice can be a natural orifice or an artificially created orifice. Accomplished by stretching a tubular body part using intraluminal pressure or by cutting part of the orifice or wall of the tubular body part.

Body Part Character 4	Approach Character 5	Device Character 6	Qualifier Character 7

0 Inferior Vena Cava
  Postcava
  Right inferior phrenic vein
  Right ovarian vein
  Right second lumbar vein
  Right suprarenal vein
  Right testicular vein
1 Splenic Vein
  Left gastroepiploic vein
  Pancreatic vein
2 Gastric Vein
3 Esophageal Vein
4 Hepatic Vein
5 Superior Mesenteric Vein
  Right gastroepiploic vein
6 Inferior Mesenteric Vein
  Sigmoid vein
  Superior rectal vein
7 Colic Vein
  Ileocolic vein
  Left colic vein
  Middle colic vein
  Right colic vein
8 Portal Vein
  Hepatic portal vein
9 Renal Vein, Right
B Renal Vein, Left
  Left inferior phrenic vein
  Left ovarian vein
  Left second lumbar vein
  Left suprarenal vein
  Left testicular vein
C Common Iliac Vein, Right
D Common Iliac Vein, Left
F External Iliac Vein, Right
G External Iliac Vein, Left
H Hypogastric Vein, Right
  Gluteal vein
  Internal iliac vein
  Internal pudendal vein
  Lateral sacral vein
  Middle hemorrhoidal vein
  Obturator vein
  Uterine vein
  Vaginal vein
  Vesical vein
J Hypogastric Vein, Left
  See H Hypogastric Vein, Right
M Femoral Vein, Right
  Deep femoral (profunda femoris) vein
  Popliteal vein
  Profunda femoris (deep femoral) vein
N Femoral Vein, Left
  See M Femoral Vein, Right
P Saphenous Vein, Right
  External pudendal vein
  Great(er) saphenous vein
  Lesser saphenous vein
  Small saphenous vein
  Superficial circumflex iliac vein
  Superficial epigastric vein
Q Saphenous Vein, Left
  See P Saphenous Vein, Right
T Foot Vein, Right
  Common digital vein
  Dorsal metatarsal vein
  Dorsal venous arch
  Plantar digital vein
  Plantar metatarsal vein
  Plantar venous arch
V Foot Vein, Left
  See T Foot Vein, Right
Y Lower Vein
	0 Open
	3 Percutaneous
	4 Percutaneous Endoscopic
		D Intraluminal Device
		Z No Device
			Z No Qualifier

Lower Veins

ICD-10-PCS 2025

0 Medical and Surgical
6 Lower Veins
9 Drainage

Definition: Taking or letting out fluids and/or gases from a body part
Explanation: The qualifier DIAGNOSTIC is used to identify drainage procedures that are biopsies

Body Part Character 4	Approach Character 5	Device Character 6	Qualifier Character 7
0 Inferior Vena Cava 　Postcava 　Right inferior phrenic vein 　Right ovarian vein 　Right second lumbar vein 　Right suprarenal vein 　Right testicular vein **1** Splenic Vein 　Left gastroepiploic vein 　Pancreatic vein **2** Gastric Vein **3** Esophageal Vein **4** Hepatic Vein **5** Superior Mesenteric Vein 　Right gastroepiploic vein **6** Inferior Mesenteric Vein 　Sigmoid vein 　Superior rectal vein **7** Colic Vein 　Ileocolic vein 　Left colic vein 　Middle colic vein 　Right colic vein **8** Portal Vein 　Hepatic portal vein **9** Renal Vein, Right **B** Renal Vein, Left 　Left inferior phrenic vein 　Left ovarian vein 　Left second lumbar vein 　Left suprarenal vein 　Left testicular vein **C** Common Iliac Vein, Right **D** Common Iliac Vein, Left **F** External Iliac Vein, Right **G** External Iliac Vein, Left **H** Hypogastric Vein, Right 　Gluteal vein 　Internal iliac vein 　Internal pudendal vein 　Lateral sacral vein 　Middle hemorrhoidal vein 　Obturator vein 　Uterine vein 　Vaginal vein 　Vesical vein **J** Hypogastric Vein, Left 　See H Hypogastric Vein, Right **M** Femoral Vein, Right 　Deep femoral (profunda femoris) vein 　Popliteal vein 　Profunda femoris (deep femoral) vein **N** Femoral Vein, Left 　See M Femoral Vein, Right **P** Saphenous Vein, Right 　External pudendal vein 　Great(er) saphenous vein 　Lesser saphenous vein 　Small saphenous vein 　Superficial circumflex iliac vein 　Superficial epigastric vein **Q** Saphenous Vein, Left 　See P Saphenous Vein, Right **T** Foot Vein, Right 　Common digital vein 　Dorsal metatarsal vein 　Dorsal venous arch 　Plantar digital vein 　Plantar metatarsal vein 　Plantar venous arch **V** Foot Vein, Left 　See T Foot Vein, Right **Y** Lower Vein	**0** Open **3** Percutaneous **4** Percutaneous Endoscopic	**0** Drainage Device	**Z** No Qualifier

Non-OR　069[0,1,2,4,5,6,7,8,9,B,C,D,F,G,H,J,M,N,P,Q,T,V,Y][0,3,4]0Z
Non-OR　069330Z

069 Continued on next page

Non-OR Procedure　DRG Non-OR Procedure　Valid OR Procedure　HAC Associated Procedure　Combination Only　New/Revised April　New/Revised October

ICD-10-PCS 2025 — Lower Veins — 069–069

0 Medical and Surgical
6 Lower Veins
9 Drainage   Definition: Taking or letting out fluids and/or gases from a body part
Explanation: The qualifier DIAGNOSTIC is used to identify drainage procedures that are biopsies

Body Part Character 4	Approach Character 5	Device Character 6	Qualifier Character 7
0 Inferior Vena Cava Postcava Right inferior phrenic vein Right ovarian vein Right second lumbar vein Right suprarenal vein Right testicular vein **1 Splenic Vein** Left gastroepiploic vein Pancreatic vein **2 Gastric Vein** **3 Esophageal Vein** **4 Hepatic Vein** **5 Superior Mesenteric Vein** Right gastroepiploic vein **6 Inferior Mesenteric Vein** Sigmoid vein Superior rectal vein **7 Colic Vein** Ileocolic vein Left colic vein Middle colic vein Right colic vein **8 Portal Vein** Hepatic portal vein **9 Renal Vein, Right** **B Renal Vein, Left** Left inferior phrenic vein Left ovarian vein Left second lumbar vein Left suprarenal vein Left testicular vein **C Common Iliac Vein, Right** **D Common Iliac Vein, Left** **F External Iliac Vein, Right** **G External Iliac Vein, Left** **H Hypogastric Vein, Right** Gluteal vein Internal iliac vein Internal pudendal vein Lateral sacral vein Middle hemorrhoidal vein Obturator vein Uterine vein Vaginal vein Vesical vein **J Hypogastric Vein, Left** See H Hypogastric Vein, Right **M Femoral Vein, Right** Deep femoral (profunda femoris) vein Popliteal vein Profunda femoris (deep femoral) vein **N Femoral Vein, Left** See M Femoral Vein, Right **P Saphenous Vein, Right** External pudendal vein Great(er) saphenous vein Lesser saphenous vein Small saphenous vein Superficial circumflex iliac vein Superficial epigastric vein **Q Saphenous Vein, Left** See P Saphenous Vein, Right **T Foot Vein, Right** Common digital vein Dorsal metatarsal vein Dorsal venous arch Plantar digital vein Plantar metatarsal vein Plantar venous arch **V Foot Vein, Left** See T Foot Vein, Right **Y Lower Vein**	**0** Open **3** Percutaneous **4** Percutaneous Endoscopic	**Z** No Device	**X** Diagnostic **Z** No Qualifier

Non-OR   069[0,1,2,3,4,5,6,7,8,9,B,C,D,F,G,H,J,M,N,P,Q,T,V,Y]3ZX
Non-OR   069[0,1,2,4,5,6,7,8,9,B,C,D,F,G,H,J,M,N,P,Q,T,V,Y][0,3,4]ZZ
Non-OR   06933ZZ

NC Noncovered Procedure   **LC** Limited Coverage   **QA** Questionable OB Admit   **NT** New Tech Add-on   **+** Combination Member   ♂ Male   ♀ Female

0 Medical and Surgical
6 Lower Veins
B Excision

Definition: Cutting out or off, without replacement, a portion of a body part
Explanation: The qualifier DIAGNOSTIC is used to identify excision procedures that are biopsies

Body Part Character 4	Approach Character 5	Device Character 6	Qualifier Character 7
0 Inferior Vena Cava Postcava Right inferior phrenic vein Right ovarian vein Right second lumbar vein Right suprarenal vein Right testicular vein **1 Splenic Vein** Left gastroepiploic vein Pancreatic vein **2 Gastric Vein** **3 Esophageal Vein** **4 Hepatic Vein** **5 Superior Mesenteric Vein** Right gastroepiploic vein **6 Inferior Mesenteric Vein** Sigmoid vein Superior rectal vein **7 Colic Vein** Ileocolic vein Left colic vein Middle colic vein Right colic vein **8 Portal Vein** Hepatic portal vein **9 Renal Vein, Right** **B Renal Vein, Left** Left inferior phrenic vein Left ovarian vein Left second lumbar vein Left suprarenal vein Left testicular vein **C Common Iliac Vein, Right** **D Common Iliac Vein, Left** **F External Iliac Vein, Right** **G External Iliac Vein, Left** **H Hypogastric Vein, Right** Gluteal vein Internal iliac vein Internal pudendal vein Lateral sacral vein Middle hemorrhoidal vein Obturator vein Uterine vein Vaginal vein Vesical vein **J Hypogastric Vein, Left** See H Hypogastric Vein, Right **M Femoral Vein, Right** Deep femoral (profunda femoris) vein Popliteal vein Profunda femoris (deep femoral) vein **N Femoral Vein, Left** See M Femoral Vein, Right **P Saphenous Vein, Right** External pudendal vein Great(er) saphenous vein Lesser saphenous vein Small saphenous vein Superficial circumflex iliac vein Superficial epigastric vein **Q Saphenous Vein, Left** See P Saphenous Vein, Right **T Foot Vein, Right** Common digital vein Dorsal metatarsal vein Dorsal venous arch Plantar digital vein Plantar metatarsal vein Plantar venous arch **V Foot Vein, Left** See T Foot Vein, Right	**0** Open **3** Percutaneous **4** Percutaneous Endoscopic	**Z** No Device	**X** Diagnostic **Z** No Qualifier
Y Lower Vein	**0** Open **3** Percutaneous **4** Percutaneous Endoscopic	**Z** No Device	**C** Hemorrhoidal Plexus **X** Diagnostic **Z** No Qualifier

Non-OR Procedure   DRG Non-OR Procedure   Valid OR Procedure   HAC Associated Procedure   Combination Only   New/Revised April   New/Revised October

ICD-10-PCS 2025 — Lower Veins — 06C–06C

- **0** Medical and Surgical
- **6** Lower Veins
- **C** Extirpation — Definition: Taking or cutting out solid matter from a body part
  Explanation: The solid matter may be an abnormal byproduct of a biological function or a foreign body; it may be imbedded in a body part or in the lumen of a tubular body part. The solid matter may or may not have been previously broken into pieces.

Body Part Character 4	Approach Character 5	Device Character 6	Qualifier Character 7

0 Inferior Vena Cava
  Postcava
  Right inferior phrenic vein
  Right ovarian vein
  Right second lumbar vein
  Right suprarenal vein
  Right testicular vein
1 Splenic Vein
  Left gastroepiploic vein
  Pancreatic vein
2 Gastric Vein
3 Esophageal Vein
4 Hepatic Vein
5 Superior Mesenteric Vein
  Right gastroepiploic vein
6 Inferior Mesenteric Vein
  Sigmoid vein
  Superior rectal vein
7 Colic Vein
  Ileocolic vein
  Left colic vein
  Middle colic vein
  Right colic vein
8 Portal Vein
  Hepatic portal vein
9 Renal Vein, Right
B Renal Vein, Left
  Left inferior phrenic vein
  Left ovarian vein
  Left second lumbar vein
  Left suprarenal vein
  Left testicular vein
C Common Iliac Vein, Right
D Common Iliac Vein, Left
F External Iliac Vein, Right
G External Iliac Vein, Left
H Hypogastric Vein, Right
  Gluteal vein
  Internal iliac vein
  Internal pudendal vein
  Lateral sacral vein
  Middle hemorrhoidal vein
  Obturator vein
  Uterine vein
  Vaginal vein
  Vesical vein
J Hypogastric Vein, Left
  See H Hypogastric Vein, Right
M Femoral Vein, Right
  Deep femoral (profunda femoris) vein
  Popliteal vein
  Profunda femoris (deep femoral) vein
N Femoral Vein, Left
  See M Femoral Vein, Right
P Saphenous Vein, Right
  External pudendal vein
  Great(er) saphenous vein
  Lesser saphenous vein
  Small saphenous vein
  Superficial circumflex iliac vein
  Superficial epigastric vein
Q Saphenous Vein, Left
  See P Saphenous Vein, Right
T Foot Vein, Right
  Common digital vein
  Dorsal metatarsal vein
  Dorsal venous arch
  Plantar digital vein
  Plantar metatarsal vein
  Plantar venous arch
V Foot Vein, Left
  See T Foot Vein, Right
Y Lower Vein
	0 Open
	3 Percutaneous
	4 Percutaneous Endoscopic
		Z No Device	**Z** No Qualifier

NC Noncovered Procedure **LC** Limited Coverage **QA** Questionable OB Admit **NT** New Tech Add-on ✚ Combination Member ♂ Male ♀ Female

0 Medical and Surgical
6 Lower Veins
D Extraction

Definition: Pulling or stripping out or off all or a portion of a body part by the use of force
Explanation: The qualifier DIAGNOSTIC is used to identify extraction procedures that are biopsies

Body Part Character 4	Approach Character 5	Device Character 6	Qualifier Character 7
M Femoral Vein, Right Deep femoral (profunda femoris) vein Popliteal vein Profunda femoris (deep femoral) vein **N Femoral Vein, Left** See M Femoral Vein, Right **P Saphenous Vein, Right** External pudendal vein Great(er) saphenous vein Lesser saphenous vein Small saphenous vein Superficial circumflex iliac vein Superficial epigastric vein **Q Saphenous Vein, Left** See P Saphenous Vein, Right **T Foot Vein, Right** Common digital vein Dorsal metatarsal vein Dorsal venous arch Plantar digital vein Plantar metatarsal vein Plantar venous arch **V Foot Vein, Left** See T Foot Vein, Right **Y Lower Vein**	**0** Open **3** Percutaneous **4** Percutaneous Endoscopic	**Z** No Device	**Z** No Qualifier

0 Medical and Surgical
6 Lower Veins
F Fragmentation

Definition: Breaking solid matter in a body part into pieces
Explanation: Physical force (e.g., manual, ultrasonic) applied directly or indirectly is used to break the solid matter into pieces. The solid matter may be an abnormal byproduct of a biological function or a foreign body. The pieces of solid matter are not taken out.

Body Part Character 4	Approach Character 5	Device Character 6	Qualifier Character 7
C Common Iliac Vein, Right **D Common Iliac Vein, Left** **F External Iliac Vein, Right** **G External Iliac Vein, Left** **H Hypogastric Vein, Right** Gluteal vein Internal iliac vein Internal pudendal vein Lateral sacral vein Middle hemorrhoidal vein Obturator vein Uterine vein Vaginal vein Vesical vein **J Hypogastric Vein, Left** See H Hypogastric Vein, Right **M Femoral Vein, Right** Deep femoral (profunda femoris) vein Popliteal vein Profunda femoris (deep femoral) vein **N Femoral Vein, Left** See M Femoral Vein, Right **P Saphenous Vein, Right** External pudendal vein Great(er) saphenous vein Lesser saphenous vein Small saphenous vein Superficial circumflex iliac vein Superficial epigastric vein **Q Saphenous Vein, Left** See P Saphenous Vein, Right **Y Lower Vein**	**3** Percutaneous	**Z** No Device	**0** Ultrasonic **Z** No Qualifier

ICD-10-PCS 2025 — Lower Veins — 06H–06H

- 0 Medical and Surgical
- 6 Lower Veins
- H Insertion

Definition: Putting in a nonbiological appliance that monitors, assists, performs, or prevents a physiological function but does not physically take the place of a body part

Explanation: None

Body Part — Character 4	Approach — Character 5	Device — Character 6	Qualifier — Character 7

0 Inferior Vena Cava
  Postcava
  Right inferior phrenic vein
  Right ovarian vein
  Right second lumbar vein
  Right suprarenal vein
  Right testicular vein
	0 Open
	3 Percutaneous
		3 Infusion Device	T Via Umbilical Vein
			Z No Qualifier

0 Inferior Vena Cava
  Postcava
  Right inferior phrenic vein
  Right ovarian vein
  Right second lumbar vein
  Right suprarenal vein
  Right testicular vein
	0 Open
	3 Percutaneous
		D Intraluminal Device	Z No Qualifier

0 Inferior Vena Cava
  Postcava
  Right inferior phrenic vein
  Right ovarian vein
  Right second lumbar vein
  Right suprarenal vein
  Right testicular vein
	4 Percutaneous Endoscopic	3 Infusion Device
		D Intraluminal Device
			Z No Qualifier

1 Splenic Vein
  Left gastroepiploic vein
  Pancreatic vein
2 Gastric Vein
3 Esophageal Vein
4 Hepatic Vein
5 Superior Mesenteric Vein
  Right gastroepiploic vein
6 Inferior Mesenteric Vein
  Sigmoid vein
  Superior rectal vein
7 Colic Vein
  Ileocolic vein
  Left colic vein
  Middle colic vein
  Right colic vein
8 Portal Vein
  Hepatic portal vein
9 Renal Vein, Right
B Renal Vein, Left
  Left inferior phrenic vein
  Left ovarian vein
  Left second lumbar vein
  Left suprarenal vein
  Left testicular vein
C Common Iliac Vein, Right
D Common Iliac Vein, Left
F External Iliac Vein, Right
G External Iliac Vein, Left
H Hypogastric Vein, Right
  Gluteal vein
  Internal iliac vein
  Internal pudendal vein
  Lateral sacral vein
  Middle hemorrhoidal vein
  Obturator vein
  Uterine vein
  Vaginal vein
  Vesical vein
J Hypogastric Vein, Left
  See H Hypogastric Vein, Right
M Femoral Vein, Right
  Deep femoral (profunda femoris) vein
  Popliteal vein
  Profunda femoris (deep femoral) vein
N Femoral Vein, Left
  See M Femoral Vein, Right
P Saphenous Vein, Right
  External pudendal vein
  Great(er) saphenous vein
  Lesser saphenous vein
  Small saphenous vein
  Superficial circumflex iliac vein
  Superficial epigastric vein
Q Saphenous Vein, Left
  See P Saphenous Vein, Right
T Foot Vein, Right
  Common digital vein
  Dorsal metatarsal vein
  Dorsal venous arch
  Plantar digital vein
  Plantar metatarsal vein
  Plantar venous arch
V Foot Vein, Left
  See T Foot Vein, Right
	0 Open
	3 Percutaneous
	4 Percutaneous Endoscopic
		3 Infusion Device
		D Intraluminal Device
			Z No Qualifier

Y Lower Vein	0 Open 3 Percutaneous 4 Percutaneous Endoscopic	2 Monitoring Device 3 Infusion Device D Intraluminal Device Y Other Device	Z No Qualifier

Non-OR	06H0[0,3]3[T,Z]
Non-OR	06H03DZ
Non-OR	06H043Z
Non-OR	06H[1,2,3,4,5,6,7,8,9,B,C,D,F,G,H,J,M,N,P,Q,T,V][0,3,4]3Z
Non-OR	06HY[0,3,4]3Z
Non-OR	06HY32Z
Non-OR	06HY[3,4]YZ

06J–06L Lower Veins ICD-10-PCS 2025

0 Medical and Surgical
6 Lower Veins
J Inspection

Definition: Visually and/or manually exploring a body part
Explanation: Visual exploration may be performed with or without optical instrumentation. Manual exploration may be performed directly or through intervening body layers.

Body Part Character 4	Approach Character 5	Device Character 6	Qualifier Character 7
Y Lower Vein	0 Open 3 Percutaneous 4 Percutaneous Endoscopic X External	Z No Device	Z No Qualifier

Non-OR 06JY[3,X]ZZ

---

0 Medical and Surgical
6 Lower Veins
L Occlusion

Definition: Completely closing an orifice or the lumen of a tubular body part
Explanation: The orifice can be a natural orifice or an artificially created orifice

Body Part Character 4	Approach Character 5	Device Character 6	Qualifier Character 7

0 **Inferior Vena Cava**
   Postcava
   Right inferior phrenic vein
   Right ovarian vein
   Right second lumbar vein
   Right suprarenal vein
   Right testicular vein
1 **Splenic Vein**
   Left gastroepiploic vein
   Pancreatic vein
4 **Hepatic Vein**
5 **Superior Mesenteric Vein**
   Right gastroepiploic vein
6 **Inferior Mesenteric Vein**
   Sigmoid vein
   Superior rectal vein
7 **Colic Vein**
   Ileocolic vein
   Left colic vein
   Middle colic vein
   Right colic vein
8 **Portal Vein**
   Hepatic portal vein
9 **Renal Vein, Right**
B **Renal Vein, Left**
   Left inferior phrenic vein
   Left ovarian vein
   Left second lumbar vein
   Left suprarenal vein
   Left testicular vein
C **Common Iliac Vein, Right**
D **Common Iliac Vein, Left**
F **External Iliac Vein, Right**
G **External Iliac Vein, Left**
	H **Hypogastric Vein, Right**
	   Gluteal vein
	   Internal iliac vein
	   Internal pudendal vein
	   Lateral sacral vein
	   Middle hemorrhoidal vein
	   Obturator vein
	   Uterine vein
	   Vaginal vein
	   Vesical vein
	J **Hypogastric Vein, Left**
	   See H Hypogastric Vein, Right
	M **Femoral Vein, Right**
	   Deep femoral (profunda femoris) vein
	   Popliteal vein
	   Profunda femoris (deep femoral) vein
	N **Femoral Vein, Left**
	   See M Femoral Vein, Right
	P **Saphenous Vein, Right**
	   External pudendal vein
	   Great(er) saphenous vein
	   Lesser saphenous vein
	   Small saphenous vein
	   Superficial circumflex iliac vein
	   Superficial epigastric vein
	Q **Saphenous Vein, Left**
	   See P Saphenous Vein, Right
	T **Foot Vein, Right**
	   Common digital vein
	   Dorsal metatarsal vein
	   Dorsal venous arch
	   Plantar digital vein
	   Plantar metatarsal vein
	   Plantar venous arch
	V **Foot Vein, Left**
	   See T Foot Vein, Right
		0 Open
		3 Percutaneous
		4 Percutaneous Endoscopic
			C Extraluminal Device
			D Intraluminal Device
			Z No Device
				Z No Qualifier

2 Gastric Vein 3 Esophageal Vein	0 Open 3 Percutaneous 4 Percutaneous Endoscopic 7 Via Natural or Artificial Opening 8 Via Natural or Artificial Opening Endoscopic	C Extraluminal Device D Intraluminal Device Z No Device	Z No Qualifier
Y Lower Vein	0 Open 3 Percutaneous 4 Percutaneous Endoscopic 7 Via Natural or Artificial Opening 8 Via Natural or Artificial Opening Endoscopic	C Extraluminal Device D Intraluminal Device Z No Device	C Hemorrhoidal Plexus Z No Qualifier

Non-OR 06L2[7,8][C,D,Z]Z
Non-OR 06L3[3,4,7,8][C,D,Z]Z

ICD-10-PCS 2025 — Lower Veins — 06N–06P

- **0** Medical and Surgical
- **6** Lower Veins
- **N** Release

Definition: Freeing a body part from an abnormal physical constraint by cutting or by the use of force
Explanation: Some of the restraining tissue may be taken out but none of the body part is taken out

Body Part — Character 4	Approach — Character 5	Device — Character 6	Qualifier — Character 7

0 Inferior Vena Cava
  Postcava
  Right inferior phrenic vein
  Right ovarian vein
  Right second lumbar vein
  Right suprarenal vein
  Right testicular vein
1 Splenic Vein
  Left gastroepiploic vein
  Pancreatic vein
2 Gastric Vein
3 Esophageal Vein
4 Hepatic Vein
5 Superior Mesenteric Vein
  Right gastroepiploic vein
6 Inferior Mesenteric Vein
  Sigmoid vein
  Superior rectal vein
7 Colic Vein
  Ileocolic vein
  Left colic vein
  Middle colic vein
  Right colic vein
8 Portal Vein
  Hepatic portal vein
9 Renal Vein, Right
B Renal Vein, Left
  Left inferior phrenic vein
  Left ovarian vein
  Left second lumbar vein
  Left suprarenal vein
  Left testicular vein
C Common Iliac Vein, Right
D Common Iliac Vein, Left
F External Iliac Vein, Right
G External Iliac Vein, Left
H Hypogastric Vein, Right
  Gluteal vein
  Internal iliac vein
  Internal pudendal vein
  Lateral sacral vein
  Middle hemorrhoidal vein
  Obturator vein
  Uterine vein
  Vaginal vein
  Vesical vein
J Hypogastric Vein, Left
  See *H Hypogastric Vein, Right*
M Femoral Vein, Right
  Deep femoral (profunda femoris) vein
  Popliteal vein
  Profunda femoris (deep femoral) vein
N Femoral Vein, Left
  See *M Femoral Vein, Right*
P Saphenous Vein, Right
  External pudendal vein
  Great(er) saphenous vein
  Lesser saphenous vein
  Small saphenous vein
  Superficial circumflex iliac vein
  Superficial epigastric vein
Q Saphenous Vein, Left
  See *P Saphenous Vein, Right*
T Foot Vein, Right
  Common digital vein
  Dorsal metatarsal vein
  Dorsal venous arch
  Plantar digital vein
  Plantar metatarsal vein
  Plantar venous arch
V Foot Vein, Left
  See *T Foot Vein, Right*
Y Lower Vein
	0 Open
	3 Percutaneous
	4 Percutaneous Endoscopic
		Z No Device	**Z** No Qualifier

- **0** Medical and Surgical
- **6** Lower Veins
- **P** Removal

Definition: Taking out or off a device from a body part
Explanation: If a device is taken out and a similar device put in without cutting or puncturing the skin or mucous membrane, the procedure is coded to the root operation CHANGE. Otherwise, the procedure for taking out a device is coded to the root operation REMOVAL.

Body Part — Character 4	Approach — Character 5	Device — Character 6	Qualifier — Character 7
Y Lower Vein	**0** Open **3** Percutaneous **4** Percutaneous Endoscopic	**0** Drainage Device **2** Monitoring Device **3** Infusion Device **7** Autologous Tissue Substitute **C** Extraluminal Device **D** Intraluminal Device **J** Synthetic Substitute **K** Nonautologous Tissue Substitute **Y** Other Device	**Z** No Qualifier
Y Lower Vein	**X** External	**0** Drainage Device **2** Monitoring Device **3** Infusion Device **D** Intraluminal Device	**Z** No Qualifier

Non-OR 06PY3[0,2,3]Z
Non-OR 06PY[3,4]YZ
Non-OR 06PYX[0,2,3,D]Z

0 Medical and Surgical
6 Lower Veins
Q Repair

Definition: Restoring, to the extent possible, a body part to its normal anatomic structure and function
Explanation: Used only when the method to accomplish the repair is not one of the other root operations

Body Part Character 4	Approach Character 5	Device Character 6	Qualifier Character 7
0 Inferior Vena Cava Postcava Right inferior phrenic vein Right ovarian vein Right second lumbar vein Right suprarenal vein Right testicular vein **1 Splenic Vein** Left gastroepiploic vein Pancreatic vein **2 Gastric Vein** **3 Esophageal Vein** **4 Hepatic Vein** **5 Superior Mesenteric Vein** Right gastroepiploic vein **6 Inferior Mesenteric Vein** Sigmoid vein Superior rectal vein **7 Colic Vein** Ileocolic vein Left colic vein Middle colic vein Right colic vein **8 Portal Vein** Hepatic portal vein **9 Renal Vein, Right** **B Renal Vein, Left** Left inferior phrenic vein Left ovarian vein Left second lumbar vein Left suprarenal vein Left testicular vein **C Common Iliac Vein, Right** **D Common Iliac Vein, Left** **F External Iliac Vein, Right** **G External Iliac Vein, Left** **H Hypogastric Vein, Right** Gluteal vein Internal iliac vein Internal pudendal vein Lateral sacral vein Middle hemorrhoidal vein Obturator vein Uterine vein Vaginal vein Vesical vein **J Hypogastric Vein, Left** *See H Hypogastric Vein, Right* **M Femoral Vein, Right** Deep femoral (profunda femoris) vein Popliteal vein Profunda femoris (deep femoral) vein **N Femoral Vein, Left** *See M Femoral Vein, Right* **P Saphenous Vein, Right** External pudendal vein Great(er) saphenous vein Lesser saphenous vein Small saphenous vein Superficial circumflex iliac vein Superficial epigastric vein **Q Saphenous Vein, Left** *See P Saphenous Vein, Right* **T Foot Vein, Right** Common digital vein Dorsal metatarsal vein Dorsal venous arch Plantar digital vein Plantar metatarsal vein Plantar venous arch **V Foot Vein, Left** *See T Foot Vein, Right* **Y Lower Vein**	**0** Open **3** Percutaneous **4** Percutaneous Endoscopic	**Z** No Device	**Z** No Qualifier

ICD-10-PCS 2025 — Lower Veins — 06R–06R

- **0 Medical and Surgical**
- **6 Lower Veins**
- **R Replacement**

Definition: Putting in or on biological or synthetic material that physically takes the place and/or function of all or a portion of a body part

Explanation: The body part may have been taken out or replaced, or may be taken out, physically eradicated, or rendered nonfunctional during the REPLACEMENT procedure. A REMOVAL procedure is coded for taking out the device used in a previous replacement procedure.

Body Part Character 4	Approach Character 5	Device Character 6	Qualifier Character 7

0 Inferior Vena Cava
   Postcava
   Right inferior phrenic vein
   Right ovarian vein
   Right second lumbar vein
   Right suprarenal vein
   Right testicular vein
1 Splenic Vein
   Left gastroepiploic vein
   Pancreatic vein
2 Gastric Vein
3 Esophageal Vein
4 Hepatic Vein
5 Superior Mesenteric Vein
   Right gastroepiploic vein
6 Inferior Mesenteric Vein
   Sigmoid vein
   Superior rectal vein
7 Colic Vein
   Ileocolic vein
   Left colic vein
   Middle colic vein
   Right colic vein
8 Portal Vein
   Hepatic portal vein
9 Renal Vein, Right
B Renal Vein, Left
   Left inferior phrenic vein
   Left ovarian vein
   Left second lumbar vein
   Left suprarenal vein
   Left testicular vein
C Common Iliac Vein, Right
D Common Iliac Vein, Left
F External Iliac Vein, Right
G External Iliac Vein, Left
H Hypogastric Vein, Right
   Gluteal vein
   Internal iliac vein
   Internal pudendal vein
   Lateral sacral vein
   Middle hemorrhoidal vein
   Obturator vein
   Uterine vein
   Vaginal vein
   Vesical vein
J Hypogastric Vein, Left
   See H Hypogastric Vein, Right
M Femoral Vein, Right
   Deep femoral (profunda femoris) vein
   Popliteal vein
   Profunda femoris (deep femoral) vein
N Femoral Vein, Left
   See M Femoral Vein, Right
P Saphenous Vein, Right
   External pudendal vein
   Great(er) saphenous vein
   Lesser saphenous vein
   Small saphenous vein
   Superficial circumflex iliac vein
   Superficial epigastric vein
Q Saphenous Vein, Left
   See P Saphenous Vein, Right
T Foot Vein, Right
   Common digital vein
   Dorsal metatarsal vein
   Dorsal venous arch
   Plantar digital vein
   Plantar metatarsal vein
   Plantar venous arch
V Foot Vein, Left
   See T Foot Vein, Right
Y Lower Vein
	0 Open
	4 Percutaneous Endoscopic
		7 Autologous Tissue Substitute
		J Synthetic Substitute
		K Nonautologous Tissue Substitute
			Z No Qualifier

NC Noncovered Procedure **LC** Limited Coverage **QA** Questionable OB Admit **NT** New Tech Add-on ✚ Combination Member ♂ Male ♀ Female

0 Medical and Surgical
6 Lower Veins
S Reposition

Definition: Moving to its normal location, or other suitable location, all or a portion of a body part
Explanation: The body part is moved to a new location from an abnormal location, or from a normal location where it is not functioning correctly. The body part may or may not be cut out or off to be moved to the new location.

Body Part Character 4	Approach Character 5	Device Character 6	Qualifier Character 7
0 Inferior Vena Cava Postcava Right inferior phrenic vein Right ovarian vein Right second lumbar vein Right suprarenal vein Right testicular vein **1 Splenic Vein** Left gastroepiploic vein Pancreatic vein **2 Gastric Vein** **3 Esophageal Vein** **4 Hepatic Vein** **5 Superior Mesenteric Vein** Right gastroepiploic vein **6 Inferior Mesenteric Vein** Sigmoid vein Superior rectal vein **7 Colic Vein** Ileocolic vein Left colic vein Middle colic vein Right colic vein **8 Portal Vein** Hepatic portal vein **9 Renal Vein, Right** **B Renal Vein, Left** Left inferior phrenic vein Left ovarian vein Left second lumbar vein Left suprarenal vein Left testicular vein **C Common Iliac Vein, Right** **D Common Iliac Vein, Left** **F External Iliac Vein, Right** **G External Iliac Vein, Left** **H Hypogastric Vein, Right** Gluteal vein Internal iliac vein Internal pudendal vein Lateral sacral vein Middle hemorrhoidal vein Obturator vein Uterine vein Vaginal vein Vesical vein **J Hypogastric Vein, Left** See H Hypogastric Vein, Right **M Femoral Vein, Right** Deep femoral (profunda femoris) vein Popliteal vein Profunda femoris (deep femoral) vein **N Femoral Vein, Left** See M Femoral Vein, Right **P Saphenous Vein, Right** External pudendal vein Great(er) saphenous vein Lesser saphenous vein Small saphenous vein Superficial circumflex iliac vein Superficial epigastric vein **Q Saphenous Vein, Left** See P Saphenous Vein, Right **T Foot Vein, Right** Common digital vein Dorsal metatarsal vein Dorsal venous arch Plantar digital vein Plantar metatarsal vein Plantar venous arch **V Foot Vein, Left** See T Foot Vein, Right **Y Lower Vein**	**0** Open **3** Percutaneous **4** Percutaneous Endoscopic	**Z** No Device	**Z** No Qualifier

ICD-10-PCS 2025 — Lower Veins

- **0** Medical and Surgical
- **6** Lower Veins
- **U** Supplement

Definition: Putting in or on biological or synthetic material that physically reinforces and/or augments the function of a portion of a body part
Explanation: The biological material is non-living, or is living and from the same individual. The body part may have been previously replaced, and the SUPPLEMENT procedure is performed to physically reinforce and/or augment the function of the replaced body part.

Body Part Character 4	Approach Character 5	Device Character 6	Qualifier Character 7

0 Inferior Vena Cava
  Postcava
  Right inferior phrenic vein
  Right ovarian vein
  Right second lumbar vein
  Right suprarenal vein
  Right testicular vein
1 Splenic Vein
  Left gastroepiploic vein
  Pancreatic vein
2 Gastric Vein
3 Esophageal Vein
4 Hepatic Vein
5 Superior Mesenteric Vein
  Right gastroepiploic vein
6 Inferior Mesenteric Vein
  Sigmoid vein
  Superior rectal vein
7 Colic Vein
  Ileocolic vein
  Left colic vein
  Middle colic vein
  Right colic vein
8 Portal Vein
  Hepatic portal vein
9 Renal Vein, Right
B Renal Vein, Left
  Left inferior phrenic vein
  Left ovarian vein
  Left second lumbar vein
  Left suprarenal vein
  Left testicular vein
C Common Iliac Vein, Right
D Common Iliac Vein, Left
F External Iliac Vein, Right
G External Iliac Vein, Left
H Hypogastric Vein, Right
  Gluteal vein
  Internal iliac vein
  Internal pudendal vein
  Lateral sacral vein
  Middle hemorrhoidal vein
  Obturator vein
  Uterine vein
  Vaginal vein
  Vesical vein
J Hypogastric Vein, Left
  See H Hypogastric Vein, Right
M Femoral Vein, Right
  Deep femoral (profunda femoris) vein
  Popliteal vein
  Profunda femoris (deep femoral) vein
N Femoral Vein, Left
  See M Femoral Vein, Right
P Saphenous Vein, Right
  External pudendal vein
  Great(er) saphenous vein
  Lesser saphenous vein
  Small saphenous vein
  Superficial circumflex iliac vein
  Superficial epigastric vein
Q Saphenous Vein, Left
  See P Saphenous Vein, Right
T Foot Vein, Right
  Common digital vein
  Dorsal metatarsal vein
  Dorsal venous arch
  Plantar digital vein
  Plantar metatarsal vein
  Plantar venous arch
V Foot Vein, Left
  See T Foot Vein, Right
Y Lower Vein
	0 Open
	3 Percutaneous
	4 Percutaneous Endoscopic
		7 Autologous Tissue Substitute
		J Synthetic Substitute
		K Nonautologous Tissue Substitute
			Z No Qualifier

NC Noncovered Procedure   **LC** Limited Coverage   **QA** Questionable OB Admit   **NT** New Tech Add-on   ✚ Combination Member   ♂ Male   ♀ Female

Lower Veins

0 Medical and Surgical
6 Lower Veins
V Restriction

Definition: Partially closing an orifice or the lumen of a tubular body part
Explanation: The orifice can be a natural orifice or an artificially created orifice

Body Part – Character 4	Approach – Character 5	Device – Character 6	Qualifier – Character 7

0 Inferior Vena Cava
  Postcava
  Right inferior phrenic vein
  Right ovarian vein
  Right second lumbar vein
  Right suprarenal vein
  Right testicular vein
1 Splenic Vein
  Left gastroepiploic vein
  Pancreatic vein
2 Gastric Vein
3 Esophageal Vein
4 Hepatic Vein
5 Superior Mesenteric Vein
  Right gastroepiploic vein
6 Inferior Mesenteric Vein
  Sigmoid vein
  Superior rectal vein
7 Colic Vein
  Ileocolic vein
  Left colic vein
  Middle colic vein
  Right colic vein
8 Portal Vein
  Hepatic portal vein
9 Renal Vein, Right
B Renal Vein, Left
  Left inferior phrenic vein
  Left ovarian vein
  Left second lumbar vein
  Left suprarenal vein
  Left testicular vein
C Common Iliac Vein, Right
D Common Iliac Vein, Left
F External Iliac Vein, Right
G External Iliac Vein, Left
H Hypogastric Vein, Right
  Gluteal vein
  Internal iliac vein
  Internal pudendal vein
  Lateral sacral vein
  Middle hemorrhoidal vein
  Obturator vein
  Uterine vein
  Vaginal vein
  Vesical vein
J Hypogastric Vein, Left
  See H Hypogastric Vein, Right
M Femoral Vein, Right
  Deep femoral (profunda femoris) vein
  Popliteal vein
  Profunda femoris (deep femoral) vein
N Femoral Vein, Left
  See M Femoral Vein, Right
P Saphenous Vein, Right
  External pudendal vein
  Great(er) saphenous vein
  Lesser saphenous vein
  Small saphenous vein
  Superficial circumflex iliac vein
  Superficial epigastric vein
Q Saphenous Vein, Left
  See P Saphenous Vein, Right
T Foot Vein, Right
  Common digital vein
  Dorsal metatarsal vein
  Dorsal venous arch
  Plantar digital vein
  Plantar metatarsal vein
  Plantar venous arch
V Foot Vein, Left
  See T Foot Vein, Right
Y Lower Vein
	0 Open
	3 Percutaneous
	4 Percutaneous Endoscopic
		C Extraluminal Device
		D Intraluminal Device
		Z No Device
			Z No Qualifier

0 Medical and Surgical
6 Lower Veins
W Revision: Correcting, to the extent possible, a portion of a malfunctioning device or the position of a displaced device

Explanation: Revision can include correcting a malfunctioning or displaced device by taking out or putting in components of the device such as a screw or pin

Body Part Character 4	Approach Character 5	Device Character 6	Qualifier Character 7
Y Lower Vein	0 Open 3 Percutaneous 4 Percutaneous Endoscopic	0 Drainage Device 2 Monitoring Device 3 Infusion Device 7 Autologous Tissue Substitute C Extraluminal Device D Intraluminal Device J Synthetic Substitute K Nonautologous Tissue Substitute Y Other Device	Z No Qualifier
Y Lower Vein	X External	0 Drainage Device 2 Monitoring Device 3 Infusion Device 7 Autologous Tissue Substitute C Extraluminal Device D Intraluminal Device J Synthetic Substitute K Nonautologous Tissue Substitute	Z No Qualifier

Non-OR 06WY3[0,2,3]Z
Non-OR 06WY[3,4]YZ
Non-OR 06WYX[0,2,3,7,C,D,J,K]Z

Lymphatic and Hemic Systems Ø71–Ø7Y

Character Meanings*

This Character Meaning table is provided as a guide to assist the user in the identification of character members that may be found in this section of code tables. It **SHOULD NOT** be used to build a PCS code.

Operation–Character 3	Body Part–Character 4	Approach–Character 5	Device–Character 6	Qualifier–Character 7
1 Bypass	Ø Lymphatic, Head	Ø Open	Ø Drainage Device	Ø Allogeneic
2 Change	1 Lymphatic, Right Neck	3 Percutaneous	1 Radioactive Element	1 Syngeneic
5 Destruction	2 Lymphatic, Left Neck	4 Percutaneous Endoscopic	3 Infusion Device	2 Zooplastic
9 Drainage	3 Lymphatic, Right Upper Extremity	8 Via Natural or Artificial Opening Endoscopic	7 Autologous Tissue Substitute	3 Peripheral Vein
B Excision	4 Lymphatic, Left Upper Extremity	X External	C Extraluminal Device	4 Central Vein
C Extirpation	5 Lymphatic, Right Axillary		D Intraluminal Device	7 Lymphatic
D Extraction	6 Lymphatic, Left Axillary		J Synthetic Substitute	G Hand-Assisted
H Insertion	7 Lymphatic, Thorax		K Nonautologous Tissue Substitute	K Thoracic Duct
J Inspection	8 Lymphatic, Internal Mammary, Right		Y Other Device	L Cisterna Chyli
L Occlusion	9 Lymphatic, Internal Mammary, Left		Z No Device	X Diagnostic
N Release	B Lymphatic, Mesenteric			Z No Qualifier
P Removal	C Lymphatic, Pelvis			
Q Repair	D Lymphatic, Aortic			
S Reposition	F Lymphatic, Right Lower Extremity			
T Resection	G Lymphatic, Left Lower Extremity			
U Supplement	H Lymphatic, Right Inguinal			
V Restriction	J Lymphatic, Left Inguinal			
W Revision	K Thoracic Duct			
Y Transplantation	L Cisterna Chyli			
	M Thymus			
	N Lymphatic			
	P Spleen			
	Q Bone Marrow, Sternum			
	R Bone Marrow, Iliac			
	S Bone Marrow, Vertebral			
	T Bone Marrow			

* Includes lymph vessels and lymph nodes.

AHA Coding Clinic for table Ø79
2021, 4Q, 47 Extraction of bone marrow from other sites
2018, 4Q, 84 Fine needle aspiration biopsy of lymphatic tissue
2017, 1Q, 34 Lymphovenous bypass following mastectomy
2014, 1Q, 26 Transbronchial needle aspiration lymph node biopsy
2013, 4Q, 111 Transbronchial needle aspiration lymph node biopsy

AHA Coding Clinic for table Ø7B
2022, 1Q, 14 Reduction mammoplasty for breast symmetry
2019, 1Q, 3-8 Whipple procedure
2018, 4Q, 84 Fine needle aspiration biopsy of lymphatic tissue
2018, 1Q, 22 Resection of lymph node chains
2016, 1Q, 30 Axillary lymph node resection with modified radical mastectomy
2014, 3Q, 10 Selective excision of paratracheal lymph nodes
2014, 1Q, 20 Fiducial marker placement
2014, 1Q, 26 Transbronchial endoscopic lymph node aspiration biopsy

AHA Coding Clinic for table Ø7D
2022, 1Q, 54 Extraction of bone marrow from other sites
2021, 4Q, 47 Extraction of bone marrow from other sites
2018, 4Q, 84 Fine needle aspiration biopsy of lymphatic tissue
2013, 4Q, 111 Root operation for bone marrow biopsy

AHA Coding Clinic for table Ø7H
2020, 4Q, 43-44 Insertion of radioactive element
2020, 4Q, 53 Bone marrow body part

AHA Coding Clinic for table Ø7Q
2017, 1Q, 34 Lymphovenous bypass following mastectomy

AHA Coding Clinic for table Ø7S
2019, 3Q, 29 Thymus transplant for T-Cell production

AHA Coding Clinic for table Ø7T
2024, 1Q, 7 Percutaneous endoscopic hand-assisted approach
2023, 2Q, 22 Norwood procedure with excision of thymus
2018, 1Q, 22 Resection of lymph node chains
2016, 2Q, 12 Resection of malignant neoplasm of infratemporal fossa
2016, 1Q, 30 Axillary lymph node resection with modified radical mastectomy
2015, 4Q, 13 New Section X codes—New Technology procedures
2014, 3Q, 9 Radical resection of level I lymph nodes
2014, 3Q, 16 Repair of Tetralogy of Fallot

AHA Coding Clinic for table Ø7Y
2023, 2Q, 32 Preparation of donor organ before transplantation
2019, 3Q, 29 Thymus transplant for T-Cell production

Lymphatic and Hemic Systems

ICD-10-PCS 2025

Lymphatic System

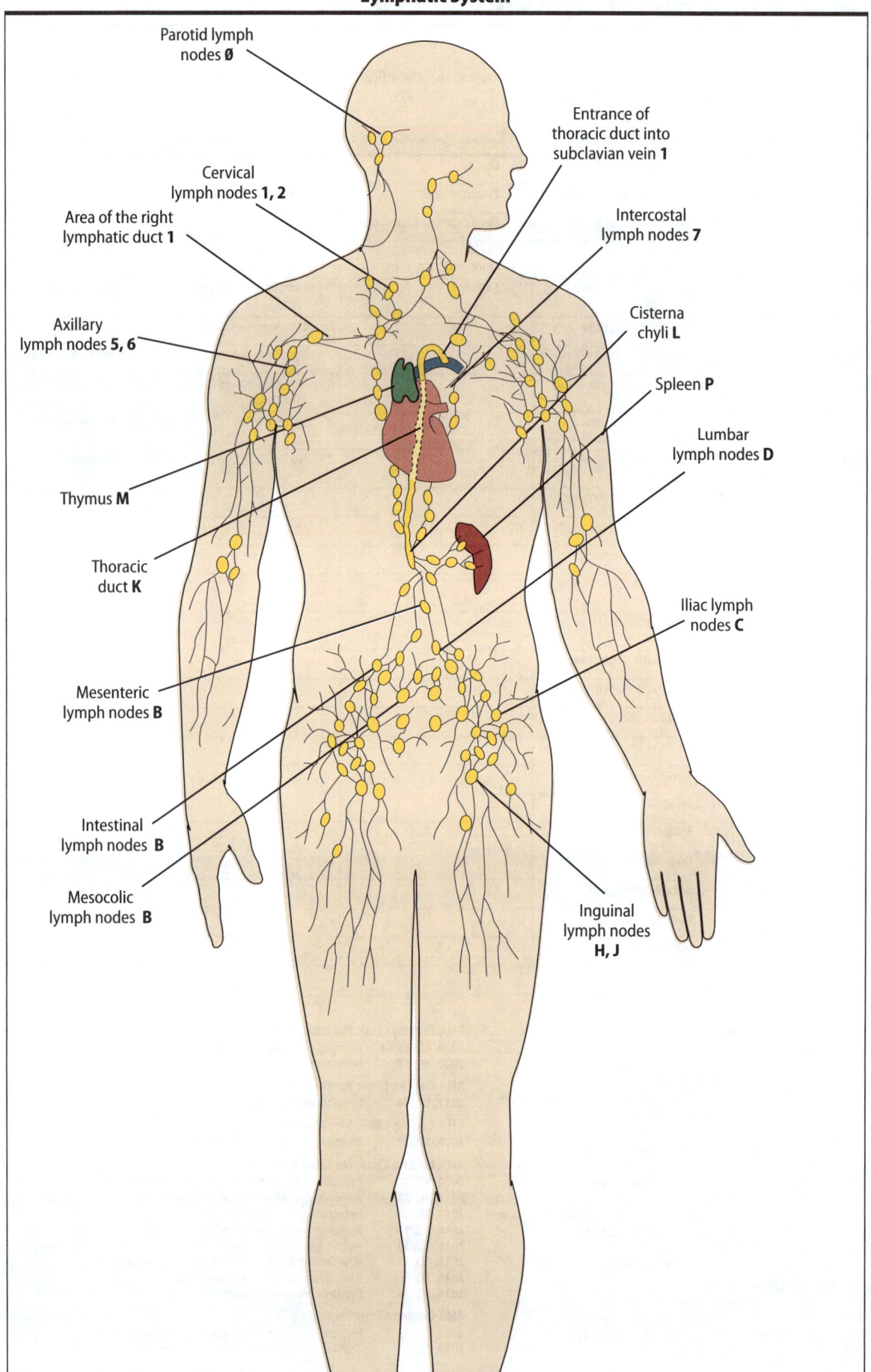

- Parotid lymph nodes **0**
- Cervical lymph nodes **1, 2**
- Area of the right lymphatic duct **1**
- Axillary lymph nodes **5, 6**
- Thymus **M**
- Thoracic duct **K**
- Mesenteric lymph nodes **B**
- Intestinal lymph nodes **B**
- Mesocolic lymph nodes **B**
- Entrance of thoracic duct into subclavian vein **1**
- Intercostal lymph nodes **7**
- Cisterna chyli **L**
- Spleen **P**
- Lumbar lymph nodes **D**
- Iliac lymph nodes **C**
- Inguinal lymph nodes **H, J**

ICD-10-PCS 2025 — Lymphatic and Hemic Systems — 071–072

- **0 Medical and Surgical**
- **7 Lymphatic and Hemic Systems**
- **1 Bypass** — Definition: Bypass: Altering the route of passage of the contents of a tubular body part

Explanation: Rerouting contents of a body part to a downstream area of the normal route, to a similar route and body part, or to an abnormal route and dissimilar body part. Includes one or more anastomoses, with or without the use of a device.

Body Part Character 4	Approach Character 5	Device Character 6	Qualifier Character 7
0 Lymphatic, Head Buccinator lymph node Infraauricular lymph node Infraparotid lymph node Parotid lymph node Preauricular lymph node Submandibular lymph node Submaxillary lymph node Submental lymph node Subparotid lymph node Suprahyoid lymph node **1 Lymphatic, Right Neck** Cervical lymph node Jugular lymph node Mastoid (postauricular) lymph node Occipital lymph node Postauricular (mastoid) lymph node Retropharyngeal lymph node Right jugular trunk Right lymphatic duct Right subclavian trunk Supraclavicular (Virchow's) lymph node Virchow's (supraclavicular) lymph node **2 Lymphatic, Left Neck** Cervical lymph node Jugular lymph node Mastoid (postauricular) lymph node Occipital lymph node Postauricular (mastoid) lymph node Retropharyngeal lymph node Supraclavicular (Virchow's) lymph node Virchow's (supraclavicular) lymph node **3 Lymphatic, Right Upper Extremity** Cubital lymph node Deltopectoral (infraclavicular) lymph node Epitrochlear lymph node Infraclavicular (deltopectoral) lymph node Supratrochlear lymph node **4 Lymphatic, Left Upper Extremity** See 3 Lymphatic, Right Upper Extremity **5 Lymphatic, Right Axillary** Anterior (pectoral) lymph node Apical (subclavicular) lymph node Brachial (lateral) lymph node Central axillary lymph node Lateral (brachial) lymph node Pectoral (anterior) lymph node Posterior (subscapular) lymph node Subclavicular (apical) lymph node Subscapular (posterior) lymph node	**0 Open** **4 Percutaneous Endoscopic**	**Z No Device**	**3 Peripheral Vein** **4 Central Vein** **7 Lymphatic** **K Thoracic Duct** **L Cisterna Chyli**
6 Lymphatic, Left Axillary See 5 Lymphatic, Right Axillary **7 Lymphatic, Thorax** Intercostal lymph node Mediastinal lymph node Parasternal lymph node Paratracheal lymph node Tracheobronchial lymph node **8 Lymphatic, Internal Mammary, Right** **9 Lymphatic, Internal Mammary, Left** **B Lymphatic, Mesenteric** Inferior mesenteric lymph node Pararectal lymph node Superior mesenteric lymph node **C Lymphatic, Pelvis** Common iliac (subaortic) lymph node Gluteal lymph node Iliac lymph node Inferior epigastric lymph node Obturator lymph node Sacral lymph node Subaortic (common iliac) lymph node Suprainguinal lymph node **D Lymphatic, Aortic** Celiac lymph node Gastric lymph node Hepatic lymph node Lumbar lymph node Pancreaticosplenic lymph node Paraaortic lymph node Retroperitoneal lymph node **F Lymphatic, Right Lower Extremity** Femoral lymph node Popliteal lymph node **G Lymphatic, Left Lower Extremity** See F Lymphatic, Right Lower Extremity **H Lymphatic, Right Inguinal** **J Lymphatic, Left Inguinal** **K Thoracic Duct** Left jugular trunk Left subclavian trunk **L Cisterna Chyli** Intestinal lymphatic trunk Lumbar lymphatic trunk			

- **0 Medical and Surgical**
- **7 Lymphatic and Hemic Systems**
- **2 Change** — Definition: Taking out or off a device from a body part and putting back an identical or similar device in or on the same body part without cutting or puncturing the skin or a mucous membrane

Explanation: All CHANGE procedures are coded using the approach EXTERNAL

Body Part Character 4	Approach Character 5	Device Character 6	Qualifier Character 7
K Thoracic Duct Left jugular trunk Left subclavian trunk **L Cisterna Chyli** Intestinal lymphatic trunk Lumbar lymphatic trunk **M Thymus** Thymus gland **N Lymphatic** **P Spleen** Accessory spleen **T Bone Marrow**	**X External**	**0 Drainage Device** **Y Other Device**	**Z No Qualifier**

Non-OR All body part, approach, device, and qualifier values

0 Medical and Surgical
7 Lymphatic and Hemic Systems
5 Destruction   Definition: Physical eradication of all or a portion of a body part by the direct use of energy, force, or a destructive agent
                 Explanation: None of the body part is physically taken out

Body Part — Character 4	Approach — Character 5	Device — Character 6	Qualifier — Character 7
0 Lymphatic, Head Buccinator lymph node Infraauricular lymph node Infraparotid lymph node Parotid lymph node Preauricular lymph node Submandibular lymph node Submaxillary lymph node Submental lymph node Subparotid lymph node Suprahyoid lymph node **1 Lymphatic, Right Neck** Cervical lymph node Jugular lymph node Mastoid (postauricular) lymph node Occipital lymph node Postauricular (mastoid) lymph node Retropharyngeal lymph node Right jugular trunk Right lymphatic duct Right subclavian trunk Supraclavicular (Virchow's) lymph node Virchow's (supraclavicular) lymph node **2 Lymphatic, Left Neck** Cervical lymph node Jugular lymph node Mastoid (postauricular) lymph node Occipital lymph node Postauricular (mastoid) lymph node Retropharyngeal lymph node Supraclavicular (Virchow's) lymph node Virchow's (supraclavicular) lymph node **3 Lymphatic, Right Upper Extremity** Cubital lymph node Deltopectoral (infraclavicular) lymph node Epitrochlear lymph node Infraclavicular (deltopectoral) lymph node Supratrochlear lymph node **4 Lymphatic, Left Upper Extremity** See 3 Lymphatic, Right Upper Extremity **5 Lymphatic, Right Axillary** Anterior (pectoral) lymph node Apical (subclavicular) lymph node Brachial (lateral) lymph node Central axillary lymph node Lateral (brachial) lymph node Pectoral (anterior) lymph node Posterior (subscapular) lymph node Subclavicular (apical) lymph node Subscapular (posterior) lymph node	**0** Open **3** Percutaneous **4** Percutaneous Endoscopic	**Z** No Device	**Z** No Qualifier
6 Lymphatic, Left Axillary See 5 Lymphatic, Right Axillary **7 Lymphatic, Thorax** Intercostal lymph node Mediastinal lymph node Parasternal lymph node Paratracheal lymph node Tracheobronchial lymph node **8 Lymphatic, Internal Mammary, Right** **9 Lymphatic, Internal Mammary, Left** **B Lymphatic, Mesenteric** Inferior mesenteric lymph node Pararectal lymph node Superior mesenteric lymph node **C Lymphatic, Pelvis** Common iliac (subaortic) lymph node Gluteal lymph node Iliac lymph node Inferior epigastric lymph node Obturator lymph node Sacral lymph node Subaortic (common iliac) lymph node Suprainguinal lymph node **D Lymphatic, Aortic** Celiac lymph node Gastric lymph node Hepatic lymph node Lumbar lymph node Pancreaticosplenic lymph node Paraaortic lymph node Retroperitoneal lymph node **F Lymphatic, Right Lower Extremity** Femoral lymph node Popliteal lymph node **G Lymphatic, Left Lower Extremity** See F Lymphatic, Right Lower Extremity **H Lymphatic, Right Inguinal** **J Lymphatic, Left Inguinal** **K Thoracic Duct** Left jugular trunk Left subclavian trunk **L Cisterna Chyli** Intestinal lymphatic trunk Lumbar lymphatic trunk **M Thymus** Thymus gland **P Spleen** Accessory spleen			

ICD-10-PCS 2025 — Lymphatic and Hemic Systems — 0Ø79–0Ø79

- **0** Medical and Surgical
- **7** Lymphatic and Hemic Systems
- **9** Drainage   Definition: Taking or letting out fluids and/or gases from a body part
  Explanation: The qualifier DIAGNOSTIC is used to identify drainage procedures that are biopsies

Body Part — Character 4	Approach — Character 5	Device — Character 6	Qualifier — Character 7
0 Lymphatic, Head Buccinator lymph node Infraauricular lymph node Infraparotid lymph node Parotid lymph node Preauricular lymph node Submandibular lymph node Submaxillary lymph node Submental lymph node Subparotid lymph node Suprahyoid lymph node **1 Lymphatic, Right Neck** Cervical lymph node Jugular lymph node Mastoid (postauricular) lymph node Occipital lymph node Postauricular (mastoid) lymph node Retropharyngeal lymph node Right jugular trunk Right lymphatic duct Right subclavian trunk Supraclavicular (Virchow's) lymph node Virchow's (supraclavicular) lymph node **2 Lymphatic, Left Neck** Cervical lymph node Jugular lymph node Mastoid (postauricular) lymph node Occipital lymph node Postauricular (mastoid) lymph node Retropharyngeal lymph node Supraclavicular (Virchow's) lymph node Virchow's (supraclavicular) lymph node **3 Lymphatic, Right Upper Extremity** Cubital lymph node Deltopectoral (infraclavicular) lymph node Epitrochlear lymph node Infraclavicular (deltopectoral) lymph node Supratrochlear lymph node **4 Lymphatic, Left Upper Extremity** See 3 Lymphatic, Right Upper Extremity **5 Lymphatic, Right Axillary** Anterior (pectoral) lymph node Apical (subclavicular) lymph node Brachial (lateral) lymph node Central axillary lymph node Lateral (brachial) lymph node Pectoral (anterior) lymph node Posterior (subscapular) lymph node Subclavicular (apical) lymph node Subscapular (posterior) lymph node **6 Lymphatic, Left Axillary** See 5 Lymphatic, Right Axillary **7 Lymphatic, Thorax** Intercostal lymph node Mediastinal lymph node Parasternal lymph node Paratracheal lymph node Tracheobronchial lymph node **8 Lymphatic, Internal Mammary, Right** **9 Lymphatic, Internal Mammary, Left** **B Lymphatic, Mesenteric** Inferior mesenteric lymph node Pararectal lymph node Superior mesenteric lymph node **C Lymphatic, Pelvis** Common iliac (subaortic) lymph node Gluteal lymph node Iliac lymph node Inferior epigastric lymph node Obturator lymph node Sacral lymph node Subaortic (common iliac) lymph node Suprainguinal lymph node **D Lymphatic, Aortic** Celiac lymph node Gastric lymph node Hepatic lymph node Lumbar lymph node Pancreaticosplenic lymph node Paraaortic lymph node Retroperitoneal lymph node **F Lymphatic, Right Lower Extremity** Femoral lymph node Popliteal lymph node **G Lymphatic, Left Lower Extremity** See F Lymphatic, Right Lower Extremity **H Lymphatic, Right Inguinal** **J Lymphatic, Left Inguinal** **K Thoracic Duct** Left jugular trunk Left subclavian trunk **L Cisterna Chyli** Intestinal lymphatic trunk Lumbar lymphatic trunk	**0** Open **3** Percutaneous **4** Percutaneous Endoscopic **8** Via Natural or Artificial Opening Endoscopic	**0** Drainage Device	**Z** No Qualifier

Non-OR 0Ø79[0,1,2,3,4,5,6,7,8,9,B,C,D,F,G,H,J,K,L][3,8]0Z

0Ø79 Continued on next page

Ø79–Ø79   Lymphatic and Hemic Systems   ICD-10-PCS 2025

Ø79 Continued

Ø Medical and Surgical
7 Lymphatic and Hemic Systems
9 Drainage   Definition: Taking or letting out fluids and/or gases from a body part
               Explanation: The qualifier DIAGNOSTIC is used to identify drainage procedures that are biopsies

Body Part Character 4	Approach Character 5	Device Character 6	Qualifier Character 7

Ø **Lymphatic, Head**
   Buccinator lymph node
   Infraauricular lymph node
   Infraparotid lymph node
   Parotid lymph node
   Preauricular lymph node
   Submandibular lymph node
   Submaxillary lymph node
   Submental lymph node
   Subparotid lymph node
   Suprahyoid lymph node
1 **Lymphatic, Right Neck**
   Cervical lymph node
   Jugular lymph node
   Mastoid (postauricular) lymph node
   Occipital lymph node
   Postauricular (mastoid) lymph node
   Retropharyngeal lymph node
   Right jugular trunk
   Right lymphatic duct
   Right subclavian trunk
   Supraclavicular (Virchow's) lymph node
   Virchow's (supraclavicular) lymph node
2 **Lymphatic, Left Neck**
   Cervical lymph node
   Jugular lymph node
   Mastoid (postauricular) lymph node
   Occipital lymph node
   Postauricular (mastoid) lymph node
   Retropharyngeal lymph node
   Supraclavicular (Virchow's) lymph node
   Virchow's (supraclavicular) lymph node
3 **Lymphatic, Right Upper Extremity**
   Cubital lymph node
   Deltopectoral (infraclavicular) lymph node
   Epitrochlear lymph node
   Infraclavicular (deltopectoral) lymph node
   Supratrochlear lymph node
4 **Lymphatic, Left Upper Extremity**
   See 3 Lymphatic, Right Upper Extremity
5 **Lymphatic, Right Axillary**
   Anterior (pectoral) lymph node
   Apical (subclavicular) lymph node
   Brachial (lateral) lymph node
   Central axillary lymph node
   Lateral (brachial) lymph node
   Pectoral (anterior) lymph node
   Posterior (subscapular) lymph node
   Subclavicular (apical) lymph node
   Subscapular (posterior) lymph node
	6 **Lymphatic, Left Axillary**
	   See 5 Lymphatic, Right Axillary
	7 **Lymphatic, Thorax**
	   Intercostal lymph node
	   Mediastinal lymph node
	   Parasternal lymph node
	   Paratracheal lymph node
	   Tracheobronchial lymph node
	8 **Lymphatic, Internal Mammary, Right**
	9 **Lymphatic, Internal Mammary, Left**
	B **Lymphatic, Mesenteric**
	   Inferior mesenteric lymph node
	   Pararectal lymph node
	   Superior mesenteric lymph node
	C **Lymphatic, Pelvis**
	   Common iliac (subaortic) lymph node
	   Gluteal lymph node
	   Iliac lymph node
	   Inferior epigastric lymph node
	   Obturator lymph node
	   Sacral lymph node
	   Subaortic (common iliac) lymph node
	   Suprainguinal lymph node
	D **Lymphatic, Aortic**
	   Celiac lymph node
	   Gastric lymph node
	   Hepatic lymph node
	   Lumbar lymph node
	   Pancreaticosplenic lymph node
	   Paraaortic lymph node
	   Retroperitoneal lymph node
	F **Lymphatic, Right Lower Extremity**
	   Femoral lymph node
	   Popliteal lymph node
	G **Lymphatic, Left Lower Extremity**
	   See F Lymphatic, Right Lower Extremity
	H **Lymphatic, Right Inguinal**
	J **Lymphatic, Left Inguinal**
	K **Thoracic Duct**
	   Left jugular trunk
	   Left subclavian trunk
	L **Cisterna Chyli**
	   Intestinal lymphatic trunk
	   Lumbar lymphatic trunk
		Ø Open
		3 Percutaneous
		4 Percutaneous Endoscopic
		8 Via Natural or Artificial Opening Endoscopic
			Z No Device	**X** Diagnostic
				Z No Qualifier

M **Thymus**
   Thymus gland
P **Spleen**
   Accessory spleen
T **Bone Marrow**
	Ø Open
	3 Percutaneous
	4 Percutaneous Endoscopic
		Ø Drainage Device	**Z** No Qualifier

M **Thymus**
   Thymus gland
P **Spleen**
   Accessory spleen
T **Bone Marrow**
	Ø Open
	3 Percutaneous
	4 Percutaneous Endoscopic
		Z No Device	**X** Diagnostic
			Z No Qualifier

Non-OR   Ø79[Ø,1,2,3,4,5,6,7,8,9,B,C,D,F,G,H,J,K,L]8ZX
Non-OR   Ø79[Ø,1,2,3,4,5,6,7,8,9,B,C,D,F,G,H,J,K,L][3,8]ZZ
Non-OR   Ø79M3ØZ
Non-OR   Ø79P[3,4]ØZ
Non-OR   Ø79T[Ø,3,4]ØZ
Non-OR   Ø79M3ZZ
Non-OR   Ø79P[3,4]Z[X,Z]
Non-OR   Ø79T[Ø,3,4]Z[X,Z]

Non-OR Procedure   DRG Non-OR Procedure   Valid OR Procedure   HAC Associated Procedure   Combination Only   New/Revised April   New/Revised October

ICD-10-PCS 2025 — Lymphatic and Hemic Systems — 07B–07B

0 Medical and Surgical
7 Lymphatic and Hemic Systems
B Excision   Definition: Cutting out or off, without replacement, a portion of a body part
           Explanation: The qualifier DIAGNOSTIC is used to identify excision procedures that are biopsies

Body Part — Character 4		Approach — Character 5	Device — Character 6	Qualifier — Character 7

0 Lymphatic, Head
  Buccinator lymph node
  Infraauricular lymph node
  Infraparotid lymph node
  Parotid lymph node
  Preauricular lymph node
  Submandibular lymph node
  Submaxillary lymph node
  Submental lymph node
  Subparotid lymph node
  Suprahyoid lymph node
1 Lymphatic, Right Neck
  Cervical lymph node
  Jugular lymph node
  Mastoid (postauricular) lymph node
  Occipital lymph node
  Postauricular (mastoid) lymph node
  Retropharyngeal lymph node
  Right jugular trunk
  Right lymphatic duct
  Right subclavian trunk
  Supraclavicular (Virchow's) lymph node
  Virchow's (supraclavicular) lymph node
2 Lymphatic, Left Neck
  Cervical lymph node
  Jugular lymph node
  Mastoid (postauricular) lymph node
  Occipital lymph node
  Postauricular (mastoid) lymph node
  Retropharyngeal lymph node
  Supraclavicular (Virchow's) lymph node
  Virchow's (supraclavicular) lymph node
3 Lymphatic, Right Upper Extremity
  Cubital lymph node
  Deltopectoral (infraclavicular) lymph node
  Epitrochlear lymph node
  Infraclavicular (deltopectoral) lymph node
  Supratrochlear lymph node
4 Lymphatic, Left Upper Extremity
  See 3 Lymphatic, Right Upper Extremity
5 Lymphatic, Right Axillary
  Anterior (pectoral) lymph node
  Apical (subclavicular) lymph node
  Brachial (lateral) lymph node
  Central axillary lymph node
  Lateral (brachial) lymph node
  Pectoral (anterior) lymph node
  Posterior (subscapular) lymph node
  Subclavicular (apical) lymph node
  Subscapular (posterior) lymph node
	6 Lymphatic, Left Axillary
	  See 5 Lymphatic, Right Axillary
	7 Lymphatic, Thorax
	  Intercostal lymph node
	  Mediastinal lymph node
	  Parasternal lymph node
	  Paratracheal lymph node
	  Tracheobronchial lymph node
	8 Lymphatic, Internal Mammary, Right
	9 Lymphatic, Internal Mammary, Left
	B Lymphatic, Mesenteric
	  Inferior mesenteric lymph node
	  Pararectal lymph node
	  Superior mesenteric lymph node
	C Lymphatic, Pelvis
	  Common iliac (subaortic) lymph node
	  Gluteal lymph node
	  Iliac lymph node
	  Inferior epigastric lymph node
	  Obturator lymph node
	  Sacral lymph node
	  Subaortic (common iliac) lymph node
	  Suprainguinal lymph node
	D Lymphatic, Aortic
	  Celiac lymph node
	  Gastric lymph node
	  Hepatic lymph node
	  Lumbar lymph node
	  Pancreaticosplenic lymph node
	  Paraaortic lymph node
	  Retroperitoneal lymph node
	F Lymphatic, Right Lower Extremity
	  Femoral lymph node
	  Popliteal lymph node
	G Lymphatic, Left Lower Extremity
	  See F Lymphatic, Right Lower Extremity
	H Lymphatic, Right Inguinal ✚
	J Lymphatic, Left Inguinal ✚
	K Thoracic Duct
	  Left jugular trunk
	  Left subclavian trunk
	L Cisterna Chyli
	  Intestinal lymphatic trunk
	  Lumbar lymphatic trunk
	M Thymus
	  Thymus gland
	P Spleen
	  Accessory spleen
		0 Open
		3 Percutaneous
		4 Percutaneous Endoscopic
			Z No Device	**X** Diagnostic
				Z No Qualifier

Non-OR 07BP[3,4]ZX

See Appendix L for Procedure Combinations
✚   07B[H,J][0,4]ZZ

0 Medical and Surgical
7 Lymphatic and Hemic Systems
C Extirpation Definition: Taking or cutting out solid matter from a body part
Explanation: The solid matter may be an abnormal byproduct of a biological function or a foreign body; it may be imbedded in a body part or in the lumen of a tubular body part. The solid matter may or may not have been previously broken into pieces.

Body Part Character 4	Approach Character 5	Device Character 6	Qualifier Character 7
0 Lymphatic, Head Buccinator lymph node Infraauricular lymph node Infraparotid lymph node Parotid lymph node Preauricular lymph node Submandibular lymph node Submaxillary lymph node Submental lymph node Subparotid lymph node Suprahyoid lymph node **1 Lymphatic, Right Neck** Cervical lymph node Jugular lymph node Mastoid (postauricular) lymph node Occipital lymph node Postauricular (mastoid) lymph node Retropharyngeal lymph node Right jugular trunk Right lymphatic duct Right subclavian trunk Supraclavicular (Virchow's) lymph node Virchow's (supraclavicular) lymph node **2 Lymphatic, Left Neck** Cervical lymph node Jugular lymph node Mastoid (postauricular) lymph node Occipital lymph node Postauricular (mastoid) lymph node Retropharyngeal lymph node Supraclavicular (Virchow's) lymph node Virchow's (supraclavicular) lymph node **3 Lymphatic, Right Upper Extremity** Cubital lymph node Deltopectoral (infraclavicular) lymph node Epitrochlear lymph node Infraclavicular (deltopectoral) lymph node Supratrochlear lymph node **4 Lymphatic, Left Upper Extremity** See 3 Lymphatic, Right Upper Extremity **5 Lymphatic, Right Axillary** Anterior (pectoral) lymph node Apical (subclavicular) lymph node Brachial (lateral) lymph node Central axillary lymph node Lateral (brachial) lymph node Pectoral (anterior) lymph node Posterior (subscapular) lymph node Subclavicular (apical) lymph node Subscapular (posterior) lymph node	**6 Lymphatic, Left Axillary** See 5 Lymphatic, Right Axillary **7 Lymphatic, Thorax** Intercostal lymph node Mediastinal lymph node Parasternal lymph node Paratracheal lymph node Tracheobronchial lymph node **8 Lymphatic, Internal Mammary, Right** **9 Lymphatic, Internal Mammary, Left** **B Lymphatic, Mesenteric** Inferior mesenteric lymph node Pararectal lymph node Superior mesenteric lymph node **C Lymphatic, Pelvis** Common iliac (subaortic) lymph node Gluteal lymph node Iliac lymph node Inferior epigastric lymph node Obturator lymph node Sacral lymph node Subaortic (common iliac) lymph node Suprainguinal lymph node **D Lymphatic, Aortic** Celiac lymph node Gastric lymph node Hepatic lymph node Lumbar lymph node Pancreaticosplenic lymph node Paraaortic lymph node Retroperitoneal lymph node **F Lymphatic, Right Lower Extremity** Femoral lymph node Popliteal lymph node **G Lymphatic, Left Lower Extremity** See F Lymphatic, Right Lower Extremity **H Lymphatic, Right Inguinal** **J Lymphatic, Left Inguinal** **K Thoracic Duct** Left jugular trunk Left subclavian trunk **L Cisterna Chyli** Intestinal lymphatic trunk Lumbar lymphatic trunk **M Thymus** Thymus gland **P Spleen** Accessory spleen	**0** Open **3** Percutaneous **4** Percutaneous Endoscopic	**Z** No Device	**Z** No Qualifier

Non-OR 07CP[3,4]ZZ

0 Medical and Surgical
7 Lymphatic and Hemic Systems
D Extraction   Definition: Pulling or stripping out or off all or a portion of a body part by the use of force
Explanation: The qualifier DIAGNOSTIC is used to identify extraction procedures that are biopsies

Body Part Character 4	Approach Character 5	Device Character 6	Qualifier Character 7

0 Lymphatic, Head
   Buccinator lymph node
   Infraauricular lymph node
   Infraparotid lymph node
   Parotid lymph node
   Preauricular lymph node
   Submandibular lymph node
   Submaxillary lymph node
   Submental lymph node
   Subparotid lymph node
   Suprahyoid lymph node
1 Lymphatic, Right Neck
   Cervical lymph node
   Jugular lymph node
   Mastoid (postauricular) lymph node
   Occipital lymph node
   Postauricular (mastoid) lymph node
   Retropharyngeal lymph node
   Right jugular trunk
   Right lymphatic duct
   Right subclavian trunk
   Supraclavicular (Virchow's) lymph node
   Virchow's (supraclavicular) lymph node
2 Lymphatic, Left Neck
   Cervical lymph node
   Jugular lymph node
   Mastoid (postauricular) lymph node
   Occipital lymph node
   Postauricular (mastoid) lymph node
   Retropharyngeal lymph node
   Supraclavicular (Virchow's) lymph   node
   Virchow's (supraclavicular) lymph   node
3 Lymphatic, Right Upper Extremity
   Cubital lymph node
   Deltopectoral (infraclavicular) lymph node
   Epitrochlear lymph node
   Infraclavicular (deltopectoral) lymph node
   Supratrochlear lymph node
4 Lymphatic, Left Upper Extremity
   See 3 Lymphatic, Right Upper Extremity
5 Lymphatic, Right Axillary
   Anterior (pectoral) lymph node
   Apical (subclavicular) lymph node
   Brachial (lateral) lymph node
   Central axillary lymph node
   Lateral (brachial) lymph node
   Pectoral (anterior) lymph node
   Posterior (subscapular) lymph node
   Subclavicular (apical) lymph node
   Subscapular (posterior) lymph node
	6 Lymphatic, Left Axillary
	   See 5 Lymphatic, Right Axillary
	7 Lymphatic, Thorax
	   Intercostal lymph node
	   Mediastinal lymph node
	   Parasternal lymph node
	   Paratracheal lymph node
	   Tracheobronchial lymph node
	8 Lymphatic, Internal Mammary, Right
	9 Lymphatic, Internal Mammary, Left
	B Lymphatic, Mesenteric
	   Inferior mesenteric lymph node
	   Pararectal lymph node
	   Superior mesenteric lymph node
	C Lymphatic, Pelvis
	   Common iliac (subaortic) lymph node
	   Gluteal lymph node
	   Iliac lymph node
	   Inferior epigastric lymph node
	   Obturator lymph node
	   Sacral lymph node
	   Subaortic (common iliac) lymph node
	   Suprainguinal lymph node
	D Lymphatic, Aortic
	   Celiac lymph node
	   Gastric lymph node
	   Hepatic lymph node
	   Lumbar lymph node
	   Pancreaticosplenic lymph node
	   Paraaortic lymph node
	   Retroperitoneal lymph node
	F Lymphatic, Right Lower Extremity
	   Femoral lymph node
	   Popliteal lymph node
	G Lymphatic, Left Lower Extremity
	   See F Lymphatic, Right Lower Extremity
	H Lymphatic, Right Inguinal
	J Lymphatic, Left Inguinal
	K Thoracic Duct
	   Left jugular trunk
	   Left subclavian trunk
	L Cisterna Chyli
	   Intestinal lymphatic trunk
	   Lumbar lymphatic trunk
		3 Percutaneous
		4 Percutaneous Endoscopic
		8 Via Natural or Artificial Opening Endoscopic
			Z No Device	**X** Diagnostic

M Thymus
   Thymus gland
P Spleen
   Accessory spleen
	3 Percutaneous
	4 Percutaneous Endoscopic
		Z No Device	**X** Diagnostic

Q Bone Marrow, Sternum **R Bone Marrow, Iliac** **S Bone Marrow, Vertebral** **T Bone Marrow**	**0** Open **3** Percutaneous	**Z** No Device	**X** Diagnostic **Z** No Qualifier

Non-OR   All body part, approach, device, and qualifier values

0 Medical and Surgical
7 Lymphatic and Hemic Systems
H Insertion

Definition: Putting in a nonbiological appliance that monitors, assists, performs, or prevents a physiological function but does not physically take the place of a body part

Explanation: None

Body Part Character 4	Approach Character 5	Device Character 6	Qualifier Character 7

K Thoracic Duct
   Left jugular trunk
   Left subclavian trunk
L Cisterna Chyli
   Intestinal lymphatic trunk
   Lumbar lymphatic trunk
M Thymus
   Thymus gland
N Lymphatic
P Spleen
   Accessory spleen
T Bone Marrow
	0 Open
	3 Percutaneous
	4 Percutaneous Endoscopic
		1 Radioactive Element
		3 Infusion Device
		Y Other Device
			Z No Qualifier

Non-OR 07H[K,L,M,N,P][0,4]3Z
Non-OR 07H[K,L,M,N,P,T]3[1,3,Y]Z
Non-OR 07H[N,P]4YZ
Non-OR 07HT[0,4][1,3,Y]Z

0 Medical and Surgical
7 Lymphatic and Hemic Systems
J Inspection

Definition: Visually and/or manually exploring a body part

Explanation: Visual exploration may be performed with or without optical instrumentation. Manual exploration may be performed directly or through intervening body layers.

Body Part Character 4	Approach Character 5	Device Character 6	Qualifier Character 7

K Thoracic Duct
   Left jugular trunk
   Left subclavian trunk
L Cisterna Chyli
   Intestinal lymphatic trunk
   Lumbar lymphatic trunk
M Thymus
   Thymus gland
T Bone Marrow
	0 Open
	3 Percutaneous
	4 Percutaneous Endoscopic
		Z No Device	Z No Qualifier

N Lymphatic	0 Open 3 Percutaneous 4 Percutaneous Endoscopic 8 Via Natural or Artificial Opening Endoscopic X External	Z No Device	Z No Qualifier
P Spleen Accessory spleen	0 Open 3 Percutaneous 4 Percutaneous Endoscopic X External	Z No Device	Z No Qualifier

Non-OR 07J[K,L,M]3ZZ
Non-OR 07JT[0,3,4]ZZ
Non-OR 07JN[3,8,X]ZZ
Non-OR 07JP[3,4,X]ZZ

0 Medical and Surgical
7 Lymphatic and Hemic Systems
L Occlusion   Definition: Completely closing an orifice or the lumen of a tubular body part
                     Explanation: The orifice can be a natural orifice or an artificially created orifice

Body Part Character 4	Approach Character 5	Device Character 6	Qualifier Character 7

0 Lymphatic, Head
   Buccinator lymph node
   Infraauricular lymph node
   Infraparotid lymph node
   Parotid lymph node
   Preauricular lymph node
   Submandibular lymph node
   Submaxillary lymph node
   Submental lymph node
   Subparotid lymph node
   Suprahyoid lymph node
1 Lymphatic, Right Neck
   Cervical lymph node
   Jugular lymph node
   Mastoid (postauricular) lymph node
   Occipital lymph node
   Postauricular (mastoid) lymph node
   Retropharyngeal lymph node
   Right jugular trunk
   Right lymphatic duct
   Right subclavian trunk
   Supraclavicular (Virchow's) lymph node
   Virchow's (supraclavicular) lymph node
2 Lymphatic, Left Neck
   Cervical lymph node
   Jugular lymph node
   Mastoid (postauricular) lymph node
   Occipital lymph node
   Postauricular (mastoid) lymph node
   Retropharyngeal lymph node
   Supraclavicular (Virchow's) lymph node
   Virchow's (supraclavicular) lymph node
3 Lymphatic, Right Upper Extremity
   Cubital lymph node
   Deltopectoral (infraclavicular) lymph node
   Epitrochlear lymph node
   Infraclavicular (deltopectoral) lymph node
   Supratrochlear lymph node
4 Lymphatic, Left Upper Extremity
   See 3 Lymphatic, Right Upper Extremity
5 Lymphatic, Right Axillary
   Anterior (pectoral) lymph node
   Apical (subclavicular) lymph node
   Brachial (lateral) lymph node
   Central axillary lymph node
   Lateral (brachial) lymph node
   Pectoral (anterior) lymph node
   Posterior (subscapular) lymph node
   Subclavicular (apical) lymph node
   Subscapular (posterior) lymph node
	6 Lymphatic, Left Axillary
	   See 5 Lymphatic, Right Axillary
	7 Lymphatic, Thorax
	   Intercostal lymph node
	   Mediastinal lymph node
	   Parasternal lymph node
	   Paratracheal lymph node
	   Tracheobronchial lymph node
	8 Lymphatic, Internal Mammary, Right
	9 Lymphatic, Internal Mammary, Left
	B Lymphatic, Mesenteric
	   Inferior mesenteric lymph node
	   Pararectal lymph node
	   Superior mesenteric lymph node
	C Lymphatic, Pelvis
	   Common iliac (subaortic) lymph node
	   Gluteal lymph node
	   Iliac lymph node
	   Inferior epigastric lymph node
	   Obturator lymph node
	   Sacral lymph node
	   Subaortic (common iliac) lymph node
	   Suprainguinal lymph node
	D Lymphatic, Aortic
	   Celiac lymph node
	   Gastric lymph node
	   Hepatic lymph node
	   Lumbar lymph node
	   Pancreaticosplenic lymph node
	   Paraaortic lymph node
	   Retroperitoneal lymph node
	F Lymphatic, Right Lower Extremity
	   Femoral lymph node
	   Popliteal lymph node
	G Lymphatic, Left Lower Extremity
	   See F Lymphatic, Right Lower Extremity
	H Lymphatic, Right Inguinal
	J Lymphatic, Left Inguinal
	K Thoracic Duct
	   Left jugular trunk
	   Left subclavian trunk
	L Cisterna Chyli
	   Intestinal lymphatic trunk
	   Lumbar lymphatic trunk
		0 Open
		3 Percutaneous
		4 Percutaneous Endoscopic
			C Extraluminal Device
			D Intraluminal Device
			Z No Device
				Z No Qualifier

0 Medical and Surgical
7 Lymphatic and Hemic Systems
N Release Definition: Freeing a body part from an abnormal physical constraint by cutting or by the use of force
Explanation: Some of the restraining tissue may be taken out but none of the body part is taken out

Body Part Character 4	Approach Character 5	Device Character 6	Qualifier Character 7
0 Lymphatic, Head Buccinator lymph node Infraauricular lymph node Infraparotid lymph node Parotid lymph node Preauricular lymph node Submandibular lymph node Submaxillary lymph node Submental lymph node Subparotid lymph node Suprahyoid lymph node **1 Lymphatic, Right Neck** Cervical lymph node Jugular lymph node Mastoid (postauricular) lymph node Occipital lymph node Postauricular (mastoid) lymph node Retropharyngeal lymph node Right jugular trunk Right lymphatic duct Right subclavian trunk Supraclavicular (Virchow's) lymph node Virchow's (supraclavicular) lymph node **2 Lymphatic, Left Neck** Cervical lymph node Jugular lymph node Mastoid (postauricular) lymph node Occipital lymph node Postauricular (mastoid) lymph node Retropharyngeal lymph node Supraclavicular (Virchow's) lymph node Virchow's (supraclavicular) lymph node **3 Lymphatic, Right Upper Extremity** Cubital lymph node Deltopectoral (infraclavicular) lymph node Epitrochlear lymph node Infraclavicular (deltopectoral) lymph node Supratrochlear lymph node **4 Lymphatic, Left Upper Extremity** See 3 Lymphatic, Right Upper Extremity **5 Lymphatic, Right Axillary** Anterior (pectoral) lymph node Apical (subclavicular) lymph node Brachial (lateral) lymph node Central axillary lymph node Lateral (brachial) lymph node Pectoral (anterior) lymph node Posterior (subscapular) lymph node Subclavicular (apical) lymph node Subscapular (posterior) lymph node	**6 Lymphatic, Left Axillary** See 5 Lymphatic, Right Axillary **7 Lymphatic, Thorax** Intercostal lymph node Mediastinal lymph node Parasternal lymph node Paratracheal lymph node Tracheobronchial lymph node **8 Lymphatic, Internal Mammary, Right** **9 Lymphatic, Internal Mammary, Left** **B Lymphatic, Mesenteric** Inferior mesenteric lymph node Pararectal lymph node Superior mesenteric lymph node **C Lymphatic, Pelvis** Common iliac (subaortic) lymph node Gluteal lymph node Iliac lymph node Inferior epigastric lymph node Obturator lymph node Sacral lymph node Subaortic (common iliac) lymph node Suprainguinal lymph node **D Lymphatic, Aortic** Celiac lymph node Gastric lymph node Hepatic lymph node Lumbar lymph node Pancreaticosplenic lymph node Paraaortic lymph node Retroperitoneal lymph node **F Lymphatic, Right Lower Extremity** Femoral lymph node Popliteal lymph node **G Lymphatic, Left Lower Extremity** See F Lymphatic, Right Lower Extremity **H Lymphatic, Right Inguinal** **J Lymphatic, Left Inguinal** **K Thoracic Duct** Left jugular trunk Left subclavian trunk **L Cisterna Chyli** Intestinal lymphatic trunk Lumbar lymphatic trunk **M Thymus** Thymus gland **P Spleen** Accessory spleen	**0** Open **3** Percutaneous **4** Percutaneous Endoscopic	**Z** No Device	**Z** No Qualifier

ICD-10-PCS 2025 — Lymphatic and Hemic Systems — 07P–07P

- **0** Medical and Surgical
- **7** Lymphatic and Hemic Systems
- **P** Removal   Definition: Taking out or off a device from a body part

Explanation: If a device is taken out and a similar device put in without cutting or puncturing the skin or mucous membrane, the procedure is coded to the root operation CHANGE. Otherwise, the procedure for taking out a device is coded to the root operation REMOVAL.

Body Part Character 4	Approach Character 5	Device Character 6	Qualifier Character 7

K Thoracic Duct
   Left jugular trunk
   Left subclavian trunk
L Cisterna Chyli
   Intestinal lymphatic trunk
   Lumbar lymphatic trunk
N Lymphatic
	0 Open
	3 Percutaneous
	4 Percutaneous Endoscopic
		0 Drainage Device
		3 Infusion Device
		7 Autologous Tissue Substitute
		C Extraluminal Device
		D Intraluminal Device
		J Synthetic Substitute
		K Nonautologous Tissue Substitute
		Y Other Device
			Z No Qualifier

K Thoracic Duct
   Left jugular trunk
   Left subclavian trunk
L Cisterna Chyli
   Intestinal lymphatic trunk
   Lumbar lymphatic trunk
N Lymphatic
	X External	**0** Drainage Device
		3 Infusion Device
		D Intraluminal Device
			Z No Qualifier

M Thymus
   Thymus gland
P Spleen
   Accessory spleen
	0 Open
	3 Percutaneous
	4 Percutaneous Endoscopic
		0 Drainage Device
		3 Infusion Device
		Y Other Device
			Z No Qualifier

M Thymus
   Thymus gland
P Spleen
   Accessory spleen
	X External	**0** Drainage Device
		3 Infusion Device
			Z No Qualifier

T Bone Marrow	**0** Open **3** Percutaneous **4** Percutaneous Endoscopic **X** External	**0** Drainage Device	**Z** No Qualifier

Non-OR   07P[K,L,N][3,4]YZ
Non-OR   07P[K,L,N]X[0,3,D]Z
Non-OR   07P[M,P][3,4]YZ
Non-OR   07P[M,P]X[0,3]Z
Non-OR   07PT[0,3,4,X]0Z

Lymphatic and Hemic Systems

0 Medical and Surgical
7 Lymphatic and Hemic Systems
Q Repair **Definition:** Restoring, to the extent possible, a body part to its normal anatomic structure and function
Explanation: Used only when the method to accomplish the repair is not one of the other root operations

Body Part — Character 4	Approach — Character 5	Device — Character 6	Qualifier — Character 7
0 Lymphatic, Head Buccinator lymph node Infraauricular lymph node Infraparotid lymph node Parotid lymph node Preauricular lymph node Submandibular lymph node Submaxillary lymph node Submental lymph node Subparotid lymph node Suprahyoid lymph node **1 Lymphatic, Right Neck** Cervical lymph node Jugular lymph node Mastoid (postauricular) lymph node Occipital lymph node Postauricular (mastoid) lymph node Retropharyngeal lymph node Right jugular trunk Right lymphatic duct Right subclavian trunk Supraclavicular (Virchow's) lymph node Virchow's (supraclavicular) lymph node **2 Lymphatic, Left Neck** Cervical lymph node Jugular lymph node Mastoid (postauricular) lymph node Occipital lymph node Postauricular (mastoid) lymph node Retropharyngeal lymph node Supraclavicular (Virchow's) lymph node Virchow's (supraclavicular) lymph node **3 Lymphatic, Right Upper Extremity** Cubital lymph node Deltopectoral (infraclavicular) lymph node Epitrochlear lymph node Infraclavicular (deltopectoral) lymph node Supratrochlear lymph node **4 Lymphatic, Left Upper Extremity** See 3 Lymphatic, Right Upper Extremity **5 Lymphatic, Right Axillary** Anterior (pectoral) lymph node Apical (subclavicular) lymph node Brachial (lateral) lymph node Central axillary lymph node Lateral (brachial) lymph node Pectoral (anterior) lymph node Posterior (subscapular) lymph node Subclavicular (apical) lymph node Subscapular (posterior) lymph node **6 Lymphatic, Left Axillary** See 5 Lymphatic, Right Axillary **7 Lymphatic, Thorax** Intercostal lymph node Mediastinal lymph node Parasternal lymph node Paratracheal lymph node Tracheobronchial lymph node **8 Lymphatic, Internal Mammary, Right** **9 Lymphatic, Internal Mammary, Left** **B Lymphatic, Mesenteric** Inferior mesenteric lymph node Pararectal lymph node Superior mesenteric lymph node **C Lymphatic, Pelvis** Common iliac (subaortic) lymph node Gluteal lymph node Iliac lymph node Inferior epigastric lymph node Obturator lymph node Sacral lymph node Subaortic (common iliac) lymph node Suprainguinal lymph node **D Lymphatic, Aortic** Celiac lymph node Gastric lymph node Hepatic lymph node Lumbar lymph node Pancreaticosplenic lymph node Paraaortic lymph node Retroperitoneal lymph node **F Lymphatic, Right Lower Extremity** Femoral lymph node Popliteal lymph node **G Lymphatic, Left Lower Extremity** See F Lymphatic, Right Lower Extremity **H Lymphatic, Right Inguinal** **J Lymphatic, Left Inguinal** **K Thoracic Duct** Left jugular trunk Left subclavian trunk **L Cisterna Chyli** Intestinal lymphatic trunk Lumbar lymphatic trunk	**0** Open **3** Percutaneous **4** Percutaneous Endoscopic **8** Via Natural or Artificial Opening Endoscopic	**Z** No Device	**Z** No Qualifier
M Thymus Thymus gland **P Spleen** Accessory spleen	**0** Open **3** Percutaneous **4** Percutaneous Endoscopic	**Z** No Device	**Z** No Qualifier

Non-OR Procedure DRG Non-OR Procedure Valid OR Procedure HAC Associated Procedure Combination Only New/Revised April New/Revised October

Lymphatic and Hemic Systems

0 Medical and Surgical
7 Lymphatic and Hemic Systems
S Reposition   Definition: Moving to its normal location, or other suitable location, all or a portion of a body part
           Explanation: The body part is moved to a new location from an abnormal location, or from a normal location where it is not functioning correctly. The body part may or may not be cut out or off to be moved to the new location.

Body Part Character 4	Approach Character 5	Device Character 6	Qualifier Character 7

M Thymus
    Thymus gland
P Spleen
    Accessory spleen
	0 Open	**Z** No Device	**Z** No Qualifier

0 Medical and Surgical
7 Lymphatic and Hemic Systems
T Resection   Definition: Cutting out or off, without replacement, all of a body part
           Explanation: None

Body Part Character 4	Approach Character 5	Device Character 6	Qualifier Character 7

0 Lymphatic, Head
    Buccinator lymph node
    Infraauricular lymph node
    Infraparotid lymph node
    Parotid lymph node
    Preauricular lymph node
    Submandibular lymph node
    Submaxillary lymph node
    Submental lymph node
    Subparotid lymph node
    Suprahyoid lymph node
1 Lymphatic, Right Neck
    Cervical lymph node
    Jugular lymph node
    Mastoid (postauricular) lymph node
    Occipital lymph node
    Postauricular (mastoid) lymph node
    Retropharyngeal lymph node
    Right jugular trunk
    Right lymphatic duct
    Right subclavian trunk
    Supraclavicular (Virchow's) lymph node
    Virchow's (supraclavicular) lymph node
2 Lymphatic, Left Neck
    Cervical lymph node
    Jugular lymph node
    Mastoid (postauricular) lymph node
    Occipital lymph node
    Postauricular (mastoid) lymph node
    Retropharyngeal lymph node
    Supraclavicular (Virchow's) lymph node
    Virchow's (supraclavicular) lymph node
3 Lymphatic, Right Upper Extremity
    Cubital lymph node
    Deltopectoral (infraclavicular) lymph node
    Epitrochlear lymph node
    Infraclavicular (deltopectoral) lymph node
    Supratrochlear lymph node
4 Lymphatic, Left Upper Extremity
    See 3 Lymphatic, Right Upper Extremity
5 Lymphatic, Right Axillary ➕
    Anterior (pectoral) lymph node
    Apical (subclavicular) lymph node
    Brachial (lateral) lymph node
    Central axillary lymph node
    Lateral (brachial) lymph node
    Pectoral (anterior) lymph node
    Posterior (subscapular) lymph node
    Subclavicular (apical) lymph node
    Subscapular (posterior) lymph node
6 Lymphatic, Left Axillary ➕
    See 5 Lymphatic, Right Axillary
7 Lymphatic, Thorax ➕
    Intercostal lymph node
    Mediastinal lymph node
    Parasternal lymph node
    Paratracheal lymph node
    Tracheobronchial lymph node
8 Lymphatic, Internal Mammary, Right ➕
9 Lymphatic, Internal Mammary, Left ➕
B Lymphatic, Mesenteric
    Inferior mesenteric lymph node
    Pararectal lymph node
    Superior mesenteric lymph node
C Lymphatic, Pelvis
    Common iliac (subaortic) lymph node
    Gluteal lymph node
    Iliac lymph node
    Inferior epigastric lymph node
    Obturator lymph node
    Sacral lymph node
    Subaortic (common iliac) lymph node
    Suprainguinal lymph node
D Lymphatic, Aortic
    Celiac lymph node
    Gastric lymph node
    Hepatic lymph node
    Lumbar lymph node
    Pancreaticosplenic lymph node
    Paraaortic lymph node
    Retroperitoneal lymph node
F Lymphatic, Right Lower Extremity
    Femoral lymph node
    Popliteal lymph node
G Lymphatic, Left Lower Extremity
    See F Lymphatic, Right Lower Extremity
H Lymphatic, Right Inguinal
J Lymphatic, Left Inguinal
K Thoracic Duct
    Left jugular trunk
    Left subclavian trunk
L Cisterna Chyli
    Intestinal lymphatic trunk
    Lumbar lymphatic trunk
M Thymus
    Thymus gland
	0 Open
	4 Percutaneous Endoscopic
		Z No Device	**Z** No Qualifier

P Spleen Accessory spleen	**0** Open	**Z** No Device	**Z** No Qualifier
P Spleen Accessory spleen	**4** Percutaneous Endoscopic	**Z** No Device	**G** Hand-Assisted **Z** No Qualifier

See Appendix L for Procedure Combinations
    ➕   07T[5,6,7,8,9]0ZZ

0 Medical and Surgical
7 Lymphatic and Hemic Systems
U Supplement Definition: Putting in or on biological or synthetic material that physically reinforces and/or augments the function of a portion of a body part
Explanation: The biological material is non-living, or is living and from the same individual. The body part may have been previously replaced, and the SUPPLEMENT procedure is performed to physically reinforce and/or augment the function of the replaced body part.

Body Part — Character 4	Approach — Character 5	Device — Character 6	Qualifier — Character 7
0 Lymphatic, Head Buccinator lymph node Infraauricular lymph node Infraparotid lymph node Parotid lymph node Preauricular lymph node Submandibular lymph node Submaxillary lymph node Submental lymph node Subparotid lymph node Suprahyoid lymph node **1 Lymphatic, Right Neck** Cervical lymph node Jugular lymph node Mastoid (postauricular) lymph node Occipital lymph node Postauricular (mastoid) lymph node Retropharyngeal lymph node Right jugular trunk Right lymphatic duct Right subclavian trunk Supraclavicular (Virchow's) lymph node Virchow's (supraclavicular) lymph node **2 Lymphatic, Left Neck** Cervical lymph node Jugular lymph node Mastoid (postauricular) lymph node Occipital lymph node Postauricular (mastoid) lymph node Retropharyngeal lymph node Supraclavicular (Virchow's) lymph node Virchow's (supraclavicular) lymph node **3 Lymphatic, Right Upper Extremity** Cubital lymph node Deltopectoral (infraclavicular) lymph node Epitrochlear lymph node Infraclavicular (deltopectoral) lymph node Supratrochlear lymph node **4 Lymphatic, Left Upper Extremity** See 3 Lymphatic, Right Upper Extremity **5 Lymphatic, Right Axillary** Anterior (pectoral) lymph node Apical (subclavicular) lymph node Brachial (lateral) lymph node Central axillary lymph node Lateral (brachial) lymph node Pectoral (anterior) lymph node Posterior (subscapular) lymph node Subclavicular (apical) lymph node Subscapular (posterior) lymph node	**0** Open **4** Percutaneous Endoscopic	**7** Autologous Tissue Substitute **J** Synthetic Substitute **K** Nonautologous Tissue Substitute	**Z** No Qualifier
6 Lymphatic, Left Axillary See 5 Lymphatic, Right Axillary **7 Lymphatic, Thorax** Intercostal lymph node Mediastinal lymph node Parasternal lymph node Paratracheal lymph node Tracheobronchial lymph node **8 Lymphatic, Internal Mammary, Right** **9 Lymphatic, Internal Mammary, Left** **B Lymphatic, Mesenteric** Inferior mesenteric lymph node Pararectal lymph node Superior mesenteric lymph node **C Lymphatic, Pelvis** Common iliac (subaortic) lymph node Gluteal lymph node Iliac lymph node Inferior epigastric lymph node Obturator lymph node Sacral lymph node Subaortic (common iliac) lymph node Suprainguinal lymph node **D Lymphatic, Aortic** Celiac lymph node Gastric lymph node Hepatic lymph node Lumbar lymph node Pancreaticosplenic lymph node Paraaortic lymph node Retroperitoneal lymph node **F Lymphatic, Right Lower Extremity** Femoral lymph node Popliteal lymph node **G Lymphatic, Left Lower Extremity** See F Lymphatic, Right Lower Extremity **H Lymphatic, Right Inguinal** **J Lymphatic, Left Inguinal** **K Thoracic Duct** Left jugular trunk Left subclavian trunk **L Cisterna Chyli** Intestinal lymphatic trunk Lumbar lymphatic trunk			

ICD-10-PCS 2025 — Lymphatic and Hemic Systems — 07V–07V

- **0** Medical and Surgical
- **7** Lymphatic and Hemic Systems
- **V** Restriction
  Definition: Partially closing an orifice or the lumen of a tubular body part
  Explanation: The orifice can be a natural orifice or an artificially created orifice

Body Part Character 4	Approach Character 5	Device Character 6	Qualifier Character 7

0 Lymphatic, Head
  Buccinator lymph node
  Infraauricular lymph node
  Infraparotid lymph node
  Parotid lymph node
  Preauricular lymph node
  Submandibular lymph node
  Submaxillary lymph node
  Submental lymph node
  Subparotid lymph node
  Suprahyoid lymph node
1 Lymphatic, Right Neck
  Cervical lymph node
  Jugular lymph node
  Mastoid (postauricular) lymph node
  Occipital lymph node
  Postauricular (mastoid) lymph node
  Retropharyngeal lymph node
  Right jugular trunk
  Right lymphatic duct
  Right subclavian trunk
  Supraclavicular (Virchow's) lymph node
  Virchow's (supraclavicular) lymph node
2 Lymphatic, Left Neck
  Cervical lymph node
  Jugular lymph node
  Mastoid (postauricular) lymph node
  Occipital lymph node
  Postauricular (mastoid) lymph node
  Retropharyngeal lymph node
  Supraclavicular (Virchow's) lymph node
  Virchow's (supraclavicular) lymph node
3 Lymphatic, Right Upper Extremity
  Cubital lymph node
  Deltopectoral (infraclavicular) lymph node
  Epitrochlear lymph node
  Infraclavicular (deltopectoral) lymph node
  Supratrochlear lymph node
4 Lymphatic, Left Upper Extremity
  See 3 Lymphatic, Right Upper Extremity
5 Lymphatic, Right Axillary
  Anterior (pectoral) lymph node
  Apical (subclavicular) lymph node
  Brachial (lateral) lymph node
  Central axillary lymph node
  Lateral (brachial) lymph node
  Pectoral (anterior) lymph node
  Posterior (subscapular) lymph node
  Subclavicular (apical) lymph node
  Subscapular (posterior) lymph node
	6 Lymphatic, Left Axillary
	  See 5 Lymphatic, Right Axillary
	7 Lymphatic, Thorax
	  Intercostal lymph node
	  Mediastinal lymph node
	  Parasternal lymph node
	  Paratracheal lymph node
	  Tracheobronchial lymph node
	8 Lymphatic, Internal Mammary, Right
	9 Lymphatic, Internal Mammary, Left
	B Lymphatic, Mesenteric
	  Inferior mesenteric lymph node
	  Pararectal lymph node
	  Superior mesenteric lymph node
	C Lymphatic, Pelvis
	  Common iliac (subaortic) lymph node
	  Gluteal lymph node
	  Iliac lymph node
	  Inferior epigastric lymph node
	  Obturator lymph node
	  Sacral lymph node
	  Subaortic (common iliac) lymph node
	  Suprainguinal lymph node
	D Lymphatic, Aortic
	  Celiac lymph node
	  Gastric lymph node
	  Hepatic lymph node
	  Lumbar lymph node
	  Pancreaticosplenic lymph node
	  Paraaortic lymph node
	  Retroperitoneal lymph node
	F Lymphatic, Right Lower Extremity
	  Femoral lymph node
	  Popliteal lymph node
	G Lymphatic, Left Lower Extremity
	  See F Lymphatic, Right Lower Extremity
	H Lymphatic, Right Inguinal
	J Lymphatic, Left Inguinal
	K Thoracic Duct
	  Left jugular trunk
	  Left subclavian trunk
	L Cisterna Chyli
	  Intestinal lymphatic trunk
	  Lumbar lymphatic trunk
		0 Open
		3 Percutaneous
		4 Percutaneous Endoscopic
			C Extraluminal Device
			D Intraluminal Device
			Z No Device
				Z No Qualifier

0 Medical and Surgical
7 Lymphatic and Hemic Systems
W Revision

Definition: Correcting, to the extent possible, a portion of a malfunctioning device or the position of a displaced device

Explanation: Revision can include correcting a malfunctioning or displaced device by taking out or putting in components of the device such as a screw or pin

Body Part Character 4	Approach Character 5	Device Character 6	Qualifier Character 7

K Thoracic Duct
  Left jugular trunk
  Left subclavian trunk
L Cisterna Chyli
  Intestinal lymphatic trunk
  Lumbar lymphatic trunk
N Lymphatic
	0 Open
	3 Percutaneous
	4 Percutaneous Endoscopic
		0 Drainage Device
		3 Infusion Device
		7 Autologous Tissue Substitute
		C Extraluminal Device
		D Intraluminal Device
		J Synthetic Substitute
		K Nonautologous Tissue Substitute
		Y Other Device
			Z No Qualifier

K Thoracic Duct
  Left jugular trunk
  Left subclavian trunk
L Cisterna Chyli
  Intestinal lymphatic trunk
  Lumbar lymphatic trunk
N Lymphatic
	X External	0 Drainage Device
		3 Infusion Device
		7 Autologous Tissue Substitute
		C Extraluminal Device
		D Intraluminal Device
		J Synthetic Substitute
		K Nonautologous Tissue Substitute
			Z No Qualifier

M Thymus
  Thymus gland
P Spleen
  Accessory spleen
	0 Open
	3 Percutaneous
	4 Percutaneous Endoscopic
		0 Drainage Device
		3 Infusion Device
		Y Other Device
			Z No Qualifier

M Thymus
  Thymus gland
P Spleen
  Accessory spleen
	X External	0 Drainage Device
		3 Infusion Device
			Z No Qualifier

T Bone Marrow	0 Open 3 Percutaneous 4 Percutaneous Endoscopic X External	0 Drainage Device	Z No Qualifier

Non-OR 07W[K,L,N][3,4]YZ
Non-OR 07W[K,L,N]X[0,3,7,C,D,J,K]Z
Non-OR 07W[M,P][3,4]YZ
Non-OR 07W[M,P]X[0,3]Z
Non-OR 07WT[0,3,4,X]0Z

0 Medical and Surgical
7 Lymphatic and Hemic Systems
Y Transplantation

Definition: Putting in or on all or a portion of a living body part taken from another individual or animal to physically take the place and/or function of all or a portion of a similar body part

Explanation: The native body part may or may not be taken out, and the transplanted body part may take over all or a portion of its function

Body Part Character 4	Approach Character 5	Device Character 6	Qualifier Character 7

M Thymus
  Thymus gland
P Spleen
  Accessory spleen
	0 Open	Z No Device	0 Allogeneic
			1 Syngeneic
			2 Zooplastic

Eye 080-08X

Character Meanings

This Character Meaning table is provided as a guide to assist the user in the identification of character members that may be found in this section of code tables. It **SHOULD NOT** be used to build a PCS code.

Operation–Character 3	Body Part–Character 4	Approach–Character 5	Device–Character 6	Qualifier–Character 7
0 Alteration	0 Eye, Right	0 Open	0 Drainage Device OR Synthetic Substitute, Intraocular Telescope	3 Nasal Cavity
1 Bypass	1 Eye, Left	3 Percutaneous	1 Radioactive Element	4 Sclera
2 Change	2 Anterior Chamber, Right	7 Via Natural or Artificial Opening	3 Infusion Device	X Diagnostic
5 Destruction	3 Anterior Chamber, Left	8 Via Natural or Artificial Opening Endoscopic	5 Epiretinal Visual Prosthesis	Z No Qualifier
7 Dilation	4 Vitreous, Right	X External	7 Autologous Tissue Substitute	
9 Drainage	5 Vitreous, Left		C Extraluminal Device	
B Excision	6 Sclera, Right		D Intraluminal Device	
C Extirpation	7 Sclera, Left		J Synthetic Substitute	
D Extraction	8 Cornea, Right		K Nonautologous Tissue Substitute	
F Fragmentation	9 Cornea, Left		Y Other Device	
H Insertion	A Choroid, Right		Z No Device	
J Inspection	B Choroid, Left			
L Occlusion	C Iris, Right			
M Reattachment	D Iris, Left			
N Release	E Retina, Right			
P Removal	F Retina, Left			
Q Repair	G Retinal Vessel, Right			
R Replacement	H Retinal Vessel, Left			
S Reposition	J Lens, Right			
T Resection	K Lens, Left			
U Supplement	L Extraocular Muscle, Right			
V Restriction	M Extraocular Muscle, Left			
W Revision	N Upper Eyelid, Right			
X Transfer	P Upper Eyelid, Left			
	Q Lower Eyelid, Right			
	R Lower Eyelid, Left			
	S Conjunctiva, Right			
	T Conjunctiva, Left			
	V Lacrimal Gland, Right			
	W Lacrimal Gland, Left			
	X Lacrimal Duct, Right			
	Y Lacrimal Duct, Left			

AHA Coding Clinic for table 081
2019, 1Q, 27   Glaucoma tube shunt

AHA Coding Clinic for table 089
2016, 2Q, 21   Laser trabeculoplasty

AHA Coding Clinic for table 08B
2014, 4Q, 35   Vitrectomy with air/fluid exchange
2014, 4Q, 36   Pars plans vitrectomy without mention of instillation of oil, air or fluid

AHA Coding Clinic for table 08J
2015, 1Q, 35   Attempted removal of foreign body from cornea

AHA Coding Clinic for table 08N
2015, 2Q, 24   Penetrating keratoplasty and anterior segment reconstruction

AHA Coding Clinic for table 08Q
2018, 3Q, 13   Repair of ruptured globe

AHA Coding Clinic for table 08R
2015, 2Q, 24   Penetrating keratoplasty and anterior segment reconstruction
2015, 2Q, 25   Penetrating keratoplasty and placement of viscoelastic eye with paracentesis

AHA Coding Clinic for table 08T
2015, 2Q, 12   Orbital exenteration

AHA Coding Clinic for table 08U
2014, 3Q, 31   Corneal amniotic membrane transplantation

Eye

Eye

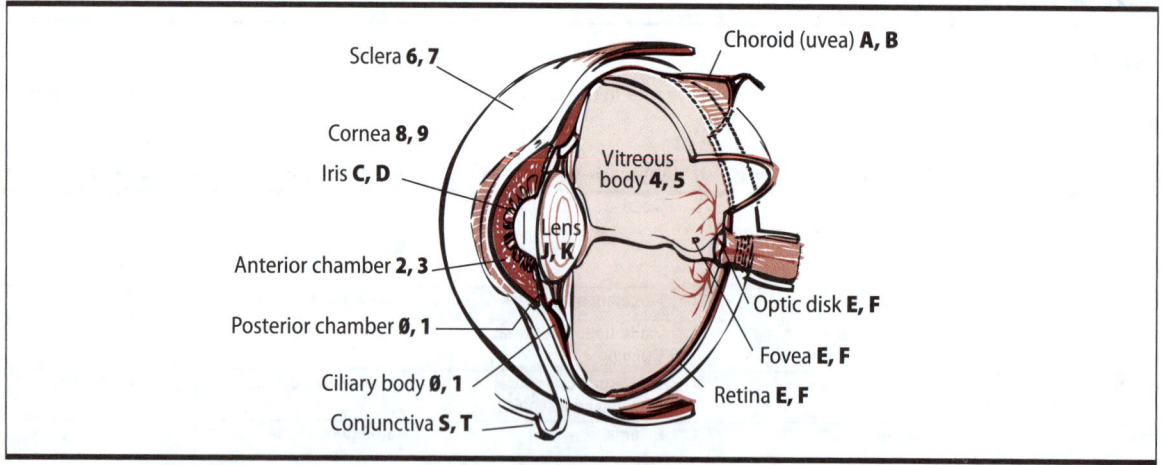

- Sclera **6, 7**
- Cornea **8, 9**
- Iris **C, D**
- Anterior chamber **2, 3**
- Posterior chamber **Ø, 1**
- Ciliary body **Ø, 1**
- Conjunctiva **S, T**
- Choroid (uvea) **A, B**
- Vitreous body **4, 5**
- Lens **J, K**
- Optic disk **E, F**
- Fovea **E, F**
- Retina **E, F**

Eye Musculature

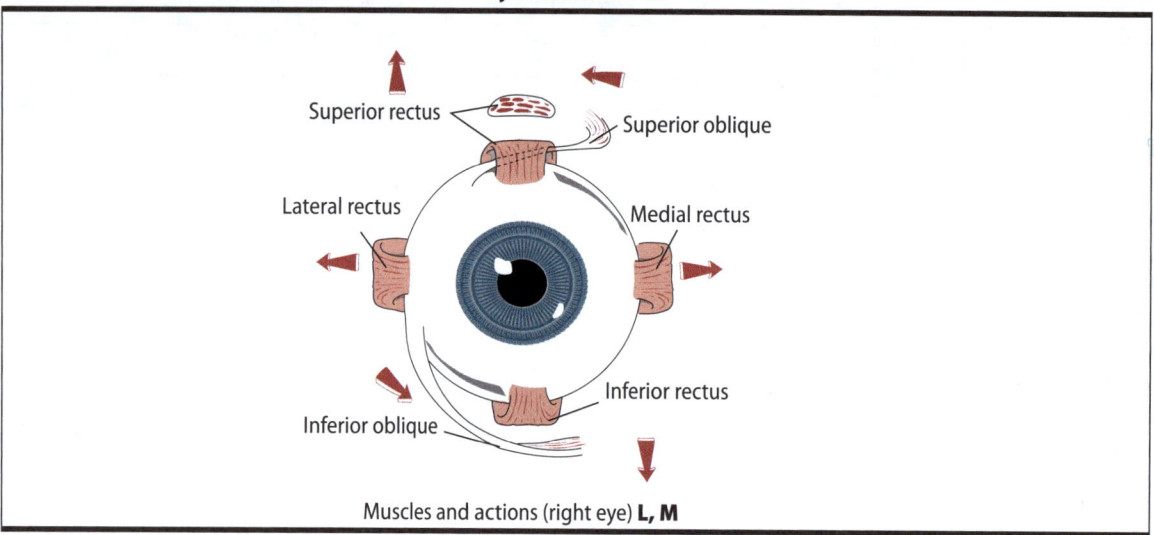

- Superior rectus
- Superior oblique
- Lateral rectus
- Medial rectus
- Inferior oblique
- Inferior rectus

Muscles and actions (right eye) **L, M**

Lacrimal System

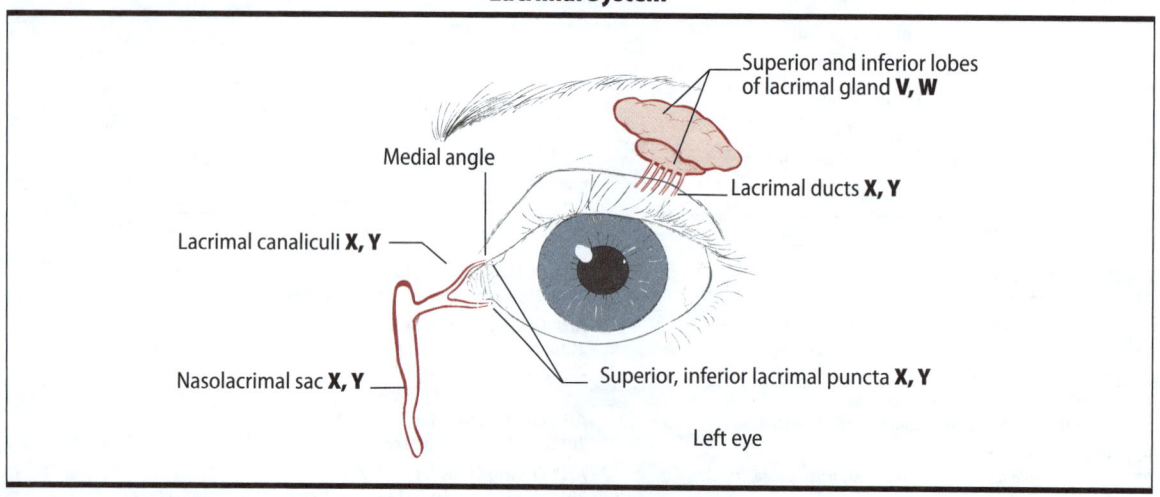

- Medial angle
- Superior and inferior lobes of lacrimal gland **V, W**
- Lacrimal ducts **X, Y**
- Lacrimal canaliculi **X, Y**
- Nasolacrimal sac **X, Y**
- Superior, inferior lacrimal puncta **X, Y**

Left eye

ICD-10-PCS 2025 — Eye — 080-082

0 Medical and Surgical
8 Eye
0 Alteration   Definition: Modifying the anatomic structure of a body part without affecting the function of the body part
Explanation: Principal purpose is to improve appearance

Body Part Character 4	Approach Character 5	Device Character 6	Qualifier Character 7
N Upper Eyelid, Right Lateral canthus Levator palpebrae superioris muscle Orbicularis oculi muscle Superior tarsal plate **P Upper Eyelid, Left** See N Upper Eyelid, Right **Q Lower Eyelid, Right** Inferior tarsal plate Medial canthus **R Lower Eyelid, Left** See Q Lower Eyelid, Right	**0** Open **3** Percutaneous **X** External	**7** Autologous Tissue Substitute **J** Synthetic Substitute **K** Nonautologous Tissue Substitute **Z** No Device	**Z** No Qualifier

Non-OR All body part, approach, device, and qualifier values

0 Medical and Surgical
8 Eye
1 Bypass   Definition: Altering the route of passage of the contents of a tubular body part
Explanation: Rerouting contents of a body part to a downstream area of the normal route, to a similar route and body part, or to an abnormal route and dissimilar body part. Includes one or more anastomoses, with or without the use of a device.

Body Part Character 4	Approach Character 5	Device Character 6	Qualifier Character 7
2 Anterior Chamber, Right Aqueous humour **3 Anterior Chamber, Left** See 2 Anterior Chamber, Right	**3** Percutaneous	**J** Synthetic Substitute **K** Nonautologous Tissue Substitute **Z** No Device	**4** Sclera
X Lacrimal Duct, Right Lacrimal canaliculus Lacrimal punctum Lacrimal sac Nasolacrimal duct **Y Lacrimal Duct, Left** See X Lacrimal Duct, Right	**0** Open **3** Percutaneous	**J** Synthetic Substitute **K** Nonautologous Tissue Substitute **Z** No Device	**3** Nasal Cavity

0 Medical and Surgical
8 Eye
2 Change   Definition: Taking out or off a device from a body part and putting back an identical or similar device in or on the same body part without cutting or puncturing the skin or a mucous membrane
Explanation: All CHANGE procedures are coded using the approach EXTERNAL

Body Part Character 4	Approach Character 5	Device Character 6	Qualifier Character 7
0 Eye, Right Ciliary body Posterior chamber **1 Eye, Left** See 0 Eye, Right	**X** External	**0** Drainage Device **Y** Other Device	**Z** No Qualifier

Non-OR All body part, approach, device, and qualifier values

Eye

0 Medical and Surgical
8 Eye
5 Destruction

Definition: Physical eradication of all or a portion of a body part by the direct use of energy, force, or a destructive agent
Explanation: None of the body part is physically taken out

Body Part Character 4	Approach Character 5	Device Character 6	Qualifier Character 7

0 Eye, Right
    Ciliary body
    Posterior chamber
1 Eye, Left
    See 0 Eye, Right
6 Sclera, Right
7 Sclera, Left
8 Cornea, Right
9 Cornea, Left
S Conjunctiva, Right
    Plica semilunaris
T Conjunctiva, Left
    See S Conjunctiva, Right
	X External	**Z** No Device	**Z** No Qualifier

2 Anterior Chamber, Right
    Aqueous humour
3 Anterior Chamber, Left
    See 2 Anterior Chamber, Right
4 Vitreous, Right
    Vitreous body
5 Vitreous, Left
    See 4 Vitreous, Right
C Iris, Right
D Iris, Left
E Retina, Right
    Fovea
    Macula
    Optic disc
F Retina, Left
    See E Retina, Right
G Retinal Vessel, Right
H Retinal Vessel, Left
J Lens, Right
    Zonule of Zinn
K Lens, Left
    See J Lens, Right
	3 Percutaneous	**Z** No Device	**Z** No Qualifier

A Choroid, Right
B Choroid, Left
L Extraocular Muscle, Right
    Inferior oblique muscle
    Inferior rectus muscle
    Lateral rectus muscle
    Medial rectus muscle
    Superior oblique muscle
    Superior rectus muscle
M Extraocular Muscle, Left
    See L Extraocular Muscle, Right
V Lacrimal Gland, Right
W Lacrimal Gland, Left
	0 Open
	3 Percutaneous
		Z No Device	**Z** No Qualifier

N Upper Eyelid, Right
    Lateral canthus
    Levator palpebrae superioris muscle
    Orbicularis oculi muscle
    Superior tarsal plate
P Upper Eyelid, Left
    See N Upper Eyelid, Right
Q Lower Eyelid, Right
    Inferior tarsal plate
    Medial canthus
R Lower Eyelid, Left
    See Q Lower Eyelid, Right
	0 Open
	3 Percutaneous
	X External
		Z No Device	**Z** No Qualifier

X Lacrimal Duct, Right
    Lacrimal canaliculus
    Lacrimal punctum
    Lacrimal sac
    Nasolacrimal duct
Y Lacrimal Duct, Left
    See X Lacrimal Duct, Right
	0 Open
	3 Percutaneous
	7 Via Natural or Artificial Opening
	8 Via Natural or Artificial Opening Endoscopic
		Z No Device	**Z** No Qualifier

Non-OR 085[E,F]3ZZ

---

0 Medical and Surgical
8 Eye
7 Dilation

Definition: Expanding an orifice or the lumen of a tubular body part
Explanation: The orifice can be a natural orifice or an artificially created orifice. Accomplished by stretching a tubular body part using intraluminal pressure or by cutting part of the orifice or wall of the tubular body part.

Body Part Character 4	Approach Character 5	Device Character 6	Qualifier Character 7

X Lacrimal Duct, Right
    Lacrimal canaliculus
    Lacrimal punctum
    Lacrimal sac
    Nasolacrimal duct
Y Lacrimal Duct, Left
    See X Lacrimal Duct, Right
	0 Open
	3 Percutaneous
	7 Via Natural or Artificial Opening
	8 Via Natural or Artificial Opening Endoscopic
		D Intraluminal Device
		Z No Device
			Z No Qualifier

ICD-10-PCS 2025   Eye   089–089

0 Medical and Surgical
8 Eye
9 Drainage   Definition: Taking or letting out fluids and/or gases from a body part
            Explanation: The qualifier DIAGNOSTIC is used to identify drainage procedures that are biopsies

Body Part Character 4		Approach Character 5	Device Character 6	Qualifier Character 7

0 Eye, Right
   Ciliary body
   Posterior chamber
1 Eye, Left
   See 0 Eye, Right
6 Sclera, Right
7 Sclera, Left
	8 Cornea, Right
	9 Cornea, Left
	S Conjunctiva, Right
	   Plica semilunaris
	T Conjunctiva, Left
	   See S Conjunctiva, Right
		X External	**0** Drainage Device	**Z** No Qualifier

0 Eye, Right
   Ciliary body
   Posterior chamber
1 Eye, Left
   See 0 Eye, Right
6 Sclera, Right
7 Sclera, Left
	8 Cornea, Right
	9 Cornea, Left
	S Conjunctiva, Right
	   Plica semilunaris
	T Conjunctiva, Left
	   See S Conjunctiva, Right
		X External	**Z** No Device	**X** Diagnostic
				Z No Qualifier

2 Anterior Chamber, Right
   Aqueous humour
3 Anterior Chamber, Left
   See 2 Anterior Chamber, Right
4 Vitreous, Right
   Vitreous body
5 Vitreous, Left
   See 4 Vitreous, Right
C Iris, Right
D Iris, Left
	E Retina, Right
	   Fovea
	   Macula
	   Optic disc
	F Retina, Left
	   See E Retina, Right
	G Retinal Vessel, Right
	H Retinal Vessel, Left
	J Lens, Right
	   Zonule of Zinn
	K Lens, Left
	   See J Lens, Right
		3 Percutaneous	**0** Drainage Device	**Z** No Qualifier

2 Anterior Chamber, Right
   Aqueous humour
3 Anterior Chamber, Left
   See 2 Anterior Chamber, Right
4 Vitreous, Right
   Vitreous body
5 Vitreous, Left
   See 4 Vitreous, Right
C Iris, Right
D Iris, Left
	E Retina, Right
	   Fovea
	   Macula
	   Optic disc
	F Retina, Left
	   See E Retina, Right
	G Retinal Vessel, Right
	H Retinal Vessel, Left
	J Lens, Right
	   Zonule of Zinn
	K Lens, Left
	   See J Lens, Right
		3 Percutaneous	**Z** No Device	**X** Diagnostic
				Z No Qualifier

A Choroid, Right
B Choroid, Left
L Extraocular Muscle, Right
   Inferior oblique muscle
   Inferior rectus muscle
   Lateral rectus muscle
   Medial rectus muscle
   Superior oblique muscle
   Superior rectus muscle
	M Extraocular Muscle, Left
	   See L Extraocular Muscle, Right
	V Lacrimal Gland, Right
	W Lacrimal Gland, Left
		0 Open
		3 Percutaneous
			0 Drainage Device	**Z** No Qualifier

A Choroid, Right
B Choroid, Left
L Extraocular Muscle, Right
   Inferior oblique muscle
   Inferior rectus muscle
   Lateral rectus muscle
   Medial rectus muscle
   Superior oblique muscle
   Superior rectus muscle
	M Extraocular Muscle, Left
	   See L Extraocular Muscle, Right
	V Lacrimal Gland, Right
	W Lacrimal Gland, Left
		0 Open
		3 Percutaneous
			Z No Device	**X** Diagnostic
				Z No Qualifier

N Upper Eyelid, Right
   Lateral canthus
   Levator palpebrae superioris muscle
   Orbicularis oculi muscle
   Superior tarsal plate
P Upper Eyelid, Left
   See N Upper Eyelid, Right
	Q Lower Eyelid, Right
	   Inferior tarsal plate
	   Medial canthus
	R Lower Eyelid, Left
	   See Q Lower Eyelid, Right
		0 Open
		3 Percutaneous
		X External
			0 Drainage Device	**Z** No Qualifier

Non-OR   089[0,1,6,7,8,9,S,T]XZ[X,Z]
Non-OR   089[N,P,Q,R][0,3,X]0Z

089 Continued on next page

0 Medical and Surgical
8 Eye
9 Drainage

Definition: Taking or letting out fluids and/or gases from a body part
Explanation: The qualifier DIAGNOSTIC is used to identify drainage procedures that are biopsies

089 Continued

Body Part Character 4	Approach Character 5	Device Character 6	Qualifier Character 7

N Upper Eyelid, Right
  Lateral canthus
  Levator palpebrae superioris muscle
  Orbicularis oculi muscle
  Superior tarsal plate
P Upper Eyelid, Left
  See N Upper Eyelid, Right
Q Lower Eyelid, Right
  Inferior tarsal plate
  Medial canthus
R Lower Eyelid, Left
  See Q Lower Eyelid, Right
	0 Open
	3 Percutaneous
	X External
		Z No Device	X Diagnostic
			Z No Qualifier

X Lacrimal Duct, Right
  Lacrimal canaliculus
  Lacrimal punctum
  Lacrimal sac
  Nasolacrimal duct
Y Lacrimal Duct, Left
  See X Lacrimal Duct, Right
	0 Open
	3 Percutaneous
	7 Via Natural or Artificial Opening
	8 Via Natural or Artificial Opening Endoscopic
		0 Drainage Device	Z No Qualifier

X Lacrimal Duct, Right
  Lacrimal canaliculus
  Lacrimal punctum
  Lacrimal sac
  Nasolacrimal duct
Y Lacrimal Duct, Left
  See X Lacrimal Duct, Right
	0 Open
	3 Percutaneous
	7 Via Natural or Artificial Opening
	8 Via Natural or Artificial Opening Endoscopic
		Z No Device	X Diagnostic
			Z No Qualifier

Non-OR   089[N,P,Q,R]0ZZ
Non-OR   089[N,P,Q,R][3,X]Z[X,Z]

0 Medical and Surgical
8 Eye
B Excision

Definition: Cutting out or off, without replacement, a portion of a body part
Explanation: The qualifier DIAGNOSTIC is used to identify excision procedures that are biopsies

Body Part Character 4	Approach Character 5	Device Character 6	Qualifier Character 7

0 Eye, Right
  Ciliary body
  Posterior chamber
1 Eye, Left
  See 0 Eye, Right
N Upper Eyelid, Right
  Lateral canthus
  Levator palpebrae superioris muscle
  Orbicularis oculi muscle
  Superior tarsal plate
P Upper Eyelid, Left
  See N Upper Eyelid, Right
Q Lower Eyelid, Right
  Inferior tarsal plate
  Medial canthus
R Lower Eyelid, Left
  See Q Lower Eyelid, Right
	0 Open
	3 Percutaneous
	X External
		Z No Device	X Diagnostic
			Z No Qualifier

4 Vitreous, Right
  Vitreous body
5 Vitreous, Left
  See 4 Vitreous, Right
C Iris, Right
D Iris, Left
E Retina, Right
  Fovea
  Macula
  Optic disc
F Retina, Left
  See E Retina, Right
J Lens, Right
  Zonule of Zinn
K Lens, Left
  See J Lens, Right
	3 Percutaneous	Z No Device	X Diagnostic
			Z No Qualifier

6 Sclera, Right
7 Sclera, Left
8 Cornea, Right
9 Cornea, Left
S Conjunctiva, Right
  Plica semilunaris
T Conjunctiva, Left
  See S Conjunctiva, Right
	X External	Z No Device	X Diagnostic
			Z No Qualifier

A Choroid, Right
B Choroid, Left
L Extraocular Muscle, Right
  Inferior oblique muscle
  Inferior rectus muscle
  Lateral rectus muscle
  Medial rectus muscle
  Superior oblique muscle
  Superior rectus muscle
M Extraocular Muscle, Left
  See L Extraocular Muscle, Right
V Lacrimal Gland, Right
W Lacrimal Gland, Left
	0 Open
	3 Percutaneous
		Z No Device	X Diagnostic
			Z No Qualifier

X Lacrimal Duct, Right
  Lacrimal canaliculus
  Lacrimal punctum
  Lacrimal sac
  Nasolacrimal duct
Y Lacrimal Duct, Left
  See X Lacrimal Duct, Right
	0 Open
	3 Percutaneous
	7 Via Natural or Artificial Opening
	8 Via Natural or Artificial Opening Endoscopic
		Z No Device	X Diagnostic
			Z No Qualifier

ICD-10-PCS 2025 — Eye — 08C–08C

- **0** Medical and Surgical
- **8** Eye
- **C** Extirpation

Definition: Taking or cutting out solid matter from a body part

Explanation: The solid matter may be an abnormal byproduct of a biological function or a foreign body; it may be imbedded in a body part or in the lumen of a tubular body part. The solid matter may or may not have been previously broken into pieces.

Body Part Character 4	Approach Character 5	Device Character 6	Qualifier Character 7

0 Eye, Right
  Ciliary body
  Posterior chamber
1 Eye, Left
  See 0 Eye, Right
6 Sclera, Right
7 Sclera, Left
8 Cornea, Right
9 Cornea, Left
S Conjunctiva, Right
  Plica semilunaris
T Conjunctiva, Left
  See S Conjunctiva, Right
	X External	**Z** No Device	**Z** No Qualifier

2 Anterior Chamber, Right
  Aqueous humour
3 Anterior Chamber, Left
  See 2 Anterior Chamber, Right
4 Vitreous, Right
  Vitreous body
5 Vitreous, Left
  See 4 Vitreous, Right
C Iris, Right
D Iris, Left
E Retina, Right
  Fovea
  Macula
  Optic disc
F Retina, Left
  See E Retina, Right
G Retinal Vessel, Right
H Retinal Vessel, Left
J Lens, Right
  Zonule of Zinn
K Lens, Left
  See J Lens, Right
	3 Percutaneous
	X External
		Z No Device	**Z** No Qualifier

A Choroid, Right
B Choroid, Left
L Extraocular Muscle, Right
  Inferior oblique muscle
  Inferior rectus muscle
  Lateral rectus muscle
  Medial rectus muscle
  Superior oblique muscle
  Superior rectus muscle
M Extraocular Muscle, Left
  See L Extraocular Muscle, Right
N Upper Eyelid, Right
  Lateral canthus
  Levator palpebrae superioris muscle
  Orbicularis oculi muscle
  Superior tarsal plate
P Upper Eyelid, Left
  See N Upper Eyelid, Right
Q Lower Eyelid, Right
  Inferior tarsal plate
  Medial canthus
R Lower Eyelid, Left
  See Q Lower Eyelid, Right
V Lacrimal Gland, Right
W Lacrimal Gland, Left
	0 Open
	3 Percutaneous
	X External
		Z No Device	**Z** No Qualifier

X Lacrimal Duct, Right
  Lacrimal canaliculus
  Lacrimal punctum
  Lacrimal sac
  Nasolacrimal duct
Y Lacrimal Duct, Left
  See X Lacrimal Duct, Right
	0 Open
	3 Percutaneous
	7 Via Natural or Artificial Opening
	8 Via Natural or Artificial Opening Endoscopic
		Z No Device	**Z** No Qualifier

Non-OR 08C[0,1,6,7,S,T]XZZ
Non-OR 08C[2,3]XZZ
Non-OR 08C[N,P,Q,R][0,3,X]ZZ

0 Medical and Surgical
8 Eye
D Extraction

Definition: Pulling or stripping out or off all or a portion of a body part by the use of force
Explanation: The qualifier DIAGNOSTIC is used to identify extraction procedures that are biopsies

Body Part Character 4	Approach Character 5	Device Character 6	Qualifier Character 7
8 Cornea, Right 9 Cornea, Left	X External	Z No Device	X Diagnostic Z No Qualifier

J Lens, Right
    Zonule of Zinn
K Lens, Left
    See J Lens, Right
	3 Percutaneous	Z No Device	Z No Qualifier

0 Medical and Surgical
8 Eye
F Fragmentation

Definition: Breaking solid matter in a body part into pieces
Explanation: Physical force (e.g., manual, ultrasonic) applied directly or indirectly is used to break the solid matter into pieces. The solid matter may be an abnormal byproduct of a biological function or a foreign body. The pieces of solid matter are not taken out.

Body Part Character 4	Approach Character 5	Device Character 6	Qualifier Character 7

4 Vitreous, Right   **NC**
    Vitreous body
5 Vitreous, Left   **NC**
    See 4 Vitreous, Right
	3 Percutaneous
	X External
		Z No Device	Z No Qualifier

Non-OR 08F[4,5]XZZ
NC 08F[4,5]XZZ

0 Medical and Surgical
8 Eye
H Insertion

Definition: Putting in a nonbiological appliance that monitors, assists, performs, or prevents a physiological function but does not physically take the place of a body part
Explanation: None

Body Part Character 4	Approach Character 5	Device Character 6	Qualifier Character 7

0 Eye, Right
    Ciliary body
    Posterior chamber
1 Eye, Left
    See 0 Eye, Right
	0 Open	5 Epiretinal Visual Prosthesis
		Y Other Device
			Z No Qualifier

0 Eye, Right
    Ciliary body
    Posterior chamber
1 Eye, Left
    See 0 Eye, Right
	3 Percutaneous	1 Radioactive Element
		3 Infusion Device
		Y Other Device
			Z No Qualifier

0 Eye, Right
    Ciliary body
    Posterior chamber
1 Eye, Left
    See 0 Eye, Right
	7 Via Natural or Artificial Opening
	8 Via Natural or Artificial Opening Endoscopic
		Y Other Device	Z No Qualifier

0 Eye, Right
    Ciliary body
    Posterior chamber
1 Eye, Left
    See 0 Eye, Right
	X External	1 Radioactive Element
		3 Infusion Device
			Z No Qualifier

Non-OR 08H[0,1]3YZ
Non-OR 08H[0,1][7,8]YZ

ICD-10-PCS 2025 — Eye — 08J–08M

0 Medical and Surgical
8 Eye
J Inspection

Definition: Visually and/or manually exploring a body part

Explanation: Visual exploration may be performed with or without optical instrumentation. Manual exploration may be performed directly or through intervening body layers.

Body Part Character 4	Approach Character 5	Device Character 6	Qualifier Character 7

0 Eye, Right
  Ciliary body
  Posterior chamber
1 Eye, Left
  See 0 Eye, Right
J Lens, Right
  Zonule of Zinn
K Lens, Left
  See J Lens, Right
	X External	Z No Device	Z No Qualifier

L Extraocular Muscle, Right
  Inferior oblique muscle
  Inferior rectus muscle
  Lateral rectus muscle
  Medial rectus muscle
  Superior oblique muscle
  Superior rectus muscle
M Extraocular Muscle, Left
  See L Extraocular Muscle, Right
	0 Open
	X External
		Z No Device	Z No Qualifier

Non-OR 08J[0,1,J,K]XZZ
Non-OR 08J[L,M]XZZ

0 Medical and Surgical
8 Eye
L Occlusion

Definition: Completely closing an orifice or the lumen of a tubular body part

Explanation: The orifice can be a natural orifice or an artificially created orifice

Body Part Character 4	Approach Character 5	Device Character 6	Qualifier Character 7

X Lacrimal Duct, Right
  Lacrimal canaliculus
  Lacrimal punctum
  Lacrimal sac
  Nasolacrimal duct
Y Lacrimal Duct, Left
  See X Lacrimal Duct, Right
	0 Open
	3 Percutaneous
		C Extraluminal Device
		D Intraluminal Device
		Z No Device
			Z No Qualifier

X Lacrimal Duct, Right
  Lacrimal canaliculus
  Lacrimal punctum
  Lacrimal sac
  Nasolacrimal duct
Y Lacrimal Duct, Left
  See X Lacrimal Duct, Right
	7 Via Natural or Artificial Opening
	8 Via Natural or Artificial Opening Endoscopic
		D Intraluminal Device
		Z No Device
			Z No Qualifier

0 Medical and Surgical
8 Eye
M Reattachment

Definition: Putting back in or on all or a portion of a separated body part to its normal location or other suitable location

Explanation: Vascular circulation and nervous pathways may or may not be reestablished

Body Part Character 4	Approach Character 5	Device Character 6	Qualifier Character 7

N Upper Eyelid, Right
  Lateral canthus
  Levator palpebrae superioris muscle
  Orbicularis oculi muscle
  Superior tarsal plate
P Upper Eyelid, Left
  See N Upper Eyelid, Right
Q Lower Eyelid, Right
  Inferior tarsal plate
  Medial canthus
R Lower Eyelid, Left
  See Q Lower Eyelid, Right
	X External	Z No Device	Z No Qualifier

0 Medical and Surgical
8 Eye
N Release — Definition: Freeing a body part from an abnormal physical constraint by cutting or by the use of force
Explanation: Some of the restraining tissue may be taken out but none of the body part is taken out

Body Part Character 4	Approach Character 5	Device Character 6	Qualifier Character 7

0 Eye, Right
  Ciliary body
  Posterior chamber
1 Eye, Left
  See 0 Eye, Right
6 Sclera, Right
7 Sclera, Left
8 Cornea, Right
9 Cornea, Left
S Conjunctiva, Right
  Plica semilunaris
T Conjunctiva, Left
  See S Conjunctiva, Right
	X External	Z No Device	Z No Qualifier

2 Anterior Chamber, Right
  Aqueous humour
3 Anterior Chamber, Left
  See 2 Anterior Chamber, Right
4 Vitreous, Right
  Vitreous body
5 Vitreous, Left
  See 4 Vitreous, Right
C Iris, Right
D Iris, Left
E Retina, Right
  Fovea
  Macula
  Optic disc
F Retina, Left
  See E Retina, Right
G Retinal Vessel, Right
H Retinal Vessel, Left
J Lens, Right
  Zonule of Zinn
K Lens, Left
  See J Lens, Right
	3 Percutaneous	Z No Device	Z No Qualifier

A Choroid, Right
B Choroid, Left
L Extraocular Muscle, Right
  Inferior oblique muscle
  Inferior rectus muscle
  Lateral rectus muscle
  Medial rectus muscle
  Superior oblique muscle
  Superior rectus muscle
M Extraocular Muscle, Left
  See L Extraocular Muscle, Right
V Lacrimal Gland, Right
W Lacrimal Gland, Left
	0 Open
	3 Percutaneous
		Z No Device	Z No Qualifier

N Upper Eyelid, Right
  Lateral canthus
  Levator palpebrae superioris muscle
  Orbicularis oculi muscle
  Superior tarsal plate
P Upper Eyelid, Left
  See N Upper Eyelid, Right
Q Lower Eyelid, Right
  Inferior tarsal plate
  Medial canthus
R Lower Eyelid, Left
  See Q Lower Eyelid, Right
	0 Open
	3 Percutaneous
	X External
		Z No Device	Z No Qualifier

X Lacrimal Duct, Right
  Lacrimal canaliculus
  Lacrimal punctum
  Lacrimal sac
  Nasolacrimal duct
Y Lacrimal Duct, Left
  See X Lacrimal Duct, Right
	0 Open
	3 Percutaneous
	7 Via Natural or Artificial Opening
	8 Via Natural or Artificial Opening Endoscopic
		Z No Device	Z No Qualifier

Non-OR Procedure   DRG Non-OR Procedure   Valid OR Procedure   HAC Associated Procedure   Combination Only   New/Revised April   New/Revised October

ICD-10-PCS 2025 — Eye

0 Medical and Surgical
8 Eye
P Removal

Definition: Taking out or off a device from a body part

Explanation: If a device is taken out and a similar device put in without cutting or puncturing the skin or mucous membrane, the procedure is coded to the root operation CHANGE. Otherwise, the procedure for taking out a device is coded to the root operation REMOVAL.

Body Part Character 4	Approach Character 5	Device Character 6	Qualifier Character 7
0 Eye, Right Ciliary body Posterior chamber **1 Eye, Left** See 0 Eye, Right	**0** Open **3** Percutaneous **7** Via Natural or Artificial Opening **8** Via Natural or Artificial Opening Endoscopic	**0** Drainage Device **1** Radioactive Element **3** Infusion Device **7** Autologous Tissue Substitute **C** Extraluminal Device **D** Intraluminal Device **J** Synthetic Substitute **K** Nonautologous Tissue Substitute **Y** Other Device	**Z** No Qualifier
0 Eye, Right Ciliary body Posterior chamber **1 Eye, Left** See 0 Eye, Right	**X** External	**0** Drainage Device **1** Radioactive Element **3** Infusion Device **7** Autologous Tissue Substitute **C** Extraluminal Device **D** Intraluminal Device **J** Synthetic Substitute **K** Nonautologous Tissue Substitute	**Z** No Qualifier
J Lens, Right Zonule of Zinn **K Lens, Left** See J Lens, Right	**3** Percutaneous	**J** Synthetic Substitute **Y** Other Device	**Z** No Qualifier
L Extraocular Muscle, Right Inferior oblique muscle Inferior rectus muscle Lateral rectus muscle Medial rectus muscle Superior oblique muscle Superior rectus muscle **M Extraocular Muscle, Left** See L Extraocular Muscle, Right	**0** Open **3** Percutaneous	**0** Drainage Device **7** Autologous Tissue Substitute **J** Synthetic Substitute **K** Nonautologous Tissue Substitute **Y** Other Device	**Z** No Qualifier

Non-OR 08P[0,1]3YZ
Non-OR 08P[0,1][7,8][0,3,D,Y]Z
Non-OR 08P[0,1]X[0,1,3,C,D,J]Z
Non-OR 08P[J,K]3YZ
Non-OR 08P[L,M]3YZ

0 Medical and Surgical
8 Eye
Q Repair Definition: Restoring, to the extent possible, a body part to its normal anatomic structure and function
Explanation: Used only when the method to accomplish the repair is not one of the other root operations

Body Part Character 4	Approach Character 5	Device Character 6	Qualifier Character 7

0 Eye, Right
   Ciliary body
   Posterior chamber
1 Eye, Left
   See 0 Eye, Right
6 Sclera, Right
7 Sclera, Left
8 Cornea, Right   NC
9 Cornea, Left   NC
S Conjunctiva, Right
   Plica semilunaris
T Conjunctiva, Left
   See S Conjunctiva, Right
	X External	Z No Device	Z No Qualifier

2 Anterior Chamber, Right
   Aqueous humour
3 Anterior Chamber, Left
   See 2 Anterior Chamber, Right
4 Vitreous, Right
   Vitreous body
5 Vitreous, Left
   See 4 Vitreous, Right
C Iris, Right
D Iris, Left
E Retina, Right
   Fovea
   Macula
   Optic disc
F Retina, Left
   See E Retina, Right
G Retinal Vessel, Right
H Retinal Vessel, Left
J Lens, Right
   Zonule of Zinn
K Lens, Left
   See J Lens, Right
	3 Percutaneous	Z No Device	Z No Qualifier

A Choroid, Right
B Choroid, Left
L Extraocular Muscle, Right
   Inferior oblique muscle
   Inferior rectus muscle
   Lateral rectus muscle
   Medial rectus muscle
   Superior oblique muscle
   Superior rectus muscle
M Extraocular Muscle, Left
   See L Extraocular Muscle, Right
V Lacrimal Gland, Right
W Lacrimal Gland, Left
	0 Open
	3 Percutaneous
		Z No Device	Z No Qualifier

N Upper Eyelid, Right
   Lateral canthus
   Levator palpebrae superioris muscle
   Orbicularis oculi muscle
   Superior tarsal plate
P Upper Eyelid, Left
   See N Upper Eyelid, Right
Q Lower Eyelid, Right
   Inferior tarsal plate
   Medial canthus
R Lower Eyelid, Left
   See Q Lower Eyelid, Right
	0 Open
	3 Percutaneous
	X External
		Z No Device	Z No Qualifier

X Lacrimal Duct, Right
   Lacrimal canaliculus
   Lacrimal punctum
   Lacrimal sac
   Nasolacrimal duct
Y Lacrimal Duct, Left
   See X Lacrimal Duct, Right
	0 Open
	3 Percutaneous
	7 Via Natural or Artificial Opening
	8 Via Natural or Artificial Opening Endoscopic
		Z No Device	Z No Qualifier

Non-OR   08Q[N,P,Q,R][0,3,X]ZZ
NC   08Q[8,9]XZZ

Non-OR Procedure   DRG Non-OR Procedure   Valid OR Procedure   HAC Associated Procedure   Combination Only   New/Revised April   New/Revised October

0 **Medical and Surgical**
8 **Eye**
R **Replacement** Definition: Putting in or on biological or synthetic material that physically takes the place and/or function of all or a portion of a body part
Explanation: The body part may have been taken out or replaced, or may be taken out, physically eradicated, or rendered nonfunctional during the REPLACEMENT procedure. A REMOVAL procedure is coded for taking out the device used in a previous replacement procedure.

Body Part Character 4	Approach Character 5	Device Character 6	Qualifier Character 7

0 Eye, Right
   Ciliary body
   Posterior chamber
1 Eye, Left
   See 0 Eye, Right
A Choroid, Right
B Choroid, Left
	0 Open
	3 Percutaneous
		7 Autologous Tissue Substitute
		J Synthetic Substitute
		K Nonautologous Tissue Substitute
			Z No Qualifier

4 Vitreous, Right
   Vitreous body
5 Vitreous, Left
   See 4 Vitreous, Right
C Iris, Right
D Iris, Left
G Retinal Vessel, Right
H Retinal Vessel, Left
	3 Percutaneous	7 Autologous Tissue Substitute
		J Synthetic Substitute
		K Nonautologous Tissue Substitute
			Z No Qualifier

6 Sclera, Right
7 Sclera, Left
S Conjunctiva, Right
   Plica semilunaris
T Conjunctiva, Left
   See S Conjunctiva, Right
	X External	7 Autologous Tissue Substitute
		J Synthetic Substitute
		K Nonautologous Tissue Substitute
			Z No Qualifier

8 Cornea, Right 9 Cornea, Left	3 Percutaneous X External	7 Autologous Tissue Substitute J Synthetic Substitute K Nonautologous Tissue Substitute	Z No Qualifier

J Lens, Right
   Zonule of Zinn
K Lens, Left
   See J Lens, Right
	3 Percutaneous	0 Synthetic Substitute, Intraocular Telescope
		7 Autologous Tissue Substitute
		J Synthetic Substitute
		K Nonautologous Tissue Substitute
			Z No Qualifier

N Upper Eyelid, Right
   Lateral canthus
   Levator palpebrae superioris muscle
   Orbicularis oculi muscle
   Superior tarsal plate
P Upper Eyelid, Left
   See N Upper Eyelid, Right
Q Lower Eyelid, Right
   Inferior tarsal plate
   Medial canthus
R Lower Eyelid, Left
   See Q Lower Eyelid, Right
	0 Open
	3 Percutaneous
	X External
		7 Autologous Tissue Substitute
		J Synthetic Substitute
		K Nonautologous Tissue Substitute
			Z No Qualifier

X Lacrimal Duct, Right
   Lacrimal canaliculus
   Lacrimal punctum
   Lacrimal sac
   Nasolacrimal duct
Y Lacrimal Duct, Left
   See X Lacrimal Duct, Right
	0 Open
	3 Percutaneous
	7 Via Natural or Artificial Opening
	8 Via Natural or Artificial Opening Endoscopic
		7 Autologous Tissue Substitute
		J Synthetic Substitute
		K Nonautologous Tissue Substitute
			Z No Qualifier

0 Medical and Surgical
8 Eye
S Reposition — Definition: Moving to its normal location, or other suitable location, all or a portion of a body part

Explanation: The body part is moved to a new location from an abnormal location, or from a normal location where it is not functioning correctly. The body part may or may not be cut out or off to be moved to the new location.

Body Part Character 4	Approach Character 5	Device Character 6	Qualifier Character 7

C Iris, Right
D Iris, Left
G Retinal Vessel, Right
H Retinal Vessel, Left
J Lens, Right
   Zonule of Zinn
K Lens, Left
   See J Lens, Right
	3 Percutaneous	Z No Device	Z No Qualifier

L Extraocular Muscle, Right
   Inferior oblique muscle
   Inferior rectus muscle
   Lateral rectus muscle
   Medial rectus muscle
   Superior oblique muscle
   Superior rectus muscle
M Extraocular Muscle, Left
   See L Extraocular Muscle, Right
V Lacrimal Gland, Right
W Lacrimal Gland, Left
	0 Open
	3 Percutaneous
		Z No Device	Z No Qualifier

N Upper Eyelid, Right
   Lateral canthus
   Levator palpebrae superioris muscle
   Orbicularis oculi muscle
   Superior tarsal plate
P Upper Eyelid, Left
   See N Upper Eyelid, Right
Q Lower Eyelid, Right
   Inferior tarsal plate
   Medial canthus
R Lower Eyelid, Left
   See Q Lower Eyelid, Right
	0 Open
	3 Percutaneous
	X External
		Z No Device	Z No Qualifier

X Lacrimal Duct, Right
   Lacrimal canaliculus
   Lacrimal punctum
   Lacrimal sac
   Nasolacrimal duct
Y Lacrimal Duct, Left
   See X Lacrimal Duct, Right
	0 Open
	3 Percutaneous
	7 Via Natural or Artificial Opening
	8 Via Natural or Artificial Opening Endoscopic
		Z No Device	Z No Qualifier

ICD-10-PCS 2025 — Eye — 08T-08T

0 Medical and Surgical
8 Eye
T Resection Definition: Cutting out or off, without replacement, all of a body part
Explanation: None

Body Part Character 4	Approach Character 5	Device Character 6	Qualifier Character 7

0 Eye, Right
  Ciliary body
  Posterior chamber
1 Eye, Left
  See 0 Eye, Right
8 Cornea, Right
9 Cornea, Left
	X External	Z No Device	Z No Qualifier

4 Vitreous, Right
  Vitreous body
5 Vitreous, Left
  See 4 Vitreous, Right
C Iris, Right
D Iris, Left
J Lens, Right
  Zonule of Zinn
K Lens, Left
  See J Lens, Right
	3 Percutaneous	Z No Device	Z No Qualifier

L Extraocular Muscle, Right
  Inferior oblique muscle
  Inferior rectus muscle
  Lateral rectus muscle
  Medial rectus muscle
  Superior oblique muscle
  Superior rectus muscle
M Extraocular Muscle, Left
  See L Extraocular Muscle, Right
V Lacrimal Gland, Right
W Lacrimal Gland, Left
	0 Open
	3 Percutaneous
		Z No Device	Z No Qualifier

N Upper Eyelid, Right
  Lateral canthus
  Levator palpebrae superioris muscle
  Orbicularis oculi muscle
  Superior tarsal plate
P Upper Eyelid, Left
  See N Upper Eyelid, Right
Q Lower Eyelid, Right
  Inferior tarsal plate
  Medial canthus
R Lower Eyelid, Left
  See Q Lower Eyelid, Right
	0 Open
	X External
		Z No Device	Z No Qualifier

X Lacrimal Duct, Right
  Lacrimal canaliculus
  Lacrimal punctum
  Lacrimal sac
  Nasolacrimal duct
Y Lacrimal Duct, Left
  See X Lacrimal Duct, Right
	0 Open
	3 Percutaneous
	7 Via Natural or Artificial Opening
	8 Via Natural or Artificial Opening Endoscopic
		Z No Device	Z No Qualifier

Eye

0 Medical and Surgical
8 Eye
U Supplement

Definition: Putting in or on biological or synthetic material that physically reinforces and/or augments the function of a portion of a body part

Explanation: The biological material is non-living, or is living and from the same individual. The body part may have been previously replaced, and the SUPPLEMENT procedure is performed to physically reinforce and/or augment the function of the replaced body part.

Body Part Character 4	Approach Character 5	Device Character 6	Qualifier Character 7

0 Eye, Right
   Ciliary body
   Posterior chamber
1 Eye, Left
   See 0 Eye, Right
C Iris, Right
D Iris, Left
E Retina, Right
   Fovea
   Macula
   Optic disc
F Retina, Left
   See E Retina, Right
G Retinal Vessel, Right
H Retinal Vessel, Left
L Extraocular Muscle, Right
   Inferior oblique muscle
   Inferior rectus muscle
   Lateral rectus muscle
   Medial rectus muscle
   Superior oblique muscle
   Superior rectus muscle
M Extraocular Muscle, Left
   See L Extraocular Muscle, Right
	0 Open
	3 Percutaneous
		7 Autologous Tissue Substitute
		J Synthetic Substitute
		K Nonautologous Tissue Substitute
			Z No Qualifier

8 Cornea, Right   [NC]
9 Cornea, Left   [NC]
N Upper Eyelid, Right
   Lateral canthus
   Levator palpebrae superioris muscle
   Orbicularis oculi muscle
   Superior tarsal plate
P Upper Eyelid, Left
   See N Upper Eyelid, Right
Q Lower Eyelid, Right
   Inferior tarsal plate
   Medial canthus
R Lower Eyelid, Left
   See Q Lower Eyelid, Right
	0 Open
	3 Percutaneous
	X External
		7 Autologous Tissue Substitute
		J Synthetic Substitute
		K Nonautologous Tissue Substitute
			Z No Qualifier

X Lacrimal Duct, Right
   Lacrimal canaliculus
   Lacrimal punctum
   Lacrimal sac
   Nasolacrimal duct
Y Lacrimal Duct, Left
   See X Lacrimal Duct, Right
	0 Open
	3 Percutaneous
	7 Via Natural or Artificial Opening
	8 Via Natural or Artificial Opening Endoscopic
		7 Autologous Tissue Substitute
		J Synthetic Substitute
		K Nonautologous Tissue Substitute
			Z No Qualifier

[NC] 08U[8,9][0,3,X]KZ

0 Medical and Surgical
8 Eye
V Restriction

Definition: Partially closing an orifice or the lumen of a tubular body part

Explanation: The orifice can be a natural orifice or an artificially created orifice

Body Part Character 4	Approach Character 5	Device Character 6	Qualifier Character 7

X Lacrimal Duct, Right
   Lacrimal canaliculus
   Lacrimal punctum
   Lacrimal sac
   Nasolacrimal duct
Y Lacrimal Duct, Left
   See X Lacrimal Duct, Right
	0 Open
	3 Percutaneous
		C Extraluminal Device
		D Intraluminal Device
		Z No Device
			Z No Qualifier

X Lacrimal Duct, Right
   Lacrimal canaliculus
   Lacrimal punctum
   Lacrimal sac
   Nasolacrimal duct
Y Lacrimal Duct, Left
   See X Lacrimal Duct, Right
	7 Via Natural or Artificial Opening
	8 Via Natural or Artificial Opening Endoscopic
		D Intraluminal Device
		Z No Device
			Z No Qualifier

Non-OR Procedure | DRG Non-OR Procedure | Valid OR Procedure | HAC Associated Procedure | Combination Only | New/Revised April | New/Revised October

0 Medical and Surgical
8 Eye
W Revision

Definition: Correcting, to the extent possible, a portion of a malfunctioning device or the position of a displaced device

Explanation: Revision can include correcting a malfunctioning or displaced device by taking out or putting in components of the device such as a screw or pin

Body Part Character 4	Approach Character 5	Device Character 6	Qualifier Character 7

0 **Eye, Right**
   Ciliary body
   Posterior chamber
1 **Eye, Left**
   See 0 Eye, Right
	0 Open
	3 Percutaneous
	7 Via Natural or Artificial Opening
	8 Via Natural or Artificial Opening Endoscopic
		0 Drainage Device
		3 Infusion Device
		7 Autologous Tissue Substitute
		C Extraluminal Device
		D Intraluminal Device
		J Synthetic Substitute
		K Nonautologous Tissue Substitute
		Y Other Device
			Z No Qualifier

0 **Eye, Right**
   Ciliary body
   Posterior chamber
1 **Eye, Left**
   See 0 Eye, Right
	X External	0 Drainage Device
		3 Infusion Device
		7 Autologous Tissue Substitute
		C Extraluminal Device
		D Intraluminal Device
		J Synthetic Substitute
		K Nonautologous Tissue Substitute
			Z No Qualifier

J **Lens, Right**
   Zonule of Zinn
K **Lens, Left**
   See J Lens, Right
	3 Percutaneous	J Synthetic Substitute
		Y Other Device
			Z No Qualifier

J **Lens, Right**
   Zonule of Zinn
K **Lens, Left**
   See J Lens, Right
	X External	J Synthetic Substitute	Z No Qualifier

L **Extraocular Muscle, Right**
   Inferior oblique muscle
   Inferior rectus muscle
   Lateral rectus muscle
   Medial rectus muscle
   Superior oblique muscle
   Superior rectus muscle
M **Extraocular Muscle, Left**
   See L Extraocular Muscle, Right
	0 Open
	3 Percutaneous
		0 Drainage Device
		7 Autologous Tissue Substitute
		J Synthetic Substitute
		K Nonautologous Tissue Substitute
		Y Other Device
			Z No Qualifier

Non-OR 08W[0,1][3,7,8]YZ
Non-OR 08W[0,1]X[0,3,7,C,D,J,K]Z
Non-OR 08W[J,K]3YZ
Non-OR 08W[J,K]XJZ
Non-OR 08W[L,M]3YZ

0 Medical and Surgical
8 Eye
X Transfer

Definition: Moving, without taking out, all or a portion of a body part to another location to take over the function of all or a portion of a body part

Explanation: The body part transferred remains connected to its vascular and nervous supply

Body Part Character 4	Approach Character 5	Device Character 6	Qualifier Character 7

L **Extraocular Muscle, Right**
   Inferior oblique muscle
   Inferior rectus muscle
   Lateral rectus muscle
   Medial rectus muscle
   Superior oblique muscle
   Superior rectus muscle
M **Extraocular Muscle, Left**
   See L Extraocular Muscle, Right
	0 Open
	3 Percutaneous
		Z No Device	Z No Qualifier

Ear, Nose, Sinus Ø9Ø–Ø9W

Character Meanings*
This Character Meaning table is provided as a guide to assist the user in the identification of character members that may be found in this section of code tables. It **SHOULD NOT** be used to build a PCS code.

	Operation–Character 3		Body Part–Character 4		Approach–Character 5		Device–Character 6		Qualifier–Character 7
Ø	Alteration	Ø	External Ear, Right	Ø	Open	Ø	Drainage Device	Ø	Endolymphatic
1	Bypass	1	External Ear, Left	3	Percutaneous	1	Radioactive Element	X	Diagnostic
2	Change	2	External Ear, Bilateral	4	Percutaneous Endoscopic	4	Hearing Device, Bone Conduction	Z	No Qualifier
3	Control	3	External Auditory Canal, Right	7	Via Natural or Artificial Opening	5	Hearing Device, Single Channel Cochlear Prosthesis		
5	Destruction	4	External Auditory Canal, Left	8	Via Natural or Artificial Opening Endoscopic	6	Hearing Device, Multiple Channel Cochlear Prosthesis		
7	Dilation	5	Middle Ear, Right	X	External	7	Autologous Tissue Substitute		
8	Division	6	Middle Ear, Left			B	Intraluminal Device, Airway		
9	Drainage	7	Tympanic Membrane, Right			D	Intraluminal Device		
B	Excision	8	Tympanic Membrane, Left			J	Synthetic Substitute		
C	Extirpation	9	Auditory Ossicle, Right			K	Nonautologous Tissue Substitute		
D	Extraction	A	Auditory Ossicle, Left			S	Hearing Device		
H	Insertion	B	Mastoid Sinus, Right			Y	Other Device		
J	Inspection	C	Mastoid Sinus, Left			Z	No Device		
M	Reattachment	D	Inner Ear, Right						
N	Release	E	Inner Ear, Left						
P	Removal	F	Eustachian Tube, Right						
Q	Repair	G	Eustachian Tube, Left						
R	Replacement	H	Ear, Right						
S	Reposition	J	Ear, Left						
T	Resection	K	Nasal Mucosa and Soft Tissue						
U	Supplement	L	Nasal Turbinate						
W	Revision	M	Nasal Septum						
		N	Nasopharynx						
		P	Accessory Sinus						
		Q	Maxillary Sinus, Right						
		R	Maxillary Sinus, Left						
		S	Frontal Sinus, Right						
		T	Frontal Sinus, Left						
		U	Ethmoid Sinus, Right						
		V	Ethmoid Sinus, Left						
		W	Sphenoid Sinus, Right						
		X	Sphenoid Sinus, Left						
		Y	Sinus						

* Includes sinus ducts.

AHA Coding Clinic for table Ø93
2018, 4Q, 38 — Control of epistaxis

AHA Coding Clinic for table Ø95
2018, 1Q, 19 — Control of epistaxis via silver nitrate cauterization

AHA Coding Clinic for table Ø97
2024, 1Q, 8 — Dilation of nasopharynx

AHA Coding Clinic for table Ø9B
2023, 2Q, 19 — Sigmoid sinus dehiscence with mastoidectomy with resurfacing

AHA Coding Clinic for table Ø9H
2022, 2Q, 17 — Congenital nasal pyriform aperture stenosis and repair
2020, 4Q, 43-44 — Insertion of radioactive element

AHA Coding Clinic for table Ø9Q
2018, 1Q, 19 — Control of epistaxis via silver nitrate cauterization
2017, 4Q, 106 — Control of bleeding of external naris using suture
2014, 4Q, 20 — Control of epistaxis
2014, 3Q, 22 — Transsphenoidal removal of pituitary tumor and fat graft placement
2013, 4Q, 114 — Balloon sinuplasty

AHA Coding Clinic for table Ø9U
2022, 1Q, 48 — Repair of facial fractures of frontal sinus and orbital roof
2019, 4Q, 28-29 — Sinus supplement

Ear, Nose, Sinus

Ear Anatomy

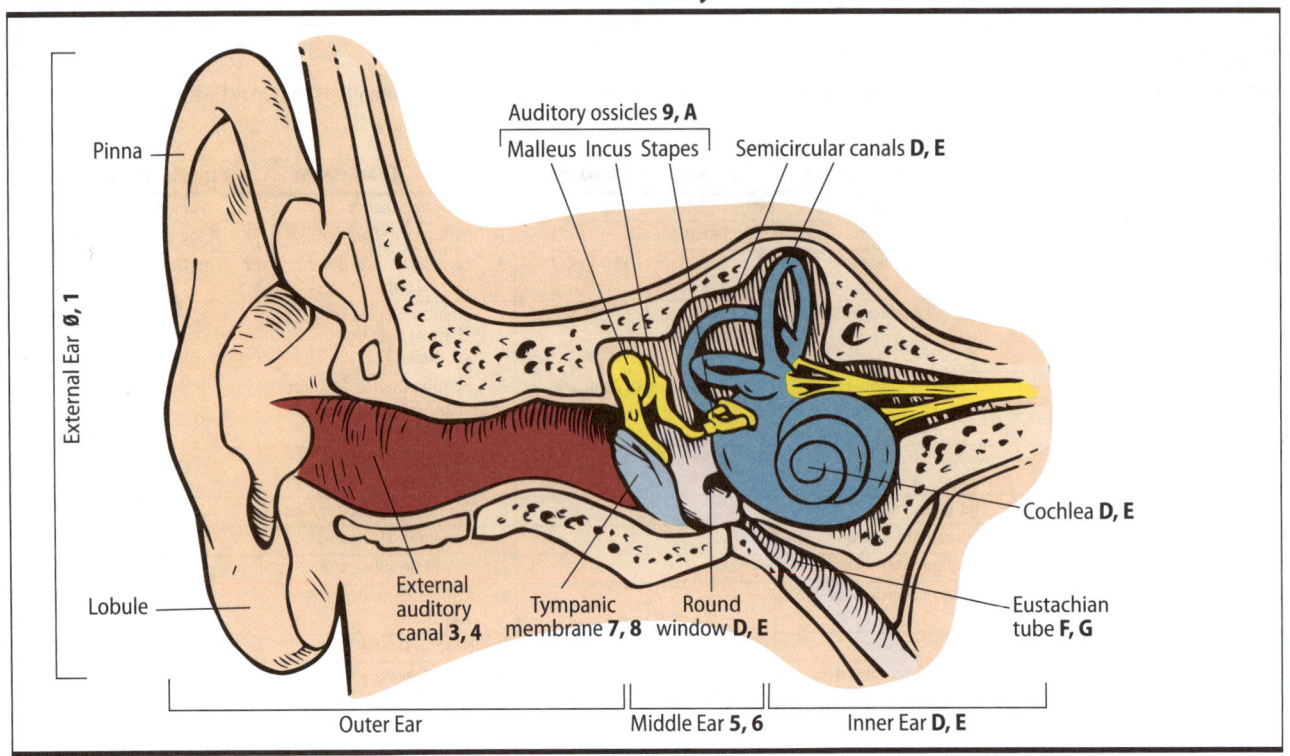

- Pinna
- Auditory ossicles **9, A**
  - Malleus
  - Incus
  - Stapes
- Semicircular canals **D, E**
- External Ear **0, 1**
- Lobule
- External auditory canal **3, 4**
- Tympanic membrane **7, 8**
- Round window **D, E**
- Cochlea **D, E**
- Eustachian tube **F, G**
- Outer Ear
- Middle Ear **5, 6**
- Inner Ear **D, E**

Nasal Turbinates

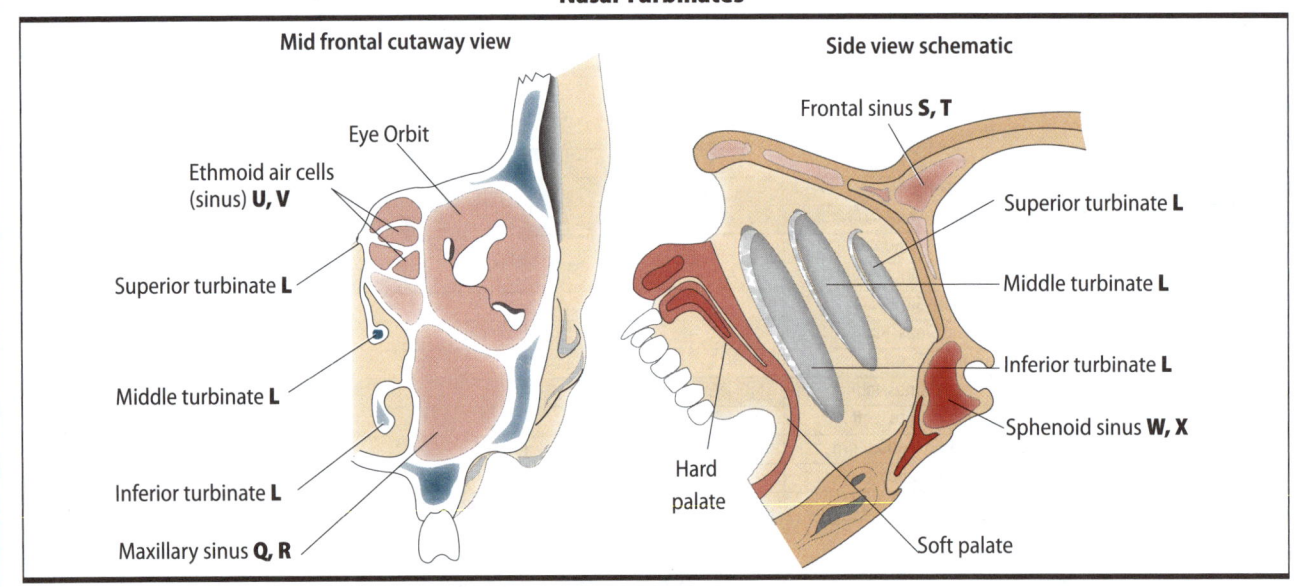

Mid frontal cutaway view
- Eye Orbit
- Ethmoid air cells (sinus) **U, V**
- Superior turbinate **L**
- Middle turbinate **L**
- Inferior turbinate **L**
- Maxillary sinus **Q, R**

Side view schematic
- Frontal sinus **S, T**
- Superior turbinate **L**
- Middle turbinate **L**
- Inferior turbinate **L**
- Sphenoid sinus **W, X**
- Hard palate
- Soft palate

Paranasal Sinuses

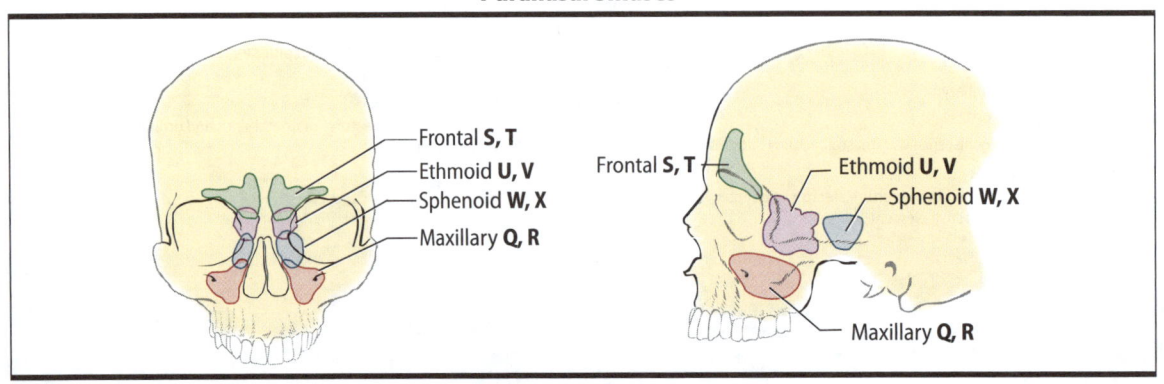

- Frontal **S, T**
- Ethmoid **U, V**
- Sphenoid **W, X**
- Maxillary **Q, R**

ICD-10-PCS 2025 — Ear, Nose, Sinus — 090–093

0 Medical and Surgical
9 Ear, Nose, Sinus
0 Alteration Definition: Modifying the anatomic structure of a body part without affecting the function of the body part
Explanation: Principal purpose is to improve appearance

Body Part Character 4	Approach Character 5	Device Character 6	Qualifier Character 7

0 External Ear, Right
  Antihelix
  Antitragus
  Auricle
  Earlobe
  Helix
  Pinna
  Tragus
1 External Ear, Left
  See 0 External Ear, Right
2 External Ear, Bilateral
  See 0 External Ear, Right
K Nasal Mucosa and Soft Tissue
  Columella
  External naris
  Greater alar cartilage
  Internal naris
  Lateral nasal cartilage
  Lesser alar cartilage
  Nasal cavity
  Nostril
	0 Open
	3 Percutaneous
	4 Percutaneous Endoscopic
	X External
		7 Autologous Tissue Substitute
		J Synthetic Substitute
		K Nonautologous Tissue Substitute
		Z No Device
			Z No Qualifier

0 Medical and Surgical
9 Ear, Nose, Sinus
1 Bypass Definition: Altering the route of passage of the contents of a tubular body part
Explanation: Rerouting contents of a body part to a downstream area of the normal route, to a similar route and body part, or to an abnormal route and dissimilar body part. Includes one or more anastomoses, with or without the use of a device.

Body Part Character 4	Approach Character 5	Device Character 6	Qualifier Character 7

D Inner Ear, Right
  Bony labyrinth
  Bony vestibule
  Cochlea
  Round window
  Semicircular canal
E Inner Ear, Left
  See D Inner Ear, Right
	0 Open	7 Autologous Tissue Substitute
		J Synthetic Substitute
		K Nonautologous Tissue Substitute
		Z No Device
			0 Endolymphatic

0 Medical and Surgical
9 Ear, Nose, Sinus
2 Change Definition: Taking out or off a device from a body part and putting back an identical or similar device in or on the same body part without cutting or puncturing the skin or a mucous membrane
Explanation: All CHANGE procedures are coded using the approach EXTERNAL

Body Part Character 4	Approach Character 5	Device Character 6	Qualifier Character 7

H Ear, Right
J Ear, Left
K Nasal Mucosa and Soft Tissue
  Columella
  External naris
  Greater alar cartilage
  Internal naris
  Lateral nasal cartilage
  Lesser alar cartilage
  Nasal cavity
  Nostril
Y Sinus
	X External	0 Drainage Device
		Y Other Device
			Z No Qualifier

Non-OR   All body part, approach, device, and qualifier values

0 Medical and Surgical
9 Ear, Nose, Sinus
3 Control Definition: Stopping, or attempting to stop, postprocedural or other acute bleeding
Explanation: None

Body Part Character 4	Approach Character 5	Device Character 6	Qualifier Character 7

K Nasal Mucosa and Soft Tissue
  Columella
  External naris
  Greater alar cartilage
  Internal naris
  Lateral nasal cartilage
  Lesser alar cartilage
  Nasal cavity
  Nostril
	7 Via Natural or Artificial Opening
	8 Via Natural or Artificial Opening Endoscopic
		Z No Device	Z No Qualifier

Non-OR   093K[7,8]ZZ

0 Medical and Surgical
9 Ear, Nose, Sinus
5 Destruction Definition: Physical eradication of all or a portion of a body part by the direct use of energy, force, or a destructive agent
Explanation: None of the body part is physically taken out

Body Part Character 4	Approach Character 5	Device Character 6	Qualifier Character 7
0 External Ear, Right Antihelix Antitragus Auricle Earlobe Helix Pinna Tragus **1 External Ear, Left** See 0 External Ear, Right	**0** Open **3** Percutaneous **4** Percutaneous Endoscopic **X** External	**Z** No Device	**Z** No Qualifier
3 External Auditory Canal, Right External auditory meatus **4 External Auditory Canal, Left** See 3 External Auditory Canal, Right	**0** Open **3** Percutaneous **4** Percutaneous Endoscopic **7** Via Natural or Artificial Opening **8** Via Natural or Artificial Opening Endoscopic **X** External	**Z** No Device	**Z** No Qualifier
5 Middle Ear, Right Oval window Tympanic cavity **6 Middle Ear, Left** See 5 Middle Ear, Right **9 Auditory Ossicle, Right** Incus Malleus Stapes **A Auditory Ossicle, Left** See 9 Auditory Ossicle, Right **D Inner Ear, Right** Bony labyrinth Bony vestibule Cochlea Round window Semicircular canal **E Inner Ear, Left** See D Inner Ear, Right	**0** Open **8** Via Natural or Artificial Opening Endoscopic	**Z** No Device	**Z** No Qualifier
7 Tympanic Membrane, Right Pars flaccida **8 Tympanic Membrane, Left** See 7 Tympanic Membrane, Right **F Eustachian Tube, Right** Auditory tube Pharyngotympanic tube **G Eustachian Tube, Left** See F Eustachian Tube, Right **L Nasal Turbinate** Inferior turbinate Middle turbinate Nasal concha Superior turbinate **N Nasopharynx** Choana Fossa of Rosenmuller Pharyngeal recess Rhinopharynx	**0** Open **3** Percutaneous **4** Percutaneous Endoscopic **7** Via Natural or Artificial Opening **8** Via Natural or Artificial Opening Endoscopic	**Z** No Device	**Z** No Qualifier
B Mastoid Sinus, Right Mastoid air cells **C Mastoid Sinus, Left** See B Mastoid Sinus, Right **M Nasal Septum** Quadrangular cartilage Septal cartilage Vomer bone **P Accessory Sinus** **Q Maxillary Sinus, Right** Antrum of Highmore **R Maxillary Sinus, Left** See Q Maxillary Sinus, Right **S Frontal Sinus, Right** **T Frontal Sinus, Left** **U Ethmoid Sinus, Right** Ethmoidal air cell **V Ethmoid Sinus, Left** See U Ethmoid Sinus, Right **W Sphenoid Sinus, Right** **X Sphenoid Sinus, Left**	**0** Open **3** Percutaneous **4** Percutaneous Endoscopic **8** Via Natural or Artificial Opening Endoscopic	**Z** No Device	**Z** No Qualifier
K Nasal Mucosa and Soft Tissue Columella External naris Greater alar cartilage Internal naris Lateral nasal cartilage Lesser alar cartilage Nasal cavity Nostril	**0** Open **3** Percutaneous **4** Percutaneous Endoscopic **8** Via Natural or Artificial Opening Endoscopic **X** External	**Z** No Device	**Z** No Qualifier

Non-OR 095[0,1][0,3,4,X]ZZ
Non-OR 095[3,4][0,3,4,7,8,X]ZZ
Non-OR 095[F,G][0,3,4,7,8]ZZ
Non-OR 095M[0,3,4,8]ZZ
Non-OR 095K[0,3,4,8,X]ZZ

0 Medical and Surgical
9 Ear, Nose, Sinus
7 Dilation — Definition: Expanding an orifice or the lumen of a tubular body part

Explanation: The orifice can be a natural orifice or an artificially created orifice. Accomplished by stretching a tubular body part using intraluminal pressure or by cutting part of the orifice or wall of the tubular body part.

Body Part Character 4	Approach Character 5	Device Character 6	Qualifier Character 7

F Eustachian Tube, Right
  Auditory tube
  Pharyngotympanic tube
G Eustachian Tube, Left
  See F Eustachian Tube, Right
	0 Open
	7 Via Natural or Artificial Opening
	8 Via Natural or Artificial Opening Endoscopic
		D Intraluminal Device
		Z No Device
			Z No Qualifier

F Eustachian Tube, Right
  Auditory tube
  Pharyngotympanic tube
G Eustachian Tube, Left
  See F Eustachian Tube, Right
	3 Percutaneous
	4 Percutaneous Endoscopic
		Z No Device	Z No Qualifier

N Nasopharynx	0 Open 7 Via Natural or Artificial Opening 8 Via Natural or Artificial Opening Endoscopic	Z No Device	Z No Qualifier

Non-OR All body part, approach, device, and qualifier values

0 Medical and Surgical
9 Ear, Nose, Sinus
8 Division — Definition: Cutting into a body part, without draining fluids and/or gases from the body part, in order to separate or transect a body part

Explanation: All or a portion of the body part is separated into two or more portions

Body Part Character 4	Approach Character 5	Device Character 6	Qualifier Character 7

L Nasal Turbinate
  Inferior turbinate
  Middle turbinate
  Nasal concha
  Superior turbinate
	0 Open
	3 Percutaneous
	4 Percutaneous Endoscopic
	7 Via Natural or Artificial Opening
	8 Via Natural or Artificial Opening Endoscopic
		Z No Device	Z No Qualifier

0 Medical and Surgical
9 Ear, Nose, Sinus
9 Drainage

Definition: Taking or letting out fluids and/or gases from a body part
Explanation: The qualifier DIAGNOSTIC is used to identify drainage procedures that are biopsies

Body Part – Character 4	Approach – Character 5	Device – Character 6	Qualifier – Character 7
0 External Ear, Right Antihelix Antitragus Auricle Earlobe Helix Pinna Tragus **1 External Ear, Left** See 0 External Ear, Right	0 Open 3 Percutaneous 4 Percutaneous Endoscopic X External	0 Drainage Device	Z No Qualifier
0 External Ear, Right Antihelix Antitragus Auricle Earlobe Helix Pinna Tragus **1 External Ear, Left** See 0 External Ear, Right	0 Open 3 Percutaneous 4 Percutaneous Endoscopic X External	Z No Device	X Diagnostic Z No Qualifier
3 External Auditory Canal, Right External auditory meatus **4 External Auditory Canal, Left** See 3 External Auditory Canal, Right **K Nasal Mucosa and Soft Tissue** Columella External naris Greater alar cartilage Internal naris Lateral nasal cartilage Lesser alar cartilage Nasal cavity Nostril	0 Open 3 Percutaneous 4 Percutaneous Endoscopic 7 Via Natural or Artificial Opening 8 Via Natural or Artificial Opening Endoscopic X External	0 Drainage Device	Z No Qualifier
3 External Auditory Canal, Right External auditory meatus **4 External Auditory Canal, Left** See 3 External Auditory Canal, Right **K Nasal Mucosa and Soft Tissue** Columella External naris Greater alar cartilage Internal naris Lateral nasal cartilage Lesser alar cartilage Nasal cavity Nostril	0 Open 3 Percutaneous 4 Percutaneous Endoscopic 7 Via Natural or Artificial Opening 8 Via Natural or Artificial Opening Endoscopic X External	Z No Device	X Diagnostic Z No Qualifier
5 Middle Ear, Right Oval window Tympanic cavity **6 Middle Ear, Left** See 5 Middle Ear, Right **9 Auditory Ossicle, Right** Incus Malleus Stapes **A Auditory Ossicle, Left** See 9 Auditory Ossicle, Right **D Inner Ear, Right** Bony labyrinth Bony vestibule Cochlea Round window Semicircular canal **E Inner Ear, Left** See D Inner Ear, Right	0 Open 7 Via Natural or Artificial Opening 8 Via Natural or Artificial Opening Endoscopic	0 Drainage Device	Z No Qualifier
5 Middle Ear, Right Oval window Tympanic cavity **6 Middle Ear, Left** See 5 Middle Ear, Right **9 Auditory Ossicle, Right** Incus Malleus Stapes **A Auditory Ossicle, Left** See 9 Auditory Ossicle, Right **D Inner Ear, Right** Bony labyrinth Bony vestibule Cochlea Round window Semicircular canal **E Inner Ear, Left** See D Inner Ear, Right	0 Open 7 Via Natural or Artificial Opening 8 Via Natural or Artificial Opening Endoscopic	Z No Device	X Diagnostic Z No Qualifier

Non-OR 099[0,1][0,3,4,X]0Z
Non-OR 099[0,1][0,3,4,X]Z[X,Z]
Non-OR 099[3,4,K][0,3,4,7,8,X]0Z
Non-OR 099[3,4,K][0,3,4,7,8,X]Z[X,Z]
Non-OR 099[5,6]80Z
Non-OR 099[9,A,D,E][7,8]0Z
Non-OR 099[5,6]0ZZ
Non-OR 099[5,6,9,A,D,E][7,8]Z[X,Z]

099 Continued on next page

ICD-10-PCS 2025 — Ear, Nose, Sinus — 099–099

099 Continued

0	Medical and Surgical
9	Ear, Nose, Sinus
9	Drainage

Definition: Taking or letting out fluids and/or gases from a body part
Explanation: The qualifier DIAGNOSTIC is used to identify drainage procedures that are biopsies

Body Part Character 4	Approach Character 5	Device Character 6	Qualifier Character 7

7 Tympanic Membrane, Right
  Pars flaccida
8 Tympanic Membrane, Left
  See 7 Tympanic Membrane, Right
B Mastoid Sinus, Right
  Mastoid air cells
C Mastoid Sinus, Left
  See B Mastoid Sinus, Right
F Eustachian Tube, Right
  Auditory tube
  Pharyngotympanic tube
G Eustachian Tube, Left
  See F Eustachian Tube, Right
L Nasal Turbinate
  Inferior turbinate
  Middle turbinate
  Nasal concha
  Superior turbinate
M Nasal Septum
  Quadrangular cartilage
  Septal cartilage
  Vomer bone
N Nasopharynx
  Choana
  Fossa of Rosenmuller
  Pharyngeal recess
  Rhinopharynx
P Accessory Sinus
Q Maxillary Sinus, Right
  Antrum of Highmore
R Maxillary Sinus, Left
  See Q Maxillary Sinus, Right
S Frontal Sinus, Right
T Frontal Sinus, Left
U Ethmoid Sinus, Right
  Ethmoidal air cell
V Ethmoid Sinus, Left
  See U Ethmoid Sinus, Right
W Sphenoid Sinus, Right
X Sphenoid Sinus, Left
	0 Open
	3 Percutaneous
	4 Percutaneous Endoscopic
	7 Via Natural or Artificial Opening
	8 Via Natural or Artificial Opening Endoscopic
		0 Drainage Device	Z No Qualifier

7 Tympanic Membrane, Right
  Pars flaccida
8 Tympanic Membrane, Left
  See 7 Tympanic Membrane, Right
B Mastoid Sinus, Right
  Mastoid air cells
C Mastoid Sinus, Left
  See B Mastoid Sinus, Right
F Eustachian Tube, Right
  Auditory tube
  Pharyngotympanic tube
G Eustachian Tube, Left
  See F Eustachian Tube, Right
L Nasal Turbinate
  Inferior turbinate
  Middle turbinate
  Nasal concha
  Superior turbinate
M Nasal Septum
  Quadrangular cartilage
  Septal cartilage
  Vomer bone
N Nasopharynx
  Choana
  Fossa of Rosenmuller
  Pharyngeal recess
  Rhinopharynx
P Accessory Sinus
Q Maxillary Sinus, Right
  Antrum of Highmore
R Maxillary Sinus, Left
  See Q Maxillary Sinus, Right
S Frontal Sinus, Right
T Frontal Sinus, Left
U Ethmoid Sinus, Right
  Ethmoidal air cell
V Ethmoid Sinus, Left
  See U Ethmoid Sinus, Right
W Sphenoid Sinus, Right
X Sphenoid Sinus, Left
	0 Open
	3 Percutaneous
	4 Percutaneous Endoscopic
	7 Via Natural or Artificial Opening
	8 Via Natural or Artificial Opening Endoscopic
		Z No Device	X Diagnostic
			Z No Qualifier

Non-OR 099[B,C][3,7,8]0Z
Non-OR 099[F,G,L,M][0,3,4,7,8]0Z
Non-OR 099N30Z
Non-OR 099[P,Q,R,S,T,U,V,W,X][3,4,7,8]0Z
Non-OR 099[7,8][0,3,4,7,8]ZZ
Non-OR 099[7,8][7,8]ZX
Non-OR 099[B,C]3ZZ
Non-OR 099[B,C][7,8]Z[X,Z]
Non-OR 099[F,G][0,3,4,7,8]ZZ
Non-OR 099[F,G][7,8]ZX
Non-OR 099[L,M][0,3,4,7,8]Z[X,Z]
Non-OR 099N[0,3,4,7,8]ZX
Non-OR 099N3ZZ
Non-OR 099[P,Q,R,S,T,U,V,W,X][3,4,7,8]Z[X,Z]

Ear, Nose, Sinus

0 Medical and Surgical
9 Ear, Nose, Sinus
B Excision

Definition: Cutting out or off, without replacement, a portion of a body part
Explanation: The qualifier DIAGNOSTIC is used to identify excision procedures that are biopsies

Body Part — Character 4	Approach — Character 5	Device — Character 6	Qualifier — Character 7
0 External Ear, Right Antihelix Antitragus Auricle Earlobe Helix Pinna Tragus **1 External Ear, Left** *See 0 External Ear, Right*	**0** Open **3** Percutaneous **4** Percutaneous Endoscopic **X** External	**Z** No Device	**X** Diagnostic **Z** No Qualifier
3 External Auditory Canal, Right External auditory meatus **4 External Auditory Canal, Left** *See 3 External Auditory Canal, Right*	**0** Open **3** Percutaneous **4** Percutaneous Endoscopic **7** Via Natural or Artificial Opening **8** Via Natural or Artificial Opening Endoscopic **X** External	**Z** No Device	**X** Diagnostic **Z** No Qualifier
5 Middle Ear, Right Oval window Tympanic cavity **6 Middle Ear, Left** *See 5 Middle Ear, Right* **9 Auditory Ossicle, Right** Incus Malleus Stapes **A Auditory Ossicle, Left** *See 9 Auditory Ossicle, Right* **D Inner Ear, Right** Bony labyrinth Bony vestibule Cochlea Round window Semicircular canal **E Inner Ear, Left** *See D Inner Ear, Right*	**0** Open **8** Via Natural or Artificial Opening Endoscopic	**Z** No Device	**X** Diagnostic **Z** No Qualifier
7 Tympanic Membrane, Right Pars flaccida **8 Tympanic Membrane, Left** *See 7 Tympanic Membrane, Right* **F Eustachian Tube, Right** Auditory tube Pharyngotympanic tube **G Eustachian Tube, Left** *See F Eustachian Tube, Right* **L Nasal Turbinate** Inferior turbinate Middle turbinate Nasal concha Superior turbinate **N Nasopharynx** Choana Fossa of Rosenmuller Pharyngeal recess Rhinopharynx	**0** Open **3** Percutaneous **4** Percutaneous Endoscopic **7** Via Natural or Artificial Opening **8** Via Natural or Artificial Opening Endoscopic	**Z** No Device	**X** Diagnostic **Z** No Qualifier
B Mastoid Sinus, Right Mastoid air cells **C Mastoid Sinus, Left** *See B Mastoid Sinus, Right* **M Nasal Septum** Quadrangular cartilage Septal cartilage Vomer bone **P Accessory Sinus** **Q Maxillary Sinus, Right** Antrum of Highmore **R Maxillary Sinus, Left** *See Q Maxillary Sinus, Right* **S Frontal Sinus, Right** **T Frontal Sinus, Left** **U Ethmoid Sinus, Right** Ethmoidal air cell **V Ethmoid Sinus, Left** *See U Ethmoid Sinus, Right* **W Sphenoid Sinus, Right** **X Sphenoid Sinus, Left**	**0** Open **3** Percutaneous **4** Percutaneous Endoscopic **8** Via Natural or Artificial Opening Endoscopic	**Z** No Device	**X** Diagnostic **Z** No Qualifier
K Nasal Mucosa and Soft Tissue Columella External naris Greater alar cartilage Internal naris Lateral nasal cartilage Lesser alar cartilage Nasal cavity Nostril	**0** Open **3** Percutaneous **4** Percutaneous Endoscopic **8** Via Natural or Artificial Opening Endoscopic **X** External	**Z** No Device	**X** Diagnostic **Z** No Qualifier

Non-OR 09B[0,1][0,3,4,X]Z[X,Z]
Non-OR 09B[3,4][0,3,4,7,8,X]Z[X,Z]
Non-OR 09B[F,G,L,N][0,3,4,7,8]Z[X,Z]
Non-OR 09BM[0,3,4,8]ZX
Non-OR 09B[P,Q,R,S,T,U,V,W,X][3,4,8]ZX
Non-OR 09BK8Z[X,Z]

ICD-10-PCS 2025 — Ear, Nose, Sinus — 09C–09C

- 0 Medical and Surgical
- 9 Ear, Nose, Sinus
- C Extirpation

Definition: Taking or cutting out solid matter from a body part
Explanation: The solid matter may be an abnormal byproduct of a biological function or a foreign body; it may be imbedded in a body part or in the lumen of a tubular body part. The solid matter may or may not have been previously broken into pieces.

Body Part Character 4	Approach Character 5	Device Character 6	Qualifier Character 7

0 External Ear, Right
  Antihelix
  Antitragus
  Auricle
  Earlobe
  Helix
  Pinna
  Tragus
1 External Ear, Left
  See 0 External Ear, Right
	0 Open
	3 Percutaneous
	4 Percutaneous Endoscopic
	X External
		Z No Device	Z No Qualifier

3 External Auditory Canal, Right
  External auditory meatus
4 External Auditory Canal, Left
  See 3 External Auditory Canal, Right
	0 Open
	3 Percutaneous
	4 Percutaneous Endoscopic
	7 Via Natural or Artificial Opening
	8 Via Natural or Artificial Opening Endoscopic
	X External
		Z No Device	Z No Qualifier

5 Middle Ear, Right
  Oval window
  Tympanic cavity
6 Middle Ear, Left
  See 5 Middle Ear, Right
9 Auditory Ossicle, Right
  Incus
  Malleus
  Stapes
A Auditory Ossicle, Left
  See 9 Auditory Ossicle, Right
D Inner Ear, Right
  Bony labyrinth
  Bony vestibule
  Cochlea
  Round window
  Semicircular canal
E Inner Ear, Left
  See D Inner Ear, Right
	0 Open
	8 Via Natural or Artificial Opening Endoscopic
		Z No Device	Z No Qualifier

7 Tympanic Membrane, Right
  Pars flaccida
8 Tympanic Membrane, Left
  See 7 Tympanic Membrane, Right
F Eustachian Tube, Right
  Auditory tube
  Pharyngotympanic tube
G Eustachian Tube, Left
  See F Eustachian Tube, Right
L Nasal Turbinate
  Inferior turbinate
  Middle turbinate
  Nasal concha
  Superior turbinate
N Nasopharynx
  Choana
  Fossa of Rosenmuller
  Pharyngeal recess
  Rhinopharynx
	0 Open
	3 Percutaneous
	4 Percutaneous Endoscopic
	7 Via Natural or Artificial Opening
	8 Via Natural or Artificial Opening Endoscopic
		Z No Device	Z No Qualifier

B Mastoid Sinus, Right
  Mastoid air cells
C Mastoid Sinus, Left
  See B Mastoid Sinus, Right
M Nasal Septum
  Quadrangular cartilage
  Septal cartilage
  Vomer bone
P Accessory Sinus
Q Maxillary Sinus, Right
  Antrum of Highmore
R Maxillary Sinus, Left
  See Q Maxillary Sinus, Right
S Frontal Sinus, Right
T Frontal Sinus, Left
U Ethmoid Sinus, Right
  Ethmoidal air cell
V Ethmoid Sinus, Left
  See U Ethmoid Sinus, Right
W Sphenoid Sinus, Right
X Sphenoid Sinus, Left
	0 Open
	3 Percutaneous
	4 Percutaneous Endoscopic
	8 Via Natural or Artificial Opening Endoscopic
		Z No Device	Z No Qualifier

K Nasal Mucosa and Soft Tissue
  Columella
  External naris
  Greater alar cartilage
  Internal naris
  Lateral nasal cartilage
  Lesser alar cartilage
  Nasal cavity
  Nostril
	0 Open
	3 Percutaneous
	4 Percutaneous Endoscopic
	8 Via Natural or Artificial Opening Endoscopic
	X External
		Z No Device	Z No Qualifier

Non-OR 09C[0,1][0,3,4,X]ZZ
Non-OR 09C[3,4][0,3,4,7,8,X]ZZ
Non-OR 09C[7,8,F,G,L][0,3,4,7,8]ZZ
Non-OR 09CM[0,3,4,8]ZZ
Non-OR 09CK8ZZ

09D–09H | EAR, NOSE, SINUS | ICD-10-PCS 2025

0 Medical and Surgical
9 Ear, Nose, Sinus
D Extraction Definition: Pulling or stripping out or off all or a portion of a body part by the use of force
Explanation: The qualifier DIAGNOSTIC is used to identify extraction procedures that are biopsies

Body Part Character 4	Approach Character 5	Device Character 6	Qualifier Character 7

7 Tympanic Membrane, Right
  Pars flaccida
8 Tympanic Membrane, Left
  See 7 Tympanic Membrane, Right
L Nasal Turbinate
  Inferior turbinate
  Middle turbinate
  Nasal concha
  Superior turbinate
	0 Open
	3 Percutaneous
	4 Percutaneous Endoscopic
	7 Via Natural or Artificial Opening
	8 Via Natural or Artificial Opening Endoscopic
		Z No Device	Z No Qualifier

9 Auditory Ossicle, Right
  Incus
  Malleus
  Stapes
A Auditory Ossicle, Left
  See 9 Auditory Ossicle, Right
	0 Open	Z No Device	Z No Qualifier

B Mastoid Sinus, Right
  Mastoid air cells
C Mastoid Sinus, Left
  See B Mastoid Sinus, Right
M Nasal Septum
  Quadrangular cartilage
  Septal cartilage
  Vomer bone
P Accessory Sinus
Q Maxillary Sinus, Right
  Antrum of Highmore
R Maxillary Sinus, Left
  See Q Maxillary Sinus, Right
S Frontal Sinus, Right
T Frontal Sinus, Left
U Ethmoid Sinus, Right
  Ethmoidal air cell
V Ethmoid Sinus, Left
  See U Ethmoid Sinus, Right
W Sphenoid Sinus, Right
X Sphenoid Sinus, Left
	0 Open
	3 Percutaneous
	4 Percutaneous Endoscopic
		Z No Device	Z No Qualifier

0 Medical and Surgical
9 Ear, Nose, Sinus
H Insertion Definition: Putting in a nonbiological appliance that monitors, assists, performs, or prevents a physiological function but does not physically take the place of a body part
Explanation: None

Body Part Character 4	Approach Character 5	Device Character 6	Qualifier Character 7

D Inner Ear, Right
  Bony labyrinth
  Bony vestibule
  Cochlea
  Round window
  Semicircular canal
E Inner Ear, Left
  See D Inner Ear, Right
	0 Open
	3 Percutaneous
	4 Percutaneous Endoscopic
		1 Radioactive Element
		4 Hearing Device, Bone Conduction
		5 Hearing Device, Single Channel Cochlear Prosthesis
		6 Hearing Device, Multiple Channel Cochlear Prosthesis
		S Hearing Device
			Z No Qualifier

H Ear, Right
J Ear, Left
K Nasal Mucosa and Soft Tissue
  Columella
  External naris
  Greater alar cartilage
  Internal naris
  Lateral nasal cartilage
  Lesser alar cartilage
  Nasal cavity
  Nostril
Y Sinus
	0 Open
	3 Percutaneous
	4 Percutaneous Endoscopic
	7 Via Natural or Artificial Opening
	8 Via Natural or Artificial Opening Endoscopic
		1 Radioactive Element
		Y Other Device
			Z No Qualifier

N Nasopharynx
  Choana
  Fossa of Rosenmuller
  Pharyngeal recess
  Rhinopharynx
	7 Via Natural or Artificial Opening
	8 Via Natural or Artificial Opening Endoscopic
		1 Radioactive Element
		B Intraluminal Device, Airway
			Z No Qualifier

Non-OR 09H[H,J,K]01Z
Non-OR 09HK0YZ
Non-OR 09H[H,J,K,Y][3,4,7,8][1,Y]Z
Non-OR 09HN[7,8][1,B]Z

Non-OR Procedure | DRG Non-OR Procedure | Valid OR Procedure | HAC Associated Procedure | Combination Only | New/Revised April | New/Revised October

0 Medical and Surgical
9 Ear, Nose, Sinus
J Inspection

Definition: Visually and/or manually exploring a body part

Explanation: Visual exploration may be performed with or without optical instrumentation. Manual exploration may be performed directly or through intervening body layers.

Body Part Character 4	Approach Character 5	Device Character 6	Qualifier Character 7

7 **Tympanic Membrane, Right**
  Pars flaccida
8 **Tympanic Membrane, Left**
  See 7 Tympanic Membrane, Right
H **Ear, Right**
J **Ear, Left**
	0 Open
	3 Percutaneous
	4 Percutaneous Endoscopic
	7 Via Natural or Artificial Opening
	8 Via Natural or Artificial Opening Endoscopic
	X External
		Z No Device	Z No Qualifier

D **Inner Ear, Right**
  Bony labyrinth
  Bony vestibule
  Cochlea
  Round window
  Semicircular canal
E **Inner Ear, Left**
  See D Inner Ear, Right
K **Nasal Mucosa and Soft Tissue**
  Columella
  External naris
  Greater alar cartilage
  Internal naris
  Lateral nasal cartilage
  Lesser alar cartilage
  Nasal cavity
  Nostril
Y **Sinus**
	0 Open
	3 Percutaneous
	4 Percutaneous Endoscopic
	8 Via Natural or Artificial Opening Endoscopic
	X External
		Z No Device	Z No Qualifier

Non-OR 09J[7,8][3,7,8,X]ZZ
Non-OR 09J[H,J][0,3,4,7,8,X]ZZ
Non-OR 09J[D,E][3,8,X]ZZ
Non-OR 09J[K,Y][0,3,4,8,X]ZZ

0 Medical and Surgical
9 Ear, Nose, Sinus
M Reattachment

Definition: Putting back in or on all or a portion of a separated body part to its normal location or other suitable location

Explanation: Vascular circulation and nervous pathways may or may not be reestablished

Body Part Character 4	Approach Character 5	Device Character 6	Qualifier Character 7

0 **External Ear, Right**
  Antihelix
  Antitragus
  Auricle
  Earlobe
  Helix
  Pinna
  Tragus
1 **External Ear, Left**
  See 0 External Ear, Right
K **Nasal Mucosa and Soft Tissue**
  Columella
  External naris
  Greater alar cartilage
  Internal naris
  Lateral nasal cartilage
  Lesser alar cartilage
  Nasal cavity
  Nostril
	X External	Z No Device	Z No Qualifier

0 Medical and Surgical
9 Ear, Nose, Sinus
N Release   Definition: Freeing a body part from an abnormal physical constraint by cutting or by the use of force
Explanation: Some of the restraining tissue may be taken out but none of the body part is taken out

Body Part Character 4	Approach Character 5	Device Character 6	Qualifier Character 7
0 External Ear, Right Antihelix Antitragus Auricle Earlobe Helix Pinna Tragus **1 External Ear, Left** See 0 External Ear, Right	0 Open 3 Percutaneous 4 Percutaneous Endoscopic X External	Z No Device	Z No Qualifier
3 External Auditory Canal, Right External auditory meatus **4 External Auditory Canal, Left** See 3 External Auditory Canal, Right	0 Open 3 Percutaneous 4 Percutaneous Endoscopic 7 Via Natural or Artificial Opening 8 Via Natural or Artificial Opening Endoscopic X External	Z No Device	Z No Qualifier
5 Middle Ear, Right Oval window Tympanic cavity **6 Middle Ear, Left** See 5 Middle Ear, Right **9 Auditory Ossicle, Right** Incus Malleus Stapes **A Auditory Ossicle, Left** See 9 Auditory Ossicle, Right **D Inner Ear, Right** Bony labyrinth Bony vestibule Cochlea Round window Semicircular canal **E Inner Ear, Left** See D Inner Ear, Right	0 Open 8 Via Natural or Artificial Opening Endoscopic	Z No Device	Z No Qualifier
7 Tympanic Membrane, Right Pars flaccida **8 Tympanic Membrane, Left** See 7 Tympanic Membrane, Right **F Eustachian Tube, Right** Auditory tube Pharyngotympanic tube **G Eustachian Tube, Left** See F Eustachian Tube, Right **L Nasal Turbinate** Inferior turbinate Middle turbinate Nasal concha Superior turbinate **N Nasopharynx** Choana Fossa of Rosenmuller Pharyngeal recess Rhinopharynx	0 Open 3 Percutaneous 4 Percutaneous Endoscopic 7 Via Natural or Artificial Opening 8 Via Natural or Artificial Opening Endoscopic	Z No Device	Z No Qualifier
B Mastoid Sinus, Right Mastoid air cells **C Mastoid Sinus, Left** See B Mastoid Sinus, Right **M Nasal Septum** Quadrangular cartilage Septal cartilage Vomer bone **P Accessory Sinus** **Q Maxillary Sinus, Right** Antrum of Highmore **R Maxillary Sinus, Left** See Q Maxillary Sinus, Right **S Frontal Sinus, Right** **T Frontal Sinus, Left** **U Ethmoid Sinus, Right** Ethmoidal air cell **V Ethmoid Sinus, Left** See U Ethmoid Sinus, Right **W Sphenoid Sinus, Right** **X Sphenoid Sinus, Left**	0 Open 3 Percutaneous 4 Percutaneous Endoscopic 8 Via Natural or Artificial Opening Endoscopic	Z No Device	Z No Qualifier
K Nasal Mucosa and Soft Tissue Columella External naris Greater alar cartilage Internal naris Lateral nasal cartilage Lesser alar cartilage Nasal cavity Nostril	0 Open 3 Percutaneous 4 Percutaneous Endoscopic 8 Via Natural or Artificial Opening Endoscopic X External	Z No Device	Z No Qualifier

Non-OR 09N[0,1]XZZ
Non-OR 09N[3,4]XZZ
Non-OR 09N[F,G,L][0,3,4,7,8]ZZ
Non-OR 09NM[0,3,4,8]ZZ
Non-OR 09NK[0,3,4,8,X]ZZ

0 Medical and Surgical
9 Ear, Nose, Sinus
P Removal

Definition: Taking out or off a device from a body part

Explanation: If a device is taken out and a similar device put in without cutting or puncturing the skin or mucous membrane, the procedure is coded to the root operation CHANGE. Otherwise, the procedure for taking out a device is coded to the root operation REMOVAL.

Body Part Character 4	Approach Character 5	Device Character 6	Qualifier Character 7

7 Tympanic Membrane, Right
   Pars flaccida
8 Tympanic Membrane, Left
   See 7 Tympanic Membrane, Right
	0 Open
	7 Via Natural or Artificial Opening
	8 Via Natural or Artificial Opening Endoscopic
	X External
		0 Drainage Device	Z No Qualifier

D Inner Ear, Right
   Bony labyrinth
   Bony vestibule
   Cochlea
   Round window
   Semicircular canal
E Inner Ear, Left
   See D Inner Ear, Right
	0 Open
	7 Via Natural or Artificial Opening
	8 Via Natural or Artificial Opening Endoscopic
		S Hearing Device	Z No Qualifier

H Ear, Right
J Ear, Left
K Nasal Mucosa and Soft Tissue
   Columella
   External naris
   Greater alar cartilage
   Internal naris
   Lateral nasal cartilage
   Lesser alar cartilage
   Nasal cavity
   Nostril
	0 Open
	3 Percutaneous
	4 Percutaneous Endoscopic
	7 Via Natural or Artificial Opening
	8 Via Natural or Artificial Opening Endoscopic
		0 Drainage Device
		7 Autologous Tissue Substitute
		D Intraluminal Device
		J Synthetic Substitute
		K Nonautologous Tissue Substitute
		Y Other Device
			Z No Qualifier

H Ear, Right
J Ear, Left
K Nasal Mucosa and Soft Tissue
   Columella
   External naris
   Greater alar cartilage
   Internal naris
   Lateral nasal cartilage
   Lesser alar cartilage
   Nasal cavity
   Nostril
	X External	0 Drainage Device
		7 Autologous Tissue Substitute
		D Intraluminal Device
		J Synthetic Substitute
		K Nonautologous Tissue Substitute
			Z No Qualifier

Y Sinus	0 Open 3 Percutaneous 4 Percutaneous Endoscopic	0 Drainage Device Y Other Device	Z No Qualifier
Y Sinus	7 Via Natural or Artificial Opening 8 Via Natural or Artificial Opening Endoscopic	Y Other Device	Z No Qualifier
Y Sinus	X External	0 Drainage Device	Z No Qualifier

Non-OR 09P[7,8][0,7,8,X]0Z
Non-OR 09P[H,J][3,4][0,J,K,Y]Z
Non-OR 09P[H,J][7,8][0,D,Y]Z
Non-OR 09PK[0,3,4,7,8][0,7,D,J,K,Y]Z
Non-OR 09P[H,J]X[0,7,D,J,K]Z
Non-OR 09PKX[0,7,D,J,K]Z
Non-OR 09PY[3,4]YZ
Non-OR 09PY[7,8]YZ
Non-OR 09PYX0Z

Ear, Nose, Sinus

0 Medical and Surgical
9 Ear, Nose, Sinus
Q Repair Definition: Restoring, to the extent possible, a body part to its normal anatomic structure and function
Explanation: Used only when the method to accomplish the repair is not one of the other root operations

Body Part — Character 4	Approach — Character 5	Device — Character 6	Qualifier — Character 7
0 External Ear, Right Antihelix Antitragus Auricle Earlobe Helix Pinna Tragus **1 External Ear, Left** *See 0 External Ear, Right* **2 External Ear, Bilateral** *See 0 External Ear, Right*	0 Open 3 Percutaneous 4 Percutaneous Endoscopic X External	Z No Device	Z No Qualifier
3 External Auditory Canal, Right External auditory meatus **4 External Auditory Canal, Left** *See 3 External Auditory Canal, Right* **F Eustachian Tube, Right** Auditory tube Pharyngotympanic tube **G Eustachian Tube, Left** *See F Eustachian Tube, Right*	0 Open 3 Percutaneous 4 Percutaneous Endoscopic 7 Via Natural or Artificial Opening 8 Via Natural or Artificial Opening Endoscopic X External	Z No Device	Z No Qualifier
5 Middle Ear, Right Oval window Tympanic cavity **6 Middle Ear, Left** *See 5 Middle Ear, Right* **9 Auditory Ossicle, Right** Incus Malleus Stapes **A Auditory Ossicle, Left** *See 9 Auditory Ossicle, Right* **D Inner Ear, Right** Bony labyrinth Bony vestibule Cochlea Round window Semicircular canal **E Inner Ear, Left** *See D Inner Ear, Right*	0 Open 8 Via Natural or Artificial Opening Endoscopic	Z No Device	Z No Qualifier
7 Tympanic Membrane, Right Pars flaccida **8 Tympanic Membrane, Left** *See 7 Tympanic Membrane, Right* **L Nasal Turbinate** Inferior turbinate Middle turbinate Nasal concha Superior turbinate **N Nasopharynx** Choana Fossa of Rosenmuller Pharyngeal recess Rhinopharynx	0 Open 3 Percutaneous 4 Percutaneous Endoscopic 7 Via Natural or Artificial Opening 8 Via Natural or Artificial Opening Endoscopic	Z No Device	Z No Qualifier
B Mastoid Sinus, Right Mastoid air cells **C Mastoid Sinus, Left** *See B Mastoid Sinus, Right* **M Nasal Septum** Quadrangular cartilage Septal cartilage Vomer bone **P Accessory Sinus** **Q Maxillary Sinus, Right** Antrum of Highmore **R Maxillary Sinus, Left** *See Q Maxillary Sinus, Right* **S Frontal Sinus, Right** **T Frontal Sinus, Left** **U Ethmoid Sinus, Right** Ethmoidal air cell **V Ethmoid Sinus, Left** *See U Ethmoid Sinus, Right* **W Sphenoid Sinus, Right** **X Sphenoid Sinus, Left**	0 Open 3 Percutaneous 4 Percutaneous Endoscopic 8 Via Natural or Artificial Opening Endoscopic	Z No Device	Z No Qualifier
K Nasal Mucosa and Soft Tissue Columella External naris Greater alar cartilage Internal naris Lateral nasal cartilage Lesser alar cartilage Nasal cavity Nostril	0 Open 3 Percutaneous 4 Percutaneous Endoscopic 8 Via Natural or Artificial Opening Endoscopic X External	Z No Device	Z No Qualifier

Non-OR 09Q[0,1,2]XZZ
Non-OR 09Q[3,4]XZZ
Non-OR 09Q[F,G][0,3,4,7,8,X]ZZ
Non-OR 09QKXZZ

ICD-10-PCS 2025 — Ear, Nose, Sinus — 09R–09R

0 Medical and Surgical
9 Ear, Nose, Sinus
R Replacement

Definition: Putting in or on biological or synthetic material that physically takes the place and/or function of all or a portion of a body part
Explanation: The body part may have been taken out or replaced, or may be taken out, physically eradicated, or rendered nonfunctional during the REPLACEMENT procedure. A REMOVAL procedure is coded for taking out the device used in a previous replacement procedure.

Body Part Character 4	Approach Character 5	Device Character 6	Qualifier Character 7
0 External Ear, Right Antihelix Antitragus Auricle Earlobe Helix Pinna Tragus **1 External Ear, Left** *See 0 External Ear, Right* **2 External Ear, Bilateral** *See 0 External Ear, Right* **K Nasal Mucosa and Soft Tissue** Columella External naris Greater alar cartilage Internal naris Lateral nasal cartilage Lesser alar cartilage Nasal cavity Nostril	0 Open X External	7 Autologous Tissue Substitute J Synthetic Substitute K Nonautologous Tissue Substitute	Z No Qualifier
5 Middle Ear, Right Oval window Tympanic cavity **6 Middle Ear, Left** *See 5 Middle Ear, Right* **9 Auditory Ossicle, Right** Incus Malleus Stapes **A Auditory Ossicle, Left** *See 9 Auditory Ossicle, Right* **D Inner Ear, Right** Bony labyrinth Bony vestibule Cochlea Round window Semicircular canal **E Inner Ear, Left** *See D Inner Ear, Right*	0 Open	7 Autologous Tissue Substitute J Synthetic Substitute K Nonautologous Tissue Substitute	Z No Qualifier
7 Tympanic Membrane, Right Pars flaccida **8 Tympanic Membrane, Left** *See 7 Tympanic Membrane, Right* **N Nasopharynx** Choana Fossa of Rosenmuller Pharyngeal recess Rhinopharynx	0 Open 7 Via Natural or Artificial Opening 8 Via Natural or Artificial Opening Endoscopic	7 Autologous Tissue Substitute J Synthetic Substitute K Nonautologous Tissue Substitute	Z No Qualifier
L Nasal Turbinate Inferior turbinate Middle turbinate Nasal concha Superior turbinate	0 Open 3 Percutaneous 4 Percutaneous Endoscopic 7 Via Natural or Artificial Opening 8 Via Natural or Artificial Opening Endoscopic	7 Autologous Tissue Substitute J Synthetic Substitute K Nonautologous Tissue Substitute	Z No Qualifier
M Nasal Septum Quadrangular cartilage Septal cartilage Vomer bone	0 Open 3 Percutaneous 4 Percutaneous Endoscopic	7 Autologous Tissue Substitute J Synthetic Substitute K Nonautologous Tissue Substitute	Z No Qualifier

0 Medical and Surgical
9 Ear, Nose, Sinus
S Reposition Definition: Moving to its normal location, or other suitable location, all or a portion of a body part
Explanation: The body part is moved to a new location from an abnormal location, or from a normal location where it is not functioning correctly. The body part may or may not be cut out or off to be moved to the new location.

Body Part Character 4	Approach Character 5	Device Character 6	Qualifier Character 7

0 External Ear, Right
    Antihelix
    Antitragus
    Auricle
    Earlobe
    Helix
    Pinna
    Tragus
1 External Ear, Left
    See 0 External Ear, Right
2 External Ear, Bilateral
    See 0 External Ear, Right
K Nasal Mucosa and Soft Tissue
    Columella
    External naris
    Greater alar cartilage
    Internal naris
    Lateral nasal cartilage
    Lesser alar cartilage
    Nasal cavity
    Nostril
	0 Open
	4 Percutaneous Endoscopic
	X External
		Z No Device	**Z** No Qualifier

7 Tympanic Membrane, Right
    Pars flaccida
8 Tympanic Membrane, Left
    See 7 Tympanic Membrane, Right
F Eustachian Tube, Right
    Auditory tube
    Pharyngotympanic tube
G Eustachian Tube, Left
    See F Eustachian Tube, Right
L Nasal Turbinate
    Inferior turbinate
    Middle turbinate
    Nasal concha
    Superior turbinate
	0 Open
	4 Percutaneous Endoscopic
	7 Via Natural or Artificial Opening
	8 Via Natural or Artificial Opening Endoscopic
		Z No Device	**Z** No Qualifier

9 Auditory Ossicle, Right
    Incus
    Malleus
    Stapes
A Auditory Ossicle, Left
    See 9 Auditory Ossicle, Right
M Nasal Septum
    Quadrangular cartilage
    Septal cartilage
    Vomer bone
	0 Open
	4 Percutaneous Endoscopic
		Z No Device	**Z** No Qualifier

Non-OR 09S[F,G][0,4,7,8]ZZ

0	Medical and Surgical								
9	Ear, Nose, Sinus								
T	Resection	Definition: Cutting out or off, without replacement, all of a body part							
		Explanation: None							

Body Part Character 4		Approach Character 5	Device Character 6	Qualifier Character 7

0 External Ear, Right
  Antihelix
  Antitragus
  Auricle
  Earlobe
  Helix
  Pinna
  Tragus
	1 External Ear, Left
	  See 0 External Ear, Right
		0 Open
		4 Percutaneous Endoscopic
		X External
			Z No Device	Z No Qualifier

5 Middle Ear, Right
  Oval window
  Tympanic cavity
6 Middle Ear, Left
  See 5 Middle Ear, Right
9 Auditory Ossicle, Right
  Incus
  Malleus
  Stapes
	A Auditory Ossicle, Left
	  See 9 Auditory Ossicle, Right
	D Inner Ear, Right
	  Bony labyrinth
	  Bony vestibule
	  Cochlea
	  Round window
	  Semicircular canal
	E Inner Ear, Left
	  See D Inner Ear, Right
		0 Open
		8 Via Natural or Artificial Opening Endoscopic
			Z No Device	Z No Qualifier

7 Tympanic Membrane, Right
  Pars flaccida
8 Tympanic Membrane, Left
  See 7 Tympanic Membrane, Right
F Eustachian Tube, Right
  Auditory tube
  Pharyngotympanic tube
G Eustachian Tube, Left
  See F Eustachian Tube, Right
	L Nasal Turbinate
	  Inferior turbinate
	  Middle turbinate
	  Nasal concha
	  Superior turbinate
	N Nasopharynx
	  Choana
	  Fossa of Rosenmuller
	  Pharyngeal recess
	  Rhinopharynx
		0 Open
		4 Percutaneous Endoscopic
		7 Via Natural or Artificial Opening
		8 Via Natural or Artificial Opening Endoscopic
			Z No Device	Z No Qualifier

B Mastoid Sinus, Right
  Mastoid air cells
C Mastoid Sinus, Left
  See B Mastoid Sinus, Right
M Nasal Septum
  Quadrangular cartilage
  Septal cartilage
  Vomer bone
P Accessory Sinus
Q Maxillary Sinus, Right
  Antrum of Highmore
	R Maxillary Sinus, Left
	  See Q Maxillary Sinus, Right
	S Frontal Sinus, Right
	T Frontal Sinus, Left
	U Ethmoid Sinus, Right
	  Ethmoidal air cell
	V Ethmoid Sinus, Left
	  See U Ethmoid Sinus, Right
	W Sphenoid Sinus, Right
	X Sphenoid Sinus, Left
		0 Open
		4 Percutaneous Endoscopic
		8 Via Natural or Artificial Opening Endoscopic
			Z No Device	Z No Qualifier

K Nasal Mucosa and Soft Tissue
  Columella
  External naris
  Greater alar cartilage
  Internal naris
  Lateral nasal cartilage
  Lesser alar cartilage
  Nasal cavity
  Nostril
		0 Open
		4 Percutaneous Endoscopic
		8 Via Natural or Artificial Opening Endoscopic
		X External
			Z No Device	Z No Qualifier

Non-OR   09T[F,G][0,4,7,8]ZZ

0 Medical and Surgical
9 Ear, Nose, Sinus
U Supplement

Definition: Putting in or on biological or synthetic material that physically reinforces and/or augments the function of a portion of a body part

Explanation: The biological material is non-living, or is living and from the same individual. The body part may have been previously replaced, and the SUPPLEMENT procedure is performed to physically reinforce and/or augment the function of the replaced body part.

Body Part — Character 4	Approach — Character 5	Device — Character 6	Qualifier — Character 7

0 External Ear, Right
  Antihelix
  Antitragus
  Auricle
  Earlobe
  Helix
  Pinna
  Tragus
1 External Ear, Left
  See 0 External Ear, Right
2 External Ear, Bilateral
  See 0 External Ear, Right
	0 Open
	X External
		7 Autologous Tissue Substitute
		J Synthetic Substitute
		K Nonautologous Tissue Substitute
			Z No Qualifier

5 Middle Ear, Right
  Oval window
  Tympanic cavity
6 Middle Ear, Left
  See 5 Middle Ear, Right
9 Auditory Ossicle, Right
  Incus
  Malleus
  Stapes
A Auditory Ossicle, Left
  See 9 Auditory Ossicle, Right
D Inner Ear, Right
  Bony labyrinth
  Bony vestibule
  Cochlea
  Round window
  Semicircular canal
E Inner Ear, Left
  See D Inner Ear, Right
	0 Open
	8 Via Natural or Artificial Opening Endoscopic
		7 Autologous Tissue Substitute
		J Synthetic Substitute
		K Nonautologous Tissue Substitute
			Z No Qualifier

7 Tympanic Membrane, Right
  Pars flaccida
8 Tympanic Membrane, Left
  See 7 Tympanic Membrane, Right
N Nasopharynx
  Choana
  Fossa of Rosenmuller
  Pharyngeal recess
  Rhinopharynx
	0 Open
	7 Via Natural or Artificial Opening
	8 Via Natural or Artificial Opening Endoscopic
		7 Autologous Tissue Substitute
		J Synthetic Substitute
		K Nonautologous Tissue Substitute
			Z No Qualifier

B Mastoid Sinus, Right
  Mastoid air cells
C Mastoid Sinus, Left
  See B Mastoid Sinus, Right
L Nasal Turbinate
  Inferior turbinate
  Middle turbinate
  Nasal concha
  Superior turbinate
P Accessory Sinus
Q Maxillary Sinus, Right
  Antrum of Highmore
R Maxillary Sinus, Left
  See Q Maxillary Sinus, Right
S Frontal Sinus, Right
T Frontal Sinus, Left
U Ethmoid Sinus, Right
  Ethmoidal air cell
V Ethmoid Sinus, Left
  See U Ethmoid Sinus, Right
W Sphenoid Sinus, Right
X Sphenoid Sinus, Left
	0 Open
	3 Percutaneous
	4 Percutaneous Endoscopic
	7 Via Natural or Artificial Opening
	8 Via Natural or Artificial Opening Endoscopic
		7 Autologous Tissue Substitute
		J Synthetic Substitute
		K Nonautologous Tissue Substitute
			Z No Qualifier

K Nasal Mucosa and Soft Tissue
  Columella
  External naris
  Greater alar cartilage
  Internal naris
  Lateral nasal cartilage
  Lesser alar cartilage
  Nasal cavity
  Nostril
	0 Open
	8 Via Natural or Artificial Opening Endoscopic
	X External
		7 Autologous Tissue Substitute
		J Synthetic Substitute
		K Nonautologous Tissue Substitute
			Z No Qualifier

M Nasal Septum
  Quadrangular cartilage
  Septal cartilage
  Vomer bone
	0 Open
	3 Percutaneous
	4 Percutaneous Endoscopic
	8 Via Natural or Artificial Opening Endoscopic
		7 Autologous Tissue Substitute
		J Synthetic Substitute
		K Nonautologous Tissue Substitute
			Z No Qualifier

ICD-10-PCS 2025 — Ear, Nose, Sinus — 09W–09W

- **0** Medical and Surgical
- **9** Ear, Nose, Sinus
- **W** Revision

Definition: Correcting, to the extent possible, a portion of a malfunctioning device or the position of a displaced device

Explanation: Revision can include correcting a malfunctioning or displaced device by taking out or putting in components of the device such as a screw or pin

Body Part Character 4	Approach Character 5	Device Character 6	Qualifier Character 7

7 Tympanic Membrane, Right
    Pars flaccida
8 Tympanic Membrane, Left
    See 7 Tympanic Membrane, Right
9 Auditory Ossicle, Right
    Incus
    Malleus
    Stapes
A Auditory Ossicle, Left
    See 9 Auditory Ossicle, Right
	0 Open
	7 Via Natural or Artificial Opening
	8 Via Natural or Artificial Opening Endoscopic
		7 Autologous Tissue Substitute
		J Synthetic Substitute
		K Nonautologous Tissue Substitute
			Z No Qualifier

D Inner Ear, Right
    Bony labyrinth
    Bony vestibule
    Cochlea
    Round window
    Semicircular canal
E Inner Ear, Left
    See D Inner Ear, Right
	0 Open
	7 Via Natural or Artificial Opening
	8 Via Natural or Artificial Opening Endoscopic
		S Hearing Device	**Z** No Qualifier

H Ear, Right
J Ear, Left
K Nasal Mucosa and Soft Tissue
    Columella
    External naris
    Greater alar cartilage
    Internal naris
    Lateral nasal cartilage
    Lesser alar cartilage
    Nasal cavity
    Nostril
	0 Open
	3 Percutaneous
	4 Percutaneous Endoscopic
	7 Via Natural or Artificial Opening
	8 Via Natural or Artificial Opening Endoscopic
		0 Drainage Device
		7 Autologous Tissue Substitute
		D Intraluminal Device
		J Synthetic Substitute
		K Nonautologous Tissue Substitute
		Y Other Device
			Z No Qualifier

H Ear, Right
J Ear, Left
K Nasal Mucosa and Soft Tissue
    Columella
    External naris
    Greater alar cartilage
    Internal naris
    Lateral nasal cartilage
    Lesser alar cartilage
    Nasal cavity
    Nostril
	X External	**0** Drainage Device
		7 Autologous Tissue Substitute
		D Intraluminal Device
		J Synthetic Substitute
		K Nonautologous Tissue Substitute
			Z No Qualifier

Y Sinus	**0** Open **3** Percutaneous **4** Percutaneous Endoscopic	**0** Drainage Device **Y** Other Device	**Z** No Qualifier
Y Sinus	**7** Via Natural or Artificial Opening **8** Via Natural or Artificial Opening Endoscopic	**Y** Other Device	**Z** No Qualifier
Y Sinus	**X** External	**0** Drainage Device	**Z** No Qualifier

Non-OR   09W[H,J][3,4][J,K,Y]Z
Non-OR   09W[H,J][7,8][D,Y]Z
Non-OR   09WK[0,3,4,7,8][0,7,D,J,K,Y]Z
Non-OR   09W[H,J,K]X[0,7,D,J,K]Z
Non-OR   09WY[3,4]YZ
Non-OR   09WY[7,8]YZ
Non-OR   09WYX0Z

Respiratory System ØB1–ØBY

Character Meanings
This Character Meaning table is provided as a guide to assist the user in the identification of character members that may be found in this section of code tables. It **SHOULD NOT** be used to build a PCS code.

Operation–Character 3		Body Part–Character 4		Approach–Character 5		Device–Character 6		Qualifier–Character 7	
1	Bypass	Ø	Tracheobronchial Tree	Ø	Open	Ø	Drainage Device	Ø	Allogeneic
2	Change	1	Trachea	3	Percutaneous	1	Radioactive Element	1	Syngeneic
5	Destruction	2	Carina	4	Percutaneous Endoscopic	2	Monitoring Device	2	Zooplastic
7	Dilation	3	Main Bronchus, Right	7	Via Natural or Artificial Opening	3	Infusion Device	3	Laser Interstitial Thermal Therapy
9	Drainage	4	Upper Lobe Bronchus, Right	8	Via Natural or Artificial Opening Endoscopic	7	Autologous Tissue Substitute	4	Cutaneous
B	Excision	5	Middle Lobe Bronchus, Right	X	External	C	Extraluminal Device	6	Esophagus
C	Extirpation	6	Lower Lobe Bronchus, Right			D	Intraluminal Device	X	Diagnostic
D	Extraction	7	Main Bronchus, Left			E	Intraluminal Device, Endotracheal Airway	Z	No Qualifier
F	Fragmentation	8	Upper Lobe Bronchus, Left			F	Tracheostomy Device		
H	Insertion	9	Lingula Bronchus			G	Intraluminal Device, Endobronchial Valve		
J	Inspection	B	Lower Lobe Bronchus, Left			J	Synthetic Substitute		
L	Occlusion	C	Upper Lung Lobe, Right			K	Nonautologous Tissue Substitute		
M	Reattachment	D	Middle Lung Lobe, Right			M	Diaphragmatic Pacemaker Lead		
N	Release	F	Lower Lung Lobe, Right			Y	Other Device		
P	Removal	G	Upper Lung Lobe, Left			Z	No Device		
Q	Repair	H	Lung Lingula						
R	Replacement	J	Lower Lung Lobe, Left						
S	Reposition	K	Lung, Right						
T	Resection	L	Lung, Left						
U	Supplement	M	Lungs, Bilateral						
V	Restriction	N	Pleura, Right						
W	Revision	P	Pleura, Left						
Y	Transplantation	Q	Pleura						
		T	Diaphragm						

AHA Coding Clinic for table ØB5
2022, 4Q, 53-54   Laser interstitial thermal therapy
2016, 2Q, 17   Photodynamic therapy for treatment of malignant mesothelioma
2015, 2Q, 31   Thoracoscopic talc pleurodesis

AHA Coding Clinic for table ØB7
2020, 3Q, 43   Tracheobronchomalacia with placement of tracheobronchial stent

AHA Coding Clinic for table ØB9
2017, 3Q, 15   Bronchoscopy with suctioning for removal of retained secretions
2017, 1Q, 51   Bronchoalveolar lavage
2016, 1Q, 26   Bronchoalveolar lavage, endobronchial biopsy and transbronchial biopsy
2016, 1Q, 27   Fiberoptic bronchoscopy with brushings and bronchoalveolar lavage

AHA Coding Clinic for table ØBB
2022, 2Q, 19   Transbronchial lung biopsy using alligator forceps
2016, 1Q, 26   Bronchoalveolar lavage, endobronchial biopsy and transbronchial biopsy
2016, 1Q, 27   Fiberoptic bronchoscopy with brushings and bronchoalveolar lavage
2014, 1Q, 20   Fiducial marker placement

AHA Coding Clinic for table ØBC
2017, 3Q, 14   Bronchoscopy with suctioning and washings for removal of mucus plug

AHA Coding Clinic for table ØBD
2020, 3Q, 40   Transbronchial cryobiopsy of upper, middle and lower lobes of lung
2018, 3Q, 28   Lung decortication for empyema

AHA Coding Clinic for table ØBH
2022, 3Q, 22   Approach value for placement of endotracheal tube
2019, 3Q, 33   Insertion of endobronchial valve
2014, 4Q, 3-10   Mechanical ventilation

AHA Coding Clinic for table ØBJ
2015, 2Q, 31   Thoracoscopic talc pleurodesis
2014, 1Q, 20   Fiducial marker placement

AHA Coding Clinic for table ØBL
2019, 3Q, 33   Insertion of endobronchial valve

AHA Coding Clinic for table ØBN
2019, 2Q, 20   Pericardiectomy for constrictive pericarditis
2018, 3Q, 28   Lung decortication
2018, 3Q, 28   Lung decortication for empyema
2015, 3Q, 15   Vascular ring surgery with release of esophagus and trachea

AHA Coding Clinic for table ØBQ
2020, 3Q, 41   Plication of diaphragm
2016, 2Q, 22   Esophageal lengthening Collis gastroplasty with Nissen fundoplication and hiatal hernia
2014, 3Q, 28   Laparoscopic Nissen fundoplication and diaphragmatic hernia repair

AHA Coding Clinic for table ØBU
2020, 3Q, 43   Tracheobronchomalacia with placement of tracheobronchial stent
2015, 1Q, 28   Repair of bronchopleural fistula using omental pedicle graft

AHA Coding Clinic for table ØBV
2020, 3Q, 41   Plication of diaphragm

AHA Coding Clinic for table ØBY
2023, 2Q, 32   Preparation of donor organ before transplantation

Respiratory System

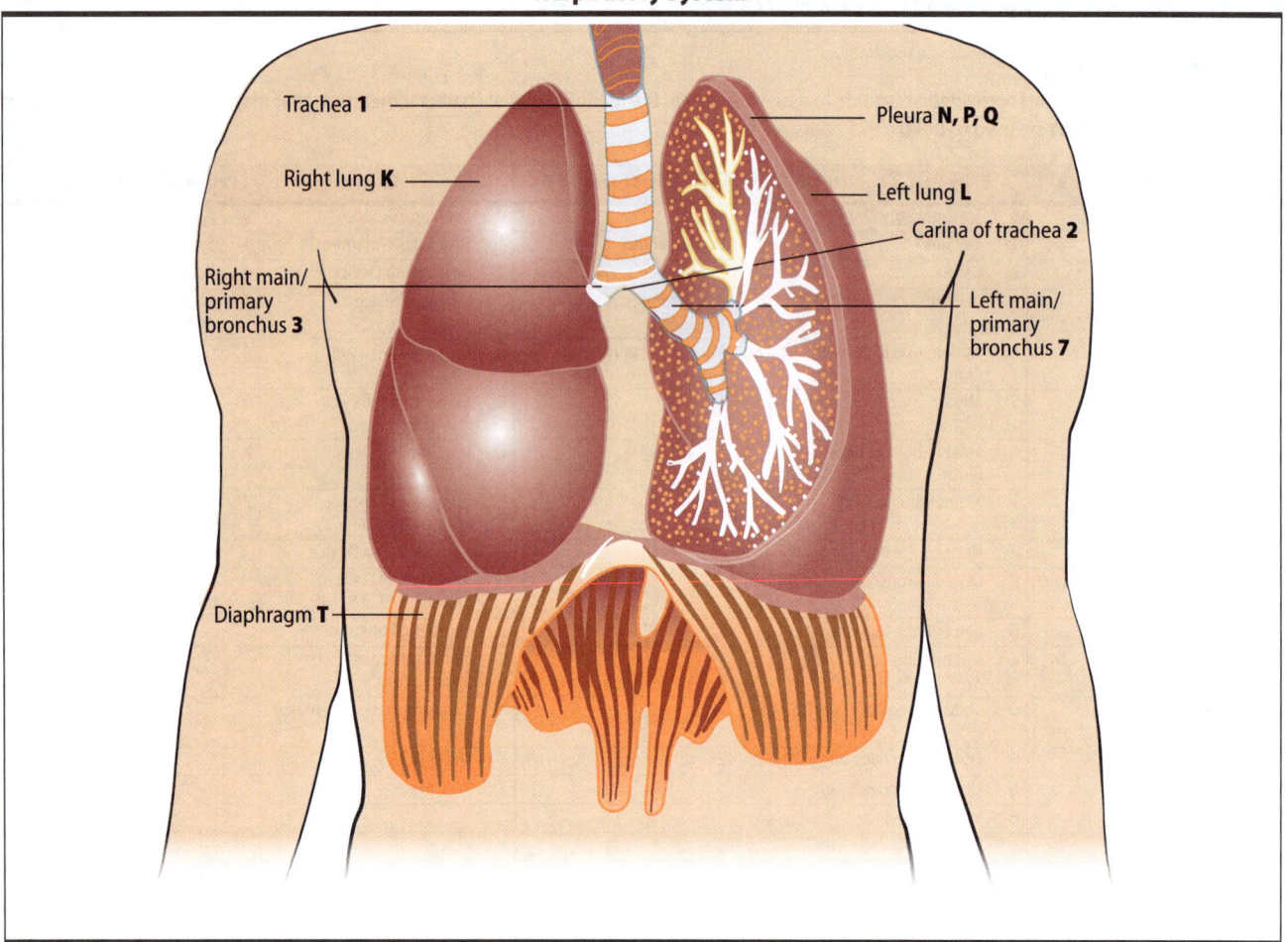

Right Lung Bronchi

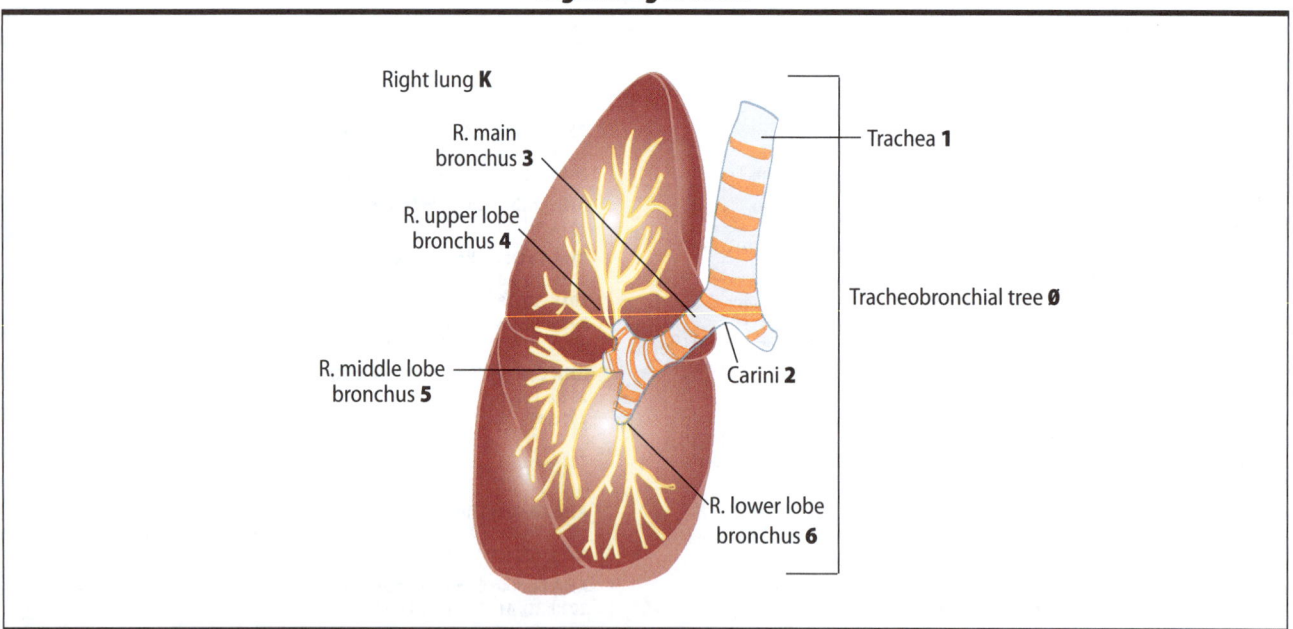

ICD-10-PCS 2025 — Respiratory System — 0B1–0B2

0 Medical and Surgical
B Respiratory System
1 Bypass

Definition: Altering the route of passage of the contents of a tubular body part

Explanation: Rerouting contents of a body part to a downstream area of the normal route, to a similar route and body part, or to an abnormal route and dissimilar body part. Includes one or more anastomoses, with or without the use of a device.

Body Part Character 4	Approach Character 5	Device Character 6	Qualifier Character 7
1 Trachea Cricoid cartilage	0 Open	D Intraluminal Device	6 Esophagus
1 Trachea Cricoid cartilage	0 Open	F Tracheostomy Device Z No Device	4 Cutaneous
1 Trachea Cricoid cartilage	3 Percutaneous 4 Percutaneous Endoscopic	F Tracheostomy Device Z No Device	4 Cutaneous

DRG Non-OR 0B113[F,Z]4
Non-OR 0B110D6

---

0 Medical and Surgical
B Respiratory System
2 Change

Definition: Taking out or off a device from a body part and putting back an identical or similar device in or on the same body part without cutting or puncturing the skin or a mucous membrane

Explanation: All CHANGE procedures are coded using the approach EXTERNAL

Body Part Character 4	Approach Character 5	Device Character 6	Qualifier Character 7
0 Tracheobronchial Tree K Lung, Right L Lung, Left Q Pleura T Diaphragm	X External	0 Drainage Device Y Other Device	Z No Qualifier
1 Trachea Cricoid cartilage	X External	0 Drainage Device E Intraluminal Device, Endotracheal Airway F Tracheostomy Device Y Other Device	Z No Qualifier

Non-OR All body part, approach, device, and qualifier values

Respiratory System

0B5–0B7   Respiratory System   ICD-10-PCS 2025

0 Medical and Surgical
B Respiratory System
5 Destruction   **Definition:** Physical eradication of all or a portion of a body part by the direct use of energy, force, or a destructive agent
                             Explanation: None of the body part is physically taken out

Body Part Character 4	Approach Character 5	Device Character 6	Qualifier Character 7

1 Trachea
   Cricoid cartilage
2 Carina
3 Main Bronchus, Right
   Bronchus intermedius
   Intermediate bronchus
4 Upper Lobe Bronchus, Right
5 Middle Lobe Bronchus, Right
6 Lower Lobe Bronchus, Right
7 Main Bronchus, Left
8 Upper Lobe Bronchus, Left
9 Lingula Bronchus
B Lower Lobe Bronchus, Left
	0 Open
	3 Percutaneous
	4 Percutaneous Endoscopic
	7 Via Natural or Artificial Opening
	8 Via Natural or Artificial Opening Endoscopic
		Z No Device	Z No Qualifier

C Upper Lung Lobe, Right D Middle Lung Lobe, Right F Lower Lung Lobe, Right G Upper Lung Lobe, Left H Lung Lingula J Lower Lung Lobe, Left K Lung, Right L Lung, Left M Lungs, Bilateral	0 Open 3 Percutaneous 4 Percutaneous Endoscopic	Z No Device	3 Laser Interstitial Thermal Therapy Z No Qualifier
C Upper Lung Lobe, Right D Middle Lung Lobe, Right F Lower Lung Lobe, Right G Upper Lung Lobe, Left H Lung Lingula J Lower Lung Lobe, Left K Lung, Right L Lung, Left M Lungs, Bilateral	7 Via Natural or Artificial Opening 8 Via Natural or Artificial Opening Endoscopic	Z No Device	Z No Qualifier
N Pleura, Right P Pleura, Left T Diaphragm	0 Open 3 Percutaneous 4 Percutaneous Endoscopic	Z No Device	Z No Qualifier

Non-OR   0B5[3,4,5,6,7,8,9,B]4ZZ
Non-OR   0B5[C,D,F,G,H,J,K,L,M]8ZZ

0 Medical and Surgical
B Respiratory System
7 Dilation   **Definition:** Expanding an orifice or the lumen of a tubular body part
                   Explanation: The orifice can be a natural orifice or an artificially created orifice. Accomplished by stretching a tubular body part using intraluminal pressure or by cutting part of the orifice or wall of the tubular body part.

Body Part Character 4	Approach Character 5	Device Character 6	Qualifier Character 7

1 Trachea
   Cricoid cartilage
2 Carina
3 Main Bronchus, Right
   Bronchus intermedius
   Intermediate bronchus
4 Upper Lobe Bronchus, Right
5 Middle Lobe Bronchus, Right
6 Lower Lobe Bronchus, Right
7 Main Bronchus, Left
8 Upper Lobe Bronchus, Left
9 Lingula Bronchus
B Lower Lobe Bronchus, Left
	0 Open
	3 Percutaneous
	4 Percutaneous Endoscopic
	7 Via Natural or Artificial Opening
	8 Via Natural or Artificial Opening Endoscopic
		D Intraluminal Device
		Z No Device
			Z No Qualifier

Non-OR   0B7[3,4,5,6,7,8,9,B][0,3,4,7,8][D,Z]Z

Non-OR Procedure   DRG Non-OR Procedure   Valid OR Procedure   HAC Associated Procedure   Combination Only   New/Revised April   New/Revised October

0 Medical and Surgical
B Respiratory System
9 Drainage   Definition: Taking or letting out fluids and/or gases from a body part
              Explanation: The qualifier DIAGNOSTIC is used to identify drainage procedures that are biopsies

Body Part Character 4	Approach Character 5	Device Character 6	Qualifier Character 7

1 Trachea
   Cricoid cartilage
2 Carina
3 Main Bronchus, Right
   Bronchus intermedius
   Intermediate bronchus
4 Upper Lobe Bronchus, Right
5 Middle Lobe Bronchus, Right
6 Lower Lobe Bronchus, Right
7 Main Bronchus, Left
8 Upper Lobe Bronchus, Left
9 Lingula Bronchus
B Lower Lobe Bronchus, Left
C Upper Lung Lobe, Right
D Middle Lung Lobe, Right
F Lower Lung Lobe, Right
G Upper Lung Lobe, Left
H Lung Lingula
J Lower Lung Lobe, Left
K Lung, Right
L Lung, Left
M Lungs, Bilateral
	0 Open
	3 Percutaneous
	4 Percutaneous Endoscopic
	7 Via Natural or Artificial Opening
	8 Via Natural or Artificial Opening Endoscopic
		0 Drainage Device	Z No Qualifier

1 Trachea
   Cricoid cartilage
2 Carina
3 Main Bronchus, Right
   Bronchus intermedius
   Intermediate bronchus
4 Upper Lobe Bronchus, Right
5 Middle Lobe Bronchus, Right
6 Lower Lobe Bronchus, Right
7 Main Bronchus, Left
8 Upper Lobe Bronchus, Left
9 Lingula Bronchus
B Lower Lobe Bronchus, Left
C Upper Lung Lobe, Right
D Middle Lung Lobe, Right
F Lower Lung Lobe, Right
G Upper Lung Lobe, Left
H Lung Lingula
J Lower Lung Lobe, Left
K Lung, Right
L Lung, Left
M Lungs, Bilateral
	0 Open
	3 Percutaneous
	4 Percutaneous Endoscopic
	7 Via Natural or Artificial Opening
	8 Via Natural or Artificial Opening Endoscopic
		Z No Device	X Diagnostic
			Z No Qualifier

N Pleura, Right P Pleura, Left	0 Open 3 Percutaneous 4 Percutaneous Endoscopic 8 Via Natural or Artificial Opening Endoscopic	0 Drainage Device	Z No Qualifier
N Pleura, Right P Pleura, Left	0 Open 3 Percutaneous 4 Percutaneous Endoscopic 8 Via Natural or Artificial Opening Endoscopic	Z No Device	X Diagnostic Z No Qualifier
T Diaphragm	0 Open 3 Percutaneous 4 Percutaneous Endoscopic	0 Drainage Device	Z No Qualifier
T Diaphragm	0 Open 3 Percutaneous 4 Percutaneous Endoscopic	Z No Device	X Diagnostic Z No Qualifier

Non-OR 0B9[1,2,3,4,5,6,7,8,9,B][7,8]0Z
Non-OR 0B9[1,2,3,4,5,6,7,8,9,B][3,4]ZX
Non-OR 0B9[1,2,3,4,5,6,7,8,9,B][7,8]Z[X,Z]
Non-OR 0B9[C,D,F,G,H,J,K,L,M][3,4,7]ZX
Non-OR 0B9[C,D,F,G,H,J,K,L,M]8Z[X,Z]
Non-OR 0B9[N,P][0,3,8]0Z
Non-OR 0B9[N,P][0,3,8]Z[X,Z]
Non-OR 0B9[N,P]4ZX
Non-OR 0B9T[3,4]0Z
Non-OR 0B9T[3,4]Z[X,Z]

Respiratory System

0BB–0BC   Respiratory System   ICD-10-PCS 2025

0 Medical and Surgical
B Respiratory System
B Excision   Definition: Cutting out or off, without replacement, a portion of a body part
Explanation: The qualifier DIAGNOSTIC is used to identify excision procedures that are biopsies

Body Part Character 4	Approach Character 5	Device Character 6	Qualifier Character 7

1 Trachea
  Cricoid cartilage
2 Carina
3 Main Bronchus, Right
  Bronchus intermedius
  Intermediate bronchus
4 Upper Lobe Bronchus, Right
5 Middle Lobe Bronchus, Right
6 Lower Lobe Bronchus, Right
7 Main Bronchus, Left
8 Upper Lobe Bronchus, Left
9 Lingula Bronchus
B Lower Lobe Bronchus, Left
C Upper Lung Lobe, Right
D Middle Lung Lobe, Right
F Lower Lung Lobe, Right
G Upper Lung Lobe, Left
H Lung Lingula
J Lower Lung Lobe, Left
K Lung, Right
L Lung, Left
M Lungs, Bilateral
	0 Open
	3 Percutaneous
	4 Percutaneous Endoscopic
	7 Via Natural or Artificial Opening
	8 Via Natural or Artificial Opening Endoscopic
		Z No Device	X Diagnostic
			Z No Qualifier

N Pleura, Right P Pleura, Left	0 Open 3 Percutaneous 4 Percutaneous Endoscopic 8 Via Natural or Artificial Opening Endoscopic	Z No Device	X Diagnostic Z No Qualifier
T Diaphragm	0 Open 3 Percutaneous 4 Percutaneous Endoscopic	Z No Device	X Diagnostic Z No Qualifier

Non-OR   0BB[1,2,3,4,5,6,7,8,9,B][3,4,7,8]ZX
Non-OR   0BB[3,4,5,6,7,8,9,B,M][4,8]ZZ
Non-OR   0BB[C,D,F,G,H,J,K,L,M]3ZX
Non-OR   0BB[C,D,F,G,H,J,K,L]8ZZ
Non-OR   0BB[N,P]3ZX

0 Medical and Surgical
B Respiratory System
C Extirpation   Definition: Taking or cutting out solid matter from a body part
Explanation: The solid matter may be an abnormal byproduct of a biological function or a foreign body; it may be imbedded in a body part or in the lumen of a tubular body part. The solid matter may or may not have been previously broken into pieces.

Body Part Character 4	Approach Character 5	Device Character 6	Qualifier Character 7

1 Trachea
  Cricoid cartilage
2 Carina
3 Main Bronchus, Right
  Bronchus intermedius
  Intermediate bronchus
4 Upper Lobe Bronchus, Right
5 Middle Lobe Bronchus, Right
6 Lower Lobe Bronchus, Right
7 Main Bronchus, Left
8 Upper Lobe Bronchus, Left
9 Lingula Bronchus
B Lower Lobe Bronchus, Left
C Upper Lung Lobe, Right
D Middle Lung Lobe, Right
F Lower Lung Lobe, Right
G Upper Lung Lobe, Left
H Lung Lingula
J Lower Lung Lobe, Left
K Lung, Right
L Lung, Left
M Lungs, Bilateral
	0 Open
	3 Percutaneous
	4 Percutaneous Endoscopic
	7 Via Natural or Artificial Opening
	8 Via Natural or Artificial Opening Endoscopic
		Z No Device	Z No Qualifier

N Pleura, Right P Pleura, Left T Diaphragm	0 Open 3 Percutaneous 4 Percutaneous Endoscopic	Z No Device	Z No Qualifier

Non-OR   0BC[1,2,3,4,5,6,7,8,9,B][7,8]ZZ
Non-OR   0BC[N,P]3ZZ

Non-OR Procedure   DRG Non-OR Procedure   Valid OR Procedure   HAC Associated Procedure   Combination Only   New/Revised April   New/Revised October

Respiratory System

0 Medical and Surgical
B Respiratory System
D Extraction — Definition: Pulling or stripping out or off all or a portion of a body part by the use of force
Explanation: The qualifier DIAGNOSTIC is used to identify extraction procedures that are biopsies

Body Part Character 4	Approach Character 5	Device Character 6	Qualifier Character 7

1 Trachea
  Cricoid cartilage
2 Carina
3 Main Bronchus, Right
  Bronchus intermedius
  Intermediate bronchus
4 Upper Lobe Bronchus, Right
5 Middle Lobe Bronchus, Right
6 Lower Lobe Bronchus, Right
7 Main Bronchus, Left
8 Upper Lobe Bronchus, Left
9 Lingula Bronchus
B Lower Lobe Bronchus, Left
C Upper Lung Lobe, Right
D Middle Lung Lobe, Right
F Lower Lung Lobe, Right
G Upper Lung Lobe, Left
H Lung Lingula
J Lower Lung Lobe, Left
K Lung, Right
L Lung, Left
M Lungs, Bilateral
	4 Percutaneous Endoscopic
	8 Via Natural or Artificial Opening Endoscopic
		Z No Device	X Diagnostic

N Pleura, Right P Pleura, Left	0 Open 3 Percutaneous 4 Percutaneous Endoscopic	Z No Device	X Diagnostic Z No Qualifier

Non-OR 0BD[1,2,3,4,5,6,7,8,9,B,C,D,F,G,H,J,K,L,M][4,8]ZX

0 Medical and Surgical
B Respiratory System
F Fragmentation — Definition: Breaking solid matter in a body part into pieces
Explanation: Physical force (e.g., manual, ultrasonic) applied directly or indirectly is used to break the solid matter into pieces. The solid matter may be an abnormal byproduct of a biological function or a foreign body. The pieces of solid matter are not taken out.

Body Part Character 4	Approach Character 5	Device Character 6	Qualifier Character 7

1 Trachea   NC
  Cricoid cartilage
2 Carina   NC
3 Main Bronchus, Right   NC
  Bronchus intermedius
  Intermediate bronchus
4 Upper Lobe Bronchus, Right   NC
5 Middle Lobe Bronchus, Right   NC
6 Lower Lobe Bronchus, Right   NC
7 Main Bronchus, Left   NC
8 Upper Lobe Bronchus, Left   NC
9 Lingula Bronchus   NC
B Lower Lobe Bronchus, Left   NC
	0 Open
	3 Percutaneous
	4 Percutaneous Endoscopic
	7 Via Natural or Artificial Opening
	8 Via Natural or Artificial Opening Endoscopic
	X External
		Z No Device	Z No Qualifier

Non-OR 0BF[1,2,3,4,5,6,7,8,9,B]XZZ
Non-OR 0BF[3,4,5,6,7,8,9,B][7,8]ZZ
NC 0BF[1,2,3,4,5,6,7,8,9,B]XZZ

Respiratory System

ØBH–ØBH Respiratory System ICD-10-PCS 2025

Ø Medical and Surgical
B Respiratory System
H Insertion Definition: Putting in a nonbiological appliance that monitors, assists, performs, or prevents a physiological function but does not physically take the place of a body part
Explanation: None

Body Part Character 4	Approach Character 5	Device Character 6	Qualifier Character 7
Ø Tracheobronchial Tree	Ø Open 3 Percutaneous 4 Percutaneous Endoscopic 7 Via Natural or Artificial Opening 8 Via Natural or Artificial Opening Endoscopic	1 Radioactive Element 2 Monitoring Device 3 Infusion Device D Intraluminal Device Y Other Device	Z No Qualifier
1 Trachea Cricoid cartilage	Ø Open	2 Monitoring Device D Intraluminal Device Y Other Device	Z No Qualifier
1 Trachea Cricoid cartilage	3 Percutaneous	D Intraluminal Device E Intraluminal Device, Endotracheal Airway Y Other Device	Z No Qualifier
1 Trachea Cricoid cartilage	4 Percutaneous Endoscopic	D Intraluminal Device Y Other Device	Z No Qualifier
1 Trachea Cricoid cartilage	7 Via Natural or Artificial Opening 8 Via Natural or Artificial Opening Endoscopic	2 Monitoring Device D Intraluminal Device E Intraluminal Device, Endotracheal Airway Y Other Device	Z No Qualifier

3 Main Bronchus, Right
   Bronchus intermedius
   Intermediate bronchus
4 Upper Lobe Bronchus, Right
5 Middle Lobe Bronchus, Right
6 Lower Lobe Bronchus, Right
7 Main Bronchus, Left
8 Upper Lobe Bronchus, Left
9 Lingula Bronchus
B Lower Lobe Bronchus, Left
	Ø Open
	3 Percutaneous
	4 Percutaneous Endoscopic
	7 Via Natural or Artificial Opening
	8 Via Natural or Artificial Opening Endoscopic
		G Intraluminal Device, Endobronchial Valve	Z No Qualifier

K Lung, Right L Lung, Left	Ø Open 3 Percutaneous 4 Percutaneous Endoscopic 7 Via Natural or Artificial Opening 8 Via Natural or Artificial Opening Endoscopic	1 Radioactive Element 2 Monitoring Device 3 Infusion Device Y Other Device	Z No Qualifier
Q Pleura	Ø Open 3 Percutaneous 4 Percutaneous Endoscopic 7 Via Natural or Artificial Opening 8 Via Natural or Artificial Opening Endoscopic	Y Other Device	Z No Qualifier
T Diaphragm	Ø Open 3 Percutaneous 4 Percutaneous Endoscopic	2 Monitoring Device M Diaphragmatic Pacemaker Lead Y Other Device	Z No Qualifier
T Diaphragm	7 Via Natural or Artificial Opening 8 Via Natural or Artificial Opening Endoscopic	Y Other Device	Z No Qualifier

DRG Non-OR ØBH[3,4,5,6,7,8,9,B]8GZ
Non-OR ØBHØ3YZ
Non-OR ØBHØ[7,8][2,3,D,Y]Z
Non-OR ØBH13[E,Y]Z
Non-OR ØBH1[7,8][2,D,E,Y]Z
Non-OR ØBH[K,L]3YZ
Non-OR ØBH[K,L]7[2,3,Y]Z
Non-OR ØBH[K,L]8[2,3]Z
Non-OR ØBHQ[3,7]YZ
Non-OR ØBHT3YZ
Non-OR ØBHT[7,8]YZ

ICD-10-PCS 2025 — Respiratory System — 0BJ–0BL

0 Medical and Surgical
B Respiratory System
J Inspection   Definition: Visually and/or manually exploring a body part
Explanation: Visual exploration may be performed with or without optical instrumentation. Manual exploration may be performed directly or through intervening body layers.

Body Part Character 4	Approach Character 5	Device Character 6	Qualifier Character 7
0 Tracheobronchial Tree 1 Trachea Cricoid cartilage K Lung, Right L Lung, Left Q Pleura T Diaphragm	0 Open 3 Percutaneous 4 Percutaneous Endoscopic 7 Via Natural or Artificial Opening 8 Via Natural or Artificial Opening Endoscopic X External	Z No Device	Z No Qualifier

Non-OR   0BJ[0,K,L,Q,T][3,7,8,X]ZZ
Non-OR   0BJ1[3,4,7,8,X]ZZ

0 Medical and Surgical
B Respiratory System
L Occlusion   Definition: Completely closing an orifice or the lumen of a tubular body part
Explanation: The orifice can be a natural orifice or an artificially created orifice

Body Part Character 4	Approach Character 5	Device Character 6	Qualifier Character 7

1 Trachea
   Cricoid cartilage
2 Carina
3 Main Bronchus, Right
   Bronchus intermedius
   Intermediate bronchus
4 Upper Lobe Bronchus, Right
5 Middle Lobe Bronchus, Right
6 Lower Lobe Bronchus, Right
7 Main Bronchus, Left
8 Upper Lobe Bronchus, Left
9 Lingula Bronchus
B Lower Lobe Bronchus, Left
	0 Open
	3 Percutaneous
	4 Percutaneous Endoscopic
		C Extraluminal Device
		D Intraluminal Device
		Z No Device
			Z No Qualifier

1 Trachea
   Cricoid cartilage
2 Carina
3 Main Bronchus, Right
   Bronchus intermedius
   Intermediate bronchus
4 Upper Lobe Bronchus, Right
5 Middle Lobe Bronchus, Right
6 Lower Lobe Bronchus, Right
7 Main Bronchus, Left
8 Upper Lobe Bronchus, Left
9 Lingula Bronchus
B Lower Lobe Bronchus, Left
	7 Via Natural or Artificial Opening
	8 Via Natural or Artificial Opening Endoscopic
		D Intraluminal Device
		Z No Device
			Z No Qualifier

Respiratory System

0BM–0BN

0 Medical and Surgical
B Respiratory System
M Reattachment   Definition: Putting back in or on all or a portion of a separated body part to its normal location or other suitable location
Explanation: Vascular circulation and nervous pathways may or may not be reestablished

Body Part – Character 4	Approach – Character 5	Device – Character 6	Qualifier – Character 7

1 Trachea
  Cricoid cartilage
2 Carina
3 Main Bronchus, Right
  Bronchus intermedius
  Intermediate bronchus
4 Upper Lobe Bronchus, Right
5 Middle Lobe Bronchus, Right
6 Lower Lobe Bronchus, Right
7 Main Bronchus, Left
8 Upper Lobe Bronchus, Left
9 Lingula Bronchus
B Lower Lobe Bronchus, Left
C Upper Lung Lobe, Right
D Middle Lung Lobe, Right
F Lower Lung Lobe, Right
G Upper Lung Lobe, Left
H Lung Lingula
J Lower Lung Lobe, Left
K Lung, Right
L Lung, Left
T Diaphragm
	0 Open	Z No Device	Z No Qualifier

0 Medical and Surgical
B Respiratory System
N Release   Definition: Freeing a body part from an abnormal physical constraint by cutting or by the use of force
Explanation: Some of the restraining tissue may be taken out but none of the body part is taken out

Body Part – Character 4	Approach – Character 5	Device – Character 6	Qualifier – Character 7

1 Trachea
  Cricoid cartilage
2 Carina
3 Main Bronchus, Right
  Bronchus intermedius
  Intermediate bronchus
4 Upper Lobe Bronchus, Right
5 Middle Lobe Bronchus, Right
6 Lower Lobe Bronchus, Right
7 Main Bronchus, Left
8 Upper Lobe Bronchus, Left
9 Lingula Bronchus
B Lower Lobe Bronchus, Left
C Upper Lung Lobe, Right
D Middle Lung Lobe, Right
F Lower Lung Lobe, Right
G Upper Lung Lobe, Left
H Lung Lingula
J Lower Lung Lobe, Left
K Lung, Right
L Lung, Left
M Lungs, Bilateral
	0 Open
	3 Percutaneous
	4 Percutaneous Endoscopic
	7 Via Natural or Artificial Opening
	8 Via Natural or Artificial Opening Endoscopic
		Z No Device	Z No Qualifier

N Pleura, Right P Pleura, Left T Diaphragm	0 Open 3 Percutaneous 4 Percutaneous Endoscopic	Z No Device	Z No Qualifier

Non-OR Procedure   DRG Non-OR Procedure   Valid OR Procedure   HAC Associated Procedure   Combination Only   New/Revised April   New/Revised October

ICD-10-PCS 2025 Respiratory System 0BP–0BP

0 Medical and Surgical
B Respiratory System
P Removal   Definition: Taking out or off a device from a body part
Explanation: If a device is taken out and a similar device put in without cutting or puncturing the skin or mucous membrane, the procedure is coded to the root operation CHANGE. Otherwise, the procedure for taking out a device is coded to the root operation REMOVAL.

Body Part Character 4	Approach Character 5	Device Character 6	Qualifier Character 7
0 Tracheobronchial Tree	0 Open 3 Percutaneous 4 Percutaneous Endoscopic 7 Via Natural or Artificial Opening 8 Via Natural or Artificial Opening Endoscopic	0 Drainage Device 1 Radioactive Element 2 Monitoring Device 3 Infusion Device 7 Autologous Tissue Substitute C Extraluminal Device D Intraluminal Device J Synthetic Substitute K Nonautologous Tissue Substitute Y Other Device	Z No Qualifier
0 Tracheobronchial Tree	X External	0 Drainage Device 1 Radioactive Element 2 Monitoring Device 3 Infusion Device D Intraluminal Device	Z No Qualifier
1 Trachea Cricoid cartilage	0 Open 3 Percutaneous 4 Percutaneous Endoscopic 7 Via Natural or Artificial Opening 8 Via Natural or Artificial Opening Endoscopic	0 Drainage Device 2 Monitoring Device 7 Autologous Tissue Substitute C Extraluminal Device D Intraluminal Device F Tracheostomy Device J Synthetic Substitute K Nonautologous Tissue Substitute	Z No Qualifier
1 Trachea Cricoid cartilage	X External	0 Drainage Device 2 Monitoring Device D Intraluminal Device F Tracheostomy Device	Z No Qualifier
K Lung, Right L Lung, Left	0 Open 3 Percutaneous 4 Percutaneous Endoscopic 7 Via Natural or Artificial Opening 8 Via Natural or Artificial Opening Endoscopic	0 Drainage Device 1 Radioactive Element 2 Monitoring Device 3 Infusion Device Y Other Device	Z No Qualifier
K Lung, Right L Lung, Left	X External	0 Drainage Device 1 Radioactive Element 2 Monitoring Device 3 Infusion Device	Z No Qualifier
Q Pleura	0 Open 3 Percutaneous 4 Percutaneous Endoscopic 7 Via Natural or Artificial Opening 8 Via Natural or Artificial Opening Endoscopic	0 Drainage Device 1 Radioactive Element 2 Monitoring Device Y Other Device	Z No Qualifier
Q Pleura	X External	0 Drainage Device 1 Radioactive Element 2 Monitoring Device	Z No Qualifier
T Diaphragm	0 Open 3 Percutaneous 4 Percutaneous Endoscopic 7 Via Natural or Artificial Opening 8 Via Natural or Artificial Opening Endoscopic	0 Drainage Device 2 Monitoring Device 7 Autologous Tissue Substitute J Synthetic Substitute K Nonautologous Tissue Substitute M Diaphragmatic Pacemaker Lead Y Other Device	Z No Qualifier
T Diaphragm	X External	0 Drainage Device 2 Monitoring Device M Diaphragmatic Pacemaker Lead	Z No Qualifier

Non-OR 0BP0[3,4]YZ
Non-OR 0BP0[7,8][0,2,3,D,Y]Z
Non-OR 0BP0X[0,1,2,3,D]Z
Non-OR 0BP1[0,3,4]FZ
Non-OR 0BP1[7,8][0,2,D,F]Z
Non-OR 0BP1X[0,2,D,F]Z
Non-OR 0BP[K,L]3YZ
Non-OR 0BPK7[0,1,2,3,Y]Z
Non-OR 0BPK8[0,1,2,3]Z
Non-OR 0BPL7[0,2,3,Y]Z
Non-OR 0BPL8[0,2,3]Z
Non-OR 0BP[K,L]X[0,1,2,3]Z
Non-OR 0BPQ[0,3,4,7,8][0,1,2,]Z
Non-OR 0BPQ[3,7]YZ
Non-OR 0BPQX[0,1,2]Z
Non-OR 0BPT3YZ
Non-OR 0BPT[7,8][0,2,Y]Z
Non-OR 0BPTX[0,2,M]Z

NC Noncovered Procedure   LC Limited Coverage   QA Questionable OB Admit   NT New Tech Add-on   ✚ Combination Member   ♂ Male   ♀ Female

Respiratory System

0BQ–0BR

ICD-10-PCS 2025

0 Medical and Surgical
B Respiratory System
Q Repair Definition: Restoring, to the extent possible, a body part to its normal anatomic structure and function
  Explanation: Used only when the method to accomplish the repair is not one of the other root operations

Body Part Character 4	Approach Character 5	Device Character 6	Qualifier Character 7

1 Trachea
  Cricoid cartilage
2 Carina
3 Main Bronchus, Right
  Bronchus intermedius
  Intermediate bronchus
4 Upper Lobe Bronchus, Right
5 Middle Lobe Bronchus, Right
6 Lower Lobe Bronchus, Right
7 Main Bronchus, Left
8 Upper Lobe Bronchus, Left
9 Lingula Bronchus
B Lower Lobe Bronchus, Left
C Upper Lung Lobe, Right
D Middle Lung Lobe, Right
F Lower Lung Lobe, Right
G Upper Lung Lobe, Left
H Lung Lingula
J Lower Lung Lobe, Left
K Lung, Right
L Lung, Left
M Lungs, Bilateral
	0 Open
	3 Percutaneous
	4 Percutaneous Endoscopic
	7 Via Natural or Artificial Opening
	8 Via Natural or Artificial Opening Endoscopic
		Z No Device	Z No Qualifier

N Pleura, Right P Pleura, Left T Diaphragm	0 Open 3 Percutaneous 4 Percutaneous Endoscopic	Z No Device	Z No Qualifier

0 Medical and Surgical
B Respiratory System
R Replacement Definition: Putting in or on biological or synthetic material that physically takes the place and/or function of all or a portion of a body part
  Explanation: The body part may have been taken out or replaced, or may be taken out, physically eradicated, or rendered nonfunctional during the REPLACEMENT procedure. A REMOVAL procedure is coded for taking out the device used in a previous replacement procedure.

Body Part Character 4	Approach Character 5	Device Character 6	Qualifier Character 7

1 Trachea
  Cricoid cartilage
2 Carina
3 Main Bronchus, Right
  Bronchus intermedius
  Intermediate bronchus
4 Upper Lobe Bronchus, Right
5 Middle Lobe Bronchus, Right
6 Lower Lobe Bronchus, Right
7 Main Bronchus, Left
8 Upper Lobe Bronchus, Left
9 Lingula Bronchus
B Lower Lobe Bronchus, Left
T Diaphragm
	0 Open
	4 Percutaneous Endoscopic
		7 Autologous Tissue Substitute
		J Synthetic Substitute
		K Nonautologous Tissue Substitute
			Z No Qualifier

Non-OR Procedure   DRG Non-OR Procedure   Valid OR Procedure   HAC Associated Procedure   Combination Only   New/Revised April   New/Revised October

Respiratory System

0 Medical and Surgical
B Respiratory System
S Reposition

Definition: Moving to its normal location, or other suitable location, all or a portion of a body part

Explanation: The body part is moved to a new location from an abnormal location, or from a normal location where it is not functioning correctly. The body part may or may not be cut out or off to be moved to the new location.

Body Part Character 4	Approach Character 5	Device Character 6	Qualifier Character 7

1 Trachea
    Cricoid cartilage
2 Carina
3 Main Bronchus, Right
    Bronchus intermedius
    Intermediate bronchus
4 Upper Lobe Bronchus, Right
5 Middle Lobe Bronchus, Right
6 Lower Lobe Bronchus, Right
7 Main Bronchus, Left
8 Upper Lobe Bronchus, Left
9 Lingula Bronchus
B Lower Lobe Bronchus, Left
C Upper Lung Lobe, Right
D Middle Lung Lobe, Right
F Lower Lung Lobe, Right
G Upper Lung Lobe, Left
H Lung Lingula
J Lower Lung Lobe, Left
K Lung, Right
L Lung, Left
T Diaphragm
	0 Open	**Z** No Device	**Z** No Qualifier

0 Medical and Surgical
B Respiratory System
T Resection

Definition: Cutting out or off, without replacement, all of a body part

Explanation: None

Body Part Character 4	Approach Character 5	Device Character 6	Qualifier Character 7

1 Trachea
    Cricoid cartilage
2 Carina
3 Main Bronchus, Right
    Bronchus intermedius
    Intermediate bronchus
4 Upper Lobe Bronchus, Right
5 Middle Lobe Bronchus, Right
6 Lower Lobe Bronchus, Right
7 Main Bronchus, Left
8 Upper Lobe Bronchus, Left
9 Lingula Bronchus
B Lower Lobe Bronchus, Left
C Upper Lung Lobe, Right
D Middle Lung Lobe, Right
F Lower Lung Lobe, Right
G Upper Lung Lobe, Left
H Lung Lingula
J Lower Lung Lobe, Left
K Lung, Right
L Lung, Left
M Lungs, Bilateral
T Diaphragm
	0 Open
	4 Percutaneous Endoscopic
		Z No Device	**Z** No Qualifier

0 Medical and Surgical
B Respiratory System
U Supplement

Definition: Putting in or on biological or synthetic material that physically reinforces and/or augments the function of a portion of a body part
Explanation: The biological material is non-living, or is living and from the same individual. The body part may have been previously replaced, and the SUPPLEMENT procedure is performed to physically reinforce and/or augment the function of the replaced body part.

Body Part Character 4	Approach Character 5	Device Character 6	Qualifier Character 7

1 Trachea
   Cricoid cartilage
2 Carina
3 Main Bronchus, Right
   Bronchus intermedius
   Intermediate bronchus
4 Upper Lobe Bronchus, Right
5 Middle Lobe Bronchus, Right
6 Lower Lobe Bronchus, Right
7 Main Bronchus, Left
8 Upper Lobe Bronchus, Left
9 Lingula Bronchus
B Lower Lobe Bronchus, Left
	0 Open
	4 Percutaneous Endoscopic
	8 Via Natural or Artificial Opening Endoscopic
		7 Autologous Tissue Substitute
		J Synthetic Substitute
		K Nonautologous Tissue Substitute
			Z No Qualifier

T Diaphragm	0 Open 4 Percutaneous Endoscopic	7 Autologous Tissue Substitute J Synthetic Substitute K Nonautologous Tissue Substitute	Z No Qualifier

0 Medical and Surgical
B Respiratory System
V Restriction

Definition: Partially closing an orifice or the lumen of a tubular body part
Explanation: The orifice can be a natural orifice or an artificially created orifice

Body Part Character 4	Approach Character 5	Device Character 6	Qualifier Character 7

1 Trachea
   Cricoid cartilage
2 Carina
3 Main Bronchus, Right
   Bronchus intermedius
   Intermediate bronchus
4 Upper Lobe Bronchus, Right
5 Middle Lobe Bronchus, Right
6 Lower Lobe Bronchus, Right
7 Main Bronchus, Left
8 Upper Lobe Bronchus, Left
9 Lingula Bronchus
B Lower Lobe Bronchus, Left
	0 Open
	3 Percutaneous
	4 Percutaneous Endoscopic
		C Extraluminal Device
		D Intraluminal Device
		Z No Device
			Z No Qualifier

1 Trachea
   Cricoid cartilage
2 Carina
3 Main Bronchus, Right
   Bronchus intermedius
   Intermediate bronchus
4 Upper Lobe Bronchus, Right
5 Middle Lobe Bronchus, Right
6 Lower Lobe Bronchus, Right
7 Main Bronchus, Left
8 Upper Lobe Bronchus, Left
9 Lingula Bronchus
B Lower Lobe Bronchus, Left
	7 Via Natural or Artificial Opening
	8 Via Natural or Artificial Opening Endoscopic
		D Intraluminal Device
		Z No Device
			Z No Qualifier

ICD-10-PCS 2025 — Respiratory System — 0BW–0BW

- **0** Medical and Surgical
- **B** Respiratory System
- **W** Revision — Definition: Correcting, to the extent possible, a portion of a malfunctioning device or the position of a displaced device
  Explanation: Revision can include correcting a malfunctioning or displaced device by taking out or putting in components of the device such as a screw or pin

Body Part Character 4	Approach Character 5	Device Character 6	Qualifier Character 7
0 Tracheobronchial Tree	**0** Open **3** Percutaneous **4** Percutaneous Endoscopic **7** Via Natural or Artificial Opening **8** Via Natural or Artificial Opening Endoscopic	**0** Drainage Device **2** Monitoring Device **3** Infusion Device **7** Autologous Tissue Substitute **C** Extraluminal Device **D** Intraluminal Device **J** Synthetic Substitute **K** Nonautologous Tissue Substitute **Y** Other Device	**Z** No Qualifier
0 Tracheobronchial Tree	**X** External	**0** Drainage Device **2** Monitoring Device **3** Infusion Device **7** Autologous Tissue Substitute **C** Extraluminal Device **D** Intraluminal Device **J** Synthetic Substitute **K** Nonautologous Tissue Substitute	**Z** No Qualifier
1 Trachea Cricoid cartilage	**0** Open **3** Percutaneous **4** Percutaneous Endoscopic **7** Via Natural or Artificial Opening **8** Via Natural or Artificial Opening Endoscopic **X** External	**0** Drainage Device **2** Monitoring Device **7** Autologous Tissue Substitute **C** Extraluminal Device **D** Intraluminal Device **F** Tracheostomy Device **J** Synthetic Substitute **K** Nonautologous Tissue Substitute	**Z** No Qualifier
K Lung, Right **L** Lung, Left	**0** Open **3** Percutaneous **4** Percutaneous Endoscopic **7** Via Natural or Artificial Opening **8** Via Natural or Artificial Opening Endoscopic	**0** Drainage Device **2** Monitoring Device **3** Infusion Device **Y** Other Device	**Z** No Qualifier
K Lung, Right **L** Lung, Left	**X** External	**0** Drainage Device **2** Monitoring Device **3** Infusion Device	**Z** No Qualifier
Q Pleura	**0** Open **3** Percutaneous **4** Percutaneous Endoscopic **7** Via Natural or Artificial Opening **8** Via Natural or Artificial Opening Endoscopic	**0** Drainage Device **2** Monitoring Device **Y** Other Device	**Z** No Qualifier
Q Pleura	**X** External	**0** Drainage Device **2** Monitoring Device	**Z** No Qualifier
T Diaphragm	**0** Open **3** Percutaneous **4** Percutaneous Endoscopic **7** Via Natural or Artificial Opening **8** Via Natural or Artificial Opening Endoscopic	**0** Drainage Device **2** Monitoring Device **7** Autologous Tissue Substitute **J** Synthetic Substitute **K** Nonautologous Tissue Substitute **M** Diaphragmatic Pacemaker Lead **Y** Other Device	**Z** No Qualifier
T Diaphragm	**X** External	**0** Drainage Device **2** Monitoring Device **7** Autologous Tissue Substitute **J** Synthetic Substitute **K** Nonautologous Tissue Substitute **M** Diaphragmatic Pacemaker Lead	**Z** No Qualifier

Non-OR 0BW0[3,4]YZ
Non-OR 0BW0[7,8][2,3,D,Y]Z
Non-OR 0BW0X[0,2,3,7,C,D,J,K]Z
Non-OR 0BW1X[0,2,7,C,D,F,J,K]Z
Non-OR 0BW[K,L]3YZ
Non-OR 0BW[K,L]7[0,2,3,Y]Z
Non-OR 0BW[K,L]8[0,2,3]Z
Non-OR 0BW[K,L]X[0,2,3]Z
Non-OR 0BWQ[0,3,4,7,8][0,2]Z
Non-OR 0BWQ[0,3,7]YZ
Non-OR 0BWQX[0,2]Z
Non-OR 0BWT[3,7,8]YZ
Non-OR 0BWTX[0,2,7,J,K,M]Z

0 Medical and Surgical
B Respiratory System
Y Transplantation — Definition: Putting in or on all or a portion of a living body part taken from another individual or animal to physically take the place and/or function of all or a portion of a similar body part
Explanation: The native body part may or may not be taken out, and the transplanted body part may take over all or a portion of its function

Body Part Character 4	Approach Character 5	Device Character 6	Qualifier Character 7
C Upper Lung Lobe, Right LC D Middle Lung Lobe, Right LC F Lower Lung Lobe, Right LC G Upper Lung Lobe, Left LC H Lung Lingula LC J Lower Lung Lobe, Left LC K Lung, Right LC L Lung, Left LC M Lungs, Bilateral LC	0 Open	Z No Device	0 Allogeneic 1 Syngeneic 2 Zooplastic

LC 0BY[C,D,F,G,H,J,K,L,M]0Z[0,1,2]

Mouth and Throat ØCØ–ØCX

Character Meanings

This Character Meaning table is provided as a guide to assist the user in the identification of character members that may be found in this section of code tables. It **SHOULD NOT** be used to build a PCS code.

Operation–Character 3		Body Part–Character 4		Approach–Character 5		Device–Character 6		Qualifier–Character 7	
Ø	Alteration	Ø	Upper Lip	Ø	Open	Ø	Drainage Device	Ø	Single
2	Change	1	Lower Lip	3	Percutaneous	1	Radioactive Element	1	Multiple
5	Destruction	2	Hard Palate	4	Percutaneous Endoscopic	5	External Fixation Device	2	All
7	Dilation	3	Soft Palate	7	Via Natural or Artificial Opening	7	Autologous Tissue Substitute	X	Diagnostic
9	Drainage	4	Buccal Mucosa	8	Via Natural or Artificial Opening Endoscopic	B	Intraluminal Device, Airway	Z	No Qualifier
B	Excision	5	Upper Gingiva	X	External	C	Extraluminal Device		
C	Extirpation	6	Lower Gingiva			D	Intraluminal Device		
D	Extraction	7	Tongue			J	Synthetic Substitute		
F	Fragmentation	8	Parotid Gland, Right			K	Nonautologous Tissue Substitute		
H	Insertion	9	Parotid Gland, Left			Y	Other Device		
J	Inspection	A	Salivary Gland			Z	No Device		
L	Occlusion	B	Parotid Duct, Right						
M	Reattachment	C	Parotid Duct, Left						
N	Release	D	Sublingual Gland, Right						
P	Removal	F	Sublingual Gland, Left						
Q	Repair	G	Submaxillary Gland, Right						
R	Replacement	H	Submaxillary Gland, Left						
S	Reposition	J	Minor Salivary Gland						
T	Resection	M	Pharynx						
U	Supplement	N	Uvula						
V	Restriction	P	Tonsils						
W	Revision	Q	Adenoids						
X	Transfer	R	Epiglottis						
		S	Larynx						
		T	Vocal Cord, Right						
		V	Vocal Cord, Left						
		W	Upper Tooth						
		X	Lower Tooth						
		Y	Mouth and Throat						

AHA Coding Clinic for table ØC9
2017, 2Q, 16   Incision and drainage of floor of mouth

AHA Coding Clinic for table ØCB
2017, 2Q, 16   Excision of floor of mouth
2016, 3Q, 28   Lingual tonsillectomy, tongue base excision and epiglottopexy
2016, 2Q, 19   Biopsy of the base of tongue
2014, 3Q, 21   Superficial parotidectomy

AHA Coding Clinic for table ØCC
2016, 2Q, 20   Sialendoscopy with stone removal

AHA Coding Clinic for table ØCH
2020, 4Q, 43-44   Insertion of radioactive element

AHA Coding Clinic for table ØCQ
2017, 1Q, 20   Preparatory nasal adhesion repair before definitive cleft palate repair

AHA Coding Clinic for table ØCR
2014, 3Q, 25   Excision of soft palate with placement of surgical obturator
2014, 2Q, 5   Oasis acellular matrix graft
2014, 2Q, 6   Composite grafting (synthetic versus nonautologous tissue substitute)

AHA Coding Clinic for table ØCS
2023, 4Q, 52-53   Reposition of larynx
2022, 2Q, 24   Palatoplasty with intravelar veloplasty
2016, 3Q, 28   Lingual tonsillectomy, tongue base excision and epiglottopexy

AHA Coding Clinic for table ØCT
2016, 2Q, 12   Resection of malignant neoplasm of infratemporal fossa
2014, 3Q, 21   Superficial parotidectomy
2014, 3Q, 23   Le Fort I osteotomy

Mouth and Throat

Salivary Glands

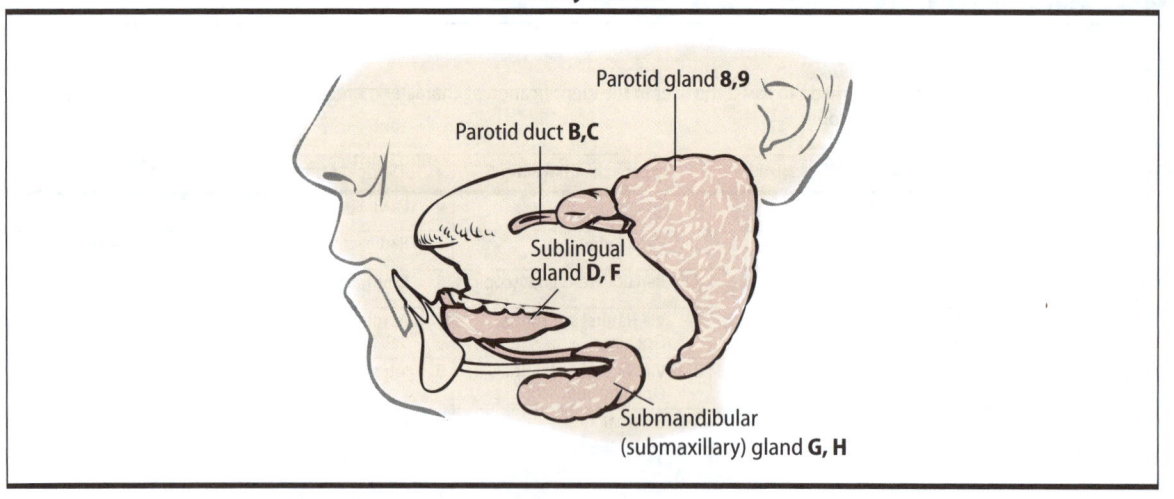

- Parotid gland **8,9**
- Parotid duct **B,C**
- Sublingual gland **D, F**
- Submandibular (submaxillary) gland **G, H**

Oral Anatomy

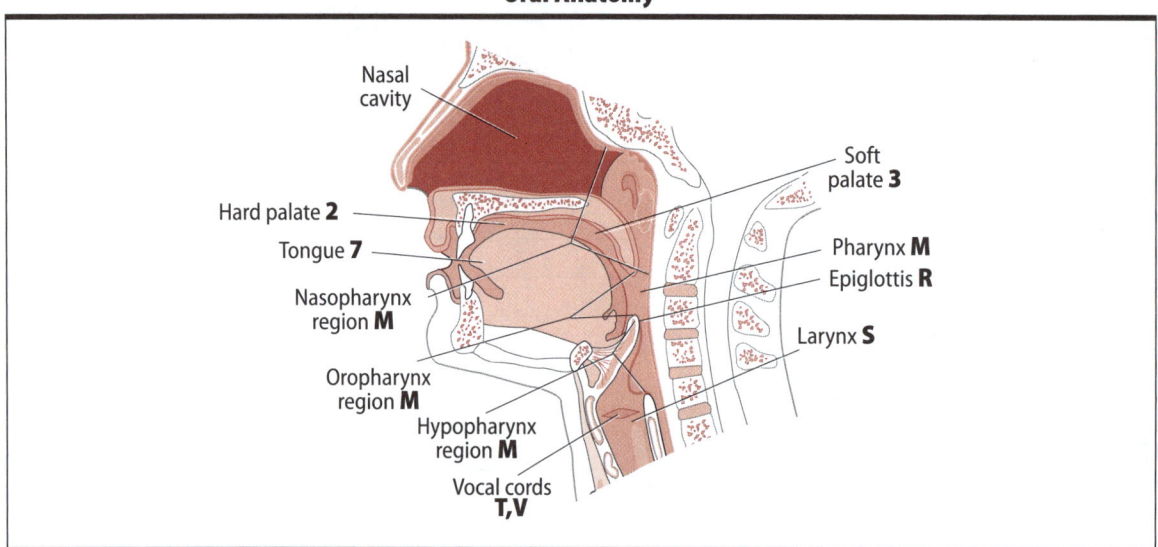

- Nasal cavity
- Hard palate **2**
- Tongue **7**
- Nasopharynx region **M**
- Oropharynx region **M**
- Hypopharynx region **M**
- Vocal cords **T,V**
- Soft palate **3**
- Pharynx **M**
- Epiglottis **R**
- Larynx **S**

Mouth Frontal View (Upper)

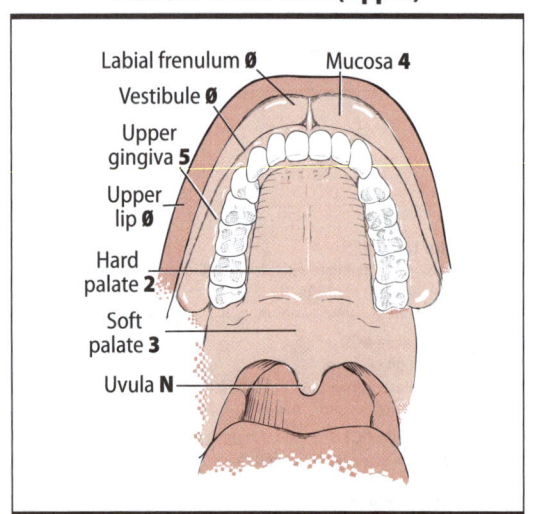

- Labial frenulum **0**
- Mucosa **4**
- Vestibule **0**
- Upper gingiva **5**
- Upper lip **0**
- Hard palate **2**
- Soft palate **3**
- Uvula **N**

Mouth Frontal View (Lower)

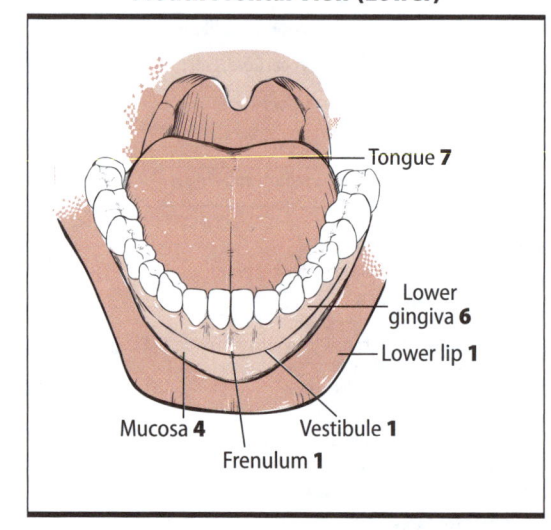

- Tongue **7**
- Lower gingiva **6**
- Lower lip **1**
- Mucosa **4**
- Vestibule **1**
- Frenulum **1**

0 Medical and Surgical
C Mouth and Throat
0 Alteration Definition: Modifying the anatomic structure of a body part without affecting the function of the body part
Explanation: Principal purpose is to improve appearance

Body Part Character 4	Approach Character 5	Device Character 6	Qualifier Character 7

0 Upper Lip
  Frenulum labii superioris
  Labial gland
  Vermilion border
1 Lower Lip
  Frenulum labii inferioris
  Labial gland
  Vermilion border
	X External	**7** Autologous Tissue Substitute
		J Synthetic Substitute
		K Nonautologous Tissue Substitute
		Z No Device
			Z No Qualifier

0 Medical and Surgical
C Mouth and Throat
2 Change Definition: Taking out or off a device from a body part and putting back an identical or similar device in or on the same body part without cutting or puncturing the skin or a mucous membrane
Explanation: All CHANGE procedures are coded using the approach EXTERNAL

Body Part Character 4	Approach Character 5	Device Character 6	Qualifier Character 7

A Salivary Gland
S Larynx
  Aryepiglottic fold
  Arytenoid cartilage
  Corniculate cartilage
  Cuneiform cartilage
  False vocal cord
  Glottis
  Rima glottidis
  Thyroid cartilage
  Ventricular fold
Y Mouth and Throat
	X External	**0** Drainage Device
		Y Other Device
			Z No Qualifier

Non-OR All body part, approach, device, and qualifier values

0C5–0C7   Mouth and Throat   ICD-10-PCS 2025

0 Medical and Surgical
C Mouth and Throat
5 Destruction   Definition: Physical eradication of all or a portion of a body part by the direct use of energy, force, or a destructive agent
Explanation: None of the body part is physically taken out

Body Part Character 4	Approach Character 5	Device Character 6	Qualifier Character 7

0 Upper Lip
  Frenulum labii superioris
  Labial gland
  Vermilion border
1 Lower Lip
  Frenulum labii inferioris
  Labial gland
  Vermilion border
2 Hard Palate
3 Soft Palate
4 Buccal Mucosa
  Buccal gland
  Molar gland
  Palatine gland
5 Upper Gingiva
6 Lower Gingiva
7 Tongue
  Frenulum linguae
N Uvula
  Palatine uvula
P Tonsils
  Palatine tonsil
Q Adenoids
  Pharyngeal tonsil
	0 Open
	3 Percutaneous
	X External
		Z No Device	Z No Qualifier

8 Parotid Gland, Right
9 Parotid Gland, Left
B Parotid Duct, Right
  Stensen's duct
C Parotid Duct, Left
  See B Parotid Duct, Right
D Sublingual Gland, Right
F Sublingual Gland, Left
G Submaxillary Gland, Right
  Submandibular gland
H Submaxillary Gland, Left
  See G Submaxillary Gland, Right
J Minor Salivary Gland
  Anterior lingual gland
	0 Open
	3 Percutaneous
		Z No Device	Z No Qualifier

M Pharynx
  Base of tongue
  Hypopharynx
  Laryngopharynx
  Lingual tonsil
  Oropharynx
  Piriform recess (sinus)
  Tongue, base of
R Epiglottis
  Glossoepiglottic fold
S Larynx
  Aryepiglottic fold
  Arytenoid cartilage
  Corniculate cartilage
  Cuneiform cartilage
  False vocal cord
  Glottis
  Rima glottidis
  Thyroid cartilage
  Ventricular fold
T Vocal Cord, Right
  Vocal fold
V Vocal Cord, Left
  See T Vocal Cord, Right
	0 Open
	3 Percutaneous
	4 Percutaneous Endoscopic
	7 Via Natural or Artificial Opening
	8 Via Natural or Artificial Opening Endoscopic
		Z No Device	Z No Qualifier

W Upper Tooth X Lower Tooth	0 Open X External	Z No Device	0 Single 1 Multiple 2 All

Non-OR   0C5[5,6][0,3,X]ZZ
Non-OR   0C5[W,X][0,X]Z[0,1,2]

0 Medical and Surgical
C Mouth and Throat
7 Dilation   Definition: Expanding an orifice or the lumen of a tubular body part
Explanation: The orifice can be a natural orifice or an artificially created orifice. Accomplished by stretching a tubular body part using intraluminal pressure or by cutting part of the orifice or wall of the tubular body part.

Body Part Character 4	Approach Character 5	Device Character 6	Qualifier Character 7

B Parotid Duct, Right
  Stensen's duct
C Parotid Duct, Left
  See B Parotid Duct, Right
	0 Open
	3 Percutaneous
	7 Via Natural or Artificial Opening
		D Intraluminal Device
		Z No Device
			Z No Qualifier

M Pharynx
  Base of tongue
  Hypopharynx
  Laryngopharynx
  Lingual tonsil
  Oropharynx
  Piriform recess (sinus)
  Tongue, base of
	7 Via Natural or Artificial Opening
	8 Via Natural or Artificial Opening Endoscopic
		D Intraluminal Device
		Z No Device
			Z No Qualifier

S Larynx
  Aryepiglottic fold
  Arytenoid cartilage
  Corniculate cartilage
  Cuneiform cartilage
  False vocal cord
  Glottis
  Rima glottidis
  Thyroid cartilage
  Ventricular fold
	0 Open
	3 Percutaneous
	4 Percutaneous Endoscopic
	7 Via Natural or Artificial Opening
	8 Via Natural or Artificial Opening Endoscopic
		D Intraluminal Device
		Z No Device
			Z No Qualifier

Non-OR   0C7[B,C][0,3,7][D,Z]Z
Non-OR   0C7M[7,8][D,Z]Z

Non-OR Procedure   DRG Non-OR Procedure   Valid OR Procedure   HAC Associated Procedure   Combination Only   New/Revised April   New/Revised October

ICD-10-PCS 2025 — Mouth and Throat — 0C9–0C9

- **0** Medical and Surgical
- **C** Mouth and Throat
- **9** Drainage
  Definition: Taking or letting out fluids and/or gases from a body part
  Explanation: The qualifier DIAGNOSTIC is used to identify drainage procedures that are biopsies

Body Part Character 4		Approach Character 5	Device Character 6	Qualifier Character 7
0 Upper Lip 　Frenulum labii superioris 　Labial gland 　Vermilion border **1** Lower Lip 　Frenulum labii inferioris 　Labial gland 　Vermilion border **2** Hard Palate **3** Soft Palate **4** Buccal Mucosa 　Buccal gland 　Molar gland 　Palatine gland	**5** Upper Gingiva **6** Lower Gingiva **7** Tongue 　Frenulum linguae **N** Uvula 　Palatine uvula **P** Tonsils 　Palatine tonsil **Q** Adenoids 　Pharyngeal tonsil	**0** Open **3** Percutaneous **X** External	**0** Drainage Device	**Z** No Qualifier
0 Upper Lip 　Frenulum labii superioris 　Labial gland 　Vermilion border **1** Lower Lip 　Frenulum labii inferioris 　Labial gland 　Vermilion border **2** Hard Palate **3** Soft Palate **4** Buccal Mucosa 　Buccal gland 　Molar gland 　Palatine gland	**5** Upper Gingiva **6** Lower Gingiva **7** Tongue 　Frenulum linguae **N** Uvula 　Palatine uvula **P** Tonsils 　Palatine tonsil **Q** Adenoids 　Pharyngeal tonsil	**0** Open **3** Percutaneous **X** External	**Z** No Device	**X** Diagnostic **Z** No Qualifier
8 Parotid Gland, Right **9** Parotid Gland, Left **B** Parotid Duct, Right 　Stensen's duct **C** Parotid Duct, Left 　See B Parotid Duct, Right **D** Sublingual Gland, Right	**F** Sublingual Gland, Left **G** Submaxillary Gland, Right 　Submandibular gland **H** Submaxillary Gland, Left 　See G Submaxillary Gland, Right **J** Minor Salivary Gland 　Anterior lingual gland	**0** Open **3** Percutaneous	**0** Drainage Device	**Z** No Qualifier
8 Parotid Gland, Right **9** Parotid Gland, Left **B** Parotid Duct, Right 　Stensen's duct **C** Parotid Duct, Left 　See B Parotid Duct, Right	**D** Sublingual Gland, Right **F** Sublingual Gland, Left **G** Submaxillary Gland, Right 　Submandibular gland **H** Submaxillary Gland, Left 　See G Submaxillary Gland, Right **J** Minor Salivary Gland 　Anterior lingual gland	**0** Open **3** Percutaneous	**Z** No Device	**X** Diagnostic **Z** No Qualifier
M Pharynx 　Base of tongue 　Hypopharynx 　Laryngopharynx 　Lingual tonsil 　Oropharynx 　Piriform recess (sinus) 　Tongue, base of **R** Epiglottis 　Glossoepiglottic fold	**S** Larynx 　Aryepiglottic fold 　Arytenoid cartilage 　Corniculate cartilage 　Cuneiform cartilage 　False vocal cord 　Glottis 　Rima glottidis 　Thyroid cartilage 　Ventricular fold **T** Vocal Cord, Right 　Vocal fold **V** Vocal Cord, Left 　See T Vocal Cord, Right	**0** Open **3** Percutaneous **4** Percutaneous Endoscopic **7** Via Natural or Artificial Opening **8** Via Natural or Artificial Opening Endoscopic	**0** Drainage Device	**Z** No Qualifier

Non-OR　0C9[0,1,2,3,4,7,N,P,Q]30Z
Non-OR　0C9[5,6][0,3,X]0Z
Non-OR　0C9[0,1,4][0,3,X]ZX
Non-OR　0C9[0,1,2,3,4,7,N,P,Q]3ZZ
Non-OR　0C9[5,6][0,3,X]Z[X,Z]
Non-OR　0C97[3,X]ZX
Non-OR　0C9[8,9,B,C,D,F,G,H,J][0,3]0Z
Non-OR　0C9[8,9,B,C,D,F,G,H,J]3ZX
Non-OR　0C9[8,9,G,H]3ZZ
Non-OR　0C9[B,C,D,F,J][0,3]ZZ
Non-OR　0C9[M,R,S,T,V]30Z

0C9 Continued on next page

Mouth and Throat

ICD-10-PCS 2025

0 Medical and Surgical
C Mouth and Throat
9 Drainage

0C9 Continued

Definition: Taking or letting out fluids and/or gases from a body part
Explanation: The qualifier DIAGNOSTIC is used to identify drainage procedures that are biopsies

Body Part Character 4	Approach Character 5	Device Character 6	Qualifier Character 7
M Pharynx Base of tongue Hypopharynx Laryngopharynx Lingual tonsil Oropharynx Piriform recess (sinus) Tongue, base of **R Epiglottis** Glossoepiglottic fold	**S Larynx** Aryepiglottic fold Arytenoid cartilage Corniculate cartilage Cuneiform cartilage False vocal cord Glottis Rima glottidis Thyroid cartilage Ventricular fold **T Vocal Cord, Right** Vocal fold **V Vocal Cord, Left** *See T Vocal Cord, Right*	0 Open 3 Percutaneous 4 Percutaneous Endoscopic 7 Via Natural or Artificial Opening 8 Via Natural or Artificial Opening Endoscopic	Z No Device	X Diagnostic Z No Qualifier
W Upper Tooth **X Lower Tooth**		0 Open X External	0 Drainage Device Z No Device	0 Single 1 Multiple 2 All

Non-OR 0C9M[0,3,4,7,8]ZX
Non-OR 0C9[M,R,S,T,V]3ZZ
Non-OR 0C9[R,S,T,V][3,4,7,8]ZX
Non-OR 0C9[W,X][0,X][0,Z][0,1,2]

---

0 Medical and Surgical
C Mouth and Throat
B Excision

Definition: Cutting out or off, without replacement, a portion of a body part
Explanation: The qualifier DIAGNOSTIC is used to identify excision procedures that are biopsies

Body Part Character 4	Approach Character 5	Device Character 6	Qualifier Character 7
0 Upper Lip Frenulum labii superioris Labial gland Vermilion border **1 Lower Lip** Frenulum labii inferioris Labial gland Vermilion border **2 Hard Palate** **3 Soft Palate** **4 Buccal Mucosa** Buccal gland Molar gland Palatine gland	**5 Upper Gingiva** **6 Lower Gingiva** **7 Tongue** Frenulum linguae **N Uvula** Palatine uvula **P Tonsils** Palatine tonsil **Q Adenoids** Pharyngeal tonsil	0 Open 3 Percutaneous X External	Z No Device	X Diagnostic Z No Qualifier
8 Parotid Gland, Right **9 Parotid Gland, Left** **B Parotid Duct, Right** Stensen's duct **C Parotid Duct, Left** *See B Parotid Duct, Right* **D Sublingual Gland, Right**	**F Sublingual Gland, Left** **G Submaxillary Gland, Right** Submandibular gland **H Submaxillary Gland, Left** *See G Submaxillary Gland, Right* **J Minor Salivary Gland** Anterior lingual gland	0 Open 3 Percutaneous	Z No Device	X Diagnostic Z No Qualifier
M Pharynx Base of tongue Hypopharynx Laryngopharynx Lingual tonsil Oropharynx Piriform recess (sinus) Tongue, base of **R Epiglottis** Glossoepiglottic fold	**S Larynx** Aryepiglottic fold Arytenoid cartilage Corniculate cartilage Cuneiform cartilage False vocal cord Glottis Rima glottidis Thyroid cartilage Ventricular fold **T Vocal Cord, Right** Vocal fold **V Vocal Cord, Left** *See T Vocal Cord, Right*	0 Open 3 Percutaneous 4 Percutaneous Endoscopic 7 Via Natural or Artificial Opening 8 Via Natural or Artificial Opening Endoscopic	Z No Device	X Diagnostic Z No Qualifier
W Upper Tooth **X Lower Tooth**		0 Open X External	Z No Device	0 Single 1 Multiple 2 All

Non-OR 0CB[0,1,4][0,3,X]ZX
Non-OR 0CB[5,6][0,3,X]Z[X,Z]
Non-OR 0CB7[3,X]ZX
Non-OR 0CB[8,9,B,C,D,F,G,H,J]3ZX

Non-OR 0CBM[0,3,4,7,8]ZX
Non-OR 0CB[R,S,T,V][3,4,7,8]ZX
Non-OR 0CB[W,X][0,X]Z[0,1,2]

Non-OR Procedure | DRG Non-OR Procedure | Valid OR Procedure | HAC Associated Procedure | Combination Only | New/Revised April | New/Revised October

0	Medical and Surgical
C	Mouth and Throat
C	Extirpation

Definition: Taking or cutting out solid matter from a body part

Explanation: The solid matter may be an abnormal byproduct of a biological function or a foreign body; it may be imbedded in a body part or in the lumen of a tubular body part. The solid matter may or may not have been previously broken into pieces.

Body Part Character 4	Approach Character 5	Device Character 6	Qualifier Character 7

0 Upper Lip
   Frenulum labii superioris
   Labial gland
   Vermilion border
1 Lower Lip
   Frenulum labii inferioris
   Labial gland
   Vermilion border
2 Hard Palate
3 Soft Palate
4 Buccal Mucosa
   Buccal gland
   Molar gland
   Palatine gland
5 Upper Gingiva
6 Lower Gingiva
7 Tongue
   Frenulum linguae
N Uvula
   Palatine uvula
P Tonsils
   Palatine tonsil
Q Adenoids
   Pharyngeal tonsil
	0 Open
	3 Percutaneous
	X External
		Z No Device	Z No Qualifier

8 Parotid Gland, Right
9 Parotid Gland, Left
B Parotid Duct, Right
   Stensen's duct
C Parotid Duct, Left
   See B Parotid Duct, Right
D Sublingual Gland, Right
F Sublingual Gland, Left
G Submaxillary Gland, Right
   Submandibular gland
H Submaxillary Gland, Left
   See G Submaxillary Gland, Right
J Minor Salivary Gland
   Anterior lingual gland
	0 Open
	3 Percutaneous
		Z No Device	Z No Qualifier

M Pharynx
   Base of tongue
   Hypopharynx
   Laryngopharynx
   Lingual tonsil
   Oropharynx
   Piriform recess (sinus)
   Tongue, base of
R Epiglottis
   Glossoepiglottic fold
S Larynx
   Aryepiglottic fold
   Arytenoid cartilage
   Corniculate cartilage
   Cuneiform cartilage
   False vocal cord
   Glottis
   Rima glottidis
   Thyroid cartilage
   Ventricular fold
T Vocal Cord, Right
   Vocal fold
V Vocal Cord, Left
   See T Vocal Cord, Right
	0 Open
	3 Percutaneous
	4 Percutaneous Endoscopic
	7 Via Natural or Artificial Opening
	8 Via Natural or Artificial Opening Endoscopic
		Z No Device	Z No Qualifier

W Upper Tooth X Lower Tooth	0 Open X External	Z No Device	0 Single 1 Multiple 2 All

Non-OR	0CC[0,1,2,3,4,7,N,P,Q]XZZ
Non-OR	0CC[5,6][0,3,X]ZZ
Non-OR	0CC[8,9,G,H]3ZZ
Non-OR	0CC[B,C,D,F,J][0,3]ZZ
Non-OR	0CC[M,S][7,8]ZZ
Non-OR	0CC[W,X][0,X]Z[0,1,2]

0	Medical and Surgical
C	Mouth and Throat
D	Extraction

Definition: Pulling or stripping out or off all or a portion of a body part by the use of force

Explanation: The qualifier DIAGNOSTIC is used to identify extraction procedures that are biopsies

Body Part Character 4	Approach Character 5	Device Character 6	Qualifier Character 7

T Vocal Cord, Right
   Vocal fold
V Vocal Cord, Left
   See T Vocal Cord, Right
	0 Open
	3 Percutaneous
	4 Percutaneous Endoscopic
	7 Via Natural or Artificial Opening
	8 Via Natural or Artificial Opening Endoscopic
		Z No Device	Z No Qualifier

W Upper Tooth X Lower Tooth	X External	Z No Device	0 Single 1 Multiple 2 All

Non-OR	0CD[W,X]XZ[0,1,2]

0CF–0CJ Mouth and Throat ICD-10-PCS 2025

0 Medical and Surgical
C Mouth and Throat
F Fragmentation **Definition:** Breaking solid matter in a body part into pieces
Explanation: Physical force (e.g., manual, ultrasonic) applied directly or indirectly is used to break the solid matter into pieces. The solid matter may be an abnormal byproduct of a biological function or a foreign body. The pieces of solid matter are not taken out.

Body Part Character 4	Approach Character 5	Device Character 6	Qualifier Character 7
B Parotid Duct, Right [NC] Stensen's duct C Parotid Duct, Left [NC] See B Parotid Duct, Right	0 Open 3 Percutaneous 7 Via Natural or Artificial Opening X External	Z No Device	Z No Qualifier

Non-OR All body part, approach, device, and qualifier values
[NC] 0CF[B,C]XZZ

---

0 Medical and Surgical
C Mouth and Throat
H Insertion **Definition:** Putting in a nonbiological appliance that monitors, assists, performs, or prevents a physiological function but does not physically take the place of a body part
Explanation: None

Body Part Character 4	Approach Character 5	Device Character 6	Qualifier Character 7
7 Tongue Frenulum linguae	0 Open 3 Percutaneous X External	1 Radioactive Element	Z No Qualifier
A Salivary Gland S Larynx Aryepiglottic fold Arytenoid cartilage Corniculate cartilage Cuneiform cartilage False vocal cord Glottis Rima glottidis Thyroid cartilage Ventricular fold	0 Open 3 Percutaneous 7 Via Natural or Artificial Opening 8 Via Natural or Artificial Opening Endoscopic	1 Radioactive Element Y Other Device	Z No Qualifier
Y Mouth and Throat	0 Open 3 Percutaneous	1 Radioactive Element Y Other Device	Z No Qualifier
Y Mouth and Throat	7 Via Natural or Artificial Opening 8 Via Natural or Artificial Opening Endoscopic	1 Radioactive Element B Intraluminal Device, Airway Y Other Device	Z No Qualifier

Non-OR 0CH[A,S]01Z
Non-OR 0CHS0YZ
Non-OR 0CH[A,S][3,7,8][1,Y]Z
Non-OR 0CHY[0,3][1,Y]Z
Non-OR 0CHY[7,8][1,B,Y]Z

---

0 Medical and Surgical
C Mouth and Throat
J Inspection **Definition:** Visually and/or manually exploring a body part
Explanation: Visual exploration may be performed with or without optical instrumentation. Manual exploration may be performed directly or through intervening body layers.

Body Part Character 4	Approach Character 5	Device Character 6	Qualifier Character 7
A Salivary Gland	0 Open 3 Percutaneous X External	Z No Device	Z No Qualifier
S Larynx Aryepiglottic fold Arytenoid cartilage Corniculate cartilage Cuneiform cartilage False vocal cord Glottis Rima glottidis Thyroid cartilage Ventricular fold Y Mouth and Throat	0 Open 3 Percutaneous 4 Percutaneous Endoscopic 7 Via Natural or Artificial Opening 8 Via Natural or Artificial Opening Endoscopic X External	Z No Device	Z No Qualifier

Non-OR All body part, approach, device, and qualifier values

0 Medical and Surgical
C Mouth and Throat
L Occlusion Definition: Completely closing an orifice or the lumen of a tubular body part
Explanation: The orifice can be a natural orifice or an artificially created orifice

Body Part Character 4	Approach Character 5	Device Character 6	Qualifier Character 7
B Parotid Duct, Right Stensen's duct **C** Parotid Duct, Left See B Parotid Duct, Right	**0** Open **3** Percutaneous **4** Percutaneous Endoscopic	**C** Extraluminal Device **D** Intraluminal Device **Z** No Device	**Z** No Qualifier
B Parotid Duct, Right Stensen's duct **C** Parotid Duct, Left See B Parotid Duct, Right	**7** Via Natural or Artificial Opening **8** Via Natural or Artificial Opening Endoscopic	**D** Intraluminal Device **Z** No Device	**Z** No Qualifier

0 Medical and Surgical
C Mouth and Throat
M Reattachment Definition: Putting back in or on all or a portion of a separated body part to its normal location or other suitable location
Explanation: Vascular circulation and nervous pathways may or may not be reestablished

Body Part Character 4	Approach Character 5	Device Character 6	Qualifier Character 7
0 Upper Lip Frenulum labii superioris Labial gland Vermilion border **1** Lower Lip Frenulum labii inferioris Labial gland Vermilion border **3** Soft Palate **7** Tongue Frenulum linguae **N** Uvula Palatine uvula	**0** Open	**Z** No Device	**Z** No Qualifier
W Upper Tooth **X** Lower Tooth	**0** Open **X** External	**Z** No Device	**0** Single **1** Multiple **2** All

Non-OR 0CM[W,X][0,X]Z[0,1,2]

Mouth and Throat

0 Medical and Surgical
C Mouth and Throat
N Release

Definition: Freeing a body part from an abnormal physical constraint by cutting or by the use of force
Explanation: Some of the restraining tissue may be taken out but none of the body part is taken out

Body Part Character 4	Approach Character 5	Device Character 6	Qualifier Character 7

0 Upper Lip
    Frenulum labii superioris
    Labial gland
    Vermilion border
1 Lower Lip
    Frenulum labii inferioris
    Labial gland
    Vermilion border
2 Hard Palate
3 Soft Palate
4 Buccal Mucosa
    Buccal gland
    Molar gland
    Palatine gland
5 Upper Gingiva
6 Lower Gingiva
7 Tongue
    Frenulum linguae
N Uvula
    Palatine uvula
P Tonsils
    Palatine tonsil
Q Adenoids
    Pharyngeal tonsil
	0 Open
	3 Percutaneous
	X External
		Z No Device	**Z** No Qualifier

8 Parotid Gland, Right
9 Parotid Gland, Left
B Parotid Duct, Right
    Stensen's duct
C Parotid Duct, Left
    See B Parotid Duct, Right
D Sublingual Gland, Right
F Sublingual Gland, Left
G Submaxillary Gland, Right
    Submandibular gland
H Submaxillary Gland, Left
    See G Submaxillary Gland, Right
J Minor Salivary Gland
    Anterior lingual gland
	0 Open
	3 Percutaneous
		Z No Device	**Z** No Qualifier

M Pharynx
    Base of tongue
    Hypopharynx
    Laryngopharynx
    Lingual tonsil
    Oropharynx
    Piriform recess (sinus)
    Tongue, base of
R Epiglottis
    Glossoepiglottic fold
S Larynx
    Aryepiglottic fold
    Arytenoid cartilage
    Corniculate cartilage
    Cuneiform cartilage
    False vocal cord
    Glottis
    Rima glottidis
    Thyroid cartilage
    Ventricular fold
T Vocal Cord, Right
    Vocal fold
V Vocal Cord, Left
    See T Vocal Cord, Right
	0 Open
	3 Percutaneous
	4 Percutaneous Endoscopic
	7 Via Natural or Artificial Opening
	8 Via Natural or Artificial Opening Endoscopic
		Z No Device	**Z** No Qualifier

W Upper Tooth **X** Lower Tooth	**0** Open **X** External	**Z** No Device	**0** Single **1** Multiple **2** All

Non-OR   0CN[0,1,5,6,7][0,3,X]ZZ
Non-OR   0CN[W,X][0,X]Z[0,1,2]

0 Medical and Surgical
C Mouth and Throat
P Removal Definition: Taking out or off a device from a body part
Explanation: If a device is taken out and a similar device put in without cutting or puncturing the skin or mucous membrane, the procedure is coded to the root operation CHANGE. Otherwise, the procedure for taking out a device is coded to the root operation REMOVAL.

Body Part Character 4	Approach Character 5	Device Character 6	Qualifier Character 7
A Salivary Gland	0 Open 3 Percutaneous	0 Drainage Device C Extraluminal Device Y Other Device	Z No Qualifier
A Salivary Gland	7 Via Natural or Artificial Opening 8 Via Natural or Artificial Opening Endoscopic	Y Other Device	Z No Qualifier

S Larynx
  Aryepiglottic fold
  Arytenoid cartilage
  Corniculate cartilage
  Cuneiform cartilage
  False vocal cord
  Glottis
  Rima glottidis
  Thyroid cartilage
  Ventricular fold
	0 Open
	3 Percutaneous
	7 Via Natural or Artificial Opening
	8 Via Natural or Artificial Opening Endoscopic
		0 Drainage Device
		7 Autologous Tissue Substitute
		D Intraluminal Device
		J Synthetic Substitute
		K Nonautologous Tissue Substitute
		Y Other Device
			Z No Qualifier

S Larynx
  Aryepiglottic fold
  Arytenoid cartilage
  Corniculate cartilage
  Cuneiform cartilage
  False vocal cord
  Glottis
  Rima glottidis
  Thyroid cartilage
  Ventricular fold
	X External	0 Drainage Device
		7 Autologous Tissue Substitute
		D Intraluminal Device
		J Synthetic Substitute
		K Nonautologous Tissue Substitute
			Z No Qualifier

Y Mouth and Throat	0 Open 3 Percutaneous 7 Via Natural or Artificial Opening 8 Via Natural or Artificial Opening Endoscopic	0 Drainage Device 1 Radioactive Element 7 Autologous Tissue Substitute D Intraluminal Device J Synthetic Substitute K Nonautologous Tissue Substitute Y Other Device	Z No Qualifier
Y Mouth and Throat	X External	0 Drainage Device 1 Radioactive Element 7 Autologous Tissue Substitute D Intraluminal Device J Synthetic Substitute K Nonautologous Tissue Substitute	Z No Qualifier

Non-OR   0CPA[0,3][0,C,Y]Z
Non-OR   0CPA[7,8]YZ
Non-OR   0CPS3YZ
Non-OR   0CPS[7,8][0,D,Y]Z
Non-OR   0CPSX[0,7,D,J,K]Z
Non-OR   0CPY3YZ
Non-OR   0CPY[7,8][0,D,Y]Z
Non-OR   0CPYX[0,1,7,D,J,K]Z

ØCQ–ØCQ Mouth and Throat

Ø Medical and Surgical
C Mouth and Throat
Q Repair — Definition: Restoring, to the extent possible, a body part to its normal anatomic structure and function
Explanation: Used only when the method to accomplish the repair is not one of the other root operations

Body Part – Character 4	Approach – Character 5	Device – Character 6	Qualifier – Character 7
Ø Upper Lip 　Frenulum labii superioris 　Labial gland 　Vermilion border 1 Lower Lip 　Frenulum labii inferioris 　Labial gland 　Vermilion border 2 Hard Palate 3 Soft Palate 4 Buccal Mucosa 　Buccal gland 　Molar gland 　Palatine gland 5 Upper Gingiva 6 Lower Gingiva 7 Tongue 　Frenulum linguae N Uvula 　Palatine uvula P Tonsils 　Palatine tonsil Q Adenoids 　Pharyngeal tonsil	Ø Open 3 Percutaneous X External	Z No Device	Z No Qualifier
8 Parotid Gland, Right 9 Parotid Gland, Left B Parotid Duct, Right 　Stensen's duct C Parotid Duct, Left 　*See B Parotid Duct, Right* D Sublingual Gland, Right F Sublingual Gland, Left G Submaxillary Gland, Right 　Submandibular gland H Submaxillary Gland, Left 　*See G Submaxillary Gland, Right* J Minor Salivary Gland 　Anterior lingual gland	Ø Open 3 Percutaneous	Z No Device	Z No Qualifier
M Pharynx 　Base of tongue 　Hypopharynx 　Laryngopharynx 　Lingual tonsil 　Oropharynx 　Piriform recess (sinus) 　Tongue, base of R Epiglottis 　Glossoepiglottic fold S Larynx 　Aryepiglottic fold 　Arytenoid cartilage 　Corniculate cartilage 　Cuneiform cartilage 　False vocal cord 　Glottis 　Rima glottidis 　Thyroid cartilage 　Ventricular fold T Vocal Cord, Right 　Vocal fold V Vocal Cord, Left 　*See T Vocal Cord, Right*	Ø Open 3 Percutaneous 4 Percutaneous Endoscopic 7 Via Natural or Artificial Opening 8 Via Natural or Artificial Opening Endoscopic	Z No Device	Z No Qualifier
W Upper Tooth X Lower Tooth	Ø Open X External	Z No Device	Ø Single 1 Multiple 2 All

Non-OR ØCQ[Ø,1,4,7]XZZ
Non-OR ØCQ[5,6][Ø,3,X]ZZ
Non-OR ØCQ[W,X][Ø,X]Z[Ø,1,2]

ICD-10-PCS 2025 Mouth and Throat 0CR–0CR

- **0** Medical and Surgical
- **C** Mouth and Throat
- **R** Replacement Definition: Putting in or on biological or synthetic material that physically takes the place and/or function of all or a portion of a body part
Explanation: The body part may have been taken out or replaced, or may be taken out, physically eradicated, or rendered nonfunctional during the REPLACEMENT procedure. A REMOVAL procedure is coded for taking out the device used in a previous replacement procedure.

Body Part Character 4	Approach Character 5	Device Character 6	Qualifier Character 7
0 Upper Lip Frenulum labii superioris Labial gland Vermilion border **1** Lower Lip Frenulum labii inferioris Labial gland Vermilion border **2** Hard Palate **3** Soft Palate **4** Buccal Mucosa Buccal gland Molar gland Palatine gland **5** Upper Gingiva **6** Lower Gingiva **7** Tongue Frenulum linguae **N** Uvula Palatine uvula	**0** Open **3** Percutaneous **X** External	**7** Autologous Tissue Substitute **J** Synthetic Substitute **K** Nonautologous Tissue Substitute	**Z** No Qualifier
B Parotid Duct, Right Stensen's duct **C** Parotid Duct, Left See B Parotid Duct, Right	**0** Open **3** Percutaneous	**7** Autologous Tissue Substitute **J** Synthetic Substitute **K** Nonautologous Tissue Substitute	**Z** No Qualifier
M Pharynx Base of tongue Hypopharynx Laryngopharynx Lingual tonsil Oropharynx Piriform recess (sinus) Tongue, base of **R** Epiglottis Glossoepiglottic fold **S** Larynx Aryepiglottic fold Arytenoid cartilage Corniculate cartilage Cuneiform cartilage False vocal cord Glottis Rima glottidis Thyroid cartilage Ventricular fold **T** Vocal Cord, Right Vocal fold **V** Vocal Cord, Left See T Vocal Cord, Right	**0** Open **7** Via Natural or Artificial Opening **8** Via Natural or Artificial Opening Endoscopic	**7** Autologous Tissue Substitute **J** Synthetic Substitute **K** Nonautologous Tissue Substitute	**Z** No Qualifier
W Upper Tooth **X** Lower Tooth	**0** Open **X** External	**7** Autologous Tissue Substitute **J** Synthetic Substitute **K** Nonautologous Tissue Substitute	**0** Single **1** Multiple **2** All

Non-OR 0CR[W,X][0,X][7,J,K][0,1,2]

Mouth and Throat

0 Medical and Surgical
C Mouth and Throat
S Reposition

Definition: Moving to its normal location, or other suitable location, all or a portion of a body part

Explanation: The body part is moved to a new location from an abnormal location, or from a normal location where it is not functioning correctly. The body part may or may not be cut out or off to be moved to the new location.

Body Part Character 4	Approach Character 5	Device Character 6	Qualifier Character 7
0 Upper Lip Frenulum labii superioris, Labial gland, Vermilion border **1 Lower Lip** Frenulum labii inferioris, Labial gland, Vermilion border **2 Hard Palate** **3 Soft Palate** **7 Tongue** Frenulum linguae **N Uvula** Palatine uvula	**0** Open **X** External	**Z** No Device	**Z** No Qualifier
B Parotid Duct, Right Stensen's duct **C Parotid Duct, Left** See B Parotid Duct, Right	**0** Open **3** Percutaneous	**Z** No Device	**Z** No Qualifier
R Epiglottis Glossoepiglottic fold **S Larynx** **T Vocal Cord, Right** Vocal fold **V Vocal Cord, Left** See T Vocal Cord, Right	**0** Open **7** Via Natural or Artificial Opening **8** Via Natural or Artificial Opening Endoscopic	**Z** No Device	**Z** No Qualifier
W Upper Tooth **X Lower Tooth**	**0** Open **X** External	**5** External Fixation Device **Z** No Device	**0** Single **1** Multiple **2** All

Non-OR 0CS[W,X][0,X][5,Z][0,1,2]

0 Medical and Surgical
C Mouth and Throat
T Resection Definition: Cutting out or off, without replacement, all of a body part
  Explanation: None

Body Part Character 4	Approach Character 5	Device Character 6	Qualifier Character 7
0 Upper Lip 　Frenulum labii superioris 　Labial gland 　Vermilion border **1** Lower Lip 　Frenulum labii inferioris 　Labial gland 　Vermilion border **2** Hard Palate **3** Soft Palate **7** Tongue 　Frenulum linguae **N** Uvula 　Palatine uvula **P** Tonsils 　Palatine tonsil **Q** Adenoids 　Pharyngeal tonsil	**0** Open **X** External	**Z** No Device	**Z** No Qualifier
8 Parotid Gland, Right **9** Parotid Gland, Left **B** Parotid Duct, Right 　Stensen's duct **C** Parotid Duct, Left 　See B Parotid Duct, Right **D** Sublingual Gland, Right **F** Sublingual Gland, Left **G** Submaxillary Gland, Right 　Submandibular gland **H** Submaxillary Gland, Left 　See G Submaxillary Gland, Right **J** Minor Salivary Gland 　Anterior lingual gland	**0** Open	**Z** No Device	**Z** No Qualifier
M Pharynx 　Base of tongue 　Hypopharynx 　Laryngopharynx 　Lingual tonsil 　Oropharynx 　Piriform recess (sinus) 　Tongue, base of **R** Epiglottis 　Glossoepiglottic fold **S** Larynx 　Aryepiglottic fold 　Arytenoid cartilage 　Corniculate cartilage 　Cuneiform cartilage 　False vocal cord 　Glottis 　Rima glottidis 　Thyroid cartilage 　Ventricular fold **T** Vocal Cord, Right 　Vocal fold **V** Vocal Cord, Left 　See T Vocal Cord, Right	**0** Open **4** Percutaneous Endoscopic **7** Via Natural or Artificial Opening **8** Via Natural or Artificial Opening Endoscopic	**Z** No Device	**Z** No Qualifier
W Upper Tooth **X** Lower Tooth	**0** Open	**Z** No Device	**0** Single **1** Multiple **2** All

Non-OR 0CT[W,X]0Z[0,1,2]

0 Medical and Surgical
C Mouth and Throat
U Supplement — Definition: Putting in or on biological or synthetic material that physically reinforces and/or augments the function of a portion of a body part
Explanation: The biological material is non-living, or is living and from the same individual. The body part may have been previously replaced, and the SUPPLEMENT procedure is performed to physically reinforce and/or augment the function of the replaced body part.

Body Part Character 4	Approach Character 5	Device Character 6	Qualifier Character 7

0 Upper Lip
  Frenulum labii superioris
  Labial gland
  Vermilion border
1 Lower Lip
  Frenulum labii inferioris
  Labial gland
  Vermilion border
2 Hard Palate
3 Soft Palate
4 Buccal Mucosa
  Buccal gland
  Molar gland
  Palatine gland
5 Upper Gingiva
6 Lower Gingiva
7 Tongue
  Frenulum linguae
N Uvula
  Palatine uvula
	0 Open
	3 Percutaneous
	X External
		7 Autologous Tissue Substitute
		J Synthetic Substitute
		K Nonautologous Tissue Substitute
			Z No Qualifier

M Pharynx
  Base of tongue
  Hypopharynx
  Laryngopharynx
  Lingual tonsil
  Oropharynx
  Piriform recess (sinus)
  Tongue, base of
R Epiglottis
  Glossoepiglottic fold
S Larynx
  Aryepiglottic fold
  Arytenoid cartilage
  Corniculate cartilage
  Cuneiform cartilage
  False vocal cord
  Glottis
  Rima glottidis
  Thyroid cartilage
  Ventricular fold
T Vocal Cord, Right
  Vocal fold
V Vocal Cord, Left
  See T Vocal Cord, Right
	0 Open
	7 Via Natural or Artificial Opening
	8 Via Natural or Artificial Opening Endoscopic
		7 Autologous Tissue Substitute
		J Synthetic Substitute
		K Nonautologous Tissue Substitute
			Z No Qualifier

Non-OR   0CU2[0,3]JZ

0 Medical and Surgical
C Mouth and Throat
V Restriction — Definition: Partially closing an orifice or the lumen of a tubular body part
Explanation: The orifice can be a natural orifice or an artificially created orifice

Body Part Character 4	Approach Character 5	Device Character 6	Qualifier Character 7

B Parotid Duct, Right
  Stensen's duct
C Parotid Duct, Left
  See B Parotid Duct, Right
	0 Open
	3 Percutaneous
		C Extraluminal Device
		D Intraluminal Device
		Z No Device
			Z No Qualifier

B Parotid Duct, Right
  Stensen's duct
C Parotid Duct, Left
  See B Parotid Duct, Right
	7 Via Natural or Artificial Opening
	8 Via Natural or Artificial Opening Endoscopic
		D Intraluminal Device
		Z No Device
			Z No Qualifier

ICD-10-PCS 2025 — Mouth and Throat — 0CW–0CW

- **0** Medical and Surgical
- **C** Mouth and Throat
- **W** Revision

Definition: Correcting, to the extent possible, a portion of a malfunctioning device or the position of a displaced device

Explanation: Revision can include correcting a malfunctioning or displaced device by taking out or putting in components of the device such as a screw or pin

Body Part Character 4	Approach Character 5	Device Character 6	Qualifier Character 7
A Salivary Gland	0 Open 3 Percutaneous	0 Drainage Device C Extraluminal Device Y Other Device	Z No Qualifier
A Salivary Gland	7 Via Natural or Artificial Opening 8 Via Natural or Artificial Opening Endoscopic	Y Other Device	Z No Qualifier
A Salivary Gland	X External	0 Drainage Device C Extraluminal Device	Z No Qualifier

S Larynx
  Aryepiglottic fold
  Arytenoid cartilage
  Corniculate cartilage
  Cuneiform cartilage
  False vocal cord
  Glottis
  Rima glottidis
  Thyroid cartilage
  Ventricular fold
	0 Open
	3 Percutaneous
	7 Via Natural or Artificial Opening
	8 Via Natural or Artificial Opening Endoscopic
		0 Drainage Device
		7 Autologous Tissue Substitute
		D Intraluminal Device
		J Synthetic Substitute
		K Nonautologous Tissue Substitute
		Y Other Device
			Z No Qualifier

S Larynx
  Aryepiglottic fold
  Arytenoid cartilage
  Corniculate cartilage
  Cuneiform cartilage
  False vocal cord
  Glottis
  Rima glottidis
  Thyroid cartilage
  Ventricular fold
	X External	0 Drainage Device
		7 Autologous Tissue Substitute
		D Intraluminal Device
		J Synthetic Substitute
		K Nonautologous Tissue Substitute
			Z No Qualifier

Y Mouth and Throat	0 Open 3 Percutaneous 7 Via Natural or Artificial Opening 8 Via Natural or Artificial Opening Endoscopic	0 Drainage Device 1 Radioactive Element 7 Autologous Tissue Substitute D Intraluminal Device J Synthetic Substitute K Nonautologous Tissue Substitute Y Other Device	Z No Qualifier
Y Mouth and Throat	X External	0 Drainage Device 1 Radioactive Element 7 Autologous Tissue Substitute D Intraluminal Device J Synthetic Substitute K Nonautologous Tissue Substitute	Z No Qualifier

Non-OR 0CWA[0,3][0,C,Y]Z
Non-OR 0CWA[7,8]YZ
Non-OR 0CWAX[0,C]Z
Non-OR 0CWS[3,7,8]YZ
Non-OR 0CWSX[0,7,D,J,K]Z
Non-OR 0CWY07Z
Non-OR 0CWY[3,7,8]YZ
Non-OR 0CWYX[0,1,7,D,J,K]Z

0 Medical and Surgical
C Mouth and Throat
X Transfer   Definition: Moving, without taking out, all or a portion of a body part to another location to take over the function of all or a portion of a body part
Explanation: The body part transferred remains connected to its vascular and nervous supply

| Body Part
Character 4 | Approach
Character 5 | Device
Character 6 | Qualifier
Character 7 |
|---|---|---|---|
| 0 Upper Lip
  Frenulum labii superioris
  Labial gland
  Vermilion border
1 Lower Lip
  Frenulum labii inferioris
  Labial gland
  Vermilion border
3 Soft Palate
4 Buccal Mucosa
  Buccal gland
  Molar gland
  Palatine gland
5 Upper Gingiva
6 Lower Gingiva
7 Tongue
  Frenulum linguae | 0 Open
X External | Z No Device | Z No Qualifier |

Gastrointestinal System ØD1–ØDY

Character Meanings

This Character Meaning table is provided as a guide to assist the user in the identification of character members that may be found in this section of code tables. It **SHOULD NOT** be used to build a PCS code.

Operation–Character 3		Body Part–Character 4		Approach–Character 5		Device–Character 6		Qualifier–Character 7	
1	Bypass	Ø	Upper Intestinal Tract	Ø	Open	Ø	Drainage Device	Ø	Allogeneic
2	Change	1	Esophagus, Upper	3	Percutaneous	1	Radioactive Element	1	Syngeneic
5	Destruction	2	Esophagus, Middle	4	Percutaneous Endoscopic	2	Monitoring Device	2	Zooplastic
7	Dilation	3	Esophagus, Lower	7	Via Natural or Artificial Opening	3	Infusion Device	3	Vertical OR Laser Interstitial Thermal Therapy
8	Division	4	Esophagogastric Junction	8	Via Natural or Artificial Opening Endoscopic	7	Autologous Tissue Substitute	4	Cutaneous
9	Drainage	5	Esophagus	F	Via Natural or Artificial Opening with Percutaneous Endoscopic Assistance	B	Intraluminal Device, Airway	5	Esophagus
B	Excision	6	Stomach	X	External	C	Extraluminal Device	6	Stomach
C	Extirpation	7	Stomach, Pylorus			D	Intraluminal Device	7	Vagina
D	Extraction	8	Small Intestine			J	Synthetic Substitute OR Magnetic Lengthening Device	8	Small Intestine
F	Fragmentation	9	Duodenum			K	Nonautologous Tissue Substitute	9	Duodenum
H	Insertion	A	Jejunum			L	Artificial Sphincter	A	Jejunum
J	Inspection	B	Ileum			M	Stimulator Lead	B	Ileum OR Bladder
L	Occlusion	C	Ileocecal Valve			U	Feeding Device	C	Ureter, Right
M	Reattachment	D	Lower Intestinal Tract			Y	Other Device	D	Ureter, Left
N	Release	E	Large Intestine			Z	No Device	E	Large Intestine
P	Removal	F	Large Intestine, Right					F	Ureters, Bilateral
Q	Repair	G	Large Intestine, Left					G	Hand-Assisted
R	Replacement	H	Cecum					H	Cecum
S	Reposition	J	Appendix					K	Ascending Colon
T	Resection	K	Ascending Colon					L	Transverse Colon
U	Supplement	L	Transverse Colon					M	Descending Colon
V	Restriction	M	Descending Colon					N	Sigmoid Colon
W	Revision	N	Sigmoid Colon					P	Rectum
X	Transfer	P	Rectum					Q	Anus
Y	Transplantation	Q	Anus					V	Thoracic Region
		R	Anal Sphincter					W	Abdominal Region
		U	Omentum					X	Diagnostic OR Pelvic Region
		V	Mesentery					Y	Inguinal Region
		W	Peritoneum					Z	No Qualifier

Gastrointestinal System

AHA Coding Clinic for Gastrointestinal System
2022, 1Q, 11	Procedures performed on a continuous vessel, ICD-10-PCS Guideline B4.1c

AHA Coding Clinic for table 0D1
2021, 1Q, 19	Kock pouch revision surgery
2019, 4Q, 29	Intestinal bypass
2017, 2Q, 17	Billroth II (distal gastrectomy and gastrojejunostomy)
2016, 2Q, 31	Laparoscopic biliopancreatic diversion with duodenal switch
2014, 4Q, 41	Abdominoperineal resection (APR) with flap closure of perineum and colostomy

AHA Coding Clinic for table 0D2
2022, 1Q, 45	Insertion, removal and replacement of endoluminal vacuum application
2019, 1Q, 26	Exchange of clogged gastrojejunostomy tube

AHA Coding Clinic for table 0D5
2022, 4Q, 53-54	Laser interstitial thermal therapy
2017, 1Q, 34	Debulking of tumor and peritoneum ablation

AHA Coding Clinic for table 0D7
2020, 3Q, 45	Dilation versus drainage of perirectal cyst
2017, 3Q, 23	Laparoscopic pyloromyotomy
2014, 4Q, 40	Dilation of gastrojejunostomy anastomosis stricture

AHA Coding Clinic for table 0D8
2019, 2Q, 15	Reversal of Roux-en-Y bypass
2017, 3Q, 22	Laparoscopic esophagomyotomy (Heller type) and Toupet fundoplication
2017, 3Q, 23	Laparoscopic pyloromyotomy

AHA Coding Clinic for table 0D9
2024, 1Q, 29	Seton placement
2020, 3Q, 45	Dilation versus drainage of perirectal cyst
2015, 2Q, 29	Insertion of nasogastric tube for drainage and feeding

AHA Coding Clinic for table 0DB
2024, 1Q, 7	Percutaneous endoscopic hand-assisted approach
2023, 2Q, 23	V-Y anoplasty and excision of mucosal ectropion
2023, 1Q, 32	Zenker's diverticulectomy
2021, 3Q, 28	Retrieval of capsule via small bowel excision
2021, 2Q, 11	Serosal injury with excision of small intestine
2021, 1Q, 20	Rectal suction biopsy
2021, 1Q, 22	Total proctocolectomy with creation of J-pouch
2019, 2Q, 15	Reversal of Roux-en-Y bypass
2019, 1Q, 3-8	Whipple procedure
2019, 1Q, 27	Excision of pelvic sidewall mass
2017, 2Q, 17	Billroth II (distal gastrectomy and gastrojejunostomy)
2017, 1Q, 16	Hepatic flexure versus transverse colon
2016, 3Q, 3-7	Stoma creation & takedown procedures
2016, 2Q, 31	Laparoscopic biliopancreatic diversion with duodenal switch
2016, 1Q, 22	Perineal proctectomy
2016, 1Q, 24	Endoscopic brush biopsy of esophagus
2014, 4Q, 40	Abdominoperineal resection (APR) with flap closure of perineum and colostomy
2014, 3Q, 28	Ileostomy takedown and parastomal hernia repair
2014, 3Q, 32	Pyloric-sparing Whipple procedure

AHA Coding Clinic for table 0DD
2021, 1Q, 20	Rectal suction biopsy
2017, 4Q, 41-42	Extraction procedures

AHA Coding Clinic for table 0DH
2023, 4Q, 53-54	Magnetic lengthening device for esophagus
2023, 3Q, 6	Tracheal agenesis with tracheostomy placement
2022, 1Q, 44	Insertion, removal and replacement of endoluminal vacuum application
2020, 4Q, 43-44	Insertion of radioactive element
2020, 3Q, 43	Staged laparoscopic gastric conduit and placement of feeding tube
2019, 2Q, 18	Endoscopic wound VAC placement
2016, 3Q, 26	Insertion of gastrostomy tube
2013, 4Q, 117	Percutaneous endoscopic placement of gastrostomy tube

AHA Coding Clinic for table 0DJ
2019, 1Q, 25	Laparoscopic appendectomy converted to open procedure
2019, 1Q, 25	Milking of inspissated material from ileum to colon
2017, 2Q, 15	Low anterior resection with sigmoidoscopy
2016, 2Q, 20	Capsule endoscopy of small intestine
2015, 3Q, 24	Esophagogastroduodenoscopy with epinephrine injection for control of bleeding

AHA Coding Clinic for table 0DL
2013, 4Q, 112	Endoscopic banding of esophageal varices

AHA Coding Clinic for table 0DN
2017, 4Q, 49-50	New and revised body part values - Repositioning of the intestine
2017, 1Q, 35	Lysis of omental and peritoneal adhesions
2015, 3Q, 15	Vascular ring surgery with release of esophagus and trachea
2015, 3Q, 16	Vascular ring surgery and double aortic arch

AHA Coding Clinic for table 0DP
2019, 2Q, 18	Removal of wound VAC

AHA Coding Clinic for table 0DQ
2024, 1Q, 28	Modified Graham patch repair of gastric perforation
2023, 2Q, 23	V-Y anoplasty and excision of mucosal ectropion
2019, 2Q, 15	Reversal of Roux-en-Y bypass
2018, 2Q, 25	Third and fourth degree obstetric lacerations
2018, 1Q, 11	Repair of internal hernia at Petersen space
2017, 3Q, 17	Posterior sagittal anorectoplasty
2016, 3Q, 3-7	Stoma creation & takedown procedures
2016, 3Q, 26	Insertion of gastrostomy tube
2016, 1Q, 7	Obstetrical perineal laceration repair
2016, 1Q, 8	Obstetrical perineal laceration repair
2014, 4Q, 20	Control of bleeding duodenal ulcer

AHA Coding Clinic for table 0DS
2019, 1Q, 30	Laparoscopic-assisted rectopexy with manual reduction of prolapse
2017, 4Q, 49-50	New and revised body part values - Repositioning of the intestine
2017, 3Q, 9	Ileocolic intussusception reduction via air enema
2017, 3Q, 17	Posterior sagittal anorectoplasty
2016, 3Q, 3-5	Stoma creation & takedown procedures

AHA Coding Clinic for table 0DT
2024, 1Q, 7	Percutaneous endoscopic hand-assisted approach
2022, 1Q, 49	Robotic-assisted low anterior resection of colon
2021, 1Q, 22	Total proctocolectomy with creation of J-pouch
2020, 4Q, 100	Robotic-assisted sigmoid colectomy with extension of incision for specimen removal
2019, 1Q, 3-8	Whipple procedure
2019, 1Q, 14	Esophagectomy with colon interposition
2017, 4Q, 49-50	New and revised body part values - Repositioning of the intestine
2014, 4Q, 40	Abdominoperineal resection (APR) with flap closure of perineum and colostomy
2014, 4Q, 42	Right colectomy with side-to-side functional end-to-end anastomosis
2014, 3Q, 6	Ileocecectomy including cecum, terminal ileum and appendix
2014, 3Q, 6	Right colectomy

AHA Coding Clinic for table 0DU
2023, 2Q, 23	V-Y anoplasty and excision of mucosal ectropion
2021, 2Q, 20	Malone antegrade continence enema procedure
2021, 1Q, 22	Total proctocolectomy with creation of J-pouch
2019, 1Q, 30	Laparoscopic-assisted rectopexy with manual reduction of prolapse

AHA Coding Clinic for table 0DV
2017, 3Q, 22	Laparoscopic esophagomyotomy (Heller type) and Toupet fundoplication
2016, 2Q, 22	Esophageal lengthening Collis gastroplasty with Nissen fundoplication and hiatal hernia
2014, 3Q, 28	Laparoscopic Nissen fundoplication and diaphragmatic hernia repair

AHA Coding Clinic for table 0DW
2021, 1Q, 19	Kock pouch revision surgery
2018, 1Q, 20	Adjustment of gastric band

AHA Coding Clinic for table 0DX
2024, 1Q, 8-9	Transfer of omentum
2022, 4Q, 56-57	Bladder augmentation
2022, 4Q, 58	Ileal ureter
2019, 4Q, 29-30	Transfer large intestine to vagina
2019, 1Q, 14	Esophagectomy with colon interposition
2017, 2Q, 18	Esophagectomy and esophagogastrectomy with cervical esophagogastrostomy
2016, 2Q, 22	Esophageal lengthening Collis gastroplasty with Nissen fundoplication and hiatal hernia
2015, 1Q, 28	Repair of bronchopleural fistula using omental pedicle graft

AHA Coding Clinic for table 0DY
2023, 2Q, 32	Preparation of donor organ before transplantation

Upper Intestinal Tract (Ø) and Lower Intestinal Tract (D)

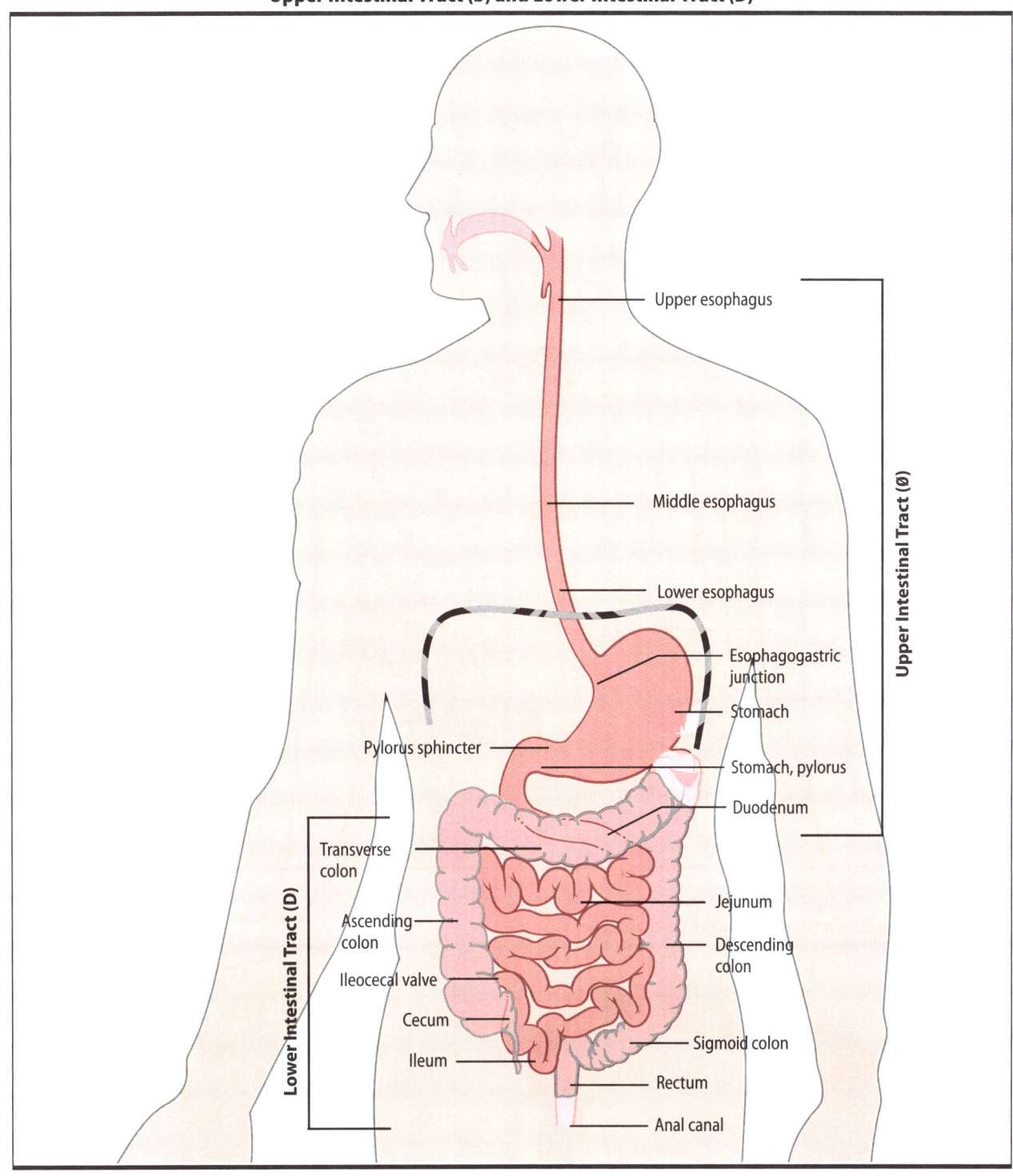

Gastrointestinal System

ICD-10-PCS 2025

Upper Intestinal Tract

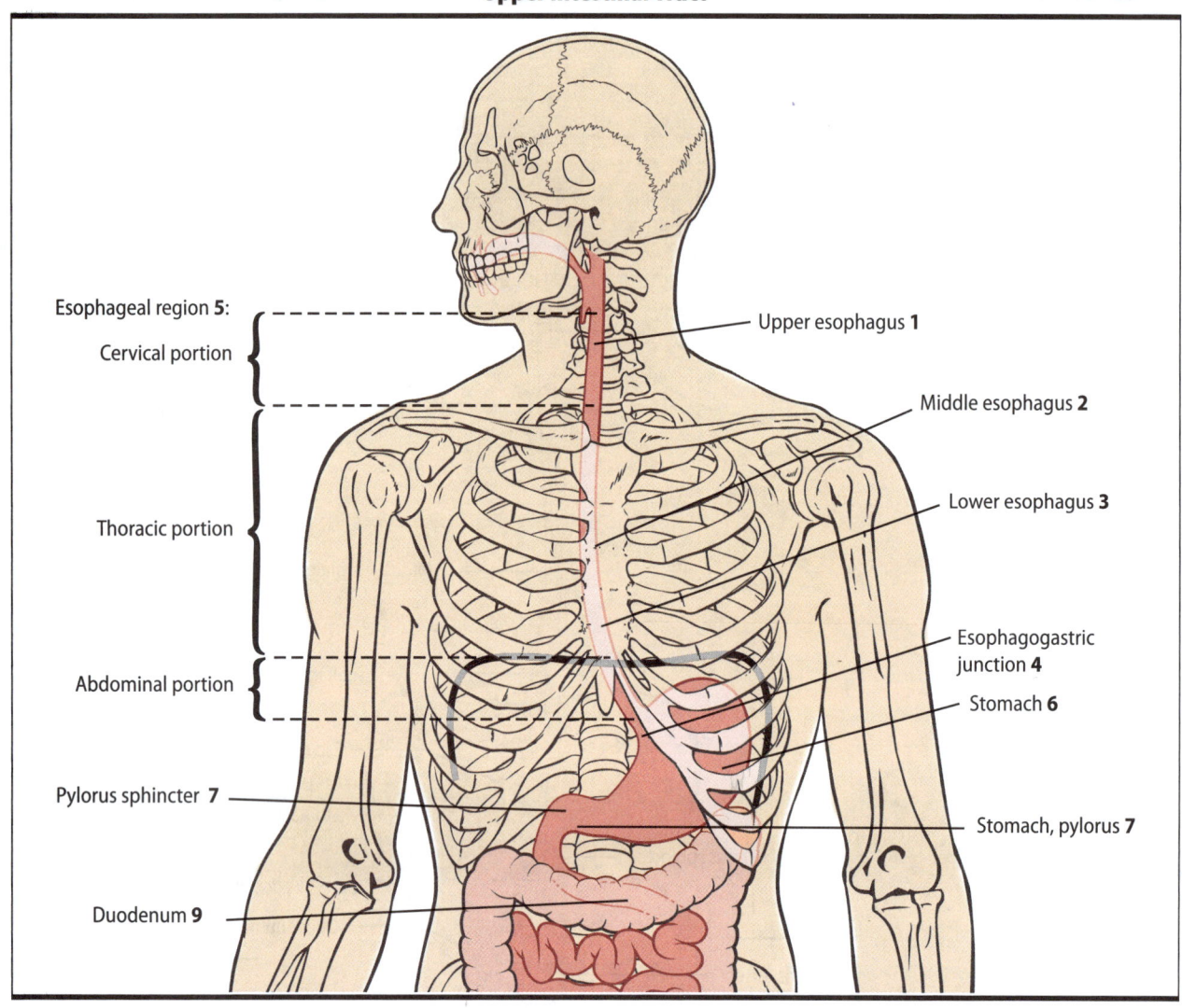

- Esophageal region 5:
  - Cervical portion
  - Thoracic portion
  - Abdominal portion
- Upper esophagus 1
- Middle esophagus 2
- Lower esophagus 3
- Esophagogastric junction 4
- Stomach 6
- Pylorus sphincter 7
- Stomach, pylorus 7
- Duodenum 9

Lower Intestinal Tract
(Jejunum Down to and Including Rectum/Anus)

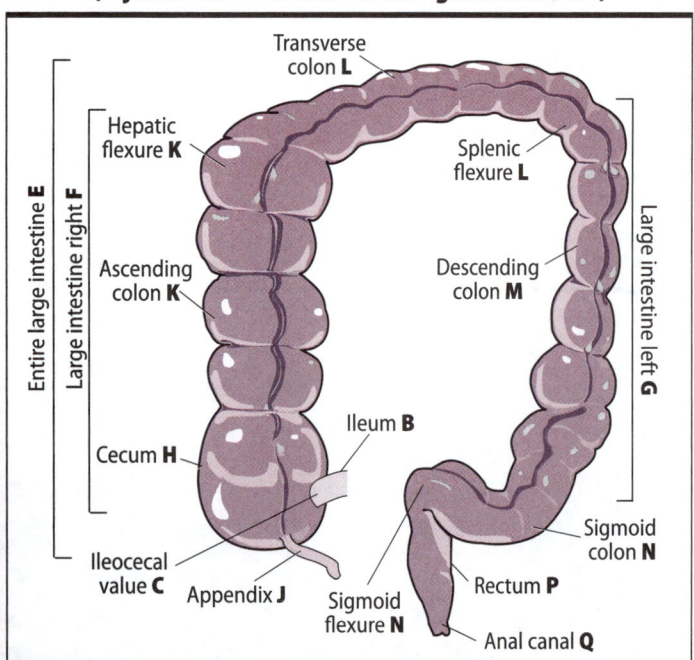

- Transverse colon L
- Hepatic flexure K
- Splenic flexure L
- Ascending colon K
- Descending colon M
- Entire large intestine E
- Large intestine right F
- Large intestine left G
- Cecum H
- Ileum B
- Ileocecal value C
- Appendix J
- Sigmoid flexure N
- Sigmoid colon N
- Rectum P
- Anal canal Q

Rectum and Anus

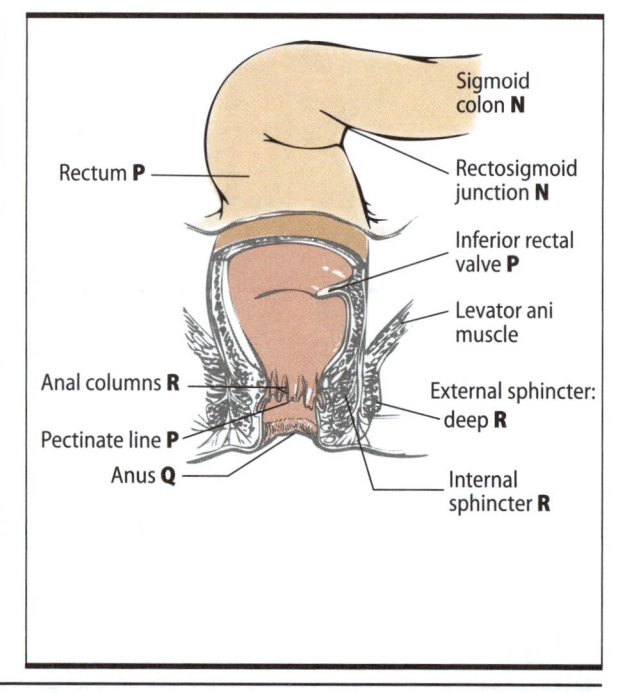

- Sigmoid colon N
- Rectum P
- Rectosigmoid junction N
- Inferior rectal valve P
- Levator ani muscle
- Anal columns R
- External sphincter: deep R
- Pectinate line P
- Anus Q
- Internal sphincter R

380

ICD-10-PCS 2025　　　　　　　　　　　　　　　　　　　Gastrointestinal System　　　　　　　　　　　　　　　　　　　0D1–0D1

0 **Medical and Surgical**
D **Gastrointestinal System**
1 **Bypass**　　　Definition: Altering the route of passage of the contents of a tubular body part
　　　　　　　　Explanation: Rerouting contents of a body part to a downstream area of the normal route, to a similar route and body part, or to an abnormal route and dissimilar body part. Includes one or more anastomoses, with or without the use of a device.

Body Part Character 4	Approach Character 5	Device Character 6	Qualifier Character 7
1 Esophagus, Upper 　Cervical esophagus 2 Esophagus, Middle 　Thoracic esophagus 3 Esophagus, Lower 　Abdominal esophagus 5 Esophagus	0 Open 4 Percutaneous Endoscopic 8 Via Natural or Artificial Opening Endoscopic	7 Autologous Tissue Substitute J Synthetic Substitute K Nonautologous Tissue Substitute Z No Device	4 Cutaneous 6 Stomach 9 Duodenum A Jejunum B Ileum
1 Esophagus, Upper 　Cervical esophagus 2 Esophagus, Middle 　Thoracic esophagus 3 Esophagus, Lower 　Abdominal esophagus 5 Esophagus	3 Percutaneous	J Synthetic Substitute	4 Cutaneous
6 Stomach 9 Duodenum	0 Open 4 Percutaneous Endoscopic 8 Via Natural or Artificial Opening Endoscopic	7 Autologous Tissue Substitute J Synthetic Substitute K Nonautologous Tissue Substitute Z No Device	4 Cutaneous 9 Duodenum A Jejunum B Ileum L Transverse Colon
6 Stomach 9 Duodenum	3 Percutaneous	J Synthetic Substitute	4 Cutaneous
8 Small Intestine	0 Open 4 Percutaneous Endoscopic 8 Via Natural or Artificial Opening Endoscopic	7 Autologous Tissue Substitute J Synthetic Substitute K Nonautologous Tissue Substitute Z No Device	4 Cutaneous 8 Small Intestine H Cecum K Ascending Colon L Transverse Colon M Descending Colon N Sigmoid Colon P Rectum Q Anus
A Jejunum 　Duodenojejunal flexure	0 Open 4 Percutaneous Endoscopic 8 Via Natural or Artificial Opening Endoscopic	7 Autologous Tissue Substitute J Synthetic Substitute K Nonautologous Tissue Substitute Z No Device	4 Cutaneous A Jejunum B Ileum H Cecum K Ascending Colon L Transverse Colon M Descending Colon N Sigmoid Colon P Rectum Q Anus
A Jejunum 　Duodenojejunal flexure	3 Percutaneous	J Synthetic Substitute	4 Cutaneous
B Ileum	0 Open 4 Percutaneous Endoscopic 8 Via Natural or Artificial Opening Endoscopic	7 Autologous Tissue Substitute J Synthetic Substitute K Nonautologous Tissue Substitute Z No Device	4 Cutaneous B Ileum H Cecum K Ascending Colon L Transverse Colon M Descending Colon N Sigmoid Colon P Rectum Q Anus
B Ileum	3 Percutaneous	J Synthetic Substitute	4 Cutaneous
E Large Intestine	0 Open 4 Percutaneous Endoscopic 8 Via Natural or Artificial Opening Endoscopic	7 Autologous Tissue Substitute J Synthetic Substitute K Nonautologous Tissue Substitute Z No Device	4 Cutaneous E Large Intestine P Rectum
H Cecum	0 Open 4 Percutaneous Endoscopic 8 Via Natural or Artificial Opening Endoscopic	7 Autologous Tissue Substitute J Synthetic Substitute K Nonautologous Tissue Substitute Z No Device	4 Cutaneous H Cecum K Ascending Colon L Transverse Colon M Descending Colon N Sigmoid Colon P Rectum
H Cecum	3 Percutaneous	J Synthetic Substitute	4 Cutaneous

　　Non-OR　　0D16[0,4,8][7,J,K,Z]4
　　Non-OR　　0D163J4
　　HAC　　　0D16[0,4,8][7,J,K,Z][9,A,B,L] when reported with PDx E66.01 and SDx K68.11, K95.01, K95.81 or T81.40–T81.49 with 7th character A

0D1 Continued on next page

NC Noncovered Procedure　　LC Limited Coverage　　QA Questionable OB Admit　　NT New Tech Add-on　　+ Combination Member　　♂ Male　　♀ Female

0 Medical and Surgical
D Gastrointestinal System
1 Bypass Definition: Altering the route of passage of the contents of a tubular body part

Explanation: Rerouting contents of a body part to a downstream area of the normal route, to a similar route and body part, or to an abnormal route and dissimilar body part. Includes one or more anastomoses, with or without the use of a device.

0D1 Continued

Body Part Character 4	Approach Character 5	Device Character 6	Qualifier Character 7
K Ascending Colon	0 Open 4 Percutaneous Endoscopic 8 Via Natural or Artificial Opening Endoscopic	7 Autologous Tissue Substitute J Synthetic Substitute K Nonautologous Tissue Substitute Z No Device	4 Cutaneous K Ascending Colon L Transverse Colon M Descending Colon N Sigmoid Colon P Rectum
K Ascending Colon	3 Percutaneous	J Synthetic Substitute	4 Cutaneous

L Transverse Colon
   Hepatic flexure
   Splenic flexure
	0 Open
	4 Percutaneous Endoscopic
	8 Via Natural or Artificial Opening Endoscopic
		7 Autologous Tissue Substitute
		J Synthetic Substitute
		K Nonautologous Tissue Substitute
		Z No Device
			4 Cutaneous
			L Transverse Colon
			M Descending Colon
			N Sigmoid Colon
			P Rectum

L Transverse Colon
   Hepatic flexure
   Splenic flexure
	3 Percutaneous	J Synthetic Substitute	4 Cutaneous

M Descending Colon	0 Open 4 Percutaneous Endoscopic 8 Via Natural or Artificial Opening Endoscopic	7 Autologous Tissue Substitute J Synthetic Substitute K Nonautologous Tissue Substitute Z No Device	4 Cutaneous M Descending Colon N Sigmoid Colon P Rectum
M Descending Colon	3 Percutaneous	J Synthetic Substitute	4 Cutaneous

N Sigmoid Colon
   Rectosigmoid junction
   Sigmoid flexure
	0 Open
	4 Percutaneous Endoscopic
	8 Via Natural or Artificial Opening Endoscopic
		7 Autologous Tissue Substitute
		J Synthetic Substitute
		K Nonautologous Tissue Substitute
		Z No Device
			4 Cutaneous
			N Sigmoid Colon
			P Rectum

N Sigmoid Colon
   Rectosigmoid junction
   Sigmoid flexure
	3 Percutaneous	J Synthetic Substitute	4 Cutaneous

0 Medical and Surgical
D Gastrointestinal System
2 Change Definition: Taking out or off a device from a body part and putting back an identical or similar device in or on the same body part without cutting or puncturing the skin or a mucous membrane

Explanation: All CHANGE procedures are coded using the approach EXTERNAL

Body Part Character 4	Approach Character 5	Device Character 6	Qualifier Character 7
0 Upper Intestinal Tract D Lower Intestinal Tract	X External	0 Drainage Device U Feeding Device Y Other Device	Z No Qualifier

U Omentum
   Gastrocolic ligament
   Gastrocolic omentum
   Gastrohepatic omentum
   Gastrophrenic ligament
   Gastrosplenic ligament
   Greater Omentum
   Hepatogastric ligament
   Lesser Omentum
V Mesentery
   Mesoappendix
   Mesocolon
W Peritoneum
   Epiploic foramen
	X External	0 Drainage Device
		Y Other Device
			Z No Qualifier

Non-OR All body part, approach, device, and qualifier values

ICD-10-PCS 2025 — Gastrointestinal System — 0D5–0D5

- **0** Medical and Surgical
- **D** Gastrointestinal System
- **5** Destruction — Definition: Physical eradication of all or a portion of a body part by the direct use of energy, force, or a destructive agent
  - Explanation: None of the body part is physically taken out

Body Part — Character 4	Approach — Character 5	Device — Character 6	Qualifier — Character 7
1 Esophagus, Upper — Cervical esophagus **2** Esophagus, Middle — Thoracic esophagus **3** Esophagus, Lower — Abdominal esophagus **4** Esophagogastric Junction — Cardia, Cardioesophageal junction, Gastroesophageal (GE) junction **5** Esophagus **6** Stomach **7** Stomach, Pylorus — Pyloric antrum, Pyloric canal, Pyloric sphincter **8** Small Intestine **9** Duodenum **A** Jejunum — Duodenojejunal flexure **B** Ileum **C** Ileocecal Valve **E** Large Intestine **F** Large Intestine, Right **G** Large Intestine, Left **H** Cecum **J** Appendix — Appendiceal orifice, Vermiform appendix **K** Ascending Colon **L** Transverse Colon — Hepatic flexure, Splenic flexure **M** Descending Colon **N** Sigmoid Colon — Rectosigmoid junction, Sigmoid flexure **P** Rectum — Anorectal junction	**0** Open **3** Percutaneous **4** Percutaneous Endoscopic	**Z** No Device	**3** Laser Interstitial Thermal Therapy **Z** No Qualifier
1 Esophagus, Upper — Cervical esophagus **2** Esophagus, Middle — Thoracic esophagus **3** Esophagus, Lower — Abdominal esophagus **4** Esophagogastric Junction — Cardia, Cardioesophageal junction, Gastroesophageal (GE) junction **5** Esophagus **6** Stomach **7** Stomach, Pylorus — Pyloric antrum, Pyloric canal, Pyloric sphincter **8** Small Intestine **9** Duodenum **A** Jejunum — Duodenojejunal flexure **B** Ileum **C** Ileocecal Valve **E** Large Intestine **F** Large Intestine, Right **G** Large Intestine, Left **H** Cecum **J** Appendix — Appendiceal orifice, Vermiform appendix **K** Ascending Colon **L** Transverse Colon — Hepatic flexure, Splenic flexure **M** Descending Colon **N** Sigmoid Colon — Rectosigmoid junction, Sigmoid flexure **P** Rectum — Anorectal junction	**7** Via Natural or Artificial Opening **8** Via Natural or Artificial Opening Endoscopic	**Z** No Device	**Z** No Qualifier
Q Anus — Anal orifice	**0** Open **3** Percutaneous **4** Percutaneous Endoscopic	**Z** No Device	**3** Laser Interstitial Thermal Therapy **Z** No Qualifier
Q Anus — Anal orifice	**7** Via Natural or Artificial Opening **8** Via Natural or Artificial Opening Endoscopic **X** External	**Z** No Device	**Z** No Qualifier
R Anal Sphincter — External anal sphincter, Internal anal sphincter **U** Omentum — Gastrocolic ligament, Gastrocolic omentum, Gastrohepatic omentum, Gastrophrenic ligament, Gastrosplenic ligament, Greater Omentum, Hepatogastric ligament, Lesser Omentum **V** Mesentery — Mesoappendix, Mesocolon **W** Peritoneum — Epiploic foramen	**0** Open **3** Percutaneous **4** Percutaneous Endoscopic	**Z** No Device	**Z** No Qualifier

DRG Non-OR 0D5[1,2,3,4,5,6,7,9,E,F,G,H,K,L,M,N]4Z3
DRG Non-OR 0D5P[0,3,4]Z3
DRG Non-OR 0D5Q4Z3

Non-OR 0D5[1,2,3,4,5,6,7,9,E,F,G,H,K,L,M,N]4ZZ
Non-OR 0D5P[0,3,4]ZZ
Non-OR 0D5[1,2,3,4,5,6,7,8,9,A,B,C,E,F,G,H,K,L,M,N]8ZZ
Non-OR 0D5P[7,8]ZZ
Non-OR 0D5Q4ZZ
Non-OR 0D5Q8ZZ
Non-OR 0D5R4ZZ

0 Medical and Surgical
D Gastrointestinal System
7 Dilation Definition: Expanding an orifice or the lumen of a tubular body part
Explanation: The orifice can be a natural orifice or an artificially created orifice. Accomplished by stretching a tubular body part using intraluminal pressure or by cutting part of the orifice or wall of the tubular body part.

Body Part Character 4	Approach Character 5	Device Character 6	Qualifier Character 7

1 Esophagus, Upper
  Cervical esophagus
2 Esophagus, Middle
  Thoracic esophagus
3 Esophagus, Lower
  Abdominal esophagus
4 Esophagogastric Junction
  Cardia
  Cardioesophageal junction
  Gastroesophageal (GE) junction
5 Esophagus
6 Stomach
7 Stomach, Pylorus
  Pyloric antrum
  Pyloric canal
  Pyloric sphincter
8 Small Intestine
9 Duodenum
A Jejunum
  Duodenojejunal flexure
B Ileum
C Ileocecal Valve
E Large Intestine
F Large Intestine, Right
G Large Intestine, Left
H Cecum
K Ascending Colon
L Transverse Colon
  Hepatic flexure
  Splenic flexure
M Descending Colon
N Sigmoid Colon
  Rectosigmoid junction
  Sigmoid flexure
P Rectum
  Anorectal junction
Q Anus
  Anal orifice
	0 Open
	3 Percutaneous
	4 Percutaneous Endoscopic
	7 Via Natural or Artificial Opening
	8 Via Natural or Artificial Opening Endoscopic
		D Intraluminal Device
		Z No Device
			Z No Qualifier

Non-OR 0D7[1,2,3,4,5,6,8,9,A,B,C,E,F,G,H,K,L,M,N,P,Q][7,8][D,Z]Z
Non-OR 0D77[4,8]DZ
Non-OR 0D777[D,Z]Z
Non-OR 0D7[8,9,A,B,C,E,F,G,H,K,L,M,N][0,3,4]DZ

0 Medical and Surgical
D Gastrointestinal System
8 Division Definition: Cutting into a body part, without draining fluids and/or gases from the body part, in order to separate or transect a body part
Explanation: All or a portion of the body part is separated into two or more portions

Body Part Character 4	Approach Character 5	Device Character 6	Qualifier Character 7

4 Esophagogastric Junction
  Cardia
  Cardioesophageal junction
  Gastroesophageal (GE) junction
7 Stomach, Pylorus
  Pyloric antrum
  Pyloric canal
  Pyloric sphincter
	0 Open
	3 Percutaneous
	4 Percutaneous Endoscopic
	7 Via Natural or Artificial Opening
	8 Via Natural or Artificial Opening Endoscopic
		Z No Device	Z No Qualifier

R Anal Sphincter
  External anal sphincter
  Internal anal sphincter
	0 Open
	3 Percutaneous
		Z No Device	Z No Qualifier

ICD-10-PCS 2025 — Gastrointestinal System — 0D9–0D9

- **0** Medical and Surgical
- **D** Gastrointestinal System
- **9** Drainage
  Definition: Taking or letting out fluids and/or gases from a body part
  Explanation: The qualifier DIAGNOSTIC is used to identify drainage procedures that are biopsies

Body Part — Character 4	Approach — Character 5	Device — Character 6	Qualifier — Character 7
1 Esophagus, Upper Cervical esophagus **2 Esophagus, Middle** Thoracic esophagus **3 Esophagus, Lower** Abdominal esophagus **4 Esophagogastric Junction** Cardia Cardioesophageal junction Gastroesophageal (GE) junction **5 Esophagus** **6 Stomach** **7 Stomach, Pylorus** Pyloric antrum Pyloric canal Pyloric sphincter **8 Small Intestine** **9 Duodenum** **A Jejunum** Duodenojejunal flexure **B Ileum** **C Ileocecal Valve** **E Large Intestine** **F Large Intestine, Right** **G Large Intestine, Left** **H Cecum** **J Appendix** Appendiceal orifice Vermiform appendix **K Ascending Colon** **L Transverse Colon** Hepatic flexure Splenic flexure **M Descending Colon** **N Sigmoid Colon** Rectosigmoid junction Sigmoid flexure **P Rectum** Anorectal junction	**0** Open **3** Percutaneous **4** Percutaneous Endoscopic **7** Via Natural or Artificial Opening **8** Via Natural or Artificial Opening Endoscopic	**0** Drainage Device	**Z** No Qualifier
1 Esophagus, Upper Cervical esophagus **2 Esophagus, Middle** Thoracic esophagus **3 Esophagus, Lower** Abdominal esophagus **4 Esophagogastric Junction** Cardia Cardioesophageal junction Gastroesophageal (GE) junction **5 Esophagus** **6 Stomach** **7 Stomach, Pylorus** Pyloric antrum Pyloric canal Pyloric sphincter **8 Small Intestine** **9 Duodenum** **A Jejunum** Duodenojejunal flexure **B Ileum** **C Ileocecal Valve** **E Large Intestine** **F Large Intestine, Right** **G Large Intestine, Left** **H Cecum** **J Appendix** Appendiceal orifice Vermiform appendix **K Ascending Colon** **L Transverse Colon** Hepatic flexure Splenic flexure **M Descending Colon** **N Sigmoid Colon** Rectosigmoid junction Sigmoid flexure **P Rectum** Anorectal junction	**0** Open **3** Percutaneous **4** Percutaneous Endoscopic **7** Via Natural or Artificial Opening **8** Via Natural or Artificial Opening Endoscopic	**Z** No Device	**X** Diagnostic **Z** No Qualifier
Q Anus Anal orifice	**0** Open **3** Percutaneous **4** Percutaneous Endoscopic **7** Via Natural or Artificial Opening **8** Via Natural or Artificial Opening Endoscopic **X** External	**0** Drainage Device	**Z** No Qualifier
Q Anus Anal orifice	**0** Open **3** Percutaneous **4** Percutaneous Endoscopic **7** Via Natural or Artificial Opening **8** Via Natural or Artificial Opening Endoscopic **X** External	**Z** No Device	**X** Diagnostic **Z** No Qualifier

Non-OR 0D9[1,2,3,4,5,C,J]30Z
Non-OR 0D9[6,7,8,9,A,B,E,F,G,H,K,L,M,N,P][3,7,8]0Z
Non-OR 0D9[1,2,3,4,5,6,7,8,9,A,B,C,E,F,G,H,K,L,M,N,P][3,4,7,8]ZX
Non-OR 0D9[1,2,3,4,5,6,7,8,9,A,B,C,E,F,G,H,J,K,L,M,N,P]3ZZ
Non-OR 0D9Q30Z
Non-OR 0D9Q[0,3,4,7,8,X]ZX
Non-OR 0D9Q3ZZ

0D9 Continued on next page

Gastrointestinal System — ØD9 Continued

0 Medical and Surgical
D Gastrointestinal System
9 Drainage   Definition: Taking or letting out fluids and/or gases from a body part
Explanation: The qualifier DIAGNOSTIC is used to identify drainage procedures that are biopsies

Body Part Character 4	Approach Character 5	Device Character 6	Qualifier Character 7
R Anal Sphincter External anal sphincter Internal anal sphincter **U Omentum** Gastrocolic ligament Gastrocolic omentum Gastrohepatic omentum Gastrophrenic ligament Gastrosplenic ligament Greater Omentum Hepatogastric ligament Lesser Omentum **V Mesentery** Mesoappendix Mesocolon **W Peritoneum** Epiploic foramen	0 Open 3 Percutaneous 4 Percutaneous Endoscopic	0 Drainage Device	Z No Qualifier
R Anal Sphincter External anal sphincter Internal anal sphincter **U Omentum** Gastrocolic ligament Gastrocolic omentum Gastrohepatic omentum Gastrophrenic ligament Gastrosplenic ligament Greater Omentum Hepatogastric ligament Lesser Omentum **V Mesentery** Mesoappendix Mesocolon **W Peritoneum** Epiploic foramen	0 Open 3 Percutaneous 4 Percutaneous Endoscopic	Z No Device	X Diagnostic Z No Qualifier

Non-OR   ØD9[R,W]3ØZ
Non-OR   ØD9[U,V][3,4]ØZ
Non-OR   ØD9[R,U,V,W]3Z[X,Z]
Non-OR   ØD9R[Ø,4]ZX
Non-OR   ØD9[U,V]4ZZ

ICD-10-PCS 2025 — Gastrointestinal System — ØDB–ØDB

- **Ø** Medical and Surgical
- **D** Gastrointestinal System
- **B** Excision **Definition:** Cutting out or off, without replacement, a portion of a body part
  Explanation: The qualifier DIAGNOSTIC is used to identify excision procedures that are biopsies

Body Part Character 4	Approach Character 5	Device Character 6	Qualifier Character 7
1 Esophagus, Upper Cervical esophagus **2 Esophagus, Middle** Thoracic esophagus **3 Esophagus, Lower** Abdominal esophagus **4 Esophagogastric Junction** Cardia Cardioesophageal junction Gastroesophageal (GE) junction **5 Esophagus** **7 Stomach, Pylorus** Pyloric antrum Pyloric canal Pyloric sphincter **8 Small Intestine** **9 Duodenum** **A Jejunum** Duodenojejunal flexure **B Ileum** **C Ileocecal Valve** **E Large Intestine** **H Cecum** **K Ascending Colon** **P Rectum** Anorectal junction	**Ø** Open **3** Percutaneous **4** Percutaneous Endoscopic **7** Via Natural or Artificial Opening **8** Via Natural or Artificial Opening Endoscopic	**Z** No Device	**X** Diagnostic **Z** No Qualifier
6 Stomach	**Ø** Open **3** Percutaneous **4** Percutaneous Endoscopic **7** Via Natural or Artificial Opening **8** Via Natural or Artificial Opening Endoscopic	**Z** No Device	**3** Vertical **X** Diagnostic **Z** No Qualifier
F Large Intestine, Right **J Appendix** Appendiceal orifice Vermiform appendix	**Ø** Open **3** Percutaneous **7** Via Natural or Artificial Opening **8** Via Natural or Artificial Opening Endoscopic	**Z** No Device	**X** Diagnostic **Z** No Qualifier
F Large Intestine, Right **J Appendix** Appendiceal orifice Vermiform appendix	**4** Percutaneous Endoscopic	**Z** No Device	**G** Hand-Assisted **X** Diagnostic **Z** No Qualifier
G Large Intestine, Left **L Transverse Colon** Hepatic flexure Splenic flexure **M Descending Colon** **N Sigmoid Colon** Rectosigmoid junction Sigmoid flexure	**Ø** Open **3** Percutaneous **7** Via Natural or Artificial Opening **8** Via Natural or Artificial Opening Endoscopic	**Z** No Device	**X** Diagnostic **Z** No Qualifier
G Large Intestine, Left **L Transverse Colon** Hepatic flexure Splenic flexure **M Descending Colon** **N Sigmoid Colon** Rectosigmoid junction Sigmoid flexure	**4** Percutaneous Endoscopic	**Z** No Device	**G** Hand-Assisted **X** Diagnostic **Z** No Qualifier
G Large Intestine, Left **L Transverse Colon** Hepatic flexure Splenic flexure **M Descending Colon** **N Sigmoid Colon** Rectosigmoid junction Sigmoid flexure	**F** Via Natural or Artificial Opening with Percutaneous Endoscopic Assistance	**Z** No Device	**Z** No Qualifier
Q Anus Anal orifice	**Ø** Open **3** Percutaneous **4** Percutaneous Endoscopic **7** Via Natural or Artificial Opening **8** Via Natural or Artificial Opening Endoscopic **X** External	**Z** No Device	**X** Diagnostic **Z** No Qualifier
R Anal Sphincter External anal sphincter Internal anal sphincter **U Omentum** Gastrocolic ligament Gastrocolic omentum Gastrohepatic omentum Gastrophrenic ligament Gastrosplenic ligament Greater Omentum Hepatogastric ligament Lesser Omentum **V Mesentery** Mesoappendix Mesocolon **W Peritoneum** Epiploic foramen	**Ø** Open **3** Percutaneous **4** Percutaneous Endoscopic	**Z** No Device	**X** Diagnostic **Z** No Qualifier

Non-OR ØDB[1,2,3,4,5,7,8,9,A,B,C,E,H,K,P][3,4,7,8]ZX
Non-OR ØDB[1,2,3,5,7,9][4,8]ZZ
Non-OR ØDB[4,E,H,K,P]8ZZ
Non-OR ØDB6[3,7,8]ZX
Non-OR ØDB68ZZ
Non-OR ØDBF[3,7,8]ZX
Non-OR ØDBF8ZZ
Non-OR ØDB[G,L,M,N][3,7,8]ZX
Non-OR ØDB[G,L,M,N]8ZZ
Non-OR ØDBQ[0,3,4,7,8,X]ZX
Non-OR ØDBQ8ZZ
Non-OR ØDBR[0,3,4]ZX
Non-OR ØDB[U,V,W][3,4]ZX

Gastrointestinal System

ØDC–ØDC — Gastrointestinal System — ICD-10-PCS 2025

Ø Medical and Surgical
D Gastrointestinal System
C Extirpation — Definition: Taking or cutting out solid matter from a body part
Explanation: The solid matter may be an abnormal byproduct of a biological function or a foreign body; it may be imbedded in a body part or in the lumen of a tubular body part. The solid matter may or may not have been previously broken into pieces.

Body Part Character 4	Approach Character 5	Device Character 6	Qualifier Character 7
1 Esophagus, Upper — Cervical esophagus 2 Esophagus, Middle — Thoracic esophagus 3 Esophagus, Lower — Abdominal esophagus 4 Esophagogastric Junction — Cardia, Cardioesophageal junction, Gastroesophageal (GE) junction 5 Esophagus 6 Stomach 7 Stomach, Pylorus — Pyloric antrum, Pyloric canal, Pyloric sphincter 8 Small Intestine 9 Duodenum A Jejunum — Duodenojejunal flexure B Ileum C Ileocecal Valve E Large Intestine F Large Intestine, Right G Large Intestine, Left H Cecum J Appendix — Appendiceal orifice, Vermiform appendix K Ascending Colon L Transverse Colon — Hepatic flexure, Splenic flexure M Descending Colon N Sigmoid Colon — Rectosigmoid junction, Sigmoid flexure P Rectum — Anorectal junction	Ø Open 3 Percutaneous 4 Percutaneous Endoscopic 7 Via Natural or Artificial Opening 8 Via Natural or Artificial Opening Endoscopic	Z No Device	Z No Qualifier
Q Anus — Anal orifice	Ø Open 3 Percutaneous 4 Percutaneous Endoscopic 7 Via Natural or Artificial Opening 8 Via Natural or Artificial Opening Endoscopic X External	Z No Device	Z No Qualifier
R Anal Sphincter — External anal sphincter, Internal anal sphincter U Omentum — Gastrocolic ligament, Gastrocolic omentum, Gastrohepatic omentum, Gastrophrenic ligament, Gastrosplenic ligament, Greater Omentum, Hepatogastric ligament, Lesser Omentum V Mesentery — Mesoappendix, Mesocolon W Peritoneum — Epiploic foramen	Ø Open 3 Percutaneous 4 Percutaneous Endoscopic	Z No Device	Z No Qualifier

Non-OR ØDC[1,2,3,4,5,6,7,8,9,A,B,C,E,F,G,H,K,L,M,N,P][7,8]ZZ
Non-OR ØDCQ[7,8,X]ZZ

ICD-10-PCS 2025 — Gastrointestinal System — ØDD–ØDD

Ø Medical and Surgical
D Gastrointestinal System
D Extraction Definition: Pulling or stripping out or off all or a portion of a body part by the use of force
Explanation: The qualifier DIAGNOSTIC is used to identify extraction procedures that are biopsies

Body Part — Character 4	Approach — Character 5	Device — Character 6	Qualifier — Character 7
1 Esophagus, Upper Cervical esophagus **2 Esophagus, Middle** Thoracic esophagus **3 Esophagus, Lower** Abdominal esophagus **4 Esophagogastric Junction** Cardia Cardioesophageal junction Gastroesophageal (GE) junction **5 Esophagus** **6 Stomach** **7 Stomach, Pylorus** Pyloric antrum Pyloric canal Pyloric sphincter **8 Small Intestine** **9 Duodenum** **A Jejunum** Duodenojejunal flexure **B Ileum** **C Ileocecal Valve** **E Large Intestine** **F Large Intestine, Right** **G Large Intestine, Left** **H Cecum** **J Appendix** Appendiceal orifice Vermiform appendix **K Ascending Colon** **L Transverse Colon** Hepatic flexure Splenic flexure **M Descending Colon** **N Sigmoid Colon** Rectosigmoid junction Sigmoid flexure **P Rectum** Anorectal junction	3 Percutaneous 4 Percutaneous Endoscopic 8 Via Natural or Artificial Opening Endoscopic	Z No Device	X Diagnostic
Q Anus Anal orifice	3 Percutaneous 4 Percutaneous Endoscopic 8 Via Natural or Artificial Opening Endoscopic X External	Z No Device	X Diagnostic

Non-OR ØDD[1,2,3,4,5,6,7,8,9,A,B,C,E,F,G,H,K,L,M,N,P][3,4,8]ZX
Non-OR ØDDQ[3,4,8,X]ZX

Gastrointestinal System

0 Medical and Surgical
D Gastrointestinal System
F Fragmentation — **Definition:** Breaking solid matter in a body part into pieces
Explanation: Physical force (e.g., manual, ultrasonic) applied directly or indirectly is used to break the solid matter into pieces. The solid matter may be an abnormal byproduct of a biological function or a foreign body. The pieces of solid matter are not taken out.

Body Part Character 4	Approach Character 5	Device Character 6	Qualifier Character 7

5 Esophagus [NC]
6 Stomach [NC]
8 Small Intestine [NC]
9 Duodenum [NC]
A Jejunum [NC]
   Duodenojejunal flexure
B Ileum [NC]
E Large Intestine [NC]
F Large Intestine, Right [NC]
G Large Intestine, Left [NC]
H Cecum [NC]
J Appendix
   Appendiceal orifice
   Vermiform appendix
K Ascending Colon [NC]
L Transverse Colon [NC]
   Hepatic flexure
   Splenic flexure
M Descending Colon [NC]
N Sigmoid Colon [NC]
   Rectosigmoid junction
   Sigmoid flexure
P Rectum [NC]
   Anorectal junction
Q Anus [NC]
   Anal orifice
	0 Open
	3 Percutaneous
	4 Percutaneous Endoscopic
	7 Via Natural or Artificial Opening
	8 Via Natural or Artificial Opening Endoscopic
	X External
		Z No Device	Z No Qualifier

Non-OR 0DF[5,6,8,9,A,B,E,F,G,H,J,K,L,M,N,P,Q]XZZ
NC 0DF[5,6,8,9,A,B,E,F,G,H,J,K,L,M,N,P,Q]XZZ

ICD-10-PCS 2025 — Gastrointestinal System — 0DH–0DH

- 0 Medical and Surgical
- D Gastrointestinal System
- H Insertion — Definition: Putting in a nonbiological appliance that monitors, assists, performs, or prevents a physiological function but does not physically take the place of a body part
  - Explanation: None

Body Part Character 4	Approach Character 5	Device Character 6	Qualifier Character 7
0 Upper Intestinal Tract D Lower Intestinal Tract	0 Open 3 Percutaneous 4 Percutaneous Endoscopic 7 Via Natural or Artificial Opening 8 Via Natural or Artificial Opening Endoscopic	Y Other Device	Z No Qualifier
1 Esophagus, Upper 2 Esophagus, Middle 3 Esophagus, Lower	7 Via Natural or Artificial Opening	J Magnetic Lengthening Device	Z No Qualifier
5 Esophagus	0 Open 3 Percutaneous 4 Percutaneous Endoscopic	1 Radioactive Element 2 Monitoring Device 3 Infusion Device D Intraluminal Device U Feeding Device Y Other Device	Z No Qualifier
5 Esophagus	7 Via Natural or Artificial Opening 8 Via Natural or Artificial Opening Endoscopic	1 Radioactive Element 2 Monitoring Device 3 Infusion Device B Intraluminal Device, Airway D Intraluminal Device U Feeding Device Y Other Device	Z No Qualifier
6 Stomach ✚	0 Open 3 Percutaneous 4 Percutaneous Endoscopic	1 Radioactive Element 2 Monitoring Device 3 Infusion Device D Intraluminal Device M Stimulator Lead U Feeding Device Y Other Device	Z No Qualifier
6 Stomach	7 Via Natural or Artificial Opening 8 Via Natural or Artificial Opening Endoscopic	1 Radioactive Element 2 Monitoring Device 3 Infusion Device D Intraluminal Device U Feeding Device Y Other Device	Z No Qualifier
8 Small Intestine 9 Duodenum A Jejunum Duodenojejunal flexure B Ileum	0 Open 3 Percutaneous 4 Percutaneous Endoscopic 7 Via Natural or Artificial Opening 8 Via Natural or Artificial Opening Endoscopic	1 Radioactive Element 2 Monitoring Device 3 Infusion Device D Intraluminal Device U Feeding Device	Z No Qualifier
E Large Intestine P Rectum Anorectal junction	0 Open 3 Percutaneous 4 Percutaneous Endoscopic 7 Via Natural or Artificial Opening 8 Via Natural or Artificial Opening Endoscopic	1 Radioactive Element D Intraluminal Device	Z No Qualifier
Q Anus Anal orifice	0 Open 3 Percutaneous 4 Percutaneous Endoscopic	D Intraluminal Device L Artificial Sphincter	Z No Qualifier
Q Anus Anal orifice	7 Via Natural or Artificial Opening 8 Via Natural or Artificial Opening Endoscopic	D Intraluminal Device	Z No Qualifier

R Anal Sphincter
   External anal sphincter
   Internal anal sphincter
	0 Open
	3 Percutaneous
	4 Percutaneous Endoscopic
		M Stimulator Lead	Z No Qualifier

Non-OR 0DH[0,D][0,3,4,7,8]YZ
Non-OR 0DH[1,2,3]7JZ
Non-OR 0DH5[0,3,4][D,U]Z
Non-OR 0DH5[3,4]YZ
Non-OR 0DH5[7,8][2,3,B,D,U,Y]Z
Non-OR 0DH631Z
Non-OR 0DH6[0,3,4]UZ
Non-OR 0DH6[3,4]YZ
Non-OR 0DH6[7,8][1,2,3,D,U,Y]Z
Non-OR 0DH[8,9,A,B][0,3,4,7,8][1,D,U]Z
Non-OR 0DH[8,9,A,B][7,8][2,3]Z
Non-OR 0DHE[0,3,4,7,8][1,D]Z
Non-OR 0DHP[0,3,4,7,8]DZ

See Appendix L for Procedure Combinations
✚ 0DH6[0,3,4]MZ

0 Medical and Surgical
D Gastrointestinal System
J Inspection Definition: Visually and/or manually exploring a body part
Explanation: Visual exploration may be performed with or without optical instrumentation. Manual exploration may be performed directly or through intervening body layers.

Body Part Character 4	Approach Character 5	Device Character 6	Qualifier Character 7
0 Upper Intestinal Tract **6** Stomach **D** Lower Intestinal Tract	**0** Open **3** Percutaneous **4** Percutaneous Endoscopic **7** Via Natural or Artificial Opening **8** Via Natural or Artificial Opening Endoscopic **X** External	**Z** No Device	**Z** No Qualifier

U Omentum
  Gastrocolic ligament
  Gastrocolic omentum
  Gastrohepatic omentum
  Gastrophrenic ligament
  Gastrosplenic ligament
  Greater Omentum
  Hepatogastric ligament
  Lesser Omentum
V Mesentery
  Mesoappendix
  Mesocolon
W Peritoneum
  Epiploic foramen
	0 Open
	3 Percutaneous
	4 Percutaneous Endoscopic
	X External
		Z No Device	**Z** No Qualifier

Non-OR 0DJ[0,6,D][3,7,8,X]ZZ
Non-OR 0DJ[U,V,W][3,X]ZZ

ICD-10-PCS 2025 — Gastrointestinal System — 0DL–0DL

0 Medical and Surgical
D Gastrointestinal System
L Occlusion   Definition: Completely closing an orifice or the lumen of a tubular body part
                     Explanation: The orifice can be a natural orifice or an artificially created orifice

Body Part – Character 4	Approach – Character 5	Device – Character 6	Qualifier – Character 7
1 Esophagus, Upper Cervical esophagus **2 Esophagus, Middle** Thoracic esophagus **3 Esophagus, Lower** Abdominal esophagus **4 Esophagogastric Junction** Cardia Cardioesophageal junction Gastroesophageal (GE) junction **5 Esophagus** **6 Stomach** **7 Stomach, Pylorus** Pyloric antrum Pyloric canal Pyloric sphincter **8 Small Intestine** **9 Duodenum** **A Jejunum** Duodenojejunal flexure **B Ileum** **C Ileocecal Valve** **E Large Intestine** **F Large Intestine, Right** **G Large Intestine, Left** **H Cecum** **K Ascending Colon** **L Transverse Colon** Hepatic flexure Splenic flexure **M Descending Colon** **N Sigmoid Colon** Rectosigmoid junction Sigmoid flexure **P Rectum** Anorectal junction	**0** Open **3** Percutaneous **4** Percutaneous Endoscopic	**C** Extraluminal Device **D** Intraluminal Device **Z** No Device	**Z** No Qualifier
1 Esophagus, Upper Cervical esophagus **2 Esophagus, Middle** Thoracic esophagus **3 Esophagus, Lower** Abdominal esophagus **4 Esophagogastric Junction** Cardia Cardioesophageal junction Gastroesophageal (GE) junction **5 Esophagus** **6 Stomach** **7 Stomach, Pylorus** Pyloric antrum Pyloric canal Pyloric sphincter **8 Small Intestine** **9 Duodenum** **A Jejunum** Duodenojejunal flexure **B Ileum** **C Ileocecal Valve** **E Large Intestine** **F Large Intestine, Right** **G Large Intestine, Left** **H Cecum** **K Ascending Colon** **L Transverse Colon** Hepatic flexure Splenic flexure **M Descending Colon** **N Sigmoid Colon** Rectosigmoid junction Sigmoid flexure **P Rectum** Anorectal junction	**7** Via Natural or Artificial Opening **8** Via Natural or Artificial Opening Endoscopic	**D** Intraluminal Device **Z** No Device	**Z** No Qualifier
Q Anus Anal orifice	**0** Open **3** Percutaneous **4** Percutaneous Endoscopic **X** External	**C** Extraluminal Device **D** Intraluminal Device **Z** No Device	**Z** No Qualifier
Q Anus Anal orifice	**7** Via Natural or Artificial Opening **8** Via Natural or Artificial Opening Endoscopic	**D** Intraluminal Device **Z** No Device	**Z** No Qualifier

Non-OR 0DL[1,2,3,4,5][0,3,4][C,D,Z]Z
Non-OR 0DL[1,2,3,4,5][7,8][D,Z]Z

0 Medical and Surgical
D Gastrointestinal System
M Reattachment Definition: Putting back in or on all or a portion of a separated body part to its normal location or other suitable location
Explanation: Vascular circulation and nervous pathways may or may not be reestablished

Body Part Character 4	Approach Character 5	Device Character 6	Qualifier Character 7

5 Esophagus
6 Stomach
8 Small Intestine
9 Duodenum
A Jejunum
  Duodenojejunal flexure
B Ileum
E Large Intestine
F Large Intestine, Right
G Large Intestine, Left
H Cecum
K Ascending Colon
L Transverse Colon
  Hepatic flexure
  Splenic flexure
M Descending Colon
N Sigmoid Colon
  Rectosigmoid junction
  Sigmoid flexure
P Rectum
  Anorectal junction
	0 Open
	4 Percutaneous Endoscopic
		Z No Device	Z No Qualifier

0 Medical and Surgical
D Gastrointestinal System
N Release Definition: Freeing a body part from an abnormal physical constraint by cutting or by the use of force
Explanation: Some of the restraining tissue may be taken out but none of the body part is taken out

Body Part Character 4	Approach Character 5	Device Character 6	Qualifier Character 7

1 Esophagus, Upper
  Cervical esophagus
2 Esophagus, Middle
  Thoracic esophagus
3 Esophagus, Lower
  Abdominal esophagus
4 Esophagogastric Junction
  Cardia
  Cardioesophageal junction
  Gastroesophageal (GE) junction
5 Esophagus
6 Stomach
7 Stomach, Pylorus
  Pyloric antrum
  Pyloric canal
  Pyloric sphincter
8 Small Intestine
9 Duodenum
A Jejunum
  Duodenojejunal flexure
B Ileum
C Ileocecal Valve
E Large Intestine
F Large Intestine, Right
G Large Intestine, Left
H Cecum
J Appendix
  Appendiceal orifice
  Vermiform appendix
K Ascending Colon
L Transverse Colon
  Hepatic flexure
  Splenic flexure
M Descending Colon
N Sigmoid Colon
  Rectosigmoid junction
  Sigmoid flexure
P Rectum
  Anorectal junction
	0 Open
	3 Percutaneous
	4 Percutaneous Endoscopic
	7 Via Natural or Artificial Opening
	8 Via Natural or Artificial Opening Endoscopic
		Z No Device	Z No Qualifier

Q Anus Anal orifice	0 Open 3 Percutaneous 4 Percutaneous Endoscopic 7 Via Natural or Artificial Opening 8 Via Natural or Artificial Opening Endoscopic X External	Z No Device	Z No Qualifier

R Anal Sphincter
  External anal sphincter
  Internal anal sphincter
U Omentum
  Gastrocolic ligament
  Gastrocolic omentum
  Gastrohepatic omentum
  Gastrophrenic ligament
  Gastrosplenic ligament
  Greater Omentum
  Hepatogastric ligament
  Lesser Omentum
V Mesentery
  Mesoappendix
  Mesocolon
W Peritoneum
  Epiploic foramen
	0 Open
	3 Percutaneous
	4 Percutaneous Endoscopic
		Z No Device	Z No Qualifier

Non-OR 0DN[8,9,A,B,E,F,G,H,K,L,M,N][7,8]ZZ

0 Medical and Surgical
D Gastrointestinal System
P Removal   Definition: Taking out or off a device from a body part
Explanation: If a device is taken out and a similar device put in without cutting or puncturing the skin or mucous membrane, the procedure is coded to the root operation CHANGE. Otherwise, the procedure for taking out a device is coded to the root operation REMOVAL.

Body Part Character 4	Approach Character 5	Device Character 6	Qualifier Character 7
0 Upper Intestinal Tract D Lower Intestinal Tract	0 Open 3 Percutaneous 4 Percutaneous Endoscopic 7 Via Natural or Artificial Opening 8 Via Natural or Artificial Opening Endoscopic	0 Drainage Device 2 Monitoring Device 3 Infusion Device 7 Autologous Tissue Substitute C Extraluminal Device D Intraluminal Device J Synthetic Substitute K Nonautologous Tissue Substitute U Feeding Device Y Other Device	Z No Qualifier
0 Upper Intestinal Tract D Lower Intestinal Tract	X External	0 Drainage Device 2 Monitoring Device 3 Infusion Device D Intraluminal Device U Feeding Device	Z No Qualifier
5 Esophagus	0 Open 3 Percutaneous 4 Percutaneous Endoscopic	1 Radioactive Element 2 Monitoring Device 3 Infusion Device U Feeding Device Y Other Device	Z No Qualifier
5 Esophagus	7 Via Natural or Artificial Opening 8 Via Natural or Artificial Opening Endoscopic	1 Radioactive Element D Intraluminal Device Y Other Device	Z No Qualifier
5 Esophagus	X External	1 Radioactive Element 2 Monitoring Device 3 Infusion Device D Intraluminal Device U Feeding Device	Z No Qualifier
6 Stomach	0 Open 3 Percutaneous 4 Percutaneous Endoscopic	0 Drainage Device 2 Monitoring Device 3 Infusion Device 7 Autologous Tissue Substitute C Extraluminal Device D Intraluminal Device J Synthetic Substitute K Nonautologous Tissue Substitute M Stimulator Lead U Feeding Device Y Other Device	Z No Qualifier
6 Stomach	7 Via Natural or Artificial Opening 8 Via Natural or Artificial Opening Endoscopic	0 Drainage Device 2 Monitoring Device 3 Infusion Device 7 Autologous Tissue Substitute C Extraluminal Device D Intraluminal Device J Synthetic Substitute K Nonautologous Tissue Substitute U Feeding Device Y Other Device	Z No Qualifier
6 Stomach	X External	0 Drainage Device 2 Monitoring Device 3 Infusion Device D Intraluminal Device U Feeding Device	Z No Qualifier

Non-OR   0DP[0,D][3,4]YZ
Non-OR   0DP[0,D][7,8][0,2,3,D,U,Y]Z
Non-OR   0DP[0,D]X[0,2,3,D,U]Z
Non-OR   0DP5[3,4]YZ
Non-OR   0DP5[7,8][1,D,Y]Z
Non-OR   0DP5X[1,2,3,D,U]Z
Non-OR   0DP6[3,4]YZ
Non-OR   0DP6[7,8][0,2,3,D,U,Y]Z
Non-OR   0DP6X[0,2,3,D,U]Z

0DP Continued on next page

0DP–0DP   Gastrointestinal System   ICD-10-PCS 2025

0DP Continued

- **0** Medical and Surgical
- **D** Gastrointestinal System
- **P** Removal   Definition: Taking out or off a device from a body part

Explanation: If a device is taken out and a similar device put in without cutting or puncturing the skin or mucous membrane, the procedure is coded to the root operation CHANGE. Otherwise, the procedure for taking out a device is coded to the root operation REMOVAL.

Body Part Character 4	Approach Character 5	Device Character 6	Qualifier Character 7
P Rectum Anorectal junction	**0** Open **3** Percutaneous **4** Percutaneous Endoscopic **7** Via Natural or Artificial Opening **8** Via Natural or Artificial Opening Endoscopic **X** External	**1** Radioactive Element	**Z** No Qualifier
Q Anus Anal orifice	**0** Open **3** Percutaneous **4** Percutaneous Endoscopic **7** Via Natural or Artificial Opening **8** Via Natural or Artificial Opening Endoscopic	**L** Artificial Sphincter	**Z** No Qualifier

R Anal Sphincter
    External anal sphincter
    Internal anal sphincter
	0 Open
	3 Percutaneous
	4 Percutaneous Endoscopic
		M Stimulator Lead	**Z** No Qualifier

U Omentum
    Gastrocolic ligament
    Gastrocolic omentum
    Gastrohepatic omentum
    Gastrophrenic ligament
    Gastrosplenic ligament
    Greater Omentum
    Hepatogastric ligament
    Lesser Omentum
V Mesentery
    Mesoappendix
    Mesocolon
W Peritoneum
    Epiploic foramen
	0 Open
	3 Percutaneous
	4 Percutaneous Endoscopic
		0 Drainage Device
		1 Radioactive Element
		7 Autologous Tissue Substitute
		J Synthetic Substitute
		K Nonautologous Tissue Substitute
			Z No Qualifier

Non-OR   0DPP[7,8,X]1Z

ICD-10-PCS 2025 — Gastrointestinal System — 0DQ–0DQ

- 0 Medical and Surgical
- D Gastrointestinal System
- Q Repair Definition: Restoring, to the extent possible, a body part to its normal anatomic structure and function
  Explanation: Used only when the method to accomplish the repair is not one of the other root operations

Body Part Character 4	Approach Character 5	Device Character 6	Qualifier Character 7
1 Esophagus, Upper 　Cervical esophagus 2 Esophagus, Middle 　Thoracic esophagus 3 Esophagus, Lower 　Abdominal esophagus 4 Esophagogastric Junction 　Cardia 　Cardioesophageal junction 　Gastroesophageal (GE) junction 5 Esophagus 6 Stomach 7 Stomach, Pylorus 　Pyloric antrum 　Pyloric canal 　Pyloric sphincter 8 Small Intestine ✚ 9 Duodenum ✚ A Jejunum ✚ 　Duodenojejunal flexure B Ileum ✚ C Ileocecal Valve E Large Intestine ✚ F Large Intestine, Right ✚ G Large Intestine, Left ✚ H Cecum J Appendix 　Appendiceal orifice 　Vermiform appendix K Ascending Colon ✚ L Transverse Colon ✚ 　Hepatic flexure 　Splenic flexure M Descending Colon ✚ N Sigmoid Colon ✚ 　Rectosigmoid junction 　Sigmoid flexure P Rectum 　Anorectal junction	0 Open 3 Percutaneous 4 Percutaneous Endoscopic 7 Via Natural or Artificial Opening 8 Via Natural or Artificial Opening Endoscopic	Z No Device	Z No Qualifier
Q Anus 　Anal orifice	0 Open 3 Percutaneous 4 Percutaneous Endoscopic 7 Via Natural or Artificial Opening 8 Via Natural or Artificial Opening Endoscopic X External	Z No Device	Z No Qualifier
R Anal Sphincter 　External anal sphincter 　Internal anal sphincter U Omentum 　Gastrocolic ligament 　Gastrocolic omentum 　Gastrohepatic omentum 　Gastrophrenic ligament 　Gastrosplenic ligament 　Greater Omentum 　Hepatogastric ligament 　Lesser Omentum V Mesentery 　Mesoappendix 　Mesocolon W Peritoneum 　Epiploic foramen	0 Open 3 Percutaneous 4 Percutaneous Endoscopic	Z No Device	Z No Qualifier

See Appendix L for Procedure Combinations
✚　0DQ[8,9,A,B,E,F,G,H,K,L,M,N]0ZZ

0DR–0DS — Gastrointestinal System — ICD-10-PCS 2025

0 Medical and Surgical
D Gastrointestinal System
R Replacement

Definition: Putting in or on biological or synthetic material that physically takes the place and/or function of all or a portion of a body part
Explanation: The body part may have been taken out or replaced, or may be taken out, physically eradicated, or rendered nonfunctional during the REPLACEMENT procedure. A REMOVAL procedure is coded for taking out the device used in a previous replacement procedure.

Body Part Character 4	Approach Character 5	Device Character 6	Qualifier Character 7
5 Esophagus	**0** Open **4** Percutaneous Endoscopic **7** Via Natural or Artificial Opening **8** Via Natural or Artificial Opening Endoscopic	**7** Autologous Tissue Substitute **J** Synthetic Substitute **K** Nonautologous Tissue Substitute	**Z** No Qualifier

R Anal Sphincter
  External anal sphincter
  Internal anal sphincter
U Omentum
  Gastrocolic ligament
  Gastrocolic omentum
  Gastrohepatic omentum
  Gastrophrenic ligament
  Gastrosplenic ligament
  Greater Omentum
  Hepatogastric ligament
  Lesser Omentum
V Mesentery
  Mesoappendix
  Mesocolon
W Peritoneum
  Epiploic foramen
	0 Open
	4 Percutaneous Endoscopic
		7 Autologous Tissue Substitute
		J Synthetic Substitute
		K Nonautologous Tissue Substitute
			Z No Qualifier

0 Medical and Surgical
D Gastrointestinal System
S Reposition

Definition: Moving to its normal location, or other suitable location, all or a portion of a body part
Explanation: The body part is moved to a new location from an abnormal location, or from a normal location where it is not functioning correctly. The body part may or may not be cut out or off to be moved to the new location.

Body Part Character 4	Approach Character 5	Device Character 6	Qualifier Character 7

5 Esophagus
6 Stomach
9 Duodenum
A Jejunum
  Duodenojejunal flexure
B Ileum
H Cecum
K Ascending Colon
L Transverse Colon
  Hepatic flexure
  Splenic flexure
M Descending Colon
N Sigmoid Colon
  Rectosigmoid junction
  Sigmoid flexure
P Rectum
  Anorectal junction
Q Anus
  Anal orifice
	0 Open
	4 Percutaneous Endoscopic
	7 Via Natural or Artificial Opening
	8 Via Natural or Artificial Opening Endoscopic
	X External
		Z No Device	**Z** No Qualifier

8 Small Intestine **E** Large Intestine	**0** Open **4** Percutaneous Endoscopic **7** Via Natural or Artificial Opening **8** Via Natural or Artificial Opening Endoscopic	**Z** No Device	**Z** No Qualifier

Non-OR   0DS[5,6,9,A,B,H,K,L,M,N,P,Q]XZZ

0	Medical and Surgical		
D	Gastrointestinal System		
T	Resection	Definition: Cutting out or off, without replacement, all of a body part	
		Explanation: None	

Body Part Character 4	Approach Character 5	Device Character 6	Qualifier Character 7
1 Esophagus, Upper 　Cervical esophagus **2** Esophagus, Middle 　Thoracic esophagus **3** Esophagus, Lower 　Abdominal esophagus **4** Esophagogastric Junction 　Cardia 　Cardioesophageal junction 　Gastroesophageal (GE) junction **5** Esophagus **6** Stomach **7** Stomach, Pylorus 　Pyloric antrum 　Pyloric canal 　Pyloric sphincter **8** Small Intestine **9** Duodenum ✚ **A** Jejunum 　Duodenojejunal flexure **B** Ileum **C** Ileocecal Valve **E** Large Intestine **H** Cecum **K** Ascending Colon **P** Rectum 　Anorectal junction **Q** Anus 　Anal orifice	**0** Open **4** Percutaneous Endoscopic **7** Via Natural or Artificial Opening **8** Via Natural or Artificial Opening Endoscopic	**Z** No Device	**Z** No Qualifier
F Large Intestine, Right **J** Appendix 　Appendiceal orifice 　Vermiform appendix	**0** Open **7** Via Natural or Artificial Opening **8** Via Natural or Artificial Opening Endoscopic	**Z** No Device	**Z** No Qualifier
F Large Intestine, Right **J** Appendix 　Appendiceal orifice 　Vermiform appendix	**4** Percutaneous Endoscopic	**Z** No Device	**G** Hand-Assisted **Z** No Qualifier
G Large Intestine, Left **L** Transverse Colon 　Hepatic flexure 　Splenic flexure **M** Descending Colon **N** Sigmoid Colon 　Rectosigmoid junction 　Sigmoid flexure	**0** Open **7** Via Natural or Artificial Opening **8** Via Natural or Artificial Opening Endoscopic **F** Via Natural or Artificial Opening with Percutaneous Endoscopic Assistance	**Z** No Device	**Z** No Qualifier
G Large Intestine, Left **L** Transverse Colon 　Hepatic flexure 　Splenic flexure **M** Descending Colon **N** Sigmoid Colon 　Rectosigmoid junction 　Sigmoid flexure	**4** Percutaneous Endoscopic	**Z** No Device	**G** Hand-Assisted **Z** No Qualifier
R Anal Sphincter 　External anal sphincter 　Internal anal sphincter **U** Omentum 　Gastrocolic ligament 　Gastrocolic omentum 　Gastrohepatic omentum 　Gastrophrenic ligament 　Gastrosplenic ligament 　Greater Omentum 　Hepatogastric ligament 　Lesser Omentum	**0** Open **4** Percutaneous Endoscopic	**Z** No Device	**Z** No Qualifier

See Appendix L for Procedure Combinations
　✚　0DT90ZZ

ØDU–ØDU Gastrointestinal System ICD-10-PCS 2025

Ø Medical and Surgical
D Gastrointestinal System
U Supplement — Definition: Putting in or on biological or synthetic material that physically reinforces and/or augments the function of a portion of a body part
Explanation: The biological material is non-living, or is living and from the same individual. The body part may have been previously replaced, and the SUPPLEMENT procedure is performed to physically reinforce and/or augment the function of the replaced body part.

Body Part Character 4	Approach Character 5	Device Character 6	Qualifier Character 7

1 Esophagus, Upper
  Cervical esophagus
2 Esophagus, Middle
  Thoracic esophagus
3 Esophagus, Lower
  Abdominal esophagus
4 Esophagogastric Junction
  Cardia
  Cardioesophageal junction
  Gastroesophageal (GE) junction
5 Esophagus
6 Stomach
7 Stomach, Pylorus
  Pyloric antrum
  Pyloric canal
  Pyloric sphincter
8 Small Intestine
9 Duodenum
A Jejunum
  Duodenojejunal flexure
B Ileum
C Ileocecal Valve
E Large Intestine
F Large Intestine, Right
G Large Intestine, Left
H Cecum
K Ascending Colon
L Transverse Colon
  Hepatic flexure
  Splenic flexure
M Descending Colon
N Sigmoid Colon
  Rectosigmoid junction
  Sigmoid flexure
P Rectum
  Anorectal junction
	Ø Open
	4 Percutaneous Endoscopic
	7 Via Natural or Artificial Opening
	8 Via Natural or Artificial Opening Endoscopic
		7 Autologous Tissue Substitute
		J Synthetic Substitute
		K Nonautologous Tissue Substitute
			Z No Qualifier

Q Anus Anal orifice	Ø Open 4 Percutaneous Endoscopic 7 Via Natural or Artificial Opening 8 Via Natural or Artificial Opening Endoscopic X External	7 Autologous Tissue Substitute J Synthetic Substitute K Nonautologous Tissue Substitute	Z No Qualifier

R Anal Sphincter
  External anal sphincter
  Internal anal sphincter
U Omentum
  Gastrocolic ligament
  Gastrocolic omentum
  Gastrohepatic omentum
  Gastrophrenic ligament
  Gastrosplenic ligament
  Greater Omentum
  Hepatogastric ligament
  Lesser Omentum
V Mesentery
  Mesoappendix
  Mesocolon
W Peritoneum
  Epiploic foramen
	Ø Open
	4 Percutaneous Endoscopic
		7 Autologous Tissue Substitute
		J Synthetic Substitute
		K Nonautologous Tissue Substitute
			Z No Qualifier

Non-OR Procedure   DRG Non-OR Procedure   Valid OR Procedure   HAC Associated Procedure   Combination Only   New/Revised April   New/Revised October

ICD-10-PCS 2025 — Gastrointestinal System — 0DV–0DV

- **0** Medical and Surgical
- **D** Gastrointestinal System
- **V** Restriction
  Definition: Partially closing an orifice or the lumen of a tubular body part
  Explanation: The orifice can be a natural orifice or an artificially created orifice

Body Part — Character 4	Approach — Character 5	Device — Character 6	Qualifier — Character 7
1 Esophagus, Upper — Cervical esophagus 2 Esophagus, Middle — Thoracic esophagus 3 Esophagus, Lower — Abdominal esophagus 4 Esophagogastric Junction — Cardia, Cardioesophageal junction, Gastroesophageal (GE) junction 5 Esophagus 6 Stomach 7 Stomach, Pylorus — Pyloric antrum, Pyloric canal, Pyloric sphincter 8 Small Intestine 9 Duodenum A Jejunum — Duodenojejunal flexure B Ileum C Ileocecal Valve E Large Intestine F Large Intestine, Right G Large Intestine, Left H Cecum K Ascending Colon L Transverse Colon — Hepatic flexure, Splenic flexure M Descending Colon N Sigmoid Colon — Rectosigmoid junction, Sigmoid flexure P Rectum — Anorectal junction	0 Open 3 Percutaneous 4 Percutaneous Endoscopic	C Extraluminal Device D Intraluminal Device Z No Device	Z No Qualifier
1 Esophagus, Upper — Cervical esophagus 2 Esophagus, Middle — Thoracic esophagus 3 Esophagus, Lower — Abdominal esophagus 4 Esophagogastric Junction — Cardia, Cardioesophageal junction, Gastroesophageal (GE) junction 5 Esophagus 6 Stomach **NC** 7 Stomach, Pylorus — Pyloric antrum, Pyloric canal, Pyloric sphincter 8 Small Intestine 9 Duodenum A Jejunum — Duodenojejunal flexure B Ileum C Ileocecal Valve E Large Intestine F Large Intestine, Right G Large Intestine, Left H Cecum K Ascending Colon L Transverse Colon — Hepatic flexure, Splenic flexure M Descending Colon N Sigmoid Colon — Rectosigmoid junction, Sigmoid flexure P Rectum — Anorectal junction	7 Via Natural or Artificial Opening 8 Via Natural or Artificial Opening Endoscopic	D Intraluminal Device Z No Device	Z No Qualifier
Q Anus — Anal orifice	0 Open 3 Percutaneous 4 Percutaneous Endoscopic X External	C Extraluminal Device D Intraluminal Device Z No Device	Z No Qualifier
Q Anus — Anal orifice	7 Via Natural or Artificial Opening 8 Via Natural or Artificial Opening Endoscopic	D Intraluminal Device Z No Device	Z No Qualifier

Non-OR 0DV6[7,8]DZ
HAC 0DV64CZ when reported with PDx E66.01 and SDx K68.11, K95.01, K95.81, or T81.40–T81.49 with 7th character A
NC 0DV6[7,8]DZ

NC Noncovered Procedure **LC** Limited Coverage **QA** Questionable OB Admit **NT** New Tech Add-on ✚ Combination Member ♂ Male ♀ Female

Gastrointestinal System

0 Medical and Surgical
D Gastrointestinal System
W Revision Definition: Correcting, to the extent possible, a portion of a malfunctioning device or the position of a displaced device
Explanation: Revision can include correcting a malfunctioning or displaced device by taking out or putting in components of the device such as a screw or pin

Body Part Character 4	Approach Character 5	Device Character 6	Qualifier Character 7
0 Upper Intestinal Tract D Lower Intestinal Tract	0 Open 3 Percutaneous 4 Percutaneous Endoscopic 7 Via Natural or Artificial Opening 8 Via Natural or Artificial Opening Endoscopic	0 Drainage Device 2 Monitoring Device 3 Infusion Device 7 Autologous Tissue Substitute C Extraluminal Device D Intraluminal Device J Synthetic Substitute K Nonautologous Tissue Substitute U Feeding Device Y Other Device	Z No Qualifier
0 Upper Intestinal Tract D Lower Intestinal Tract	X External	0 Drainage Device 2 Monitoring Device 3 Infusion Device 7 Autologous Tissue Substitute C Extraluminal Device D Intraluminal Device J Synthetic Substitute K Nonautologous Tissue Substitute U Feeding Device	Z No Qualifier
5 Esophagus	0 Open 3 Percutaneous 4 Percutaneous Endoscopic	Y Other Device	Z No Qualifier
5 Esophagus	7 Via Natural or Artificial Opening 8 Via Natural or Artificial Opening Endoscopic	D Intraluminal Device Y Other Device	Z No Qualifier
5 Esophagus	X External	D Intraluminal Device	Z No Qualifier
6 Stomach	0 Open 3 Percutaneous 4 Percutaneous Endoscopic	0 Drainage Device 2 Monitoring Device 3 Infusion Device 7 Autologous Tissue Substitute C Extraluminal Device D Intraluminal Device J Synthetic Substitute K Nonautologous Tissue Substitute M Stimulator Lead U Feeding Device Y Other Device	Z No Qualifier
6 Stomach	7 Via Natural or Artificial Opening 8 Via Natural or Artificial Opening Endoscopic	0 Drainage Device 2 Monitoring Device 3 Infusion Device 7 Autologous Tissue Substitute C Extraluminal Device D Intraluminal Device J Synthetic Substitute K Nonautologous Tissue Substitute U Feeding Device Y Other Device	Z No Qualifier
6 Stomach	X External	0 Drainage Device 2 Monitoring Device 3 Infusion Device 7 Autologous Tissue Substitute C Extraluminal Device D Intraluminal Device J Synthetic Substitute K Nonautologous Tissue Substitute U Feeding Device	Z No Qualifier

Non-OR 0DW[0,D][3,4,7,8]YZ
Non-OR 0DW[0,D]8UZ
Non-OR 0DW[0,D]X[0,2,3,7,C,D,J,K,U]Z
Non-OR 0DW5[0,3,4]YZ
Non-OR 0DW5[7,8]YZ
Non-OR 0DW5XDZ
Non-OR 0DW6[3,4]YZ
Non-OR 0DW68UZ
Non-OR 0DW6[7,8]YZ
Non-OR 0DW6X[0,2,3,7,C,D,J,K,U]Z

0DW Continued on next page

0 Medical and Surgical
D Gastrointestinal System
W Revision

Definition: Correcting, to the extent possible, a portion of a malfunctioning device or the position of a displaced device

Explanation: Revision can include correcting a malfunctioning or displaced device by taking out or putting in components of the device such as a screw or pin

Body Part Character 4	Approach Character 5	Device Character 6	Qualifier Character 7
8 Small Intestine E Large Intestine	0 Open 4 Percutaneous Endoscopic 7 Via Natural or Artificial Opening 8 Via Natural or Artificial Opening Endoscopic	7 Autologous Tissue Substitute J Synthetic Substitute K Nonautologous Tissue Substitute	Z No Qualifier
Q Anus Anal orifice	0 Open 3 Percutaneous 4 Percutaneous Endoscopic 7 Via Natural or Artificial Opening 8 Via Natural or Artificial Opening Endoscopic	L Artificial Sphincter	Z No Qualifier

R Anal Sphincter
   External anal sphincter
   Internal anal sphincter
	0 Open
	3 Percutaneous
	4 Percutaneous Endoscopic
		M Stimulator Lead	Z No Qualifier

U Omentum
   Gastrocolic ligament
   Gastrocolic omentum
   Gastrohepatic omentum
   Gastrophrenic ligament
   Gastrosplenic ligament
   Greater Omentum
   Hepatogastric ligament
   Lesser Omentum
V Mesentery
   Mesoappendix
   Mesocolon
W Peritoneum
   Epiploic foramen
	0 Open
	3 Percutaneous
	4 Percutaneous Endoscopic
		0 Drainage Device
		7 Autologous Tissue Substitute
		J Synthetic Substitute
		K Nonautologous Tissue Substitute
			Z No Qualifier

Non-OR 0DW[U,V,W][0,3,4]0Z

0 Medical and Surgical
D Gastrointestinal System
X Transfer

Definition: Moving, without taking out, all or a portion of a body part to another location to take over the function of all or a portion of a body part

Explanation: The body part transferred remains connected to its vascular and nervous supply

Body Part Character 4	Approach Character 5	Device Character 6	Qualifier Character 7
6 Stomach	0 Open 4 Percutaneous Endoscopic	Z No Device	5 Esophagus
8 Small Intestine	0 Open 4 Percutaneous Endoscopic	Z No Device	5 Esophagus B Bladder C Ureter, Right D Ureter, Left F Ureters, Bilateral
E Large Intestine	0 Open 4 Percutaneous Endoscopic	Z No Device	5 Esophagus 7 Vagina B Bladder

U Omentum
   Gastrocolic ligament
   Gastrocolic omentum
   Gastrohepatic omentum
   Gastrophrenic ligament
   Gastrosplenic ligament
   Greater omentum
   Hepatogastric ligament
   Lesser omentum
	0 Open
	4 Percutaneous Endoscopic
		Z No Device	V Thoracic Region
			W Abdominal Region
			X Pelvic Region
			Y Inguinal Region

0 **Medical and Surgical**
D **Gastrointestinal System**
Y **Transplantation** Definition: Putting in or on all or a portion of a living body part taken from another individual or animal to physically take the place and/or function of all or a portion of a similar body part
Explanation: The native body part may or may not be taken out, and the transplanted body part may take over all or a portion of its function

Body Part Character 4	Approach Character 5	Device Character 6	Qualifier Character 7
5 Esophagus 6 Stomach 8 Small Intestine LC E Large Intestine LC	0 Open	Z No Device	0 Allogeneic 1 Syngeneic 2 Zooplastic

Non-OR 0DY50Z[0,1,2]
LC 0DY[8,E]0Z[0,1,2]

Hepatobiliary System and Pancreas 0F1–0FY

Character Meanings

This Character Meaning table is provided as a guide to assist the user in the identification of character members that may be found in this section of code tables. It **SHOULD NOT** be used to build a PCS code.

Operation–Character 3		Body Part–Character 4		Approach–Character 5		Device–Character 6		Qualifier–Character 7	
1	Bypass	0	Liver	0	Open	0	Drainage Device	0	Allogeneic
2	Change	1	Liver, Right Lobe	3	Percutaneous	1	Radioactive Element	1	Syngeneic
5	Destruction	2	Liver, Left Lobe	4	Percutaneous Endoscopic	2	Monitoring Device	2	Zooplastic
7	Dilation	4	Gallbladder	7	Via Natural or Artificial Opening	3	Infusion Device	3	Duodenum OR Laser Interstitial Thermal Therapy
8	Division	5	Hepatic Duct, Right	8	Via Natural or Artificial Opening Endoscopic	7	Autologous Tissue Substitute	4	Stomach
9	Drainage	6	Hepatic Duct, Left	X	External	C	Extraluminal Device	5	Hepatic Duct, Right
B	Excision	7	Hepatic Duct, Common			D	Intraluminal Device	6	Hepatic Duct, Left
C	Extirpation	8	Cystic Duct			J	Synthetic Substitute	7	Hepatic Duct, Caudate
D	Extraction	9	Common Bile Duct			K	Nonautologous Tissue Substitute	8	Cystic Duct
F	Fragmentation	B	Hepatobiliary Duct			Y	Other Device	9	Common Bile Duct
H	Insertion	C	Ampulla of Vater			Z	No Device	B	Small Intestine
J	Inspection	D	Pancreatic Duct					C	Large Intestine
L	Occlusion	F	Pancreatic Duct, Accessory					F	Irreversible Electroporation
M	Reattachment	G	Pancreas					G	Hand-Assisted
N	Release							X	Diagnostic
P	Removal							Z	No Qualifier
Q	Repair								
R	Replacement								
S	Reposition								
T	Resection								
U	Supplement								
V	Restriction								
W	Revision								
Y	Transplantation								

AHA Coding Clinic for table 0F1
2020, 4Q, 53   Bypass pancreatic duct to stomach

AHA Coding Clinic for table 0F5
2022, 4Q, 53-54   Laser interstitial thermal therapy
2018, 4Q, 39   Irreversible electroporation

AHA Coding Clinic for table 0F7
2016, 3Q, 27   Endoscopic retrograde cholangiopancreatography with sphincterotomy and insertion of pancreatic stent
2016, 1Q, 25   Endoscopic retrograde cholangiopancreatography with brush biopsy of pancreatic and common bile ducts
2015, 1Q, 32   Percutaneous transhepatic biliary drainage catheter placement
2014, 3Q, 15   Drainage of pancreatic pseudocyst

AHA Coding Clinic for table 0F8
2021, 4Q, 48-49   Division of liver for staged hepatectomy

AHA Coding Clinic for table 0F9
2023, 2Q, 22   Direct endoscopic necrosectomy
2020, 3Q, 34   Cystogastrostomy with stent insertion
2015, 1Q, 32   Percutaneous transhepatic biliary drainage catheter placement
2014, 3Q, 15   Drainage of pancreatic pseudocyst

AHA Coding Clinic for table 0FB
2024, 1Q, 7   Percutaneous endoscopic hand-assisted approach
2023, 2Q, 22   Direct endoscopic necrosectomy
2023, 1Q, 38   Ex-vivo liver tumor resection and autotransplantation
2019, 1Q, 3-8   Whipple procedure
2016, 3Q, 41   Open cholecystectomy with needle biopsy of liver
2016, 1Q, 23   Endoscopic ultrasound with aspiration biopsy of common hepatic duct
2016, 1Q, 25   Endoscopic retrograde cholangiopancreatography with brush biopsy of pancreatic and common bile ducts
2014, 3Q, 32   Pyloric-sparing Whipple procedure

AHA Coding Clinic for table 0FC
2023, 2Q, 22   Direct endoscopic necrosectomy
2016, 3Q, 27   Endoscopic retrograde cholangiopancreatography with sphincterotomy and insertion of pancreatic stent

AHA Coding Clinic for table 0FD
2023, 2Q, 22   Direct endoscopic necrosectomy

AHA Coding Clinic for table 0FH
2022, 2Q, 26   Radioembolization of right hepatic lobe
2020, 4Q, 43-44   Insertion of radioactive element

AHA Coding Clinic for table 0FQ
2016, 3Q, 27   Revision of common bile duct anastomosis
2013, 4Q, 109   Separating conjoined twins

AHA Coding Clinic for table 0FT
2024, 1Q, 7   Percutaneous endoscopic hand-assisted approach
2021, 4Q, 49   Division of liver for staged hepatectomy
2019, 1Q, 3-8   Whipple procedure
2012, 4Q, 99   Domino liver transplant

AHA Coding Clinic for table 0FY
2023, 2Q, 32   Preparation of donor organ before transplantation
2023, 1Q, 38   Ex-vivo liver tumor resection and autotransplantation
2014, 3Q, 13   Orthotopic liver transplant with end to side cavoplasty
2012, 4Q, 99   Domino liver transplant

Hepatobiliary System and Pancreas

Liver

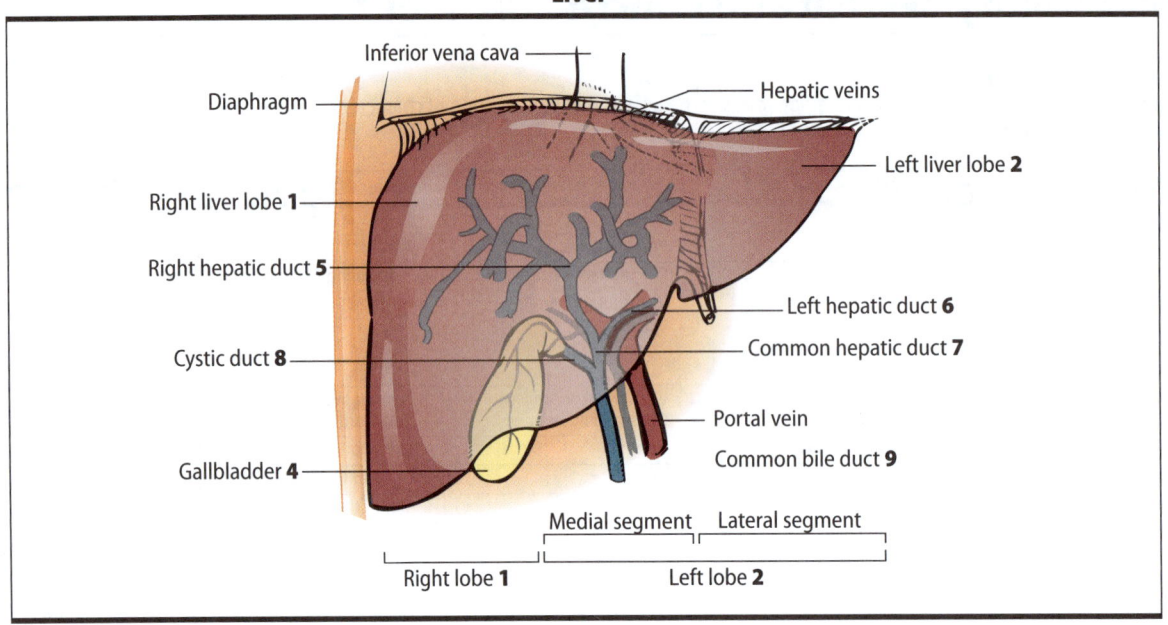

- Inferior vena cava
- Diaphragm
- Hepatic veins
- Right liver lobe 1
- Left liver lobe 2
- Right hepatic duct 5
- Left hepatic duct 6
- Cystic duct 8
- Common hepatic duct 7
- Gallbladder 4
- Portal vein
- Common bile duct 9
- Medial segment
- Lateral segment
- Right lobe 1
- Left lobe 2

Pancreas

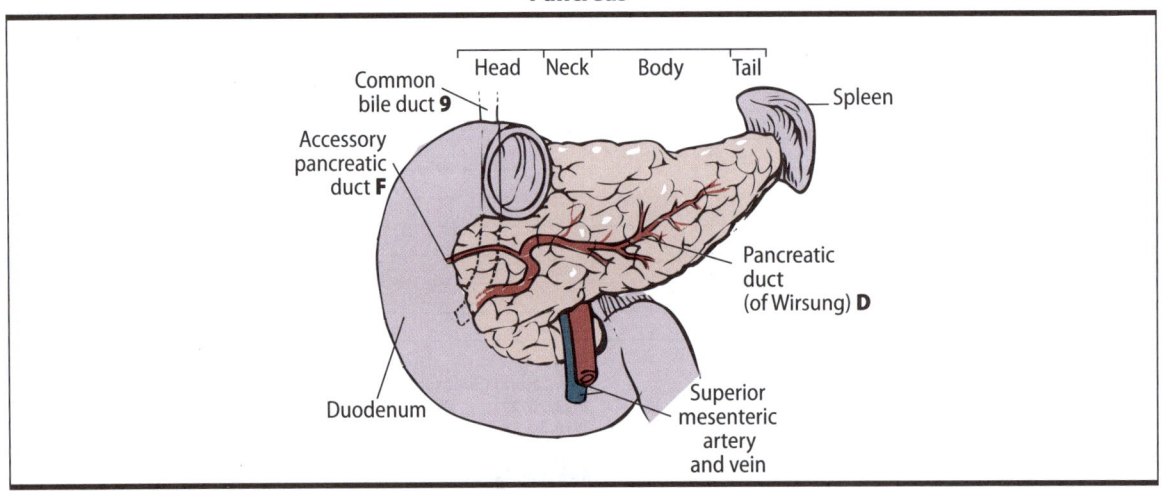

- Head, Neck, Body, Tail
- Common bile duct 9
- Spleen
- Accessory pancreatic duct F
- Pancreatic duct (of Wirsung) D
- Duodenum
- Superior mesenteric artery and vein

Gallbladder and Ducts

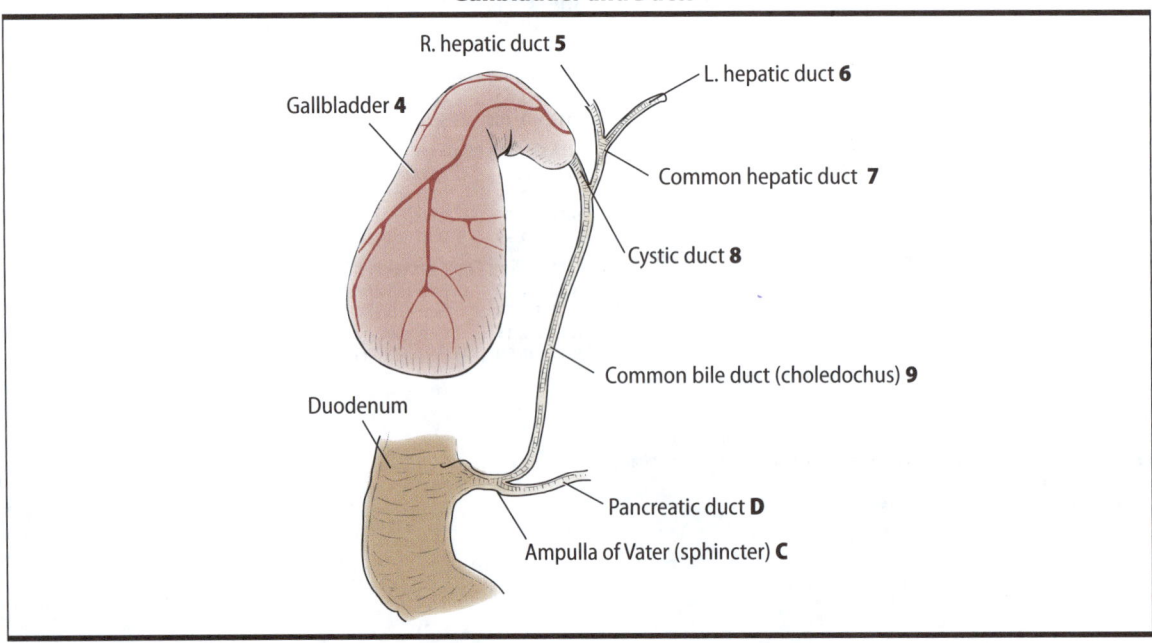

- R. hepatic duct 5
- L. hepatic duct 6
- Gallbladder 4
- Common hepatic duct 7
- Cystic duct 8
- Common bile duct (choledochus) 9
- Duodenum
- Pancreatic duct D
- Ampulla of Vater (sphincter) C

Hepatobiliary System and Pancreas

0 Medical and Surgical
F Hepatobiliary System and Pancreas
1 Bypass   Definition: Altering the route of passage of the contents of a tubular body part

Explanation: Rerouting contents of a body part to a downstream area of the normal route, to a similar route and body part, or to an abnormal route and dissimilar body part. Includes one or more anastomoses, with or without the use of a device.

Body Part Character 4	Approach Character 5	Device Character 6	Qualifier Character 7
4 Gallbladder 5 Hepatic Duct, Right 6 Hepatic Duct, Left 7 Hepatic Duct, Common 8 Cystic Duct 9 Common Bile Duct	0 Open 4 Percutaneous Endoscopic	D Intraluminal Device Z No Device	3 Duodenum 4 Stomach 5 Hepatic Duct, Right 6 Hepatic Duct, Left 7 Hepatic Duct, Caudate 8 Cystic Duct 9 Common Bile Duct B Small Intestine
D Pancreatic Duct Duct of Wirsung	0 Open 4 Percutaneous Endoscopic	D Intraluminal Device Z No Device	3 Duodenum 4 Stomach B Small Intestine C Large Intestine
F Pancreatic Duct, Accessory Duct of Santorini G Pancreas	0 Open 4 Percutaneous Endoscopic	D Intraluminal Device Z No Device	3 Duodenum B Small Intestine C Large Intestine

0 Medical and Surgical
F Hepatobiliary System and Pancreas
2 Change   Definition: Taking out or off a device from a body part and putting back an identical or similar device in or on the same body part without cutting or puncturing the skin or a mucous membrane

Explanation: All CHANGE procedures are coded using the approach EXTERNAL

Body Part Character 4	Approach Character 5	Device Character 6	Qualifier Character 7

0 Liver
   Quadrate lobe
4 Gallbladder
B Hepatobiliary Duct
D Pancreatic Duct
   Duct of Wirsung
G Pancreas
	X External	0 Drainage Device
		Y Other Device
			Z No Qualifier

Non-OR All body part, approach, device, and qualifier values

0F5–0F7 Hepatobiliary System and Pancreas ICD-10-PCS 2025

0 Medical and Surgical
F Hepatobiliary System and Pancreas
5 Destruction Definition: Physical eradication of all or a portion of a body part by the direct use of energy, force, or a destructive agent
Explanation: None of the body part is physically taken out

Body Part Character 4	Approach Character 5	Device Character 6	Qualifier Character 7
0 Liver Quadrate lobe **1** Liver, Right Lobe **2** Liver, Left Lobe	**0** Open **3** Percutaneous **4** Percutaneous Endoscopic	**Z** No Device	**3** Laser Interstitial Thermal Therapy **F** Irreversible Electroporation **Z** No Qualifier
4 Gallbladder	**0** Open **3** Percutaneous **4** Percutaneous Endoscopic	**Z** No Device	**3** Laser Interstitial Thermal Therapy **Z** No Qualifier
4 Gallbladder	**8** Via Natural or Artificial Opening Endoscopic	**Z** No Device	**Z** No Qualifier

5 Hepatic Duct, Right
6 Hepatic Duct, Left
7 Hepatic Duct, Common
8 Cystic Duct
9 Common Bile Duct
C Ampulla of Vater
   Duodenal ampulla
   Hepatopancreatic ampulla
D Pancreatic Duct
   Duct of Wirsung
F Pancreatic Duct, Accessory
   Duct of Santorini
	0 Open
	3 Percutaneous
	4 Percutaneous Endoscopic
		Z No Device	**3** Laser Interstitial Thermal Therapy
			Z No Qualifier

5 Hepatic Duct, Right
6 Hepatic Duct, Left
7 Hepatic Duct, Common
8 Cystic Duct
9 Common Bile Duct
C Ampulla of Vater
   Duodenal ampulla
   Hepatopancreatic ampulla
D Pancreatic Duct
   Duct of Wirsung
F Pancreatic Duct, Accessory
   Duct of Santorini
	7 Via Natural or Artificial Opening
	8 Via Natural or Artificial Opening Endoscopic
		Z No Device	**Z** No Qualifier

G Pancreas	**0** Open **3** Percutaneous **4** Percutaneous Endoscopic	**Z** No Device	**3** Laser Interstitial Thermal Therapy **F** Irreversible Electroporation **Z** No Qualifier
G Pancreas	**8** Via Natural or Artificial Opening Endoscopic	**Z** No Device	**Z** No Qualifier

DRG Non-OR   0F5[5,6,7,8,9,C,D,F]4Z3
DRG Non-OR   0F5G4Z3
Non-OR   0F5[5,6,7,8,9,C,D,F]4ZZ
Non-OR   0F5[5,6,7,8,9,C,D,F]8ZZ
Non-OR   0F5G4Z[F,Z]
Non-OR   0F5G8ZZ

0 Medical and Surgical
F Hepatobiliary System and Pancreas
7 Dilation Definition: Expanding an orifice or the lumen of a tubular body part
Explanation: The orifice can be a natural orifice or an artificially created orifice. Accomplished by stretching a tubular body part using intraluminal pressure or by cutting part of the orifice or wall of the tubular body part.

Body Part Character 4	Approach Character 5	Device Character 6	Qualifier Character 7

5 Hepatic Duct, Right
6 Hepatic Duct, Left
7 Hepatic Duct, Common
8 Cystic Duct
9 Common Bile Duct
C Ampulla of Vater
   Duodenal ampulla
   Hepatopancreatic ampulla
D Pancreatic Duct
   Duct of Wirsung
F Pancreatic Duct, Accessory
   Duct of Santorini
	0 Open
	3 Percutaneous
	4 Percutaneous Endoscopic
	7 Via Natural or Artificial Opening
	8 Via Natural or Artificial Opening Endoscopic
		D Intraluminal Device
		Z No Device
			Z No Qualifier

Non-OR   0F7[5,6,7,8,9][3,4,8][D,Z]Z
Non-OR   0F7[5,6,7,8,9,D]]7DZ
Non-OR   0F7C8[D,Z]Z
Non-OR   0F7[D,F][4,8][D,Z]Z

Non-OR Procedure   DRG Non-OR Procedure   Valid OR Procedure   HAC Associated Procedure   Combination Only   New/Revised April   New/Revised October

ICD-10-PCS 2025 — Hepatobiliary System and Pancreas — 0F8–0F9

0 Medical and Surgical
F Hepatobiliary System and Pancreas
8 Division — Definition: Cutting into a body part, without draining fluids and/or gases from the body part, in order to separate or transect a body part
Explanation: All or a portion of the body part is separated into two or more portions

Body Part — Character 4	Approach — Character 5	Device — Character 6	Qualifier — Character 7
0 Liver 1 Liver, Right Lobe 2 Liver, Left Lobe G Pancreas	0 Open 3 Percutaneous 4 Percutaneous Endoscopic	Z No Device	Z No Qualifier

Non-OR 0F8[0,1,2]3ZZ

---

0 Medical and Surgical
F Hepatobiliary System and Pancreas
9 Drainage — Definition: Taking or letting out fluids and/or gases from a body part
Explanation: The qualifier DIAGNOSTIC is used to identify drainage procedures that are biopsies

Body Part — Character 4	Approach — Character 5	Device — Character 6	Qualifier — Character 7
0 Liver Quadrate lobe 1 Liver, Right Lobe 2 Liver, Left Lobe	0 Open 3 Percutaneous 4 Percutaneous Endoscopic	0 Drainage Device	Z No Qualifier
0 Liver Quadrate lobe 1 Liver, Right Lobe 2 Liver, Left Lobe	0 Open 3 Percutaneous 4 Percutaneous Endoscopic	Z No Device	X Diagnostic Z No Qualifier
4 Gallbladder G Pancreas	0 Open 3 Percutaneous 4 Percutaneous Endoscopic 8 Via Natural or Artificial Opening Endoscopic	0 Drainage Device	Z No Qualifier
4 Gallbladder G Pancreas	0 Open 3 Percutaneous 4 Percutaneous Endoscopic 8 Via Natural or Artificial Opening Endoscopic	Z No Device	X Diagnostic Z No Qualifier

5 Hepatic Duct, Right
6 Hepatic Duct, Left
7 Hepatic Duct, Common
8 Cystic Duct
9 Common Bile Duct
C Ampulla of Vater
  Duodenal ampulla
  Hepatopancreatic ampulla
D Pancreatic Duct
  Duct of Wirsung
F Pancreatic Duct, Accessory
  Duct of Santorini
	0 Open
	3 Percutaneous
	4 Percutaneous Endoscopic
	7 Via Natural or Artificial Opening
	8 Via Natural or Artificial Opening Endoscopic
		0 Drainage Device	Z No Qualifier

5 Hepatic Duct, Right
6 Hepatic Duct, Left
7 Hepatic Duct, Common
8 Cystic Duct
9 Common Bile Duct
C Ampulla of Vater
  Duodenal ampulla
  Hepatopancreatic ampulla
D Pancreatic Duct
  Duct of Wirsung
F Pancreatic Duct, Accessory
  Duct of Santorini
	0 Open
	3 Percutaneous
	4 Percutaneous Endoscopic
	7 Via Natural or Artificial Opening
	8 Via Natural or Artificial Opening Endoscopic
		Z No Device	X Diagnostic
			Z No Qualifier

Non-OR 0F9[0,1,2][3,4]0Z
Non-OR 0F9[0,1,2][3,4]Z[X,Z]
Non-OR 0F9[4,G]80Z
Non-OR 0F9G30Z
Non-OR 0F9[4,G]8Z[X,Z]
Non-OR 0F9G3Z[XZ]
Non-OR 0F9G4ZX
Non-OR 0F9[5,6,8][3,8]0Z
Non-OR 0F97[3,4,7,8]0Z
Non-OR 0F99[3,8]0Z
Non-OR 0F9C[3,4,8]0Z
Non-OR 0F9[D,F][3,8]0Z
Non-OR 0F9[5,6,8,9,C,D,F]3Z[X,Z]
Non-OR 0F9[5,6,8,9,C,D,F][4,7,8]ZX
Non-OR 0F9[5,6,8,D,F]8ZZ
Non-OR 0F97[3,4,7,8]Z[X,Z]
Non-OR 0F99[4,7,8]ZZ
Non-OR 0F9C[4,8]ZZ

ØFB–ØFC Hepatobiliary System and Pancreas ICD-10-PCS 2025

Ø Medical and Surgical
F Hepatobiliary System and Pancreas
B Excision Definition: Cutting out or off, without replacement, a portion of a body part
  Explanation: The qualifier DIAGNOSTIC is used to identify excision procedures that are biopsies

Body Part Character 4	Approach Character 5	Device Character 6	Qualifier Character 7
Ø Liver Quadrate lobe **1** Liver, Right Lobe **2** Liver, Left Lobe	**Ø** Open **3** Percutaneous	**Z** No Device	**X** Diagnostic **Z** No Qualifier
Ø Liver Quadrate lobe **1** Liver, Right Lobe **2** Liver, Left Lobe	**4** Percutaneous Endoscopic	**Z** No Device	**G** Hand-assisted **X** Diagnostic **Z** No Qualifier
4 Gallbladder	**Ø** Open **3** Percutaneous **4** Percutaneous Endoscopic **8** Via Natural or Artificial Opening Endoscopic	**Z** No Device	**X** Diagnostic **Z** No Qualifier

5 Hepatic Duct, Right
6 Hepatic Duct, Left
7 Hepatic Duct, Common
8 Cystic Duct
9 Common Bile Duct
C Ampulla of Vater
    Duodenal ampulla
    Hepatopancreatic ampulla
D Pancreatic Duct
    Duct of Wirsung
F Pancreatic Duct, Accessory
    Duct of Santorini
	Ø Open
	3 Percutaneous
	4 Percutaneous Endoscopic
	7 Via Natural or Artificial Opening
	8 Via Natural or Artificial Opening Endoscopic
		Z No Device	**X** Diagnostic
			Z No Qualifier

G Pancreas	**Ø** Open **3** Percutaneous **8** Via Natural or Artificial Opening Endoscopic	**Z** No Device	**X** Diagnostic **Z** No Qualifier
G Pancreas	**4** Percutaneous Endoscopic	**Z** No Devic	**G** Hand-assisted **X** Diagnostic **Z** No Qualifier

Non-OR ØFB[Ø,1,2]3ZX
Non-OR ØFB4[3,8]ZX
Non-OR ØFB[5,6,7,8,9,C,D,F][3,4,7,8]ZX
Non-OR ØFB[5,6,7,8,9,C,D,F][4,8]ZZ
Non-OR ØFBG[3,8]ZX

Ø Medical and Surgical
F Hepatobiliary System and Pancreas
C Extirpation Definition: Taking or cutting out solid matter from a body part
  Explanation: The solid matter may be an abnormal byproduct of a biological function or a foreign body; it may be imbedded in a body part or in the lumen of a tubular body part. The solid matter may or may not have been previously broken into pieces.

Body Part Character 4	Approach Character 5	Device Character 6	Qualifier Character 7
Ø Liver Quadrate lobe **1** Liver, Right Lobe **2** Liver, Left Lobe	**Ø** Open **3** Percutaneous **4** Percutaneous Endoscopic	**Z** No Device	**Z** No Qualifier
4 Gallbladder **G** Pancreas	**Ø** Open **3** Percutaneous **4** Percutaneous Endoscopic **8** Via Natural or Artificial Opening Endoscopic	**Z** No Device	**Z** No Qualifier

5 Hepatic Duct, Right
6 Hepatic Duct, Left
7 Hepatic Duct, Common
8 Cystic Duct
9 Common Bile Duct
C Ampulla of Vater
    Duodenal ampulla
    Hepatopancreatic ampulla
D Pancreatic Duct
    Duct of Wirsung
F Pancreatic Duct, Accessory
    Duct of Santorini
	Ø Open
	3 Percutaneous
	4 Percutaneous Endoscopic
	7 Via Natural or Artificial Opening
	8 Via Natural or Artificial Opening Endoscopic
		Z No Device	**Z** No Qualifier

Non-OR ØFC[5,6,7,8][3,4,7,8]ZZ
Non-OR ØFC9[3,7,8]ZZ
Non-OR ØFCC[4,8]ZZ
Non-OR ØFC[D,F][3,4,8]ZZ

Non-OR Procedure   DRG Non-OR Procedure   Valid OR Procedure   HAC Associated Procedure   Combination Only   New/Revised April   New/Revised October

0 Medical and Surgical
F Hepatobiliary System and Pancreas
D Extraction Definition: Pulling or stripping out or off all or a portion of a body part by the use of force
Explanation: The qualifier DIAGNOSTIC is used to identify extraction procedures that are biopsies

Body Part Character 4	Approach Character 5	Device Character 6	Qualifier Character 7
0 Liver Quadrate lobe 1 Liver, Right Lobe 2 Liver, Left Lobe	3 Percutaneous 4 Percutaneous Endoscopic	Z No Device	X Diagnostic

4 Gallbladder
5 Hepatic Duct, Right
6 Hepatic Duct, Left
7 Hepatic Duct, Common
8 Cystic Duct
9 Common Bile Duct
C Ampulla of Vater
   Duodenal ampulla
   Hepatopancreatic ampulla
D Pancreatic Duct
   Duct of Wirsung
F Pancreatic Duct, Accessory
   Duct of Santorini
G Pancreas
	3 Percutaneous
	4 Percutaneous Endoscopic
	8 Via Natural or Artificial Opening Endoscopic
		Z No Device	X Diagnostic

Non-OR 0FD[0,1,2]3ZX
Non-OR 0FD[4,5,6,7,8,9,C,D,F,G][3,4,8]ZX

0 Medical and Surgical
F Hepatobiliary System and Pancreas
F Fragmentation Definition: Breaking solid matter in a body part into pieces
Explanation: Physical force (e.g., manual, ultrasonic) applied directly or indirectly is used to break the solid matter into pieces. The solid matter may be an abnormal byproduct of a biological function or a foreign body. The pieces of solid matter are not taken out.

Body Part Character 4	Approach Character 5	Device Character 6	Qualifier Character 7

4 Gallbladder [NC]
5 Hepatic Duct, Right [NC]
6 Hepatic Duct, Left [NC]
7 Hepatic Duct, Common
8 Cystic Duct [NC]
9 Common Bile Duct [NC]
C Ampulla of Vater [NC]
   Duodenal ampulla
   Hepatopancreatic ampulla
D Pancreatic Duct [NC]
   Duct of Wirsung
F Pancreatic Duct, Accessory [NC]
   Duct of Santorini
	0 Open
	3 Percutaneous
	4 Percutaneous Endoscopic
	7 Via Natural or Artificial Opening
	8 Via Natural or Artificial Opening Endoscopic
	X External
		Z No Device	Z No Qualifier

Non-OR 0FF[4,5,6,7,8,9,C,D,F][8,X]ZZ
NC 0FF[4,5,6,8,9,C,D,F]XZZ

0 Medical and Surgical
F Hepatobiliary System and Pancreas
H Insertion Definition: Putting in a nonbiological appliance that monitors, assists, performs, or prevents a physiological function but does not physically take the place of a body part
Explanation: None

Body Part Character 4	Approach Character 5	Device Character 6	Qualifier Character 7
0 Liver Quadrate lobe 4 Gallbladder G Pancreas	0 Open 3 Percutaneous 4 Percutaneous Endoscopic	1 Radioactive Element 2 Monitoring Device 3 Infusion Device Y Other Device	Z No Qualifier
1 Liver, Right Lobe 2 Liver, Left Lobe	0 Open 3 Percutaneous 4 Percutaneous Endoscopic	2 Monitoring Device 3 Infusion Device	Z No Qualifier
B Hepatobiliary Duct ⊕ D Pancreatic Duct Duct of Wirsung	0 Open 3 Percutaneous 4 Percutaneous Endoscopic 7 Via Natural or Artificial Opening 8 Via Natural or Artificial Opening Endoscopic	1 Radioactive Element 2 Monitoring Device 3 Infusion Device D Intraluminal Device Y Other Device	Z No Qualifier

Non-OR 0FH[0,4,G]31Z
Non-OR 0FH[0,4,G][0,3,4]3Z
Non-OR 0FH[0,4,G][3,4]YZ
Non-OR 0FH[1,2][0,3,4]3Z

Non-OR 0FH[B,D][0,3,4]3Z
Non-OR 0FH[B,D][4,8]DZ
Non-OR 0FH[B,D][7,8][2,3]Z
Non-OR 0FH[B,D][3,4,7,8]YZ

See Appendix L for Procedure Combinations
⊕ 0FHB7DZ

NC Noncovered Procedure   **LC** Limited Coverage   **QA** Questionable OB Admit   **NT** New Tech Add-on   ⊕ Combination Member   ♂ Male   ♀ Female

Hepatobiliary System and Pancreas

0 Medical and Surgical
F Hepatobiliary System and Pancreas
J Inspection Definition: Visually and/or manually exploring a body part
Explanation: Visual exploration may be performed with or without optical instrumentation. Manual exploration may be performed directly or through intervening body layers.

Body Part Character 4	Approach Character 5	Device Character 6	Qualifier Character 7
0 Liver Quadrate lobe	**0** Open **3** Percutaneous **4** Percutaneous Endoscopic **X** External	**Z** No Device	**Z** No Qualifier
4 Gallbladder **G** Pancreas	**0** Open **3** Percutaneous **4** Percutaneous Endoscopic **8** Via Natural or Artificial Opening Endoscopic **X** External	**Z** No Device	**Z** No Qualifier
B Hepatobiliary Duct **D** Pancreatic Duct Duct of Wirsung	**0** Open **3** Percutaneous **4** Percutaneous Endoscopic **7** Via Natural or Artificial Opening **8** Via Natural or Artificial Opening Endoscopic	**Z** No Device	**Z** No Qualifier

Non-OR 0FJ0[3,X]ZZ
Non-OR 0FJ[4,G][3,8,X]ZZ
Non-OR 0FJ[B,D][3,7,8]ZZ

0 Medical and Surgical
F Hepatobiliary System and Pancreas
L Occlusion Definition: Completely closing an orifice or the lumen of a tubular body part
Explanation: The orifice can be a natural orifice or an artificially created orifice

Body Part Character 4	Approach Character 5	Device Character 6	Qualifier Character 7
5 Hepatic Duct, Right **6** Hepatic Duct, Left **7** Hepatic Duct, Common **8** Cystic Duct **9** Common Bile Duct **C** Ampulla of Vater Duodenal ampulla Hepatopancreatic ampulla **D** Pancreatic Duct Duct of Wirsung **F** Pancreatic Duct, Accessory Duct of Santorini	**0** Open **3** Percutaneous **4** Percutaneous Endoscopic	**C** Extraluminal Device **D** Intraluminal Device **Z** No Device	**Z** No Qualifier
5 Hepatic Duct, Right **6** Hepatic Duct, Left **7** Hepatic Duct, Common **8** Cystic Duct **9** Common Bile Duct **C** Ampulla of Vater Duodenal ampulla Hepatopancreatic ampulla **D** Pancreatic Duct Duct of Wirsung **F** Pancreatic Duct, Accessory Duct of Santorini	**7** Via Natural or Artificial Opening **8** Via Natural or Artificial Opening Endoscopic	**D** Intraluminal Device **Z** No Device	**Z** No Qualifier

Non-OR 0FL[5,6,7,8,9][3,4][C,D,Z]Z
Non-OR 0FL[5,6,7,8,9][7,8][D,Z]Z

0 Medical and Surgical
F Hepatobiliary System and Pancreas
M Reattachment
Definition: Putting back in or on all or a portion of a separated body part to its normal location or other suitable location
Explanation: Vascular circulation and nervous pathways may or may not be reestablished

Body Part — Character 4	Approach — Character 5	Device — Character 6	Qualifier — Character 7

0 Liver
   Quadrate lobe
1 Liver, Right Lobe
2 Liver, Left Lobe
4 Gallbladder
5 Hepatic Duct, Right
6 Hepatic Duct, Left
7 Hepatic Duct, Common
8 Cystic Duct
9 Common Bile Duct
C Ampulla of Vater
   Duodenal ampulla
   Hepatopancreatic ampulla
D Pancreatic Duct
   Duct of Wirsung
F Pancreatic Duct, Accessory
   Duct of Santorini
G Pancreas
	0 Open
	4 Percutaneous Endoscopic
		Z No Device	Z No Qualifier

Non-OR 0FM[4,5,6,7,8,9]4ZZ

0 Medical and Surgical
F Hepatobiliary System and Pancreas
N Release
Definition: Freeing a body part from an abnormal physical constraint by cutting or by the use of force
Explanation: Some of the restraining tissue may be taken out but none of the body part is taken out

Body Part — Character 4	Approach — Character 5	Device — Character 6	Qualifier — Character 7
0 Liver Quadrate lobe 1 Liver, Right Lobe 2 Liver, Left Lobe	0 Open 3 Percutaneous 4 Percutaneous Endoscopic	Z No Device	Z No Qualifier
4 Gallbladder G Pancreas	0 Open 3 Percutaneous 4 Percutaneous Endoscopic 8 Via Natural or Artificial Opening Endoscopic	Z No Device	Z No Qualifier

5 Hepatic Duct, Right
6 Hepatic Duct, Left
7 Hepatic Duct, Common
8 Cystic Duct
9 Common Bile Duct
C Ampulla of Vater
   Duodenal ampulla
   Hepatopancreatic ampulla
D Pancreatic Duct
   Duct of Wirsung
F Pancreatic Duct, Accessory
   Duct of Santorini
	0 Open
	3 Percutaneous
	4 Percutaneous Endoscopic
	7 Via Natural or Artificial Opening
	8 Via Natural or Artificial Opening Endoscopic
		Z No Device	Z No Qualifier

ØFP–ØFP Hepatobiliary System and Pancreas ICD-10-PCS 2025

Ø Medical and Surgical
F Hepatobiliary System and Pancreas
P Removal   Definition: Taking out or off a device from a body part

Explanation: If a device is taken out and a similar device put in without cutting or puncturing the skin or mucous membrane, the procedure is coded to the root operation CHANGE. Otherwise, the procedure for taking out a device is coded to the root operation REMOVAL.

Body Part Character 4	Approach Character 5	Device Character 6	Qualifier Character 7
Ø Liver Quadrate lobe	Ø Open 3 Percutaneous 4 Percutaneous Endoscopic	Ø Drainage Device 2 Monitoring Device 3 Infusion Device Y Other Device	Z No Qualifier
Ø Liver Quadrate lobe	X External	Ø Drainage Device 2 Monitoring Device 3 Infusion Device	Z No Qualifier
4 Gallbladder G Pancreas	Ø Open 3 Percutaneous 4 Percutaneous Endoscopic	Ø Drainage Device 2 Monitoring Device 3 Infusion Device D Intraluminal Device Y Other Device	Z No Qualifier
4 Gallbladder G Pancreas	8 Via Natural or Artificial Opening Endoscopic	Ø Drainage Device	Z No Qualifier
4 Gallbladder G Pancreas	X External	Ø Drainage Device 2 Monitoring Device 3 Infusion Device D Intraluminal Device	Z No Qualifier
B Hepatobiliary Duct D Pancreatic Duct Duct of Wirsung	Ø Open 3 Percutaneous 4 Percutaneous Endoscopic 7 Via Natural or Artificial Opening 8 Via Natural or Artificial Opening Endoscopic	Ø Drainage Device 1 Radioactive Element 2 Monitoring Device 3 Infusion Device 7 Autologous Tissue Substitute C Extraluminal Device D Intraluminal Device J Synthetic Substitute K Nonautologous Tissue Substitute Y Other Device	Z No Qualifier
B Hepatobiliary Duct D Pancreatic Duct Duct of Wirsung	X External	Ø Drainage Device 1 Radioactive Element 2 Monitoring Device 3 Infusion Device D Intraluminal Device	Z No Qualifier

Non-OR   ØFPØ[3,4]YZ
Non-OR   ØFPØX[Ø,2,3]Z
Non-OR   ØFPG3ØZ
Non-OR   ØFP[4,G][3,4]YZ
Non-OR   ØFP4X[Ø,2,3,D]Z
Non-OR   ØFPGX[Ø,2,3]Z
Non-OR   ØFP[B,D][3,4]YZ
Non-OR   ØFP[B,D][7,8][Ø,2,3,D,Y]Z
Non-OR   ØFP[B,D]X[Ø,1,2,3,D]Z

See Appendix L for Procedure Combinations
Combo-only   ØFP[B,D][7,8]DZ
Combo-only   ØFP[B,D]XDZ

ICD-10-PCS 2025 — Hepatobiliary System and Pancreas — 0FQ–0FS

- **0** Medical and Surgical
- **F** Hepatobiliary System and Pancreas
- **Q** Repair
  Definition: Restoring, to the extent possible, a body part to its normal anatomic structure and function
  Explanation: Used only when the method to accomplish the repair is not one of the other root operations

Body Part Character 4	Approach Character 5	Device Character 6	Qualifier Character 7
0 Liver Quadrate lobe **1** Liver, Right Lobe **2** Liver, Left Lobe	**0** Open **3** Percutaneous **4** Percutaneous Endoscopic	**Z** No Device	**Z** No Qualifier
4 Gallbladder **G** Pancreas	**0** Open **3** Percutaneous **4** Percutaneous Endoscopic **8** Via Natural or Artificial Opening Endoscopic	**Z** No Device	**Z** No Qualifier

5 Hepatic Duct, Right
6 Hepatic Duct, Left
7 Hepatic Duct, Common
8 Cystic Duct
9 Common Bile Duct
C Ampulla of Vater
    Duodenal ampulla
    Hepatopancreatic ampulla
D Pancreatic Duct
    Duct of Wirsung
F Pancreatic Duct, Accessory
    Duct of Santorini
	0 Open
	3 Percutaneous
	4 Percutaneous Endoscopic
	7 Via Natural or Artificial Opening
	8 Via Natural or Artificial Opening Endoscopic
		Z No Device	**Z** No Qualifier

- **0** Medical and Surgical
- **F** Hepatobiliary System and Pancreas
- **R** Replacement
  Definition: Putting in or on biological or synthetic material that physically takes the place and/or function of all or a portion of a body part
  Explanation: The body part may have been taken out or replaced, or may be taken out, physically eradicated, or rendered nonfunctional during the REPLACEMENT procedure. A REMOVAL procedure is coded for taking out the device used in a previous replacement procedure.

Body Part Character 4	Approach Character 5	Device Character 6	Qualifier Character 7

5 Hepatic Duct, Right
6 Hepatic Duct, Left
7 Hepatic Duct, Common
8 Cystic Duct
9 Common Bile Duct
C Ampulla of Vater
    Duodenal ampulla
    Hepatopancreatic ampulla
D Pancreatic Duct
    Duct of Wirsung
F Pancreatic Duct, Accessory
    Duct of Santorini
	0 Open
	4 Percutaneous Endoscopic
	8 Via Natural or Artificial Opening Endoscopic
		7 Autologous Tissue Substitute
		J Synthetic Substitute
		K Nonautologous Tissue Substitute
			Z No Qualifier

- **0** Medical and Surgical
- **F** Hepatobiliary System and Pancreas
- **S** Reposition
  Definition: Moving to its normal location, or other suitable location, all or a portion of a body part
  Explanation: The body part is moved to a new location from an abnormal location, or from a normal location where it is not functioning correctly. The body part may or may not be cut out or off to be moved to the new location.

Body Part Character 4	Approach Character 5	Device Character 6	Qualifier Character 7

0 Liver
    Quadrate lobe
4 Gallbladder
5 Hepatic Duct, Right
6 Hepatic Duct, Left
7 Hepatic Duct, Common
8 Cystic Duct
9 Common Bile Duct
C Ampulla of Vater
    Duodenal ampulla
    Hepatopancreatic ampulla
D Pancreatic Duct
    Duct of Wirsung
F Pancreatic Duct, Accessory
    Duct of Santorini
G Pancreas
	0 Open
	4 Percutaneous Endoscopic
		Z No Device	**Z** No Qualifier

NC Noncovered Procedure   **LC** Limited Coverage   **QA** Questionable OB Admit   **NT** New Tech Add-on   ✚ Combination Member   ♂ Male   ♀ Female

0FT–0FU Hepatobiliary System and Pancreas ICD-10-PCS 2025

0 Medical and Surgical
F Hepatobiliary System and Pancreas
T Resection Definition: Cutting out or off, without replacement, all of a body part
  Explanation: None

Body Part Character 4	Approach Character 5	Device Character 6	Qualifier Character 7
0 Liver Quadrate lobe **1** Liver, Right Lobe **2** Liver, Left Lobe **4** Gallbladder **G** Pancreas	**0** Open	**Z** No Device	**Z** No Qualifier
0 Liver Quadrate lobe **1** Liver, Right Lobe **2** Liver, Left Lobe **4** Gallbladder **G** Pancreas	**4** Percutaneous Endoscopic	**Z** No Device	**G** Hand-assisted **Z** No Qualifier

5 Hepatic Duct, Right
6 Hepatic Duct, Left
7 Hepatic Duct, Common
8 Cystic Duct
9 Common Bile Duct
C Ampulla of Vater
  Duodenal ampulla
  Hepatopancreatic ampulla
D Pancreatic Duct
  Duct of Wirsung
F Pancreatic Duct, Accessory
  Duct of Santorini
	0 Open
	4 Percutaneous Endoscopic
	7 Via Natural or Artificial Opening
	8 Via Natural or Artificial Opening Endoscopic
		Z No Device	**Z** No Qualifier

Non-OR 0FT[D,F][4,8]ZZ

See Appendix L for Procedure Combinations
 0FTG0ZZ

0 Medical and Surgical
F Hepatobiliary System and Pancreas
U Supplement Definition: Putting in or on biological or synthetic material that physically reinforces and/or augments the function of a portion of a body part
  Explanation: The biological material is non-living, or is living and from the same individual. The body part may have been previously replaced, and the SUPPLEMENT procedure is performed to physically reinforce and/or augment the function of the replaced body part.

Body Part Character 4	Approach Character 5	Device Character 6	Qualifier Character 7

5 Hepatic Duct, Right
6 Hepatic Duct, Left
7 Hepatic Duct, Common
8 Cystic Duct
9 Common Bile Duct
C Ampulla of Vater
  Duodenal ampulla
  Hepatopancreatic ampulla
D Pancreatic Duct
  Duct of Wirsung
F Pancreatic Duct, Accessory
  Duct of Santorini
	0 Open
	3 Percutaneous
	4 Percutaneous Endoscopic
	8 Via Natural or Artificial Opening Endoscopic
		7 Autologous Tissue Substitute
		J Synthetic Substitute
		K Nonautologous Tissue Substitute
			Z No Qualifier

ICD-10-PCS 2025 — Hepatobiliary System and Pancreas — 0FV–0FV

- **0** Medical and Surgical
- **F** Hepatobiliary System and Pancreas
- **V** Restriction Definition: Partially closing an orifice or the lumen of a tubular body part
  Explanation: The orifice can be a natural orifice or an artificially created orifice

Body Part Character 4	Approach Character 5	Device Character 6	Qualifier Character 7

5 Hepatic Duct, Right
6 Hepatic Duct, Left
7 Hepatic Duct, Common
8 Cystic Duct
9 Common Bile Duct
C Ampulla of Vater
     Duodenal ampulla
     Hepatopancreatic ampulla
D Pancreatic Duct
     Duct of Wirsung
F Pancreatic Duct, Accessory
     Duct of Santorini
	0 Open
	3 Percutaneous
	4 Percutaneous Endoscopic
		C Extraluminal Device
		D Intraluminal Device
		Z No Device
			Z No Qualifier

5 Hepatic Duct, Right
6 Hepatic Duct, Left
7 Hepatic Duct, Common
8 Cystic Duct
9 Common Bile Duct
C Ampulla of Vater
     Duodenal ampulla
     Hepatopancreatic ampulla
D Pancreatic Duct
     Duct of Wirsung
F Pancreatic Duct, Accessory
     Duct of Santorini
	7 Via Natural or Artificial Opening
	8 Via Natural or Artificial Opening Endoscopic
		D Intraluminal Device
		Z No Device
			Z No Qualifier

Non-OR 0FV[5,6,7,8,9][3,4][C,D,Z]Z
Non-OR 0FV[5,6,7,8,9][7,8][D,Z]Z

ØFW–ØFY — Hepatobiliary System and Pancreas — ICD-10-PCS 2025

Ø Medical and Surgical
F Hepatobiliary System and Pancreas
W Revision — Definition: Correcting, to the extent possible, a portion of a malfunctioning device or the position of a displaced device
Explanation: Revision can include correcting a malfunctioning or displaced device by taking out or putting in components of the device such as a screw or pin

Body Part Character 4	Approach Character 5	Device Character 6	Qualifier Character 7
Ø Liver Quadrate lobe	Ø Open 3 Percutaneous 4 Percutaneous Endoscopic	Ø Drainage Device 2 Monitoring Device 3 Infusion Device Y Other Device	Z No Qualifier
Ø Liver Quadrate lobe	X External	Ø Drainage Device 2 Monitoring Device 3 Infusion Device	Z No Qualifier
4 Gallbladder G Pancreas	Ø Open 3 Percutaneous 4 Percutaneous Endoscopic	Ø Drainage Device 2 Monitoring Device 3 Infusion Device D Intraluminal Device Y Other Device	Z No Qualifier
4 Gallbladder G Pancreas	8 Via Natural or Artificial Opening Endoscopic	Ø Drainage Device	Z No Qualifier
4 Gallbladder G Pancreas	X External	Ø Drainage Device 2 Monitoring Device 3 Infusion Device D Intraluminal Device	Z No Qualifier
B Hepatobiliary Duct D Pancreatic Duct Duct of Wirsung	Ø Open 3 Percutaneous 4 Percutaneous Endoscopic 7 Via Natural or Artificial Opening 8 Via Natural or Artificial Opening Endoscopic	Ø Drainage Device 2 Monitoring Device 3 Infusion Device 7 Autologous Tissue Substitute C Extraluminal Device D Intraluminal Device J Synthetic Substitute K Nonautologous Tissue Substitute Y Other Device	Z No Qualifier
B Hepatobiliary Duct D Pancreatic Duct Duct of Wirsung	X External	Ø Drainage Device 2 Monitoring Device 3 Infusion Device 7 Autologous Tissue Substitute C Extraluminal Device D Intraluminal Device J Synthetic Substitute K Nonautologous Tissue Substitute	Z No Qualifier

Non-OR ØFWØ[3,4]YZ
Non-OR ØFWØX[Ø,2,3]Z
Non-OR ØFW[4,G][3,4]YZ
Non-OR ØFW[4,G]X[Ø,2,3,D]Z
Non-OR ØFW[B,D][3,4,7,8]YZ
Non-OR ØFW[B,D]X[Ø,2,3,7,C,D,J,K]Z

Ø Medical and Surgical
F Hepatobiliary System and Pancreas
Y Transplantation — Definition: Putting in or on all or a portion of a living body part taken from another individual or animal to physically take the place and/or function of all or a portion of a similar body part
Explanation: The native body part may or may not be taken out, and the transplanted body part may take over all or a portion of its function

Body Part Character 4	Approach Character 5	Device Character 6	Qualifier Character 7
Ø Liver LC Quadrate lobe G Pancreas LC NC ✚	Ø Open	Z No Device	Ø Allogeneic 1 Syngeneic 2 Zooplastic

LC ØFYØØZ[Ø,1,2]
LC ØFYGØZ[Ø,1]
NC ØFYGØZ2
NC ØFYGØZ[Ø,1] If reported alone without one of the following procedures ØTYØØZ[Ø,1,2], ØTY1ØZ[Ø,1,2] and without one of the following diagnoses E1Ø.1Ø-E1Ø.9, E89.1

See Appendix L for Procedure Combinations
✚ ØFYGØZ[Ø,1,2]

Endocrine System 0G2–0GW

Character Meanings

This Character Meaning table is provided as a guide to assist the user in the identification of character members that may be found in this section of code tables. It **SHOULD NOT** be used to build a PCS code.

Operation–Character 3	Body Part–Character 4	Approach–Character 5	Device–Character 6	Qualifier–Character 7
2 Change	0 Pituitary Gland	0 Open	0 Drainage Device	3 Laser Interstitial Thermal Therapy
5 Destruction	1 Pineal Body	3 Percutaneous	1 Radioactive Element	X Diagnostic
8 Division	2 Adrenal Gland, Left	4 Percutaneous Endoscopic	2 Monitoring Device	Z No Qualifier
9 Drainage	3 Adrenal Gland, Right	X External	3 Infusion Device	
B Excision	4 Adrenal Glands, Bilateral		Y Other Device	
C Extirpation	5 Adrenal Gland		Z No Device	
H Insertion	6 Carotid Body, Left			
J Inspection	7 Carotid Body, Right			
M Reattachment	8 Carotid Bodies, Bilateral			
N Release	9 Para-aortic Body			
P Removal	B Coccygeal Glomus			
Q Repair	C Glomus Jugulare			
S Reposition	D Aortic Body			
T Resection	F Paraganglion Extremity			
W Revision	G Thyroid Gland Lobe, Left			
	H Thyroid Gland Lobe, Right			
	J Thyroid Gland Isthmus			
	K Thyroid Gland			
	L Superior Parathyroid Gland, Right			
	M Superior Parathyroid Gland, Left			
	N Inferior Parathyroid Gland, Right			
	P Inferior Parathyroid Gland, Left			
	Q Parathyroid Glands, Multiple			
	R Parathyroid Gland			
	S Endocrine Gland			

AHA Coding Clinic for table 0G5
2022, 4Q, 53-54   Laser interstitial thermal therapy

AHA Coding Clinic for table 0GB
2021, 2Q, 7   Infrarenal para-aortic paraganglioma with excision
2017, 2Q, 20   Near total thyroidectomy
2014, 3Q, 22   Transsphenoidal removal of pituitary tumor and fat graft placement

AHA Coding Clinic for table 0GH
2020, 4Q, 43-44   Insertion of radioactive element

AHA Coding Clinic for table 0GT
2017, 2Q, 20   Near total thyroidectomy

Endocrine System

Endocrine System

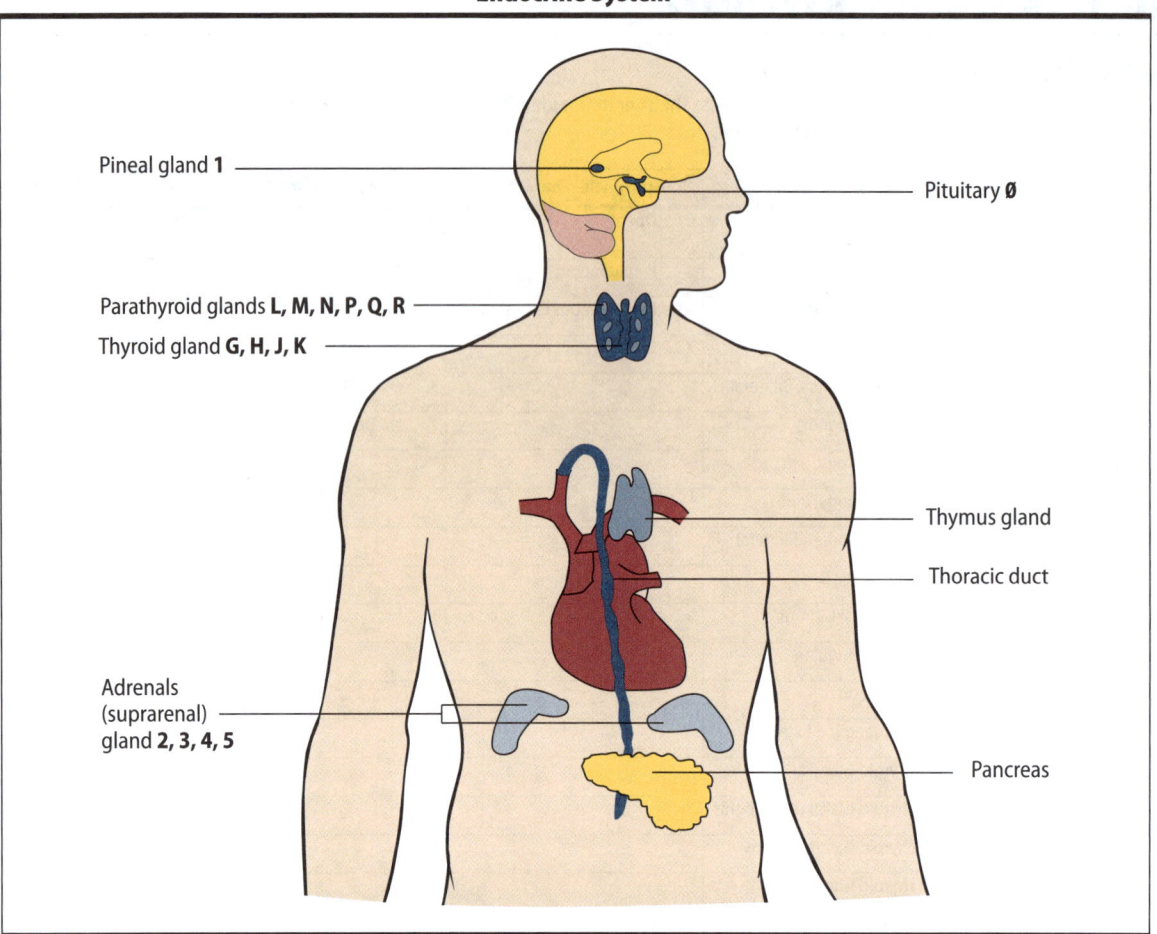

- Pineal gland **1**
- Pituitary **Ø**
- Parathyroid glands **L, M, N, P, Q, R**
- Thyroid gland **G, H, J, K**
- Thymus gland
- Thoracic duct
- Adrenals (suprarenal) gland **2, 3, 4, 5**
- Pancreas

Left Adrenal Gland

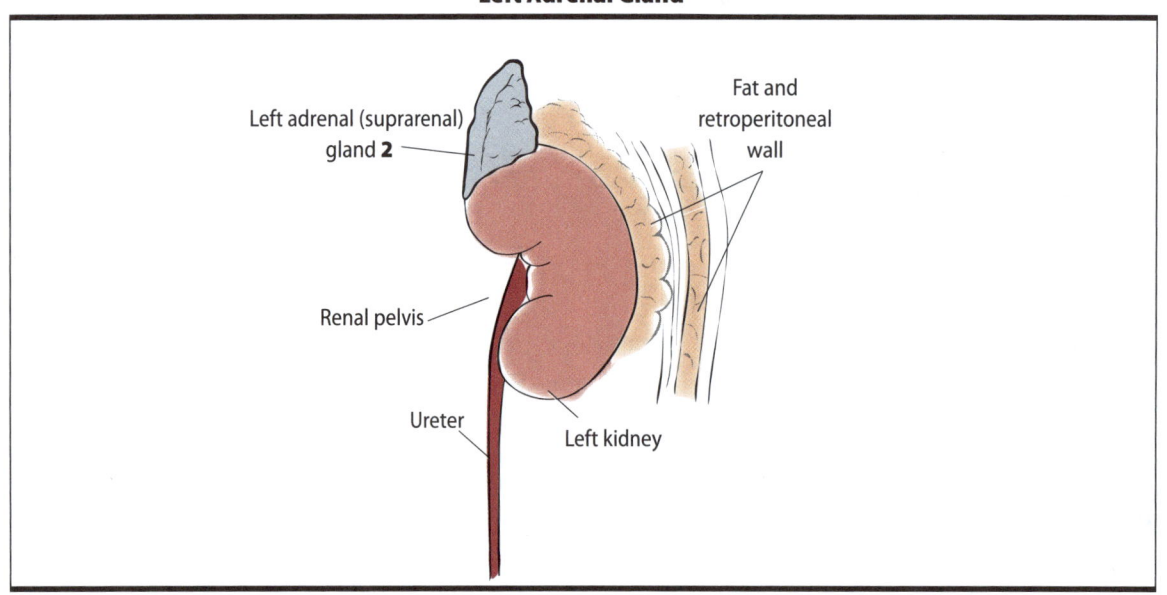

- Left adrenal (suprarenal) gland **2**
- Fat and retroperitoneal wall
- Renal pelvis
- Ureter
- Left kidney

Thyroid

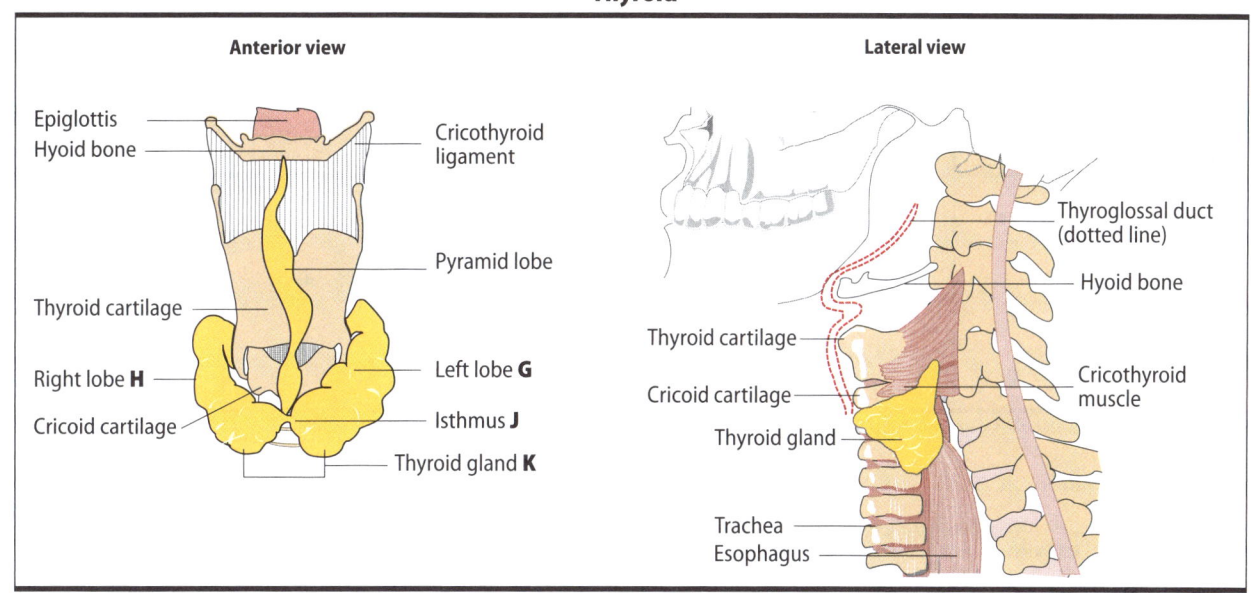

Anterior view

- Epiglottis
- Hyoid bone
- Cricothyroid ligament
- Pyramid lobe
- Thyroid cartilage
- Right lobe **H**
- Left lobe **G**
- Cricoid cartilage
- Isthmus **J**
- Thyroid gland **K**

Lateral view

- Thyroglossal duct (dotted line)
- Hyoid bone
- Thyroid cartilage
- Cricothyroid muscle
- Cricoid cartilage
- Thyroid gland
- Trachea
- Esophagus

Thyroid and Parathyroid Glands

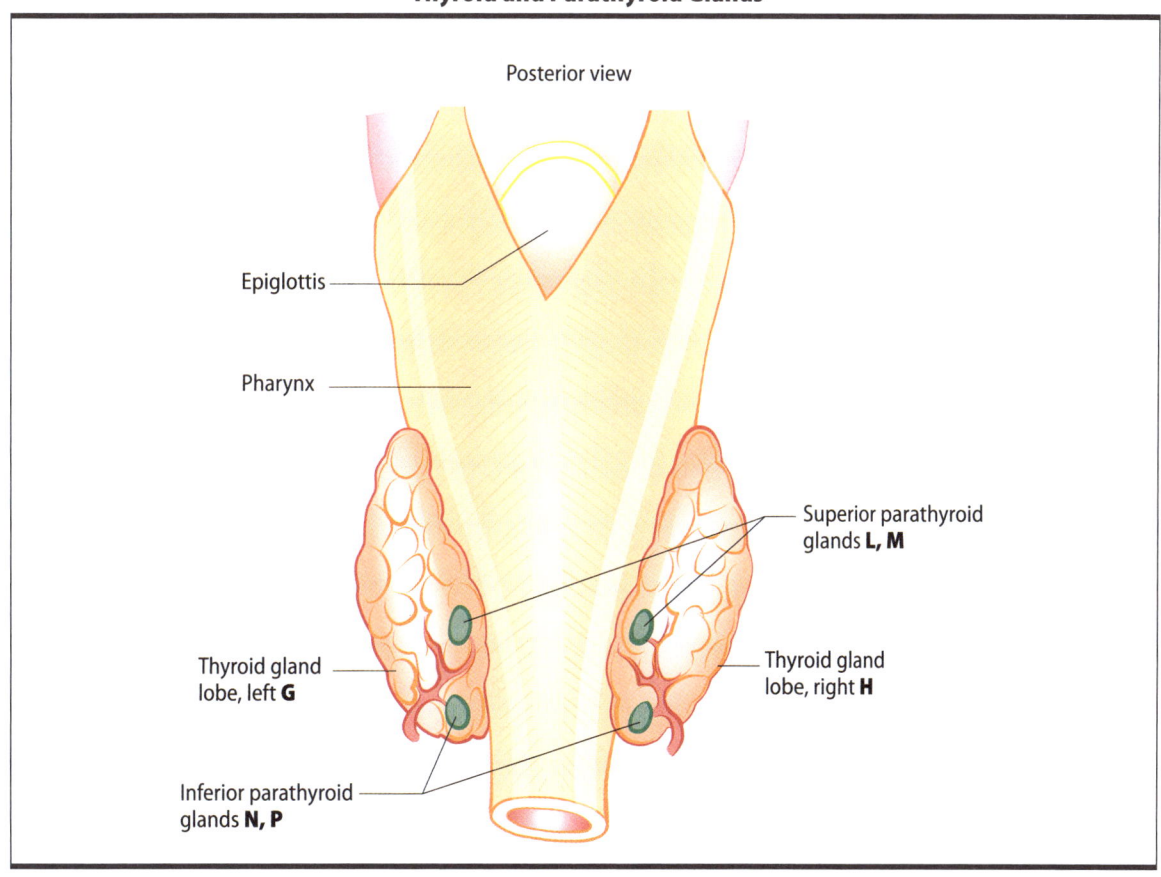

Posterior view

- Epiglottis
- Pharynx
- Superior parathyroid glands **L, M**
- Thyroid gland lobe, left **G**
- Thyroid gland lobe, right **H**
- Inferior parathyroid glands **N, P**

Endocrine System

0G2–0G8   Endocrine System   ICD-10-PCS 2025

0 Medical and Surgical
G Endocrine System
2 Change   Definition: Taking out or off a device from a body part and putting back an identical or similar device in or on the same body part without cutting or puncturing the skin or a mucous membrane
Explanation: All CHANGE procedures are coded using the approach EXTERNAL

Body Part Character 4	Approach Character 5	Device Character 6	Qualifier Character 7

0 Pituitary Gland
   Adenohypophysis
   Hypophysis
   Neurohypophysis
1 Pineal Body
5 Adrenal Gland
   Suprarenal gland
K Thyroid Gland
R Parathyroid Gland
S Endocrine Gland
	X External	0 Drainage Device
		Y Other Device
			Z No Qualifier

Non-OR   All body part, approach, device, and qualifier values

---

0 Medical and Surgical
G Endocrine System
5 Destruction   Definition: Physical eradication of all or a portion of a body part by the direct use of energy, force, or a destructive agent
Explanation: None of the body part is physically taken out

Body Part Character 4	Approach Character 5	Device Character 6	Qualifier Character 7

0 Pituitary Gland
   Adenohypophysis
   Hypophysis
   Neurohypophysis
1 Pineal Body
2 Adrenal Gland, Left
   Suprarenal gland
3 Adrenal Gland, Right
   See 2 Adrenal Gland, Left
4 Adrenal Glands, Bilateral
   See 2 Adrenal Gland, Left
6 Carotid Body, Left
   Carotid glomus
7 Carotid Body, Right
   See 6 Carotid Body, Left
8 Carotid Bodies, Bilateral
   See 6 Carotid Body, Left
9 Para-aortic Body
B Coccygeal Glomus
   Coccygeal body
C Glomus Jugulare
   Jugular body
D Aortic Body
F Paraganglion Extremity
G Thyroid Gland Lobe, Left
H Thyroid Gland Lobe, Right
K Thyroid Gland
L Superior Parathyroid Gland, Right
M Superior Parathyroid Gland, Left
N Inferior Parathyroid Gland, Right
P Inferior Parathyroid Gland, Left
Q Parathyroid Glands, Multiple
R Parathyroid Gland
	0 Open
	3 Percutaneous
	4 Percutaneous Endoscopic
		Z No Device	3 Laser Interstitial Thermal Therapy
			Z No Qualifier

---

0 Medical and Surgical
G Endocrine System
8 Division   Definition: Cutting into a body part, without draining fluids and/or gases from the body part, in order to separate or transect a body part
Explanation: All or a portion of the body part is separated into two or more portions

Body Part Character 4	Approach Character 5	Device Character 6	Qualifier Character 7

0 Pituitary Gland
   Adenohypophysis
   Hypophysis
   Neurohypophysis
J Thyroid Gland Isthmus
	0 Open
	3 Percutaneous
	4 Percutaneous Endoscopic
		Z No Device	Z No Qualifier

Non-OR Procedure   DRG Non-OR Procedure   Valid OR Procedure   HAC Associated Procedure   Combination Only   New/Revised April   New/Revised October

ICD-10-PCS 2025 — Endocrine System — 0G9–0G9

- 0 Medical and Surgical
- G Endocrine System
- 9 Drainage
  Definition: Taking or letting out fluids and/or gases from a body part
  Explanation: The qualifier DIAGNOSTIC is used to identify drainage procedures that are biopsies

Body Part Character 4	Approach Character 5	Device Character 6	Qualifier Character 7

0 Pituitary Gland
  Adenohypophysis
  Hypophysis
  Neurohypophysis
1 Pineal Body
2 Adrenal Gland, Left
  Suprarenal gland
3 Adrenal Gland, Right
  See 2 Adrenal Gland, Left
4 Adrenal Glands, Bilateral
  See 2 Adrenal Gland, Left
6 Carotid Body, Left
  Carotid glomus
7 Carotid Body, Right
  See 6 Carotid Body, Left
8 Carotid Bodies, Bilateral
  See 6 Carotid Body, Left
9 Para-aortic Body
B Coccygeal Glomus
  Coccygeal body
C Glomus Jugulare
  Jugular body
D Aortic Body
F Paraganglion Extremity
G Thyroid Gland Lobe, Left
H Thyroid Gland Lobe, Right
K Thyroid Gland
L Superior Parathyroid Gland, Right
M Superior Parathyroid Gland, Left
N Inferior Parathyroid Gland, Right
P Inferior Parathyroid Gland, Left
Q Parathyroid Glands, Multiple
R Parathyroid Gland
	0 Open
	3 Percutaneous
	4 Percutaneous Endoscopic
		0 Drainage Device	Z No Qualifier

0 Pituitary Gland
  Adenohypophysis
  Hypophysis
  Neurohypophysis
1 Pineal Body
2 Adrenal Gland, Left
  Suprarenal gland
3 Adrenal Gland, Right
  See 2 Adrenal Gland, Left
4 Adrenal Glands, Bilateral
  See 2 Adrenal Gland, Left
6 Carotid Body, Left
  Carotid glomus
7 Carotid Body, Right
  See 6 Carotid Body, Left
8 Carotid Bodies, Bilateral
  See 6 Carotid Body, Left
9 Para-aortic Body
B Coccygeal Glomus
  Coccygeal body
C Glomus Jugulare
  Jugular body
D Aortic Body
F Paraganglion Extremity
G Thyroid Gland Lobe, Left
H Thyroid Gland Lobe, Right
K Thyroid Gland
L Superior Parathyroid Gland, Right
M Superior Parathyroid Gland, Left
N Inferior Parathyroid Gland, Right
P Inferior Parathyroid Gland, Left
Q Parathyroid Glands, Multiple
R Parathyroid Gland
	0 Open
	3 Percutaneous
	4 Percutaneous Endoscopic
		Z No Device	X Diagnostic
			Z No Qualifier

Non-OR 0G9[0,1,2,3,4,6,7,8,9,B,C,D,F,G,H,K,L,M,N,P,Q,R]30Z
Non-OR 0G9[G,H,K,L,M,N,P,Q,R]40Z
Non-OR 0G9[2,3,4,G,H,K][3,4]ZX
Non-OR 0G9[0,1,2,3,4,6,7,8,9,B,C,D,F,G,H,K,L,M,N,P,Q,R]3ZZ
Non-OR 0G9[G,H,K,L,M,N,P,Q,R]4ZZ

0 Medical and Surgical
G Endocrine System
B Excision   Definition: Cutting out or off, without replacement, a portion of a body part
Explanation: The qualifier DIAGNOSTIC is used to identify excision procedures that are biopsies

Body Part Character 4	Approach Character 5	Device Character 6	Qualifier Character 7

0 Pituitary Gland
  Adenohypophysis
  Hypophysis
  Neurohypophysis
1 Pineal Body
2 Adrenal Gland, Left
  Suprarenal gland
3 Adrenal Gland, Right
  See 2 Adrenal Gland, Left
4 Adrenal Glands, Bilateral
  See 2 Adrenal Gland, Left
6 Carotid Body, Left
  Carotid glomus
7 Carotid Body, Right
  See 6 Carotid Body, Left
8 Carotid Bodies, Bilateral
  See 6 Carotid Body, Left
9 Para-aortic Body
B Coccygeal Glomus
  Coccygeal body
C Glomus Jugulare
  Jugular body
D Aortic Body
F Paraganglion Extremity
G Thyroid Gland Lobe, Left
H Thyroid Gland Lobe, Right
J Thyroid Gland Isthmus
L Superior Parathyroid Gland, Right
M Superior Parathyroid Gland, Left
N Inferior Parathyroid Gland, Right
P Inferior Parathyroid Gland, Left
Q Parathyroid Glands, Multiple
R Parathyroid Gland
	0 Open
	3 Percutaneous
	4 Percutaneous Endoscopic
		Z No Device	**X** Diagnostic
			Z No Qualifier

Non-OR   0GB[2,3,4,G,H,J][3,4]ZX

ICD-10-PCS 2025   Endocrine System   0GC–0GJ

0 Medical and Surgical
G Endocrine System
C Extirpation   Definition: Taking or cutting out solid matter from a body part

Explanation: The solid matter may be an abnormal byproduct of a biological function or a foreign body; it may be imbedded in a body part or in the lumen of a tubular body part. The solid matter may or may not have been previously broken into pieces.

Body Part Character 4	Approach Character 5	Device Character 6	Qualifier Character 7

0 Pituitary Gland
   Adenohypophysis
   Hypophysis
   Neurohypophysis
1 Pineal Body
2 Adrenal Gland, Left
   Suprarenal gland
3 Adrenal Gland, Right
   See 2 Adrenal Gland, Left
4 Adrenal Glands, Bilateral
   See 2 Adrenal Gland, Left
6 Carotid Body, Left
   Carotid glomus
7 Carotid Body, Right
   See 6 Carotid Body, Left
8 Carotid Bodies, Bilateral
   See 6 Carotid Body, Left
9 Para-aortic Body
B Coccygeal Glomus
   Coccygeal body
C Glomus Jugulare
   Jugular body
D Aortic Body
F Paraganglion Extremity
G Thyroid Gland Lobe, Left
H Thyroid Gland Lobe, Right
K Thyroid Gland
L Superior Parathyroid Gland, Right
M Superior Parathyroid Gland, Left
N Inferior Parathyroid Gland, Right
P Inferior Parathyroid Gland, Left
Q Parathyroid Glands, Multiple
R Parathyroid Gland
	0 Open
	3 Percutaneous
	4 Percutaneous Endoscopic
		Z No Device	Z No Qualifier

0 Medical and Surgical
G Endocrine System
H Insertion   Definition: Putting in a nonbiological appliance that monitors, assists, performs, or prevents a physiological function but does not physically take the place of a body part

Explanation: None

Body Part Character 4	Approach Character 5	Device Character 6	Qualifier Character 7
S Endocrine Gland	0 Open 3 Percutaneous 4 Percutaneous Endoscopic	1 Radioactive Element 2 Monitoring Device 3 Infusion Device Y Other Device	Z No Qualifier

Non-OR   0GHS31Z
Non-OR   0GHS[3,4]YZ

0 Medical and Surgical
G Endocrine System
J Inspection   Definition: Visually and/or manually exploring a body part

Explanation: Visual exploration may be performed with or without optical instrumentation. Manual exploration may be performed directly or through intervening body layers.

Body Part Character 4	Approach Character 5	Device Character 6	Qualifier Character 7

0 Pituitary Gland
   Adenohypophysis
   Hypophysis
   Neurohypophysis
1 Pineal Body
5 Adrenal Gland
   Suprarenal gland
K Thyroid Gland
R Parathyroid Gland
S Endocrine Gland
	0 Open
	3 Percutaneous
	4 Percutaneous Endoscopic
		Z No Device	Z No Qualifier

Non-OR   0GJ[0,1,5,K,R,S]3ZZ

0 Medical and Surgical
G Endocrine System
M Reattachment   Definition: Putting back in or on all or a portion of a separated body part to its normal location or other suitable location
                     Explanation: Vascular circulation and nervous pathways may or may not be reestablished

Body Part Character 4	Approach Character 5	Device Character 6	Qualifier Character 7

2 Adrenal Gland, Left
    Suprarenal gland
3 Adrenal Gland, Right
    See 2 Adrenal Gland, Left
G Thyroid Gland Lobe, Left
H Thyroid Gland Lobe, Right
L Superior Parathyroid Gland, Right
M Superior Parathyroid Gland, Left
N Inferior Parathyroid Gland, Right
P Inferior Parathyroid Gland, Left
Q Parathyroid Glands, Multiple
R Parathyroid Gland
	0 Open
	4 Percutaneous Endoscopic
		Z No Device	**Z** No Qualifier

0 Medical and Surgical
G Endocrine System
N Release   Definition: Freeing a body part from an abnormal physical constraint by cutting or by the use of force
                Explanation: Some of the restraining tissue may be taken out but none of the body part is taken out

Body Part Character 4	Approach Character 5	Device Character 6	Qualifier Character 7

0 Pituitary Gland
    Adenohypophysis
    Hypophysis
    Neurohypophysis
1 Pineal Body
2 Adrenal Gland, Left
    Suprarenal gland
3 Adrenal Gland, Right
    See 2 Adrenal Gland, Left
4 Adrenal Glands, Bilateral
    See 2 Adrenal Gland, Left
6 Carotid Body, Left
    Carotid glomus
7 Carotid Body, Right
    See 6 Carotid Body, Left
8 Carotid Bodies, Bilateral
    See 6 Carotid Body, Left
9 Para-aortic Body
B Coccygeal Glomus
    Coccygeal body
C Glomus Jugulare
    Jugular body
D Aortic Body
F Paraganglion Extremity
G Thyroid Gland Lobe, Left
H Thyroid Gland Lobe, Right
K Thyroid Gland
L Superior Parathyroid Gland, Right
M Superior Parathyroid Gland, Left
N Inferior Parathyroid Gland, Right
P Inferior Parathyroid Gland, Left
Q Parathyroid Glands, Multiple
R Parathyroid Gland
	0 Open
	3 Percutaneous
	4 Percutaneous Endoscopic
		Z No Device	**Z** No Qualifier

Non-OR   0GN[6,7,8,9,B,C,D,F][0,3,4]ZZ

ICD-10-PCS 2025 — Endocrine System — 0GP–0GQ

0 Medical and Surgical
G Endocrine System
P Removal   Definition: Taking out or off a device from a body part
Explanation: If a device is taken out and a similar device put in without cutting or puncturing the skin or mucous membrane, the procedure is coded to the root operation CHANGE. Otherwise, the procedure for taking out a device is coded to the root operation REMOVAL.

Body Part Character 4	Approach Character 5	Device Character 6	Qualifier Character 7

0 Pituitary Gland
  Adenohypophysis
  Hypophysis
  Neurohypophysis
1 Pineal Body
5 Adrenal Gland
  Suprarenal gland
K Thyroid Gland
R Parathyroid Gland
	0 Open
	3 Percutaneous
	4 Percutaneous Endoscopic
	X External
		0 Drainage Device	Z No Qualifier

S Endocrine Gland	0 Open 3 Percutaneous 4 Percutaneous Endoscopic	0 Drainage Device 2 Monitoring Device 3 Infusion Device Y Other Device	Z No Qualifier
S Endocrine Gland	X External	0 Drainage Device 2 Monitoring Device 3 Infusion Device	Z No Qualifier

Non-OR 0GP[0,1,5,K,R]X0Z
Non-OR 0GPS[3,4]YZ
Non-OR 0GPSX[0,2,3]Z

0 Medical and Surgical
G Endocrine System
Q Repair   Definition: Restoring, to the extent possible, a body part to its normal anatomic structure and function
Explanation: Used only when the method to accomplish the repair is not one of the other root operations

Body Part Character 4	Approach Character 5	Device Character 6	Qualifier Character 7

0 Pituitary Gland
  Adenohypophysis
  Hypophysis
  Neurohypophysis
1 Pineal Body
2 Adrenal Gland, Left
  Suprarenal gland
3 Adrenal Gland, Right
  See 2 Adrenal Gland, Left
4 Adrenal Glands, Bilateral
  See 2 Adrenal Gland, Left
6 Carotid Body, Left
  Carotid glomus
7 Carotid Body, Right
  See 6 Carotid Body, Left
8 Carotid Bodies, Bilateral
  See 6 Carotid Body, Left
9 Para-aortic Body
B Coccygeal Glomus
  Coccygeal body
C Glomus Jugulare
  Jugular body
D Aortic Body
F Paraganglion Extremity
G Thyroid Gland Lobe, Left
H Thyroid Gland Lobe, Right
J Thyroid Gland Isthmus
K Thyroid Gland
L Superior Parathyroid Gland, Right
M Superior Parathyroid Gland, Left
N Inferior Parathyroid Gland, Right
P Inferior Parathyroid Gland, Left
Q Parathyroid Glands, Multiple
R Parathyroid Gland
	0 Open
	3 Percutaneous
	4 Percutaneous Endoscopic
		Z No Device	Z No Qualifier

0 Medical and Surgical
G Endocrine System
S Reposition

Definition: Moving to its normal location, or other suitable location, all or a portion of a body part

Explanation: The body part is moved to a new location from an abnormal location, or from a normal location where it is not functioning correctly. The body part may or may not be cut out or off to be moved to the new location.

Body Part Character 4	Approach Character 5	Device Character 6	Qualifier Character 7

2 Adrenal Gland, Left
   Suprarenal gland
3 Adrenal Gland, Right
   See 2 Adrenal Gland, Left
G Thyroid Gland Lobe, Left
H Thyroid Gland Lobe, Right
L Superior Parathyroid Gland, Right
M Superior Parathyroid Gland, Left
N Inferior Parathyroid Gland, Right
P Inferior Parathyroid Gland, Left
Q Parathyroid Glands, Multiple
R Parathyroid Gland
	0 Open
	4 Percutaneous Endoscopic
		Z No Device	Z No Qualifier

0 Medical and Surgical
G Endocrine System
T Resection

Definition: Cutting out or off, without replacement, all of a body part

Explanation: None

Body Part Character 4	Approach Character 5	Device Character 6	Qualifier Character 7

0 Pituitary Gland
   Adenohypophysis
   Hypophysis
   Neurohypophysis
1 Pineal Body
2 Adrenal Gland, Left
   Suprarenal gland
3 Adrenal Gland, Right
   See 2 Adrenal Gland, Left
4 Adrenal Glands, Bilateral
   See 2 Adrenal Gland, Left
6 Carotid Body, Left
   Carotid glomus
7 Carotid Body, Right
   See 6 Carotid Body, Left
8 Carotid Bodies, Bilateral
   See 6 Carotid Body, Left
9 Para-aortic Body
B Coccygeal Glomus
   Coccygeal body
C Glomus Jugulare
   Jugular body
D Aortic Body
F Paraganglion Extremity
G Thyroid Gland Lobe, Left
H Thyroid Gland Lobe, Right
J Thyroid Gland Isthmus
K Thyroid Gland
L Superior Parathyroid Gland, Right
M Superior Parathyroid Gland, Left
N Inferior Parathyroid Gland, Right
P Inferior Parathyroid Gland, Left
Q Parathyroid Glands, Multiple
R Parathyroid Gland
	0 Open
	4 Percutaneous Endoscopic
		Z No Device	Z No Qualifier

Non-OR 0GT[6,7,8,9,B,C,D,F][0,4]ZZ

ICD-10-PCS 2025 — Endocrine System — 0GW–0GW

0 Medical and Surgical
G Endocrine System
W Revision

Definition: Correcting, to the extent possible, a portion of a malfunctioning device or the position of a displaced device

Explanation: Revision can include correcting a malfunctioning or displaced device by taking out or putting in components of the device such as a screw or pin

Body Part Character 4	Approach Character 5	Device Character 6	Qualifier Character 7

0 Pituitary Gland
    Adenohypophysis
    Hypophysis
    Neurohypophysis
1 Pineal Body
5 Adrenal Gland
    Suprarenal gland
K Thyroid Gland
R Parathyroid Gland
	0 Open
	3 Percutaneous
	4 Percutaneous Endoscopic
	X External
		0 Drainage Device	**Z** No Qualifier

S Endocrine Gland	**0** Open **3** Percutaneous **4** Percutaneous Endoscopic	**0** Drainage Device **2** Monitoring Device **3** Infusion Device **Y** Other Device	**Z** No Qualifier
S Endocrine Gland	**X** External	**0** Drainage Device **2** Monitoring Device **3** Infusion Device	**Z** No Qualifier

Non-OR   0GW[0,1,5,K,R]X0Z
Non-OR   0GWS[3,4]YZ
Non-OR   0GWSX[0,2,3]Z

Skin and Breast ØHØ–ØHX

Character Meanings*

This Character Meaning table is provided as a guide to assist the user in the identification of character members that may be found in this section of code tables. It **SHOULD NOT** be used to build a PCS code.

Operation–Character 3	Body Part–Character 4	Approach–Character 5	Device–Character 6	Qualifier–Character 7
Ø Alteration	Ø Skin, Scalp	Ø Open	Ø Drainage Device	2 Cell Suspension Technique
2 Change	1 Skin, Face	3 Percutaneous	1 Radioactive Element	3 Full Thickness OR Laser Interstitial Thermal Therapy
5 Destruction	2 Skin, Right Ear	7 Via Natural or Artificial Opening	7 Autologous Tissue Substitute	4 Partial Thickness
8 Division	3 Skin, Left Ear	8 Via Natural or Artificial Opening Endoscopic	J Synthetic Substitute	5 Latissimus Dorsi Myocutaneous Flap
9 Drainage	4 Skin, Neck	X External	K Nonautologous Tissue Substitute	6 Transverse Rectus Abdominis Myocutaneous Flap
B Excision	5 Skin, Chest		N Tissue Expander	7 Deep Inferior Epigastric Artery Perforator Flap
C Extirpation	6 Skin, Back		Y Other Device	8 Superficial Inferior Epigastric Artery Flap
D Extraction	7 Skin, Abdomen		Z No Device	9 Gluteal Artery Perforator Flap
H Insertion	8 Skin, Buttock			B Lumbar Artery Perforator Flap
J Inspection	9 Skin, Perineum			D Multiple
M Reattachment	A Skin, Inguinal			X Diagnostic
N Release	B Skin, Right Upper Arm			Z No Qualifier
P Removal	C Skin, Left Upper Arm			
Q Repair	D Skin, Right Lower Arm			
R Replacement	E Skin, Left Lower Arm			
S Reposition	F Skin, Right Hand			
T Resection	G Skin, Left Hand			
U Supplement	H Skin, Right Upper Leg			
W Revision	J Skin, Left Upper Leg			
X Transfer	K Skin, Right Lower Leg			
	L Skin, Left Lower Leg			
	M Skin, Right Foot			
	N Skin, Left Foot			
	P Skin			
	Q Finger Nail			
	R Toe Nail			
	S Hair			
	T Breast, Right			
	U Breast, Left			
	V Breast, Bilateral			
	W Nipple, Right			
	X Nipple, Left			
	Y Supernumerary Breast			

* Includes skin and breast glands and ducts.

Skin and Breast

AHA Coding Clinic for table 0H0
- 2022, 1Q, 14 — Reduction mammoplasty for breast symmetry
- 2022, 1Q, 15 — Nipple reconstruction and breast reduction
- 2019, 4Q, 30-31 — Breast procedures

AHA Coding Clinic for table 0H5
- 2022, 4Q, 53-54 — Laser interstitial thermal therapy
- 2019, 4Q, 30-31 — Breast procedures

AHA Coding Clinic for table 0H9
- 2019, 4Q, 30-31 — Breast procedures

AHA Coding Clinic for table 0HB
- 2022, 1Q, 14 — Reduction mammoplasty for breast symmetry
- 2020, 1Q, 31 — Repair of buried penis
- 2019, 4Q, 30-31 — Breast procedures
- 2018, 1Q, 14 — Excisional debridement of breast tissue and skin
- 2016, 3Q, 29 — Closure of bilateral alveolar clefts
- 2015, 3Q, 3-8 — Excisional and nonexcisional debridement

AHA Coding Clinic for table 0HC
- 2019, 4Q, 30-31 — Breast procedures

AHA Coding Clinic for table 0HD
- 2019, 4Q, 30-31 — Breast procedures
- 2016, 1Q, 40 — Nonexcisional debridement of skin and subcutaneous tissue
- 2015, 3Q, 3-8 — Excisional and nonexcisional debridement

AHA Coding Clinic for table 0HH
- 2019, 4Q, 30-31 — Breast procedures
- 2017, 4Q, 67 — New qualifier values - Pedicle flap procedures
- 2014, 2Q, 12 — Pedicle latissimus myocutaneous flap with placement of breast tissue expanders
- 2013, 4Q, 107 — Breast tissue expander placement using acellular dermal matrix

AHA Coding Clinic for table 0HJ
- 2019, 4Q, 30-31 — Breast procedures

AHA Coding Clinic for table 0HN
- 2019, 4Q, 30-31 — Breast procedures

AHA Coding Clinic for table 0HP
- 2022, 3Q, 20 — Bilateral breast capsulectomy and tissue expander removal
- 2019, 4Q, 30-31 — Breast procedures
- 2018, 3Q, 13 — Deep inferior epigastric artery perforator flap breast reconstruction
- 2016, 2Q, 27 — Removal of nonviable transverse rectus abdominis myocutaneous (TRAM) flaps

AHA Coding Clinic for table 0HQ
- 2019, 4Q, 30-31 — Breast procedures
- 2018, 2Q, 25 — Third and fourth degree obstetric lacerations
- 2016, 1Q, 7 — Obstetrical perineal laceration repair
- 2014, 4Q, 31 — Delayed wound closure following fracture treatment

AHA Coding Clinic for table 0HR
- 2023, 2Q, 30 — Inframammary fold adjacent tissue transfer and deep inferior epigastric perforator flap breast reconstruction
- 2022, 1Q, 15 — Nipple reconstruction and breast reduction
- 2020, 1Q, 27 — Delayed reconstruction following mastectomy using gracilis musculocutaneous free flap
- 2020, 1Q, 28 — Free flap microvascular breast reconstruction
- 2020, 1Q, 30 — Polarity Skin TE™ application
- 2019, 4Q, 30-31 — Breast procedures
- 2019, 4Q, 32 — Cell suspension epithelial autograft
- 2019, 3Q, 32 — Breast reconstruction with neurotization
- 2018, 3Q, 13 — Deep inferior epigastric artery perforator flap breast reconstruction
- 2017, 1Q, 35 — Epifix® allograft
- 2014, 3Q, 14 — Application of TheraSkin® and excisional debridement

AHA Coding Clinic for table 0HT
- 2021, 2Q, 16 — Goldilocks breast reconstruction
- 2018, 3Q, 13 — Deep inferior epigastric artery perforator flap breast reconstruction
- 2014, 4Q, 34 — Skin-sparing mastectomy

AHA Coding Clinic for table 0HU
- 2019, 4Q, 30-31 — Breast procedures

AHA Coding Clinic for table 0HW
- 2019, 4Q, 30-31 — Breast procedures

AHA Coding Clinic for table 0HX
- 2023, 2Q, 23 — V-Y anoplasty and excision of mucosal ectropion
- 2023, 2Q, 30 — Inframammary fold adjacent tissue transfer and deep inferior epigastric perforator flap breast reconstruction
- 2022, 3Q, 13 — Repair of prolapsed neovaginal graft

Skin and Breast

Integumentary Anatomy

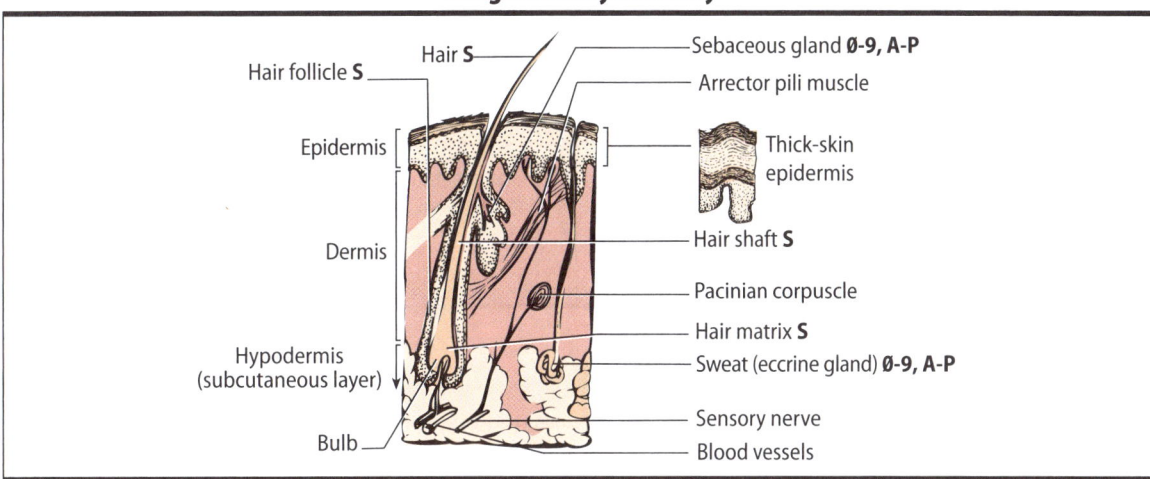

- Hair follicle **S**
- Hair **S**
- Sebaceous gland **Ø-9, A-P**
- Arrector pili muscle
- Epidermis
- Thick-skin epidermis
- Dermis
- Hair shaft **S**
- Pacinian corpuscle
- Hair matrix **S**
- Hypodermis (subcutaneous layer)
- Sweat (eccrine gland) **Ø-9, A-P**
- Sensory nerve
- Bulb
- Blood vessels

Nail Anatomy

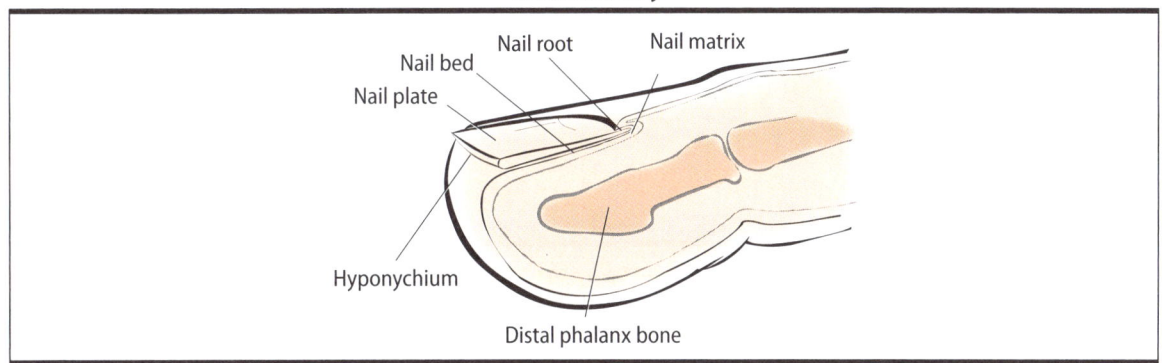

- Nail bed
- Nail root
- Nail matrix
- Nail plate
- Hyponychium
- Distal phalanx bone

Breast

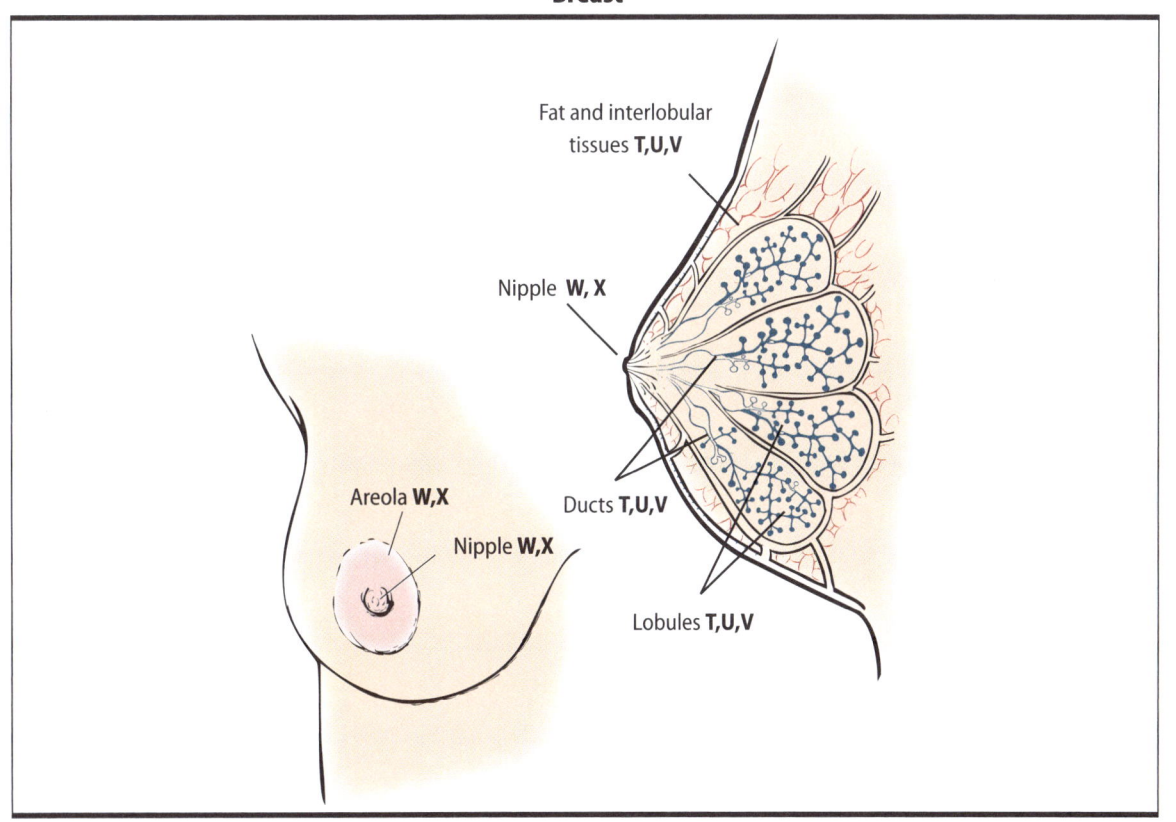

- Fat and interlobular tissues **T, U, V**
- Nipple **W, X**
- Areola **W, X**
- Nipple **W, X**
- Ducts **T, U, V**
- Lobules **T, U, V**

Skin and Breast

0 Medical and Surgical
H Skin and Breast
0 Alteration

Definition: Modifying the anatomic structure of a body part without affecting the function of the body part
Explanation: Principal purpose is to improve appearance

Body Part Character 4	Approach Character 5	Device Character 6	Qualifier Character 7

T Breast, Right
  Mammary duct
  Mammary gland
U Breast, Left
  See T Breast, Right
V Breast, Bilateral
  See T Breast, Right
	0 Open
	3 Percutaneous
		7 Autologous Tissue Substitute
		J Synthetic Substitute
		K Nonautologous Tissue Substitute
		Z No Device
			Z No Qualifier

Non-OR 0H0[T,U,V]3JZ

0 Medical and Surgical
H Skin and Breast
2 Change

Definition: Taking out or off a device from a body part and putting back an identical or similar device in or on the same body part without cutting or puncturing the skin or a mucous membrane
Explanation: All CHANGE procedures are coded using the approach EXTERNAL

Body Part Character 4	Approach Character 5	Device Character 6	Qualifier Character 7

P Skin
  Dermis
  Epidermis
  Sebaceous gland
  Sweat gland
T Breast, Right
  Mammary duct
  Mammary gland
U Breast, Left
  See T Breast, Right
	X External	0 Drainage Device
		Y Other Device
			Z No Qualifier

Non-OR All body part, approach, device, and qualifier values

0 Medical and Surgical
H Skin and Breast
5 Destruction   Definition: Physical eradication of all or a portion of a body part by the direct use of energy, force, or a destructive agent
Explanation: None of the body part is physically taken out

Body Part Character 4	Approach Character 5	Device Character 6	Qualifier Character 7

0 Skin, Scalp
1 Skin, Face
2 Skin, Right Ear
3 Skin, Left Ear
4 Skin, Neck
5 Skin, Chest
    Breast procedures, skin only
6 Skin, Back
7 Skin, Abdomen
8 Skin, Buttock
9 Skin, Perineum
    Perianal skin
A Skin, Inguinal
B Skin, Right Upper Arm
C Skin, Left Upper Arm
D Skin, Right Lower Arm
E Skin, Left Lower Arm
F Skin, Right Hand
G Skin, Left Hand
H Skin, Right Upper Leg
J Skin, Left Upper Leg
K Skin, Right Lower Leg
L Skin, Left Lower Leg
M Skin, Right Foot
N Skin, Left Foot
	X External	**Z** No Device	**D** Multiple
			Z No Qualifier

Q Finger Nail
    Nail bed
    Nail plate
R Toe Nail
    See Q Finger Nail
	X External	**Z** No Device	**Z** No Qualifier

T Breast, Right
    Mammary duct
    Mammary gland
U Breast, Left
    See T Breast, Right
V Breast, Bilateral
    See T Breast, Right
	0 Open
	3 Percutaneous
		Z No Device	**3** Laser Interstitial Thermal Therapy
			Z No Qualifier

T Breast, Right
    Mammary duct
    Mammary gland
U Breast, Left
    See T Breast, Right
V Breast, Bilateral
    See T Breast, Right
	7 Via Natural or Artificial Opening
	8 Via Natural or Artificial Opening Endoscopic
		Z No Device	**Z** No Qualifier

W Nipple, Right
    Areola
X Nipple, Left
    See W Nipple, Right
	0 Open
	3 Percutaneous
	7 Via Natural or Artificial Opening
	8 Via Natural or Artificial Opening Endoscopic
	X External
		Z No Device	**Z** No Qualifier

DRG Non-OR 0H5[0,1,4,5,6,7,8,9,A,B,C,D,E,F,G,H,J,K,L,M,N]XZ[D,Z]
DRG Non-OR 0H5[Q,R]XZZ
Non-OR 0H5[2,3]XZ[D,Z]

0 Medical and Surgical
H Skin and Breast
8 Division

Definition: Cutting into a body part, without draining fluids and/or gases from the body part, in order to separate or transect a body part
Explanation: All or a portion of the body part is separated into two or more portions

Body Part Character 4	Approach Character 5	Device Character 6	Qualifier Character 7

0 Skin, Scalp
1 Skin, Face
2 Skin, Right Ear
3 Skin, Left Ear
4 Skin, Neck
5 Skin, Chest
   Breast procedures, skin only
6 Skin, Back
7 Skin, Abdomen
8 Skin, Buttock
9 Skin, Perineum
   Perianal skin
A Skin, Inguinal
B Skin, Right Upper Arm
C Skin, Left Upper Arm
D Skin, Right Lower Arm
E Skin, Left Lower Arm
F Skin, Right Hand
G Skin, Left Hand
H Skin, Right Upper Leg
J Skin, Left Upper Leg
K Skin, Right Lower Leg
L Skin, Left Lower Leg
M Skin, Right Foot
N Skin, Left Foot
	X External	Z No Device	Z No Qualifier

Non-OR All body part, approach, device, and qualifier values

| ICD-10-PCS 2025 | Skin and Breast | 0H9–0H9 |

0 Medical and Surgical
H Skin and Breast
9 Drainage   Definition: Taking or letting out fluids and/or gases from a body part
Explanation: The qualifier DIAGNOSTIC is used to identify drainage procedures that are biopsies

Body Part Character 4	Approach Character 5	Device Character 6	Qualifier Character 7

0 Skin, Scalp
1 Skin, Face
2 Skin, Right Ear
3 Skin, Left Ear
4 Skin, Neck
5 Skin, Chest
   Breast procedures, skin only
6 Skin, Back
7 Skin, Abdomen
8 Skin, Buttock
9 Skin, Perineum
   Perianal skin
A Skin, Inguinal
B Skin, Right Upper Arm
C Skin, Left Upper Arm
D Skin, Right Lower Arm
E Skin, Left Lower Arm
F Skin, Right Hand
G Skin, Left Hand
H Skin, Right Upper Leg
J Skin, Left Upper Leg
K Skin, Right Lower Leg
L Skin, Left Lower Leg
M Skin, Right Foot
N Skin, Left Foot
Q Finger Nail
   Nail bed
   Nail plate
R Toe Nail
   See Q Finger Nail
	X External	**0** Drainage Device	**Z** No Qualifier

0 Skin, Scalp
1 Skin, Face
2 Skin, Right Ear
3 Skin, Left Ear
4 Skin, Neck
5 Skin, Chest
   Breast procedures, skin only
6 Skin, Back
7 Skin, Abdomen
8 Skin, Buttock
9 Skin, Perineum
   Perianal skin
A Skin, Inguinal
B Skin, Right Upper Arm
C Skin, Left Upper Arm
D Skin, Right Lower Arm
E Skin, Left Lower Arm
F Skin, Right Hand
G Skin, Left Hand
H Skin, Right Upper Leg
J Skin, Left Upper Leg
K Skin, Right Lower Leg
L Skin, Left Lower Leg
M Skin, Right Foot
N Skin, Left Foot
Q Finger Nail
   Nail bed
   Nail plate
R Toe Nail
   See Q Finger Nail
	X External	**Z** No Device	**X** Diagnostic
			Z No Qualifier

T Breast, Right
   Mammary duct
   Mammary gland
U Breast, Left
   See T Breast, Right
V Breast, Bilateral
   See T Breast, Right
	0 Open
	3 Percutaneous
	7 Via Natural or Artificial Opening
	8 Via Natural or Artificial Opening Endoscopic
		0 Drainage Device	**Z** No Qualifier

T Breast, Right
   Mammary duct
   Mammary gland
U Breast, Left
   See T Breast, Right
V Breast, Bilateral
   See T Breast, Right
	0 Open
	3 Percutaneous
	7 Via Natural or Artificial Opening
	8 Via Natural or Artificial Opening Endoscopic
		Z No Device	**X** Diagnostic
			Z No Qualifier

W Nipple, Right
   Areola
X Nipple, Left
   See W Nipple, Right
	0 Open
	3 Percutaneous
	7 Via Natural or Artificial Opening
	8 Via Natural or Artificial Opening Endoscopic
	X External
		0 Drainage Device	**Z** No Qualifier

W Nipple, Right
   Areola
X Nipple, Left
   See W Nipple, Right
	0 Open
	3 Percutaneous
	7 Via Natural or Artificial Opening
	8 Via Natural or Artificial Opening Endoscopic
	X External
		Z No Device	**X** Diagnostic
			Z No Qualifier

Non-OR 0H9[0,1,2,3,4,5,6,7,8,A,B,C,D,E,F,G,H,J,K,L,M,N,Q,R]X0Z
Non-OR 0H9[0,1,2,3,4,5,6,7,8,A,B,C,D,E,F,G,H,J,K,L,M,N,Q,R]XZ[X,Z]
Non-OR 0H99XZX
Non-OR 0H9[T,U,V][0,3,7,8]0Z
Non-OR 0H9[T,U,V][3,7,8]Z[X,Z]
Non-OR 0H9[W,X][0,3,7,8,X]0Z
Non-OR 0H9[W,X][3,7,8,X]Z[X,Z]

NC Noncovered Procedure   **LC** Limited Coverage   **QA** Questionable OB Admit   **NT** New Tech Add-on   ✚ Combination Member   ♂ Male   ♀ Female

0HB–0HB   Skin and Breast   ICD-10-PCS 2025

0 Medical and Surgical
H Skin and Breast
B Excision   Definition: Cutting out or off, without replacement, a portion of a body part
               Explanation: The qualifier DIAGNOSTIC is used to identify excision procedures that are biopsies

Body Part Character 4	Approach Character 5	Device Character 6	Qualifier Character 7

0 Skin, Scalp
1 Skin, Face
2 Skin, Right Ear
3 Skin, Left Ear
4 Skin, Neck
5 Skin, Chest
    Breast procedures, skin only
6 Skin, Back
7 Skin, Abdomen
8 Skin, Buttock
9 Skin, Perineum
    Perianal skin
A Skin, Inguinal
B Skin, Right Upper Arm
C Skin, Left Upper Arm
D Skin, Right Lower Arm
E Skin, Left Lower Arm
F Skin, Right Hand
G Skin, Left Hand
H Skin, Right Upper Leg
J Skin, Left Upper Leg
K Skin, Right Lower Leg
L Skin, Left Lower Leg
M Skin, Right Foot
N Skin, Left Foot
Q Finger Nail
    Nail bed
    Nail plate
R Toe Nail
    See Q Finger Nail
	X External	Z No Device	X Diagnostic
			Z No Qualifier

T Breast, Right
    Mammary duct
    Mammary gland
U Breast, Left
    See T Breast, Right
V Breast, Bilateral
    See T Breast, Right
Y Supernumerary Breast
	0 Open
	3 Percutaneous
	7 Via Natural or Artificial Opening
	8 Via Natural or Artificial Opening Endoscopic
		Z No Device	X Diagnostic
			Z No Qualifier

W Nipple, Right
    Areola
X Nipple, Left
    See W Nipple, Right
	0 Open
	3 Percutaneous
	7 Via Natural or Artificial Opening
	8 Via Natural or Artificial Opening Endoscopic
	X External
		Z No Device	X Diagnostic
			Z No Qualifier

DRG Non-OR   0HB9XZZ
Non-OR   0HB[0,1,2,3,4,5,6,7,8,A,B,C,D,E,F,G,H,J,K,L,M,N,Q,R]XZ[X,Z]
Non-OR   0HB9XZX
Non-OR   0HB[T,U,V,Y][3,7,8]ZX
Non-OR   0HB[W,X][3,7,8,X]ZX

ICD-10-PCS 2025 — Skin and Breast — 0HC–0HC

0 Medical and Surgical
H Skin and Breast
C Extirpation

Definition: Taking or cutting out solid matter from a body part
Explanation: The solid matter may be an abnormal byproduct of a biological function or a foreign body; it may be imbedded in a body part or in the lumen of a tubular body part. The solid matter may or may not have been previously broken into pieces.

Body Part Character 4	Approach Character 5	Device Character 6	Qualifier Character 7

0 Skin, Scalp
1 Skin, Face
2 Skin, Right Ear
3 Skin, Left Ear
4 Skin, Neck
5 Skin, Chest
   Breast procedures, skin only
6 Skin, Back
7 Skin, Abdomen
8 Skin, Buttock
9 Skin, Perineum
   Perianal skin
A Skin, Inguinal
B Skin, Right Upper Arm
C Skin, Left Upper Arm
D Skin, Right Lower Arm
E Skin, Left Lower Arm
F Skin, Right Hand
G Skin, Left Hand
H Skin, Right Upper Leg
J Skin, Left Upper Leg
K Skin, Right Lower Leg
L Skin, Left Lower Leg
M Skin, Right Foot
N Skin, Left Foot
Q Finger Nail
   Nail bed
   Nail plate
R Toe Nail
   See Q Finger Nail
	X External	Z No Device	Z No Qualifier

T Breast, Right
   Mammary duct
   Mammary gland
U Breast, Left
   See T Breast, Right
V Breast, Bilateral
   See T Breast, Right
	0 Open
	3 Percutaneous
	7 Via Natural or Artificial Opening
	8 Via Natural or Artificial Opening Endoscopic
		Z No Device	Z No Qualifier

W Nipple, Right
   Areola
X Nipple, Left
   See W Nipple, Right
	0 Open
	3 Percutaneous
	7 Via Natural or Artificial Opening
	8 Via Natural or Artificial Opening Endoscopic
	X External
		Z No Device	Z No Qualifier

Non-OR   0HC[0,1,2,3,4,5,6,7,8,9,A,B,C,D,E,F,G,H,J,K,L,M,N,Q,R]XZZ
Non-OR   0HC[T,U,V][3,7,8]ZZ
Non-OR   0HC[W,X][3,7,8,X]ZZ

Skin and Breast

0 Medical and Surgical
H Skin and Breast
D Extraction Definition: Pulling or stripping out or off all or a portion of a body part by the use of force
Explanation: The qualifier DIAGNOSTIC is used to identify extraction procedures that are biopsies

Body Part Character 4	Approach Character 5	Device Character 6	Qualifier Character 7

0 Skin, Scalp
1 Skin, Face
2 Skin, Right Ear
3 Skin, Left Ear
4 Skin, Neck
5 Skin, Chest
    Breast procedures, skin only
6 Skin, Back
7 Skin, Abdomen
8 Skin, Buttock
9 Skin, Perineum
    Perianal skin
A Skin, Inguinal
B Skin, Right Upper Arm
C Skin, Left Upper Arm
D Skin, Right Lower Arm
E Skin, Left Lower Arm
F Skin, Right Hand
G Skin, Left Hand
H Skin, Right Upper Leg
J Skin, Left Upper Leg
K Skin, Right Lower Leg
L Skin, Left Lower Leg
M Skin, Right Foot
N Skin, Left Foot
Q Finger Nail
    Nail bed
    Nail plate
R Toe Nail
    See Q Finger Nail
S Hair
	X External	**Z** No Device	**Z** No Qualifier

T Breast, Right
    Mammary duct
    Mammary gland
U Breast, Left
    See T Breast, Right
V Breast, Bilateral
    See T Breast, Right
Y Supernumerary Breast
	0 Open	**Z** No Device	**Z** No Qualifier

Non-OR All body part, approach, device, and qualifier values

0 Medical and Surgical
H Skin and Breast
H Insertion Definition: Putting in a nonbiological appliance that monitors, assists, performs, or prevents a physiological function but does not physically take the place of a body part
Explanation: None

Body Part Character 4	Approach Character 5	Device Character 6	Qualifier Character 7
P Skin	X External	Y Other Device	Z No Qualifier

T Breast, Right
  Mammary duct
  Mammary gland
U Breast, Left
  See T Breast, Right
	0 Open
	3 Percutaneous
	7 Via Natural or Artificial Opening
	8 Via Natural or Artificial Opening Endoscopic
		1 Radioactive Element
		N Tissue Expander
		Y Other Device
			Z No Qualifier

V Breast, Bilateral
  Mammary duct
  Mammary gland
	0 Open
	3 Percutaneous
	7 Via Natural or Artificial Opening
	8 Via Natural or Artificial Opening Endoscopic
		1 Radioactive Element
		N Tissue Expander
			Z No Qualifier

W Nipple, Right
  Areola
X Nipple, Left
  See W Nipple, Right
	0 Open
	3 Percutaneous
	7 Via Natural or Artificial Opening
	8 Via Natural or Artificial Opening Endoscopic
		1 Radioactive Element
		N Tissue Expander
			Z No Qualifier

W Nipple, Right
  Areola
X Nipple, Left
  See W Nipple, Right
	X External	1 Radioactive Element	Z No Qualifier

Non-OR 0HHPXYZ
Non-OR 0HH[T,U][3,7,8]YZ

0 Medical and Surgical
H Skin and Breast
J Inspection Definition: Visually and/or manually exploring a body part
Explanation: Visual exploration may be performed with or without optical instrumentation. Manual exploration may be performed directly or through intervening body layers.

Body Part Character 4	Approach Character 5	Device Character 6	Qualifier Character 7

P Skin
  Dermis
  Epidermis
  Sebaceous gland
  Sweat gland
Q Finger Nail
  Nail bed
  Nail plate
R Toe Nail
  See Q Finger Nail
	X External	Z No Device	Z No Qualifier

T Breast, Right
  Mammary duct
  Mammary gland
U Breast, Left
  See T Breast, Right
	0 Open
	3 Percutaneous
	7 Via Natural or Artificial Opening
	8 Via Natural or Artificial Opening Endoscopic
		Z No Device	Z No Qualifier

Non-OR All body part, approach, device and qualifier values

ØHM–ØHM Skin and Breast ICD-10-PCS 2025

Ø Medical and Surgical
H Skin and Breast
M Reattachment   Definition: Putting back in or on all or a portion of a separated body part to its normal location or other suitable location
Explanation: Vascular circulation and nervous pathways may or may not be reestablished

Body Part Character 4	Approach Character 5	Device Character 6	Qualifier Character 7

Ø Skin, Scalp
1 Skin, Face
2 Skin, Right Ear
3 Skin, Left Ear
4 Skin, Neck
5 Skin, Chest
  Breast procedures, skin only
6 Skin, Back
7 Skin, Abdomen
8 Skin, Buttock
9 Skin, Perineum
  Perianal skin
A Skin, Inguinal
B Skin, Right Upper Arm
C Skin, Left Upper Arm
D Skin, Right Lower Arm
E Skin, Left Lower Arm
F Skin, Right Hand
G Skin, Left Hand
H Skin, Right Upper Leg
J Skin, Left Upper Leg
K Skin, Right Lower Leg
L Skin, Left Lower Leg
M Skin, Right Foot
N Skin, Left Foot
T Breast, Right
  Mammary duct
  Mammary gland
U Breast, Left
  See T Breast, Right
V Breast, Bilateral
  See T Breast, Right
W Nipple, Right
  Areola
X Nipple, Left
  See W Nipple, Right
	X External	Z No Device	Z No Qualifier

Non-OR   ØHMØXZZ

0 Medical and Surgical
H Skin and Breast
N Release Definition: Freeing a body part from an abnormal physical constraint by cutting or by the use of force
Explanation: Some of the restraining tissue may be taken out but none of the body part is taken out

Body Part Character 4	Approach Character 5	Device Character 6	Qualifier Character 7

0 Skin, Scalp
1 Skin, Face
2 Skin, Right Ear
3 Skin, Left Ear
4 Skin, Neck
5 Skin, Chest
   Breast procedures, skin only
6 Skin, Back
7 Skin, Abdomen
8 Skin, Buttock
9 Skin, Perineum
   Perianal skin
A Skin, Inguinal
B Skin, Right Upper Arm
C Skin, Left Upper Arm
D Skin, Right Lower Arm
E Skin, Left Lower Arm
F Skin, Right Hand
G Skin, Left Hand
H Skin, Right Upper Leg
J Skin, Left Upper Leg
K Skin, Right Lower Leg
L Skin, Left Lower Leg
M Skin, Right Foot
N Skin, Left Foot
Q Finger Nail
   Nail bed
   Nail plate
R Toe Nail
   See Q Finger Nail
	X External	**Z** No Device	**Z** No Qualifier

T Breast, Right
   Mammary duct
   Mammary gland
U Breast, Left
   See T Breast, Right
V Breast, Bilateral
   See T Breast, Right
	0 Open
	3 Percutaneous
	7 Via Natural or Artificial Opening
	8 Via Natural or Artificial Opening Endoscopic
		Z No Device	**Z** No Qualifier

W Nipple, Right
   Areola
X Nipple, Left
   See W Nipple, Right
	0 Open
	3 Percutaneous
	7 Via Natural or Artificial Opening
	8 Via Natural or Artificial Opening Endoscopic
	X External
		Z No Device	**Z** No Qualifier

0HP–0HP	Skin and Breast	ICD-10-PCS 2025

0 Medical and Surgical
H Skin and Breast
P Removal

Definition: Taking out or off a device from a body part

Explanation: If a device is taken out and a similar device put in without cutting or puncturing the skin or mucous membrane, the procedure is coded to the root operation CHANGE. Otherwise, the procedure for taking out a device is coded to the root operation REMOVAL.

Body Part Character 4	Approach Character 5	Device Character 6	Qualifier Character 7

P Skin
  Dermis
  Epidermis
  Sebaceous gland
  Sweat gland
	X External	**0** Drainage Device
		7 Autologous Tissue Substitute
		J Synthetic Substitute
		K Nonautologous Tissue Substitute
		Y Other Device
			Z No Qualifier

Q Finger Nail
  Nail bed
  Nail plate
R Toe Nail
  See Q Finger Nail
	X External	**0** Drainage Device
		7 Autologous Tissue Substitute
		J Synthetic Substitute
		K Nonautologous Tissue Substitute
			Z No Qualifier

S Hair	**X** External	**7** Autologous Tissue Substitute **J** Synthetic Substitute **K** Nonautologous Tissue Substitute	**Z** No Qualifier

T Breast, Right
  Mammary duct
  Mammary gland
U Breast, Left
  See T Breast, Right
	0 Open
	3 Percutaneous
	7 Via Natural or Artificial Opening
	8 Via Natural or Artificial Opening Endoscopic
		0 Drainage Device
		1 Radioactive Element
		7 Autologous Tissue Substitute
		J Synthetic Substitute
		K Nonautologous Tissue Substitute
		N Tissue Expander
		Y Other Device
			Z No Qualifier

Non-OR 0HPPX[0,7,J,K,Y]Z
Non-OR 0HP[Q,R]X[0,7,J,K]Z
Non-OR 0HPSX[7,J,K]Z
Non-OR 0HP[T,U]0[0,1,7,K]Z
Non-OR 0HP[T,U]3[0,1,7,K,Y]Z
Non-OR 0HP[T,U][7,8][0,1,7,J,K,N,Y]Z

Non-OR Procedure DRG Non-OR Procedure Valid OR Procedure HAC Associated Procedure Combination Only New/Revised April New/Revised October

0 **Medical and Surgical**
H **Skin and Breast**
Q **Repair**   Definition: Restoring, to the extent possible, a body part to its normal anatomic structure and function
          Explanation: Used only when the method to accomplish the repair is not one of the other root operations

Body Part Character 4	Approach Character 5	Device Character 6	Qualifier Character 7

0 Skin, Scalp
1 Skin, Face
2 Skin, Right Ear
3 Skin, Left Ear
4 Skin, Neck
5 Skin, Chest
   Breast procedures, skin only
6 Skin, Back
7 Skin, Abdomen
8 Skin, Buttock
9 Skin, Perineum
   Perianal skin
A Skin, Inguinal
B Skin, Right Upper Arm
C Skin, Left Upper Arm
D Skin, Right Lower Arm
E Skin, Left Lower Arm
F Skin, Right Hand
G Skin, Left Hand
H Skin, Right Upper Leg
J Skin, Left Upper Leg
K Skin, Right Lower Leg
L Skin, Left Lower Leg
M Skin, Right Foot
N Skin, Left Foot
Q Finger Nail
   Nail bed
   Nail plate
R Toe Nail
   See Q Finger Nail
	X External	Z No Device	Z No Qualifier

T Breast, Right
   Mammary duct
   Mammary gland
U Breast, Left
   See T Breast, Right
V Breast, Bilateral
   See T Breast, Right
Y Supernumerary Breast
	0 Open
	3 Percutaneous
	7 Via Natural or Artificial Opening
	8 Via Natural or Artificial Opening Endoscopic
		Z No Device	Z No Qualifier

W Nipple, Right
   Areola
X Nipple, Left
   See W Nipple, Right
	0 Open
	3 Percutaneous
	7 Via Natural or Artificial Opening
	8 Via Natural or Artificial Opening Endoscopic
	X External
		Z No Device	Z No Qualifier

DRG Non-OR   0HQ9XZZ
Non-OR   0HQ[0,1,2,3,4,5,6,7,8,A,B,C,D,E,F,G,H,J,K,L,M,N]XZZ

0HR–0HR Skin and Breast ICD-10-PCS 2025

0 Medical and Surgical
H Skin and Breast
R Replacement

Definition: Putting in or on biological or synthetic material that physically takes the place and/or function of all or a portion of a body part

Explanation: The body part may have been taken out or replaced, or may be taken out, physically eradicated, or rendered nonfunctional during the REPLACEMENT procedure. A REMOVAL procedure is coded for taking out the device used in a previous replacement procedure.

Body Part Character 4	Approach Character 5	Device Character 6	Qualifier Character 7

0 Skin, Scalp
1 Skin, Face
2 Skin, Right Ear
3 Skin, Left Ear
4 Skin, Neck
5 Skin, Chest
   Breast procedures, skin only
6 Skin, Back
7 Skin, Abdomen
8 Skin, Buttock
9 Skin, Perineum
   Perianal skin
A Skin, Inguinal
B Skin, Right Upper Arm
C Skin, Left Upper Arm
D Skin, Right Lower Arm
E Skin, Left Lower Arm
F Skin, Right Hand
G Skin, Left Hand
H Skin, Right Upper Leg
J Skin, Left Upper Leg
K Skin, Right Lower Leg
L Skin, Left Lower Leg
M Skin, Right Foot
N Skin, Left Foot
	X External	7 Autologous Tissue Substitute	2 Cell Suspension Technique
			3 Full Thickness
			4 Partial Thickness

0 Skin, Scalp
1 Skin, Face
2 Skin, Right Ear
3 Skin, Left Ear
4 Skin, Neck
5 Skin, Chest
   Breast procedures, skin only
6 Skin, Back
7 Skin, Abdomen
8 Skin, Buttock
9 Skin, Perineum
   Perianal skin
A Skin, Inguinal
B Skin, Right Upper Arm
C Skin, Left Upper Arm
D Skin, Right Lower Arm
E Skin, Left Lower Arm
F Skin, Right Hand
G Skin, Left Hand
H Skin, Right Upper Leg
J Skin, Left Upper Leg
K Skin, Right Lower Leg
L Skin, Left Lower Leg
M Skin, Right Foot
N Skin, Left Foot
	X External	J Synthetic Substitute	3 Full Thickness
			4 Partial Thickness
			Z No Qualifier

0 Skin, Scalp
1 Skin, Face
2 Skin, Right Ear
3 Skin, Left Ear
4 Skin, Neck
5 Skin, Chest
   Breast procedures, skin only
6 Skin, Back
7 Skin, Abdomen
8 Skin Buttock
9 Skin, Perineum
   Perianal skin
A Skin, Inguinal
B Skin, Right Upper Arm
C Skin, Left Upper Arm
D Skin, Right Lower Arm
E Skin, Left Lower Arm
F Skin, Right Hand
G Skin, Left Hand
H Skin, Right Upper Leg
J Skin, Left Upper Leg
K Skin, Right Lower Leg
L Skin, Left Lower Leg
M Skin, Right Foot
N Skin, Left Foot
	X External	K Nonautologous Tissue Substitute	3 Full Thickness
			4 Partial Thickness

Q Finger Nail
   Nail bed
   Nail plate
R Toe Nail
   See Q Finger Nail
S Hair
	X External	7 Autologous Tissue Substitute
		J Synthetic Substitute
		K Nonautologous Tissue Substitute
			Z No Qualifier

T Breast, Right
   Mammary duct
   Mammary gland
U Breast, Left
   See T Breast, Right
V Breast, Bilateral
   See T Breast, Right
	0 Open	7 Autologous Tissue Substitute	5 Latissimus Dorsi Myocutaneous Flap
			6 Transverse Rectus Abdominis Myocutaneous Flap
			7 Deep Inferior Epigastric Artery Perforator Flap
			8 Superficial Inferior Epigastric Artery Flap
			9 Gluteal Artery Perforator Flap
			B Lumbar Artery Perforator Flap
			Z No Qualifier

T Breast, Right
   Mammary duct
   Mammary gland
U Breast, Left
   See T Breast, Right
V Breast, Bilateral
   See T Breast, Right
	0 Open	J Synthetic Substitute
		K Nonautologous Tissue Substitute
			Z No Qualifier

T Breast, Right
   Mammary duct
   Mammary gland
U Breast, Left
   See T Breast, Right
V Breast, Bilateral
   See T Breast, Right
	3 Percutaneous	7 Autologous Tissue Substitute
		J Synthetic Substitute
		K Nonautologous Tissue Substitute
			Z No Qualifier

W Nipple, Right
   Areola
X Nipple, Left
   See W Nipple, Right
	0 Open
	3 Percutaneous
	X External
		7 Autologous Tissue Substitute
		J Synthetic Substitute
		K Nonautologous Tissue Substitute
			Z No Qualifier

Non-OR 0HRSX7Z

See Appendix L for Procedure Combinations
   0HR[T,U,V]37Z

Non-OR Procedure   DRG Non-OR Procedure   Valid OR Procedure   HAC Associated Procedure   Combination Only   New/Revised April   New/Revised October

ICD-10-PCS 2025 — Skin and Breast — 0HS–0HU

0	Medical and Surgical
H	Skin and Breast
S	Reposition

Definition: Moving to its normal location, or other suitable location, all or a portion of a body part

Explanation: The body part is moved to a new location from an abnormal location, or from a normal location where it is not functioning correctly. The body part may or may not be cut out or off to be moved to the new location.

Body Part Character 4	Approach Character 5	Device Character 6	Qualifier Character 7

S Hair
W Nipple, Right
    Areola
X Nipple, Left
    See W Nipple, Right
	X External	**Z** No Device	**Z** No Qualifier

T Breast, Right
    Mammary duct
    Mammary gland
U Breast, Left
    See T Breast, Right
V Breast, Bilateral
    See T Breast, Right
	0 Open	**Z** No Device	**Z** No Qualifier

Non-OR 0HSSXZZ

0	Medical and Surgical
H	Skin and Breast
T	Resection

Definition: Cutting out or off, without replacement, all of a body part

Explanation: None

Body Part Character 4	Approach Character 5	Device Character 6	Qualifier Character 7

Q Finger Nail
    Nail bed
    Nail plate
R Toe Nail
    See Q Finger Nail
W Nipple, Right
    Areola
X Nipple, Left
    See W Nipple, Right
	X External	**Z** No Device	**Z** No Qualifier

T Breast, Right ➕
    Mammary duct
    Mammary gland
U Breast, Left ➕
    See T Breast, Right
V Breast, Bilateral ➕
    See T Breast, Right
Y Supernumerary Breast
	0 Open	**Z** No Device	**Z** No Qualifier

Non-OR 0HT[Q,R]XZZ

See Appendix L for Procedure Combinations
➕ 0HT[T,U,V]0ZZ

0	Medical and Surgical
H	Skin and Breast
U	Supplement

Definition: Putting in or on biological or synthetic material that physically reinforces and/or augments the function of a portion of a body part

Explanation: The biological material is non-living, or is living and from the same individual. The body part may have been previously replaced, and the SUPPLEMENT procedure is performed to physically reinforce and/or augment the function of the replaced body part.

Body Part Character 4	Approach Character 5	Device Character 6	Qualifier Character 7

T Breast, Right
    Mammary duct
    Mammary gland
U Breast, Left
    See T Breast, Right
V Breast, Bilateral
    See T Breast, Right
	0 Open
	3 Percutaneous
	7 Via Natural or Artificial Opening
	8 Via Natural or Artificial Opening Endoscopic
		7 Autologous Tissue Substitute
		J Synthetic Substitute
		K Nonautologous Tissue Substitute
			Z No Qualifier

W Nipple, Right
    Areola
X Nipple, Left
    See W Nipple, Right
	0 Open
	3 Percutaneous
	7 Via Natural or Artificial Opening
	8 Via Natural or Artificial Opening Endoscopic
	X External
		7 Autologous Tissue Substitute
		J Synthetic Substitute
		K Nonautologous Tissue Substitute
			Z No Qualifier

Non-OR 0HU[T,U,V]3JZ

NC Noncovered Procedure **LC** Limited Coverage **OA** Questionable OB Admit **NT** New Tech Add-on ➕ Combination Member ♂ Male ♀ Female

0HW–0HX Skin and Breast ICD-10-PCS 2025

0 Medical and Surgical
H Skin and Breast
W Revision Definition: Correcting, to the extent possible, a portion of a malfunctioning device or the position of a displaced device
Explanation: Revision can include correcting a malfunctioning or displaced device by taking out or putting in components of the device such as a screw or pin

Body Part Character 4	Approach Character 5	Device Character 6	Qualifier Character 7
P Skin Dermis Epidermis Sebaceous gland Sweat gland	X External	0 Drainage Device 7 Autologous Tissue Substitute J Synthetic Substitute K Nonautologous Tissue Substitute Y Other Device	Z No Qualifier
Q Finger Nail Nail bed Nail plate **R Toe Nail** See Q Finger Nail	X External	0 Drainage Device 7 Autologous Tissue Substitute J Synthetic Substitute K Nonautologous Tissue Substitute	Z No Qualifier
S Hair	X External	7 Autologous Tissue Substitute J Synthetic Substitute K Nonautologous Tissue Substitute	Z No Qualifier
T Breast, Right Mammary duct Mammary gland **U Breast, Left** See T Breast, Right	0 Open 3 Percutaneous 7 Via Natural or Artificial Opening 8 Via Natural or Artificial Opening Endoscopic	0 Drainage Device 7 Autologous Tissue Substitute J Synthetic Substitute K Nonautologous Tissue Substitute N Tissue Expander Y Other Device	Z No Qualifier

Non-OR 0HWPX[0,7,J,K,Y]Z
Non-OR 0HW[Q,R]X[0,7,J,K]Z
Non-OR 0HWSX[7,J,K]Z
Non-OR 0HW[T,U]0[0,7,K,N]Z
Non-OR 0HW[T,U]3[0,7,K,N,Y]Z
Non-OR 0HW[T,U][7,8][0,7,J,K,N,Y]Z

0 Medical and Surgical
H Skin and Breast
X Transfer Definition: Moving, without taking out, all or a portion of a body part to another location to take over the function of all or a portion of a body part
Explanation: The body part transferred remains connected to its vascular and nervous supply

Body Part Character 4	Approach Character 5	Device Character 6	Qualifier Character 7

0 Skin, Scalp
 1 Skin, Face
 2 Skin, Right Ear
 3 Skin, Left Ear
 4 Skin, Neck
 5 Skin, Chest
   Breast procedures, skin only
 6 Skin, Back
 7 Skin, Abdomen
 8 Skin, Buttock
 9 Skin, Perineum
   Perianal skin
 A Skin, Inguinal
 B Skin, Right Upper Arm
 C Skin, Left Upper Arm
 D Skin, Right Lower Arm
 E Skin, Left Lower Arm
 F Skin, Right Hand
 G Skin, Left Hand
 H Skin, Right Upper Leg
 J Skin, Left Upper Leg
 K Skin, Right Lower Leg
 L Skin, Left Lower Leg
 M Skin, Right Foot
 N Skin, Left Foot
	X External	Z No Device	Z No Qualifier

Non-OR Procedure   DRG Non-OR Procedure   Valid OR Procedure   HAC Associated Procedure   Combination Only   New/Revised April   New/Revised October

Subcutaneous Tissue and Fascia ØJØ–ØJX

Character Meanings

This Character Meaning table is provided as a guide to assist the user in the identification of character members that may be found in this section of code tables. It **SHOULD NOT** be used to build a PCS code.

Operation–Character 3		Body Part–Character 4		Approach–Character 5		Device–Character 6		Qualifier–Character 7	
Ø	Alteration	Ø	Subcutaneous Tissue and Fascia, Scalp	Ø	Open	Ø	Drainage Device OR Monitoring Device, Hemodynamic	B	Skin and Subcutaneous Tissue
2	Change	1	Subcutaneous Tissue and Fascia, Face	3	Percutaneous	1	Radioactive Element	C	Skin, Subcutaneous Tissue and Fascia
5	Destruction	4	Subcutaneous Tissue and Fascia, Right Neck	X	External	2	Monitoring Device	X	Diagnostic
8	Division	5	Subcutaneous Tissue and Fascia, Left Neck			3	Infusion Device	Z	No Qualifier
9	Drainage	6	Subcutaneous Tissue and Fascia, Chest			4	Pacemaker, Single Chamber		
B	Excision	7	Subcutaneous Tissue and Fascia, Back			5	Pacemaker, Single Chamber Rate Responsive		
C	Extirpation	8	Subcutaneous Tissue and Fascia, Abdomen			6	Pacemaker, Dual Chamber		
D	Extraction	9	Subcutaneous Tissue and Fascia, Buttock			7	Autologous Tissue Substitute OR Cardiac Resynchronization Pacemaker Pulse Generator		
H	Insertion	B	Subcutaneous Tissue and Fascia, Perineum			8	Defibrillator Generator		
J	Inspection	C	Subcutaneous Tissue and Fascia, Pelvic Region			9	Cardiac Resynchronization Defibrillator Pulse Generator		
N	Release	D	Subcutaneous Tissue and Fascia, Right Upper Arm			A	Contractility Modulation Device		
P	Removal	F	Subcutaneous Tissue and Fascia, Left Upper Arm			B	Stimulator Generator, Single Array		
Q	Repair	G	Subcutaneous Tissue and Fascia, Right Lower Arm			C	Stimulator Generator, Single Array Rechargeable		
R	Replacement	H	Subcutaneous Tissue and Fascia, Left Lower Arm			D	Stimulator Generator, Multiple Array		
U	Supplement	J	Subcutaneous Tissue and Fascia, Right Hand			E	Stimulator Generator, Multiple Array Rechargeable		
W	Revision	K	Subcutaneous Tissue and Fascia, Left Hand			F	Subcutaneous Defibrillator Lead		
X	Transfer	L	Subcutaneous Tissue and Fascia, Right Upper Leg			H	Contraceptive Device		
		M	Subcutaneous Tissue and Fascia, Left Upper Leg			J	Synthetic Substitute		
		N	Subcutaneous Tissue and Fascia, Right Lower Leg			K	Nonautologous Tissue Substitute		
		P	Subcutaneous Tissue and Fascia, Left Lower Leg			M	Stimulator Generator		
		Q	Subcutaneous Tissue and Fascia, Right Foot			N	Tissue Expander		
		R	Subcutaneous Tissue and Fascia, Left Foot			P	Cardiac Rhythm Related Device		
		S	Subcutaneous Tissue and Fascia, Head and Neck			V	Infusion Device, Pump		
		T	Subcutaneous Tissue and Fascia, Trunk			W	Vascular Access Device, Totally Implantable		
		V	Subcutaneous Tissue and Fascia, Upper Extremity			X	Vascular Access Device, Tunneled		
		W	Subcutaneous Tissue and Fascia, Lower Extremity			Y	Other Device		
						Z	No Device		

Subcutaneous Tissue and Fascia

AHA Coding Clinic for table 0J2
2018, 3Q, 10	Disruption of perma-catheter fibrin sheath via angioplasty of superior vena cava
2017, 2Q, 26	Exchange of tunneled catheter

AHA Coding Clinic for table 0J5
2019, 3Q, 25	Endoscopic removal of pilonidal sinus and cyst

AHA Coding Clinic for table 0J8
2017, 3Q, 11	Bilateral escharotomy of leg, thigh and foot

AHA Coding Clinic for table 0J9
2018, 3Q, 16	Incision and drainage of submandibular space
2018, 3Q, 16	Incision and drainage of neck abscess
2015, 3Q, 23	Incision and drainage of multiple abscess cavities using vessel loop

AHA Coding Clinic for table 0JB
2023, 2Q, 30	Excisional debridement and non-excisional debridement at deeper layer same site
2022, 3Q, 11	Ulceration and soft tissue redundancy at amputation site due to osteo-integrated implant
2020, 1Q, 31	Repair of buried penis
2019, 3Q, 25	Endoscopic removal of pilonidal sinus and cyst
2018, 3Q, 17	Excisional debridement of periosteum
2018, 1Q, 7	Placement of fat graft following lumbar decompression surgery
2015, 3Q, 3-8	Excisional and nonexcisional debridement
2015, 2Q, 13	Transfer of free flap to reconstruct orbital defect
2015, 1Q, 29	Fistulectomy with placement of seton
2014, 4Q, 38	Abdominoplasty and abdominal wall plication for hernia repair
2014, 3Q, 22	Transsphenoidal removal of pituitary tumor and fat graft placement

AHA Coding Clinic for table 0JC
2017, 3Q, 22	Replacement of native skull bone flap

AHA Coding Clinic for table 0JD
2023, 2Q, 30	Excisional debridement and non-excisional debridement at deeper layer same site
2023, 1Q, 36	Maggot therapy
2016, 3Q, 20	VersaJet™ nonexcisional debridement of leg muscle
2016, 3Q, 21	Nonexcisional debridement of infected lumbar wound
2016, 3Q, 21	Nonexcisional pulsed lavage debridement
2016, 3Q, 22	Debridement of bone and tendon using Tenex ultrasound device
2016, 1Q, 40	Nonexcisional debridement of skin and subcutaneous tissue
2015, 3Q, 3-8	Excisional and nonexcisional debridement
2015, 1Q, 23	Non-Excisional debridement with lavage of wound

AHA Coding Clinic for table 0JH
2024, 2Q, 28	Deep brain stimulation with placement of extension wire during insertion of implantable pulse generator
2024, 2Q, 29	Wireless stimulation endocardially for cardiac resynchronization (WiSE®-CRT) system
2020, 4Q, 54	Insertion of other device into subcutaneous tissue and fascia
2020, 4Q, 55	Insertion of subcutaneous pump system for ascites drainage
2020, 2Q, 15	Ommaya reservoir with ventricular catheter placement
2020, 2Q, 16	Ommaya reservoir placement for cerebrospinal fluid infusion therapy
2019, 4Q, 33	Subcutaneous implantable cardioverter defibrillator lead
2017, 4Q, 63-64	Added and revised device values - Vascular access reservoir
2017, 2Q, 24	Tunneled catheter versus totally implantable catheter
2017, 2Q, 26	Exchange of tunneled catheter
2016, 4Q, 97-98	Phrenic neurostimulator
2016, 2Q, 14	Insertion of peritoneal totally implantable venous access device
2016, 2Q, 15	Removal and replacement of tunneled internal jugular catheter
2015, 4Q, 14	New Section X codes—New Technology procedures
2015, 4Q, 30-31	Vascular access devices
2015, 2Q, 33	Totally implantable central venous access device (Port-a-Cath)
2014, 3Q, 19	End of life replacement of Baclofen pump
2013, 4Q, 116	Device character for Port-A-Cath placement
2012, 4Q, 104	Placement of subcutaneous implantable cardioverter defibrillator

AHA Coding Clinic for table 0JN
2017, 3Q, 11	Bilateral escharotomy of leg, thigh and foot

AHA Coding Clinic for table 0JP
2019, 4Q, 33	Subcutaneous implantable cardioverter defibrillator lead
2018, 4Q, 86	Placement of lumboatrial shunt
2018, 3Q, 29	Decommissioning of left ventricular assist device with exploration of mediastinum
2016, 2Q, 15	Removal and replacement of tunneled internal jugular catheter
2015, 4Q, 31	Vascular access devices
2014, 3Q, 19	End of life replacement of Baclofen pump
2013, 4Q, 109	Separating conjoined twins
2012, 4Q, 104	Placement of subcutaneous implantable cardioverter defibrillator

AHA Coding Clinic for table 0JQ
2022, 3Q, 24	Leakage of cerebrospinal fluid with revision of intrathecal baclofen system
2017, 3Q, 19	Anterior repair of cystocele
2014, 4Q, 44	Posterior colporrhaphy/rectocele repair

AHA Coding Clinic for table 0JR
2015, 2Q, 13	Transfer of free flap to reconstruct orbital defect

AHA Coding Clinic for table 0JU
2018, 2Q, 20	Prelaminated free flap graft using Alloderm™
2018, 1Q, 7	Placement of fat graft following lumbar decompression surgery

AHA Coding Clinic for table 0JW
2022, 3Q, 24	Leakage of cerebrospinal fluid with revision of intrathecal baclofen system
2019, 4Q, 33	Subcutaneous implantable cardioverter defibrillator lead
2018, 1Q, 8	Ventricular peritoneal shunt ligation
2015, 4Q, 33	Externalization of peritoneal dialysis catheter
2015, 2Q, 9	Revision of ventriculoperitoneal (VP) shunt
2012, 4Q, 104	Placement of subcutaneous implantable cardioverter defibrillator

AHA Coding Clinic for table 0JX
2022, 3Q, 11	Ulceration and soft tissue redundancy at amputation site due to osteo-integrated implant
2022, 1Q, 48	Repair of facial fractures of frontal sinus and orbital roof
2021, 3Q, 19	Elbow amputation and targeted muscle reinnervation
2021, 2Q, 16	Goldilocks breast reconstruction
2018, 1Q, 10	Complex wound closure using pericranial flap
2014, 3Q, 18	Placement of reverse sural fasciocutaneous pedicle flap
2013, 4Q, 109	Separating conjoined twins

ICD-10-PCS 2025 — Subcutaneous Tissue and Fascia — 0J0–0J2

0 Medical and Surgical
J Subcutaneous Tissue and Fascia
0 Alteration — Definition: Modifying the anatomic structure of a body part without affecting the function of the body part
Explanation: Principal purpose is to improve appearance

Body Part Character 4	Approach Character 5	Device Character 6	Qualifier Character 7
1 Subcutaneous Tissue and Fascia, Face Chin Masseteric fascia Orbital fascia Submandibular space **4 Subcutaneous Tissue and Fascia, Right Neck** Deep cervical fascia Pretracheal fascia Prevertebral fascia **5 Subcutaneous Tissue and Fascia, Left Neck** *See 4 Subcutaneous Tissue and Fascia, Right Neck* **6 Subcutaneous Tissue and Fascia, Chest** Pectoral fascia **7 Subcutaneous Tissue and Fascia, Back** **8 Subcutaneous Tissue and Fascia, Abdomen** **9 Subcutaneous Tissue and Fascia, Buttock** **D Subcutaneous Tissue and Fascia, Right Upper Arm** Axillary fascia Deltoid fascia Infraspinatus fascia Subscapular aponeurosis Supraspinatus fascia **F Subcutaneous Tissue and Fascia, Left Upper Arm** *See D Subcutaneous Tissue and Fascia, Right Upper Arm* **G Subcutaneous Tissue and Fascia, Right Lower Arm** Antebrachial fascia Bicipital aponeurosis **H Subcutaneous Tissue and Fascia, Left Lower Arm** *See G Subcutaneous Tissue and Fascia, Right Lower Arm* **L Subcutaneous Tissue and Fascia, Right Upper Leg** Crural fascia Fascia lata Iliac fascia Iliotibial tract (band) **M Subcutaneous Tissue and Fascia, Left Upper Leg** *See L Subcutaneous Tissue and Fascia, Right Upper Leg* **N Subcutaneous Tissue and Fascia, Right Lower Leg** **P Subcutaneous Tissue and Fascia, Left Lower Leg**	0 Open 3 Percutaneous	Z No Device	Z No Qualifier

0 Medical and Surgical
J Subcutaneous Tissue and Fascia
2 Change — Definition: Taking out or off a device from a body part and putting back an identical or similar device in or on the same body part without cutting or puncturing the skin or a mucous membrane
Explanation: All CHANGE procedures are coded using the approach EXTERNAL

Body Part Character 4	Approach Character 5	Device Character 6	Qualifier Character 7
S Subcutaneous Tissue and Fascia, Head and Neck **T Subcutaneous Tissue and Fascia, Trunk** External oblique aponeurosis Transversalis fascia **V Subcutaneous Tissue and Fascia, Upper Extremity** **W Subcutaneous Tissue and Fascia, Lower Extremity**	X External	0 Drainage Device Y Other Device	Z No Qualifier

Non-OR All body part, approach, device, and qualifier values

0 Medical and Surgical
J Subcutaneous Tissue and Fascia
5 Destruction Definition: Physical eradication of all or a portion of a body part by the direct use of energy, force, or a destructive agent
Explanation: None of the body part is physically taken out

Body Part — Character 4	Approach — Character 5	Device — Character 6	Qualifier — Character 7

0 Subcutaneous Tissue and Fascia, Scalp
   Galea aponeurotica
1 Subcutaneous Tissue and Fascia, Face
   Chin
   Masseteric fascia
   Orbital fascia
   Submandibular space
4 Subcutaneous Tissue and Fascia, Right Neck
   Deep cervical fascia
   Pretracheal fascia
   Prevertebral fascia
5 Subcutaneous Tissue and Fascia, Left Neck
   See 4 Subcutaneous Tissue and Fascia, Right Neck
6 Subcutaneous Tissue and Fascia, Chest
   Pectoral fascia
7 Subcutaneous Tissue and Fascia, Back
8 Subcutaneous Tissue and Fascia, Abdomen
9 Subcutaneous Tissue and Fascia, Buttock
B Subcutaneous Tissue and Fascia, Perineum
C Subcutaneous Tissue and Fascia, Pelvic Region
D Subcutaneous Tissue and Fascia, Right Upper Arm
   Axillary fascia
   Deltoid fascia
   Infraspinatus fascia
   Subscapular aponeurosis
   Supraspinatus fascia
F Subcutaneous Tissue and Fascia, Left Upper Arm
   See D Subcutaneous Tissue and Fascia, Right Upper Arm
G Subcutaneous Tissue and Fascia, Right Lower Arm
   Antebrachial fascia
   Bicipital aponeurosis
H Subcutaneous Tissue and Fascia, Left Lower Arm
   See G Subcutaneous Tissue and Fascia, Right Lower Arm
J Subcutaneous Tissue and Fascia, Right Hand
   Palmar fascia (aponeurosis)
K Subcutaneous Tissue and Fascia, Left Hand
   See J Subcutaneous Tissue and Fascia, Right Hand
L Subcutaneous Tissue and Fascia, Right Upper Leg
   Crural fascia
   Fascia lata
   Iliac fascia
   Iliotibial tract (band)
M Subcutaneous Tissue and Fascia, Left Upper Leg
   See L Subcutaneous Tissue and Fascia, Right Upper Leg
N Subcutaneous Tissue and Fascia, Right Lower Leg
P Subcutaneous Tissue and Fascia, Left Lower Leg
Q Subcutaneous Tissue and Fascia, Right Foot
   Plantar fascia (aponeurosis)
R Subcutaneous Tissue and Fascia, Left Foot
   See Q Subcutaneous Tissue and Fascia, Right Foot
	0 Open
	3 Percutaneous
		Z No Device	**Z** No Qualifier

DRG Non-OR All body part, approach, device, and qualifier values

0 Medical and Surgical
J Subcutaneous Tissue and Fascia
8 Division Definition: Cutting into a body part, without draining fluids and/or gases from the body part, in order to separate or transect a body part
Explanation: All or a portion of the body part is separated into two or more portions

Body Part Character 4	Approach Character 5	Device Character 6	Qualifier Character 7

0 Subcutaneous Tissue and Fascia, Scalp
   Galea aponeurotica
1 Subcutaneous Tissue and Fascia, Face
   Chin
   Masseteric fascia
   Orbital fascia
   Submandibular space
4 Subcutaneous Tissue and Fascia, Right Neck
   Deep cervical fascia
   Pretracheal fascia
   Prevertebral fascia
5 Subcutaneous Tissue and Fascia, Left Neck
   See 4 Subcutaneous Tissue and Fascia, Right Neck
6 Subcutaneous Tissue and Fascia, Chest
   Pectoral fascia
7 Subcutaneous Tissue and Fascia, Back
8 Subcutaneous Tissue and Fascia, Abdomen
9 Subcutaneous Tissue and Fascia, Buttock
B Subcutaneous Tissue and Fascia, Perineum
C Subcutaneous Tissue and Fascia, Pelvic Region
D Subcutaneous Tissue and Fascia, Right Upper Arm
   Axillary fascia
   Deltoid fascia
   Infraspinatus fascia
   Subscapular aponeurosis
   Supraspinatus fascia
F Subcutaneous Tissue and Fascia, Left Upper Arm
   See D Subcutaneous Tissue and Fascia, Right Upper Arm
G Subcutaneous Tissue and Fascia, Right Lower Arm
   Antebrachial fascia
   Bicipital aponeurosis
H Subcutaneous Tissue and Fascia, Left Lower Arm
   See G Subcutaneous Tissue and Fascia, Right Lower Arm
J Subcutaneous Tissue and Fascia, Right Hand
   Palmar fascia (aponeurosis)
K Subcutaneous Tissue and Fascia, Left Hand
   See J Subcutaneous Tissue and Fascia, Right Hand
L Subcutaneous Tissue and Fascia, Right Upper Leg
   Crural fascia
   Fascia lata
   Iliac fascia
   Iliotibial tract (band)
M Subcutaneous Tissue and Fascia, Left Upper Leg
   See L Subcutaneous Tissue and Fascia, Right Upper Leg
N Subcutaneous Tissue and Fascia, Right Lower Leg
P Subcutaneous Tissue and Fascia, Left Lower Leg
Q Subcutaneous Tissue and Fascia, Right Foot
   Plantar fascia (aponeurosis)
R Subcutaneous Tissue and Fascia, Left Foot
   See Q Subcutaneous Tissue and Fascia, Right Foot
S Subcutaneous Tissue and Fascia, Head and Neck
T Subcutaneous Tissue and Fascia, Trunk
   External oblique aponeurosis
   Transversalis fascia
V Subcutaneous Tissue and Fascia, Upper Extremity
W Subcutaneous Tissue and Fascia, Lower Extremity
	0 Open
	3 Percutaneous
		Z No Device	Z No Qualifier

0 Medical and Surgical
J Subcutaneous Tissue and Fascia
9 Drainage Definition: Taking or letting out fluids and/or gases from a body part
Explanation: The qualifier DIAGNOSTIC is used to identify drainage procedures that are biopsies

Body Part Character 4	Approach Character 5	Device Character 6	Qualifier Character 7
0 Subcutaneous Tissue and Fascia, Scalp Galea aponeurotica **1 Subcutaneous Tissue and Fascia, Face** Chin Masseteric fascia Orbital fascia Submandibular space **4 Subcutaneous Tissue and Fascia, Right Neck** Deep cervical fascia Pretracheal fascia Prevertebral fascia **5 Subcutaneous Tissue and Fascia, Left Neck** See 4 Subcutaneous Tissue and Fascia, Right Neck **6 Subcutaneous Tissue and Fascia, Chest** Pectoral fascia **7 Subcutaneous Tissue and Fascia, Back** **8 Subcutaneous Tissue and Fascia, Abdomen** **9 Subcutaneous Tissue and Fascia, Buttock** **B Subcutaneous Tissue and Fascia, Perineum** **C Subcutaneous Tissue and Fascia, Pelvic Region** **D Subcutaneous Tissue and Fascia, Right Upper Arm** Axillary fascia Deltoid fascia Infraspinatus fascia Subscapular aponeurosis Supraspinatus fascia **F Subcutaneous Tissue and Fascia, Left Upper Arm** See D Subcutaneous Tissue and Fascia, Right Upper Arm	**G Subcutaneous Tissue and Fascia, Right Lower Arm** Antebrachial fascia Bicipital aponeurosis **H Subcutaneous Tissue and Fascia, Left Lower Arm** See G Subcutaneous Tissue and Fascia, Right Lower Arm **J Subcutaneous Tissue and Fascia, Right Hand** Palmar fascia (aponeurosis) **K Subcutaneous Tissue and Fascia, Left Hand** See J Subcutaneous Tissue and Fascia, Right Hand **L Subcutaneous Tissue and Fascia, Right Upper Leg** Crural fascia Fascia lata Iliac fascia Iliotibial tract (band) **M Subcutaneous Tissue and Fascia, Left Upper Leg** See L Subcutaneous Tissue and Fascia, Right Upper Leg **N Subcutaneous Tissue and Fascia, Right Lower Leg** **P Subcutaneous Tissue and Fascia, Left Lower Leg** **Q Subcutaneous Tissue and Fascia, Right Foot** Plantar fascia (aponeurosis) **R Subcutaneous Tissue and Fascia, Left Foot** See Q Subcutaneous Tissue and Fascia, Right Foot	**0 Open** **3 Percutaneous**	**0 Drainage Device**	**Z No Qualifier**

Non-OR All body part, approach, device, and qualifier values

0J9 Continued on next page

0 Medical and Surgical
J Subcutaneous Tissue and Fascia
9 Drainage Definition: Taking or letting out fluids and/or gases from a body part
Explanation: The qualifier DIAGNOSTIC is used to identify drainage procedures that are biopsies

0J9 Continued

Body Part Character 4	Approach Character 5	Device Character 6	Qualifier Character 7

0 Subcutaneous Tissue and Fascia, Scalp
  Galea aponeurotica
1 Subcutaneous Tissue and Fascia, Face
  Chin
  Masseteric fascia
  Orbital fascia
  Submandibular space
4 Subcutaneous Tissue and Fascia, Right Neck
  Deep cervical fascia
  Pretracheal fascia
  Prevertebral fascia
5 Subcutaneous Tissue and Fascia, Left Neck
  See 4 Subcutaneous Tissue and Fascia, Right Neck
6 Subcutaneous Tissue and Fascia, Chest
  Pectoral fascia
7 Subcutaneous Tissue and Fascia, Back
8 Subcutaneous Tissue and Fascia, Abdomen
9 Subcutaneous Tissue and Fascia, Buttock
B Subcutaneous Tissue and Fascia, Perineum
C Subcutaneous Tissue and Fascia, Pelvic Region
D Subcutaneous Tissue and Fascia, Right Upper Arm
  Axillary fascia
  Deltoid fascia
  Infraspinatus fascia
  Subscapular aponeurosis
  Supraspinatus fascia
F Subcutaneous Tissue and Fascia, Left Upper Arm
  See D Subcutaneous Tissue and Fascia, Right Upper Arm
G Subcutaneous Tissue and Fascia, Right Lower Arm
  Antebrachial fascia
  Bicipital aponeurosis
H Subcutaneous Tissue and Fascia, Left Lower Arm
  See G Subcutaneous Tissue and Fascia, Right Lower Arm
J Subcutaneous Tissue and Fascia, Right Hand
  Palmar fascia (aponeurosis)
K Subcutaneous Tissue and Fascia, Left Hand
  See J Subcutaneous Tissue and Fascia, Right Hand
L Subcutaneous Tissue and Fascia, Right Upper Leg
  Crural fascia
  Fascia lata
  Iliac fascia
  Iliotibial tract (band)
M Subcutaneous Tissue and Fascia, Left Upper Leg
  See L Subcutaneous Tissue and Fascia, Right Upper Leg
N Subcutaneous Tissue and Fascia, Right Lower Leg
P Subcutaneous Tissue and Fascia, Left Lower Leg
Q Subcutaneous Tissue and Fascia, Right Foot
  Plantar fascia (aponeurosis)
R Subcutaneous Tissue and Fascia, Left Foot
  See Q Subcutaneous Tissue and Fascia, Right Foot
	0 Open
	3 Percutaneous
		Z No Device	**X** Diagnostic
			Z No Qualifier

Non-OR All body part, approach, device, and qualifier values

/ ØJB-ØJB / Subcutaneous Tissue and Fascia / ICD-10-PCS 2025

Ø Medical and Surgical
J Subcutaneous Tissue and Fascia
B Excision Definition: Cutting out or off, without replacement, a portion of a body part
Explanation: The qualifier DIAGNOSTIC is used to identify excision procedures that are biopsies

Body Part Character 4	Approach Character 5	Device Character 6	Qualifier Character 7
Ø Subcutaneous Tissue and Fascia, Scalp Galea aponeurotica **1 Subcutaneous Tissue and Fascia, Face** Chin Masseteric fascia Orbital fascia Submandibular space **4 Subcutaneous Tissue and Fascia, Right Neck** Deep cervical fascia Pretracheal fascia Prevertebral fascia **5 Subcutaneous Tissue and Fascia, Left Neck** See 4 Subcutaneous Tissue and Fascia, Right Neck **6 Subcutaneous Tissue and Fascia, Chest** Pectoral fascia **7 Subcutaneous Tissue and Fascia, Back** **8 Subcutaneous Tissue and Fascia, Abdomen** **9 Subcutaneous Tissue and Fascia, Buttock** **B Subcutaneous Tissue and Fascia, Perineum** **C Subcutaneous Tissue and Fascia, Pelvic Region** **D Subcutaneous Tissue and Fascia, Right Upper Arm** Axillary fascia Deltoid fascia Infraspinatus fascia Subscapular aponeurosis Supraspinatus fascia **F Subcutaneous Tissue and Fascia, Left Upper Arm** See D Subcutaneous Tissue and Fascia, Right Upper Arm **G Subcutaneous Tissue and Fascia, Right Lower Arm** Antebrachial fascia Bicipital aponeurosis **H Subcutaneous Tissue and Fascia, Left Lower Arm** See G Subcutaneous Tissue and Fascia, Right Lower Arm **J Subcutaneous Tissue and Fascia, Right Hand** Palmar fascia (aponeurosis) **K Subcutaneous Tissue and Fascia, Left Hand** See J Subcutaneous Tissue and Fascia, Right Hand **L Subcutaneous Tissue and Fascia, Right Upper Leg** Crural fascia Fascia lata Iliac fascia Iliotibial tract (band) **M Subcutaneous Tissue and Fascia, Left Upper Leg** See L Subcutaneous Tissue and Fascia, Right Upper Leg **N Subcutaneous Tissue and Fascia, Right Lower Leg** **P Subcutaneous Tissue and Fascia, Left Lower Leg** **Q Subcutaneous Tissue and Fascia, Right Foot** Plantar fascia (aponeurosis) **R Subcutaneous Tissue and Fascia, Left Foot** See Q Subcutaneous Tissue and Fascia, Right Foot	**Ø** Open **3** Percutaneous	**Z** No Device	**X** Diagnostic **Z** No Qualifier

DRG Non-OR ØJB[Ø,4,5,6,7,8,9,B,C,D,F,G,H,L,M,N,P,Q,R]3ZZ
Non-OR ØJB[Ø,1,4,5,6,7,8,9,B,C,D,F,G,H,J,K,L,M,N,P,Q,R][Ø,3]ZX

Subcutaneous Tissue and Fascia

0 Medical and Surgical
J Subcutaneous Tissue and Fascia
C Extirpation Definition: Taking or cutting out solid matter from a body part
Explanation: The solid matter may be an abnormal byproduct of a biological function or a foreign body; it may be imbedded in a body part or in the lumen of a tubular body part. The solid matter may or may not have been previously broken into pieces.

Body Part Character 4	Approach Character 5	Device Character 6	Qualifier Character 7

0 Subcutaneous Tissue and Fascia, Scalp
    Galea aponeurotica
1 Subcutaneous Tissue and Fascia, Face
    Chin
    Masseteric fascia
    Orbital fascia
    Submandibular space
4 Subcutaneous Tissue and Fascia, Right Neck
    Deep cervical fascia
    Pretracheal fascia
    Prevertebral fascia
5 Subcutaneous Tissue and Fascia, Left Neck
    See 4 Subcutaneous Tissue and Fascia, Right Neck
6 Subcutaneous Tissue and Fascia, Chest
    Pectoral fascia
7 Subcutaneous Tissue and Fascia, Back
8 Subcutaneous Tissue and Fascia, Abdomen
9 Subcutaneous Tissue and Fascia, Buttock
B Subcutaneous Tissue and Fascia, Perineum
C Subcutaneous Tissue and Fascia, Pelvic Region
D Subcutaneous Tissue and Fascia, Right Upper Arm
    Axillary fascia
    Deltoid fascia
    Infraspinatus fascia
    Subscapular aponeurosis
    Supraspinatus fascia
F Subcutaneous Tissue and Fascia, Left Upper Arm
    See D Subcutaneous Tissue and Fascia, Right Upper Arm
G Subcutaneous Tissue and Fascia, Right Lower Arm
    Antebrachial fascia
    Bicipital aponeurosis
H Subcutaneous Tissue and Fascia, Left Lower Arm
    See G Subcutaneous Tissue and Fascia, Right Lower Arm
J Subcutaneous Tissue and Fascia, Right Hand
    Palmar fascia (aponeurosis)
K Subcutaneous Tissue and Fascia, Left Hand
    See J Subcutaneous Tissue and Fascia, Right Hand
L Subcutaneous Tissue and Fascia, Right Upper Leg
    Crural fascia
    Fascia lata
    Iliac fascia
    Iliotibial tract (band)
M Subcutaneous Tissue and Fascia, Left Upper Leg
    See L Subcutaneous Tissue and Fascia, Right Upper Leg
N Subcutaneous Tissue and Fascia, Right Lower Leg
P Subcutaneous Tissue and Fascia, Left Lower Leg
Q Subcutaneous Tissue and Fascia, Right Foot
    Plantar fascia (aponeurosis)
R Subcutaneous Tissue and Fascia, Left Foot
    See Q Subcutaneous Tissue and Fascia, Right Foot
	0 Open
	3 Percutaneous
		Z No Device	**Z** No Qualifier

Non-OR   0JC[0,1,4,5,6,7,8,9,B,C,D,F,G,H,J,K,L,M,N,P,Q,R]3ZZ

0 Medical and Surgical
J Subcutaneous Tissue and Fascia
D Extraction Definition: Pulling or stripping out or off all or a portion of a body part by the use of force
Explanation: The qualifier DIAGNOSTIC is used to identify extraction procedures that are biopsies

Body Part Character 4	Approach Character 5	Device Character 6	Qualifier Character 7
0 Subcutaneous Tissue and Fascia, Scalp Galea aponeurotica **1 Subcutaneous Tissue and Fascia, Face** Chin Masseteric fascia Orbital fascia Submandibular space **4 Subcutaneous Tissue and Fascia, Right Neck** Deep cervical fascia Pretracheal fascia Prevertebral fascia **5 Subcutaneous Tissue and Fascia, Left Neck** See 4 Subcutaneous Tissue and Fascia, Right Neck **6 Subcutaneous Tissue and Fascia, Chest** Pectoral fascia **7 Subcutaneous Tissue and Fascia, Back** **8 Subcutaneous Tissue and Fascia, Abdomen** **9 Subcutaneous Tissue and Fascia, Buttock** **B Subcutaneous Tissue and Fascia, Perineum** **C Subcutaneous Tissue and Fascia, Pelvic Region** **D Subcutaneous Tissue and Fascia, Right Upper Arm** Axillary fascia Deltoid fascia Infraspinatus fascia Subscapular aponeurosis Supraspinatus fascia **F Subcutaneous Tissue and Fascia, Left Upper Arm** See D Subcutaneous Tissue and Fascia, Right Upper Arm **G Subcutaneous Tissue and Fascia, Right Lower Arm** Antebrachial fascia Bicipital aponeurosis **H Subcutaneous Tissue and Fascia, Left Lower Arm** See G Subcutaneous Tissue and Fascia, Right Lower Arm **J Subcutaneous Tissue and Fascia, Right Hand** Palmar fascia (aponeurosis) **K Subcutaneous Tissue and Fascia, Left Hand** See J Subcutaneous Tissue and Fascia, Right Hand **L Subcutaneous Tissue and Fascia, Right Upper Leg** Crural fascia Fascia lata Iliac fascia Iliotibial tract (band) **M Subcutaneous Tissue and Fascia, Left Upper Leg** See L Subcutaneous Tissue and Fascia, Right Upper Leg **N Subcutaneous Tissue and Fascia, Right Lower Leg** **P Subcutaneous Tissue and Fascia, Left Lower Leg** **Q Subcutaneous Tissue and Fascia, Right Foot** Plantar fascia (aponeurosis) **R Subcutaneous Tissue and Fascia, Left Foot** See Q Subcutaneous Tissue and Fascia, Right Foot	0 Open 3 Percutaneous	Z No Device	Z No Qualifier

Non-OR 0JD[0,1,4,5,B,C,D,F,G,H,J,K,N,P,Q,R]3ZZ
See Appendix L for Procedure Combinations
Combo-only 0JD[6,7,8,9,L,M]3ZZ

ICD-10-PCS 2025 — Subcutaneous Tissue and Fascia — 0JH–0JH

- **0** Medical and Surgical
- **J** Subcutaneous Tissue and Fascia
- **H** Insertion
  Definition: Putting in a nonbiological appliance that monitors, assists, performs, or prevents a physiological function but does not physically take the place of a body part
  Explanation: None

Body Part Character 4	Approach Character 5	Device Character 6	Qualifier Character 7
0 Subcutaneous Tissue and Fascia, Scalp Galea aponeurotica **1** Subcutaneous Tissue and Fascia, Face Chin Masseteric fascia Orbital fascia Submandibular space **4** Subcutaneous Tissue and Fascia, Right Neck Deep cervical fascia Pretracheal fascia Prevertebral fascia **5** Subcutaneous Tissue and Fascia, Left Neck See 4 Subcutaneous Tissue and Fascia, Right Neck **9** Subcutaneous Tissue and Fascia, Buttock **B** Subcutaneous Tissue and Fascia, Perineum **C** Subcutaneous Tissue and Fascia, Pelvic Region **J** Subcutaneous Tissue and Fascia, Right Hand Palmar fascia (aponeurosis) **K** Subcutaneous Tissue and Fascia, Left Hand See J Subcutaneous Tissue and Fascia, Right Hand **Q** Subcutaneous Tissue and Fascia, Right Foot Plantar fascia (aponeurosis) **R** Subcutaneous Tissue and Fascia, Left Foot See Q Subcutaneous Tissue and Fascia, Right Foot	**0** Open **3** Percutaneous	**N** Tissue Expander	**Z** No Qualifier
6 Subcutaneous Tissue and Fascia, Chest ➕ Pectoral fascia	**0** Open **3** Percutaneous	**0** Monitoring Device, Hemodynamic **2** Monitoring Device **4** Pacemaker, Single Chamber **5** Pacemaker, Single Chamber Rate Responsive **6** Pacemaker, Dual Chamber **7** Cardiac Resynchronization Pacemaker Pulse Generator **8** Defibrillator Generator **9** Cardiac Resynchronization Defibrillator Pulse Generator **A** Contractility Modulation Device **B** Stimulator Generator, Single Array **C** Stimulator Generator, Single Array Rechargeable **D** Stimulator Generator, Multiple Array **E** Stimulator Generator, Multiple Array Rechargeable **F** Subcutaneous Defibrillator Lead **H** Contraceptive Device **M** Stimulator Generator **N** Tissue Expander **P** Cardiac Rhythm Related Device **V** Infusion Device, Pump **W** Vascular Access Device, Totally Implantable **X** Vascular Access Device, Tunneled **Y** Other Device	**Z** No Qualifier
7 Subcutaneous Tissue and Fascia, Back NC ➕	**0** Open **3** Percutaneous	**B** Stimulator Generator, Single Array **C** Stimulator Generator, Single Array Rechargeable **D** Stimulator Generator, Multiple Array **E** Stimulator Generator, Multiple Array Rechargeable **M** Stimulator Generator **N** Tissue Expander **V** Infusion Device, Pump **Y** Other Device	**Z** No Qualifier

DRG Non-OR 0JH6[0,3][4,5,6,7,H,P,X]Z
DRG Non-OR 0JH63WX
Non-OR 0JH63YZ
Non-OR 0JH73YZ
NC 0JH7[0,3]MZ
HAC 0JH6[0,3][4,5,6,7,8,9,F,P]Z when reported with SDx K68.11 or T81.40-T81.49, T82.7 with 7th character A
HAC 0JH63XZ when reported with SDx J95.811

See Appendix L for Procedure Combinations
➕ 0JH6[0,3][4,5,6,7,8,9,A,B,C,D,E,F,M,P]Z
➕ 0JH7[0,3][B,C,D,E,M]Z

0JH Continued on next page

NC Noncovered Procedure   **LC** Limited Coverage   **QA** Questionable OB Admit   **NT** New Tech Add-on   ➕ Combination Member   ♂ Male   ♀ Female

ØJH–ØJH Subcutaneous Tissue and Fascia ICD-10-PCS 2025

ØJH Continued

Ø Medical and Surgical
J Subcutaneous Tissue and Fascia
H Insertion
  Definition: Putting in a nonbiological appliance that monitors, assists, performs, or prevents a physiological function but does not physically take the place of a body part
  Explanation: None

Body Part Character 4	Approach Character 5	Device Character 6	Qualifier Character 7
8 Subcutaneous Tissue and Fascia, Abdomen [NC+]	**Ø** Open **3** Percutaneous	**Ø** Monitoring Device, Hemodynamic **2** Monitoring Device **4** Pacemaker, Single Chamber **5** Pacemaker, Single Chamber Rate Responsive **6** Pacemaker, Dual Chamber **7** Cardiac Resynchronization Pacemaker Pulse Generator **8** Defibrillator Generator **9** Cardiac Resynchronization Defibrillator Pulse Generator **A** Contractility Modulation Device **B** Stimulator Generator, Single Array **C** Stimulator Generator, Single Array Rechargeable **D** Stimulator Generator, Multiple Array **E** Stimulator Generator, Multiple Array Rechargeable **H** Contraceptive Device **M** Stimulator Generator **N** Tissue Expander **P** Cardiac Rhythm Related Device **V** Infusion Device, Pump **W** Vascular Access Device, Totally Implantable **X** Vascular Access Device, Tunneled **Y** Other Device	**Z** No Qualifier

D Subcutaneous Tissue and Fascia, Right Upper Arm
  Axillary fascia
  Deltoid fascia
  Infraspinatus fascia
  Subscapular aponeurosis
  Supraspinatus fascia
F Subcutaneous Tissue and Fascia, Left Upper Arm
  See D Subcutaneous Tissue and Fascia, Right Upper Arm
G Subcutaneous Tissue and Fascia, Right Lower Arm
  Antebrachial fascia
  Bicipital aponeurosis
H Subcutaneous Tissue and Fascia, Left Lower Arm
  See G Subcutaneous Tissue and Fascia, Right Lower Arm
L Subcutaneous Tissue and Fascia, Right Upper Leg
  Crural fascia
  Fascia lata
  Iliac fascia
  Iliotibial tract (band)
M Subcutaneous Tissue and Fascia, Left Upper Leg
  See L Subcutaneous Tissue and Fascia, Right Upper Leg
N Subcutaneous Tissue and Fascia, Right Lower Leg
P Subcutaneous Tissue and Fascia, Left Lower Leg
	Ø Open
	3 Percutaneous
		H Contraceptive Device
		N Tissue Expander
		V Infusion Device, Pump
		W Vascular Access Device, Totally Implantable
		X Vascular Access Device, Tunneled
			Z No Qualifier

S Subcutaneous Tissue and Fascia, Head and Neck **V** Subcutaneous Tissue and Fascia, Upper Extremity **W** Subcutaneous Tissue and Fascia, Lower Extremity	**Ø** Open **3** Percutaneous	**1** Radioactive Element **3** Infusion Device **Y** Other Device	**Z** No Qualifier

T Subcutaneous Tissue and Fascia, Trunk
  External oblique aponeurosis
  Transversalis fascia
	Ø Open
	3 Percutaneous
		1 Radioactive Element
		3 Infusion Device
		V Infusion Device, Pump
		Y Other Device
			Z No Qualifier

DRG Non-OR ØJH8[Ø,3][2,4,5,6,7,H,P,X]Z
DRG Non-OR ØJH83WX
DRG Non-OR ØJH[D,F,G,H,L,M,N,P]ØXZ
DRG Non-OR ØJH[D,F,G,H,L,M,N,P]3[W,X]Z
DRG Non-OR ØJHN3HZ
DRG Non-OR ØJHP[Ø,3]HZ

Non-OR ØJH83YZ
Non-OR ØJH[D,F,G,H,L,M][Ø,3]HZ
Non-OR ØJHNØHZ
Non-OR ØJH[S,V,W]Ø3Z
Non-OR ØJH[S,V,W]3[3,Y]Z
Non-OR ØJHTØ3Z
Non-OR ØJHT3[3,Y]Z

HAC ØJH8[Ø,3][4,5,6,7,8,9,P]Z when reported with SDx K68.11 or T81.4Ø-T81.49, T82.7 with 7th character A
NC ØJH8[Ø,3]MZ

See Appendix L for Procedure Combinations
  ØJH8[Ø,3][4,5,6,7,8,9,A,B,C,D,E,M,P]Z

Non-OR Procedure DRG Non-OR Procedure Valid OR Procedure HAC Associated Procedure Combination Only New/Revised April New/Revised October

ICD-10-PCS 2025 — Subcutaneous Tissue and Fascia — 0JJ–0JN

0 Medical and Surgical
J Subcutaneous Tissue and Fascia
J Inspection   Definition: Visually and/or manually exploring a body part
Explanation: Visual exploration may be performed with or without optical instrumentation. Manual exploration may be performed directly or through intervening body layers.

Body Part — Character 4	Approach — Character 5	Device — Character 6	Qualifier — Character 7

S Subcutaneous Tissue and Fascia, Head and Neck
T Subcutaneous Tissue and Fascia, Trunk
  External oblique aponeurosis
  Transversalis fascia
V Subcutaneous Tissue and Fascia, Upper Extremity
W Subcutaneous Tissue and Fascia, Lower Extremity
	0 Open
	3 Percutaneous
	X External
		Z No Device	**Z** No Qualifier

Non-OR   All body part, approach, device, and qualifier values

---

0 Medical and Surgical
J Subcutaneous Tissue and Fascia
N Release   Definition: Freeing a body part from an abnormal physical constraint by cutting or by the use of force
Explanation: Some of the restraining tissue may be taken out but none of the body part is taken out

Body Part — Character 4	Approach — Character 5	Device — Character 6	Qualifier — Character 7

0 Subcutaneous Tissue and Fascia, Scalp
   Galea aponeurotica
1 Subcutaneous Tissue and Fascia, Face
   Chin
   Masseteric fascia
   Orbital fascia
   Submandibular space
4 Subcutaneous Tissue and Fascia, Right Neck
   Deep cervical fascia
   Pretracheal fascia
   Prevertebral fascia
5 Subcutaneous Tissue and Fascia, Left Neck
   See 4 Subcutaneous Tissue and Fascia, Right Neck
6 Subcutaneous Tissue and Fascia, Chest
   Pectoral fascia
7 Subcutaneous Tissue and Fascia, Back
8 Subcutaneous Tissue and Fascia, Abdomen
9 Subcutaneous Tissue and Fascia, Buttock
B Subcutaneous Tissue and Fascia, Perineum
C Subcutaneous Tissue and Fascia, Pelvic Region
D Subcutaneous Tissue and Fascia, Right Upper Arm
   Axillary fascia
   Deltoid fascia
   Infraspinatus fascia
   Subscapular aponeurosis
   Supraspinatus fascia
F Subcutaneous Tissue and Fascia, Left Upper Arm
   See D Subcutaneous Tissue and Fascia, Right Upper Arm
 	
G Subcutaneous Tissue and Fascia, Right Lower Arm
   Antebrachial fascia
   Bicipital aponeurosis
H Subcutaneous Tissue and Fascia, Left Lower Arm
   See G Subcutaneous Tissue and Fascia, Right Lower Arm
J Subcutaneous Tissue and Fascia, Right Hand
   Palmar fascia (aponeurosis)
K Subcutaneous Tissue and Fascia, Left Hand
   See J Subcutaneous Tissue and Fascia, Right Hand
L Subcutaneous Tissue and Fascia, Right Upper Leg
   Crural fascia
   Fascia lata
   Iliac fascia
   Iliotibial tract (band)
M Subcutaneous Tissue and Fascia, Left Upper Leg
   See L Subcutaneous Tissue and Fascia, Right Upper Leg
N Subcutaneous Tissue and Fascia, Right Lower Leg
P Subcutaneous Tissue and Fascia, Left Lower Leg
Q Subcutaneous Tissue and Fascia, Right Foot
   Plantar fascia (aponeurosis)
R Subcutaneous Tissue and Fascia, Left Foot
   See Q Subcutaneous Tissue and Fascia, Right Foot
	0 Open
	3 Percutaneous
	X External
		Z No Device	**Z** No Qualifier

Non-OR   0JN[0,1,4,5,6,7,8,9,B,C,D,F,G,H,J,K,L,M,N,P,Q,R]XZZ

Subcutaneous Tissue and Fascia

0JP–0JP   ICD-10-PCS 2025

0 Medical and Surgical
J Subcutaneous Tissue and Fascia
P Removal   Definition: Taking out or off a device from a body part
Explanation: If a device is taken out and a similar device put in without cutting or puncturing the skin or mucous membrane, the procedure is coded to the root operation CHANGE. Otherwise, the procedure for taking out a device is coded to the root operation REMOVAL.

Body Part Character 4	Approach Character 5	Device Character 6	Qualifier Character 7
S Subcutaneous Tissue and Fascia, Head and Neck	**0** Open **3** Percutaneous	**0** Drainage Device **1** Radioactive Element **3** Infusion Device **7** Autologous Tissue Substitute **J** Synthetic Substitute **K** Nonautologous Tissue Substitute **N** Tissue Expander **Y** Other Device	**Z** No Qualifier
S Subcutaneous Tissue and Fascia, Head and Neck	**X** External	**0** Drainage Device **1** Radioactive Element **3** Infusion Device	**Z** No Qualifier
T Subcutaneous Tissue and Fascia, Trunk External oblique aponeurosis Transversalis fascia	**0** Open **3** Percutaneous	**0** Drainage Device **1** Radioactive Element **2** Monitoring Device **3** Infusion Device **7** Autologous Tissue Substitute **F** Subcutaneous Defibrillator Lead **H** Contraceptive Device **J** Synthetic Substitute **K** Nonautologous Tissue Substitute **M** Stimulator Generator **N** Tissue Expander **P** Cardiac Rhythm Related Device **V** Infusion Device, Pump **W** Vascular Access Device, Totally Implantable **X** Vascular Access Device, Tunneled **Y** Other Device	**Z** No Qualifier
T Subcutaneous Tissue and Fascia, Trunk External oblique aponeurosis Transversalis fascia	**X** External	**0** Drainage Device **1** Radioactive Element **2** Monitoring Device **3** Infusion Device **H** Contraceptive Device **V** Infusion Device, Pump **X** Vascular Access Device, Tunneled	**Z** No Qualifier
V Subcutaneous Tissue and Fascia, Upper Extremity **W** Subcutaneous Tissue and Fascia, Lower Extremity	**0** Open **3** Percutaneous	**0** Drainage Device **1** Radioactive Element **3** Infusion Device **7** Autologous Tissue Substitute **H** Contraceptive Device **J** Synthetic Substitute **K** Nonautologous Tissue Substitute **N** Tissue Expander **V** Infusion Device, Pump **W** Vascular Access Device, Totally Implantable **X** Vascular Access Device, Tunneled **Y** Other Device	**Z** No Qualifier
V Subcutaneous Tissue and Fascia, Upper Extremity **W** Subcutaneous Tissue and Fascia, Lower Extremity	**X** External	**0** Drainage Device **1** Radioactive Element **3** Infusion Device **H** Contraceptive Device **V** Infusion Device, Pump **X** Vascular Access Device, Tunneled	**Z** No Qualifier

Non-OR   0JPS[0,3][0,1,3,7,J,K,N,Y]Z
Non-OR   0JPSX[0,1,3]Z
Non-OR   0JPT[0,3][0,1,2,3,7,H,J,K,M,N,V,W,X,Y]Z
Non-OR   0JPTX[0,1,2,3,H,V,X]Z
Non-OR   0JP[V,W][0,3][0,1,3,7,H,J,K,N,V,W,X,Y]Z
Non-OR   0JP[V,W]X[0,1,3,H,V,X]Z
HAC   0JPT[0,3][F,P]Z when reported with SDx K68.11 or T81.40-T81.49, T82.7 with 7th character A

Non-OR Procedure   DRG Non-OR Procedure   Valid OR Procedure   HAC Associated Procedure   Combination Only   New/Revised April   New/Revised October

- **0** Medical and Surgical
- **J** Subcutaneous Tissue and Fascia
- **Q** Repair Definition: Restoring, to the extent possible, a body part to its normal anatomic structure and function
  Explanation: Used only when the method to accomplish the repair is not one of the other root operations

Body Part Character 4	Approach Character 5	Device Character 6	Qualifier Character 7

0 Subcutaneous Tissue and Fascia, Scalp
  Galea aponeurotica
1 Subcutaneous Tissue and Fascia, Face
  Chin
  Masseteric fascia
  Orbital fascia
  Submandibular space
4 Subcutaneous Tissue and Fascia, Right Neck
  Deep cervical fascia
  Pretracheal fascia
  Prevertebral fascia
5 Subcutaneous Tissue and Fascia, Left Neck
  See 4 Subcutaneous Tissue and Fascia, Right Neck
6 Subcutaneous Tissue and Fascia, Chest
  Pectoral fascia
7 Subcutaneous Tissue and Fascia, Back
8 Subcutaneous Tissue and Fascia, Abdomen
9 Subcutaneous Tissue and Fascia, Buttock
B Subcutaneous Tissue and Fascia, Perineum
C Subcutaneous Tissue and Fascia, Pelvic Region
D Subcutaneous Tissue and Fascia, Right Upper Arm
  Axillary fascia
  Deltoid fascia
  Infraspinatus fascia
  Subscapular aponeurosis
  Supraspinatus fascia
F Subcutaneous Tissue and Fascia, Left Upper Arm
  See D Subcutaneous Tissue and Fascia, Right Upper Arm
G Subcutaneous Tissue and Fascia, Right Lower Arm
  Antebrachial fascia
  Bicipital aponeurosis
H Subcutaneous Tissue and Fascia, Left Lower Arm
  See G Subcutaneous Tissue and Fascia, Right Lower Arm
J Subcutaneous Tissue and Fascia, Right Hand
  Palmar fascia (aponeurosis)
K Subcutaneous Tissue and Fascia, Left Hand
  See J Subcutaneous Tissue and Fascia, Right Hand
L Subcutaneous Tissue and Fascia, Right Upper Leg
  Crural fascia
  Fascia lata
  Iliac fascia
  Iliotibial tract (band)
M Subcutaneous Tissue and Fascia, Left Upper Leg
  See L Subcutaneous Tissue and Fascia, Right Upper Leg
N Subcutaneous Tissue and Fascia, Right Lower Leg
P Subcutaneous Tissue and Fascia, Left Lower Leg
Q Subcutaneous Tissue and Fascia, Right Foot
  Plantar fascia (aponeurosis)
R Subcutaneous Tissue and Fascia, Left Foot
  See Q Subcutaneous Tissue and Fascia, Right Foot
	0 Open
	3 Percutaneous
		Z No Device	**Z** No Qualifier

Non-OR   0JQ[0,1,4,5,6,7,8,9,B,C,D,F,G,H,J,K,L,M,N,P,Q,R]3ZZ

0 Medical and Surgical
J Subcutaneous Tissue and Fascia
R Replacement

Definition: Putting in or on biological or synthetic material that physically takes the place and/or function of all or a portion of a body part

Explanation: The body part may have been taken out or replaced, or may be taken out, physically eradicated, or rendered nonfunctional during the REPLACEMENT procedure. A REMOVAL procedure is coded for taking out the device used in a previous replacement procedure.

Body Part Character 4	Approach Character 5	Device Character 6	Qualifier Character 7

0 Subcutaneous Tissue and Fascia, Scalp
    Galea aponeurotica
1 Subcutaneous Tissue and Fascia, Face
    Chin
    Masseteric fascia
    Orbital fascia
    Submandibular space
4 Subcutaneous Tissue and Fascia, Right Neck
    Deep cervical fascia
    Pretracheal fascia
    Prevertebral fascia
5 Subcutaneous Tissue and Fascia, Left Neck
    See 4 Subcutaneous Tissue and Fascia, Right Neck
6 Subcutaneous Tissue and Fascia, Chest
    Pectoral fascia
7 Subcutaneous Tissue and Fascia, Back
8 Subcutaneous Tissue and Fascia, Abdomen
9 Subcutaneous Tissue and Fascia, Buttock
B Subcutaneous Tissue and Fascia, Perineum
C Subcutaneous Tissue and Fascia, Pelvic Region
D Subcutaneous Tissue and Fascia, Right Upper Arm
    Axillary fascia
    Deltoid fascia
    Infraspinatus fascia
    Subscapular aponeurosis
    Supraspinatus fascia
F Subcutaneous Tissue and Fascia, Left Upper Arm
    See D Subcutaneous Tissue and Fascia, Right Upper Arm
G Subcutaneous Tissue and Fascia, Right Lower Arm
    Antebrachial fascia
    Bicipital aponeurosis
H Subcutaneous Tissue and Fascia, Left Lower Arm
    See G Subcutaneous Tissue and Fascia, Right Lower Arm
J Subcutaneous Tissue and Fascia, Right Hand
    Palmar fascia (aponeurosis)
K Subcutaneous Tissue and Fascia, Left Hand
    See J Subcutaneous Tissue and Fascia, Right Hand
L Subcutaneous Tissue and Fascia, Right Upper Leg
    Crural fascia
    Fascia lata
    Iliac fascia
    Iliotibial tract (band)
M Subcutaneous Tissue and Fascia, Left Upper Leg
    See L Subcutaneous Tissue and Fascia, Right Upper Leg
N Subcutaneous Tissue and Fascia, Right Lower Leg
P Subcutaneous Tissue and Fascia, Left Lower Leg
Q Subcutaneous Tissue and Fascia, Right Foot
    Plantar fascia (aponeurosis)
R Subcutaneous Tissue and Fascia, Left Foot
    See Q Subcutaneous Tissue and Fascia, Right Foot
	0 Open
	3 Percutaneous
		7 Autologous Tissue Substitute
		J Synthetic Substitute
		K Nonautologous Tissue Substitute
			Z No Qualifier

0 Medical and Surgical
J Subcutaneous Tissue and Fascia
U Supplement: Definition: Putting in or on biological or synthetic material that physically reinforces and/or augments the function of a portion of a body part
Explanation: The biological material is non-living, or is living and from the same individual. The body part may have been previously replaced, and the SUPPLEMENT procedure is performed to physically reinforce and/or augment the function of the replaced body part.

Body Part Character 4	Approach Character 5	Device Character 6	Qualifier Character 7

0 Subcutaneous Tissue and Fascia, Scalp
   Galea aponeurotica
1 Subcutaneous Tissue and Fascia, Face
   Chin
   Masseteric fascia
   Orbital fascia
   Submandibular space
4 Subcutaneous Tissue and Fascia, Right Neck
   Deep cervical fascia
   Pretracheal fascia
   Prevertebral fascia
5 Subcutaneous Tissue and Fascia, Left Neck
   See 4 Subcutaneous Tissue and Fascia, Right Neck
6 Subcutaneous Tissue and Fascia, Chest
   Pectoral fascia
7 Subcutaneous Tissue and Fascia, Back
8 Subcutaneous Tissue and Fascia, Abdomen
9 Subcutaneous Tissue and Fascia, Buttock
B Subcutaneous Tissue and Fascia, Perineum
C Subcutaneous Tissue and Fascia, Pelvic Region
D Subcutaneous Tissue and Fascia, Right Upper Arm
   Axillary fascia
   Deltoid fascia
   Infraspinatus fascia
   Subscapular aponeurosis
   Supraspinatus fascia
F Subcutaneous Tissue and Fascia, Left Upper Arm
   See D Subcutaneous Tissue and Fascia, Right Upper Arm
G Subcutaneous Tissue and Fascia, Right Lower Arm
   Antebrachial fascia
   Bicipital aponeurosis
H Subcutaneous Tissue and Fascia, Left Lower Arm
   See G Subcutaneous Tissue and Fascia, Right Lower Arm
J Subcutaneous Tissue and Fascia, Right Hand
   Palmar fascia (aponeurosis)
K Subcutaneous Tissue and Fascia, Left Hand
   See J Subcutaneous Tissue and Fascia, Right Hand
L Subcutaneous Tissue and Fascia, Right Upper Leg
   Crural fascia
   Fascia lata
   Iliac fascia
   Iliotibial tract (band)
M Subcutaneous Tissue and Fascia, Left Upper Leg
   See L Subcutaneous Tissue and Fascia, Right Upper Leg
N Subcutaneous Tissue and Fascia, Right Lower Leg
P Subcutaneous Tissue and Fascia, Left Lower Leg
Q Subcutaneous Tissue and Fascia, Right Foot
   Plantar fascia (aponeurosis)
R Subcutaneous Tissue and Fascia, Left Foot
   See Q Subcutaneous Tissue and Fascia, Right Foot
	0 Open
	3 Percutaneous
		7 Autologous Tissue Substitute
		J Synthetic Substitute
		K Nonautologous Tissue Substitute
			Z No Qualifier

Subcutaneous Tissue and Fascia

0JW–0JW   Subcutaneous Tissue and Fascia   ICD-10-PCS 2025

0 Medical and Surgical
J Subcutaneous Tissue and Fascia
W Revision   Definition: Correcting, to the extent possible, a portion of a malfunctioning device or the position of a displaced device
                Explanation: Revision can include correcting a malfunctioning or displaced device by taking out or putting in components of the device such as a screw or pin

Body Part Character 4	Approach Character 5	Device Character 6	Qualifier Character 7
S Subcutaneous Tissue and Fascia, Head and Neck	**0** Open **3** Percutaneous	**0** Drainage Device **3** Infusion Device **7** Autologous Tissue Substitute **J** Synthetic Substitute **K** Nonautologous Tissue Substitute **N** Tissue Expander **Y** Other Device	**Z** No Qualifier
S Subcutaneous Tissue and Fascia, Head and Neck	**X** External	**0** Drainage Device **3** Infusion Device **7** Autologous Tissue Substitute **J** Synthetic Substitute **K** Nonautologous Tissue Substitute **N** Tissue Expander	**Z** No Qualifier
T Subcutaneous Tissue and Fascia, Trunk External oblique aponeurosis Transversalis fascia	**0** Open **3** Percutaneous	**0** Drainage Device **2** Monitoring Device **3** Infusion Device **7** Autologous Tissue Substitute **F** Subcutaneous Defibrillator Lead **H** Contraceptive Device **J** Synthetic Substitute **K** Nonautologous Tissue Substitute **M** Stimulator Generator **N** Tissue Expander **P** Cardiac Rhythm Related Device **V** Infusion Device, Pump **W** Vascular Access Device, Totally Implantable **X** Vascular Access Device, Tunneled **Y** Other Device	**Z** No Qualifier
T Subcutaneous Tissue and Fascia, Trunk External oblique aponeurosis Transversalis fascia	**X** External	**0** Drainage Device **2** Monitoring Device **3** Infusion Device **7** Autologous Tissue Substitute **F** Subcutaneous Defibrillator Lead **H** Contraceptive Device **J** Synthetic Substitute **K** Nonautologous Tissue Substitute **M** Stimulator Generator **N** Tissue Expander **P** Cardiac Rhythm Related Device **V** Infusion Device, Pump **W** Vascular Access Device, Totally Implantable **X** Vascular Access Device, Tunneled	**Z** No Qualifier
V Subcutaneous Tissue and Fascia, Upper Extremity **W** Subcutaneous Tissue and Fascia, Lower Extremity	**0** Open **3** Percutaneous	**0** Drainage Device **3** Infusion Device **7** Autologous Tissue Substitute **H** Contraceptive Device **J** Synthetic Substitute **K** Nonautologous Tissue Substitute **N** Tissue Expander **V** Infusion Device, Pump **W** Vascular Access Device, Totally Implantable **X** Vascular Access Device, Tunneled **Y** Other Device	**Z** No Qualifier
V Subcutaneous Tissue and Fascia, Upper Extremity **W** Subcutaneous Tissue and Fascia, Lower Extremity	**X** External	**0** Drainage Device **3** Infusion Device **7** Autologous Tissue Substitute **H** Contraceptive Device **J** Synthetic Substitute **K** Nonautologous Tissue Substitute **N** Tissue Expander **V** Infusion Device, Pump **W** Vascular Access Device, Totally Implantable **X** Vascular Access Device, Tunneled	**Z** No Qualifier

DRG Non-OR	0JWS[0,3][0,3,7,J,K,N,Y]Z	Non-OR	0JWTX[0,2,3,7,F,H,J,K,N,P,V,W,X]Z
DRG Non-OR	0JWT[0,3][0,3,7,H,J,K,M,N,V,W,X]Z	Non-OR	0JW[V,W]X[0,3,7,H,J,K,N,V,W,X]Z
DRG Non-OR	0JWTXMZ	HAC	0JWT[0,3][F,P]Z when reported with SDx K68.11 or T81.40-T81.49, T82.7 with 7th character A
DRG Non-OR	0JW[V,W][0,3][0,3,7,H,J,K,N,V,W,X,Y]Z	HAC	0JWTXFZ when reported with SDx K68.11, or T81.40-T81.49, T82.7 with 7th character A
Non-OR	0JWSX[0,3,7,J,K,N]Z		
Non-OR	0JWT3YZ		

Non-OR Procedure   DRG Non-OR Procedure   Valid OR Procedure   HAC Associated Procedure   Combination Only   New/Revised April   New/Revised October

0　**Medical and Surgical**
J　**Subcutaneous Tissue and Fascia**
X　**Transfer**　Definition: Moving, without taking out, all or a portion of a body part to another location to take over the function of all or a portion of a body part
　　　　Explanation: The body part transferred remains connected to its vascular and nervous supply

Body Part Character 4	Approach Character 5	Device Character 6	Qualifier Character 7
0 Subcutaneous Tissue and Fascia, Scalp 　Galea aponeurotica 1 Subcutaneous Tissue and Fascia, Face 　Chin 　Masseteric fascia 　Orbital fascia 　Submandibular space 4 Subcutaneous Tissue and Fascia, Right Neck 　Deep cervical fascia 　Pretracheal fascia 　Prevertebral fascia 5 Subcutaneous Tissue and Fascia, Left Neck 　See 4 Subcutaneous Tissue and Fascia, Right Neck 6 Subcutaneous Tissue and Fascia, Chest 　Pectoral fascia 7 Subcutaneous Tissue and Fascia, Back 8 Subcutaneous Tissue and Fascia, Abdomen 9 Subcutaneous Tissue and Fascia, Buttock B Subcutaneous Tissue and Fascia, Perineum C Subcutaneous Tissue and Fascia, Pelvic Region D Subcutaneous Tissue and Fascia, Right Upper Arm 　Axillary fascia 　Deltoid fascia 　Infraspinatus fascia 　Subscapular aponeurosis 　Supraspinatus fascia F Subcutaneous Tissue and Fascia, Left Upper Arm 　See D Subcutaneous Tissue and Fascia, Right Upper Arm G Subcutaneous Tissue and Fascia, Right Lower Arm 　Antebrachial fascia 　Bicipital aponeurosis H Subcutaneous Tissue and Fascia, Left Lower Arm 　See G Subcutaneous Tissue and Fascia, Right Lower Arm J Subcutaneous Tissue and Fascia, Right Hand 　Palmar fascia (aponeurosis) K Subcutaneous Tissue and Fascia, Left Hand 　See J Subcutaneous Tissue and Fascia, Right Hand L Subcutaneous Tissue and Fascia, Right Upper Leg 　Crural fascia 　Fascia lata 　Iliac fascia 　Iliotibial tract (band) M Subcutaneous Tissue and Fascia, Left Upper Leg 　See L Subcutaneous Tissue and Fascia, Right Upper Leg N Subcutaneous Tissue and Fascia, Right Lower Leg P Subcutaneous Tissue and Fascia, Left Lower Leg Q Subcutaneous Tissue and Fascia, Right Foot 　Plantar fascia (aponeurosis) R Subcutaneous Tissue and Fascia, Left Foot 　See Q Subcutaneous Tissue and Fascia, Right Foot	0 Open 3 Percutaneous	Z No Device	B Skin and Subcutaneous Tissue C Skin, Subcutaneous Tissue and Fascia Z No Qualifier

Muscles ØK2–ØKX

Character Meanings

This Character Meaning table is provided as a guide to assist the user in the identification of character members that may be found in this section of code tables. It **SHOULD NOT** be used to build a PCS code.

Operation–Character 3	Body Part–Character 4	Approach–Character 5	Device–Character 6	Qualifier–Character 7
2 Change	Ø Head Muscle	Ø Open	Ø Drainage Device	Ø Skin
5 Destruction	1 Facial Muscle	3 Percutaneous	7 Autologous Tissue Substitute	1 Subcutaneous Tissue
8 Division	2 Neck Muscle, Right	4 Percutaneous Endoscopic	J Synthetic Substitute	2 Skin and Subcutaneous Tissue
9 Drainage	3 Neck Muscle, Left	7 Via Natural or Artificial Opening	K Nonautologous Tissue Substitute	5 Latissimus Dorsi Myocutaneous Flap
B Excision	4 Tongue, Palate, Pharynx Muscle	8 Via Natural or Artificial Opening Endoscopic	M Stimulator Lead	6 Transverse Rectus Abdominis Myocutaneous Flap
C Extirpation	5 Shoulder Muscle, Right	X External	Y Other Device	7 Deep Inferior Epigastric Artery Perforator Flap
D Extraction	6 Shoulder Muscle, Left		Z No Device	8 Superficial Inferior Epigastric Artery Flap
H Insertion	7 Upper Arm Muscle, Right			9 Gluteal Artery Perforator Flap
J Inspection	8 Upper Arm Muscle, Left			X Diagnostic
M Reattachment	9 Lower Arm and Wrist Muscle, Right			Z No Qualifier
N Release	B Lower Arm and Wrist Muscle, Left			
P Removal	C Hand Muscle, Right			
Q Repair	D Hand Muscle, Left			
R Replacement	F Trunk Muscle, Right			
S Reposition	G Trunk Muscle, Left			
T Resection	H Thorax Muscle, Right			
U Supplement	J Thorax Muscle, Left			
W Revision	K Abdomen Muscle, Right			
X Transfer	L Abdomen Muscle, Left			
	M Perineum Muscle			
	N Hip Muscle, Right			
	P Hip Muscle, Left			
	Q Upper Leg Muscle, Right			
	R Upper Leg Muscle, Left			
	S Lower Leg Muscle, Right			
	T Lower Leg Muscle, Left			
	V Foot Muscle, Right			
	W Foot Muscle, Left			
	X Upper Muscle			
	Y Lower Muscle			

AHA Coding Clinic for table ØK8
- 2021, 4Q, 50 — Endoscopic division of tongue, palate and pharynx muscle
- 2020, 2Q, 25 — Endoscopic stapling of Zenker's diverticulum

AHA Coding Clinic for table ØKB
- 2023, 2Q, 30 — Excisional debridement and non-excisional debridement at deeper layer same site
- 2023, 1Q, 32 — Zenker's diverticulectomy
- 2020, 1Q, 27 — Delayed reconstruction following mastectomy using gracilis musculocutaneous free flap
- 2016, 3Q, 20 — Excisional debridement of sacrum
- 2015, 3Q, 3-8 — Excisional and nonexcisional debridement

AHA Coding Clinic for table ØKD
- 2023, 2Q, 30 — Excisional debridement and non-excisional debridement at deeper layer same site
- 2017, 4Q, 41-42 — Extraction procedures

AHA Coding Clinic for table ØKH
- 2020, 4Q, 63 — Intercompartmental pressure measurement

AHA Coding Clinic for table ØKN
- 2017, 2Q, 12 — Compartment syndrome and fasciotomy of foot
- 2017, 2Q, 13 — Compartment syndrome and fasciotomy of leg
- 2015, 2Q, 22 — Arthroscopic subacromial decompression
- 2014, 4Q, 39 — Abdominal component release with placement of mesh for hernia repair

AHA Coding Clinic for table ØKQ
- 2022, 3Q, 13 — Repair of prolapsed neovaginal graft
- 2018, 2Q, 25 — Third and fourth degree obstetric lacerations

AHA Coding Clinic for table ØKQ (Continued)
- 2016, 2Q, 34 — Assisted vaginal delivery
- 2016, 1Q, 7 — Obstetrical perineal laceration repair
- 2014, 4Q, 43 — Second degree obstetric perineal laceration
- 2013, 4Q, 120 — Repair of second degree perineum obstetric laceration

AHA Coding Clinic for table ØKS
- 2022, 3Q, 11 — Ulceration and soft tissue redundancy at amputation site due to osteo-integrated implant
- 2017, 1Q, 41 — Manual reduction of hernia

AHA Coding Clinic for table ØKT
- 2016, 2Q, 12 — Resection of malignant neoplasm of infratemporal fossa
- 2015, 1Q, 38 — Abdominoperineal resection with flap closure of the perineum and colostomy

AHA Coding Clinic for table ØKX
- 2023, 1Q, 34 — Repair of Stage 4 pressure ulcer and application of Amniofill®
- 2022, 3Q, 11 — Ulceration and soft tissue redundancy at amputation site due to osteo-integrated implant
- 2018, 2Q, 18 — Transverse rectus abdominis myocutaneous (TRAM) delay
- 2017, 4Q, 67 — New qualifier values - Pedicle flap procedures
- 2016, 3Q, 30 — Resection of femur with interposition arthroplasty
- 2015, 3Q, 33 — Cleft lip repair using Millard rotation advancement
- 2015, 2Q, 26 — Pharyngeal flap to soft palate
- 2014, 4Q, 41 — Abdominoperineal resection (APR) with flap closure of perineum and colostomy
- 2014, 2Q, 10 — Transverse abdominomyocutaneous (TRAM) breast reconstruction
- 2014, 2Q, 12 — Pedicle latissimus myocutaneous flap with placement of breast tissue expanders

Muscles

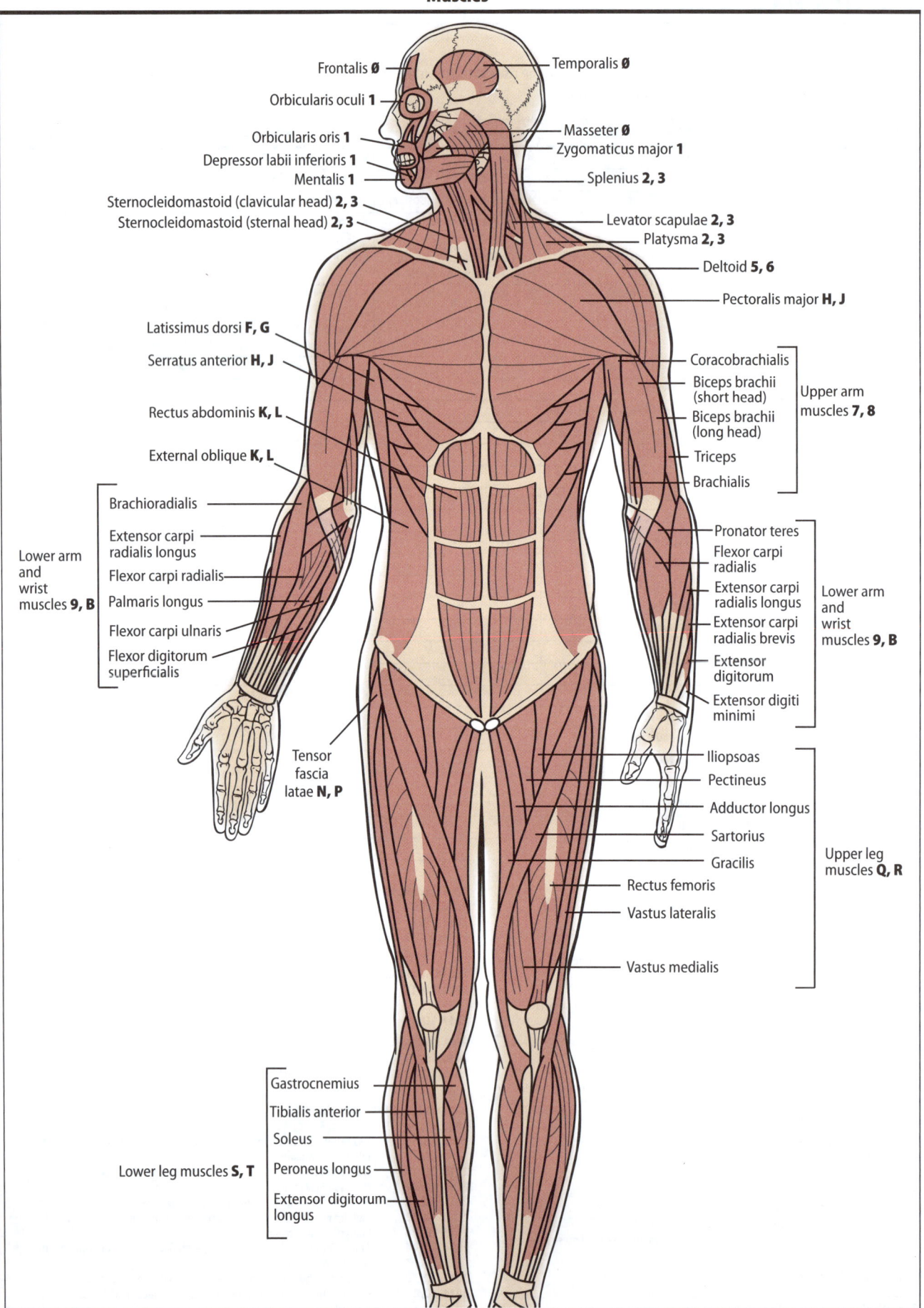

- Frontalis **0**
- Temporalis **0**
- Orbicularis oculi **1**
- Orbicularis oris **1**
- Masseter **0**
- Depressor labii inferioris **1**
- Zygomaticus major **1**
- Mentalis **1**
- Splenius **2, 3**
- Sternocleidomastoid (clavicular head) **2, 3**
- Levator scapulae **2, 3**
- Sternocleidomastoid (sternal head) **2, 3**
- Platysma **2, 3**
- Deltoid **5, 6**
- Pectoralis major **H, J**
- Latissimus dorsi **F, G**
- Coracobrachialis
- Serratus anterior **H, J**
- Biceps brachii (short head)
- Biceps brachii (long head)
- Rectus abdominis **K, L**
- Triceps
- External oblique **K, L**
- Brachialis
- Upper arm muscles **7, 8**
- Brachioradialis
- Pronator teres
- Extensor carpi radialis longus
- Flexor carpi radialis
- Flexor carpi radialis
- Extensor carpi radialis longus
- Palmaris longus
- Extensor carpi radialis brevis
- Flexor carpi ulnaris
- Extensor digitorum
- Flexor digitorum superficialis
- Extensor digiti minimi
- Lower arm and wrist muscles **9, B**
- Lower arm and wrist muscles **9, B**
- Tensor fascia latae **N, P**
- Iliopsoas
- Pectineus
- Adductor longus
- Sartorius
- Gracilis
- Rectus femoris
- Vastus lateralis
- Vastus medialis
- Upper leg muscles **Q, R**
- Gastrocnemius
- Tibialis anterior
- Soleus
- Lower leg muscles **S, T**
- Peroneus longus
- Extensor digitorum longus

0 Medical and Surgical
K Muscles
2 Change   Definition: Taking out or off a device from a body part and putting back an identical or similar device in or on the same body part without cutting or puncturing the skin or a mucous membrane
Explanation: All CHANGE procedures are coded using the approach EXTERNAL

Body Part Character 4	Approach Character 5	Device Character 6	Qualifier Character 7
X Upper Muscle **Y** Lower Muscle	**X** External	**0** Drainage Device **Y** Other Device	**Z** No Qualifier

Non-OR All body part, approach, device, and qualifier values

0 Medical and Surgical
K Muscles
5 Destruction   Definition: Physical eradication of all or a portion of a body part by the direct use of energy, force, or a destructive agent
Explanation: None of the body part is physically taken out

Body Part Character 4	Approach Character 5	Device Character 6	Qualifier Character 7

0 **Head Muscle**
    Auricularis muscle
    Masseter muscle
    Pterygoid muscle
    Splenius capitis muscle
    Temporalis muscle
    Temporoparietalis muscle
1 **Facial Muscle**
    Buccinator muscle
    Corrugator supercilii muscle
    Depressor anguli oris muscle
    Depressor labii inferioris muscle
    Depressor septi nasi muscle
    Depressor supercilii muscle
    Levator anguli oris muscle
    Levator labii superioris alaeque nasi muscle
    Levator labii superioris muscle
    Mentalis muscle
    Nasalis muscle
    Occipitofrontalis muscle
    Orbicularis oris muscle
    Procerus muscle
    Risorius muscle
    Zygomaticus muscle
2 **Neck Muscle, Right**
    Anterior vertebral muscle
    Arytenoid muscle
    Cricothyroid muscle
    Infrahyoid muscle
    Levator scapulae muscle
    Platysma muscle
    Scalene muscle
    Splenius cervicis muscle
    Sternocleidomastoid muscle
    Suprahyoid muscle
    Thyroarytenoid muscle
3 **Neck Muscle, Left**
    See 2 Neck Muscle, Right
4 **Tongue, Palate, Pharynx Muscle**
    Chondroglossus muscle
    Genioglossus muscle
    Hyoglossus muscle
    Inferior longitudinal muscle
    Levator veli palatini muscle
    Palatoglossal muscle
    Palatopharyngeal muscle
    Pharyngeal constrictor muscle
    Salpingopharyngeus muscle
    Styloglossus muscle
    Stylopharyngeus muscle
    Superior longitudinal muscle
    Tensor veli palatini muscle
5 **Shoulder Muscle, Right**
    Deltoid muscle
    Infraspinatus muscle
    Subscapularis muscle
    Supraspinatus muscle
    Teres major muscle
    Teres minor muscle
6 **Shoulder Muscle, Left**
    See 5 Shoulder Muscle, Right
7 **Upper Arm Muscle, Right**
    Biceps brachii muscle
    Brachialis muscle
    Coracobrachialis muscle
    Triceps brachii muscle
8 **Upper Arm Muscle, Left**
    See 7 Upper Arm Muscle, Right
9 **Lower Arm and Wrist Muscle, Right**
    Anatomical snuffbox
    Anconeus muscle
    Brachioradialis muscle
    Extensor carpi radialis muscle
    Extensor carpi ulnaris muscle
    Flexor carpi radialis muscle
    Flexor carpi ulnaris muscle
    Flexor pollicis longus muscle
    Palmaris longus muscle
    Pronator quadratus muscle
    Pronator teres muscle
B **Lower Arm and Wrist Muscle, Left**
    See 9 Lower Arm and Wrist Muscle, Right
C **Hand Muscle, Right**
    Adductor pollicis muscle
    Hypothenar muscle
    Palmar interosseous muscle
    Thenar muscle
D **Hand Muscle, Left**
    See C Hand Muscle, Right
F **Trunk Muscle, Right**
    Coccygeus muscle
    Erector spinae muscle
    Interspinalis muscle
    Intertransversarius muscle
    Latissimus dorsi muscle
    Quadratus lumborum muscle
    Rhomboid major muscle
    Rhomboid minor muscle
    Serratus posterior muscle
    Transversospinalis muscle
    Trapezius muscle
G **Trunk Muscle, Left**
    See F Trunk Muscle, Right
H **Thorax Muscle, Right**
    Intercostal muscle
    Levatores costarum muscle
    Pectoralis major muscle
    Pectoralis minor muscle
    Serratus anterior muscle
    Subclavius muscle
    Subcostal muscle
    Transverse thoracis muscle
J **Thorax Muscle, Left**
    See H Thorax Muscle, Right
K **Abdomen Muscle, Right**
    External oblique muscle
    Internal oblique muscle
    Pyramidalis muscle
    Rectus abdominis muscle
    Transversus abdominis muscle
L **Abdomen Muscle, Left**
    See K Abdomen Muscle, Right
M **Perineum Muscle**
    Bulbospongiosus muscle
    Cremaster muscle
    Deep transverse perineal muscle
    Ischiocavernosus muscle
    Levator ani muscle
    Superficial transverse perineal muscle
N **Hip Muscle, Right**
    Gemellus muscle
    Gluteus maximus muscle
    Gluteus medius muscle
    Gluteus minimus muscle
    Iliacus muscle
    Iliopsoas muscle
    Obturator muscle
    Piriformis muscle
    Psoas muscle
    Quadratus femoris muscle
    Tensor fasciae latae muscle
P **Hip Muscle, Left**
    See N Hip Muscle, Right
Q **Upper Leg Muscle, Right**
    Adductor brevis muscle
    Adductor longus muscle
    Adductor magnus muscle
    Biceps femoris muscle
    Gracilis muscle
    Hamstring muscle
    Pectineus muscle
    Quadriceps (femoris)
    Rectus femoris muscle
    Sartorius muscle
    Semimembranosus muscle
    Semitendinosus muscle
    Vastus intermedius muscle
    Vastus lateralis muscle
    Vastus medialis muscle
R **Upper Leg Muscle, Left**
    See Q Upper Leg Muscle, Right
S **Lower Leg Muscle, Right**
    Extensor digitorum longus muscle
    Extensor hallucis longus muscle
    Fibularis brevis muscle
    Fibularis longus muscle
    Flexor digitorum longus muscle
    Flexor hallucis longus muscle
    Gastrocnemius muscle
    Peroneus brevis muscle
    Peroneus longus muscle
    Plantaris muscle
    Popliteus muscle
    Soleus muscle
    Tibialis anterior muscle
    Tibialis posterior muscle
T **Lower Leg Muscle, Left**
    See S Lower Leg Muscle, Right
V **Foot Muscle, Right**
    Abductor hallucis muscle
    Adductor hallucis muscle
    Extensor digitorum brevis muscle
    Extensor hallucis brevis muscle
    Flexor digitorum brevis muscle
    Flexor hallucis brevis muscle
    Quadratus plantae muscle
W **Foot Muscle, Left**
    See V Foot Muscle, Right
	0 Open
	3 Percutaneous
	4 Percutaneous Endoscopic
		Z No Device	**Z** No Qualifier

0K8–0K8 Muscles ICD-10-PCS 2025

0 Medical and Surgical
K Muscles
8 Division **Definition:** Cutting into a body part, without draining fluids and/or gases from the body part, in order to separate or transect a body part
Explanation: All or a portion of the body part is separated into two or more portions

Body Part Character 4	Approach Character 5	Device Character 6	Qualifier Character 7
0 Head Muscle Auricularis muscle Masseter muscle Pterygoid muscle Splenius capitis muscle Temporalis muscle Temporoparietalis muscle **1 Facial Muscle** Buccinator muscle Corrugator supercilii muscle Depressor anguli oris muscle Depressor labii inferioris muscle Depressor septi nasi muscle Depressor supercilii muscle Levator anguli oris muscle Levator labii superioris alaeque nasi muscle Levator labii superioris muscle Mentalis muscle Nasalis muscle Occipitofrontalis muscle Orbicularis oris muscle Procerus muscle Risorius muscle Zygomaticus muscle **2 Neck Muscle, Right** Anterior vertebral muscle Arytenoid muscle Cricothyroid muscle Infrahyoid muscle Levator scapulae muscle Platysma muscle Scalene muscle Splenius cervicis muscle Sternocleidomastoid muscle Suprahyoid muscle Thyroarytenoid muscle **3 Neck Muscle, Left** See 2 Neck Muscle, Right Tensor veli palatini muscle **5 Shoulder Muscle, Right** Deltoid muscle Infraspinatus muscle Subscapularis muscle Supraspinatus muscle Teres major muscle Teres minor muscle **6 Shoulder Muscle, Left** See 5 Shoulder Muscle, Right **7 Upper Arm Muscle, Right** Biceps brachii muscle Brachialis muscle Coracobrachialis muscle Triceps brachii muscle **8 Upper Arm Muscle, Left** See 7 Upper Arm Muscle, Right	**9 Lower Arm and Wrist Muscle, Right** Anatomical snuffbox Anconeus muscle Brachioradialis muscle Extensor carpi radialis muscle Extensor carpi ulnaris muscle Flexor carpi radialis muscle Flexor carpi ulnaris muscle Flexor pollicis longus muscle Palmaris longus muscle Pronator quadratus muscle Pronator teres muscle **B Lower Arm and Wrist Muscle, Left** See 9 Lower Arm and Wrist Muscle, Right **C Hand Muscle, Right** Adductor pollicis muscle Hypothenar muscle Palmar interosseous muscle Thenar muscle **D Hand Muscle, Left** See C Hand Muscle, Right **F Trunk Muscle, Right** Coccygeus muscle Erector spinae muscle Interspinalis muscle Intertransversarius muscle Latissimus dorsi muscle Quadratus lumborum muscle Rhomboid major muscle Rhomboid minor muscle Serratus posterior muscle Transversospinalis muscle Trapezius muscle **G Trunk Muscle, Left** See F Trunk Muscle, Right **H Thorax Muscle, Right** Intercostal muscle Levatores costarum muscle Pectoralis major muscle Pectoralis minor muscle Serratus anterior muscle Subclavius muscle Subcostal muscle Transverse thoracis muscle **J Thorax Muscle, Left** See H Thorax Muscle, Right **K Abdomen Muscle, Right** External oblique muscle Internal oblique muscle Pyramidalis muscle Rectus abdominis muscle Transversus abdominis muscle **L Abdomen Muscle, Left** See K Abdomen Muscle, Right **M Perineum Muscle** Bulbospongiosus muscle Cremaster muscle Deep transverse perineal muscle Ischiocavernosus muscle Levator ani muscle Superficial transverse perineal muscle	**N Hip Muscle, Right** Gemellus muscle Gluteus maximus muscle Gluteus medius muscle Gluteus minimus muscle Iliacus muscle Iliopsoas muscle Obturator muscle Piriformis muscle Psoas muscle Quadratus femoris muscle Tensor fasciae latae muscle **P Hip Muscle, Left** See N Hip Muscle, Right **Q Upper Leg Muscle, Right** Adductor brevis muscle Adductor longus muscle Adductor magnus muscle Biceps femoris muscle Gracilis muscle Hamstring muscle Pectineus muscle Quadriceps (femoris) Rectus femoris muscle Sartorius muscle Semimembranosus muscle Semitendinosus muscle Vastus intermedius muscle Vastus lateralis muscle Vastus medialis muscle **R Upper Leg Muscle, Left** See Q Upper Leg Muscle, Right **S Lower Leg Muscle, Right** Extensor digitorum longus muscle Extensor hallucis longus muscle Fibularis brevis muscle Fibularis longus muscle Flexor digitorum longus muscle Flexor hallucis longus muscle Gastrocnemius muscle Peroneus brevis muscle Peroneus longus muscle Plantaris muscle Popliteus muscle Soleus muscle Tibialis anterior muscle Tibialis posterior muscle **T Lower Leg Muscle, Left** See S Lower Leg Muscle, Right **V Foot Muscle, Right** Abductor hallucis muscle Adductor hallucis muscle Extensor digitorum brevis muscle Extensor hallucis brevis muscle Flexor digitorum brevis muscle Flexor hallucis brevis muscle Quadratus plantae muscle **W Foot Muscle, Left** See V Foot Muscle, Right	**0** Open **3** Percutaneous **4** Percutaneous Endoscopic	**Z** No Device	**Z** No Qualifier
4 Tongue, Palate, Pharynx Muscle Chondroglossus muscle Genioglossus muscle Hyoglossus muscle Inferior longitudinal muscle Levator veli palatini muscle Palatoglossal muscle Palatopharyngeal muscle Pharyngeal constrictor muscle Salpingopharyngeus muscle Styloglossus muscle Stylopharyngeus muscle Superior longitudinal muscle Tensor veli palatini muscle			**0** Open **3** Percutaneous **4** Percutaneous Endoscopic **7** Via Natural or Artificial Opening **8** Via Natural or Artificial Opening Endoscopic	**Z** No Device	**Z** No Qualifier

Non-OR Procedure   DRG Non-OR Procedure   Valid OR Procedure   HAC Associated Procedure   Combination Only   New/Revised April   New/Revised October

ICD-10-PCS 2025 — Muscles — 0K9–0K9

0 Medical and Surgical
K Muscles
9 Drainage

Definition: Taking or letting out fluids and/or gases from a body part
Explanation: The qualifier DIAGNOSTIC is used to identify drainage procedures that are biopsies

Body Part — Character 4	Approach — Character 5	Device — Character 6	Qualifier — Character 7
0 Head Muscle Auricularis muscle Masseter muscle Pterygoid muscle Splenius capitis muscle Temporalis muscle Temporoparietalis muscle **1 Facial Muscle** Buccinator muscle Corrugator supercilii muscle Depressor anguli oris muscle Depressor labii inferioris muscle Depressor septi nasi muscle Depressor supercilii muscle Levator anguli oris muscle Levator labii superioris alaeque nasi muscle Levator labii superioris muscle Mentalis muscle Nasalis muscle Occipitofrontalis muscle Orbicularis oris muscle Procerus muscle Risorius muscle Zygomaticus muscle **2 Neck Muscle, Right** Anterior vertebral muscle Arytenoid muscle Cricothyroid muscle Infrahyoid muscle Levator scapulae muscle Platysma muscle Scalene muscle Splenius cervicis muscle Sternocleidomastoid muscle Suprahyoid muscle Thyroarytenoid muscle **3 Neck Muscle, Left** See 2 Neck Muscle, Right **4 Tongue, Palate, Pharynx Muscle** Chondroglossus muscle Genioglossus muscle Hyoglossus muscle Inferior longitudinal muscle Levator veli palatini muscle Palatoglossal muscle Palatopharyngeal muscle Pharyngeal constrictor muscle Salpingopharyngeus muscle Styloglossus muscle Stylopharyngeus muscle Superior longitudinal muscle Tensor veli palatini muscle **5 Shoulder Muscle, Right** Deltoid muscle Infraspinatus muscle Subscapularis muscle Supraspinatus muscle Teres major muscle Teres minor muscle **6 Shoulder Muscle, Left** See 5 Shoulder Muscle, Right **7 Upper Arm Muscle, Right** Biceps brachii muscle Brachialis muscle Coracobrachialis muscle Triceps brachii muscle **8 Upper Arm Muscle, Left** See 7 Upper Arm Muscle, Right **9 Lower Arm and Wrist Muscle, Right** Anatomical snuffbox Anconeus muscle Brachioradialis muscle Extensor carpi radialis muscle Extensor carpi ulnaris muscle Flexor carpi radialis muscle Flexor carpi ulnaris muscle Flexor pollicis longus muscle Palmaris longus muscle Pronator quadratus muscle Pronator teres muscle **B Lower Arm and Wrist Muscle, Left** See 9 Lower Arm and Wrist Muscle, Right **C Hand Muscle, Right** Adductor pollicis muscle Hypothenar muscle Palmar interosseous muscle Thenar muscle **D Hand Muscle, Left** See C Hand Muscle, Right **F Trunk Muscle, Right** Coccygeus muscle Erector spinae muscle Interspinalis muscle Intertransversarius muscle Latissimus dorsi muscle Quadratus lumborum muscle Rhomboid major muscle Rhomboid minor muscle Serratus posterior muscle Transversospinalis muscle Trapezius muscle **G Trunk Muscle, Left** See F Trunk Muscle, Right **H Thorax Muscle, Right** Intercostal muscle Levatores costarum muscle Pectoralis major muscle Pectoralis minor muscle Serratus anterior muscle Subclavius muscle Subcostal muscle Transverse thoracis muscle **J Thorax Muscle, Left** See H Thorax Muscle, Right **K Abdomen Muscle, Right** External oblique muscle Internal oblique muscle Pyramidalis muscle Rectus abdominis muscle Transversus abdominis muscle **L Abdomen Muscle, Left** See K Abdomen Muscle, Right **M Perineum Muscle** Bulbospongiosus muscle Cremaster muscle Deep transverse perineal muscle Ischiocavernosus muscle Levator ani muscle Superficial transverse perineal muscle **N Hip Muscle, Right** Gemellus muscle Gluteus maximus muscle Gluteus medius muscle Gluteus minimus muscle Iliacus muscle Iliopsoas muscle Obturator muscle Piriformis muscle Psoas muscle Quadratus femoris muscle Tensor fasciae latae muscle **P Hip Muscle, Left** See N Hip Muscle, Right **Q Upper Leg Muscle, Right** Adductor brevis muscle Adductor longus muscle Adductor magnus muscle Biceps femoris muscle Gracilis muscle Hamstring muscle Pectineus muscle Quadriceps (femoris) Rectus femoris muscle Sartorius muscle Semimembranosus muscle Semitendinosus muscle Vastus intermedius muscle Vastus lateralis muscle Vastus medialis muscle **R Upper Leg Muscle, Left** See Q Upper Leg Muscle, Right **S Lower Leg Muscle, Right** Extensor digitorum longus muscle Extensor hallucis longus muscle Fibularis brevis muscle Fibularis longus muscle Flexor digitorum longus muscle Flexor hallucis longus muscle Gastrocnemius muscle Peroneus brevis muscle Peroneus longus muscle Plantaris muscle Popliteus muscle Soleus muscle Tibialis anterior muscle Tibialis posterior muscle **T Lower Leg Muscle, Left** See S Lower Leg Muscle, Right **V Foot Muscle, Right** Abductor hallucis muscle Adductor hallucis muscle Extensor digitorum brevis muscle Extensor hallucis brevis muscle Flexor digitorum brevis muscle Flexor hallucis brevis muscle Quadratus plantae muscle **W Foot Muscle, Left** See V Foot Muscle, Right	**0** Open **3** Percutaneous **4** Percutaneous Endoscopic	**0** Drainage Device	**Z** No Qualifier

Non-OR 0K9[0,1,2,3,4,5,6,7,8,9,B,C,D,F,G,H,J,K,L,M,N,P,Q,R,S,T,V,W]30Z

0K9 Continued on next page

NC Noncovered Procedure   LC Limited Coverage   QA Questionable OB Admit   NT New Tech Add-on   ✚ Combination Member   ♂ Male   ♀ Female

473

ØK9 Continued

Ø Medical and Surgical
K Muscles
9 Drainage

Definition: Taking or letting out fluids and/or gases from a body part
Explanation: The qualifier DIAGNOSTIC is used to identify drainage procedures that are biopsies

Body Part Character 4		Approach Character 5	Device Character 6	Qualifier Character 7
Ø Head Muscle Auricularis muscle Masseter muscle Pterygoid muscle Splenius capitis muscle Temporalis muscle Temporoparietalis muscle **1 Facial Muscle** Buccinator muscle Corrugator supercilii muscle Depressor anguli oris muscle Depressor labii inferioris muscle Depressor septi nasi muscle Depressor supercilii muscle Levator anguli oris muscle Levator labii superioris alaeque nasi muscle Levator labii superioris muscle Mentalis muscle Nasalis muscle Occipitofrontalis muscle Orbicularis oris muscle Procerus muscle Risorius muscle Zygomaticus muscle **2 Neck Muscle, Right** Anterior vertebral muscle Arytenoid muscle Cricothyroid muscle Infrahyoid muscle Levator scapulae muscle Platysma muscle Scalene muscle Splenius cervicis muscle Sternocleidomastoid muscle Suprahyoid muscle Thyroarytenoid muscle **3 Neck Muscle, Left** See 2 Neck Muscle, Right **4 Tongue, Palate, Pharynx Muscle** Chondroglossus muscle Genioglossus muscle Hyoglossus muscle Inferior longitudinal muscle Levator veli palatini muscle Palatoglossal muscle Palatopharyngeal muscle Pharyngeal constrictor muscle Salpingopharyngeus muscle Styloglossus muscle Stylopharyngeus muscle Superior longitudinal muscle Tensor veli palatini muscle **5 Shoulder Muscle, Right** Deltoid muscle Infraspinatus muscle Subscapularis muscle Supraspinatus muscle Teres major muscle Teres minor muscle **6 Shoulder Muscle, Left** See 5 Shoulder Muscle, Right	**7 Upper Arm Muscle, Right** Biceps brachii muscle Brachialis muscle Coracobrachialis muscle Triceps brachii muscle **8 Upper Arm Muscle, Left** See 7 Upper Arm Muscle, Right **9 Lower Arm and Wrist Muscle, Right** Anatomical snuffbox Anconeus muscle Brachioradialis muscle Extensor carpi radialis muscle Extensor carpi ulnaris muscle Flexor carpi radialis muscle Flexor carpi ulnaris muscle Flexor pollicis longus muscle Palmaris longus muscle Pronator quadratus muscle Pronator teres muscle **B Lower Arm and Wrist Muscle, Left** See 9 Lower Arm and Wrist Muscle, Right **C Hand Muscle, Right** Adductor pollicis muscle Hypothenar muscle Palmar interosseous muscle Thenar muscle **D Hand Muscle, Left** See C Hand Muscle, Right **F Trunk Muscle, Right** Coccygeus muscle Erector spinae muscle Interspinalis muscle Intertransversarius muscle Latissimus dorsi muscle Quadratus lumborum muscle Rhomboid major muscle Rhomboid minor muscle Serratus posterior muscle Transversospinalis muscle Trapezius muscle **G Trunk Muscle, Left** See F Trunk Muscle, Right **H Thorax Muscle, Right** Intercostal muscle Levatores costarum muscle Pectoralis major muscle Pectoralis minor muscle Serratus anterior muscle Subclavius muscle Subcostal muscle Transverse thoracis muscle **J Thorax Muscle, Left** See H Thorax Muscle, Right **K Abdomen Muscle, Right** External oblique muscle Internal oblique muscle Pyramidalis muscle Rectus abdominis muscle Transversus abdominis muscle **L Abdomen Muscle, Left** See K Abdomen Muscle, Right	**M Perineum Muscle** Bulbospongiosus muscle Cremaster muscle Deep transverse perineal muscle Ischiocavernosus muscle Levator ani muscle Superficial transverse perineal muscle **N Hip Muscle, Right** Gemellus muscle Gluteus maximus muscle Gluteus medius muscle Gluteus minimus muscle Iliacus muscle Iliopsoas muscle Obturator muscle Piriformis muscle Psoas muscle Quadratus femoris muscle Tensor fasciae latae muscle **P Hip Muscle, Left** See N Hip Muscle, Right **Q Upper Leg Muscle, Right** Adductor brevis muscle Adductor longus muscle Adductor magnus muscle Biceps femoris muscle Gracilis muscle Hamstring muscle Pectineus muscle Quadriceps (femoris) Rectus femoris muscle Sartorius muscle Semimembranosus muscle Semitendinosus muscle Vastus intermedius muscle Vastus lateralis muscle Vastus medialis muscle **R Upper Leg Muscle, Left** See Q Upper Leg Muscle, Right **S Lower Leg Muscle, Right** Extensor digitorum longus muscle Extensor hallucis longus muscle Fibularis brevis muscle Fibularis longus muscle Flexor digitorum longus muscle Flexor hallucis longus muscle Gastrocnemius muscle Peroneus brevis muscle Peroneus longus muscle Plantaris muscle Popliteus muscle Soleus muscle Tibialis anterior muscle Tibialis posterior muscle **T Lower Leg Muscle, Left** See S Lower Leg Muscle, Right **V Foot Muscle, Right** Abductor hallucis muscle Adductor hallucis muscle Extensor digitorum brevis muscle Extensor hallucis brevis muscle Flexor digitorum brevis muscle Flexor hallucis brevis muscle Quadratus plantae muscle **W Foot Muscle, Left** See V Foot Muscle, Right	**Ø** Open **3** Percutaneous **4** Percutaneous Endoscopic	**Z** No Device	**X** Diagnostic **Z** No Qualifier

Non-OR ØK9[Ø,1,2,3,4,5,6,7,8,9,B,F,G,H,J,K,L,M,N,P,Q,R,S,T,V,W]3ZZ
Non-OR ØK9[C,D][3,4]ZZ

Non-OR Procedure | DRG Non-OR Procedure | Valid OR Procedure | HAC Associated Procedure | Combination Only | New/Revised April | New/Revised October

474 ICD-10-PCS 2025

ICD-10-PCS 2025 — Muscles — 0KB–0KB

- **0** Medical and Surgical
- **K** Muscles
- **B** Excision

Definition: Cutting out or off, without replacement, a portion of a body part
Explanation: The qualifier DIAGNOSTIC is used to identify excision procedures that are biopsies

Body Part Character 4	Approach Character 5	Device Character 6	Qualifier Character 7
(see list below)	0 Open 3 Percutaneous 4 Percutaneous Endoscopic	Z No Device	X Diagnostic Z No Qualifier

Body Part Character 4:

0 Head Muscle
- Auricularis muscle
- Masseter muscle
- Pterygoid muscle
- Splenius capitis muscle
- Temporalis muscle
- Temporoparietalis muscle

1 Facial Muscle
- Buccinator muscle
- Corrugator supercilii muscle
- Depressor anguli oris muscle
- Depressor labii inferioris muscle
- Depressor septi nasi muscle
- Depressor supercilii muscle
- Levator anguli oris muscle
- Levator labii superioris alaeque nasi muscle
- Levator labii superioris muscle
- Mentalis muscle
- Nasalis muscle
- Occipitofrontalis muscle
- Orbicularis oris muscle
- Procerus muscle
- Risorius muscle
- Zygomaticus muscle

2 Neck Muscle, Right
- Anterior vertebral muscle
- Arytenoid muscle
- Cricothyroid muscle
- Infrahyoid muscle
- Levator scapulae muscle
- Platysma muscle
- Scalene muscle
- Splenius cervicis muscle
- Sternocleidomastoid muscle
- Suprahyoid muscle
- Thyroarytenoid muscle

3 Neck Muscle, Left
- *See 2 Neck Muscle, Right*

4 Tongue, Palate, Pharynx Muscle
- Chondroglossus muscle
- Genioglossus muscle
- Hyoglossus muscle
- Inferior longitudinal muscle
- Levator veli palatini muscle
- Palatoglossal muscle
- Palatopharyngeal muscle
- Pharyngeal constrictor muscle
- Salpingopharyngeus muscle
- Styloglossus muscle
- Stylopharyngeus muscle
- Superior longitudinal muscle
- Tensor veli palatini muscle

5 Shoulder Muscle, Right
- Deltoid muscle
- Infraspinatus muscle
- Subscapularis muscle
- Supraspinatus muscle
- Teres major muscle
- Teres minor muscle

6 Shoulder Muscle, Left
- *See 5 Shoulder Muscle, Right*

7 Upper Arm Muscle, Right
- Biceps brachii muscle
- Brachialis muscle
- Coracobrachialis muscle
- Triceps brachii muscle

8 Upper Arm Muscle, Left
- *See 7 Upper Arm Muscle, Right*

9 Lower Arm and Wrist Muscle, Right
- Anatomical snuffbox
- Anconeus muscle
- Brachioradialis muscle
- Extensor carpi radialis muscle
- Extensor carpi ulnaris muscle
- Flexor carpi radialis muscle
- Flexor carpi ulnaris muscle
- Flexor pollicis longus muscle
- Palmaris longus muscle
- Pronator quadratus muscle
- Pronator teres muscle

B Lower Arm and Wrist Muscle, Left
- *See 9 Lower Arm and Wrist Muscle, Right*

C Hand Muscle, Right
- Adductor pollicis muscle
- Hypothenar muscle
- Palmar interosseous muscle
- Thenar muscle

D Hand Muscle, Left
- *See C Hand Muscle, Right*

F Trunk Muscle, Right
- Coccygeus muscle
- Erector spinae muscle
- Interspinalis muscle
- Intertransversarius muscle
- Latissimus dorsi muscle
- Quadratus lumborum muscle
- Rhomboid major muscle
- Rhomboid minor muscle
- Serratus posterior muscle
- Transversospinalis muscle
- Trapezius muscle

G Trunk Muscle, Left
- *See F Trunk Muscle, Right*

H Thorax Muscle, Right
- Intercostal muscle
- Levatores costarum muscle
- Pectoralis major muscle
- Pectoralis minor muscle
- Serratus anterior muscle
- Subclavius muscle
- Subcostal muscle
- Transverse thoracis muscle

J Thorax Muscle, Left
- *See H Thorax Muscle, Right*

K Abdomen Muscle, Right
- External oblique muscle
- Internal oblique muscle
- Pyramidalis muscle
- Rectus abdominis muscle
- Transversus abdominis muscle

L Abdomen Muscle, Left
- *See K Abdomen Muscle, Right*

M Perineum Muscle
- Bulbospongiosus muscle
- Cremaster muscle
- Deep transverse perineal muscle
- Ischiocavernosus muscle
- Levator ani muscle
- Superficial transverse perineal muscle

N Hip Muscle, Right
- Gemellus muscle
- Gluteus maximus muscle
- Gluteus medius muscle
- Gluteus minimus muscle
- Iliacus muscle
- Iliopsoas muscle
- Obturator muscle
- Piriformis muscle
- Psoas muscle
- Quadratus femoris muscle
- Tensor fasciae latae muscle

P Hip Muscle, Left
- *See N Hip Muscle, Right*

Q Upper Leg Muscle, Right
- Adductor brevis muscle
- Adductor longus muscle
- Adductor magnus muscle
- Biceps femoris muscle
- Gracilis muscle
- Hamstring muscle
- Pectineus muscle
- Quadriceps (femoris)
- Rectus femoris muscle
- Sartorius muscle
- Semimembranosus muscle
- Semitendinosus muscle
- Vastus intermedius muscle
- Vastus lateralis muscle
- Vastus medialis muscle

R Upper Leg Muscle, Left
- *See Q Upper Leg Muscle, Right*

S Lower Leg Muscle, Right
- Extensor digitorum longus muscle
- Extensor hallucis longus muscle
- Fibularis brevis muscle
- Fibularis longus muscle
- Flexor digitorum longus muscle
- Flexor hallucis longus muscle
- Gastrocnemius muscle
- Peroneus brevis muscle
- Peroneus longus muscle
- Plantaris muscle
- Popliteus muscle
- Soleus muscle
- Tibialis anterior muscle
- Tibialis posterior muscle

T Lower Leg Muscle, Left
- *See S Lower Leg Muscle, Right*

V Foot Muscle, Right
- Abductor hallucis muscle
- Adductor hallucis muscle
- Extensor digitorum brevis muscle
- Extensor hallucis brevis muscle
- Flexor digitorum brevis muscle
- Flexor hallucis brevis muscle
- Quadratus plantae muscle

W Foot Muscle, Left
- *See V Foot Muscle, Right*

Non-OR 0KB[N,P]3Z[X,Z]

Muscles

0KC–0KC

0 Medical and Surgical
K Muscles
C Extirpation   **Definition:** Taking or cutting out solid matter from a body part
Explanation: The solid matter may be an abnormal byproduct of a biological function or a foreign body; it may be imbedded in a body part or in the lumen of a tubular body part. The solid matter may or may not have been previously broken into pieces.

Body Part — Character 4	Approach — Character 5	Device — Character 6	Qualifier — Character 7
0 Head Muscle Auricularis muscle Masseter muscle Pterygoid muscle Splenius capitis muscle Temporalis muscle Temporoparietalis muscle **1 Facial Muscle** Buccinator muscle Corrugator supercilii muscle Depressor anguli oris muscle Depressor labii inferioris muscle Depressor septi nasi muscle Depressor supercilii muscle Levator anguli oris muscle Levator labii superioris alaeque nasi muscle Levator labii superioris muscle Mentalis muscle Nasalis muscle Occipitofrontalis muscle Orbicularis oris muscle Procerus muscle Risorius muscle Zygomaticus muscle **2 Neck Muscle, Right** Anterior vertebral muscle Arytenoid muscle Cricothyroid muscle Infrahyoid muscle Levator scapulae muscle Platysma muscle Scalene muscle Splenius cervicis muscle Sternocleidomastoid muscle Suprahyoid muscle Thyroarytenoid muscle **3 Neck Muscle, Left** *See 2 Neck Muscle, Right* **4 Tongue, Palate, Pharynx Muscle** Chondroglossus muscle Genioglossus muscle Hyoglossus muscle Inferior longitudinal muscle Levator veli palatini muscle Palatoglossal muscle Palatopharyngeal muscle Pharyngeal constrictor muscle Salpingopharyngeus muscle Styloglossus muscle Stylopharyngeus muscle Superior longitudinal muscle Tensor veli palatini muscle **5 Shoulder Muscle, Right** Deltoid muscle Infraspinatus muscle Subscapularis muscle Supraspinatus muscle Teres major muscle Teres minor muscle **6 Shoulder Muscle, Left** *See 5 Shoulder Muscle, Right* **7 Upper Arm Muscle, Right** Biceps brachii muscle Brachialis muscle Coracobrachialis muscle Triceps brachii muscle **8 Upper Arm Muscle, Left** *See 7 Upper Arm Muscle, Right* **9 Lower Arm and Wrist Muscle, Right** Anatomical snuffbox Anconeus muscle Brachioradialis muscle Extensor carpi radialis muscle Extensor carpi ulnaris muscle Flexor carpi radialis muscle Flexor carpi ulnaris muscle Flexor pollicis longus muscle Palmaris longus muscle Pronator quadratus muscle Pronator teres muscle **B Lower Arm and Wrist Muscle, Left** *See 9 Lower Arm and Wrist Muscle, Right* **C Hand Muscle, Right** Adductor pollicis muscle Hypothenar muscle Palmar interosseous muscle Thenar muscle **D Hand Muscle, Left** *See C Hand Muscle, Right* **F Trunk Muscle, Right** Coccygeus muscle Erector spinae muscle Interspinalis muscle Intertransversarius muscle Latissimus dorsi muscle Quadratus lumborum muscle Rhomboid major muscle Rhomboid minor muscle Serratus posterior muscle Transversospinalis muscle Trapezius muscle **G Trunk Muscle, Left** *See F Trunk Muscle, Right* **H Thorax Muscle, Right** Intercostal muscle Levatores costarum muscle Pectoralis major muscle Pectoralis minor muscle Serratus anterior muscle Subclavius muscle Subcostal muscle Transverse thoracis muscle **J Thorax Muscle, Left** *See H Thorax Muscle, Right* **K Abdomen Muscle, Right** External oblique muscle Internal oblique muscle Pyramidalis muscle Rectus abdominis muscle Transversus abdominis muscle **L Abdomen Muscle, Left** *See K Abdomen Muscle, Right* **M Perineum Muscle** Bulbospongiosus muscle Cremaster muscle Deep transverse perineal muscle Ischiocavernosus muscle Levator ani muscle Superficial transverse perineal muscle **N Hip Muscle, Right** Gemellus muscle Gluteus maximus muscle Gluteus medius muscle Gluteus minimus muscle Iliacus muscle Iliopsoas muscle Obturator muscle Piriformis muscle Psoas muscle Quadratus femoris muscle Tensor fasciae latae muscle **P Hip Muscle, Left** *See N Hip Muscle, Right* **Q Upper Leg Muscle, Right** Adductor brevis muscle Adductor longus muscle Adductor magnus muscle Biceps femoris muscle Gracilis muscle Hamstring muscle Pectineus muscle Quadriceps (femoris) Rectus femoris muscle Sartorius muscle Semimembranosus muscle Semitendinosus muscle Vastus intermedius muscle Vastus lateralis muscle Vastus medialis muscle **R Upper Leg Muscle, Left** *See Q Upper Leg Muscle, Right* **S Lower Leg Muscle, Right** Extensor digitorum longus muscle Extensor hallucis longus muscle Fibularis brevis muscle Fibularis longus muscle Flexor digitorum longus muscle Flexor hallucis longus muscle Gastrocnemius muscle Peroneus brevis muscle Peroneus longus muscle Plantaris muscle Popliteus muscle Soleus muscle Tibialis anterior muscle Tibialis posterior muscle **T Lower Leg Muscle, Left** *See S Lower Leg Muscle, Right* **V Foot Muscle, Right** Abductor hallucis muscle Adductor hallucis muscle Extensor digitorum brevis muscle Extensor hallucis brevis muscle Flexor digitorum brevis muscle Flexor hallucis brevis muscle Quadratus plantae muscle **W Foot Muscle, Left** *See V Foot Muscle, Right*	**0** Open **3** Percutaneous **4** Percutaneous Endoscopic	**Z** No Device	**Z** No Qualifier

Non-OR Procedure DRG Non-OR Procedure Valid OR Procedure HAC Associated Procedure Combination Only New/Revised April New/Revised October

0 Medical and Surgical
K Muscles
D Extraction Definition: Pulling or stripping out or off all or a portion of a body part by the use of force
Explanation: The qualifier DIAGNOSTIC is used to identify extraction procedures that are biopsies

Body Part Character 4	Approach Character 5	Device Character 6	Qualifier Character 7
0 Head Muscle Auricularis muscle Masseter muscle Pterygoid muscle Splenius capitis muscle Temporalis muscle Temporoparietalis muscle **1 Facial Muscle** Buccinator muscle Corrugator supercilii muscle Depressor anguli oris muscle Depressor labii inferioris muscle Depressor septi nasi muscle Depressor supercilii muscle Levator anguli oris muscle Levator labii superioris alaeque nasi muscle Levator labii superioris muscle Mentalis muscle Nasalis muscle Occipitofrontalis muscle Orbicularis oris muscle Procerus muscle Risorius muscle Zygomaticus muscle **2 Neck Muscle, Right** Anterior vertebral muscle Arytenoid muscle Cricothyroid muscle Infrahyoid muscle Levator scapulae muscle Platysma muscle Scalene muscle Splenius cervicis muscle Sternocleidomastoid muscle Suprahyoid muscle Thyroarytenoid muscle **3 Neck Muscle, Left** See 2 Neck Muscle, Right **4 Tongue, Palate, Pharynx Muscle** Chondroglossus muscle Genioglossus muscle Hyoglossus muscle Inferior longitudinal muscle Levator veli palatini muscle Palatoglossal muscle Palatopharyngeal muscle Pharyngeal constrictor muscle Salpingopharyngeus muscle Styloglossus muscle Stylopharyngeus muscle Superior longitudinal muscle Tensor veli palatini muscle **5 Shoulder Muscle, Right** Deltoid muscle Infraspinatus muscle Subscapularis muscle Supraspinatus muscle Teres major muscle Teres minor muscle **6 Shoulder Muscle, Left** See 5 Shoulder Muscle, Right	**7 Upper Arm Muscle, Right** Biceps brachii muscle Brachialis muscle Coracobrachialis muscle Triceps brachii muscle **8 Upper Arm Muscle, Left** See 7 Upper Arm Muscle, Right **9 Lower Arm and Wrist Muscle, Right** Anatomical snuffbox Anconeus muscle Brachioradialis muscle Extensor carpi radialis muscle Extensor carpi ulnaris muscle Flexor carpi radialis muscle Flexor carpi ulnaris muscle Flexor pollicis longus muscle Palmaris longus muscle Pronator quadratus muscle Pronator teres muscle **B Lower Arm and Wrist Muscle, Left** See 9 Lower Arm and Wrist Muscle, Right **C Hand Muscle, Right** Adductor pollicis muscle Hypothenar muscle Palmar interosseous muscle Thenar muscle **D Hand Muscle, Left** See C Hand Muscle, Right **F Trunk Muscle, Right** Coccygeus muscle Erector spinae muscle Interspinalis muscle Intertransversarius muscle Latissimus dorsi muscle Quadratus lumborum muscle Rhomboid major muscle Rhomboid minor muscle Serratus posterior muscle Transversospinalis muscle Trapezius muscle **G Trunk Muscle, Left** See F Trunk Muscle, Right **H Thorax Muscle, Right** Intercostal muscle Levatores costarum muscle Pectoralis major muscle Pectoralis minor muscle Serratus anterior muscle Subclavius muscle Subcostal muscle Transverse thoracis muscle **J Thorax Muscle, Left** See H Thorax Muscle, Right **K Abdomen Muscle, Right** External oblique muscle Internal oblique muscle Pyramidalis muscle Rectus abdominis muscle Transversus abdominis muscle **L Abdomen Muscle, Left** See K Abdomen Muscle, Right	**M Perineum Muscle** Bulbospongiosus muscle Cremaster muscle Deep transverse perineal muscle Ischiocavernosus muscle Levator ani muscle Superficial transverse perineal muscle **N Hip Muscle, Right** Gemellus muscle Gluteus maximus muscle Gluteus medius muscle Gluteus minimus muscle Iliacus muscle Iliopsoas muscle Obturator muscle Piriformis muscle Psoas muscle Quadratus femoris muscle Tensor fasciae latae muscle **P Hip Muscle, Left** See N Hip Muscle, Right **Q Upper Leg Muscle, Right** Adductor brevis muscle Adductor longus muscle Adductor magnus muscle Biceps femoris muscle Gracilis muscle Hamstring muscle Pectineus muscle Quadriceps (femoris) Rectus femoris muscle Sartorius muscle Semimembranosus muscle Semitendinosus muscle Vastus intermedius muscle Vastus lateralis muscle Vastus medialis muscle **R Upper Leg Muscle, Left** See Q Upper Leg Muscle, Right **S Lower Leg Muscle, Right** Extensor digitorum longus muscle Extensor hallucis longus muscle Fibularis brevis muscle Fibularis longus muscle Flexor digitorum longus muscle Flexor hallucis longus muscle Gastrocnemius muscle Peroneus brevis muscle Peroneus longus muscle Plantaris muscle Popliteus muscle Soleus muscle Tibialis anterior muscle Tibialis posterior muscle **T Lower Leg Muscle, Left** See S Lower Leg Muscle, Right **V Foot Muscle, Right** Abductor hallucis muscle Adductor hallucis muscle Extensor digitorum brevis muscle Extensor hallucis brevis muscle Flexor digitorum brevis muscle Flexor hallucis brevis muscle Quadratus plantae muscle **W Foot Muscle, Left** See V Foot Muscle, Right	**0** Open	**Z** No Device	**Z** No Qualifier

0 Medical and Surgical
K Muscles
H Insertion — Definition: Putting in a nonbiological appliance that monitors, assists, performs, or prevents a physiological function but does not physically take the place of a body part
Explanation: None

Body Part Character 4	Approach Character 5	Device Character 6	Qualifier Character 7
X Upper Muscle Y Lower Muscle	0 Open 3 Percutaneous 4 Percutaneous Endoscopic	M Stimulator Lead Y Other Device	Z No Qualifier

Non-OR 0KH[X,Y][3,4]YZ

0 Medical and Surgical
K Muscles
J Inspection — Definition: Visually and/or manually exploring a body part
Explanation: Visual exploration may be performed with or without optical instrumentation. Manual exploration may be performed directly or through intervening body layers.

Body Part Character 4	Approach Character 5	Device Character 6	Qualifier Character 7
X Upper Muscle Y Lower Muscle	0 Open 3 Percutaneous 4 Percutaneous Endoscopic X External	Z No Device	Z No Qualifier

Non-OR 0KJ[X,Y][3,X]ZZ

Muscles

0 Medical and Surgical
K Muscles
M Reattachment Definition: Putting back in or on all or a portion of a separated body part to its normal location or other suitable location
Explanation: Vascular circulation and nervous pathways may or may not be reestablished

Body Part Character 4			Approach Character 5	Device Character 6	Qualifier Character 7
0 Head Muscle Auricularis muscle Masseter muscle Pterygoid muscle Splenius capitis muscle Temporalis muscle Temporoparietalis muscle **1** Facial Muscle Buccinator muscle Corrugator supercilii muscle Depressor anguli oris muscle Depressor labii inferioris muscle Depressor septi nasi muscle Depressor supercilii muscle Levator anguli oris muscle Levator labii superioris alaeque nasi muscle Levator labii superioris muscle Mentalis muscle Nasalis muscle Occipitofrontalis muscle Orbicularis oris muscle Procerus muscle Risorius muscle Zygomaticus muscle **2** Neck Muscle, Right Anterior vertebral muscle Arytenoid muscle Cricothyroid muscle Infrahyoid muscle Levator scapulae muscle Platysma muscle Scalene muscle Splenius cervicis muscle Sternocleidomastoid muscle Suprahyoid muscle Thyroarytenoid muscle **3** Neck Muscle, Left *See* 2 Neck Muscle, Right **4** Tongue, Palate, Pharynx Muscle Chondroglossus muscle Genioglossus muscle Hyoglossus muscle Inferior longitudinal muscle Levator veli palatini muscle Palatoglossal muscle Palatopharyngeal muscle Pharyngeal constrictor muscle Salpingopharyngeus muscle Styloglossus muscle Stylopharyngeus muscle Superior longitudinal muscle Tensor veli palatini muscle **5** Shoulder Muscle, Right Deltoid muscle Infraspinatus muscle Subscapularis muscle Supraspinatus muscle Teres major muscle Teres minor muscle **6** Shoulder Muscle, Left *See* 5 Shoulder Muscle, Right	**7** Upper Arm Muscle, Right Biceps brachii muscle Brachialis muscle Coracobrachialis muscle Triceps brachii muscle **8** Upper Arm Muscle, Left *See* 7 Upper Arm Muscle, Right **9** Lower Arm and Wrist Muscle, Right Anatomical snuffbox Anconeus muscle Brachioradialis muscle Extensor carpi radialis muscle Extensor carpi ulnaris muscle Flexor carpi radialis muscle Flexor carpi ulnaris muscle Flexor pollicis longus muscle Palmaris longus muscle Pronator quadratus muscle Pronator teres muscle **B** Lower Arm and Wrist Muscle, Left *See* 9 Lower Arm and Wrist Muscle, Right **C** Hand Muscle, Right Adductor pollicis muscle Hypothenar muscle Palmar interosseous muscle Thenar muscle **D** Hand Muscle, Left *See* C Hand Muscle, Right **F** Trunk Muscle, Right Coccygeus muscle Erector spinae muscle Interspinalis muscle Intertransversarius muscle Latissimus dorsi muscle Quadratus lumborum muscle Rhomboid major muscle Rhomboid minor muscle Serratus posterior muscle Transversospinalis muscle Trapezius muscle **G** Trunk Muscle, Left *See* F Trunk Muscle, Right **H** Thorax Muscle, Right Intercostal muscle Levatores costarum muscle Pectoralis major muscle Pectoralis minor muscle Serratus anterior muscle Subclavius muscle Subcostal muscle Transverse thoracis muscle **J** Thorax Muscle, Left *See* H Thorax Muscle, Right **K** Abdomen Muscle, Right External oblique muscle Internal oblique muscle Pyramidalis muscle Rectus abdominis muscle Transversus abdominis muscle **L** Abdomen Muscle, Left *See* K Abdomen Muscle, Right	**M** Perineum Muscle Bulbospongiosus muscle Cremaster muscle Deep transverse perineal muscle Ischiocavernosus muscle Levator ani muscle Superficial transverse perineal muscle **N** Hip Muscle, Right Gemellus muscle Gluteus maximus muscle Gluteus medius muscle Gluteus minimus muscle Iliacus muscle Iliopsoas muscle Obturator muscle Piriformis muscle Psoas muscle Quadratus femoris muscle Tensor fasciae latae muscle **P** Hip Muscle, Left *See* N Hip Muscle, Right **Q** Upper Leg Muscle, Right Adductor brevis muscle Adductor longus muscle Adductor magnus muscle Biceps femoris muscle Gracilis muscle Hamstring muscle Pectineus muscle Quadriceps (femoris) Rectus femoris muscle Sartorius muscle Semimembranosus muscle Semitendinosus muscle Vastus intermedius muscle Vastus lateralis muscle Vastus medialis muscle **R** Upper Leg Muscle, Left *See* Q Upper Leg Muscle, Right **S** Lower Leg Muscle, Right Extensor digitorum longus muscle Extensor hallucis longus muscle Fibularis brevis muscle Fibularis longus muscle Flexor digitorum longus muscle Flexor hallucis longus muscle Gastrocnemius muscle Peroneus brevis muscle Peroneus longus muscle Plantaris muscle Popliteus muscle Soleus muscle Tibialis anterior muscle Tibialis posterior muscle **T** Lower Leg Muscle, Left *See* S Lower Leg Muscle, Right **V** Foot Muscle, Right Abductor hallucis muscle Adductor hallucis muscle Extensor digitorum brevis muscle Extensor hallucis brevis muscle Flexor digitorum brevis muscle Flexor hallucis brevis muscle Quadratus plantae muscle **W** Foot Muscle, Left *See* V Foot Muscle, Right	**0** Open **4** Percutaneous Endoscopic	**Z** No Device	**Z** No Qualifier

ØKN–ØKN Muscles

Ø Medical and Surgical
K Muscles
N Release

Definition: Freeing a body part from an abnormal physical constraint by cutting or by the use of force
Explanation: Some of the restraining tissue may be taken out but none of the body part is taken out

Body Part — Character 4	Approach — Character 5	Device — Character 6	Qualifier — Character 7
Ø Head Muscle Auricularis muscle Masseter muscle Pterygoid muscle Splenius capitis muscle Temporalis muscle Temporoparietalis muscle **1 Facial Muscle** Buccinator muscle Corrugator supercilii muscle Depressor anguli oris muscle Depressor labii inferioris muscle Depressor septi nasi muscle Depressor supercilii muscle Levator anguli oris muscle Levator labii superioris alaeque nasi muscle Levator labii superioris muscle Mentalis muscle Nasalis muscle Occipitofrontalis muscle Orbicularis oris muscle Procerus muscle Risorius muscle Zygomaticus muscle **2 Neck Muscle, Right** Anterior vertebral muscle Arytenoid muscle Cricothyroid muscle Infrahyoid muscle Levator scapulae muscle Platysma muscle Scalene muscle Splenius cervicis muscle Sternocleidomastoid muscle Suprahyoid muscle Thyroarytenoid muscle **3 Neck Muscle, Left** *See 2 Neck Muscle, Right* **4 Tongue, Palate, Pharynx Muscle** Chondroglossus muscle Genioglossus muscle Hyoglossus muscle Inferior longitudinal muscle Levator veli palatini muscle Palatoglossal muscle Palatopharyngeal muscle Pharyngeal constrictor muscle Salpingopharyngeus muscle Styloglossus muscle Stylopharyngeus muscle Superior longitudinal muscle Tensor veli palatini muscle **5 Shoulder Muscle, Right** Deltoid muscle Infraspinatus muscle Subscapularis muscle Supraspinatus muscle Teres major muscle Teres minor muscle **6 Shoulder Muscle, Left** *See 5 Shoulder Muscle, Right* **7 Upper Arm Muscle, Right** Biceps brachii muscle Brachialis muscle Coracobrachialis muscle Triceps brachii muscle **8 Upper Arm Muscle, Left** *See 7 Upper Arm Muscle, Right* **9 Lower Arm and Wrist Muscle, Right** Anatomical snuffbox Anconeus muscle Brachioradialis muscle Extensor carpi radialis muscle Extensor carpi ulnaris muscle Flexor carpi radialis muscle Flexor carpi ulnaris muscle Flexor pollicis longus muscle Palmaris longus muscle Pronator quadratus muscle Pronator teres muscle **B Lower Arm and Wrist Muscle, Left** *See 9 Lower Arm and Wrist Muscle, Right* **C Hand Muscle, Right** Adductor pollicis muscle Hypothenar muscle Palmar interosseous muscle Thenar muscle **D Hand Muscle, Left** *See C Hand Muscle, Right* **F Trunk Muscle, Right** Coccygeus muscle Erector spinae muscle Interspinalis muscle Intertransversarius muscle Latissimus dorsi muscle Quadratus lumborum muscle Rhomboid major muscle Rhomboid minor muscle Serratus posterior muscle Transversospinalis muscle Trapezius muscle **G Trunk Muscle, Left** *See F Trunk Muscle, Right* **H Thorax Muscle, Right** Intercostal muscle Levatores costarum muscle Pectoralis major muscle Pectoralis minor muscle Serratus anterior muscle Subclavius muscle Subcostal muscle Transverse thoracis muscle **J Thorax Muscle, Left** *See H Thorax Muscle, Right* **K Abdomen Muscle, Right** External oblique muscle Internal oblique muscle Pyramidalis muscle Rectus abdominis muscle Transversus abdominis muscle **L Abdomen Muscle, Left** *See K Abdomen Muscle, Right* **M Perineum Muscle** Bulbospongiosus muscle Cremaster muscle Deep transverse perineal muscle Ischiocavernosus muscle Levator ani muscle Superficial transverse perineal muscle **N Hip Muscle, Right** Gemellus muscle Gluteus maximus muscle Gluteus medius muscle Gluteus minimus muscle Iliacus muscle Iliopsoas muscle Obturator muscle Piriformis muscle Psoas muscle Quadratus femoris muscle Tensor fasciae latae muscle **P Hip Muscle, Left** *See N Hip Muscle, Right* **Q Upper Leg Muscle, Right** Adductor brevis muscle Adductor longus muscle Adductor magnus muscle Biceps femoris muscle Gracilis muscle Hamstring muscle Pectineus muscle Quadriceps (femoris) Rectus femoris muscle Sartorius muscle Semimembranosus muscle Semitendinosus muscle Vastus intermedius muscle Vastus lateralis muscle Vastus medialis muscle **R Upper Leg Muscle, Left** *See Q Upper Leg Muscle, Right* **S Lower Leg Muscle, Right** Extensor digitorum longus muscle Extensor hallucis longus muscle Fibularis brevis muscle Fibularis longus muscle Flexor digitorum longus muscle Flexor hallucis longus muscle Gastrocnemius muscle Peroneus brevis muscle Peroneus longus muscle Plantaris muscle Popliteus muscle Soleus muscle Tibialis anterior muscle Tibialis posterior muscle **T Lower Leg Muscle, Left** *See S Lower Leg Muscle, Right* **V Foot Muscle, Right** Abductor hallucis muscle Adductor hallucis muscle Extensor digitorum brevis muscle Extensor hallucis brevis muscle Flexor digitorum brevis muscle Flexor hallucis brevis muscle Quadratus plantae muscle **W Foot Muscle, Left** *See V Foot Muscle, Right*	**Ø** Open **3** Percutaneous **4** Percutaneous Endoscopic **X** External	**Z** No Device	**Z** No Qualifier

Non-OR ØKN[Ø,1,2,3,4,5,6,7,8,9,B,C,D,F,G,H,J,K,L,M,N,P,Q,R,S,T,V,W]XZZ

0 Medical and Surgical
K Muscles
P Removal

Definition: Taking out or off a device from a body part

Explanation: If a device is taken out and a similar device put in without cutting or puncturing the skin or mucous membrane, the procedure is coded to the root operation CHANGE. Otherwise, the procedure for taking out a device is coded to the root operation REMOVAL.

Body Part Character 4	Approach Character 5	Device Character 6	Qualifier Character 7
X Upper Muscle Y Lower Muscle	0 Open 3 Percutaneous 4 Percutaneous Endoscopic	0 Drainage Device 7 Autologous Tissue Substitute J Synthetic Substitute K Nonautologous Tissue Substitute M Stimulator Lead Y Other Device	Z No Qualifier
X Upper Muscle Y Lower Muscle	X External	0 Drainage Device M Stimulator Lead	Z No Qualifier

Non-OR 0KP[X,Y][3,4]YZ
Non-OR 0KP[X,Y]X[0,M]Z

0 Medical and Surgical
K Muscles
Q Repair

Definition: Restoring, to the extent possible, a body part to its normal anatomic structure and function
Explanation: Used only when the method to accomplish the repair is not one of the other root operations

Body Part Character 4	Approach Character 5	Device Character 6	Qualifier Character 7

0 **Head Muscle**
  Auricularis muscle
  Masseter muscle
  Pterygoid muscle
  Splenius capitis muscle
  Temporalis muscle
  Temporoparietalis muscle
1 **Facial Muscle**
  Buccinator muscle
  Corrugator supercilii muscle
  Depressor anguli oris muscle
  Depressor labii inferioris muscle
  Depressor septi nasi muscle
  Depressor supercilii muscle
  Levator anguli oris muscle
  Levator labii superioris alaeque nasi muscle
  Levator labii superioris muscle
  Mentalis muscle
  Nasalis muscle
  Occipitofrontalis muscle
  Orbicularis oris muscle
  Procerus muscle
  Risorius muscle
  Zygomaticus muscle
2 **Neck Muscle, Right**
  Anterior vertebral muscle
  Arytenoid muscle
  Cricothyroid muscle
  Infrahyoid muscle
  Levator scapulae muscle
  Platysma muscle
  Scalene muscle
  Splenius cervicis muscle
  Sternocleidomastoid muscle
  Suprahyoid muscle
  Thyroarytenoid muscle
3 **Neck Muscle, Left**
  See 2 Neck Muscle, Right
4 **Tongue, Palate, Pharynx Muscle**
  Chondroglossus muscle
  Genioglossus muscle
  Hyoglossus muscle
  Inferior longitudinal muscle
  Levator veli palatini muscle
  Palatoglossal muscle
  Palatopharyngeal muscle
  Pharyngeal constrictor muscle
  Salpingopharyngeus muscle
  Styloglossus muscle
  Stylopharyngeus muscle
  Superior longitudinal muscle
  Tensor veli palatini muscle
5 **Shoulder Muscle, Right**
  Deltoid muscle
  Infraspinatus muscle
  Subscapularis muscle
  Supraspinatus muscle
  Teres major muscle
  Teres minor muscle
6 **Shoulder Muscle, Left**
  See 5 Shoulder Muscle, Right
	7 **Upper Arm Muscle, Right**
	  Biceps brachii muscle
	  Brachialis muscle
	  Coracobrachialis muscle
	  Triceps brachii muscle
	8 **Upper Arm Muscle, Left**
	  See 7 Upper Arm Muscle, Right
	9 **Lower Arm and Wrist Muscle, Right**
	  Anatomical snuffbox
	  Anconeus muscle
	  Brachioradialis muscle
	  Extensor carpi radialis muscle
	  Extensor carpi ulnaris muscle
	  Flexor carpi radialis muscle
	  Flexor carpi ulnaris muscle
	  Flexor pollicis longus muscle
	  Palmaris longus muscle
	  Pronator quadratus muscle
	  Pronator teres muscle
	B **Lower Arm and Wrist Muscle, Left**
	  See 9 Lower Arm and Wrist Muscle, Right
	C **Hand Muscle, Right**
	  Adductor pollicis muscle
	  Hypothenar muscle
	  Palmar interosseous muscle
	  Thenar muscle
	D **Hand Muscle, Left**
	  See C Hand Muscle, Right
	F **Trunk Muscle, Right**
	  Coccygeus muscle
	  Erector spinae muscle
	  Interspinalis muscle
	  Intertransversarius muscle
	  Latissimus dorsi muscle
	  Quadratus lumborum muscle
	  Rhomboid major muscle
	  Rhomboid minor muscle
	  Serratus posterior muscle
	  Transversospinalis muscle
	  Trapezius muscle
	G **Trunk Muscle, Left**
	  See F Trunk Muscle, Right
	H **Thorax Muscle, Right**
	  Intercostal muscle
	  Levatores costarum muscle
	  Pectoralis major muscle
	  Pectoralis minor muscle
	  Serratus anterior muscle
	  Subclavius muscle
	  Subcostal muscle
	  Transverse thoracis muscle
	J **Thorax Muscle, Left**
	  See H Thorax Muscle, Right
	K **Abdomen Muscle, Right**
	  External oblique muscle
	  Internal oblique muscle
	  Pyramidalis muscle
	  Rectus abdominis muscle
	  Transversus abdominis muscle
	L **Abdomen Muscle, Left**
	  See K Abdomen Muscle, Right
		M **Perineum Muscle**
		  Bulbospongiosus muscle
		  Cremaster muscle
		  Deep transverse perineal muscle
		  Ischiocavernosus muscle
		  Levator ani muscle
		  Superficial transverse perineal muscle
		N **Hip Muscle, Right**
		  Gemellus muscle
		  Gluteus maximus muscle
		  Gluteus medius muscle
		  Gluteus minimus muscle
		  Iliacus muscle
		  Iliopsoas muscle
		  Obturator muscle
		  Piriformis muscle
		  Psoas muscle
		  Quadratus femoris muscle
		  Tensor fasciae latae muscle
		P **Hip Muscle, Left**
		  See N Hip Muscle, Right
		Q **Upper Leg Muscle, Right**
		  Adductor brevis muscle
		  Adductor longus muscle
		  Adductor magnus muscle
		  Biceps femoris muscle
		  Gracilis muscle
		  Hamstring muscle
		  Pectineus muscle
		  Quadriceps (femoris)
		  Rectus femoris muscle
		  Sartorius muscle
		  Semimembranosus muscle
		  Semitendinosus muscle
		  Vastus intermedius muscle
		  Vastus lateralis muscle
		  Vastus medialis muscle
		R **Upper Leg Muscle, Left**
		  See Q Upper Leg Muscle, Right
		S **Lower Leg Muscle, Right**
		  Extensor digitorum longus muscle
		  Extensor hallucis longus muscle
		  Fibularis brevis muscle
		  Fibularis longus muscle
		  Flexor digitorum longus muscle
		  Flexor hallucis longus muscle
		  Gastrocnemius muscle
		  Peroneus brevis muscle
		  Peroneus longus muscle
		  Plantaris muscle
		  Popliteus muscle
		  Soleus muscle
		  Tibialis anterior muscle
		  Tibialis posterior muscle
		T **Lower Leg Muscle, Left**
		  See S Lower Leg Muscle, Right
		V **Foot Muscle, Right**
		  Abductor hallucis muscle
		  Adductor hallucis muscle
		  Extensor digitorum brevis muscle
		  Extensor hallucis brevis muscle
		  Flexor digitorum brevis muscle
		  Flexor hallucis brevis muscle
		  Quadratus plantae muscle
		W **Foot Muscle, Left**
		  See V Foot Muscle, Right
			0 Open
			3 Percutaneous
			4 Percutaneous Endoscopic
				Z No Device	Z No Qualifier

ICD-10-PCS 2025 — Muscles — ØKR–ØKR

- **Ø** Medical and Surgical
- **K** Muscles
- **R** Replacement

Definition: Putting in or on biological or synthetic material that physically takes the place and/or function of all or a portion of a body part

Explanation: The body part may have been taken out or replaced, or may be taken out, physically eradicated, or rendered nonfunctional during the REPLACEMENT procedure. A REMOVAL procedure is coded for taking out the device used in a previous replacement procedure.

Body Part – Character 4	Approach – Character 5	Device – Character 6	Qualifier – Character 7
Ø Head Muscle Auricularis muscle Masseter muscle Pterygoid muscle Splenius capitis muscle Temporalis muscle Temporoparietalis muscle **1 Facial Muscle** Buccinator muscle Corrugator supercilii muscle Depressor anguli oris muscle Depressor labii inferioris muscle Depressor septi nasi muscle Depressor supercilii muscle Levator anguli oris muscle Levator labii superioris alaeque nasi muscle Levator labii superioris muscle Mentalis muscle Nasalis muscle Occipitofrontalis muscle Orbicularis oris muscle Procerus muscle Risorius muscle Zygomaticus muscle **2 Neck Muscle, Right** Anterior vertebral muscle Arytenoid muscle Cricothyroid muscle Infrahyoid muscle Levator scapulae muscle Platysma muscle Scalene muscle Splenius cervicis muscle Sternocleidomastoid muscle Suprahyoid muscle Thyroarytenoid muscle **3 Neck Muscle, Left** See 2 Neck Muscle, Right **4 Tongue, Palate, Pharynx Muscle** Chondroglossus muscle Genioglossus muscle Hyoglossus muscle Inferior longitudinal muscle Levator veli palatini muscle Palatoglossal muscle Palatopharyngeal muscle Pharyngeal constrictor muscle Salpingopharyngeus muscle Styloglossus muscle Stylopharyngeus muscle Superior longitudinal muscle Tensor veli palatini muscle **5 Shoulder Muscle, Right** Deltoid muscle Infraspinatus muscle Subscapularis muscle Supraspinatus muscle Teres major muscle Teres minor muscle **6 Shoulder Muscle, Left** See 5 Shoulder Muscle, Right **7 Upper Arm Muscle, Right** Biceps brachii muscle Brachialis muscle Coracobrachialis muscle Triceps brachii muscle **8 Upper Arm Muscle, Left** See 7 Upper Arm Muscle, Right **9 Lower Arm and Wrist Muscle, Right** Anatomical snuffbox Anconeus muscle Brachioradialis muscle Extensor carpi radialis muscle Extensor carpi ulnaris muscle Flexor carpi radialis muscle Flexor carpi ulnaris muscle Flexor pollicis longus muscle Palmaris longus muscle Pronator quadratus muscle Pronator teres muscle **B Lower Arm and Wrist Muscle, Left** See 9 Lower Arm and Wrist Muscle, Right **C Hand Muscle, Right** Adductor pollicis muscle Hypothenar muscle Palmar interosseous muscle Thenar muscle **D Hand Muscle, Left** See C Hand Muscle, Right **F Trunk Muscle, Right** Coccygeus muscle Erector spinae muscle Interspinalis muscle Intertransversarius muscle Latissimus dorsi muscle Quadratus lumborum muscle Rhomboid major muscle Rhomboid minor muscle Serratus posterior muscle Transversospinalis muscle Trapezius muscle **G Trunk Muscle, Left** See F Trunk Muscle, Right **H Thorax Muscle, Right** Intercostal muscle Levatores costarum muscle Pectoralis major muscle Pectoralis minor muscle Serratus anterior muscle Subclavius muscle Subcostal muscle Transverse thoracis muscle **J Thorax Muscle, Left** See H Thorax Muscle, Right **K Abdomen Muscle, Right** External oblique muscle Internal oblique muscle Pyramidalis muscle Rectus abdominis muscle Transversus abdominis muscle **L Abdomen Muscle, Left** See K Abdomen Muscle, Right **M Perineum Muscle** Bulbospongiosus muscle Cremaster muscle Deep transverse perineal muscle Ischiocavernosus muscle Levator ani muscle Superficial transverse perineal muscle **N Hip Muscle, Right** Gemellus muscle Gluteus maximus muscle Gluteus medius muscle Gluteus minimus muscle Iliacus muscle Iliopsoas muscle Obturator muscle Piriformis muscle Psoas muscle Quadratus femoris muscle Tensor fasciae latae muscle **P Hip Muscle, Left** See N Hip Muscle, Right **Q Upper Leg Muscle, Right** Adductor brevis muscle Adductor longus muscle Adductor magnus muscle Biceps femoris muscle Gracilis muscle Hamstring muscle Pectineus muscle Quadriceps (femoris) Rectus femoris muscle Sartorius muscle Semimembranosus muscle Semitendinosus muscle Vastus intermedius muscle Vastus lateralis muscle Vastus medialis muscle **R Upper Leg Muscle, Left** See Q Upper Leg Muscle, Right **S Lower Leg Muscle, Right** Extensor digitorum longus muscle Extensor hallucis longus muscle Fibularis brevis muscle Fibularis longus muscle Flexor digitorum longus muscle Flexor hallucis longus muscle Gastrocnemius muscle Peroneus brevis muscle Peroneus longus muscle Plantaris muscle Popliteus muscle Soleus muscle Tibialis anterior muscle Tibialis posterior muscle **T Lower Leg Muscle, Left** See S Lower Leg Muscle, Right **V Foot Muscle, Right** Abductor hallucis muscle Adductor hallucis muscle Extensor digitorum brevis muscle Extensor hallucis brevis muscle Flexor digitorum brevis muscle Flexor hallucis brevis muscle Quadratus plantae muscle **W Foot Muscle, Left** See V Foot Muscle, Right	**Ø** Open **4** Percutaneous Endoscopic	**7** Autologous Tissue Substitute **J** Synthetic Substitute **K** Nonautologous Tissue Substitute	**Z** No Qualifier

---

NC Noncovered Procedure **LC** Limited Coverage **QA** Questionable OB Admit **NT** New Tech Add-on ✚ Combination Member ♂ Male ♀ Female

Muscles

0KS–0KS Muscles ICD-10-PCS 2025

0 Medical and Surgical
K Muscles
S Reposition

Definition: Moving to its normal location, or other suitable location, all or a portion of a body part
Explanation: The body part is moved to a new location from an abnormal location, or from a normal location where it is not functioning correctly. The body part may or may not be cut out or off to be moved to the new location.

Body Part Character 4	Approach Character 5	Device Character 6	Qualifier Character 7
0 Head Muscle Auricularis muscle; Masseter muscle; Pterygoid muscle; Splenius capitis muscle; Temporalis muscle; Temporoparietalis muscle **1 Facial Muscle** Buccinator muscle; Corrugator supercilii muscle; Depressor anguli oris muscle; Depressor labii inferioris muscle; Depressor septi nasi muscle; Depressor supercilii muscle; Levator anguli oris muscle; Levator labii superioris alaeque nasi muscle; Levator labii superioris muscle; Mentalis muscle; Nasalis muscle; Occipitofrontalis muscle; Orbicularis oris muscle; Procerus muscle; Risorius muscle; Zygomaticus muscle **2 Neck Muscle, Right** Anterior vertebral muscle; Arytenoid muscle; Cricothyroid muscle; Infrahyoid muscle; Levator scapulae muscle; Platysma muscle; Scalene muscle; Splenius cervicis muscle; Sternocleidomastoid muscle; Suprahyoid muscle; Thyroarytenoid muscle **3 Neck Muscle, Left** See 2 Neck Muscle, Right **4 Tongue, Palate, Pharynx Muscle** Chondroglossus muscle; Genioglossus muscle; Hyoglossus muscle; Inferior longitudinal muscle; Levator veli palatini muscle; Palatoglossal muscle; Palatopharyngeal muscle; Pharyngeal constrictor muscle; Salpingopharyngeus muscle; Styloglossus muscle; Stylopharyngeus muscle; Superior longitudinal muscle; Tensor veli palatini muscle **5 Shoulder Muscle, Right** Deltoid muscle; Infraspinatus muscle; Subscapularis muscle; Supraspinatus muscle; Teres major muscle; Teres minor muscle **6 Shoulder Muscle, Left** See 5 Shoulder Muscle, Right **7 Upper Arm Muscle, Right** Biceps brachii muscle; Brachialis muscle; Coracobrachialis muscle; Triceps brachii muscle **8 Upper Arm Muscle, Left** See 7 Upper Arm Muscle, Right **9 Lower Arm and Wrist Muscle, Right** Anatomical snuffbox; Anconeus muscle; Brachioradialis muscle; Extensor carpi radialis muscle; Extensor carpi ulnaris muscle; Flexor carpi radialis muscle; Flexor carpi ulnaris muscle; Flexor pollicis longus muscle; Palmaris longus muscle; Pronator quadratus muscle; Pronator teres muscle **B Lower Arm and Wrist Muscle, Left** See 9 Lower Arm and Wrist Muscle, Right **C Hand Muscle, Right** Adductor pollicis muscle; Hypothenar muscle; Palmar interosseous muscle; Thenar muscle **D Hand Muscle, Left** See C Hand Muscle, Right **F Trunk Muscle, Right** Coccygeus muscle; Erector spinae muscle; Interspinalis muscle; Intertransversarius muscle; Latissimus dorsi muscle; Quadratus lumborum muscle; Rhomboid major muscle; Rhomboid minor muscle; Serratus posterior muscle; Transversospinalis muscle; Trapezius muscle **G Trunk Muscle, Left** See F Trunk Muscle, Right **H Thorax Muscle, Right** Intercostal muscle; Levatores costarum muscle; Pectoralis major muscle; Pectoralis minor muscle; Serratus anterior muscle; Subclavius muscle; Subcostal muscle; Transverse thoracis muscle **J Thorax Muscle, Left** See H Thorax Muscle, Right **K Abdomen Muscle, Right** External oblique muscle; Internal oblique muscle; Pyramidalis muscle; Rectus abdominis muscle; Transversus abdominis muscle **L Abdomen Muscle, Left** See K Abdomen Muscle, Right **M Perineum Muscle** Bulbospongiosus muscle; Cremaster muscle; Deep transverse perineal muscle; Ischiocavernosus muscle; Levator ani muscle; Superficial transverse perineal muscle **N Hip Muscle, Right** Gemellus muscle; Gluteus maximus muscle; Gluteus medius muscle; Gluteus minimus muscle; Iliacus muscle; Iliopsoas muscle; Obturator muscle; Piriformis muscle; Psoas muscle; Quadratus femoris muscle; Tensor fasciae latae muscle **P Hip Muscle, Left** See N Hip Muscle, Right **Q Upper Leg Muscle, Right** Adductor brevis muscle; Adductor longus muscle; Adductor magnus muscle; Biceps femoris muscle; Gracilis muscle; Hamstring muscle; Pectineus muscle; Quadriceps (femoris); Rectus femoris muscle; Sartorius muscle; Semimembranosus muscle; Semitendinosus muscle; Vastus intermedius muscle; Vastus lateralis muscle; Vastus medialis muscle **R Upper Leg Muscle, Left** See Q Upper Leg Muscle, Right **S Lower Leg Muscle, Right** Extensor digitorum longus muscle; Extensor hallucis longus muscle; Fibularis brevis muscle; Fibularis longus muscle; Flexor digitorum longus muscle; Flexor hallucis longus muscle; Gastrocnemius muscle; Peroneus brevis muscle; Peroneus longus muscle; Plantaris muscle; Popliteus muscle; Soleus muscle; Tibialis anterior muscle; Tibialis posterior muscle **T Lower Leg Muscle, Left** See S Lower Leg Muscle, Right **V Foot Muscle, Right** Abductor hallucis muscle; Adductor hallucis muscle; Extensor digitorum brevis muscle; Extensor hallucis brevis muscle; Flexor digitorum brevis muscle; Flexor hallucis brevis muscle; Quadratus plantae muscle **W Foot Muscle, Left** See V Foot Muscle, Right	**0** Open **4** Percutaneous Endoscopic	**Z** No Device	**Z** No Qualifier

Non-OR Procedure DRG Non-OR Procedure Valid OR Procedure HAC Associated Procedure Combination Only New/Revised April New/Revised October

ICD-10-PCS 2025 — Muscles — 0KT–0KT

- **0** Medical and Surgical
- **K** Muscles
- **T** Resection **Definition:** Cutting out or off, without replacement, all of a body part
  Explanation: None

Body Part Character 4	Approach Character 5	Device Character 6	Qualifier Character 7
0 Head Muscle Auricularis muscle Masseter muscle Pterygoid muscle Splenius capitis muscle Temporalis muscle Temporoparietalis muscle **1** Facial Muscle Buccinator muscle Corrugator supercilii muscle Depressor anguli oris muscle Depressor labii inferioris muscle Depressor septi nasi muscle Depressor supercilii muscle Levator anguli oris muscle Levator labii superioris alaeque nasi muscle Levator labii superioris muscle Mentalis muscle Nasalis muscle Occipitofrontalis muscle Orbicularis oris muscle Procerus muscle Risorius muscle Zygomaticus muscle **2** Neck Muscle, Right Anterior vertebral muscle Arytenoid muscle Cricothyroid muscle Infrahyoid muscle Levator scapulae muscle Platysma muscle Scalene muscle Splenius cervicis muscle Sternocleidomastoid muscle Suprahyoid muscle Thyroarytenoid muscle **3** Neck Muscle, Left *See* 2 Neck Muscle, Right **4** Tongue, Palate, Pharynx Muscle Chondroglossus muscle Genioglossus muscle Hyoglossus muscle Inferior longitudinal muscle Levator veli palatini muscle Palatoglossal muscle Palatopharyngeal muscle Pharyngeal constrictor muscle Salpingopharyngeus muscle Styloglossus muscle Stylopharyngeus muscle Superior longitudinal muscle Tensor veli palatini muscle **5** Shoulder Muscle, Right Deltoid muscle Infraspinatus muscle Subscapularis muscle Supraspinatus muscle Teres major muscle Teres minor muscle **6** Shoulder Muscle, Left *See* 5 Shoulder Muscle, Right	**0** Open **4** Percutaneous Endoscopic	**Z** No Device	**Z** No Qualifier
7 Upper Arm Muscle, Right Biceps brachii muscle Brachialis muscle Coracobrachialis muscle Triceps brachii muscle **8** Upper Arm Muscle, Left *See* 7 Upper Arm Muscle, Right **9** Lower Arm and Wrist Muscle, Right Anatomical snuffbox Anconeus muscle Brachioradialis muscle Extensor carpi radialis muscle Extensor carpi ulnaris muscle Flexor carpi radialis muscle Flexor carpi ulnaris muscle Flexor pollicis longus muscle Palmaris longus muscle Pronator quadratus muscle Pronator teres muscle **B** Lower Arm and Wrist Muscle, Left *See* 9 Lower Arm and Wrist Muscle, Right **C** Hand Muscle, Right Adductor pollicis muscle Hypothenar muscle Palmar interosseous muscle Thenar muscle **D** Hand Muscle, Left *See* C Hand Muscle, Right **F** Trunk Muscle, Right Coccygeus muscle Erector spinae muscle Interspinalis muscle Intertransversarius muscle Latissimus dorsi muscle Quadratus lumborum muscle Rhomboid major muscle Rhomboid minor muscle Serratus posterior muscle Transversospinalis muscle Trapezius muscle **G** Trunk Muscle, Left *See* F Trunk Muscle, Right **H** Thorax Muscle, Right ✚ Intercostal muscle Levatores costarum muscle Pectoralis major muscle Pectoralis minor muscle Serratus anterior muscle Subclavius muscle Subcostal muscle Transverse thoracis muscle **J** Thorax Muscle, Left ✚ *See* H Thorax Muscle, Right **K** Abdomen Muscle, Right External oblique muscle Internal oblique muscle Pyramidalis muscle Rectus abdominis muscle Transversus abdominis muscle **L** Abdomen Muscle, Left *See* K Abdomen Muscle, Right			
M Perineum Muscle Bulbospongiosus muscle Cremaster muscle Deep transverse perineal muscle Ischiocavernosus muscle Levator ani muscle Superficial transverse perineal muscle **N** Hip Muscle, Right Gemellus muscle Gluteus maximus muscle Gluteus medius muscle Gluteus minimus muscle Iliacus muscle Iliopsoas muscle Obturator muscle Piriformis muscle Psoas muscle Quadratus femoris muscle Tensor fasciae latae muscle **P** Hip Muscle, Left *See* N Hip Muscle, Right **Q** Upper Leg Muscle, Right Adductor brevis muscle Adductor longus muscle Adductor magnus muscle Biceps femoris muscle Gracilis muscle Hamstring muscle Pectineus muscle Quadriceps (femoris) Rectus femoris muscle Sartorius muscle Semimembranosus muscle Semitendinosus muscle Vastus intermedius muscle Vastus lateralis muscle Vastus medialis muscle **R** Upper Leg Muscle, Left *See* Q Upper Leg Muscle, Right **S** Lower Leg Muscle, Right Extensor digitorum longus muscle Extensor hallucis longus muscle Fibularis brevis muscle Fibularis longus muscle Flexor digitorum longus muscle Flexor hallucis longus muscle Gastrocnemius muscle Peroneus brevis muscle Peroneus longus muscle Plantaris muscle Popliteus muscle Soleus muscle Tibialis anterior muscle Tibialis posterior muscle **T** Lower Leg Muscle, Left *See* S Lower Leg Muscle, Right **V** Foot Muscle, Right Abductor hallucis muscle Adductor hallucis muscle Extensor digitorum brevis muscle Extensor hallucis brevis muscle Flexor digitorum brevis muscle Flexor hallucis brevis muscle Quadratus plantae muscle **W** Foot Muscle, Left *See* V Foot Muscle, Right			

See Appendix L for Procedure Combinations
✚ 0KT[H,J]0ZZ

NC Noncovered Procedure **LC** Limited Coverage **QA** Questionable OB Admit **NT** New Tech Add-on ✚ Combination Member ♂ Male ♀ Female

Muscles

0 Medical and Surgical
K Muscles
U Supplement

Definition: Putting in or on biological or synthetic material that physically reinforces and/or augments the function of a portion of a body part

Explanation: The biological material is non-living, or is living and from the same individual. The body part may have been previously replaced, and the SUPPLEMENT procedure is performed to physically reinforce and/or augment the function of the replaced body part.

Body Part — Character 4	Approach — Character 5	Device — Character 6	Qualifier — Character 7
0 Head Muscle Auricularis muscle Masseter muscle Pterygoid muscle Splenius capitis muscle Temporalis muscle Temporoparietalis muscle **1 Facial Muscle** Buccinator muscle Corrugator supercilii muscle Depressor anguli oris muscle Depressor labii inferioris muscle Depressor septi nasi muscle Depressor supercilii muscle Levator anguli oris muscle Levator labii superioris alaeque nasi muscle Levator labii superioris muscle Mentalis muscle Nasalis muscle Occipitofrontalis muscle Orbicularis oris muscle Procerus muscle Risorius muscle Zygomaticus muscle **2 Neck Muscle, Right** Anterior vertebral muscle Arytenoid muscle Cricothyroid muscle Infrahyoid muscle Levator scapulae muscle Platysma muscle Scalene muscle Splenius cervicis muscle Sternocleidomastoid muscle Suprahyoid muscle Thyroarytenoid muscle **3 Neck Muscle, Left** See 2 Neck Muscle, Right **4 Tongue, Palate, Pharynx Muscle** Chondroglossus muscle Genioglossus muscle Hyoglossus muscle Inferior longitudinal muscle Levator veli palatini muscle Palatoglossal muscle Palatopharyngeal muscle Pharyngeal constrictor muscle Salpingopharyngeus muscle Styloglossus muscle Stylopharyngeus muscle Superior longitudinal muscle Tensor veli palatini muscle **5 Shoulder Muscle, Right** Deltoid muscle Infraspinatus muscle Subscapularis muscle Supraspinatus muscle Teres major muscle Teres minor muscle **6 Shoulder Muscle, Left** See 5 Shoulder Muscle, Right **7 Upper Arm Muscle, Right** Biceps brachii muscle Brachialis muscle Coracobrachialis muscle Triceps brachii muscle **8 Upper Arm Muscle, Left** See 7 Upper Arm Muscle, Right **9 Lower Arm and Wrist Muscle, Right** Anatomical snuffbox Anconeus muscle Brachioradialis muscle Extensor carpi radialis muscle Extensor carpi ulnaris muscle Flexor carpi radialis muscle Flexor carpi ulnaris muscle Flexor pollicis longus muscle Palmaris longus muscle Pronator quadratus muscle Pronator teres muscle **B Lower Arm and Wrist Muscle, Left** See 9 Lower Arm and Wrist Muscle, Right **C Hand Muscle, Right** Adductor pollicis muscle Hypothenar muscle Palmar interosseous muscle Thenar muscle **D Hand Muscle, Left** See C Hand Muscle, Right **F Trunk Muscle, Right** Coccygeus muscle Erector spinae muscle Interspinalis muscle Intertransversarius muscle Latissimus dorsi muscle Quadratus lumborum muscle Rhomboid major muscle Rhomboid minor muscle Serratus posterior muscle Transversospinalis muscle Trapezius muscle **G Trunk Muscle, Left** See F Trunk Muscle, Right **H Thorax Muscle, Right** Intercostal muscle Levatores costarum muscle Pectoralis major muscle Pectoralis minor muscle Serratus anterior muscle Subclavius muscle Subcostal muscle Transverse thoracis muscle **J Thorax Muscle, Left** See H Thorax Muscle, Right **K Abdomen Muscle, Right** External oblique muscle Internal oblique muscle Pyramidalis muscle Rectus abdominis muscle Transversus abdominis muscle **L Abdomen Muscle, Left** See K Abdomen Muscle, Right **M Perineum Muscle** Bulbospongiosus muscle Cremaster muscle Deep transverse perineal muscle Ischiocavernosus muscle Levator ani muscle Superficial transverse perineal muscle **N Hip Muscle, Right** Gemellus muscle Gluteus maximus muscle Gluteus medius muscle Gluteus minimus muscle Iliacus muscle Iliopsoas muscle Obturator muscle Piriformis muscle Psoas muscle Quadratus femoris muscle Tensor fasciae latae muscle **P Hip Muscle, Left** See N Hip Muscle, Right **Q Upper Leg Muscle, Right** Adductor brevis muscle Adductor longus muscle Adductor magnus muscle Biceps femoris muscle Gracilis muscle Hamstring muscle Pectineus muscle Quadriceps (femoris) Rectus femoris muscle Sartorius muscle Semimembranosus muscle Semitendinosus muscle Vastus intermedius muscle Vastus lateralis muscle Vastus medialis muscle **R Upper Leg Muscle, Left** See Q Upper Leg Muscle, Right **S Lower Leg Muscle, Right** Extensor digitorum longus muscle Extensor hallucis longus muscle Fibularis brevis muscle Fibularis longus muscle Flexor digitorum longus muscle Flexor hallucis longus muscle Gastrocnemius muscle Peroneus brevis muscle Peroneus longus muscle Plantaris muscle Popliteus muscle Soleus muscle Tibialis anterior muscle Tibialis posterior muscle **T Lower Leg Muscle, Left** See S Lower Leg Muscle, Right **V Foot Muscle, Right** Abductor hallucis muscle Adductor hallucis muscle Extensor digitorum brevis muscle Extensor hallucis brevis muscle Flexor digitorum brevis muscle Flexor hallucis brevis muscle Quadratus plantae muscle **W Foot Muscle, Left** See V Foot Muscle, Right	**0** Open **4** Percutaneous Endoscopic	**7** Autologous Tissue Substitute **J** Synthetic Substitute **K** Nonautologous Tissue Substitute	**Z** No Qualifier

Non-OR Procedure | DRG Non-OR Procedure | Valid OR Procedure | HAC Associated Procedure | Combination Only | New/Revised April | New/Revised October

Ø Medical and Surgical
K Muscles
W Revision

Definition: Correcting, to the extent possible, a portion of a malfunctioning device or the position of a displaced device

Explanation: Revision can include correcting a malfunctioning or displaced device by taking out or putting in components of the device such as a screw or pin

Body Part Character 4	Approach Character 5	Device Character 6	Qualifier Character 7
X Upper Muscle Y Lower Muscle	Ø Open 3 Percutaneous 4 Percutaneous Endoscopic	Ø Drainage Device 7 Autologous Tissue Substitute J Synthetic Substitute K Nonautologous Tissue Substitute M Stimulator Lead Y Other Device	Z No Qualifier
X Upper Muscle Y Lower Muscle	X External	Ø Drainage Device 7 Autologous Tissue Substitute J Synthetic Substitute K Nonautologous Tissue Substitute M Stimulator Lead	Z No Qualifier

Non-OR ØKW[X,Y][3,4]YZ
Non-OR ØKW[X,Y]X[Ø,7,J,K,M]Z

Muscles

0 Medical and Surgical
K Muscles
X Transfer

Definition: Moving, without taking out, all or a portion of a body part to another location to take over the function of all or a portion of a body part

Explanation: The body part transferred remains connected to its vascular and nervous supply

Body Part — Character 4	Approach — Character 5	Device — Character 6	Qualifier — Character 7

Body Part — Character 4

- **0 Head Muscle**
  - Auricularis muscle
  - Masseter muscle
  - Pterygoid muscle
  - Splenius capitis muscle
  - Temporalis muscle
  - Temporoparietalis muscle
- **1 Facial Muscle**
  - Buccinator muscle
  - Corrugator supercilii muscle
  - Depressor anguli oris muscle
  - Depressor labii inferioris muscle
  - Depressor septi nasi muscle
  - Depressor supercilii muscle
  - Levator anguli oris muscle
  - Levator labii superioris alaeque nasi muscle
  - Levator labii superioris muscle
  - Mentalis muscle
  - Nasalis muscle
  - Occipitofrontalis muscle
  - Orbicularis oris muscle
  - Procerus muscle
  - Risorius muscle
  - Zygomaticus muscle
- **2 Neck Muscle, Right**
  - Anterior vertebral muscle
  - Arytenoid muscle
  - Cricothyroid muscle
  - Infrahyoid muscle
  - Levator scapulae muscle
  - Platysma muscle
  - Scalene muscle
  - Splenius cervicis muscle
  - Sternocleidomastoid muscle
  - Suprahyoid muscle
  - Thyroarytenoid muscle
- **3 Neck Muscle, Left**
  - See 2 Neck Muscle, Right
- **4 Tongue, Palate, Pharynx Muscle**
  - Chondroglossus muscle
  - Genioglossus muscle
  - Hyoglossus muscle
  - Inferior longitudinal muscle
  - Levator veli palatini muscle
  - Palatoglossal muscle
  - Palatopharyngeal muscle
  - Pharyngeal constrictor muscle
  - Salpingopharyngeus muscle
  - Styloglossus muscle
  - Stylopharyngeus muscle
  - Superior longitudinal muscle
  - Tensor veli palatini muscle
- **5 Shoulder Muscle, Right**
  - Deltoid muscle
  - Infraspinatus muscle
  - Subscapularis muscle
  - Supraspinatus muscle
  - Teres major muscle
  - Teres minor muscle
- **6 Shoulder Muscle, Left**
  - See 5 Shoulder Muscle, Right
- **7 Upper Arm Muscle, Right**
  - Biceps brachii muscle
  - Brachialis muscle
  - Coracobrachialis muscle
  - Triceps brachii muscle
- **8 Upper Arm Muscle, Left**
  - See 7 Upper Arm Muscle, Right
- **9 Lower Arm and Wrist Muscle, Right**
  - Anatomical snuffbox
  - Anconeus muscle
  - Brachioradialis muscle
  - Extensor carpi radialis muscle
  - Extensor carpi ulnaris muscle
  - Flexor carpi radialis muscle
  - Flexor carpi ulnaris muscle
  - Flexor pollicis longus muscle
  - Palmaris longus muscle
  - Pronator quadratus muscle
  - Pronator teres muscle
- **B Lower Arm and Wrist Muscle, Left**
  - See 9 Lower Arm and Wrist Muscle, Right
- **C Hand Muscle, Right**
  - Adductor pollicis muscle
  - Hypothenar muscle
  - Palmar interosseous muscle
  - Thenar muscle
- **D Hand Muscle, Left**
  - See C Hand Muscle, Right
- **H Thorax Muscle, Right**
  - Intercostal muscle
  - Levatores costarum muscle
  - Pectoralis major muscle
  - Pectoralis minor muscle
  - Serratus anterior muscle
  - Subclavius muscle
  - Subcostal muscle
  - Transverse thoracis muscle
- **J Thorax Muscle, Left**
  - See H Thorax Muscle, Right
- **M Perineum Muscle**
  - Bulbospongiosus muscle
  - Cremaster muscle
  - Deep transverse perineal muscle
  - Ischiocavernosus muscle
  - Levator ani muscle
  - Superficial transverse perineal muscle
- **N Hip Muscle, Right**
  - Gemellus muscle
  - Gluteus maximus muscle
  - Gluteus medius muscle
  - Gluteus minimus muscle
  - Iliacus muscle
  - Iliopsoas muscle
  - Obturator muscle
  - Piriformis muscle
  - Psoas muscle
  - Quadratus femoris muscle
  - Tensor fasciae latae muscle
- **P Hip Muscle, Left**
  - See N Hip Muscle, Right
- **Q Upper Leg Muscle, Right**
  - Adductor brevis muscle
  - Adductor longus muscle
  - Adductor magnus muscle
  - Biceps femoris muscle
  - Gracilis muscle
  - Hamstring muscle
  - Pectineus muscle
  - Quadriceps (femoris)
  - Rectus femoris muscle
  - Sartorius muscle
  - Semimembranosus muscle
  - Semitendinosus muscle
  - Vastus intermedius muscle
  - Vastus lateralis muscle
  - Vastus medialis muscle
- **R Upper Leg Muscle, Left**
  - See Q Upper Leg Muscle, Right
- **S Lower Leg Muscle, Right**
  - Extensor digitorum longus muscle
  - Extensor hallucis longus muscle
  - Fibularis brevis muscle
  - Fibularis longus muscle
  - Flexor digitorum longus muscle
  - Flexor hallucis longus muscle
  - Gastrocnemius muscle
  - Peroneus brevis muscle
  - Peroneus longus muscle
  - Plantaris muscle
  - Popliteus muscle
  - Soleus muscle
  - Tibialis anterior muscle
  - Tibialis posterior muscle
- **T Lower Leg Muscle, Left**
  - See S Lower Leg Muscle, Right
- **V Foot Muscle, Right**
  - Abductor hallucis muscle
  - Adductor hallucis muscle
  - Extensor digitorum brevis muscle
  - Extensor hallucis brevis muscle
  - Flexor digitorum brevis muscle
  - Flexor hallucis brevis muscle
  - Quadratus plantae muscle
- **W Foot Muscle, Left**
  - See V Foot Muscle, Right

Approach — Character 5

- **0** Open
- **4** Percutaneous Endoscopic

Device — Character 6

- **Z** No Device

Qualifier — Character 7

- **0** Skin
- **1** Subcutaneous Tissue
- **2** Skin and Subcutaneous Tissue
- **Z** No Qualifier

0KX Continued on next page

ICD-10-PCS 2025 — Muscles — 0KX–0KX

0KX Continued

- **0** Medical and Surgical
- **K** Muscles
- **X** Transfer

Definition: Moving, without taking out, all or a portion of a body part to another location to take over the function of all or a portion of a body part

Explanation: The body part transferred remains connected to its vascular and nervous supply

Body Part Character 4	Approach Character 5	Device Character 6	Qualifier Character 7

F Trunk Muscle, Right
  Coccygeus muscle
  Erector spinae muscle
  Interspinalis muscle
  Intertransversarius muscle
  Latissimus dorsi muscle
  Quadratus lumborum muscle
  Rhomboid major muscle
  Rhomboid minor muscle
  Serratus posterior muscle
  Transversospinalis muscle
  Trapezius muscle
G Trunk Muscle, Left
  See F Trunk Muscle, Right
	0 Open
	4 Percutaneous Endoscopic
		Z No Device	**0** Skin
			1 Subcutaneous Tissue
			2 Skin and Subcutaneous Tissue
			5 Latissimus Dorsi Myocutaneous Flap
			7 Deep Inferior Epigastric Artery Perforator Flap
			8 Superficial Inferior Epigastric Artery Flap
			9 Gluteal Artery Perforator Flap
			Z No Qualifier

K Abdomen Muscle, Right
  External oblique muscle
  Internal oblique muscle
  Pyramidalis muscle
  Rectus abdominis muscle
  Transversus abdominis muscle
L Abdomen Muscle, Left
  See K Abdomen Muscle, Right
	0 Open
	4 Percutaneous Endoscopic
		Z No Device	**0** Skin
			1 Subcutaneous Tissue
			2 Skin and Subcutaneous Tissue
			6 Transverse Rectus Abdominis Myocutaneous Flap
			Z No Qualifier

Tendons 0L2–0LX

Character Meanings*

This Character Meaning table is provided as a guide to assist the user in the identification of character members that may be found in this section of code tables. It **SHOULD NOT** be used to build a PCS code.

Operation–Character 3		Body Part–Character 4		Approach–Character 5		Device–Character 6		Qualifier–Character 7	
2	Change	0	Head and Neck Tendon	0	Open	0	Drainage Device	X	Diagnostic
5	Destruction	1	Shoulder Tendon, Right	3	Percutaneous	7	Autologous Tissue Substitute	Z	No Qualifier
8	Division	2	Shoulder Tendon, Left	4	Percutaneous Endoscopic	J	Synthetic Substitute		
9	Drainage	3	Upper Arm Tendon, Right	X	External	K	Nonautologous Tissue Substitute		
B	Excision	4	Upper Arm Tendon, Left			Y	Other Device		
C	Extirpation	5	Lower Arm and Wrist Tendon, Right			Z	No Device		
D	Extraction	6	Lower Arm and Wrist Tendon, Left						
H	Insertion	7	Hand Tendon, Right						
J	Inspection	8	Hand Tendon, Left						
M	Reattachment	9	Trunk Tendon, Right						
N	Release	B	Trunk Tendon, Left						
P	Removal	C	Thorax Tendon, Right						
Q	Repair	D	Thorax Tendon, Left						
R	Replacement	F	Abdomen Tendon, Right						
S	Reposition	G	Abdomen Tendon, Left						
T	Resection	H	Perineum Tendon						
U	Supplement	J	Hip Tendon, Right						
W	Revision	K	Hip Tendon, Left						
X	Transfer	L	Upper Leg Tendon, Right						
		M	Upper Leg Tendon, Left						
		N	Lower Leg Tendon, Right						
		P	Lower Leg Tendon, Left						
		Q	Knee Tendon, Right						
		R	Knee Tendon, Left						
		S	Ankle Tendon, Right						
		T	Ankle Tendon, Left						
		V	Foot Tendon, Right						
		W	Foot Tendon, Left						
		X	Upper Tendon						
		Y	Lower Tendon						

* Includes synovial membrane.

AHA Coding Clinic for table 0L8
2016, 3Q, 30   Resection of femur with interposition arthroplasty

AHA Coding Clinic for table 0LB
2017, 2Q, 21   Arthroscopic anterior cruciate ligament revision using autograft with anterolateral ligament reconstruction
2015, 3Q, 26   Thumb arthroplasty with resection of trapezium
2014, 3Q, 14   Application of TheraSkin® and excisional debridement
2014, 3Q, 18   Placement of reverse sural fasciocutaneous pedicle flap

AHA Coding Clinic for table 0LD
2017, 4Q, 41   Extraction procedures

AHA Coding Clinic for table 0LQ
2016, 3Q, 32   Rotator cuff repair, tenodesis, decompression, acromioplasty and coracoplasty
2015, 2Q, 11   Repair of patellar and quadriceps tendons with allograft
2013, 3Q, 20   Superior labrum anterior posterior (SLAP) repair and subacromial decompression

AHA Coding Clinic for table 0LS
2016, 3Q, 32   Rotator cuff repair, tenodesis, decompression, acromioplasty and coracoplasty
2015, 3Q, 14   Endoprosthetic replacement of humerus and tendon reattachment

AHA Coding Clinic for table 0LU
2015, 2Q, 11   Repair of patellar and quadriceps tendons with allograft

Tendons

Foot Tendons

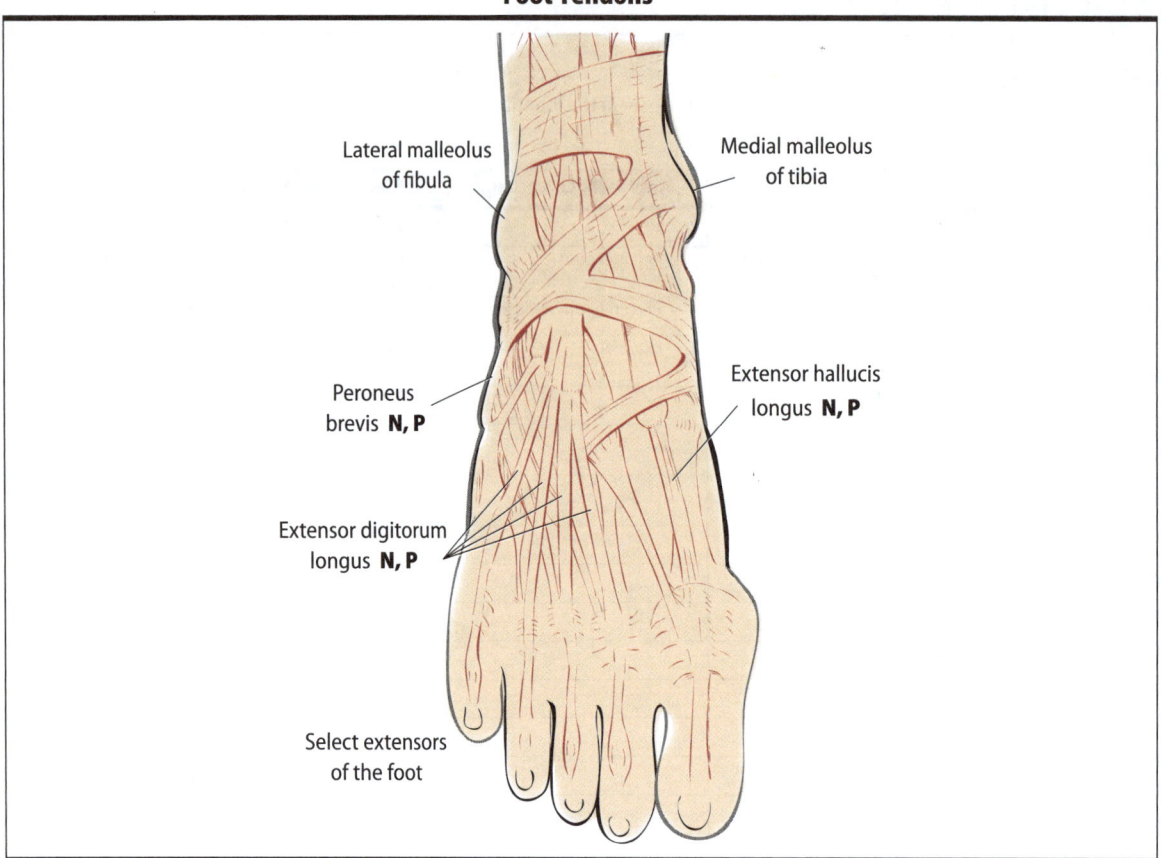

- Lateral malleolus of fibula
- Medial malleolus of tibia
- Peroneus brevis **N, P**
- Extensor hallucis longus **N, P**
- Extensor digitorum longus **N, P**
- Select extensors of the foot

Shoulder Tendons

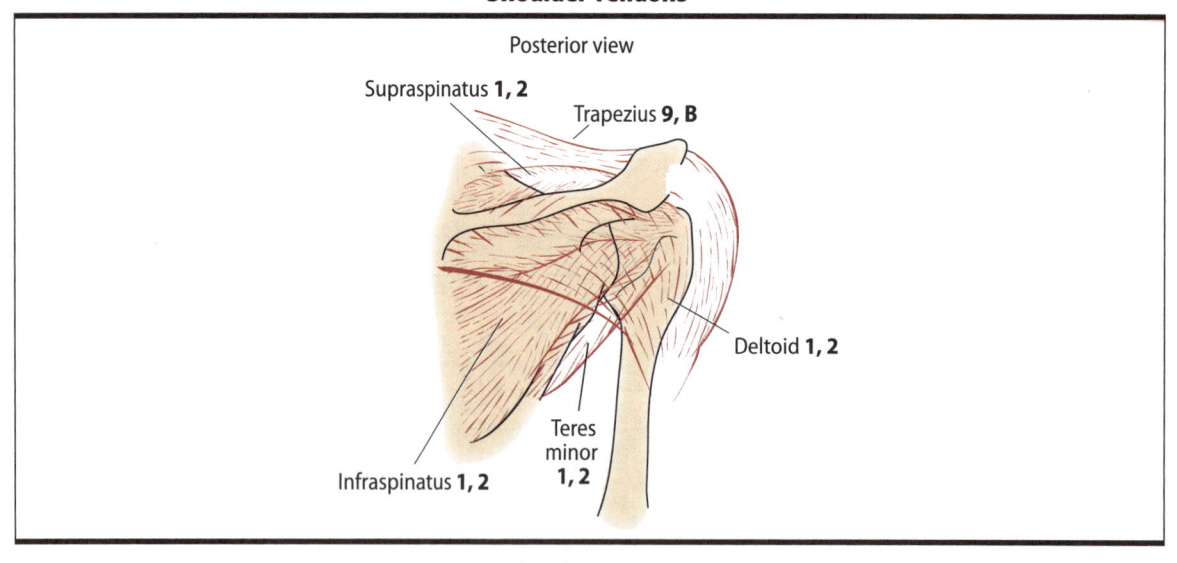

Posterior view

- Supraspinatus **1, 2**
- Trapezius **9, B**
- Deltoid **1, 2**
- Teres minor **1, 2**
- Infraspinatus **1, 2**

Tendons of Wrist and Hand

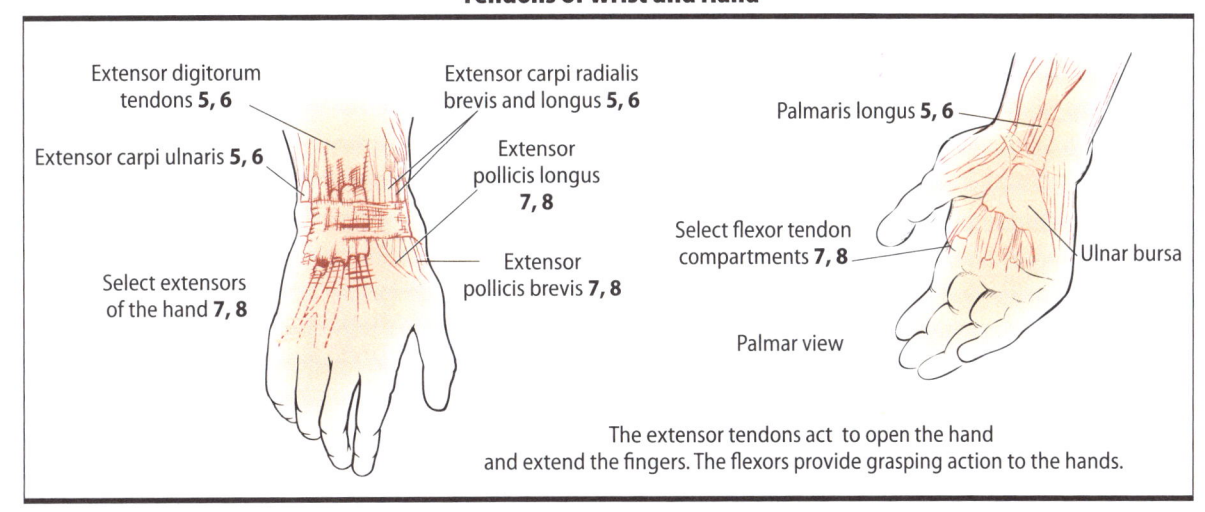

Extensor digitorum tendons **5, 6**
Extensor carpi radialis brevis and longus **5, 6**
Extensor carpi ulnaris **5, 6**
Extensor pollicis longus **7, 8**
Select extensors of the hand **7, 8**
Extensor pollicis brevis **7, 8**

Palmaris longus **5, 6**
Select flexor tendon compartments **7, 8**
Ulnar bursa
Palmar view

The extensor tendons act to open the hand and extend the fingers. The flexors provide grasping action to the hands.

Leg Muscles and Tendons

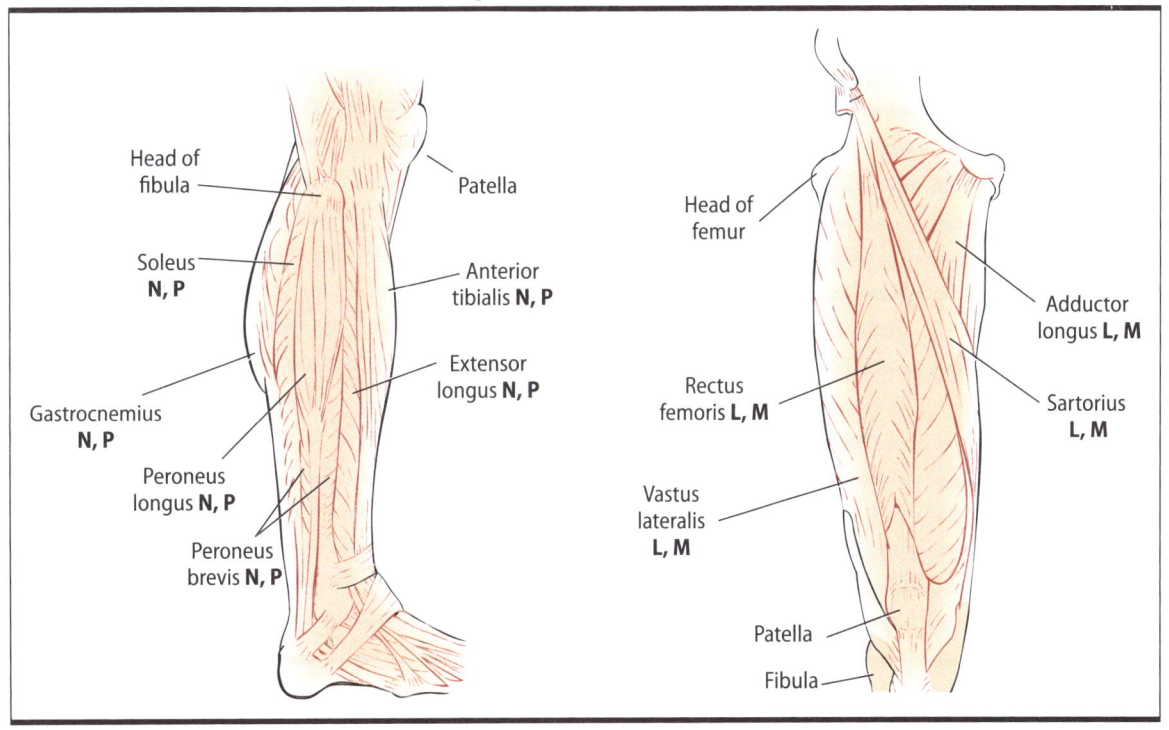

Head of fibula
Patella
Soleus **N, P**
Anterior tibialis **N, P**
Extensor longus **N, P**
Gastrocnemius **N, P**
Peroneus longus **N, P**
Peroneus brevis **N, P**

Head of femur
Adductor longus **L, M**
Rectus femoris **L, M**
Sartorius **L, M**
Vastus lateralis **L, M**
Patella
Fibula

0 Medical and Surgical
L Tendons
2 Change

Definition: Taking out or off a device from a body part and putting back an identical or similar device in or on the same body part without cutting or puncturing the skin or a mucous membrane

Explanation: All CHANGE procedures are coded using the approach EXTERNAL

Body Part Character 4	Approach Character 5	Device Character 6	Qualifier Character 7
X Upper Tendon Y Lower Tendon	X External	0 Drainage Device Y Other Device	Z No Qualifier

Non-OR All body part, approach, device, and qualifier values

0 Medical and Surgical
L Tendons
5 Destruction

Definition: Physical eradication of all or a portion of a body part by the direct use of energy, force, or a destructive agent

Explanation: None of the body part is physically taken out

Body Part Character 4	Approach Character 5	Device Character 6	Qualifier Character 7

0 Head and Neck Tendon
1 Shoulder Tendon, Right
2 Shoulder Tendon, Left
3 Upper Arm Tendon, Right
4 Upper Arm Tendon, Left
5 Lower Arm and Wrist Tendon, Right
6 Lower Arm and Wrist Tendon, Left
7 Hand Tendon, Right
8 Hand Tendon, Left
9 Trunk Tendon, Right
B Trunk Tendon, Left
C Thorax Tendon, Right
D Thorax Tendon, Left
F Abdomen Tendon, Right
G Abdomen Tendon, Left
H Perineum Tendon
J Hip Tendon, Right
K Hip Tendon, Left
L Upper Leg Tendon, Right
M Upper Leg Tendon, Left
N Lower Leg Tendon, Right
   Achilles tendon
P Lower Leg Tendon, Left
   See N Lower Leg Tendon, Right
Q Knee Tendon, Right
   Patellar tendon
R Knee Tendon, Left
   See Q Knee Tendon, Right
S Ankle Tendon, Right
T Ankle Tendon, Left
V Foot Tendon, Right
W Foot Tendon, Left
	0 Open
	3 Percutaneous
	4 Percutaneous Endoscopic
		Z No Device	Z No Qualifier

0 Medical and Surgical
L Tendons
8 Division

Definition: Cutting into a body part, without draining fluids and/or gases from the body part, in order to separate or transect a body part
Explanation: All or a portion of the body part is separated into two or more portions

Body Part Character 4	Approach Character 5	Device Character 6	Qualifier Character 7
0 Head and Neck Tendon	0 Open	Z No Device	Z No Qualifier
1 Shoulder Tendon, Right	3 Percutaneous		
2 Shoulder Tendon, Left	4 Percutaneous Endoscopic		
3 Upper Arm Tendon, Right			
4 Upper Arm Tendon, Left			
5 Lower Arm and Wrist Tendon, Right			
6 Lower Arm and Wrist Tendon, Left			
7 Hand Tendon, Right			
8 Hand Tendon, Left			
9 Trunk Tendon, Right			
B Trunk Tendon, Left			
C Thorax Tendon, Right			
D Thorax Tendon, Left			
F Abdomen Tendon, Right			
G Abdomen Tendon, Left			
H Perineum Tendon			
J Hip Tendon, Right			
K Hip Tendon, Left			
L Upper Leg Tendon, Right			
M Upper Leg Tendon, Left			
N Lower Leg Tendon, Right Achilles tendon			
P Lower Leg Tendon, Left See N Lower Leg Tendon, Right			
Q Knee Tendon, Right Patellar tendon			
R Knee Tendon, Left See Q Knee Tendon, Right			
S Ankle Tendon, Right			
T Ankle Tendon, Left			
V Foot Tendon, Right			
W Foot Tendon, Left			

0L9–0L9 Tendons

0 Medical and Surgical
L Tendons
9 Drainage

Definition: Taking or letting out fluids and/or gases from a body part
Explanation: The qualifier DIAGNOSTIC is used to identify drainage procedures that are biopsies

Body Part - Character 4	Approach - Character 5	Device - Character 6	Qualifier - Character 7

0 Head and Neck Tendon
1 Shoulder Tendon, Right
2 Shoulder Tendon, Left
3 Upper Arm Tendon, Right
4 Upper Arm Tendon, Left
5 Lower Arm and Wrist Tendon, Right
6 Lower Arm and Wrist Tendon, Left
7 Hand Tendon, Right
8 Hand Tendon, Left
9 Trunk Tendon, Right
B Trunk Tendon, Left
C Thorax Tendon, Right
D Thorax Tendon, Left
F Abdomen Tendon, Right
G Abdomen Tendon, Left
H Perineum Tendon
J Hip Tendon, Right
K Hip Tendon, Left
L Upper Leg Tendon, Right
M Upper Leg Tendon, Left
N Lower Leg Tendon, Right
    Achilles tendon
P Lower Leg Tendon, Left
    See N Lower Leg Tendon, Right
Q Knee Tendon, Right
    Patellar tendon
R Knee Tendon, Left
    See Q Knee Tendon, Right
S Ankle Tendon, Right
T Ankle Tendon, Left
V Foot Tendon, Right
W Foot Tendon, Left
	0 Open
	3 Percutaneous
	4 Percutaneous Endoscopic
		0 Drainage Device	**Z** No Qualifier

0 Head and Neck Tendon
1 Shoulder Tendon, Right
2 Shoulder Tendon, Left
3 Upper Arm Tendon, Right
4 Upper Arm Tendon, Left
5 Lower Arm and Wrist Tendon, Right
6 Lower Arm and Wrist Tendon, Left
7 Hand Tendon, Right
8 Hand Tendon, Left
9 Trunk Tendon, Right
B Trunk Tendon, Left
C Thorax Tendon, Right
D Thorax Tendon, Left
F Abdomen Tendon, Right
G Abdomen Tendon, Left
H Perineum Tendon
J Hip Tendon, Right
K Hip Tendon, Left
L Upper Leg Tendon, Right
M Upper Leg Tendon, Left
N Lower Leg Tendon, Right
    Achilles tendon
P Lower Leg Tendon, Left
    See N Lower Leg Tendon, Right
Q Knee Tendon, Right
    Patellar tendon
R Knee Tendon, Left
    See Q Knee Tendon, Right
S Ankle Tendon, Right
T Ankle Tendon, Left
V Foot Tendon, Right
W Foot Tendon, Left
	0 Open
	3 Percutaneous
	4 Percutaneous Endoscopic
		Z No Device	**X** Diagnostic
			Z No Qualifier

Non-OR 0L9[0,1,2,3,4,5,6,7,8,9,B,C,D,F,G,H,J,K,L,M,N,P,Q,R,S,T,V,W]30Z
Non-OR 0L9[0,1,2,3,4,5,6,7,8,9,B,C,D,F,G,H,J,K,L,M,N,P,Q,R,S,T,V,W]3ZZ
Non-OR 0L9[7,8]4ZZ

0 Medical and Surgical
L Tendons
B Excision

Definition: Cutting out or off, without replacement, a portion of a body part
Explanation: The qualifier DIAGNOSTIC is used to identify excision procedures that are biopsies

Body Part Character 4	Approach Character 5	Device Character 6	Qualifier Character 7

0 Head and Neck Tendon
1 Shoulder Tendon, Right
2 Shoulder Tendon, Left
3 Upper Arm Tendon, Right
4 Upper Arm Tendon, Left
5 Lower Arm and Wrist Tendon, Right
6 Lower Arm and Wrist Tendon, Left
7 Hand Tendon, Right
8 Hand Tendon, Left
9 Trunk Tendon, Right
B Trunk Tendon, Left
C Thorax Tendon, Right
D Thorax Tendon, Left
F Abdomen Tendon, Right
G Abdomen Tendon, Left
H Perineum Tendon
J Hip Tendon, Right
K Hip Tendon, Left
L Upper Leg Tendon, Right
M Upper Leg Tendon, Left
N Lower Leg Tendon, Right
   Achilles tendon
P Lower Leg Tendon, Left
   See N Lower Leg Tendon, Right
Q Knee Tendon, Right
   Patellar tendon
R Knee Tendon, Left
   See Q Knee Tendon, Right
S Ankle Tendon, Right
T Ankle Tendon, Left
V Foot Tendon, Right
W Foot Tendon, Left
	0 Open
	3 Percutaneous
	4 Percutaneous Endoscopic
		Z No Device	X Diagnostic
			Z No Qualifier

0 Medical and Surgical
L Tendons
C Extirpation

Definition: Taking or cutting out solid matter from a body part

Explanation: The solid matter may be an abnormal byproduct of a biological function or a foreign body; it may be imbedded in a body part or in the lumen of a tubular body part. The solid matter may or may not have been previously broken into pieces.

Body Part Character 4	Approach Character 5	Device Character 6	Qualifier Character 7

0 Head and Neck Tendon
1 Shoulder Tendon, Right
2 Shoulder Tendon, Left
3 Upper Arm Tendon, Right
4 Upper Arm Tendon, Left
5 Lower Arm and Wrist Tendon, Right
6 Lower Arm and Wrist Tendon, Left
7 Hand Tendon, Right
8 Hand Tendon, Left
9 Trunk Tendon, Right
B Trunk Tendon, Left
C Thorax Tendon, Right
D Thorax Tendon, Left
F Abdomen Tendon, Right
G Abdomen Tendon, Left
H Perineum Tendon
J Hip Tendon, Right
K Hip Tendon, Left
L Upper Leg Tendon, Right
M Upper Leg Tendon, Left
N Lower Leg Tendon, Right
   Achilles tendon
P Lower Leg Tendon, Left
   See N Lower Leg Tendon, Right
Q Knee Tendon, Right
   Patellar tendon
R Knee Tendon, Left
   See Q Knee Tendon, Right
S Ankle Tendon, Right
T Ankle Tendon, Left
V Foot Tendon, Right
W Foot Tendon, Left
	0 Open
	3 Percutaneous
	4 Percutaneous Endoscopic
		Z No Device	Z No Qualifier

0 Medical and Surgical
L Tendons
D Extraction

Definition: Pulling or stripping out or off all or a portion of a body part by the use of force
Explanation: The qualifier DIAGNOSTIC is used to identify extraction procedures that are biopsies

Body Part — Character 4	Approach — Character 5	Device — Character 6	Qualifier — Character 7

0 Head and Neck Tendon
1 Shoulder Tendon, Right
2 Shoulder Tendon, Left
3 Upper Arm Tendon, Right
4 Upper Arm Tendon, Left
5 Lower Arm and Wrist Tendon, Right
6 Lower Arm and Wrist Tendon, Left
7 Hand Tendon, Right
8 Hand Tendon, Left
9 Trunk Tendon, Right
B Trunk Tendon, Left
C Thorax Tendon, Right
D Thorax Tendon, Left
F Abdomen Tendon, Right
G Abdomen Tendon, Left
H Perineum Tendon
J Hip Tendon, Right
K Hip Tendon, Left
L Upper Leg Tendon, Right
M Upper Leg Tendon, Left
N Lower Leg Tendon, Right
   Achilles tendon
P Lower Leg Tendon, Left
   See N Lower Leg Tendon, Right
Q Knee Tendon, Right
   Patellar tendon
R Knee Tendon, Left
   See Q Knee Tendon, Right
S Ankle Tendon, Right
T Ankle Tendon, Left
V Foot Tendon, Right
W Foot Tendon, Left
	0 Open	Z No Device	Z No Qualifier

0 Medical and Surgical
L Tendons
H Insertion

Definition: Putting in a nonbiological appliance that monitors, assists, performs, or prevents a physiological function but does not physically take the place of a body part
Explanation: None

Body Part — Character 4	Approach — Character 5	Device — Character 6	Qualifier — Character 7
X Upper Tendon Y Lower Tendon	0 Open 3 Percutaneous 4 Percutaneous Endoscopic	Y Other Device	Z No Qualifier

Non-OR 0LH[X,Y][3,4]YZ

0 Medical and Surgical
L Tendons
J Inspection

Definition: Visually and/or manually exploring a body part
Explanation: Visual exploration may be performed with or without optical instrumentation. Manual exploration may be performed directly or through intervening body layers.

Body Part — Character 4	Approach — Character 5	Device — Character 6	Qualifier — Character 7
X Upper Tendon Y Lower Tendon	0 Open 3 Percutaneous 4 Percutaneous Endoscopic X External	Z No Device	Z No Qualifier

Non-OR 0LJ[X,Y][3,X]ZZ

0LM–0LN Tendons

0 Medical and Surgical
L Tendons
M Reattachment — Definition: Putting back in or on all or a portion of a separated body part to its normal location or other suitable location
Explanation: Vascular circulation and nervous pathways may or may not be reestablished

Body Part Character 4	Approach Character 5	Device Character 6	Qualifier Character 7

0 Head and Neck Tendon
1 Shoulder Tendon, Right
2 Shoulder Tendon, Left
3 Upper Arm Tendon, Right
4 Upper Arm Tendon, Left
5 Lower Arm and Wrist Tendon, Right
6 Lower Arm and Wrist Tendon, Left
7 Hand Tendon, Right
8 Hand Tendon, Left
9 Trunk Tendon, Right
B Trunk Tendon, Left
C Thorax Tendon, Right
D Thorax Tendon, Left
F Abdomen Tendon, Right
G Abdomen Tendon, Left
H Perineum Tendon
J Hip Tendon, Right
K Hip Tendon, Left
L Upper Leg Tendon, Right
M Upper Leg Tendon, Left
N Lower Leg Tendon, Right
   Achilles tendon
P Lower Leg Tendon, Left
   See N Lower Leg Tendon, Right
Q Knee Tendon, Right
   Patellar tendon
R Knee Tendon, Left
   See Q Knee Tendon, Right
S Ankle Tendon, Right
T Ankle Tendon, Left
V Foot Tendon, Right
W Foot Tendon, Left
	0 Open
	4 Percutaneous Endoscopic
		Z No Device	Z No Qualifier

0 Medical and Surgical
L Tendons
N Release — Definition: Freeing a body part from an abnormal physical constraint by cutting or by the use of force
Explanation: Some of the restraining tissue may be taken out but none of the body part is taken out

Body Part Character 4	Approach Character 5	Device Character 6	Qualifier Character 7

0 Head and Neck Tendon
1 Shoulder Tendon, Right
2 Shoulder Tendon, Left
3 Upper Arm Tendon, Right
4 Upper Arm Tendon, Left
5 Lower Arm and Wrist Tendon, Right
6 Lower Arm and Wrist Tendon, Left
7 Hand Tendon, Right
8 Hand Tendon, Left
9 Trunk Tendon, Right
B Trunk Tendon, Left
C Thorax Tendon, Right
D Thorax Tendon, Left
F Abdomen Tendon, Right
G Abdomen Tendon, Left
H Perineum Tendon
J Hip Tendon, Right
K Hip Tendon, Left
L Upper Leg Tendon, Right
M Upper Leg Tendon, Left
N Lower Leg Tendon, Right
   Achilles tendon
P Lower Leg Tendon, Left
   See N Lower Leg Tendon, Right
Q Knee Tendon, Right
   Patellar tendon
R Knee Tendon, Left
   See Q Knee Tendon, Right
S Ankle Tendon, Right
T Ankle Tendon, Left
V Foot Tendon, Right
W Foot Tendon, Left
	0 Open
	3 Percutaneous
	4 Percutaneous Endoscopic
	X External
		Z No Device	Z No Qualifier

Non-OR 0LN[0,1,2,3,4,5,6,7,8,9,B,C,D,F,G,H,J,K,L,M,N,P,Q,R,S,T,V,W]XZZ

ICD-10-PCS 2025   Tendons   0LP–0LQ

0 Medical and Surgical
L Tendons
P Removal   Definition: Taking out or off a device from a body part
Explanation: If a device is taken out and a similar device put in without cutting or puncturing the skin or mucous membrane, the procedure is coded to the root operation CHANGE. Otherwise, the procedure for taking out a device is coded to the root operation REMOVAL.

Body Part Character 4	Approach Character 5	Device Character 6	Qualifier Character 7
X Upper Tendon Y Lower Tendon	0 Open 3 Percutaneous 4 Percutaneous Endoscopic	0 Drainage Device 7 Autologous Tissue Substitute J Synthetic Substitute K Nonautologous Tissue Substitute Y Other Device	Z No Qualifier
X Upper Tendon Y Lower Tendon	X External	0 Drainage Device	Z No Qualifier

Non-OR   0LP[X,Y]30Z
Non-OR   0LP[X,Y][3,4]YZ
Non-OR   0LP[X,Y]X0Z

0 Medical and Surgical
L Tendons
Q Repair   Definition: Restoring, to the extent possible, a body part to its normal anatomic structure and function
Explanation: Used only when the method to accomplish the repair is not one of the other root operations

Body Part Character 4	Approach Character 5	Device Character 6	Qualifier Character 7

0 Head and Neck Tendon
1 Shoulder Tendon, Right
2 Shoulder Tendon, Left
3 Upper Arm Tendon, Right
4 Upper Arm Tendon, Left
5 Lower Arm and Wrist Tendon, Right
6 Lower Arm and Wrist Tendon, Left
7 Hand Tendon, Right
8 Hand Tendon, Left
9 Trunk Tendon, Right
B Trunk Tendon, Left
C Thorax Tendon, Right
D Thorax Tendon, Left
F Abdomen Tendon, Right
G Abdomen Tendon, Left
H Perineum Tendon
J Hip Tendon, Right
K Hip Tendon, Left
L Upper Leg Tendon, Right
M Upper Leg Tendon, Left
N Lower Leg Tendon, Right
    Achilles tendon
P Lower Leg Tendon, Left
    See N Lower Leg Tendon, Right
Q Knee Tendon, Right
    Patellar tendon
R Knee Tendon, Left
    See Q Knee Tendon, Right
S Ankle Tendon, Right
T Ankle Tendon, Left
V Foot Tendon, Right
W Foot Tendon, Left
	0 Open
	3 Percutaneous
	4 Percutaneous Endoscopic
		Z No Device	Z No Qualifier

0LR–0LS Tendons

0 Medical and Surgical
L Tendons
R Replacement

Definition: Putting in or on biological or synthetic material that physically takes the place and/or function of all or a portion of a body part

Explanation: The body part may have been taken out or replaced, or may be taken out, physically eradicated, or rendered nonfunctional during the REPLACEMENT procedure. A REMOVAL procedure is coded for taking out the device used in a previous replacement procedure.

Body Part Character 4	Approach Character 5	Device Character 6	Qualifier Character 7

0 Head and Neck Tendon
1 Shoulder Tendon, Right
2 Shoulder Tendon, Left
3 Upper Arm Tendon, Right
4 Upper Arm Tendon, Left
5 Lower Arm and Wrist Tendon, Right
6 Lower Arm and Wrist Tendon, Left
7 Hand Tendon, Right
8 Hand Tendon, Left
9 Trunk Tendon, Right
B Trunk Tendon, Left
C Thorax Tendon, Right
D Thorax Tendon, Left
F Abdomen Tendon, Right
G Abdomen Tendon, Left
H Perineum Tendon
J Hip Tendon, Right
K Hip Tendon, Left
L Upper Leg Tendon, Right
M Upper Leg Tendon, Left
N Lower Leg Tendon, Right
    Achilles tendon
P Lower Leg Tendon, Left
    See N Lower Leg Tendon, Right
Q Knee Tendon, Right
    Patellar tendon
R Knee Tendon, Left
    See Q Knee Tendon, Right
S Ankle Tendon, Right
T Ankle Tendon, Left
V Foot Tendon, Right
W Foot Tendon, Left
	0 Open
	4 Percutaneous Endoscopic
		7 Autologous Tissue Substitute
		J Synthetic Substitute
		K Nonautologous Tissue Substitute
			Z No Qualifier

0 Medical and Surgical
L Tendons
S Reposition

Definition: Moving to its normal location, or other suitable location, all or a portion of a body part

Explanation: The body part is moved to a new location from an abnormal location, or from a normal location where it is not functioning correctly. The body part may or may not be cut out or off to be moved to the new location.

Body Part Character 4	Approach Character 5	Device Character 6	Qualifier Character 7

0 Head and Neck Tendon
1 Shoulder Tendon, Right
2 Shoulder Tendon, Left
3 Upper Arm Tendon, Right
4 Upper Arm Tendon, Left
5 Lower Arm and Wrist Tendon, Right
6 Lower Arm and Wrist Tendon, Left
7 Hand Tendon, Right
8 Hand Tendon, Left
9 Trunk Tendon, Right
B Trunk Tendon, Left
C Thorax Tendon, Right
D Thorax Tendon, Left
F Abdomen Tendon, Right
G Abdomen Tendon, Left
H Perineum Tendon
J Hip Tendon, Right
K Hip Tendon, Left
L Upper Leg Tendon, Right
M Upper Leg Tendon, Left
N Lower Leg Tendon, Right
    Achilles tendon
P Lower Leg Tendon, Left
    See N Lower Leg Tendon, Right
Q Knee Tendon, Right
    Patellar tendon
R Knee Tendon, Left
    See Q Knee Tendon, Right
S Ankle Tendon, Right
T Ankle Tendon, Left
V Foot Tendon, Right
W Foot Tendon, Left
	0 Open
	4 Percutaneous Endoscopic
		Z No Device	**Z** No Qualifier

Non-OR Procedure   DRG Non-OR Procedure   Valid OR Procedure   HAC Associated Procedure   Combination Only   New/Revised April   New/Revised October

ICD-10-PCS 2025 — Tendons — 0LT–0LU

0 Medical and Surgical
L Tendons
T Resection Definition: Cutting out or off, without replacement, all of a body part
Explanation: None

Body Part Character 4	Approach Character 5	Device Character 6	Qualifier Character 7

0 Head and Neck Tendon
1 Shoulder Tendon, Right
2 Shoulder Tendon, Left
3 Upper Arm Tendon, Right
4 Upper Arm Tendon, Left
5 Lower Arm and Wrist Tendon, Right
6 Lower Arm and Wrist Tendon, Left
7 Hand Tendon, Right
8 Hand Tendon, Left
9 Trunk Tendon, Right
B Trunk Tendon, Left
C Thorax Tendon, Right
D Thorax Tendon, Left
F Abdomen Tendon, Right
G Abdomen Tendon, Left
H Perineum Tendon
J Hip Tendon, Right
K Hip Tendon, Left
L Upper Leg Tendon, Right
M Upper Leg Tendon, Left
N Lower Leg Tendon, Right
   Achilles tendon
P Lower Leg Tendon, Left
   See N Lower Leg Tendon, Right
Q Knee Tendon, Right
   Patellar tendon
R Knee Tendon, Left
   See Q Knee Tendon, Right
S Ankle Tendon, Right
T Ankle Tendon, Left
V Foot Tendon, Right
W Foot Tendon, Left
	0 Open
	4 Percutaneous Endoscopic
		Z No Device	Z No Qualifier

0 Medical and Surgical
L Tendons
U Supplement Definition: Putting in or on biological or synthetic material that physically reinforces and/or augments the function of a portion of a body part
Explanation: The biological material is non-living, or is living and from the same individual. The body part may have been previously replaced, and the SUPPLEMENT procedure is performed to physically reinforce and/or augment the function of the replaced body part.

Body Part Character 4	Approach Character 5	Device Character 6	Qualifier Character 7

0 Head and Neck Tendon
1 Shoulder Tendon, Right
2 Shoulder Tendon, Left
3 Upper Arm Tendon, Right
4 Upper Arm Tendon, Left
5 Lower Arm and Wrist Tendon, Right
6 Lower Arm and Wrist Tendon, Left
7 Hand Tendon, Right
8 Hand Tendon, Left
9 Trunk Tendon, Right
B Trunk Tendon, Left
C Thorax Tendon, Right
D Thorax Tendon, Left
F Abdomen Tendon, Right
G Abdomen Tendon, Left
H Perineum Tendon
J Hip Tendon, Right
K Hip Tendon, Left
L Upper Leg Tendon, Right
M Upper Leg Tendon, Left
N Lower Leg Tendon, Right
   Achilles tendon
P Lower Leg Tendon, Left
   See N Lower Leg Tendon, Right
Q Knee Tendon, Right
   Patellar tendon
R Knee Tendon, Left
   See Q Knee Tendon, Right
S Ankle Tendon, Right
T Ankle Tendon, Left
V Foot Tendon, Right
W Foot Tendon, Left
	0 Open
	4 Percutaneous Endoscopic
		7 Autologous Tissue Substitute
		J Synthetic Substitute
		K Nonautologous Tissue Substitute
			Z No Qualifier

NC Noncovered Procedure **LC** Limited Coverage **QA** Questionable OB Admit **NT** New Tech Add-on ✚ Combination Member ♂ Male ♀ Female

Tendons 0LW–0LX

0 Medical and Surgical
L Tendons
W Revision Definition: Correcting, to the extent possible, a portion of a malfunctioning device or the position of a displaced device
Explanation: Revision can include correcting a malfunctioning or displaced device by taking out or putting in components of the device such as a screw or pin

Body Part Character 4	Approach Character 5	Device Character 6	Qualifier Character 7
X Upper Tendon Y Lower Tendon	0 Open 3 Percutaneous 4 Percutaneous Endoscopic	0 Drainage Device 7 Autologous Tissue Substitute J Synthetic Substitute K Nonautologous Tissue Substitute Y Other Device	Z No Qualifier
X Upper Tendon Y Lower Tendon	X External	0 Drainage Device 7 Autologous Tissue Substitute J Synthetic Substitute K Nonautologous Tissue Substitute	Z No Qualifier

Non-OR 0LW[X,Y][3,4]YZ
Non-OR 0LW[X,Y]X[0,7,J,K]Z

0 Medical and Surgical
L Tendons
X Transfer Definition: Moving, without taking out, all or a portion of a body part to another location to take over the function of all or a portion of a body part
Explanation: The body part transferred remains connected to its vascular and nervous supply

Body Part Character 4	Approach Character 5	Device Character 6	Qualifier Character 7

0 Head and Neck Tendon
1 Shoulder Tendon, Right
2 Shoulder Tendon, Left
3 Upper Arm Tendon, Right
4 Upper Arm Tendon, Left
5 Lower Arm and Wrist Tendon, Right
6 Lower Arm and Wrist Tendon, Left
7 Hand Tendon, Right
8 Hand Tendon, Left
9 Trunk Tendon, Right
B Trunk Tendon, Left
C Thorax Tendon, Right
D Thorax Tendon, Left
F Abdomen Tendon, Right
G Abdomen Tendon, Left
H Perineum Tendon
J Hip Tendon, Right
K Hip Tendon, Left
L Upper Leg Tendon, Right
M Upper Leg Tendon, Left
N Lower Leg Tendon, Right
   Achilles tendon
P Lower Leg Tendon, Left
   See N Lower Leg Tendon, Right
Q Knee Tendon, Right
   Patellar tendon
R Knee Tendon, Left
   See Q Knee Tendon, Right
S Ankle Tendon, Right
T Ankle Tendon, Left
V Foot Tendon, Right
W Foot Tendon, Left
	0 Open
	4 Percutaneous Endoscopic
		Z No Device	Z No Qualifier

Bursae and Ligaments ØM2–ØMX

Character Meanings*

This Character Meaning table is provided as a guide to assist the user in the identification of character members that may be found in this section of code tables. It **SHOULD NOT** be used to build a PCS code.

Operation–Character 3		Body Part–Character 4		Approach–Character 5		Device–Character 6		Qualifier–Character 7	
2	Change	Ø	Head and Neck Bursa and Ligament	Ø	Open	Ø	Drainage Device	X	Diagnostic
5	Destruction	1	Shoulder Bursa and Ligament, Right	3	Percutaneous	7	Autologous Tissue Substitute	Z	No Qualifier
8	Division	2	Shoulder Bursa and Ligament, Left	4	Percutaneous Endoscopic	J	Synthetic Substitute		
9	Drainage	3	Elbow Bursa and Ligament, Right	X	External	K	Nonautologous Tissue Substitute		
B	Excision	4	Elbow Bursa and Ligament, Left			Y	Other Device		
C	Extirpation	5	Wrist Bursa and Ligament, Right			Z	No Device		
D	Extraction	6	Wrist Bursa and Ligament, Left						
H	Insertion	7	Hand Bursa and Ligament, Right						
J	Inspection	8	Hand Bursa and Ligament, Left						
M	Reattachment	9	Upper Extremity Bursa and Ligament, Right						
N	Release	B	Upper Extremity Bursa and Ligament, Left						
P	Removal	C	Upper Spine Bursa and Ligament						
Q	Repair	D	Lower Spine Bursa and Ligament						
R	Replacement	F	Sternum Bursa and Ligament						
S	Reposition	G	Rib(s) Bursa and Ligament						
T	Resection	H	Abdomen Bursa and Ligament, Right						
U	Supplement	J	Abdomen Bursa and Ligament, Left						
W	Revision	K	Perineum Bursa and Ligament						
X	Transfer	L	Hip Bursa and Ligament, Right						
		M	Hip Bursa and Ligament, Left						
		N	Knee Bursa and Ligament, Right						
		P	Knee Bursa and Ligament, Left						
		Q	Ankle Bursa and Ligament, Right						
		R	Ankle Bursa and Ligament, Left						
		S	Foot Bursa and Ligament, Right						
		T	Foot Bursa and Ligament, Left						
		V	Lower Extremity Bursa and Ligament, Right						
		W	Lower Extremity Bursa and Ligament, Left						
		X	Upper Bursa and Ligament						
		Y	Lower Bursa and Ligament						

* Includes synovial membrane.

AHA Coding Clinic for table ØMB
2018, 3Q, 17   Excisional debridement of periosteum

AHA Coding Clinic for table ØMM
2013, 3Q, 20   Superior labrum anterior posterior (SLAP) repair and subacromial decompression

AHA Coding Clinic for table ØMQ
2014, 3Q, 9   Interspinous ligamentoplasty

AHA Coding Clinic for table ØMT
2017, 2Q, 21   Arthroscopic anterior cruciate ligament revision using autograft with anterolateral ligament reconstruction

AHA Coding Clinic for table ØMU
2017, 2Q, 21   Arthroscopic anterior cruciate ligament revision using autograft with anterolateral ligament reconstruction

Bursae and Ligaments

Shoulder Ligaments

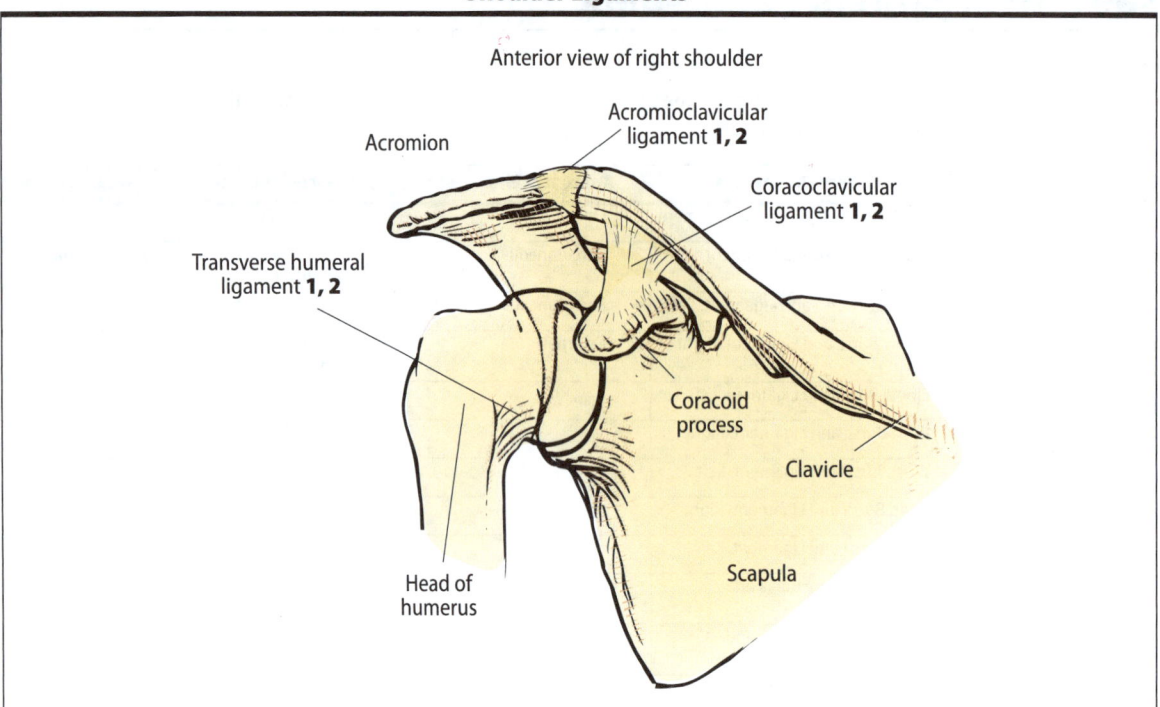

Anterior view of right shoulder

- Acromion
- Acromioclavicular ligament **1, 2**
- Coracoclavicular ligament **1, 2**
- Transverse humeral ligament **1, 2**
- Coracoid process
- Clavicle
- Head of humerus
- Scapula

Knee Bursae

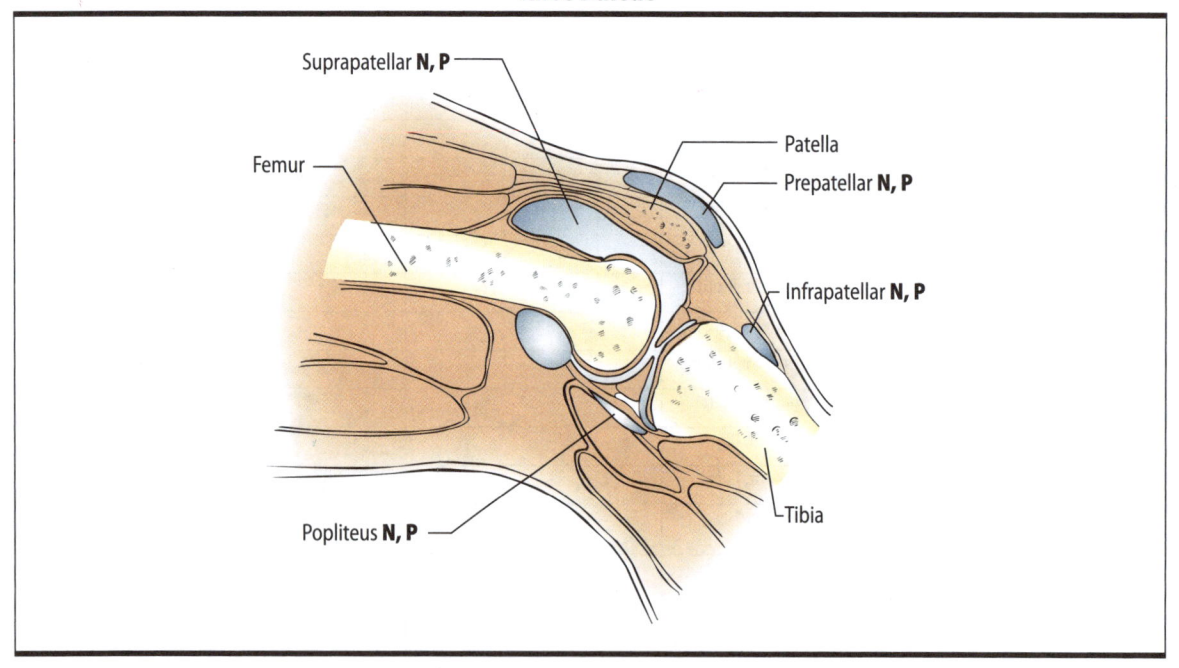

- Suprapatellar **N, P**
- Femur
- Patella
- Prepatellar **N, P**
- Infrapatellar **N, P**
- Popliteus **N, P**
- Tibia

Knee Ligaments

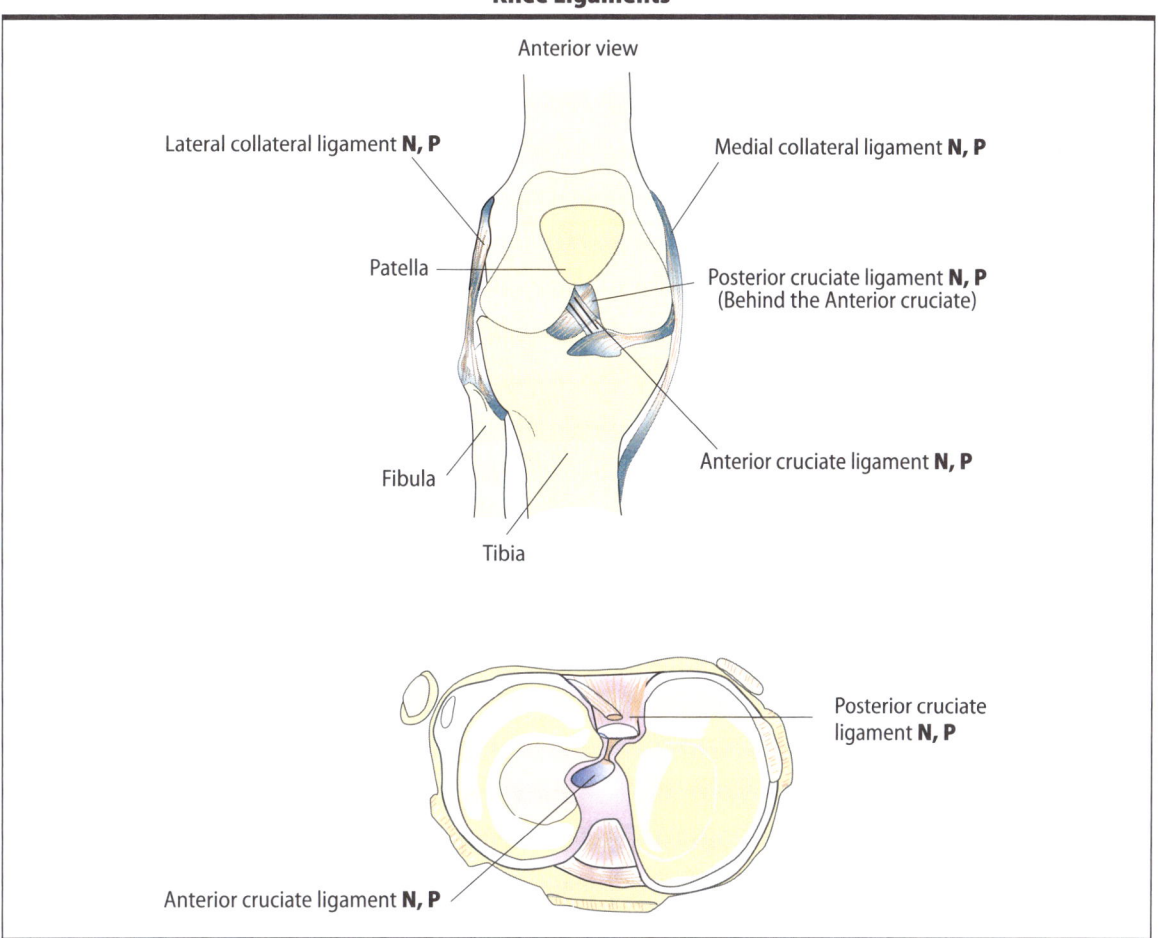

Anterior view

- Lateral collateral ligament **N, P**
- Medial collateral ligament **N, P**
- Patella
- Posterior cruciate ligament **N, P** (Behind the Anterior cruciate)
- Anterior cruciate ligament **N, P**
- Fibula
- Tibia

- Posterior cruciate ligament **N, P**
- Anterior cruciate ligament **N, P**

Wrist Ligaments

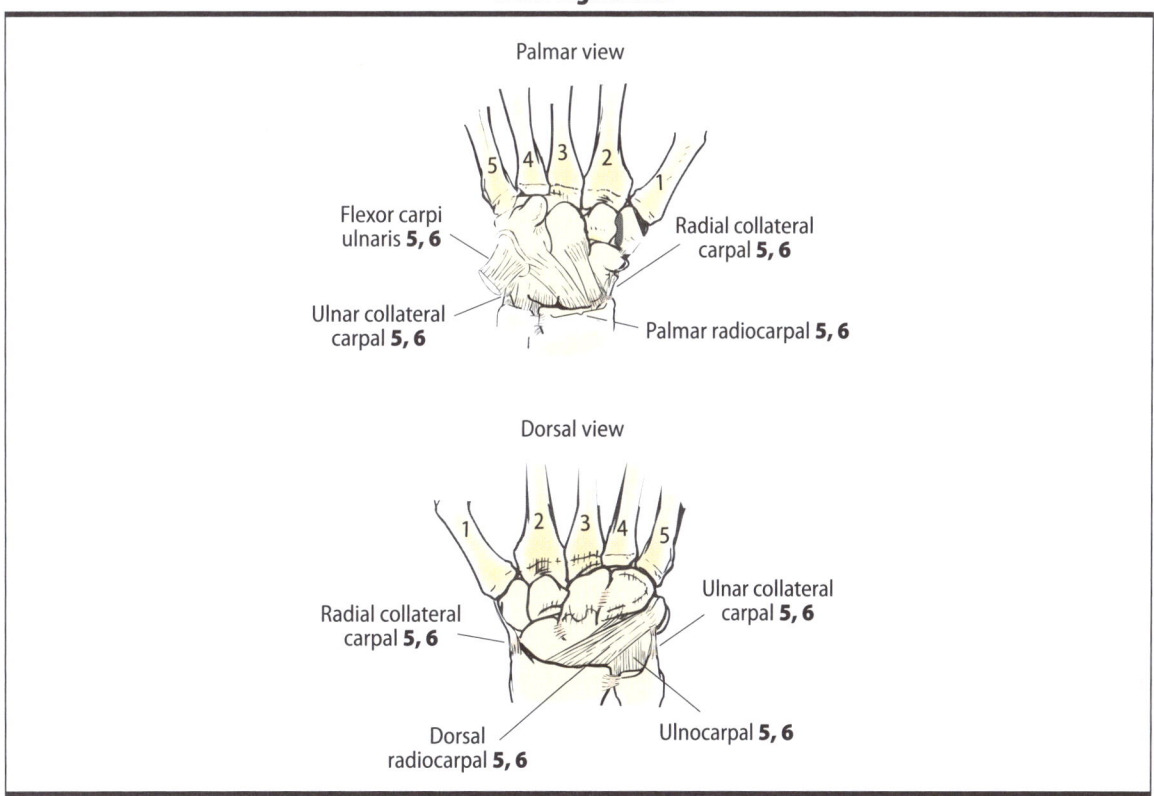

Palmar view

- Flexor carpi ulnaris **5, 6**
- Radial collateral carpal **5, 6**
- Ulnar collateral carpal **5, 6**
- Palmar radiocarpal **5, 6**

Dorsal view

- Radial collateral carpal **5, 6**
- Ulnar collateral carpal **5, 6**
- Dorsal radiocarpal **5, 6**
- Ulnocarpal **5, 6**

ØM2–ØM5 Bursae and Ligaments

Ø Medical and Surgical
M Bursae and Ligaments
2 Change — Definition: Taking out or off a device from a body part and putting back an identical or similar device in or on the same body part without cutting or puncturing the skin or a mucous membrane
Explanation: All CHANGE procedures are coded using the approach EXTERNAL

Body Part — Character 4	Approach — Character 5	Device — Character 6	Qualifier — Character 7
X Upper Bursa and Ligament Y Lower Bursa and Ligament	X External	Ø Drainage Device Y Other Device	Z No Qualifier

Non-OR   All body part, approach, device, and qualifier values

---

Ø Medical and Surgical
M Bursae and Ligaments
5 Destruction — Definition: Physical eradication of all or a portion of a body part by the direct use of energy, force, or a destructive agent
Explanation: None of the body part is physically taken out

Body Part — Character 4	Approach — Character 5	Device — Character 6	Qualifier — Character 7

Ø Head and Neck Bursa and Ligament
  Alar ligament of axis
  Cervical interspinous ligament
  Cervical intertransverse ligament
  Cervical ligamentum flavum
  Interspinous ligament, cervical
  Intertransverse ligament, cervical
  Lateral temporomandibular ligament
  Ligamentum flavum, cervical
  Sphenomandibular ligament
  Stylomandibular ligament
  Transverse ligament of atlas
1 Shoulder Bursa and Ligament, Right
  Acromioclavicular ligament
  Coracoacromial ligament
  Coracoclavicular ligament
  Coracohumeral ligament
  Costoclavicular ligament
  Glenohumeral ligament
  Interclavicular ligament
  Sternoclavicular ligament
  Subacromial bursa
  Transverse humeral ligament
  Transverse scapular ligament
2 Shoulder Bursa and Ligament, Left
  See 1 Shoulder Bursa and Ligament, Right
3 Elbow Bursa and Ligament, Right
  Annular ligament
  Olecranon bursa
  Radial collateral ligament
  Ulnar collateral ligament
4 Elbow Bursa and Ligament, Left
  See 3 Elbow Bursa and Ligament, Right
5 Wrist Bursa and Ligament, Right
  Palmar ulnocarpal ligament
  Radial collateral carpal ligament
  Radiocarpal ligament
  Radioulnar ligament
  Scapholunate ligament
  Ulnar collateral carpal ligament
6 Wrist Bursa and Ligament, Left
  See 5 Wrist Bursa and Ligament, Right
7 Hand Bursa and Ligament, Right
  Carpometacarpal ligament
  Intercarpal ligament
  Interphalangeal ligament
  Lunotriquetral ligament
  Metacarpal ligament
  Metacarpophalangeal ligament
  Pisohamate ligament
  Pisometacarpal ligament
  Scaphotrapezium ligament
8 Hand Bursa and Ligament, Left
  See 7 Hand Bursa and Ligament, Right
9 Upper Extremity Bursa and Ligament, Right
B Upper Extremity Bursa and Ligament, Left
C Upper Spine Bursa and Ligament
  Interspinous ligament, thoracic
  Intertransverse ligament, thoracic
  Ligamentum flavum, thoracic
  Supraspinous ligament
	D Lower Spine Bursa and Ligament
	  Iliolumbar ligament
	  Interspinous ligament, lumbar
	  Intertransverse ligament, lumbar
	  Ligamentum flavum, lumbar
	  Sacrococcygeal ligament
	  Sacroiliac ligament
	  Sacrospinous ligament
	  Sacrotuberous ligament
	  Supraspinous ligament
	F Sternum Bursa and Ligament
	  Costoxiphoid ligament
	  Sternocostal ligament
	G Rib(s) Bursa and Ligament
	  Costotransverse ligament
	H Abdomen Bursa and Ligament, Right
	J Abdomen Bursa and Ligament, Left
	K Perineum Bursa and Ligament
	L Hip Bursa and Ligament, Right
	  Iliofemoral ligament
	  Ischiofemoral ligament
	  Pubofemoral ligament
	  Transverse acetabular ligament
	  Trochanteric bursa
	M Hip Bursa and Ligament, Left
	  See L Hip Bursa and Ligament, Right
	N Knee Bursa and Ligament, Right
	  Anterior cruciate ligament (ACL)
	  Lateral collateral ligament (LCL)
	  Ligament of head of fibula
	  Medial collateral ligament (MCL)
	  Patellar ligament
	  Popliteal ligament
	  Posterior cruciate ligament (PCL)
	  Prepatellar bursa
	P Knee Bursa and Ligament, Left
	  See N Knee Bursa and Ligament, Right
	Q Ankle Bursa and Ligament, Right
	  Calcaneofibular ligament
	  Deltoid ligament
	  Ligament of the lateral malleolus
	  Talofibular ligament
	R Ankle Bursa and Ligament, Left
	  See Q Ankle Bursa and Ligament, Right
	S Foot Bursa and Ligament, Right
	  Calcaneocuboid ligament
	  Cuneonavicular ligament
	  Intercuneiform ligament
	  Interphalangeal ligament
	  Metatarsal ligament
	  Metatarsophalangeal ligament
	  Subtalar ligament
	  Talocalcaneal ligament
	  Talocalcaneonavicular ligament
	  Tarsometatarsal ligament
	T Foot Bursa and Ligament, Left
	  See S Foot Bursa and Ligament, Right
	V Lower Extremity Bursa and Ligament, Right
	W Lower Extremity Bursa and Ligament, Left
		Ø Open
		3 Percutaneous
		4 Percutaneous Endoscopic
			Z No Device	Z No Qualifier

0 Medical and Surgical
M Bursae and Ligaments
8 Division — Definition: Cutting into a body part, without draining fluids and/or gases from the body part, in order to separate or transect a body part
Explanation: All or a portion of the body part is separated into two or more portions

Body Part Character 4	Approach Character 5	Device Character 6	Qualifier Character 7
0 Head and Neck Bursa and Ligament Alar ligament of axis Cervical interspinous ligament Cervical intertransverse ligament Cervical ligamentum flavum Interspinous ligament, cervical Intertransverse ligament, cervical Lateral temporomandibular ligament Ligamentum flavum, cervical Sphenomandibular ligament Stylomandibular ligament Transverse ligament of atlas **1** Shoulder Bursa and Ligament, Right Acromioclavicular ligament Coracoacromial ligament Coracoclavicular ligament Coracohumeral ligament Costoclavicular ligament Glenohumeral ligament Interclavicular ligament Sternoclavicular ligament Subacromial bursa Transverse humeral ligament Transverse scapular ligament **2** Shoulder Bursa and Ligament, Left *See 1 Shoulder Bursa and Ligament, Right* **3** Elbow Bursa and Ligament, Right Annular ligament Olecranon bursa Radial collateral ligament Ulnar collateral ligament **4** Elbow Bursa and Ligament, Left *See 3 Elbow Bursa and Ligament, Right* **5** Wrist Bursa and Ligament, Right Palmar ulnocarpal ligament Radial collateral carpal ligament Radiocarpal ligament Radioulnar ligament Scapholunate ligament Ulnar collateral carpal ligament **6** Wrist Bursa and Ligament, Left *See 5 Wrist Bursa and Ligament, Right* **7** Hand Bursa and Ligament, Right Carpometacarpal ligament Intercarpal ligament Interphalangeal ligament Lunotriquetral ligament Metacarpal ligament Metacarpophalangeal ligament Pisohamate ligament Pisometacarpal ligament Scaphotrapezium ligament **8** Hand Bursa and Ligament, Left *See 7 Hand Bursa and Ligament, Right* **9** Upper Extremity Bursa and Ligament, Right **B** Upper Extremity Bursa and Ligament, Left **C** Upper Spine Bursa and Ligament Interspinous ligament, thoracic Intertransverse ligament, thoracic Ligamentum flavum, thoracic Supraspinous ligament	**D** Lower Spine Bursa and Ligament Iliolumbar ligament Interspinous ligament, lumbar Intertransverse ligament, lumbar Ligamentum flavum, lumbar Sacrococcygeal ligament Sacroiliac ligament Sacrospinous ligament Sacrotuberous ligament Supraspinous ligament **F** Sternum Bursa and Ligament Costoxiphoid ligament Sternocostal ligament **G** Rib(s) Bursa and Ligament Costotransverse ligament **H** Abdomen Bursa and Ligament, Right **J** Abdomen Bursa and Ligament, Left **K** Perineum Bursa and Ligament **L** Hip Bursa and Ligament, Right Iliofemoral ligament Ischiofemoral ligament Pubofemoral ligament Transverse acetabular ligament Trochanteric bursa **M** Hip Bursa and Ligament, Left *See L Hip Bursa and Ligament, Right* **N** Knee Bursa and Ligament, Right Anterior cruciate ligament (ACL) Lateral collateral ligament (LCL) Ligament of head of fibula Medial collateral ligament (MCL) Patellar ligament Popliteal ligament Posterior cruciate ligament (PCL) Prepatellar bursa **P** Knee Bursa and Ligament, Left *See N Knee Bursa and Ligament, Right* **Q** Ankle Bursa and Ligament, Right Calcaneofibular ligament Deltoid ligament Ligament of the lateral malleolus Talofibular ligament **R** Ankle Bursa and Ligament, Left *See Q Ankle Bursa and Ligament, Right* **S** Foot Bursa and Ligament, Right Calcaneocuboid ligament Cuneonavicular ligament Intercuneiform ligament Interphalangeal ligament Metatarsal ligament Metatarsophalangeal ligament Subtalar ligament Talocalcaneal ligament Talocalcaneonavicular ligament Tarsometatarsal ligament **T** Foot Bursa and Ligament, Left *See S Foot Bursa and Ligament, Right* **V** Lower Extremity Bursa and Ligament, Right **W** Lower Extremity Bursa and Ligament, Left	**0** Open **3** Percutaneous **4** Percutaneous Endoscopic	**Z** No Device	**Z** No Qualifier

0 Medical and Surgical
M Bursae and Ligaments
9 Drainage **Definition:** Taking or letting out fluids and/or gases from a body part
Explanation: The qualifier DIAGNOSTIC is used to identify drainage procedures that are biopsies

Body Part Character 4	Approach Character 5	Device Character 6	Qualifier Character 7
0 Head and Neck Bursa and Ligament Alar ligament of axis Cervical interspinous ligament Cervical intertransverse ligament Cervical ligamentum flavum Interspinous ligament, cervical Intertransverse ligament, cervical Lateral temporomandibular ligament Ligamentum flavum, cervical Sphenomandibular ligament Stylomandibular ligament Transverse ligament of atlas **1 Shoulder Bursa and Ligament, Right** Acromioclavicular ligament Coracoacromial ligament Coracoclavicular ligament Coracohumeral ligament Costoclavicular ligament Glenohumeral ligament Interclavicular ligament Sternoclavicular ligament Subacromial bursa Transverse humeral ligament Transverse scapular ligament **2 Shoulder Bursa and Ligament, Left** *See 1 Shoulder Bursa and Ligament, Right* **3 Elbow Bursa and Ligament, Right** Annular ligament Olecranon bursa Radial collateral ligament Ulnar collateral ligament **4 Elbow Bursa and Ligament, Left** *See 3 Elbow Bursa and Ligament, Right* **5 Wrist Bursa and Ligament, Right** Palmar ulnocarpal ligament Radial collateral carpal ligament Radiocarpal ligament Radioulnar ligament Scapholunate ligament Ulnar collateral carpal ligament **6 Wrist Bursa and Ligament, Left** *See 5 Wrist Bursa and Ligament, Right* **7 Hand Bursa and Ligament, Right** Carpometacarpal ligament Intercarpal ligament Interphalangeal ligament Lunotriquetral ligament Metacarpal ligament Metacarpophalangeal ligament Pisohamate ligament Pisometacarpal ligament Scaphotrapezium ligament **8 Hand Bursa and Ligament, Left** *See 7 Hand Bursa and Ligament, Right* **9 Upper Extremity Bursa and Ligament, Right** **B Upper Extremity Bursa and Ligament, Left** **C Upper Spine Bursa and Ligament** Interspinous ligament, thoracic Intertransverse ligament, thoracic Ligamentum flavum, thoracic Supraspinous ligament	**D Lower Spine Bursa and Ligament** Iliolumbar ligament Interspinous ligament, lumbar Intertransverse ligament, lumbar Ligamentum flavum, lumbar Sacrococcygeal ligament Sacroiliac ligament Sacrospinous ligament Sacrotuberous ligament Supraspinous ligament **F Sternum Bursa and Ligament** Costoxiphoid ligament Sternocostal ligament **G Rib(s) Bursa and Ligament** Costotransverse ligament **H Abdomen Bursa and Ligament, Right** **J Abdomen Bursa and Ligament, Left** **K Perineum Bursa and Ligament** **L Hip Bursa and Ligament, Right** Iliofemoral ligament Ischiofemoral ligament Pubofemoral ligament Transverse acetabular ligament Trochanteric bursa **M Hip Bursa and Ligament, Left** *See L Hip Bursa and Ligament, Right* **N Knee Bursa and Ligament, Right** Anterior cruciate ligament (ACL) Lateral collateral ligament (LCL) Ligament of head of fibula Medial collateral ligament (MCL) Patellar ligament Popliteal ligament Posterior cruciate ligament (PCL) Prepatellar bursa **P Knee Bursa and Ligament, Left** *See N Knee Bursa and Ligament, Right* **Q Ankle Bursa and Ligament, Right** Calcaneofibular ligament Deltoid ligament Ligament of the lateral malleolus Talofibular ligament **R Ankle Bursa and Ligament, Left** *See Q Ankle Bursa and Ligament, Right* **S Foot Bursa and Ligament, Right** Calcaneocuboid ligament Cuneonavicular ligament Intercuneiform ligament Interphalangeal ligament Metatarsal ligament Metatarsophalangeal ligament Subtalar ligament Talocalcaneal ligament Talocalcaneonavicular ligament Tarsometatarsal ligament **T Foot Bursa and Ligament, Left** *See S Foot Bursa and Ligament, Right* **V Lower Extremity Bursa and Ligament, Right** **W Lower Extremity Bursa and Ligament, Left**	**0** Open **3** Percutaneous **4** Percutaneous Endoscopic	**0** Drainage Device	**Z** No Qualifier

Non-OR 0M9[0,1,2,3,4,5,6,7,8,9,B,C,D,F,G,H,J,K,L,M,N,P,Q,R,S,T,V,W]30Z
Non-OR 0M9[1,2,3,4,7,8,9,B,C,D,F,G,H,J,K,L,M,V,W]40Z

0M9 Continued on next page

ICD-10-PCS 2025 — Bursae and Ligaments — ØM9–ØM9

ØM9 Continued

- Ø **Medical and Surgical**
- M **Bursae and Ligaments**
- 9 **Drainage**   Definition: Taking or letting out fluids and/or gases from a body part
  Explanation: The qualifier DIAGNOSTIC is used to identify drainage procedures that are biopsies

Body Part Character 4	Approach Character 5	Device Character 6	Qualifier Character 7
Ø **Head and Neck Bursa and Ligament** Alar ligament of axis Cervical interspinous ligament Cervical intertransverse ligament Cervical ligamentum flavum Interspinous ligament, cervical Intertransverse ligament, cervical Lateral temporomandibular ligament Ligamentum flavum, cervical Sphenomandibular ligament Stylomandibular ligament Transverse ligament of atlas 1 **Shoulder Bursa and Ligament, Right** Acromioclavicular ligament Coracoacromial ligament Coracoclavicular ligament Coracohumeral ligament Costoclavicular ligament Glenohumeral ligament Interclavicular ligament Sternoclavicular ligament Subacromial bursa Transverse humeral ligament Transverse scapular ligament 2 **Shoulder Bursa and Ligament, Left** See 1 Shoulder Bursa and Ligament, Right 3 **Elbow Bursa and Ligament, Right** Annular ligament Olecranon bursa Radial collateral ligament Ulnar collateral ligament 4 **Elbow Bursa and Ligament, Left** See 3 Elbow Bursa and Ligament, Right 5 **Wrist Bursa and Ligament, Right** Palmar ulnocarpal ligament Radial collateral carpal ligament Radiocarpal ligament Radioulnar ligament Scapholunate ligament Ulnar collateral carpal ligament 6 **Wrist Bursa and Ligament, Left** See 5 Wrist Bursa and Ligament, Right 7 **Hand Bursa and Ligament, Right** Carpometacarpal ligament Intercarpal ligament Interphalangeal ligament Lunotriquetral ligament Metacarpal ligament Metacarpophalangeal ligament Pisohamate ligament Pisometacarpal ligament Scaphotrapezium ligament 8 **Hand Bursa and Ligament, Left** See 7 Hand Bursa and Ligament, Right 9 **Upper Extremity Bursa and Ligament, Right** B **Upper Extremity Bursa and Ligament, Left** C **Upper Spine Bursa and Ligament** Interspinous ligament, thoracic Intertransverse ligament, thoracic Ligamentum flavum, thoracic Supraspinous ligament	Ø Open 3 Percutaneous 4 Percutaneous Endoscopic	Z No Device	X Diagnostic Z No Qualifier
D **Lower Spine Bursa and Ligament** Iliolumbar ligament Interspinous ligament, lumbar Intertransverse ligament, lumbar Ligamentum flavum, lumbar Sacrococcygeal ligament Sacroiliac ligament Sacrospinous ligament Sacrotuberous ligament Supraspinous ligament F **Sternum Bursa and Ligament** Costoxiphoid ligament Sternocostal ligament G **Rib(s) Bursa and Ligament** Costotransverse ligament H **Abdomen Bursa and Ligament, Right** J **Abdomen Bursa and Ligament, Left** K **Perineum Bursa and Ligament** L **Hip Bursa and Ligament, Right** Iliofemoral ligament Ischiofemoral ligament Pubofemoral ligament Transverse acetabular ligament Trochanteric bursa M **Hip Bursa and Ligament, Left** See L Hip Bursa and Ligament, Right N **Knee Bursa and Ligament, Right** Anterior cruciate ligament (ACL) Lateral collateral ligament (LCL) Ligament of head of fibula Medial collateral ligament (MCL) Patellar ligament Popliteal ligament Posterior cruciate ligament (PCL) Prepatellar bursa P **Knee Bursa and Ligament, Left** See N Knee Bursa and Ligament, Right Q **Ankle Bursa and Ligament, Right** Calcaneofibular ligament Deltoid ligament Ligament of the lateral malleolus Talofibular ligament R **Ankle Bursa and Ligament, Left** See Q Ankle Bursa and Ligament, Right S **Foot Bursa and Ligament, Right** Calcaneocuboid ligament Cuneonavicular ligament Intercuneiform ligament Interphalangeal ligament Metatarsal ligament Metatarsophalangeal ligament Subtalar ligament Talocalcaneal ligament Talocalcaneonavicular ligament Tarsometatarsal ligament T **Foot Bursa and Ligament, Left** See S Foot Bursa and Ligament, Right V **Lower Extremity Bursa and Ligament, Right** W **Lower Extremity Bursa and Ligament, Left**			

Non-OR   ØM9[Ø,1,2,3,4,5,6,7,8,C,D,F,G,L,M,N,P,Q,R,S,T][Ø,3,4]ZX
Non-OR   ØM9[Ø,1,2,3,4,5,6,7,8,9,B,C,D,F,G,H,J,K,L,M,N,P,Q,R,S,T,V,W]3ZZ
Non-OR   ØM9[Ø,5,6,7,8,9,B,C,D,F,G,H,J,K,N,P,Q,R,S,T,V,W]4ZZ

0 **Medical and Surgical**
M **Bursae and Ligaments**
B **Excision** Definition: Cutting out or off, without replacement, a portion of a body part
Explanation: The qualifier DIAGNOSTIC is used to identify excision procedures that are biopsies

Body Part Character 4	Approach Character 5	Device Character 6	Qualifier Character 7
0 Head and Neck Bursa and Ligament Alar ligament of axis Cervical interspinous ligament Cervical intertransverse ligament Cervical ligamentum flavum Interspinous ligament, cervical Intertransverse ligament, cervical Lateral temporomandibular ligament Ligamentum flavum, cervical Sphenomandibular ligament Stylomandibular ligament Transverse ligament of atlas **1 Shoulder Bursa and Ligament, Right** Acromioclavicular ligament Coracoacromial ligament Coracoclavicular ligament Coracohumeral ligament Costoclavicular ligament Glenohumeral ligament Interclavicular ligament Sternoclavicular ligament Subacromial bursa Transverse humeral ligament Transverse scapular ligament **2 Shoulder Bursa and Ligament, Left** See 1 Shoulder Bursa and Ligament, Right **3 Elbow Bursa and Ligament, Right** Annular ligament Olecranon bursa Radial collateral ligament Ulnar collateral ligament **4 Elbow Bursa and Ligament, Left** See 3 Elbow Bursa and Ligament, Right **5 Wrist Bursa and Ligament, Right** Palmar ulnocarpal ligament Radial collateral carpal ligament Radiocarpal ligament Radioulnar ligament Scapholunate ligament Ulnar collateral carpal ligament **6 Wrist Bursa and Ligament, Left** See 5 Wrist Bursa and Ligament, Right **7 Hand Bursa and Ligament, Right** Carpometacarpal ligament Intercarpal ligament Interphalangeal ligament Lunotriquetral ligament Metacarpal ligament Metacarpophalangeal ligament Pisohamate ligament Pisometacarpal ligament Scaphotrapezium ligament **8 Hand Bursa and Ligament, Left** See 7 Hand Bursa and Ligament, Right **9 Upper Extremity Bursa and Ligament, Right** **B Upper Extremity Bursa and Ligament, Left** **C Upper Spine Bursa and Ligament** Interspinous ligament, thoracic Intertransverse ligament, thoracic Ligamentum flavum, thoracic Supraspinous ligament **D Lower Spine Bursa and Ligament** Iliolumbar ligament Interspinous ligament, lumbar Intertransverse ligament, lumbar Ligamentum flavum, lumbar Sacrococcygeal ligament Sacroiliac ligament Sacrospinous ligament Sacrotuberous ligament Supraspinous ligament **F Sternum Bursa and Ligament** Costoxiphoid ligament Sternocostal ligament **G Rib(s) Bursa and Ligament** Costotransverse ligament **H Abdomen Bursa and Ligament, Right** **J Abdomen Bursa and Ligament, Left** **K Perineum Bursa and Ligament** **L Hip Bursa and Ligament, Right** Iliofemoral ligament Ischiofemoral ligament Pubofemoral ligament Transverse acetabular ligament Trochanteric bursa **M Hip Bursa and Ligament, Left** See L Hip Bursa and Ligament, Right **N Knee Bursa and Ligament, Right** Anterior cruciate ligament (ACL) Lateral collateral ligament (LCL) Ligament of head of fibula Medial collateral ligament (MCL) Patellar ligament Popliteal ligament Posterior cruciate ligament (PCL) Prepatellar bursa **P Knee Bursa and Ligament, Left** See N Knee Bursa and Ligament, Right **Q Ankle Bursa and Ligament, Right** Calcaneofibular ligament Deltoid ligament Ligament of the lateral malleolus Talofibular ligament **R Ankle Bursa and Ligament, Left** See Q Ankle Bursa and Ligament, Right **S Foot Bursa and Ligament, Right** Calcaneocuboid ligament Cuneonavicular ligament Intercuneiform ligament Interphalangeal ligament Metatarsal ligament Metatarsophalangeal ligament Subtalar ligament Talocalcaneal ligament Talocalcaneonavicular ligament Tarsometatarsal ligament **T Foot Bursa and Ligament, Left** See S Foot Bursa and Ligament, Right **V Lower Extremity Bursa and Ligament, Right** **W Lower Extremity Bursa and Ligament, Left**	**0** Open **3** Percutaneous **4** Percutaneous Endoscopic	**Z** No Device	**X** Diagnostic **Z** No Qualifier

Non-OR ØMB[0,1,2,3,4,5,6,7,8,B,C,D,F,G,L,M,N,P,Q,R,S,T][0,3,4]ZX
Non-OR ØMB94ZX

0　Medical and Surgical
M　Bursae and Ligaments
C　Extirpation　Definition: Taking or cutting out solid matter from a body part
　　　　　　　　　Explanation: The solid matter may be an abnormal byproduct of a biological function or a foreign body; it may be imbedded in a body part or in the lumen of a tubular body part. The solid matter may or may not have been previously broken into pieces.

Body Part Character 4	Approach Character 5	Device Character 6	Qualifier Character 7
0 Head and Neck Bursa and Ligament 　Alar ligament of axis 　Cervical interspinous ligament 　Cervical intertransverse ligament 　Cervical ligamentum flavum 　Interspinous ligament, cervical 　Intertransverse ligament, cervical 　Lateral temporomandibular ligament 　Ligamentum flavum, cervical 　Sphenomandibular ligament 　Stylomandibular ligament 　Transverse ligament of atlas **1** Shoulder Bursa and Ligament, Right 　Acromioclavicular ligament 　Coracoacromial ligament 　Coracoclavicular ligament 　Coracohumeral ligament 　Costoclavicular ligament 　Glenohumeral ligament 　Interclavicular ligament 　Sternoclavicular ligament 　Subacromial bursa 　Transverse humeral ligament 　Transverse scapular ligament **2** Shoulder Bursa and Ligament, Left 　*See* 1 Shoulder Bursa and Ligament, Right **3** Elbow Bursa and Ligament, Right 　Annular ligament 　Olecranon bursa 　Radial collateral ligament 　Ulnar collateral ligament **4** Elbow Bursa and Ligament, Left 　*See* 3 Elbow Bursa and Ligament, Right **5** Wrist Bursa and Ligament, Right 　Palmar ulnocarpal ligament 　Radial collateral carpal ligament 　Radiocarpal ligament 　Radioulnar ligament 　Scapholunate ligament 　Ulnar collateral carpal ligament **6** Wrist Bursa and Ligament, Left 　*See* 5 Wrist Bursa and Ligament, Right **7** Hand Bursa and Ligament, Right 　Carpometacarpal ligament 　Intercarpal ligament 　Interphalangeal ligament 　Lunotriquetral ligament 　Metacarpal ligament 　Metacarpophalangeal ligament 　Pisohamate ligament 　Pisometacarpal ligament 　Scaphotrapezium ligament **8** Hand Bursa and Ligament, Left 　*See* 7 Hand Bursa and Ligament, Right **9** Upper Extremity Bursa and Ligament, Right **B** Upper Extremity Bursa and Ligament, Left **C** Upper Spine Bursa and Ligament 　Interspinous ligament, thoracic 　Intertransverse ligament, thoracic 　Ligamentum flavum, thoracic 　Supraspinous ligament	**0** Open **3** Percutaneous **4** Percutaneous Endoscopic	**Z** No Device	**Z** No Qualifier

D Lower Spine Bursa and Ligament
　Iliolumbar ligament
　Interspinous ligament, lumbar
　Intertransverse ligament, lumbar
　Ligamentum flavum, lumbar
　Sacrococcygeal ligament
　Sacroiliac ligament
　Sacrospinous ligament
　Sacrotuberous ligament
　Supraspinous ligament
F Sternum Bursa and Ligament
　Costoxiphoid ligament
　Sternocostal ligament
G Rib(s) Bursa and Ligament
　Costotransverse ligament
H Abdomen Bursa and Ligament, Right
J Abdomen Bursa and Ligament, Left
K Perineum Bursa and Ligament
L Hip Bursa and Ligament, Right
　Iliofemoral ligament
　Ischiofemoral ligament
　Pubofemoral ligament
　Transverse acetabular ligament
　Trochanteric bursa
M Hip Bursa and Ligament, Left
　See L Hip Bursa and Ligament, Right
N Knee Bursa and Ligament, Right
　Anterior cruciate ligament (ACL)
　Lateral collateral ligament (LCL)
　Ligament of head of fibula
　Medial collateral ligament (MCL)
　Patellar ligament
　Popliteal ligament
　Posterior cruciate ligament (PCL)
　Prepatellar bursa
P Knee Bursa and Ligament, Left
　See N Knee Bursa and Ligament, Right
Q Ankle Bursa and Ligament, Right
　Calcaneofibular ligament
　Deltoid ligament
　Ligament of the lateral malleolus
　Talofibular ligament
R Ankle Bursa and Ligament, Left
　See Q Ankle Bursa and Ligament, Right
S Foot Bursa and Ligament, Right
　Calcaneocuboid ligament
　Cuneonavicular ligament
　Intercuneiform ligament
　Interphalangeal ligament
　Metatarsal ligament
　Metatarsophalangeal ligament
　Subtalar ligament
　Talocalcaneal ligament
　Talocalcaneonavicular ligament
　Tarsometatarsal ligament
T Foot Bursa and Ligament, Left
　See S Foot Bursa and Ligament, Right
V Lower Extremity Bursa and Ligament, Right
W Lower Extremity Bursa and Ligament, Left

0 Medical and Surgical
M Bursae and Ligaments
D Extraction

Definition: Pulling or stripping out or off all or a portion of a body part by the use of force
Explanation: The qualifier DIAGNOSTIC is used to identify extraction procedures that are biopsies

Body Part Character 4	Approach Character 5	Device Character 6	Qualifier Character 7
0 Head and Neck Bursa and Ligament Alar ligament of axis Cervical interspinous ligament Cervical intertransverse ligament Cervical ligamentum flavum Interspinous ligament, cervical Intertransverse ligament, cervical Lateral temporomandibular ligament Ligamentum flavum, cervical Sphenomandibular ligament Stylomandibular ligament Transverse ligament of atlas **1 Shoulder Bursa and Ligament, Right** Acromioclavicular ligament Coracoacromial ligament Coracoclavicular ligament Coracohumeral ligament Costoclavicular ligament Glenohumeral ligament Interclavicular ligament Sternoclavicular ligament Subacromial bursa Transverse humeral ligament Transverse scapular ligament **2 Shoulder Bursa and Ligament, Left** See 1 Shoulder Bursa and Ligament, Right **3 Elbow Bursa and Ligament, Right** Annular ligament Olecranon bursa Radial collateral ligament Ulnar collateral ligament **4 Elbow Bursa and Ligament, Left** See 3 Elbow Bursa and Ligament, Right **5 Wrist Bursa and Ligament, Right** Palmar ulnocarpal ligament Radial collateral carpal ligament Radiocarpal ligament Radioulnar ligament Scapholunate ligament Ulnar collateral carpal ligament **6 Wrist Bursa and Ligament, Left** See 5 Wrist Bursa and Ligament, Right **7 Hand Bursa and Ligament, Right** Carpometacarpal ligament Intercarpal ligament Interphalangeal ligament Lunotriquetral ligament Metacarpal ligament Metacarpophalangeal ligament Pisohamate ligament Pisometacarpal ligament Scaphotrapezium ligament **8 Hand Bursa and Ligament, Left** See 7 Hand Bursa and Ligament, Right **9 Upper Extremity Bursa and Ligament, Right** **B Upper Extremity Bursa and Ligament, Left** **C Upper Spine Bursa and Ligament** Interspinous ligament, thoracic Intertransverse ligament, thoracic Ligamentum flavum, thoracic Supraspinous ligament **D Lower Spine Bursa and Ligament** Iliolumbar ligament Interspinous ligament, lumbar Intertransverse ligament, lumbar Ligamentum flavum, lumbar Sacrococcygeal ligament Sacroiliac ligament Sacrospinous ligament Sacrotuberous ligament Supraspinous ligament **F Sternum Bursa and Ligament** Costoxiphoid ligament Sternocostal ligament **G Rib(s) Bursa and Ligament** Costotransverse ligament **H Abdomen Bursa and Ligament, Right** **J Abdomen Bursa and Ligament, Left** **K Perineum Bursa and Ligament** **L Hip Bursa and Ligament, Right** Iliofemoral ligament Ischiofemoral ligament Pubofemoral ligament Transverse acetabular ligament Trochanteric bursa **M Hip Bursa and Ligament, Left** See L Hip Bursa and Ligament, Right **N Knee Bursa and Ligament, Right** Anterior cruciate ligament (ACL) Lateral collateral ligament (LCL) Ligament of head of fibula Medial collateral ligament (MCL) Patellar ligament Popliteal ligament Posterior cruciate ligament (PCL) Prepatellar bursa **P Knee Bursa and Ligament, Left** See N Knee Bursa and Ligament, Right **Q Ankle Bursa and Ligament, Right** Calcaneofibular ligament Deltoid ligament Ligament of the lateral malleolus Talofibular ligament **R Ankle Bursa and Ligament, Left** See Q Ankle Bursa and Ligament, Right **S Foot Bursa and Ligament, Right** Calcaneocuboid ligament Cuneonavicular ligament Intercuneiform ligament Interphalangeal ligament Metatarsal ligament Metatarsophalangeal ligament Subtalar ligament Talocalcaneal ligament Talocalcaneonavicular ligament Tarsometatarsal ligament **T Foot Bursa and Ligament, Left** See S Foot Bursa and Ligament, Right **V Lower Extremity Bursa and Ligament, Right** **W Lower Extremity Bursa and Ligament, Left**	**0** Open **3** Percutaneous **4** Percutaneous Endoscopic	**Z** No Device	**Z** No Qualifier

ICD-10-PCS 2025 — Bursae and Ligaments — 0MH–0MJ

0 Medical and Surgical
M Bursae and Ligaments
H Insertion   Definition: Putting in a nonbiological appliance that monitors, assists, performs, or prevents a physiological function but does not physically take the place of a body part
Explanation: None

Body Part Character 4	Approach Character 5	Device Character 6	Qualifier Character 7
X Upper Bursa and Ligament Y Lower Bursa and Ligament	0 Open 3 Percutaneous 4 Percutaneous Endoscopic	Y Other Device	Z No Qualifier

Non-OR   0MH[X,Y][3,4]YZ

0 Medical and Surgical
M Bursae and Ligaments
J Inspection   Definition: Visually and/or manually exploring a body part
Explanation: Visual exploration may be performed with or without optical instrumentation. Manual exploration may be performed directly or through intervening body layers.

Body Part Character 4	Approach Character 5	Device Character 6	Qualifier Character 7
X Upper Bursa and Ligament Y Lower Bursa and Ligament	0 Open 3 Percutaneous 4 Percutaneous Endoscopic X External	Z No Device	Z No Qualifier

Non-OR   0MJ[X,Y][3,X]ZZ

- **0** Medical and Surgical
- **M** Bursae and Ligaments
- **M** Reattachment **Definition:** Putting back in or on all or a portion of a separated body part to its normal location or other suitable location
  Explanation: Vascular circulation and nervous pathways may or may not be reestablished

Body Part Character 4	Approach Character 5	Device Character 6	Qualifier Character 7
0 Head and Neck Bursa and Ligament 　Alar ligament of axis 　Cervical interspinous ligament 　Cervical intertransverse ligament 　Cervical ligamentum flavum 　Interspinous ligament, cervical 　Intertransverse ligament, cervical 　Lateral temporomandibular ligament 　Ligamentum flavum, cervical 　Sphenomandibular ligament 　Stylomandibular ligament 　Transverse ligament of atlas **1** Shoulder Bursa and Ligament, Right 　Acromioclavicular ligament 　Coracoacromial ligament 　Coracoclavicular ligament 　Coracohumeral ligament 　Costoclavicular ligament 　Glenohumeral ligament 　Interclavicular ligament 　Sternoclavicular ligament 　Subacromial bursa 　Transverse humeral ligament 　Transverse scapular ligament **2** Shoulder Bursa and Ligament, Left 　See **1** Shoulder Bursa and Ligament, Right **3** Elbow Bursa and Ligament, Right 　Annular ligament 　Olecranon bursa 　Radial collateral ligament 　Ulnar collateral ligament **4** Elbow Bursa and Ligament, Left 　See **3** Elbow Bursa and Ligament, Right **5** Wrist Bursa and Ligament, Right 　Palmar ulnocarpal ligament 　Radial collateral carpal ligament 　Radiocarpal ligament 　Radioulnar ligament 　Scapholunate ligament 　Ulnar collateral carpal ligament **6** Wrist Bursa and Ligament, Left 　See **5** Wrist Bursa and Ligament, Right **7** Hand Bursa and Ligament, Right 　Carpometacarpal ligament 　Intercarpal ligament 　Interphalangeal ligament 　Lunotriquetral ligament 　Metacarpal ligament 　Metacarpophalangeal ligament 　Pisohamate ligament 　Pisometacarpal ligament 　Scaphotrapezium ligament **8** Hand Bursa and Ligament, Left 　See **7** Hand Bursa and Ligament, Right **9** Upper Extremity Bursa and Ligament, Right **B** Upper Extremity Bursa and Ligament, Left **C** Upper Spine Bursa and Ligament 　Interspinous ligament, thoracic 　Intertransverse ligament, thoracic 　Ligamentum flavum, thoracic 　Supraspinous ligament **D** Lower Spine Bursa and Ligament 　Iliolumbar ligament 　Interspinous ligament, lumbar 　Intertransverse ligament, lumbar 　Ligamentum flavum, lumbar 　Sacrococcygeal ligament 　Sacroiliac ligament 　Sacrospinous ligament 　Sacrotuberous ligament 　Supraspinous ligament **F** Sternum Bursa and Ligament 　Costoxiphoid ligament 　Sternocostal ligament **G** Rib(s) Bursa and Ligament 　Costotransverse ligament **H** Abdomen Bursa and Ligament, Right **J** Abdomen Bursa and Ligament, Left **K** Perineum Bursa and Ligament **L** Hip Bursa and Ligament, Right 　Iliofemoral ligament 　Ischiofemoral ligament 　Pubofemoral ligament 　Transverse acetabular ligament 　Trochanteric bursa **M** Hip Bursa and Ligament, Left 　See **L** Hip Bursa and Ligament, Right **N** Knee Bursa and Ligament, Right 　Anterior cruciate ligament (ACL) 　Lateral collateral ligament (LCL) 　Ligament of head of fibula 　Medial collateral ligament (MCL) 　Patellar ligament 　Popliteal ligament 　Posterior cruciate ligament (PCL) 　Prepatellar bursa **P** Knee Bursa and Ligament, Left 　See **N** Knee Bursa and Ligament, Right **Q** Ankle Bursa and Ligament, Right 　Calcaneofibular ligament 　Deltoid ligament 　Ligament of the lateral malleolus 　Talofibular ligament **R** Ankle Bursa and Ligament, Left 　See **Q** Ankle Bursa and Ligament, Right **S** Foot Bursa and Ligament, Right 　Calcaneocuboid ligament 　Cuneonavicular ligament 　Intercuneiform ligament 　Interphalangeal ligament 　Metatarsal ligament 　Metatarsophalangeal ligament 　Subtalar ligament 　Talocalcaneal ligament 　Talocalcaneonavicular ligament 　Tarsometatarsal ligament **T** Foot Bursa and Ligament, Left 　See **S** Foot Bursa and Ligament, Right **V** Lower Extremity Bursa and Ligament, Right **W** Lower Extremity Bursa and Ligament, Left	**0** Open **4** Percutaneous Endoscopic	**Z** No Device	**Z** No Qualifier

0 Medical and Surgical
M Bursae and Ligaments
N Release Definition: Freeing a body part from an abnormal physical constraint by cutting or by the use of force
Explanation: Some of the restraining tissue may be taken out but none of the body part is taken out

Body Part Character 4	Approach Character 5	Device Character 6	Qualifier Character 7
0 Head and Neck Bursa and Ligament Alar ligament of axis Cervical interspinous ligament Cervical intertransverse ligament Cervical ligamentum flavum Interspinous ligament, cervical Intertransverse ligament, cervical Lateral temporomandibular ligament Ligamentum flavum, cervical Sphenomandibular ligament Stylomandibular ligament Transverse ligament of atlas **1 Shoulder Bursa and Ligament, Right** Acromioclavicular ligament Coracoacromial ligament Coracoclavicular ligament Coracohumeral ligament Costoclavicular ligament Glenohumeral ligament Interclavicular ligament Sternoclavicular ligament Subacromial bursa Transverse humeral ligament Transverse scapular ligament **2 Shoulder Bursa and Ligament, Left** *See 1 Shoulder Bursa and Ligament, Right* **3 Elbow Bursa and Ligament, Right** Annular ligament Olecranon bursa Radial collateral ligament Ulnar collateral ligament **4 Elbow Bursa and Ligament, Left** *See 3 Elbow Bursa and Ligament, Right* **5 Wrist Bursa and Ligament, Right** Palmar ulnocarpal ligament Radial collateral carpal ligament Radiocarpal ligament Radioulnar ligament Scapholunate ligament Ulnar collateral carpal ligament **6 Wrist Bursa and Ligament, Left** *See 5 Wrist Bursa and Ligament, Right* **7 Hand Bursa and Ligament, Right** Carpometacarpal ligament Intercarpal ligament Interphalangeal ligament Lunotriquetral ligament Metacarpal ligament Metacarpophalangeal ligament Pisohamate ligament Pisometacarpal ligament Scaphotrapezium ligament **8 Hand Bursa and Ligament, Left** *See 7 Hand Bursa and Ligament, Right* **9 Upper Extremity Bursa and Ligament, Right** **B Upper Extremity Bursa and Ligament, Left** **C Upper Spine Bursa and Ligament** Interspinous ligament, thoracic Intertransverse ligament, thoracic Ligamentum flavum, thoracic Supraspinous ligament **D Lower Spine Bursa and Ligament** Iliolumbar ligament Interspinous ligament, lumbar Intertransverse ligament, lumbar Ligamentum flavum, lumbar Sacrococcygeal ligament Sacroiliac ligament Sacrospinous ligament Sacrotuberous ligament Supraspinous ligament **F Sternum Bursa and Ligament** Costoxiphoid ligament Sternocostal ligament **G Rib(s) Bursa and Ligament** Costotransverse ligament **H Abdomen Bursa and Ligament, Right** **J Abdomen Bursa and Ligament, Left** **K Perineum Bursa and Ligament** **L Hip Bursa and Ligament, Right** Iliofemoral ligament Ischiofemoral ligament Pubofemoral ligament Transverse acetabular ligament Trochanteric bursa **M Hip Bursa and Ligament, Left** *See L Hip Bursa and Ligament, Right* **N Knee Bursa and Ligament, Right** Anterior cruciate ligament (ACL) Lateral collateral ligament (LCL) Ligament of head of fibula Medial collateral ligament (MCL) Patellar ligament Popliteal ligament Posterior cruciate ligament (PCL) Prepatellar bursa **P Knee Bursa and Ligament, Left** *See N Knee Bursa and Ligament, Right* **Q Ankle Bursa and Ligament, Right** Calcaneofibular ligament Deltoid ligament Ligament of the lateral malleolus Talofibular ligament **R Ankle Bursa and Ligament, Left** *See Q Ankle Bursa and Ligament, Right* **S Foot Bursa and Ligament, Right** Calcaneocuboid ligament Cuneonavicular ligament Intercuneiform ligament Interphalangeal ligament Metatarsal ligament Metatarsophalangeal ligament Subtalar ligament Talocalcaneal ligament Talocalcaneonavicular ligament Tarsometatarsal ligament **T Foot Bursa and Ligament, Left** *See S Foot Bursa and Ligament, Right* **V Lower Extremity Bursa and Ligament, Right** **W Lower Extremity Bursa and Ligament, Left**	**0** Open **3** Percutaneous **4** Percutaneous Endoscopic **X** External	**Z** No Device	**Z** No Qualifier

Non-OR 0MN[0,1,2,3,4,5,6,7,8,9,B,C,D,F,G,H,J,K,L,M,N,P,Q,R,S,T,V,W]XZZ

0MP–0MP Bursae and Ligaments ICD-10-PCS 2025

0 Medical and Surgical
M Bursae and Ligaments
P Removal Definition: Taking out or off a device from a body part
Explanation: If a device is taken out and a similar device put in without cutting or puncturing the skin or mucous membrane, the procedure is coded to the root operation CHANGE. Otherwise, the procedure for taking out a device is coded to the root operation REMOVAL.

Body Part Character 4	Approach Character 5	Device Character 6	Qualifier Character 7
X Upper Bursa and Ligament Y Lower Bursa and Ligament	0 Open 3 Percutaneous 4 Percutaneous Endoscopic	0 Drainage Device 7 Autologous Tissue Substitute J Synthetic Substitute K Nonautologous Tissue Substitute Y Other Device	Z No Qualifier
X Upper Bursa and Ligament Y Lower Bursa and Ligament	X External	0 Drainage Device	Z No Qualifier

Non-OR 0MP[X,Y]30Z
Non-OR 0MP[X,Y][3,4]YZ
Non-OR 0MP[X,Y]X0Z

ICD-10-PCS 2025 — Bursae and Ligaments — ØMQ–ØMQ

- Ø Medical and Surgical
- M Bursae and Ligaments
- Q Repair Definition: Restoring, to the extent possible, a body part to its normal anatomic structure and function
  Explanation: Used only when the method to accomplish the repair is not one of the other root operations

Body Part Character 4	Approach Character 5	Device Character 6	Qualifier Character 7
Ø Head and Neck Bursa and Ligament Alar ligament of axis Cervical interspinous ligament Cervical intertransverse ligament Cervical ligamentum flavum Interspinous ligament, cervical Intertransverse ligament, cervical Lateral temporomandibular ligament Ligamentum flavum, cervical Sphenomandibular ligament Stylomandibular ligament Transverse ligament of atlas **1 Shoulder Bursa and Ligament, Right** Acromioclavicular ligament Coracoacromial ligament Coracoclavicular ligament Coracohumeral ligament Costoclavicular ligament Glenohumeral ligament Interclavicular ligament Sternoclavicular ligament Subacromial bursa Transverse humeral ligament Transverse scapular ligament **2 Shoulder Bursa and Ligament, Left** *See 1 Shoulder Bursa and Ligament, Right* **3 Elbow Bursa and Ligament, Right** Annular ligament Olecranon bursa Radial collateral ligament Ulnar collateral ligament **4 Elbow Bursa and Ligament, Left** *See 3 Elbow Bursa and Ligament, Right* **5 Wrist Bursa and Ligament, Right** Palmar ulnocarpal ligament Radial collateral carpal ligament Radiocarpal ligament Radioulnar ligament Scapholunate ligament Ulnar collateral carpal ligament **6 Wrist Bursa and Ligament, Left** *See 5 Wrist Bursa and Ligament, Right* **7 Hand Bursa and Ligament, Right** Carpometacarpal ligament Intercarpal ligament Interphalangeal ligament Lunotriquetral ligament Metacarpal ligament Metacarpophalangeal ligament Pisohamate ligament Pisometacarpal ligament Scaphotrapezium ligament **8 Hand Bursa and Ligament, Left** *See 7 Hand Bursa and Ligament, Right* **9 Upper Extremity Bursa and Ligament, Right** **B Upper Extremity Bursa and Ligament, Left** **C Upper Spine Bursa and Ligament** Interspinous ligament, thoracic Intertransverse ligament, thoracic Ligamentum flavum, thoracic Supraspinous ligament **D Lower Spine Bursa and Ligament** Iliolumbar ligament Interspinous ligament, lumbar Intertransverse ligament, lumbar Ligamentum flavum, lumbar Sacrococcygeal ligament Sacroiliac ligament Sacrospinous ligament Sacrotuberous ligament Supraspinous ligament **F Sternum Bursa and Ligament** Costoxiphoid ligament Sternocostal ligament **G Rib(s) Bursa and Ligament** Costotransverse ligament **H Abdomen Bursa and Ligament, Right** **J Abdomen Bursa and Ligament, Left** **K Perineum Bursa and Ligament** **L Hip Bursa and Ligament, Right** Iliofemoral ligament Ischiofemoral ligament Pubofemoral ligament Transverse acetabular ligament Trochanteric bursa **M Hip Bursa and Ligament, Left** *See L Hip Bursa and Ligament, Right* **N Knee Bursa and Ligament, Right** Anterior cruciate ligament (ACL) Lateral collateral ligament (LCL) Ligament of head of fibula Medial collateral ligament (MCL) Patellar ligament Popliteal ligament Posterior cruciate ligament (PCL) Prepatellar bursa **P Knee Bursa and Ligament, Left** *See N Knee Bursa and Ligament, Right* **Q Ankle Bursa and Ligament, Right** Calcaneofibular ligament Deltoid ligament Ligament of the lateral malleolus Talofibular ligament **R Ankle Bursa and Ligament, Left** *See Q Ankle Bursa and Ligament, Right* **S Foot Bursa and Ligament, Right** Calcaneocuboid ligament Cuneonavicular ligament Intercuneiform ligament Interphalangeal ligament Metatarsal ligament Metatarsophalangeal ligament Subtalar ligament Talocalcaneal ligament Talocalcaneonavicular ligament Tarsometatarsal ligament **T Foot Bursa and Ligament, Left** *See S Foot Bursa and Ligament, Right* **V Lower Extremity Bursa and Ligament, Right** **W Lower Extremity Bursa and Ligament, Left**	Ø Open 3 Percutaneous 4 Percutaneous Endoscopic	Z No Device	Z No Qualifier

0 Medical and Surgical
M Bursae and Ligaments
R Replacement

Definition: Putting in or on biological or synthetic material that physically takes the place and/or function of all or a portion of a body part

Explanation: The body part may have been taken out or replaced, or may be taken out, physically eradicated, or rendered nonfunctional during the REPLACEMENT procedure. A REMOVAL procedure is coded for taking out the device used in a previous replacement procedure.

Body Part Character 4	Approach Character 5	Device Character 6	Qualifier Character 7
0 Head and Neck Bursa and Ligament Alar ligament of axis Cervical interspinous ligament Cervical intertransverse ligament Cervical ligamentum flavum Interspinous ligament, cervical Intertransverse ligament, cervical Lateral temporomandibular ligament Ligamentum flavum, cervical Sphenomandibular ligament Stylomandibular ligament Transverse ligament of atlas **1 Shoulder Bursa and Ligament, Right** Acromioclavicular ligament Coracoacromial ligament Coracoclavicular ligament Coracohumeral ligament Costoclavicular ligament Glenohumeral ligament Interclavicular ligament Sternoclavicular ligament Subacromial bursa Transverse humeral ligament Transverse scapular ligament **2 Shoulder Bursa and Ligament, Left** *See* 1 Shoulder Bursa and Ligament, Right **3 Elbow Bursa and Ligament, Right** Annular ligament Olecranon bursa Radial collateral ligament Ulnar collateral ligament **4 Elbow Bursa and Ligament, Left** *See* 3 Elbow Bursa and Ligament, Right **5 Wrist Bursa and Ligament, Right** Palmar ulnocarpal ligament Radial collateral carpal ligament Radiocarpal ligament Radioulnar ligament Scapholunate ligament Ulnar collateral carpal ligament **6 Wrist Bursa and Ligament, Left** *See* 5 Wrist Bursa and Ligament, Right **7 Hand Bursa and Ligament, Right** Carpometacarpal ligament Intercarpal ligament Interphalangeal ligament Lunotriquetral ligament Metacarpal ligament Metacarpophalangeal ligament Pisohamate ligament Pisometacarpal ligament Scaphotrapezium ligament **8 Hand Bursa and Ligament, Left** *See* 7 Hand Bursa and Ligament, Right **9 Upper Extremity Bursa and Ligament, Right** **B Upper Extremity Bursa and Ligament, Left** **C Upper Spine Bursa and Ligament** Interspinous ligament, thoracic Intertransverse ligament, thoracic Ligamentum flavum, thoracic Supraspinous ligament	**D Lower Spine Bursa and Ligament** Iliolumbar ligament Interspinous ligament, lumbar Intertransverse ligament, lumbar Ligamentum flavum, lumbar Sacrococcygeal ligament Sacroiliac ligament Sacrospinous ligament Sacrotuberous ligament Supraspinous ligament **F Sternum Bursa and Ligament** Costoxiphoid ligament Sternocostal ligament **G Rib(s) Bursa and Ligament** Costotransverse ligament **H Abdomen Bursa and Ligament, Right** **J Abdomen Bursa and Ligament, Left** **K Perineum Bursa and Ligament** **L Hip Bursa and Ligament, Right** Iliofemoral ligament Ischiofemoral ligament Pubofemoral ligament Transverse acetabular ligament Trochanteric bursa **M Hip Bursa and Ligament, Left** *See* L Hip Bursa and Ligament, Right **N Knee Bursa and Ligament, Right** Anterior cruciate ligament (ACL) Lateral collateral ligament (LCL) Ligament of head of fibula Medial collateral ligament (MCL) Patellar ligament Popliteal ligament Posterior cruciate ligament (PCL) Prepatellar bursa **P Knee Bursa and Ligament, Left** *See* N Knee Bursa and Ligament, Right **Q Ankle Bursa and Ligament, Right** Calcaneofibular ligament Deltoid ligament Ligament of the lateral malleolus Talofibular ligament **R Ankle Bursa and Ligament, Left** *See* Q Ankle Bursa and Ligament, Right **S Foot Bursa and Ligament, Right** Calcaneocuboid ligament Cuneonavicular ligament Intercuneiform ligament Interphalangeal ligament Metatarsal ligament Metatarsophalangeal ligament Subtalar ligament Talocalcaneal ligament Talocalcaneonavicular ligament Tarsometatarsal ligament **T Foot Bursa and Ligament, Left** *See* S Foot Bursa and Ligament, Right **V Lower Extremity Bursa and Ligament, Right** **W Lower Extremity Bursa and Ligament, Left**	**0** Open **4** Percutaneous Endoscopic	**7** Autologous Tissue Substitute **J** Synthetic Substitute **K** Nonautologous Tissue Substitute	**Z** No Qualifier

ICD-10-PCS 2025 — Bursae and Ligaments — 0MS-0MS

- **0** Medical and Surgical
- **M** Bursae and Ligaments
- **S** Reposition

Definition: Moving to its normal location, or other suitable location, all or a portion of a body part
Explanation: The body part is moved to a new location from an abnormal location, or from a normal location where it is not functioning correctly. The body part may or may not be cut out or off to be moved to the new location.

Body Part — Character 4	Approach — Character 5	Device — Character 6	Qualifier — Character 7

0 Head and Neck Bursa and Ligament
  Alar ligament of axis
  Cervical interspinous ligament
  Cervical intertransverse ligament
  Cervical ligamentum flavum
  Interspinous ligament, cervical
  Intertransverse ligament, cervical
  Lateral temporomandibular ligament
  Ligamentum flavum, cervical
  Sphenomandibular ligament
  Stylomandibular ligament
  Transverse ligament of atlas
1 Shoulder Bursa and Ligament, Right
  Acromioclavicular ligament
  Coracoacromial ligament
  Coracoclavicular ligament
  Coracohumeral ligament
  Costoclavicular ligament
  Glenohumeral ligament
  Interclavicular ligament
  Sternoclavicular ligament
  Subacromial bursa
  Transverse humeral ligament
  Transverse scapular ligament
2 Shoulder Bursa and Ligament, Left
  See 1 Shoulder Bursa and Ligament, Right
3 Elbow Bursa and Ligament, Right
  Annular ligament
  Olecranon bursa
  Radial collateral ligament
  Ulnar collateral ligament
4 Elbow Bursa and Ligament, Left
  See 3 Elbow Bursa and Ligament, Right
5 Wrist Bursa and Ligament, Right
  Palmar ulnocarpal ligament
  Radial collateral carpal ligament
  Radiocarpal ligament
  Radioulnar ligament
  Scapholunate ligament
  Ulnar collateral carpal ligament
6 Wrist Bursa and Ligament, Left
  See 5 Wrist Bursa and Ligament, Right
7 Hand Bursa and Ligament, Right
  Carpometacarpal ligament
  Intercarpal ligament
  Interphalangeal ligament
  Lunotriquetral ligament
  Metacarpal ligament
  Metacarpophalangeal ligament
  Pisohamate ligament
  Pisometacarpal ligament
  Scaphotrapezium ligament
8 Hand Bursa and Ligament, Left
  See 7 Hand Bursa and Ligament, Right
9 Upper Extremity Bursa and Ligament, Right
B Upper Extremity Bursa and Ligament, Left
C Upper Spine Bursa and Ligament
  Interspinous ligament, thoracic
  Intertransverse ligament, thoracic
  Ligamentum flavum, thoracic
  Supraspinous ligament
D Lower Spine Bursa and Ligament
  Iliolumbar ligament
  Interspinous ligament, lumbar
  Intertransverse ligament, lumbar
  Ligamentum flavum, lumbar
  Sacrococcygeal ligament
  Sacroiliac ligament
  Sacrospinous ligament
  Sacrotuberous ligament
  Supraspinous ligament
F Sternum Bursa and Ligament
  Costoxiphoid ligament
  Sternocostal ligament
G Rib(s) Bursa and Ligament
  Costotransverse ligament
H Abdomen Bursa and Ligament, Right
J Abdomen Bursa and Ligament, Left
K Perineum Bursa and Ligament
L Hip Bursa and Ligament, Right
  Iliofemoral ligament
  Ischiofemoral ligament
  Pubofemoral ligament
  Transverse acetabular ligament
  Trochanteric bursa
M Hip Bursa and Ligament, Left
  See L Hip Bursa and Ligament, Right
N Knee Bursa and Ligament, Right
  Anterior cruciate ligament (ACL)
  Lateral collateral ligament (LCL)
  Ligament of head of fibula
  Medial collateral ligament (MCL)
  Patellar ligament
  Popliteal ligament
  Posterior cruciate ligament (PCL)
  Prepatellar bursa
P Knee Bursa and Ligament, Left
  See N Knee Bursa and Ligament, Right
Q Ankle Bursa and Ligament, Right
  Calcaneofibular ligament
  Deltoid ligament
  Ligament of the lateral malleolus
  Talofibular ligament
R Ankle Bursa and Ligament, Left
  See Q Ankle Bursa and Ligament, Right
S Foot Bursa and Ligament, Right
  Calcaneocuboid ligament
  Cuneonavicular ligament
  Intercuneiform ligament
  Interphalangeal ligament
  Metatarsal ligament
  Metatarsophalangeal ligament
  Subtalar ligament
  Talocalcaneal ligament
  Talocalcaneonavicular ligament
  Tarsometatarsal ligament
T Foot Bursa and Ligament, Left
  See S Foot Bursa and Ligament, Right
V Lower Extremity Bursa and Ligament, Right
W Lower Extremity Bursa and Ligament, Left
	0 Open
	4 Percutaneous Endoscopic
		Z No Device	**Z** No Qualifier

NC Noncovered Procedure   **LC** Limited Coverage   **QA** Questionable OB Admit   **NT** New Tech Add-on   ✚ Combination Member   ♂ Male   ♀ Female

0 Medical and Surgical
M Bursae and Ligaments
T Resection

Definition: Cutting out or off, without replacement, all of a body part
Explanation: None

Body Part Character 4	Approach Character 5	Device Character 6	Qualifier Character 7
0 Head and Neck Bursa and Ligament Alar ligament of axis Cervical interspinous ligament Cervical intertransverse ligament Cervical ligamentum flavum Interspinous ligament, cervical Intertransverse ligament, cervical Lateral temporomandibular ligament Ligamentum flavum, cervical Sphenomandibular ligament Stylomandibular ligament Transverse ligament of atlas **1 Shoulder Bursa and Ligament, Right** Acromioclavicular ligament Coracoacromial ligament Coracoclavicular ligament Coracohumeral ligament Costoclavicular ligament Glenohumeral ligament Interclavicular ligament Sternoclavicular ligament Subacromial bursa Transverse humeral ligament Transverse scapular ligament **2 Shoulder Bursa and Ligament, Left** *See 1 Shoulder Bursa and Ligament, Right* **3 Elbow Bursa and Ligament, Right** Annular ligament Olecranon bursa Radial collateral ligament Ulnar collateral ligament **4 Elbow Bursa and Ligament, Left** *See 3 Elbow Bursa and Ligament, Right* **5 Wrist Bursa and Ligament, Right** Palmar ulnocarpal ligament Radial collateral carpal ligament Radiocarpal ligament Radioulnar ligament Scapholunate ligament Ulnar collateral carpal ligament **6 Wrist Bursa and Ligament, Left** *See 5 Wrist Bursa and Ligament, Right* **7 Hand Bursa and Ligament, Right** Carpometacarpal ligament Intercarpal ligament Interphalangeal ligament Lunotriquetral ligament Metacarpal ligament Metacarpophalangeal ligament Pisohamate ligament Pisometacarpal ligament Scaphotrapezium ligament **8 Hand Bursa and Ligament, Left** *See 7 Hand Bursa and Ligament, Right* **9 Upper Extremity Bursa and Ligament, Right** **B Upper Extremity Bursa and Ligament, Left** **C Upper Spine Bursa and Ligament** Interspinous ligament, thoracic Intertransverse ligament, thoracic Ligamentum flavum, thoracic Supraspinous ligament	**0 Open** **4 Percutaneous Endoscopic**	**Z No Device**	**Z No Qualifier**
D Lower Spine Bursa and Ligament Iliolumbar ligament Interspinous ligament, lumbar Intertransverse ligament, lumbar Ligamentum flavum, lumbar Sacrococcygeal ligament Sacroiliac ligament Sacrospinous ligament Sacrotuberous ligament Supraspinous ligament **F Sternum Bursa and Ligament** Costoxiphoid ligament Sternocostal ligament **G Rib(s) Bursa and Ligament** Costotransverse ligament **H Abdomen Bursa and Ligament, Right** **J Abdomen Bursa and Ligament, Left** **K Perineum Bursa and Ligament** **L Hip Bursa and Ligament, Right** Iliofemoral ligament Ischiofemoral ligament Pubofemoral ligament Transverse acetabular ligament Trochanteric bursa **M Hip Bursa and Ligament, Left** *See L Hip Bursa and Ligament, Right* **N Knee Bursa and Ligament, Right** Anterior cruciate ligament (ACL) Lateral collateral ligament (LCL) Ligament of head of fibula Medial collateral ligament (MCL) Patellar ligament Popliteal ligament Posterior cruciate ligament (PCL) Prepatellar bursa **P Knee Bursa and Ligament, Left** *See N Knee Bursa and Ligament, Right* **Q Ankle Bursa and Ligament, Right** Calcaneofibular ligament Deltoid ligament Ligament of the lateral malleolus Talofibular ligament **R Ankle Bursa and Ligament, Left** *See Q Ankle Bursa and Ligament, Right* **S Foot Bursa and Ligament, Right** Calcaneocuboid ligament Cuneonavicular ligament Intercuneiform ligament Interphalangeal ligament Metatarsal ligament Metatarsophalangeal ligament Subtalar ligament Talocalcaneal ligament Talocalcaneonavicular ligament Tarsometatarsal ligament **T Foot Bursa and Ligament, Left** *See S Foot Bursa and Ligament, Right* **V Lower Extremity Bursa and Ligament, Right** **W Lower Extremity Bursa and Ligament, Left**			

ICD-10-PCS 2025 — Bursae and Ligaments — 0MU–0MU

0 Medical and Surgical
M Bursae and Ligaments
U Supplement

Definition: Putting in or on biological or synthetic material that physically reinforces and/or augments the function of a portion of a body part
Explanation: The biological material is non-living, or is living and from the same individual. The body part may have been previously replaced, and the SUPPLEMENT procedure is performed to physically reinforce and/or augment the function of the replaced body part.

Body Part Character 4	Approach Character 5	Device Character 6	Qualifier Character 7
0 Head and Neck Bursa and Ligament Alar ligament of axis Cervical interspinous ligament Cervical intertransverse ligament Cervical ligamentum flavum Interspinous ligament, cervical Intertransverse ligament, cervical Lateral temporomandibular ligament Ligamentum flavum, cervical Sphenomandibular ligament Stylomandibular ligament Transverse ligament of atlas **1** Shoulder Bursa and Ligament, Right Acromioclavicular ligament Coracoacromial ligament Coracoclavicular ligament Coracohumeral ligament Costoclavicular ligament Glenohumeral ligament Interclavicular ligament Sternoclavicular ligament Subacromial bursa Transverse humeral ligament Transverse scapular ligament **2** Shoulder Bursa and Ligament, Left *See 1 Shoulder Bursa and Ligament, Right* **3** Elbow Bursa and Ligament, Right Annular ligament Olecranon bursa Radial collateral ligament Ulnar collateral ligament **4** Elbow Bursa and Ligament, Left *See 3 Elbow Bursa and Ligament, Right* **5** Wrist Bursa and Ligament, Right Palmar ulnocarpal ligament Radial collateral carpal ligament Radiocarpal ligament Radioulnar ligament Scapholunate ligament Ulnar collateral carpal ligament **6** Wrist Bursa and Ligament, Left *See 5 Wrist Bursa and Ligament, Right* **7** Hand Bursa and Ligament, Right Carpometacarpal ligament Intercarpal ligament Interphalangeal ligament Lunotriquetral ligament Metacarpal ligament Metacarpophalangeal ligament Pisohamate ligament Pisometacarpal ligament Scaphotrapezium ligament **8** Hand Bursa and Ligament, Left *See 7 Hand Bursa and Ligament, Right* **9** Upper Extremity Bursa and Ligament, Right **B** Upper Extremity Bursa and Ligament, Left **C** Upper Spine Bursa and Ligament Interspinous ligament, thoracic Intertransverse ligament, thoracic Ligamentum flavum, thoracic Supraspinous ligament **D** Lower Spine Bursa and Ligament Iliolumbar ligament Interspinous ligament, lumbar Intertransverse ligament, lumbar Ligamentum flavum, lumbar Sacrococcygeal ligament Sacroiliac ligament Sacrospinous ligament Sacrotuberous ligament Supraspinous ligament **F** Sternum Bursa and Ligament Costoxiphoid ligament Sternocostal ligament **G** Rib(s) Bursa and Ligament Costotransverse ligament **H** Abdomen Bursa and Ligament, Right **J** Abdomen Bursa and Ligament, Left **K** Perineum Bursa and Ligament **L** Hip Bursa and Ligament, Right Iliofemoral ligament Ischiofemoral ligament Pubofemoral ligament Transverse acetabular ligament Trochanteric bursa **M** Hip Bursa and Ligament, Left *See L Hip Bursa and Ligament, Right* **N** Knee Bursa and Ligament, Right Anterior cruciate ligament (ACL) Lateral collateral ligament (LCL) Ligament of head of fibula Medial collateral ligament (MCL) Patellar ligament Popliteal ligament Posterior cruciate ligament (PCL) Prepatellar bursa **P** Knee Bursa and Ligament, Left *See N Knee Bursa and Ligament, Right* **Q** Ankle Bursa and Ligament, Right Calcaneofibular ligament Deltoid ligament Ligament of the lateral malleolus Talofibular ligament **R** Ankle Bursa and Ligament, Left *See Q Ankle Bursa and Ligament, Right* **S** Foot Bursa and Ligament, Right Calcaneocuboid ligament Cuneonavicular ligament Intercuneiform ligament Interphalangeal ligament Metatarsal ligament Metatarsophalangeal ligament Subtalar ligament Talocalcaneal ligament Talocalcaneonavicular ligament Tarsometatarsal ligament **T** Foot Bursa and Ligament, Left *See S Foot Bursa and Ligament, Right* **V** Lower Extremity Bursa and Ligament, Right **W** Lower Extremity Bursa and Ligament, Left	**0** Open **4** Percutaneous Endoscopic	**7** Autologous Tissue Substitute **J** Synthetic Substitute **K** Nonautologous Tissue Substitute	**Z** No Qualifier

0 Medical and Surgical
M Bursae and Ligaments
W Revision — Definition: Correcting, to the extent possible, a portion of a malfunctioning device or the position of a displaced device

Explanation: Revision can include correcting a malfunctioning or displaced device by taking out or putting in components of the device such as a screw or pin

Body Part Character 4	Approach Character 5	Device Character 6	Qualifier Character 7
X Upper Bursa and Ligament Y Lower Bursa and Ligament	0 Open 3 Percutaneous 4 Percutaneous Endoscopic	0 Drainage Device 7 Autologous Tissue Substitute J Synthetic Substitute K Nonautologous Tissue Substitute Y Other Device	Z No Qualifier
X Upper Bursa and Ligament Y Lower Bursa and Ligament	X External	0 Drainage Device 7 Autologous Tissue Substitute J Synthetic Substitute K Nonautologous Tissue Substitute	Z No Qualifier

Non-OR 0MW[X,Y][3,4]YZ
Non-OR 0MW[X,Y]X[0,7,J,K]Z

0 Medical and Surgical
M Bursae and Ligaments
X Transfer

Definition: Moving, without taking out, all or a portion of a body part to another location to take over the function of all or a portion of a body part

Explanation: The body part transferred remains connected to its vascular and nervous supply

Body Part Character 4	Approach Character 5	Device Character 6	Qualifier Character 7
0 Head and Neck Bursa and Ligament 　Alar ligament of axis 　Cervical interspinous ligament 　Cervical intertransverse ligament 　Cervical ligamentum flavum 　Interspinous ligament, cervical 　Intertransverse ligament, cervical 　Lateral temporomandibular ligament 　Ligamentum flavum, cervical 　Sphenomandibular ligament 　Stylomandibular ligament 　Transverse ligament of atlas **1** Shoulder Bursa and Ligament, Right 　Acromioclavicular ligament 　Coracoacromial ligament 　Coracoclavicular ligament 　Coracohumeral ligament 　Costoclavicular ligament 　Glenohumeral ligament 　Interclavicular ligament 　Sternoclavicular ligament 　Subacromial bursa 　Transverse humeral ligament 　Transverse scapular ligament **2** Shoulder Bursa and Ligament, Left 　See 1 Shoulder Bursa and Ligament, Right **3** Elbow Bursa and Ligament, Right 　Annular ligament 　Olecranon bursa 　Radial collateral ligament 　Ulnar collateral ligament **4** Elbow Bursa and Ligament, Left 　See 3 Elbow Bursa and Ligament, Right **5** Wrist Bursa and Ligament, Right 　Palmar ulnocarpal ligament 　Radial collateral carpal ligament 　Radiocarpal ligament 　Radioulnar ligament 　Scapholunate ligament 　Ulnar collateral carpal ligament **6** Wrist Bursa and Ligament, Left 　See 5 Wrist Bursa and Ligament, Right **7** Hand Bursa and Ligament, Right 　Carpometacarpal ligament 　Intercarpal ligament 　Interphalangeal ligament 　Lunotriquetral ligament 　Metacarpal ligament 　Metacarpophalangeal ligament 　Pisohamate ligament 　Pisometacarpal ligament 　Scaphotrapezium ligament **8** Hand Bursa and Ligament, Left 　See 7 Hand Bursa and Ligament, Right **9** Upper Extremity Bursa and Ligament, Right **B** Upper Extremity Bursa and Ligament, Left **C** Upper Spine Bursa and Ligament 　Interspinous ligament, thoracic 　Intertransverse ligament, thoracic 　Ligamentum flavum, thoracic 　Supraspinous ligament	**0** Open **4** Percutaneous Endoscopic	**Z** No Device	**Z** No Qualifier

D Lower Spine Bursa and Ligament
　Iliolumbar ligament
　Interspinous ligament, lumbar
　Intertransverse ligament, lumbar
　Ligamentum flavum, lumbar
　Sacrococcygeal ligament
　Sacroiliac ligament
　Sacrospinous ligament
　Sacrotuberous ligament
　Supraspinous ligament
F Sternum Bursa and Ligament
　Costoxiphoid ligament
　Sternocostal ligament
G Rib(s) Bursa and Ligament
　Costotransverse ligament
H Abdomen Bursa and Ligament, Right
J Abdomen Bursa and Ligament, Left
K Perineum Bursa and Ligament
L Hip Bursa and Ligament, Right
　Iliofemoral ligament
　Ischiofemoral ligament
　Pubofemoral ligament
　Transverse acetabular ligament
　Trochanteric bursa
M Hip Bursa and Ligament, Left
　See L Hip Bursa and Ligament, Right
N Knee Bursa and Ligament, Right
　Anterior cruciate ligament (ACL)
　Lateral collateral ligament (LCL)
　Ligament of head of fibula
　Medial collateral ligament (MCL)
　Patellar ligament
　Popliteal ligament
　Posterior cruciate ligament (PCL)
　Prepatellar bursa
P Knee Bursa and Ligament, Left
　See N Knee Bursa and Ligament, Right
Q Ankle Bursa and Ligament, Right
　Calcaneofibular ligament
　Deltoid ligament
　Ligament of the lateral malleolus
　Talofibular ligament
R Ankle Bursa and Ligament, Left
　See Q Ankle Bursa and Ligament, Right
S Foot Bursa and Ligament, Right
　Calcaneocuboid ligament
　Cuneonavicular ligament
　Intercuneiform ligament
　Interphalangeal ligament
　Metatarsal ligament
　Metatarsophalangeal ligament
　Subtalar ligament
　Talocalcaneal ligament
　Talocalcaneonavicular ligament
　Tarsometatarsal ligament
T Foot Bursa and Ligament, Left
　See S Foot Bursa and Ligament, Right
V Lower Extremity Bursa and Ligament, Right
W Lower Extremity Bursa and Ligament, Left

Head and Facial Bones ØN2–ØNW

Character Meanings

This Character Meaning table is provided as a guide to assist the user in the identification of character members that may be found in this section of code tables. It **SHOULD NOT** be used to build a PCS code.

Operation–Character 3		Body Part–Character 4		Approach–Character 5		Device–Character 6		Qualifier–Character 7	
2	Change	Ø	Skull	Ø	Open	Ø	Drainage Device	X	Diagnostic
5	Destruction	1	Frontal Bone	3	Percutaneous	3	Infusion Device	Z	No Qualifier
8	Division	3	Parietal Bone, Right	4	Percutaneous Endoscopic	4	Internal Fixation Device		
9	Drainage	4	Parietal Bone, Left	X	External	5	External Fixation Device		
B	Excision	5	Temporal Bone, Right			7	Autologous Tissue Substitute		
C	Extirpation	6	Temporal Bone, Left			J	Synthetic Substitute		
D	Extraction	7	Occipital Bone			K	Nonautologous Tissue Substitute		
H	Insertion	B	Nasal Bone			M	Bone Growth Stimulator		
J	Inspection	C	Sphenoid Bone			N	Neurostimulator Generator		
N	Release	F	Ethmoid Bone, Right			S	Hearing Device		
P	Removal	G	Ethmoid Bone, Left			Y	Other Device		
Q	Repair	H	Lacrimal Bone, Right			Z	No Device		
R	Replacement	J	Lacrimal Bone, Left						
S	Reposition	K	Palatine Bone, Right						
T	Resection	L	Palatine Bone, Left						
U	Supplement	M	Zygomatic Bone, Right						
W	Revision	N	Zygomatic Bone, Left						
		P	Orbit, Right						
		Q	Orbit, Left						
		R	Maxilla						
		T	Mandible, Right						
		V	Mandible, Left						
		W	Facial Bone						
		X	Hyoid Bone						

AHA Coding Clinic for table ØNB
- 2024, 2Q, 17 — Resection of sellar craniopharyngioma
- 2022, 2Q, 17 — Congenital nasal pyriform aperture stenosis and repair
- 2021, 3Q, 21 — Excision of thyroglossal duct cyst
- 2021, 1Q, 21 — Maxillectomy with reconstruction of maxilla
- 2017, 1Q, 20 — Preparatory nasal adhesion repair before definitive cleft palate repair
- 2015, 3Q, 3-8 — Excisional and nonexcisional debridement
- 2015, 2Q, 12 — Orbital exenteration

AHA Coding Clinic for table ØND
- 2017, 4Q, 41 — Extraction procedures

AHA Coding Clinic for table ØNH
- 2021, 4Q, 51 — Insertion of infusion device in skull
- 2015, 3Q, 13 — Nonexcisional debridement of cranial wound with removal and replacement of hardware

AHA Coding Clinic for table ØNP
- 2023, 1Q, 31 — Removal of autologous bone flap due to bone resorption
- 2022, 4Q, 58-59 — Infusion device in head and facial bones
- 2015, 3Q, 13 — Nonexcisional debridement of cranial wound with removal and replacement of hardware

AHA Coding Clinic for table ØNQ
- 2016, 3Q, 29 — Closure of bilateral alveolar clefts

AHA Coding Clinic for table ØNR
- 2021, 3Q, 29 — Repair of superior semicircular canal dehiscence
- 2021, 1Q, 21 — Maxillectomy with reconstruction of maxilla
- 2017, 3Q, 17 — Resection of schwannoma and placement of DuraGen and Lorenz cranial plating system
- 2017, 3Q, 22 — Replacement of native skull bone flap
- 2017, 1Q, 23 — Reconstruction of mandible using titanium and bone
- 2014, 3Q, 7 — Hemi-cranioplasty for repair of cranial defect

AHA Coding Clinic for table ØNS
- 2023, 3Q, 23 — Aspiration and injection of bone marrow at fracture site
- 2022, 1Q, 48 — Repair of facial fractures of frontal sinus and orbital roof
- 2017, 3Q, 22 — Replacement of native skull bone flap
- 2017, 1Q, 20 — Preparatory nasal adhesion repair before definitive cleft palate repair
- 2016, 2Q, 30 — Clipping (occlusion) of cerebral artery, decompressive craniectomy and storage of bone flap in abdominal wall
- 2015, 3Q, 17 — Craniosynostosis with cranial vault reconstruction
- 2015, 3Q, 27 — Moyamoya disease and hemispheric pial synangiosis with craniotomy
- 2014, 3Q, 27 — Le Fort I osteotomy
- 2013, 3Q, 24 — Distraction osteogenesis
- 2013, 3Q, 25 — Fracture of frontal bone with repair and coagulation for hemostasis

AHA Coding Clinic for table ØNU
- 2023, 2Q, 19 — Sigmoid sinus dehiscence with mastoidectomy with resurfacing
- 2021, 3Q, 29 — Repair of superior semicircular canal dehiscence
- 2016, 3Q, 29 — Closure of bilateral alveolar clefts
- 2013, 3Q, 24 — Distraction osteogenesis

AHA Coding Clinic for table ØNW
- 2022, 4Q, 58-59 — Infusion device in head and facial bones

Head and Facial Bones

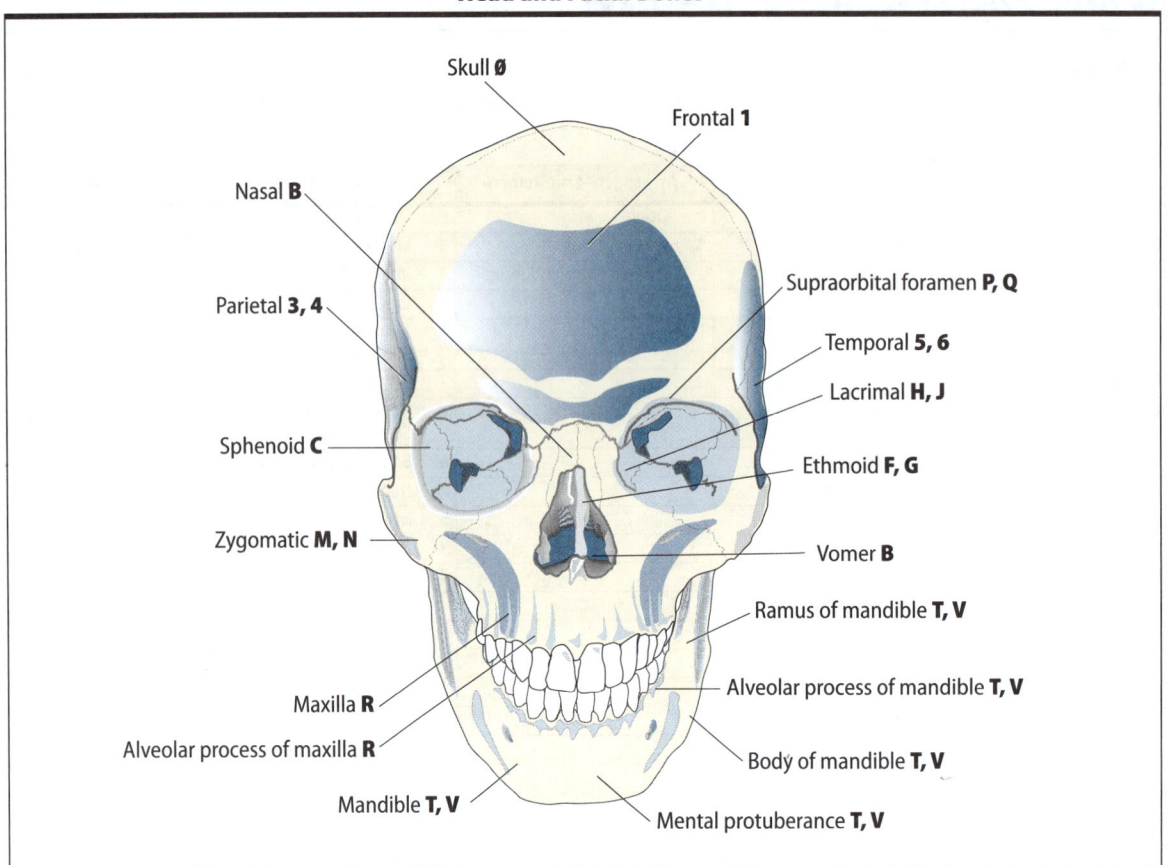

Head and Facial Bones

- Skull **0**
- Frontal **1**
- Nasal **B**
- Supraorbital foramen **P, Q**
- Parietal **3, 4**
- Temporal **5, 6**
- Lacrimal **H, J**
- Sphenoid **C**
- Ethmoid **F, G**
- Zygomatic **M, N**
- Vomer **B**
- Ramus of mandible **T, V**
- Maxilla **R**
- Alveolar process of mandible **T, V**
- Alveolar process of maxilla **R**
- Body of mandible **T, V**
- Mandible **T, V**
- Mental protuberance **T, V**

Skull Bones

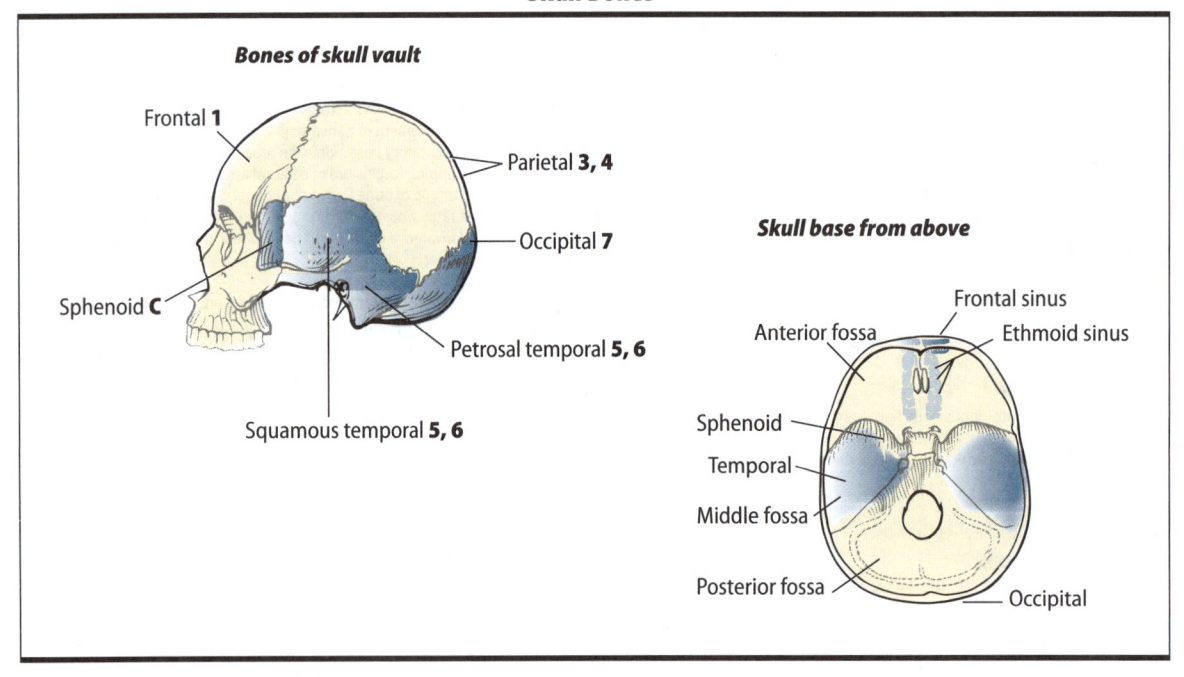

Bones of skull vault

- Frontal **1**
- Parietal **3, 4**
- Occipital **7**
- Sphenoid **C**
- Petrosal temporal **5, 6**
- Squamous temporal **5, 6**

Skull base from above

- Frontal sinus
- Ethmoid sinus
- Anterior fossa
- Sphenoid
- Temporal
- Middle fossa
- Posterior fossa
- Occipital

ICD-10-PCS 2025 — Head and Facial Bones — 0N2–0N5

- **0** Medical and Surgical
- **N** Head and Facial Bones
- **2** Change   Definition: Taking out or off a device from a body part and putting back an identical or similar device in or on the same body part without cutting or puncturing the skin or a mucous membrane
    Explanation: All CHANGE procedures are coded using the approach EXTERNAL

Body Part Character 4	Approach Character 5	Device Character 6	Qualifier Character 7
0 Skull **B** Nasal Bone Vomer of nasal septum **W** Facial Bone	**X** External	**0** Drainage Device **Y** Other Device	**Z** No Qualifier

Non-OR   All body part, approach, device, and qualifier values

- **0** Medical and Surgical
- **N** Head and Facial Bones
- **5** Destruction   Definition: Physical eradication of all or a portion of a body part by the direct use of energy, force, or a destructive agent
    Explanation: None of the body part is physically taken out

Body Part Character 4	Approach Character 5	Device Character 6	Qualifier Character 7

0 Skull
1 Frontal Bone
  Zygomatic process of frontal bone
3 Parietal Bone, Right
4 Parietal Bone, Left
5 Temporal Bone, Right
  Mastoid process
  Petrous part of temporal bone
  Tympanic part of temporal bone
  Zygomatic process of temporal bone
6 Temporal Bone, Left
  See 5 Temporal Bone, Right
7 Occipital Bone
  Foramen magnum
B Nasal Bone
  Vomer of nasal septum
C Sphenoid Bone
  Greater wing
  Lesser wing
  Optic foramen
  Pterygoid process
  Sella turcica
F Ethmoid Bone, Right
  Cribriform plate
G Ethmoid Bone, Left
  See F Ethmoid Bone, Right
H Lacrimal Bone, Right
J Lacrimal Bone, Left
K Palatine Bone, Right
L Palatine Bone, Left
M Zygomatic Bone, Right
N Zygomatic Bone, Left
P Orbit, Right
  Bony orbit
  Orbital portion of ethmoid bone
  Orbital portion of frontal bone
  Orbital portion of lacrimal bone
  Orbital portion of maxilla
  Orbital portion of palatine bone
  Orbital portion of sphenoid bone
  Orbital portion of zygomatic bone
Q Orbit, Left
  See P Orbit, Right
R Maxilla
  Alveolar process of maxilla
T Mandible, Right
  Alveolar process of mandible
  Condyloid process
  Mandibular notch
  Mental foramen
V Mandible, Left
  See T Mandible, Right
X Hyoid Bone
	0 Open
	3 Percutaneous
	4 Percutaneous Endoscopic
		Z No Device	**Z** No Qualifier

529

0N8–0N8 Head and Facial Bones ICD-10-PCS 2025

0 Medical and Surgical
N Head and Facial Bones
8 Division Definition: Cutting into a body part, without draining fluids and/or gases from the body part, in order to separate or transect a body part
Explanation: All or a portion of the body part is separated into two or more portions

Body Part Character 4	Approach Character 5	Device Character 6	Qualifier Character 7

0 Skull
1 Frontal Bone
   Zygomatic process of frontal bone
3 Parietal Bone, Right
4 Parietal Bone, Left
5 Temporal Bone, Right
   Mastoid process
   Petrous part of temporal bone
   Tympanic part of temporal bone
   Zygomatic process of temporal bone
6 Temporal Bone, Left
   See 5 Temporal Bone, Right
7 Occipital Bone
   Foramen magnum
B Nasal Bone
   Vomer of nasal septum
C Sphenoid Bone
   Greater wing
   Lesser wing
   Optic foramen
   Pterygoid process
   Sella turcica
F Ethmoid Bone, Right
   Cribriform plate
G Ethmoid Bone, Left
   See F Ethmoid Bone, Right
H Lacrimal Bone, Right
J Lacrimal Bone, Left
K Palatine Bone, Right
L Palatine Bone, Left
M Zygomatic Bone, Right
N Zygomatic Bone, Left
P Orbit, Right
   Bony orbit
   Orbital portion of ethmoid bone
   Orbital portion of frontal bone
   Orbital portion of lacrimal bone
   Orbital portion of maxilla
   Orbital portion of palatine bone
   Orbital portion of sphenoid bone
   Orbital portion of zygomatic bone
Q Orbit, Left
   See P Orbit, Right
R Maxilla
   Alveolar process of maxilla
T Mandible, Right
   Alveolar process of mandible
   Condyloid process
   Mandibular notch
   Mental foramen
V Mandible, Left
   See T Mandible, Right
X Hyoid Bone
	0 Open
	3 Percutaneous
	4 Percutaneous Endoscopic
		Z No Device	**Z** No Qualifier

Non-OR 0N8B[0,3,4]ZZ

ICD-10-PCS 2025 — Head and Facial Bones — 0N9–0N9

- **0** Medical and Surgical
- **N** Head and Facial Bones
- **9** Drainage   Definition: Taking or letting out fluids and/or gases from a body part
    Explanation: The qualifier DIAGNOSTIC is used to identify drainage procedures that are biopsies

Body Part Character 4	Approach Character 5	Device Character 6	Qualifier Character 7

0 Skull
 1 Frontal Bone
   Zygomatic process of frontal bone
 3 Parietal Bone, Right
 4 Parietal Bone, Left
 5 Temporal Bone, Right
   Mastoid process
   Petrous part of temporal bone
   Tympanic part of temporal bone
   Zygomatic process of temporal bone
 6 Temporal Bone, Left
   See 5 Temporal Bone, Right
 7 Occipital Bone
   Foramen magnum
 B Nasal Bone
   Vomer of nasal septum
 C Sphenoid Bone
   Greater wing
   Lesser wing
   Optic foramen
   Pterygoid process
   Sella turcica
 F Ethmoid Bone, Right
   Cribriform plate
 G Ethmoid Bone, Left
   See F Ethmoid Bone, Right
 H Lacrimal Bone, Right
 J Lacrimal Bone, Left
 K Palatine Bone, Right
 L Palatine Bone, Left
 M Zygomatic Bone, Right
 N Zygomatic Bone, Left
 P Orbit, Right
   Bony orbit
   Orbital portion of ethmoid bone
   Orbital portion of frontal bone
   Orbital portion of lacrimal bone
   Orbital portion of maxilla
   Orbital portion of palatine bone
   Orbital portion of sphenoid bone
   Orbital portion of zygomatic bone
 Q Orbit, Left
   See P Orbit, Right
 R Maxilla
   Alveolar process of maxilla
 T Mandible, Right
   Alveolar process of mandible
   Condyloid process
   Mandibular notch
   Mental foramen
 V Mandible, Left
   See T Mandible, Right
 X Hyoid Bone
	0 Open
	 3 Percutaneous
	 4 Percutaneous Endoscopic
		0 Drainage Device	**Z** No Qualifier

Non-OR 0N9[0,1,3,4,5,6,7,C,F,G,H,J,K,L,M,N,P,Q,X]30Z
Non-OR 0N9[B,R,T,V][0,3,4]0Z

0N9 Continued on next page

Head and Facial Bones

ØN9 Continued

0 Medical and Surgical
N Head and Facial Bones
9 Drainage   Definition: Taking or letting out fluids and/or gases from a body part
              Explanation: The qualifier DIAGNOSTIC is used to identify drainage procedures that are biopsies

Body Part Character 4	Approach Character 5	Device Character 6	Qualifier Character 7

0 Skull
1 Frontal Bone
   Zygomatic process of frontal bone
3 Parietal Bone, Right
4 Parietal Bone, Left
5 Temporal Bone, Right
   Mastoid process
   Petrous part of temporal bone
   Tympanic part of temporal bone
   Zygomatic process of temporal bone
6 Temporal Bone, Left
   See 5 Temporal Bone, Right
7 Occipital Bone
   Foramen magnum
B Nasal Bone
   Vomer of nasal septum
C Sphenoid Bone
   Greater wing
   Lesser wing
   Optic foramen
   Pterygoid process
   Sella turcica
F Ethmoid Bone, Right
   Cribriform plate
G Ethmoid Bone, Left
   See F Ethmoid Bone, Right
H Lacrimal Bone, Right
J Lacrimal Bone, Left
K Palatine Bone, Right
L Palatine Bone, Left
M Zygomatic Bone, Right
N Zygomatic Bone, Left
P Orbit, Right
   Bony orbit
   Orbital portion of ethmoid bone
   Orbital portion of frontal bone
   Orbital portion of lacrimal bone
   Orbital portion of maxilla
   Orbital portion of palatine bone
   Orbital portion of sphenoid bone
   Orbital portion of zygomatic bone
Q Orbit, Left
   See P Orbit, Right
R Maxilla
   Alveolar process of maxilla
T Mandible, Right
   Alveolar process of mandible
   Condyloid process
   Mandibular notch
   Mental foramen
V Mandible, Left
   See T Mandible, Right
X Hyoid Bone
	0 Open
	3 Percutaneous
	4 Percutaneous Endoscopic
		Z No Device	X Diagnostic
			Z No Qualifier

Non-OR   ØN9[0,1,3,4,5,6,7,C,F,G,H,J,K,L,M,N,P,Q,X]3ZZ
Non-OR   ØN9B[0,3,4]Z[X,Z]
Non-OR   ØN9[R,T,V][0,3,4]ZZ

0 Medical and Surgical
N Head and Facial Bones
B Excision Definition: Cutting out or off, without replacement, a portion of a body part
Explanation: The qualifier DIAGNOSTIC is used to identify excision procedures that are biopsies

Body Part Character 4	Approach Character 5	Device Character 6	Qualifier Character 7

0 Skull
1 Frontal Bone
  Zygomatic process of frontal bone
3 Parietal Bone, Right
4 Parietal Bone, Left
5 Temporal Bone, Right
  Mastoid process
  Petrous part of temporal bone
  Tympanic part of temporal bone
  Zygomatic process of temporal bone
6 Temporal Bone, Left
  See 5 Temporal Bone, Right
7 Occipital Bone
  Foramen magnum
B Nasal Bone
  Vomer of nasal septum
C Sphenoid Bone
  Greater wing
  Lesser wing
  Optic foramen
  Pterygoid process
  Sella turcica
F Ethmoid Bone, Right
  Cribriform plate
G Ethmoid Bone, Left
  See F Ethmoid Bone, Right
H Lacrimal Bone, Right
J Lacrimal Bone, Left
K Palatine Bone, Right
L Palatine Bone, Left
M Zygomatic Bone, Right
N Zygomatic Bone, Left
P Orbit, Right
  Bony orbit
  Orbital portion of ethmoid bone
  Orbital portion of frontal bone
  Orbital portion of lacrimal bone
  Orbital portion of maxilla
  Orbital portion of palatine bone
  Orbital portion of sphenoid bone
  Orbital portion of zygomatic bone
Q Orbit, Left
  See P Orbit, Right
R Maxilla
  Alveolar process of maxilla
T Mandible, Right
  Alveolar process of mandible
  Condyloid process
  Mandibular notch
  Mental foramen
V Mandible, Left
  See T Mandible, Right
X Hyoid Bone
	0 Open
	3 Percutaneous
	4 Percutaneous Endoscopic
		Z No Device	**X** Diagnostic
			Z No Qualifier

Non-OR 0NB[B,R,T,V][0,3,4]ZX

Head and Facial Bones

0 Medical and Surgical
N Head and Facial Bones
C Extirpation   Definition: Taking or cutting out solid matter from a body part
Explanation: The solid matter may be an abnormal byproduct of a biological function or a foreign body; it may be imbedded in a body part or in the lumen of a tubular body part. The solid matter may or may not have been previously broken into pieces.

Body Part Character 4	Approach Character 5	Device Character 6	Qualifier Character 7

1 Frontal Bone
  Zygomatic process of frontal bone
3 Parietal Bone, Right
4 Parietal Bone, Left
5 Temporal Bone, Right
  Mastoid process
  Petrous part of temporal bone
  Tympanic part of temporal bone
  Zygomatic process of temporal bone
6 Temporal Bone, Left
  See 5 Temporal Bone, Right
7 Occipital Bone
  Foramen magnum
B Nasal Bone
  Vomer of nasal septum
C Sphenoid Bone
  Greater wing
  Lesser wing
  Optic foramen
  Pterygoid process
  Sella turcica
F Ethmoid Bone, Right
  Cribriform plate
G Ethmoid Bone, Left
  See F Ethmoid Bone, Right
H Lacrimal Bone, Right
J Lacrimal Bone, Left
K Palatine Bone, Right
L Palatine Bone, Left
M Zygomatic Bone, Right
N Zygomatic Bone, Left
P Orbit, Right
  Bony orbit
  Orbital portion of ethmoid bone
  Orbital portion of frontal bone
  Orbital portion of lacrimal bone
  Orbital portion of maxilla
  Orbital portion of palatine bone
  Orbital portion of sphenoid bone
  Orbital portion of zygomatic bone
Q Orbit, Left
  See P Orbit, Right
R Maxilla
  Alveolar process of maxilla
T Mandible, Right
  Alveolar process of mandible
  Condyloid process
  Mandibular notch
  Mental foramen
V Mandible, Left
  See T Mandible, Right
X Hyoid Bone
	0 Open
	3 Percutaneous
	4 Percutaneous Endoscopic
		Z No Device	**Z** No Qualifier

Non-OR   0NC[B,R,T,V][0,3,4]ZZ

ICD-10-PCS 2025 — Head and Facial Bones — 0ND–0ND

- **0** Medical and Surgical
- **N** Head and Facial Bones
- **D** Extraction Definition: Pulling or stripping out or off all or a portion of a body part by the use of force
  Explanation: The qualifier DIAGNOSTIC is used to identify extraction procedures that are biopsies

Body Part Character 4	Approach Character 5	Device Character 6	Qualifier Character 7
0 Skull **1** Frontal Bone Zygomatic process of frontal bone **3** Parietal Bone, Right **4** Parietal Bone, Left **5** Temporal Bone, Right Mastoid process Petrous part of temporal bone Tympanic part of temporal bone Zygomatic process of temporal bone **6** Temporal Bone, Left *See 5 Temporal Bone, Right* **7** Occipital Bone Foramen magnum **B** Nasal Bone Vomer of nasal septum **C** Sphenoid Bone Greater wing Lesser wing Optic foramen Pterygoid process Sella turcica **F** Ethmoid Bone, Right Cribriform plate **G** Ethmoid Bone, Left *See F Ethmoid Bone, Right* **H** Lacrimal Bone, Right **J** Lacrimal Bone, Left **K** Palatine Bone, Right **L** Palatine Bone, Left **M** Zygomatic Bone, Right **N** Zygomatic Bone, Left **P** Orbit, Right Bony orbit Orbital portion of ethmoid bone Orbital portion of frontal bone Orbital portion of lacrimal bone Orbital portion of maxilla Orbital portion of palatine bone Orbital portion of sphenoid bone Orbital portion of zygomatic bone **Q** Orbit, Left *See P Orbit, Right* **R** Maxilla Alveolar process of maxilla **T** Mandible, Right Alveolar process of mandible Condyloid process Mandibular notch Mental foramen **V** Mandible, Left *See T Mandible, Right* **X** Hyoid Bone	**0** Open	**Z** No Device	**Z** No Qualifier

ØNH–ØNH Head and Facial Bones ICD-10-PCS 2025

Ø Medical and Surgical
N Head and Facial Bones
H Insertion Definition: Putting in a nonbiological appliance that monitors, assists, performs, or prevents a physiological function but does not physically take the place of a body part
Explanation: None

Body Part Character 4	Approach Character 5	Device Character 6	Qualifier Character 7
Ø Skull ✚	**Ø** Open	**3** Infusion Device **4** Internal Fixation Device **5** External Fixation Device **M** Bone Growth Stimulator **N** Neurostimulator Generator	**Z** No Qualifier
Ø Skull	**3** Percutaneous **4** Percutaneous Endoscopic	**3** Infusion Device **4** Internal Fixation Device **5** External Fixation Device **M** Bone Growth Stimulator	**Z** No Qualifier

1 Frontal Bone
    Zygomatic process of frontal bone
3 Parietal Bone, Right
4 Parietal Bone, Left
7 Occipital Bone
    Foramen magnum
C Sphenoid Bone
    Greater wing
    Lesser wing
    Optic foramen
    Pterygoid process
    Sella turcica
F Ethmoid Bone, Right
    Cribriform plate
G Ethmoid Bone, Left
    See F Ethmoid Bone, Right
H Lacrimal Bone, Right
J Lacrimal Bone, Left
K Palatine Bone, Right
L Palatine Bone, Left
M Zygomatic Bone, Right
N Zygomatic Bone, Left
P Orbit, Right
    Bony orbit
    Orbital portion of ethmoid bone
    Orbital portion of frontal bone
    Orbital portion of lacrimal bone
    Orbital portion of maxilla
    Orbital portion of palatine bone
    Orbital portion of sphenoid bone
    Orbital portion of zygomatic bone
Q Orbit, Left
    See P Orbit, Right
X Hyoid Bone
	Ø Open
	3 Percutaneous
	4 Percutaneous Endoscopic
		4 Internal Fixation Device	**Z** No Qualifier

5 Temporal Bone, Right
    Mastoid process
    Petrous part of temporal bone
    Tympanic part of temporal bone
    Zygomatic process of temporal bone
6 Temporal Bone, Left
    See 5 Temporal Bone, Right
	Ø Open
	3 Percutaneous
	4 Percutaneous Endoscopic
		4 Internal Fixation Device
		S Hearing Device
			Z No Qualifier

B Nasal Bone Vomer of nasal septum	**Ø** Open **3** Percutaneous **4** Percutaneous Endoscopic	**4** Internal Fixation Device **M** Bone Growth Stimulator	**Z** No Qualifier

R Maxilla
    Alveolar process of maxilla
T Mandible, Right
    Alveolar process of mandible
    Condyloid process
    Mandibular notch
    Mental foramen
V Mandible, Left
    See T Mandible, Right
	Ø Open
	3 Percutaneous
	4 Percutaneous Endoscopic
		4 Internal Fixation Device
		5 External Fixation Device
			Z No Qualifier

W Facial Bone	**Ø** Open **3** Percutaneous **4** Percutaneous Endoscopic	**M** Bone Growth Stimulator	**Z** No Qualifier

Non-OR ØNHØØ5Z
Non-OR ØNHØ[3,4]5Z
Non-OR ØNHB[Ø,3,4][4,M]Z

See Appendix L for Procedure Combinations
✚ ØNHØØNZ

Non-OR Procedure DRG Non-OR Procedure Valid OR Procedure HAC Associated Procedure Combination Only New/Revised April New/Revised October

ICD-10-PCS 2025   Head and Facial Bones   ØNJ–ØNN

Ø Medical and Surgical
N Head and Facial Bones
J Inspection   Definition: Visually and/or manually exploring a body part
     Explanation: Visual exploration may be performed with or without optical instrumentation. Manual exploration may be performed directly or through intervening body layers.

Body Part Character 4	Approach Character 5	Device Character 6	Qualifier Character 7
Ø Skull B Nasal Bone Vomer of nasal septum W Facial Bone	Ø Open 3 Percutaneous 4 Percutaneous Endoscopic X External	Z No Device	Z No Qualifier

Non-OR   ØNJ[Ø,B,W][3,X]ZZ

Ø Medical and Surgical
N Head and Facial Bones
N Release   Definition: Freeing a body part from an abnormal physical constraint by cutting or by the use of force
     Explanation: Some of the restraining tissue may be taken out but none of the body part is taken out

Body Part Character 4	Approach Character 5	Device Character 6	Qualifier Character 7

1 Frontal Bone
    Zygomatic process of frontal bone
3 Parietal Bone, Right
4 Parietal Bone, Left
5 Temporal Bone, Right
    Mastoid process
    Petrous part of temporal bone
    Tympanic part of temporal bone
    Zygomatic process of temporal bone
6 Temporal Bone, Left
    See 5 Temporal Bone, Right
7 Occipital Bone
    Foramen magnum
B Nasal Bone
    Vomer of nasal septum
C Sphenoid Bone
    Greater wing
    Lesser wing
    Optic foramen
    Pterygoid process
    Sella turcica
F Ethmoid Bone, Right
    Cribriform plate
G Ethmoid Bone, Left
    See F Ethmoid Bone, Right
H Lacrimal Bone, Right
J Lacrimal Bone, Left
K Palatine Bone, Right
L Palatine Bone, Left
M Zygomatic Bone, Right
N Zygomatic Bone, Left
P Orbit, Right
    Bony orbit
    Orbital portion of ethmoid bone
    Orbital portion of frontal bone
    Orbital portion of lacrimal bone
    Orbital portion of maxilla
    Orbital portion of palatine bone
    Orbital portion of sphenoid bone
    Orbital portion of zygomatic bone
Q Orbit, Left
    See P Orbit, Right
R Maxilla
    Alveolar process of maxilla
T Mandible, Right
    Alveolar process of mandible
    Condyloid process
    Mandibular notch
    Mental foramen
V Mandible, Left
    See T Mandible, Right
X Hyoid Bone
	Ø Open
	3 Percutaneous
	4 Percutaneous Endoscopic
		Z No Device	Z No Qualifier

Non-OR   ØNNB[Ø,3,4]ZZ

Head and Facial Bones

0NP–0NP Head and Facial Bones ICD-10-PCS 2025

- **0** Medical and Surgical
- **N** Head and Facial Bones
- **P** Removal
  Definition: Taking out or off a device from a body part
  Explanation: If a device is taken out and a similar device put in without cutting or puncturing the skin or mucous membrane, the procedure is coded to the root operation CHANGE. Otherwise, the procedure for taking out a device is coded to the root operation REMOVAL.

Body Part Character 4	Approach Character 5	Device Character 6	Qualifier Character 7
0 Skull	0 Open	0 Drainage Device 3 Infusion Device 4 Internal Fixation Device 5 External Fixation Device 7 Autologous Tissue Substitute J Synthetic Substitute K Nonautologous Tissue Substitute M Bone Growth Stimulator N Neurostimulator Generator S Hearing Device	Z No Qualifier
0 Skull	3 Percutaneous 4 Percutaneous Endoscopic	0 Drainage Device 3 Infusion Device 4 Internal Fixation Device 5 External Fixation Device 7 Autologous Tissue Substitute J Synthetic Substitute K Nonautologous Tissue Substitute M Bone Growth Stimulator S Hearing Device	Z No Qualifier
0 Skull	X External	0 Drainage Device 3 Infusion Device 4 Internal Fixation Device 5 External Fixation Device M Bone Growth Stimulator S Hearing Device	Z No Qualifier
B Nasal Bone Vomer of nasal septum W Facial Bone	0 Open 3 Percutaneous 4 Percutaneous Endoscopic	0 Drainage Device 4 Internal Fixation Device 5 External Fixation Device 7 Autologous Tissue Substitute J Synthetic Substitute K Nonautologous Tissue Substitute M Bone Growth Stimulator	Z No Qualifier
B Nasal Bone Vomer of nasal septum W Facial Bone	X External	0 Drainage Device 4 Internal Fixation Device 5 External Fixation Device M Bone Growth Stimulator	Z No Qualifier

Non-OR 0NP0[3,4]5Z
Non-OR 0NP0X[0,3,5]Z
Non-OR 0NPB[0,3,4][0,4,7,J,K,M]Z
Non-OR 0NPBX[0,4,M]Z
Non-OR 0NPWX[0,M]Z

ICD-10-PCS 2025 — Head and Facial Bones — ØNQ–ØNQ

Ø Medical and Surgical
N Head and Facial Bones
Q Repair Definition: Restoring, to the extent possible, a body part to its normal anatomic structure and function
Explanation: Used only when the method to accomplish the repair is not one of the other root operations

Body Part Character 4	Approach Character 5	Device Character 6	Qualifier Character 7

Ø Skull
1 Frontal Bone
  Zygomatic process of frontal bone
3 Parietal Bone, Right
4 Parietal Bone, Left
5 Temporal Bone, Right
  Mastoid process
  Petrous part of temporal bone
  Tympanic part of temporal bone
  Zygomatic process of temporal bone
6 Temporal Bone, Left
  See 5 Temporal Bone, Right
7 Occipital Bone
  Foramen magnum
B Nasal Bone
  Vomer of nasal septum
C Sphenoid Bone
  Greater wing
  Lesser wing
  Optic foramen
  Pterygoid process
  Sella turcica
F Ethmoid Bone, Right
  Cribriform plate
G Ethmoid Bone, Left
  See F Ethmoid Bone, Right
H Lacrimal Bone, Right
J Lacrimal Bone, Left
K Palatine Bone, Right
L Palatine Bone, Left
M Zygomatic Bone, Right
N Zygomatic Bone, Left
P Orbit, Right
  Bony orbit
  Orbital portion of ethmoid bone
  Orbital portion of frontal bone
  Orbital portion of lacrimal bone
  Orbital portion of maxilla
  Orbital portion of palatine bone
  Orbital portion of sphenoid bone
  Orbital portion of zygomatic bone
Q Orbit, Left
  See P Orbit, Right
R Maxilla
  Alveolar process of maxilla
T Mandible, Right
  Alveolar process of mandible
  Condyloid process
  Mandibular notch
  Mental foramen
V Mandible, Left
  See T Mandible, Right
X Hyoid Bone
	Ø Open
	3 Percutaneous
	4 Percutaneous Endoscopic
	X External
		Z No Device	**Z** No Qualifier

Non-OR ØNQ[Ø,1,3,4,5,6,7,B,C,F,G,H,J,K,L,M,N,P,Q,R,T,V,X]XZZ

0 Medical and Surgical
N Head and Facial Bones
R Replacement **Definition:** Putting in or on biological or synthetic material that physically takes the place and/or function of all or a portion of a body part
Explanation: The body part may have been taken out or replaced, or may be taken out, physically eradicated, or rendered nonfunctional during the REPLACEMENT procedure. A REMOVAL procedure is coded for taking out the device used in a previous replacement procedure.

Body Part Character 4	Approach Character 5	Device Character 6	Qualifier Character 7
0 Skull **1** Frontal Bone 　Zygomatic process of frontal bone **3** Parietal Bone, Right **4** Parietal Bone, Left **5** Temporal Bone, Right 　Mastoid process 　Petrous part of temporal bone 　Tympanic part of temporal bone 　Zygomatic process of temporal bone **6** Temporal Bone, Left 　*See 5 Temporal Bone, Right* **7** Occipital Bone 　Foramen magnum **B** Nasal Bone 　Vomer of nasal septum **C** Sphenoid Bone 　Greater wing 　Lesser wing 　Optic foramen 　Pterygoid process 　Sella turcica **F** Ethmoid Bone, Right 　Cribriform plate **G** Ethmoid Bone, Left 　*See F Ethmoid Bone, Right* **H** Lacrimal Bone, Right **J** Lacrimal Bone, Left **K** Palatine Bone, Right **L** Palatine Bone, Left **M** Zygomatic Bone, Right **N** Zygomatic Bone, Left **P** Orbit, Right 　Bony orbit 　Orbital portion of ethmoid bone 　Orbital portion of frontal bone 　Orbital portion of lacrimal bone 　Orbital portion of maxilla 　Orbital portion of palatine bone 　Orbital portion of sphenoid bone 　Orbital portion of zygomatic bone **Q** Orbit, Left 　*See P Orbit, Right* **R** Maxilla 　Alveolar process of maxilla **T** Mandible, Right 　Alveolar process of mandible 　Condyloid process 　Mandibular notch 　Mental foramen **V** Mandible, Left 　*See T Mandible, Right* **X** Hyoid Bone	**0** Open **3** Percutaneous **4** Percutaneous Endoscopic	**7** Autologous Tissue Substitute **J** Synthetic Substitute **K** Nonautologous Tissue Substitute	**Z** No Qualifier

ICD-10-PCS 2025   Head and Facial Bones   0NS–0NS

- **0** Medical and Surgical
- **N** Head and Facial Bones
- **S** Reposition   Definition: Moving to its normal location, or other suitable location, all or a portion of a body part
  Explanation: The body part is moved to a new location from an abnormal location, or from a normal location where it is not functioning correctly. The body part may or may not be cut out or off to be moved to the new location.

Body Part Character 4	Approach Character 5	Device Character 6	Qualifier Character 7

0 Skull
R Maxilla
   Alveolar process of maxilla
T Mandible, Right
   Alveolar process of mandible
   Condyloid process
   Mandibular notch
   Mental foramen
V Mandible, Left
   See T Mandible, Right
	0 Open
	3 Percutaneous
	4 Percutaneous Endoscopic
		4 Internal Fixation Device
		5 External Fixation Device
		Z No Device
			Z No Qualifier

0 Skull
R Maxilla
   Alveolar process of maxilla
T Mandible, Right
   Alveolar process of mandible
   Condyloid process
   Mandibular notch
   Mental foramen
V Mandible, Left
   See T Mandible, Right
	X External	**Z** No Device	**Z** No Qualifier

1 Frontal Bone
   Zygomatic process of frontal bone
3 Parietal Bone, Right
4 Parietal Bone, Left
5 Temporal Bone, Right
   Mastoid process
   Petrous part of temporal bone
   Tympanic part of temporal bone
   Zygomatic process of temporal bone
6 Temporal Bone, Left
   See 5 Temporal Bone, Right
7 Occipital Bone
   Foramen magnum
B Nasal Bone
   Vomer of nasal septum
C Sphenoid Bone
   Greater wing
   Lesser wing
   Optic foramen
   Pterygoid process
   Sella turcica
F Ethmoid Bone, Right
   Cribriform plate
G Ethmoid Bone, Left
   See F Ethmoid Bone, Right
H Lacrimal Bone, Right
J Lacrimal Bone, Left
K Palatine Bone, Right
L Palatine Bone, Left
M Zygomatic Bone, Right
N Zygomatic Bone, Left
P Orbit, Right
   Bony orbit
   Orbital portion of ethmoid bone
   Orbital portion of frontal bone
   Orbital portion of lacrimal bone
   Orbital portion of maxilla
   Orbital portion of palatine bone
   Orbital portion of sphenoid bone
   Orbital portion of zygomatic bone
Q Orbit, Left
   See P Orbit, Right
X Hyoid Bone
	0 Open
	3 Percutaneous
	4 Percutaneous Endoscopic
		4 Internal Fixation Device
		Z No Device
			Z No Qualifier

Non-OR   0NS[R,T,V][3,4][4,5,Z]Z
Non-OR   0NS[0,R,T,V]XZZ
Non-OR   0NS[B,C,F,G,H,J,K,L,M,N,P,Q,X][3,4][4,Z]Z

0NS Continued on next page

0 Medical and Surgical
N Head and Facial Bones
S Reposition Definition: Moving to its normal location, or other suitable location, all or a portion of a body part
Explanation: The body part is moved to a new location from an abnormal location, or from a normal location where it is not functioning correctly. The body part may or may not be cut out or off to be moved to the new location.

0NS Continued

Body Part Character 4	Approach Character 5	Device Character 6	Qualifier Character 7
1 Frontal Bone Zygomatic process of frontal bone **3 Parietal Bone, Right** **4 Parietal Bone, Left** **5 Temporal Bone, Right** Mastoid process Petrous part of temporal bone Tympanic part of temporal bone Zygomatic process of temporal bone **6 Temporal Bone, Left** See 5 Temporal Bone, Right **7 Occipital Bone** Foramen magnum **B Nasal Bone** Vomer of nasal septum **C Sphenoid Bone** Greater wing Lesser wing Optic foramen Pterygoid process Sella turcica **F Ethmoid Bone, Right** Cribriform plate **G Ethmoid Bone, Left** See F Ethmoid Bone, Right **H Lacrimal Bone, Right** **J Lacrimal Bone, Left** **K Palatine Bone, Right** **L Palatine Bone, Left** **M Zygomatic Bone, Right** **N Zygomatic Bone, Left** **P Orbit, Right** Bony orbit Orbital portion of ethmoid bone Orbital portion of frontal bone Orbital portion of lacrimal bone Orbital portion of maxilla Orbital portion of palatine bone Orbital portion of sphenoid bone Orbital portion of zygomatic bone **Q Orbit, Left** See P Orbit, Right **X Hyoid Bone**	**X** External	**Z** No Device	**Z** No Qualifier

Non-OR 0NS[1,3,4,5,6,7,B,C,F,G,H,J,K,L,M,N,P,Q,X]XZZ

0 Medical and Surgical
N Head and Facial Bones
T Resection   Definition: Cutting out or off, without replacement, all of a body part
                 Explanation: None

Body Part Character 4	Approach Character 5	Device Character 6	Qualifier Character 7

1 Frontal Bone
   Zygomatic process of frontal bone
3 Parietal Bone, Right
4 Parietal Bone, Left
5 Temporal Bone, Right
   Mastoid process
   Petrous part of temporal bone
   Tympanic part of temporal bone
   Zygomatic process of temporal bone
6 Temporal Bone, Left
   See *5 Temporal Bone, Right*
7 Occipital Bone
   Foramen magnum
B Nasal Bone
   Vomer of nasal septum
C Sphenoid Bone
   Greater wing
   Lesser wing
   Optic foramen
   Pterygoid process
   Sella turcica
F Ethmoid Bone, Right
   Cribriform plate
G Ethmoid Bone, Left
   See *F Ethmoid Bone, Right*
H Lacrimal Bone, Right
J Lacrimal Bone, Left
K Palatine Bone, Right
L Palatine Bone, Left
M Zygomatic Bone, Right
N Zygomatic Bone, Left
P Orbit, Right
   Bony orbit
   Orbital portion of ethmoid bone
   Orbital portion of frontal bone
   Orbital portion of lacrimal bone
   Orbital portion of maxilla
   Orbital portion of palatine bone
   Orbital portion of sphenoid bone
   Orbital portion of zygomatic bone
Q Orbit, Left
   See *P Orbit, Right*
R Maxilla
   Alveolar process of maxilla
T Mandible, Right
   Alveolar process of mandible
   Condyloid process
   Mandibular notch
   Mental foramen
V Mandible, Left
   See *T Mandible, Right*
X Hyoid Bone
	0 Open	**Z No Device**	**Z No Qualifier**

0 Medical and Surgical
N Head and Facial Bones
U Supplement   Definition: Putting in or on biological or synthetic material that physically reinforces and/or augments the function of a portion of a body part
                  Explanation: The biological material is non-living, or is living and from the same individual. The body part may have been previously replaced, and the SUPPLEMENT procedure is performed to physically reinforce and/or augment the function of the replaced body part.

Body Part Character 4	Approach Character 5	Device Character 6	Qualifier Character 7

0 Skull
1 Frontal Bone
    Zygomatic process of frontal bone
3 Parietal Bone, Right
4 Parietal Bone, Left
5 Temporal Bone, Right
    Mastoid process
    Petrous part of temporal bone
    Tympanic part of temporal bone
    Zygomatic process of temporal bone
6 Temporal Bone, Left
    See 5 Temporal Bone, Right
7 Occipital Bone
    Foramen magnum
B Nasal Bone
    Vomer of nasal septum
C Sphenoid Bone
    Greater wing
    Lesser wing
    Optic foramen
    Pterygoid process
    Sella turcica
F Ethmoid Bone, Right
    Cribriform plate
G Ethmoid Bone, Left
    See F Ethmoid Bone, Right
H Lacrimal Bone, Right
J Lacrimal Bone, Left
K Palatine Bone, Right
L Palatine Bone, Left
M Zygomatic Bone, Right
N Zygomatic Bone, Left
P Orbit, Right
    Bony orbit
    Orbital portion of ethmoid bone
    Orbital portion of frontal bone
    Orbital portion of lacrimal bone
    Orbital portion of maxilla
    Orbital portion of palatine bone
    Orbital portion of sphenoid bone
    Orbital portion of zygomatic bone
Q Orbit, Left
    See P Orbit, Right
R Maxilla
    Alveolar process of maxilla
T Mandible, Right
    Alveolar process of mandible
    Condyloid process
    Mandibular notch
    Mental foramen
V Mandible, Left
    See T Mandible, Right
X Hyoid Bone
	0 Open
	3 Percutaneous
	4 Percutaneous Endoscopic
		7 Autologous Tissue Substitute
		J Synthetic Substitute
		K Nonautologous Tissue Substitute
			Z No Qualifier

ICD-10-PCS 2025 — Head and Facial Bones — ØNW–ØNW

- **Ø** Medical and Surgical
- **N** Head and Facial Bones
- **W** Revision   Definition: Correcting, to the extent possible, a portion of a malfunctioning device or the position of a displaced device
  Explanation: Revision can include correcting a malfunctioning or displaced device by taking out or putting in components of the device such as a screw or pin

Body Part Character 4	Approach Character 5	Device Character 6	Qualifier Character 7
Ø Skull	Ø Open	Ø Drainage Device 3 Infusion Device 4 Internal Fixation Device 5 External Fixation Device 7 Autologous Tissue Substitute J Synthetic Substitute K Nonautologous Tissue Substitute M Bone Growth Stimulator N Neurostimulator Generator S Hearing Device	Z No Qualifier
Ø Skull	3 Percutaneous 4 Percutaneous Endoscopic X External	Ø Drainage Device 3 Infusion Device 4 Internal Fixation Device 5 External Fixation Device 7 Autologous Tissue Substitute J Synthetic Substitute K Nonautologous Tissue Substitute M Bone Growth Stimulator S Hearing Device	Z No Qualifier
B Nasal Bone Vomer of nasal septum W Facial Bone	Ø Open 3 Percutaneous 4 Percutaneous Endoscopic X External	Ø Drainage Device 4 Internal Fixation Device 5 External Fixation Device 7 Autologous Tissue Substitute J Synthetic Substitute K Nonautologous Tissue Substitute M Bone Growth Stimulator	Z No Qualifier

Non-OR   ØNWØX[Ø,3,4,5,7,J,K,M,S]Z
Non-OR   ØNWB[Ø,3,4,X][Ø,4,7,J,K,M]Z
Non-OR   ØNWWX[Ø,4,7,J,K,M]Z

Upper Bones ØP2–ØPW

Character Meanings

This Character Meaning table is provided as a guide to assist the user in the identification of character members that may be found in this section of code tables. It **SHOULD NOT** be used to build a PCS code.

Operation–Character 3	Body Part–Character 4	Approach–Character 5	Device–Character 6	Qualifier–Character 7
2 Change	Ø Sternum	Ø Open	Ø Drainage Device OR Internal Fixation Device, Rigid Plate	3 Laser Interstitial Thermal Therapy
5 Destruction	1 Ribs, 1 to 2	3 Percutaneous	3 Spinal Stabilization Device, Vertebral Body Tether	X Diagnostic
8 Division	2 Ribs, 3 or more	4 Percutaneous Endoscopic	4 Internal Fixation Device	Z No Qualifier
9 Drainage	3 Cervical Vertebra	X External	5 External Fixation Device	
B Excision	4 Thoracic Vertebra		6 Internal Fixation Device, Intramedullary	
C Extirpation	5 Scapula, Right		7 Autologous Tissue Substitute OR Internal Fixation Device, Intramedullary Limb Lengthening	
D Extraction	6 Scapula, Left		8 External Fixation Device, Limb Lengthening	
H Insertion	7 Glenoid Cavity, Right		B External Fixation Device, Monoplanar	
J Inspection	8 Glenoid Cavity, Left		C External Fixation Device, Ring	
N Release	9 Clavicle, Right		D External Fixation Device, Hybrid	
P Removal	B Clavicle, Left		J Synthetic Substitute	
Q Repair	C Humeral Head, Right		K Nonautologous Tissue Substitute	
R Replacement	D Humeral Head, Left		M Bone Growth Stimulator	
S Reposition	F Humeral Shaft, Right		Y Other Device	
T Resection	G Humeral Shaft, Left		Z No Device	
U Supplement	H Radius, Right			
W Revision	J Radius, Left			
	K Ulna, Right			
	L Ulna, Left			
	M Carpal, Right			
	N Carpal, Left			
	P Metacarpal, Right			
	Q Metacarpal, Left			
	R Thumb Phalanx, Right			
	S Thumb Phalanx, Left			
	T Finger Phalanx, Right			
	V Finger Phalanx, Left			
	Y Upper Bone			

AHA Coding Clinic for table ØP5
2023, 1Q, 10   Laser interstitial thermal therapy

AHA Coding Clinic for table ØPB
2023, 2Q, 30   Excisional debridement and non-excisional debridement at deeper layer same site
2015, 3Q, 3-8   Excisional and nonexcisional debridement
2015, 2Q, 34   Decompressive laminectomy
2013, 4Q, 109   Separating conjoined twins
2013, 4Q, 116   Spinal decompression
2013, 3Q, 20   Superior labrum anterior posterior (SLAP) repair and subacromial decompression
2012, 4Q, 101   Rib resection with reconstruction of anterior chest wall
2012, 2Q, 19   Multiple decompressive cervical laminectomies

AHA Coding Clinic for table ØPC
2021, 3Q, 15   Curettage of bilateral humeral head and bone graft placement
2019, 3Q, 19   Removal of sternal wire

AHA Coding Clinic for table ØPD
2023, 2Q, 30   Excisional debridement and non-excisional debridement at deeper layer same site
2017, 4Q, 41   Extraction procedures

AHA Coding Clinic for table ØPH
2020, 1Q, 29   Repair of sternal dehiscence using Sternal Talon® device
2019, 4Q, 34   Intramedullary limb lengthening internal fixation device
2019, 2Q, 40   Decompression of spinal cord and placement of instrumentation
2018, 3Q, 26   Anterior vertebral tethering using Dynesys Tethering System
2017, 2Q, 20   Exchange of intramedullary antibiotic impregnated spacer
2016, 4Q, 117   Placement of magnetic growth rods
2014, 4Q, 28   Removal and replacement of displaced growing rods

AHA Coding Clinic for table ØPP
2019, 3Q, 19   Removal of sternal wire
2017, 2Q, 20   Exchange of intramedullary antibiotic impregnated spacer
2016, 4Q, 117   Placement of magnetic growth rods
2014, 4Q, 28   Removal and replacement of displaced growing rods

AHA Coding Clinic for table ØPR
2018, 4Q, 92   Radial head arthroplasty

AHA Coding Clinic for table ØPS
2023, 3Q, 23   Aspiration and injection of bone marrow at fracture site
2021, 4Q, 51-52   Vertebral body tethering
2020, 1Q, 33   Spinal fusion without use of bone graft
2018, 3Q, 26   Anterior vertebral tethering using Dynesys Tethering System
2017, 4Q, 53   New and revised body part values - Ribs
2016, 1Q, 21   Elongation derotation flexion casting
2015, 4Q, 33   Ravitch operation
2015, 2Q, 35   Application of tongs to reduce and stabilize cervical fracture
2014, 4Q, 26   Placement of vertical expandable prosthetic titanium rib (VEPTR)
2014, 4Q, 32   Open reduction internal fixation of fracture with debridement
2014, 3Q, 33   Radial fracture treatment with open reduction internal fixation, and release of carpal ligament

AHA Coding Clinic for table ØPT
2015, 3Q, 26   Thumb arthroplasty with resection of trapezium

AHA Coding Clinic for table ØPU
2023, 2Q, 24   Remplissage of subscapularis tendon
2021, 3Q, 15   Curettage of bilateral humeral head and bone graft placement
2015, 2Q, 20   Cervical laminoplasty
2013, 4Q, 109   Separating conjoined twins

AHA Coding Clinic for table ØPW
2014, 4Q, 26   Adjustment of VEPTR lengthening mechanism
2014, 4Q, 27   Bilateral lengthening of growing rods

Upper Bones

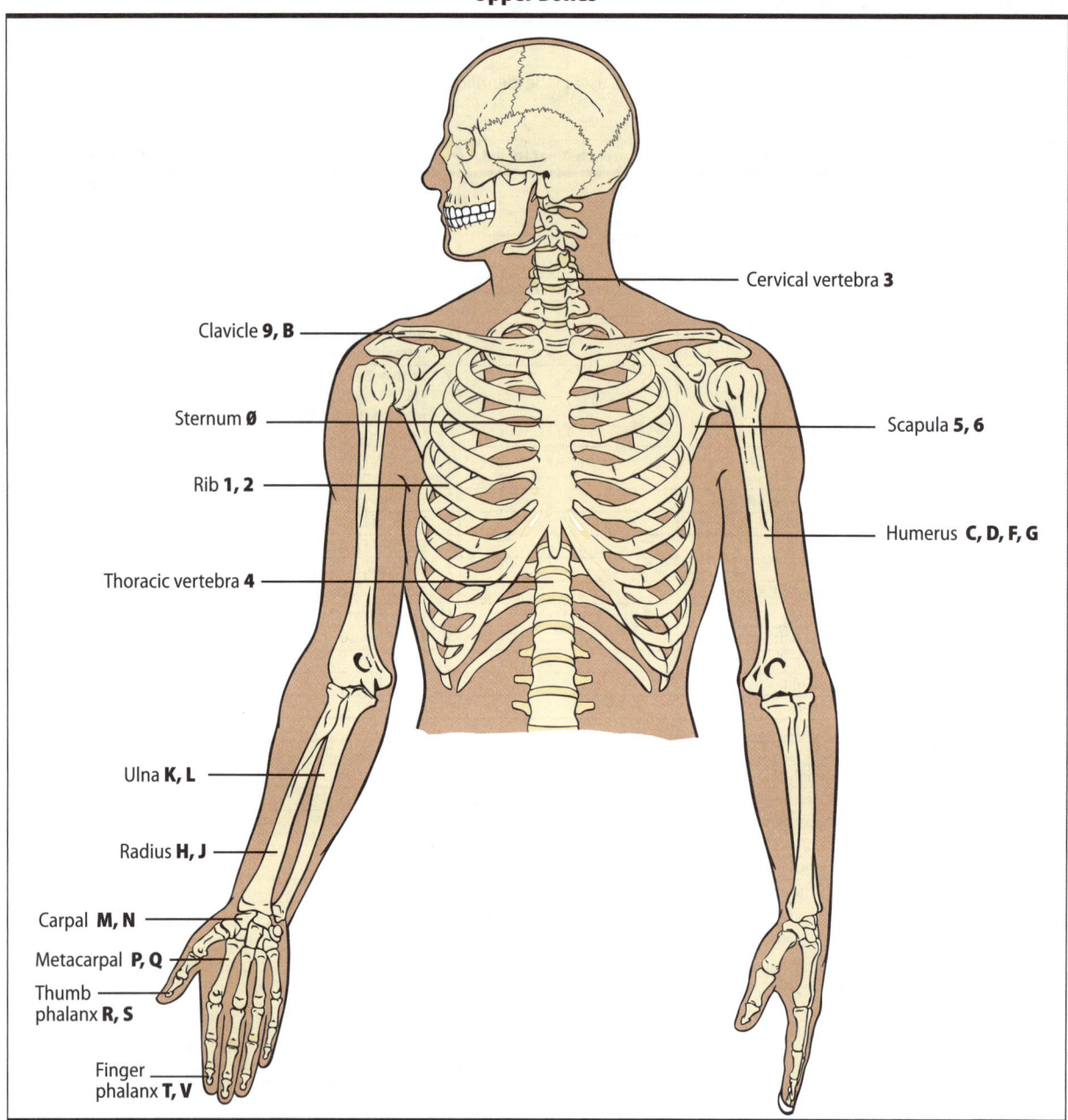

Cervical vertebra **3**
Clavicle **9, B**
Sternum **Ø**
Rib **1, 2**
Thoracic vertebra **4**
Scapula **5, 6**
Humerus **C, D, F, G**
Ulna **K, L**
Radius **H, J**
Carpal **M, N**
Metacarpal **P, Q**
Thumb phalanx **R, S**
Finger phalanx **T, V**

Upper Bones

Humerus and Scapula

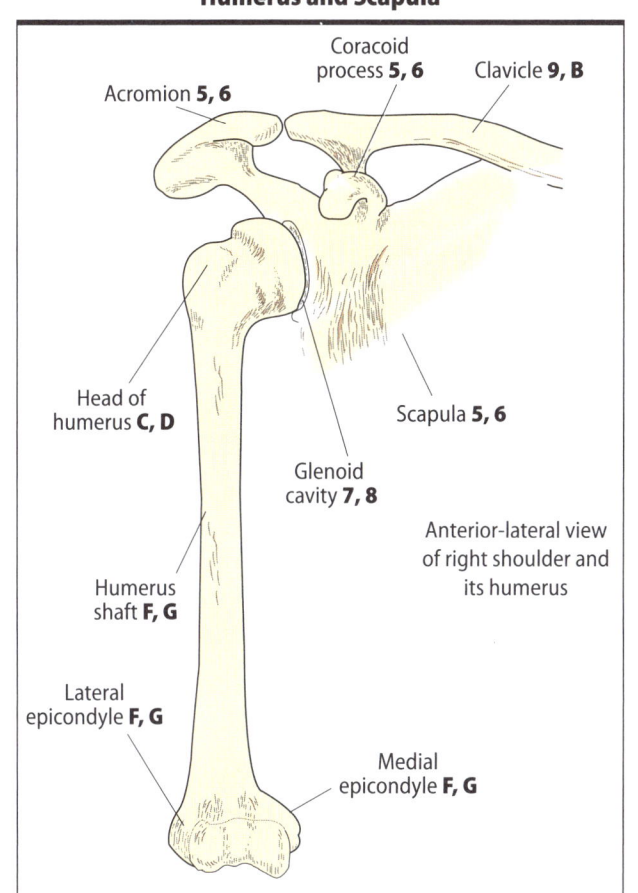

- Acromion **5, 6**
- Coracoid process **5, 6**
- Clavicle **9, B**
- Head of humerus **C, D**
- Scapula **5, 6**
- Glenoid cavity **7, 8**
- Humerus shaft **F, G**
- Lateral epicondyle **F, G**
- Medial epicondyle **F, G**

Anterior-lateral view of right shoulder and its humerus

Radius and Ulna

- Radius **H, J**
- Olecranon process **K, L**
- Coronoid process **K, L**
- Ulna **K, L**
- Shaft **H, J**
- Shaft **K, L**
- Radial styloid process **H, J**
- Ulnar styloid process **K, L**
- Carpal **M, N**

Phalanges

- Distal phalanx **T, V**
- Middle phalanx **T, V**
- Phalanges (digits) **T, V**
- Proximal phalanx **T, V**
- Distal phalanx (thumb) **R, S**
- Proximal phalanx (thumb) **R, S**
- Metacarpals **P, Q**
- Carpals **M, N**

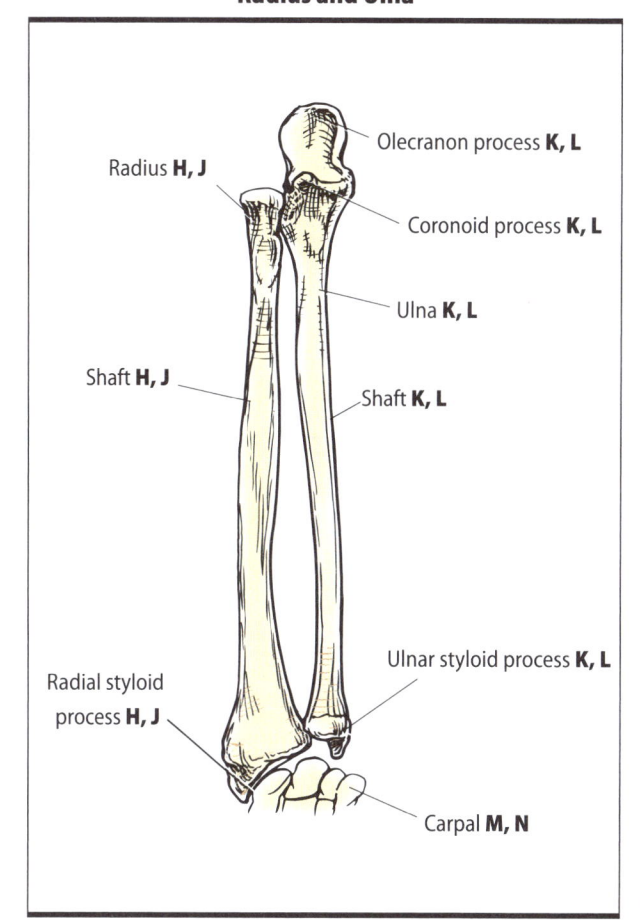

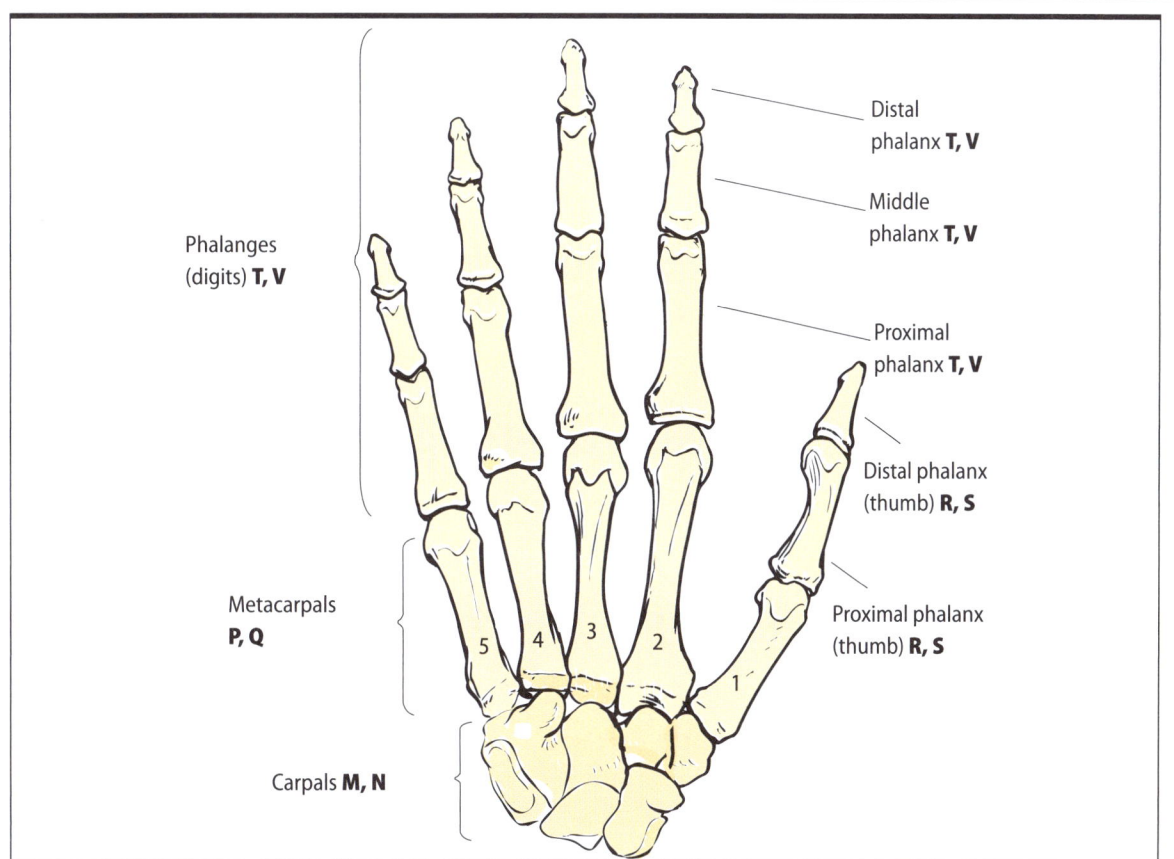

0 Medical and Surgical
P Upper Bones
2 Change

Definition: Taking out or off a device from a body part and putting back an identical or similar device in or on the same body part without cutting or puncturing the skin or a mucous membrane

Explanation: All CHANGE procedures are coded using the approach EXTERNAL

Body Part Character 4	Approach Character 5	Device Character 6	Qualifier Character 7
Y Upper Bone	X External	0 Drainage Device Y Other Device	Z No Qualifier

Non-OR All body part, approach, device, and qualifier values

---

0 Medical and Surgical
P Upper Bones
5 Destruction

Definition: Physical eradication of all or a portion of a body part by the direct use of energy, force, or a destructive agent

Explanation: None of the body part is physically taken out

Body Part Character 4	Approach Character 5	Device Character 6	Qualifier Character 7

0 Sternum
  Manubrium
  Suprasternal notch
  Xiphoid process
1 Ribs, 1 to 2
2 Ribs, 3 or More
5 Scapula, Right
  Acromion (process)
  Coracoid process
6 Scapula, Left
  See 5 Scapula, Right
7 Glenoid Cavity, Right
  Glenoid fossa (of scapula)
8 Glenoid Cavity, Left
  See 7 Glenoid Cavity, Right
9 Clavicle, Right
B Clavicle, Left
C Humeral Head, Right
  Greater tuberosity
  Lesser tuberosity
  Neck of humerus (anatomical)(surgical)
D Humeral Head, Left
  See C Humeral Head, Right
F Humeral Shaft, Right
  Distal humerus
  Humerus, distal
  Lateral epicondyle of humerus
  Medial epicondyle of humerus
G Humeral Shaft, Left
  See F Humeral Shaft, Right
H Radius, Right
  Ulnar notch
J Radius, Left
  See H Radius, Right
K Ulna, Right
  Olecranon process
  Radial notch
L Ulna, Left
  See K Ulna, Right
M Carpal, Right
  Capitate bone
  Hamate bone
  Lunate bone
  Pisiform bone
  Scaphoid bone
  Trapezium bone
  Trapezoid bone
  Triquetral bone
N Carpal, Left
  See M Carpal, Right
P Metacarpal, Right
Q Metacarpal, Left
R Thumb Phalanx, Right
S Thumb Phalanx, Left
T Finger Phalanx, Right
V Finger Phalanx, Left
	0 Open
	3 Percutaneous
	4 Percutaneous Endoscopic
		Z No Device	Z No Qualifier

3 Cervical Vertebra
  Dens
  Odontoid process
  Spinous process
  Transverse foramen
  Transverse process
  Vertebral arch
  Vertebral body
  Vertebral foramen
  Vertebral lamina
  Vertebral pedicle
4 Thoracic Vertebra
  Spinous process
  Transverse process
  Vertebral arch
  Vertebral body
  Vertebral foramen
  Vertebral lamina
  Vertebral pedicle
	0 Open
	3 Percutaneous
	4 Percutaneous Endoscopic
		Z No Device	3 Laser Interstitial Thermal Therapy
			Z No Qualifier

ICD-10-PCS 2025 — Upper Bones — 0P8–0P8

0 Medical and Surgical
P Upper Bones
8 Division

Definition: Cutting into a body part, without draining fluids and/or gases from the body part, in order to separate or transect a body part
Explanation: All or a portion of the body part is separated into two or more portions

Body Part Character 4	Approach Character 5	Device Character 6	Qualifier Character 7

0 Sternum
    Manubrium
    Suprasternal notch
    Xiphoid process
1 Ribs, 1 to 2
2 Ribs, 3 or More
3 Cervical Vertebra
    Dens
    Odontoid process
    Spinous process
    Transverse foramen
    Transverse process
    Vertebral arch
    Vertebral body
    Vertebral foramen
    Vertebral lamina
    Vertebral pedicle
4 Thoracic Vertebra
    Spinous process
    Transverse process
    Vertebral arch
    Vertebral body
    Vertebral foramen
    Vertebral lamina
    Vertebral pedicle
5 Scapula, Right
    Acromion (process)
    Coracoid process
6 Scapula, Left
    See 5 Scapula, Right
7 Glenoid Cavity, Right
    Glenoid fossa (of scapula)
8 Glenoid Cavity, Left
    See 7 Glenoid Cavity, Right
9 Clavicle, Right
B Clavicle, Left
C Humeral Head, Right
    Greater tuberosity
    Lesser tuberosity
    Neck of humerus (anatomical)(surgical)
D Humeral Head, Left
    See C Humeral Head, Right
F Humeral Shaft, Right
    Distal humerus
    Humerus, distal
    Lateral epicondyle of humerus
    Medial epicondyle of humerus
G Humeral Shaft, Left
    See F Humeral Shaft, Right
H Radius, Right
    Ulnar notch
J Radius, Left
    See H Radius, Right
K Ulna, Right
    Olecranon process
    Radial notch
L Ulna, Left
    See K Ulna, Right
M Carpal, Right
    Capitate bone
    Hamate bone
    Lunate bone
    Pisiform bone
    Scaphoid bone
    Trapezium bone
    Trapezoid bone
    Triquetral bone
N Carpal, Left
    See M Carpal, Right
P Metacarpal, Right
Q Metacarpal, Left
R Thumb Phalanx, Right
S Thumb Phalanx, Left
T Finger Phalanx, Right
V Finger Phalanx, Left
	0 Open
	3 Percutaneous
	4 Percutaneous Endoscopic
		Z No Device	Z No Qualifier

Upper Bones

0 Medical and Surgical
P Upper Bones
9 Drainage

Definition: Taking or letting out fluids and/or gases from a body part
Explanation: The qualifier DIAGNOSTIC is used to identify drainage procedures that are biopsies

Body Part Character 4	Approach Character 5	Device Character 6	Qualifier Character 7

0 Sternum
  Manubrium
  Suprasternal notch
  Xiphoid process
1 Ribs, 1 to 2
2 Ribs, 3 or More
3 Cervical Vertebra
  Dens
  Odontoid process
  Spinous process
  Transverse foramen
  Transverse process
  Vertebral arch
  Vertebral body
  Vertebral foramen
  Vertebral lamina
  Vertebral pedicle
4 Thoracic Vertebra
  Spinous process
  Transverse process
  Vertebral arch
  Vertebral body
  Vertebral foramen
  Vertebral lamina
  Vertebral pedicle
5 Scapula, Right
  Acromion (process)
  Coracoid process
6 Scapula, Left
  See 5 Scapula, Right
7 Glenoid Cavity, Right
  Glenoid fossa (of scapula)
8 Glenoid Cavity, Left
  See 7 Glenoid Cavity, Right
9 Clavicle, Right
B Clavicle, Left
C Humeral Head, Right
  Greater tuberosity
  Lesser tuberosity
  Neck of humerus (anatomical)(surgical)
D Humeral Head, Left
  See C Humeral Head, Right
F Humeral Shaft, Right
  Distal humerus
  Humerus, distal
  Lateral epicondyle of humerus
  Medial epicondyle of humerus
G Humeral Shaft, Left
  See F Humeral Shaft, Right
H Radius, Right
  Ulnar notch
J Radius, Left
  See H Radius, Right
K Ulna, Right
  Olecranon process
  Radial notch
L Ulna, Left
  See K Ulna, Right
M Carpal, Right
  Capitate bone
  Hamate bone
  Lunate bone
  Pisiform bone
  Scaphoid bone
  Trapezium bone
  Trapezoid bone
  Triquetral bone
N Carpal, Left
  See M Carpal, Right
P Metacarpal, Right
Q Metacarpal, Left
R Thumb Phalanx, Right
S Thumb Phalanx, Left
T Finger Phalanx, Right
V Finger Phalanx, Left
	0 Open
	3 Percutaneous
	4 Percutaneous Endoscopic
		0 Drainage Device	**Z** No Qualifier

Non-OR 0P9[0,1,2,3,4,5,6,7,8,9,B,C,D,F,G,H,J,K,L,M,N,P,Q,R,S,T,V]30Z

0P9 Continued on next page

ICD-10-PCS 2025 — Upper Bones — 0P9–0P9

0P9 Continued

- **0** Medical and Surgical
- **P** Upper Bones
- **9** Drainage

Definition: Taking or letting out fluids and/or gases from a body part
Explanation: The qualifier DIAGNOSTIC is used to identify drainage procedures that are biopsies

Body Part — Character 4	Approach — Character 5	Device — Character 6	Qualifier — Character 7
0 Sternum Manubrium Suprasternal notch Xiphoid process **1 Ribs, 1 to 2** **2 Ribs, 3 or More** **3 Cervical Vertebra** Dens Odontoid process Spinous process Transverse foramen Transverse process Vertebral arch Vertebral body Vertebral foramen Vertebral lamina Vertebral pedicle **4 Thoracic Vertebra** Spinous process Transverse process Vertebral arch Vertebral body Vertebral foramen Vertebral lamina Vertebral pedicle **5 Scapula, Right** Acromion (process) Coracoid process **6 Scapula, Left** *See 5 Scapula, Right* **7 Glenoid Cavity, Right** Glenoid fossa (of scapula) **8 Glenoid Cavity, Left** *See 7 Glenoid Cavity, Right* **9 Clavicle, Right** **B Clavicle, Left** **C Humeral Head, Right** Greater tuberosity Lesser tuberosity Neck of humerus (anatomical)(surgical) **D Humeral Head, Left** *See C Humeral Head, Right* **F Humeral Shaft, Right** Distal humerus Humerus, distal Lateral epicondyle of humerus Medial epicondyle of humerus **G Humeral Shaft, Left** *See F Humeral Shaft, Right* **H Radius, Right** Ulnar notch **J Radius, Left** *See H Radius, Right* **K Ulna, Right** Olecranon process Radial notch **L Ulna, Left** *See K Ulna, Right* **M Carpal, Right** Capitate bone Hamate bone Lunate bone Pisiform bone Scaphoid bone Trapezium bone Trapezoid bone Triquetral bone **N Carpal, Left** *See M Carpal, Right* **P Metacarpal, Right** **Q Metacarpal, Left** **R Thumb Phalanx, Right** **S Thumb Phalanx, Left** **T Finger Phalanx, Right** **V Finger Phalanx, Left**	**0** Open **3** Percutaneous **4** Percutaneous Endoscopic	**Z** No Device	**X** Diagnostic **Z** No Qualifier

Non-OR 0P9[0,1,2,3,4,5,6,7,8,9,B,C,D,F,G,H,J,K,L,M,N,P,Q,R,S,T,V]3ZZ

Upper Bones

ØPB–ØPB   Upper Bones   ICD-10-PCS 2025

Ø Medical and Surgical
P Upper Bones
B Excision   Definition: Cutting out or off, without replacement, a portion of a body part
                 Explanation: The qualifier DIAGNOSTIC is used to identify excision procedures that are biopsies

Body Part Character 4	Approach Character 5	Device Character 6	Qualifier Character 7

Ø **Sternum**
   Manubrium
   Suprasternal notch
   Xiphoid process
1 **Ribs, 1 to 2**
2 **Ribs, 3 or More**
3 **Cervical Vertebra**
   Dens
   Odontoid process
   Spinous process
   Transverse foramen
   Transverse process
   Vertebral arch
   Vertebral body
   Vertebral foramen
   Vertebral lamina
   Vertebral pedicle
4 **Thoracic Vertebra**
   Spinous process
   Transverse process
   Vertebral arch
   Vertebral body
   Vertebral foramen
   Vertebral lamina
   Vertebral pedicle
5 **Scapula, Right**
   Acromion (process)
   Coracoid process
6 **Scapula, Left**
   See 5 Scapula, Right
7 **Glenoid Cavity, Right**
   Glenoid fossa (of scapula)
8 **Glenoid Cavity, Left**
   See 7 Glenoid Cavity, Right
9 **Clavicle, Right**
B **Clavicle, Left**
C **Humeral Head, Right**
   Greater tuberosity
   Lesser tuberosity
   Neck of humerus (anatomical)(surgical)
D **Humeral Head, Left**
   See C Humeral Head, Right
F **Humeral Shaft, Right**
   Distal humerus
   Humerus, distal
   Lateral epicondyle of humerus
   Medial epicondyle of humerus
G **Humeral Shaft, Left**
   See F Humeral Shaft, Right
H **Radius, Right**
   Ulnar notch
J **Radius, Left**
   See H Radius, Right
K **Ulna, Right**
   Olecranon process
   Radial notch
L **Ulna, Left**
   See K Ulna, Right
M **Carpal, Right**
   Capitate bone
   Hamate bone
   Lunate bone
   Pisiform bone
   Scaphoid bone
   Trapezium bone
   Trapezoid bone
   Triquetral bone
N **Carpal, Left**
   See M Carpal, Right
P **Metacarpal, Right**
Q **Metacarpal, Left**
R **Thumb Phalanx, Right**
S **Thumb Phalanx, Left**
T **Finger Phalanx, Right**
V **Finger Phalanx, Left**
	Ø Open
	3 Percutaneous
	4 Percutaneous Endoscopic
		Z No Device	**X** Diagnostic
			Z No Qualifier

Non-OR Procedure   DRG Non-OR Procedure   Valid OR Procedure   HAC Associated Procedure   Combination Only   New/Revised April   New/Revised October

ICD-10-PCS 2025 — Upper Bones — 0PC–0PC

0 Medical and Surgical
P Upper Bones
C Extirpation — Definition: Taking or cutting out solid matter from a body part
Explanation: The solid matter may be an abnormal byproduct of a biological function or a foreign body; it may be imbedded in a body part or in the lumen of a tubular body part. The solid matter may or may not have been previously broken into pieces.

Body Part Character 4	Approach Character 5	Device Character 6	Qualifier Character 7
0 Sternum Manubrium Suprasternal notch Xiphoid process **1 Ribs, 1 to 2** **2 Ribs, 3 or More** **3 Cervical Vertebra** Dens Odontoid process Spinous process Transverse foramen Transverse process Vertebral arch Vertebral body Vertebral foramen Vertebral lamina Vertebral pedicle **4 Thoracic Vertebra** Spinous process Transverse process Vertebral arch Vertebral body Vertebral foramen Vertebral lamina Vertebral pedicle **5 Scapula, Right** Acromion (process) Coracoid process **6 Scapula, Left** See 5 Scapula, Right **7 Glenoid Cavity, Right** Glenoid fossa (of scapula) **8 Glenoid Cavity, Left** See 7 Glenoid Cavity, Right **9 Clavicle, Right** **B Clavicle, Left** **C Humeral Head, Right** Greater tuberosity Lesser tuberosity Neck of humerus (anatomical)(surgical) **D Humeral Head, Left** See C Humeral Head, Right **F Humeral Shaft, Right** Distal humerus Humerus, distal Lateral epicondyle of humerus Medial epicondyle of humerus **G Humeral Shaft, Left** See F Humeral Shaft, Right **H Radius, Right** Ulnar notch **J Radius, Left** See H Radius, Right **K Ulna, Right** Olecranon process Radial notch **L Ulna, Left** See K Ulna, Right **M Carpal, Right** Capitate bone Hamate bone Lunate bone Pisiform bone Scaphoid bone Trapezium bone Trapezoid bone Triquetral bone **N Carpal, Left** See M Carpal, Right **P Metacarpal, Right** **Q Metacarpal, Left** **R Thumb Phalanx, Right** **S Thumb Phalanx, Left** **T Finger Phalanx, Right** **V Finger Phalanx, Left**	**0** Open **3** Percutaneous **4** Percutaneous Endoscopic	**Z** No Device	**Z** No Qualifier

NC Noncovered Procedure · LC Limited Coverage · QA Questionable OB Admit · NT New Tech Add-on · Combination Member · ♂ Male · ♀ Female

0 Medical and Surgical
P Upper Bones
D Extraction

Definition: Pulling or stripping out or off all or a portion of a body part by the use of force
Explanation: The qualifier DIAGNOSTIC is used to identify extraction procedures that are biopsies

Body Part Character 4	Approach Character 5	Device Character 6	Qualifier Character 7

0 Sternum
    Manubrium
    Suprasternal notch
    Xiphoid process
1 Ribs, 1 to 2
2 Ribs, 3 or More
3 Cervical Vertebra
    Dens
    Odontoid process
    Spinous process
    Transverse foramen
    Transverse process
    Vertebral arch
    Vertebral body
    Vertebral foramen
    Vertebral lamina
    Vertebral pedicle
4 Thoracic Vertebra
    Spinous process
    Transverse process
    Vertebral arch
    Vertebral body
    Vertebral foramen
    Vertebral lamina
    Vertebral pedicle
5 Scapula, Right
    Acromion (process)
    Coracoid process
6 Scapula, Left
    See 5 Scapula, Right
7 Glenoid Cavity, Right
    Glenoid fossa (of scapula)
8 Glenoid Cavity, Left
    See 7 Glenoid Cavity, Right
9 Clavicle, Right
B Clavicle, Left
C Humeral Head, Right
    Greater tuberosity
    Lesser tuberosity
    Neck of humerus (anatomical)(surgical)
D Humeral Head, Left
    See C Humeral Head, Right
F Humeral Shaft, Right
    Distal humerus
    Humerus, distal
    Lateral epicondyle of humerus
    Medial epicondyle of humerus
G Humeral Shaft, Left
    See F Humeral Shaft, Right
H Radius, Right
    Ulnar notch
J Radius, Left
    See H Radius, Right
K Ulna, Right
    Olecranon process
    Radial notch
L Ulna, Left
    See K Ulna, Right
M Carpal, Right
    Capitate bone
    Hamate bone
    Lunate bone
    Pisiform bone
    Scaphoid bone
    Trapezium bone
    Trapezoid bone
    Triquetral bone
N Carpal, Left
    See M Carpal, Right
P Metacarpal, Right
Q Metacarpal, Left
R Thumb Phalanx, Right
S Thumb Phalanx, Left
T Finger Phalanx, Right
V Finger Phalanx, Left
	0 Open	**Z** No Device	**Z** No Qualifier

Non-OR Procedure   DRG Non-OR Procedure   Valid OR Procedure   HAC Associated Procedure   Combination Only   New/Revised April   New/Revised October

ICD-10-PCS 2025 — Upper Bones — 0PH–0PH

0 Medical and Surgical
P Upper Bones
H Insertion

Definition: Putting in a nonbiological appliance that monitors, assists, performs, or prevents a physiological function but does not physically take the place of a body part
Explanation: None

Body Part — Character 4	Approach — Character 5	Device — Character 6	Qualifier — Character 7
0 Sternum Manubrium Suprasternal notch Xiphoid process	**0** Open **3** Percutaneous **4** Percutaneous Endoscopic	**0** Internal Fixation Device, Rigid Plate **4** Internal Fixation Device	**Z** No Qualifier
1 Ribs, 1 to 2 **2** Ribs, 3 or More **3** Cervical Vertebra Dens Odontoid process Spinous process Transverse foramen Transverse process Vertebral arch Vertebral body Vertebral foramen Vertebral lamina Vertebral pedicle **4** Thoracic Vertebra Spinous process Transverse process Vertebral arch Vertebral body Vertebral foramen Vertebral lamina Vertebral pedicle **5** Scapula, Right Acromion (process) Coracoid process **6** Scapula, Left *See 5 Scapula, Right* **7** Glenoid Cavity, Right Glenoid fossa (of scapula) **8** Glenoid Cavity, Left *See 7 Glenoid Cavity, Right* **9** Clavicle, Right **B** Clavicle, Left	**0** Open **3** Percutaneous **4** Percutaneous Endoscopic	**4** Internal Fixation Device	**Z** No Qualifier
C Humeral Head, Right Greater tuberosity Lesser tuberosity Neck of humerus (anatomical)(surgical) **D** Humeral Head, Left *See C Humeral Head, Right* **H** Radius, Right Ulnar notch **J** Radius, Left *See H Radius, Right* **K** Ulna, Right Olecranon process Radial notch **L** Ulna, Left *See K Ulna, Right*	**0** Open **3** Percutaneous **4** Percutaneous Endoscopic	**4** Internal Fixation Device **5** External Fixation Device **6** Internal Fixation Device, Intramedullary **8** External Fixation Device, Limb Lengthening **B** External Fixation Device, Monoplanar **C** External Fixation Device, Ring **D** External Fixation Device, Hybrid	**Z** No Qualifier
F Humeral Shaft, Right Distal humerus Humerus, distal Lateral epicondyle of humerus Medial epicondyle of humerus **G** Humeral Shaft, Left *See F Humeral Shaft, Right*	**0** Open **3** Percutaneous **4** Percutaneous Endoscopic	**4** Internal Fixation Device **5** External Fixation Device **6** Internal Fixation Device, Intramedullary **7** Internal Fixation Device, Intramedullary Limb Lengthening **8** External Fixation Device, Limb Lengthening **B** External Fixation Device, Monoplanar **C** External Fixation Device, Ring **D** External Fixation Device, Hybrid	**Z** No Qualifier
M Carpal, Right Capitate bone Hamate bone Lunate bone Pisiform bone Scaphoid bone Trapezium bone Trapezoid bone Triquetral bone **N** Carpal, Left *See M Carpal, Right* **P** Metacarpal, Right **Q** Metacarpal, Left **R** Thumb Phalanx, Right **S** Thumb Phalanx, Left **T** Finger Phalanx, Right **V** Finger Phalanx, Left	**0** Open **3** Percutaneous **4** Percutaneous Endoscopic	**4** Internal Fixation Device **5** External Fixation Device	**Z** No Qualifier
Y Upper Bone	**0** Open **3** Percutaneous **4** Percutaneous Endoscopic	**M** Bone Growth Stimulator	**Z** No Qualifier

Non-OR 0PH[C,D,H,J,K,L][0,3,4]8Z
Non-OR 0PH[F,G][0,3,4]8Z

NC Noncovered Procedure **LC** Limited Coverage **QA** Questionable OB Admit **NT** New Tech Add-on ✚ Combination Member ♂ Male ♀ Female

Upper Bones

0PJ–0PN   Upper Bones   ICD-10-PCS 2025

0 Medical and Surgical
P Upper Bones
J Inspection   **Definition:** Visually and/or manually exploring a body part
Explanation: Visual exploration may be performed with or without optical instrumentation. Manual exploration may be performed directly or through intervening body layers.

Body Part Character 4	Approach Character 5	Device Character 6	Qualifier Character 7
Y Upper Bone	0 Open 3 Percutaneous 4 Percutaneous Endoscopic X External	Z No Device	Z No Qualifier

Non-OR   0PJY[3,X]ZZ

---

0 Medical and Surgical
P Upper Bones
N Release   **Definition:** Freeing a body part from an abnormal physical constraint by cutting or by the use of force
Explanation: Some of the restraining tissue may be taken out but none of the body part is taken out

Body Part Character 4	Approach Character 5	Device Character 6	Qualifier Character 7

0 Sternum
    Manubrium
    Suprasternal notch
    Xiphoid process
1 Ribs, 1 to 2
2 Ribs, 3 or More
3 Cervical Vertebra
    Dens
    Odontoid process
    Spinous process
    Transverse foramen
    Transverse process
    Vertebral arch
    Vertebral body
    Vertebral foramen
    Vertebral lamina
    Vertebral pedicle
4 Thoracic Vertebra
    Spinous process
    Transverse process
    Vertebral arch
    Vertebral body
    Vertebral foramen
    Vertebral lamina
    Vertebral pedicle
5 Scapula, Right
    Acromion (process)
    Coracoid process
6 Scapula, Left
    See 5 Scapula, Right
7 Glenoid Cavity, Right
    Glenoid fossa (of scapula)
8 Glenoid Cavity, Left
    See 7 Glenoid Cavity, Right
9 Clavicle, Right
B Clavicle, Left
C Humeral Head, Right
    Greater tuberosity
    Lesser tuberosity
    Neck of humerus
       (anatomical) (surgical)
D Humeral Head, Left
    See C Humeral Head, Right
	F Humeral Shaft, Right
	    Distal humerus
	    Humerus, distal
	    Lateral epicondyle of
	       humerus
	    Medial epicondyle of
	       humerus
	G Humeral Shaft, Left
	    See F Humeral Shaft, Right
	H Radius, Right
	    Ulnar notch
	J Radius, Left
	    See H Radius, Right
	K Ulna, Right
	    Olecranon process
	    Radial notch
	L Ulna, Left
	    See K Ulna, Right
	M Carpal, Right
	    Capitate bone
	    Hamate bone
	    Lunate bone
	    Pisiform bone
	    Scaphoid bone
	    Trapezium bone
	    Trapezoid bone
	    Triquetral bone
	N Carpal, Left
	    See M Carpal, Right
	P Metacarpal, Right
	Q Metacarpal, Left
	R Thumb Phalanx, Right
	S Thumb Phalanx, Left
	T Finger Phalanx, Right
	V Finger Phalanx, Left
		0 Open
		3 Percutaneous
		4 Percutaneous Endoscopic
			Z No Device	**Z** No Qualifier

ICD-10-PCS 2025 — Upper Bones — ØPP–ØPP

0 Medical and Surgical
P Upper Bones
P Removal   Definition: Taking out or off a device from a body part
Explanation: If a device is taken out and a similar device put in without cutting or puncturing the skin or mucous membrane, the procedure is coded to the root operation CHANGE. Otherwise, the procedure for taking out a device is coded to the root operation REMOVAL.

Body Part Character 4	Approach Character 5	Device Character 6	Qualifier Character 7
0 Sternum Manubrium Suprasternal notch Xiphoid process **1 Ribs, 1 to 2** **2 Ribs, 3 or More** **3 Cervical Vertebra** Dens Odontoid process Spinous process Transverse foramen Transverse process Vertebral arch Vertebral body Vertebral foramen Vertebral lamina Vertebral pedicle **4 Thoracic Vertebra** Spinous process Transverse process Vertebral arch Vertebral body Vertebral foramen Vertebral lamina Vertebral pedicle **5 Scapula, Right** Acromion (process) Coracoid process **6 Scapula, Left** See 5 Scapula, Right **7 Glenoid Cavity, Right** Glenoid fossa (of scapula) **8 Glenoid Cavity, Left** See 7 Glenoid Cavity, Right **9 Clavicle, Right** **B Clavicle, Left**	**0** Open **3** Percutaneous **4** Percutaneous Endoscopic	**4** Internal Fixation Device **7** Autologous Tissue Substitute **J** Synthetic Substitute **K** Nonautologous Tissue Substitute	**Z** No Qualifier
0 Sternum Manubrium Suprasternal notch Xiphoid process **1 Ribs, 1 to 2** **2 Ribs, 3 or More** **3 Cervical Vertebra** Dens Odontoid process Spinous process Transverse foramen Transverse process Vertebral arch Vertebral body Vertebral foramen Vertebral lamina Vertebral pedicle **4 Thoracic Vertebra** Spinous process Transverse process Vertebral arch Vertebral body Vertebral foramen Vertebral lamina Vertebral pedicle **5 Scapula, Right** Acromion (process) Coracoid process **6 Scapula, Left** See 5 Scapula, Right **7 Glenoid Cavity, Right** Glenoid fossa (of scapula) **8 Glenoid Cavity, Left** See 7 Glenoid Cavity, Right **9 Clavicle, Right** **B Clavicle, Left**	**X** External	**4** Internal Fixation Device	**Z** No Qualifier
C Humeral Head, Right Greater tuberosity Lesser tuberosity Neck of humerus (anatomical) (surgical) **D Humeral Head, Left** See C Humeral Head, Right **F Humeral Shaft, Right** Distal humerus Humerus, distal Lateral epicondyle of humerus Medial epicondyle of humerus **G Humeral Shaft, Left** See F Humeral Shaft, Right **H Radius, Right** Ulnar notch **J Radius, Left** See H Radius, Right **K Ulna, Right** Olecranon process Radial notch **L Ulna, Left** See K Ulna, Right **M Carpal, Right** Capitate bone Hamate bone Lunate bone Pisiform bone Scaphoid bone Trapezium bone Trapezoid bone Triquetral bone **N Carpal, Left** See M Carpal, Right **P Metacarpal, Right** **Q Metacarpal, Left** **R Thumb Phalanx, Right** **S Thumb Phalanx, Left** **T Finger Phalanx, Right** **V Finger Phalanx, Left**	**0** Open **3** Percutaneous **4** Percutaneous Endoscopic	**4** Internal Fixation Device **5** External Fixation Device **7** Autologous Tissue Substitute **J** Synthetic Substitute **K** Nonautologous Tissue Substitute	**Z** No Qualifier

Non-OR ØPP[Ø,1,2,3,4,5,6,7,8,9,B]X4Z

ØPP Continued on next page

Upper Bones

0PP Continued

- **0** Medical and Surgical
- **P** Upper Bones
- **P** Removal

Definition: Taking out or off a device from a body part

Explanation: If a device is taken out and a similar device put in without cutting or puncturing the skin or mucous membrane, the procedure is coded to the root operation CHANGE. Otherwise, the procedure for taking out a device is coded to the root operation REMOVAL.

Body Part Character 4	Approach Character 5	Device Character 6	Qualifier Character 7
C Humeral Head, Right Greater tuberosity Lesser tuberosity Neck of humerus (anatomical) (surgical) **D Humeral Head, Left** *See C Humeral Head, Right* **F Humeral Shaft, Right** Distal humerus Humerus, distal Lateral epicondyle of humerus Medial epicondyle of humerus **G Humeral Shaft, Left** *See F Humeral Shaft, Right* **H Radius, Right** Ulnar notch **J Radius, Left** *See H Radius, Right* **K Ulna, Right** Olecranon process Radial notch **L Ulna, Left** *See K Ulna, Right* **M Carpal, Right** Capitate bone Hamate bone Lunate bone Pisiform bone Scaphoid bone Trapezium bone Trapezoid bone Triquetral bone **N Carpal, Left** *See M Carpal, Right* **P Metacarpal, Right** **Q Metacarpal, Left** **R Thumb Phalanx, Right** **S Thumb Phalanx, Left** **T Finger Phalanx, Right** **V Finger Phalanx, Left**	**X** External	**4** Internal Fixation Device **5** External Fixation Device	**Z** No Qualifier
Y Upper Bone	**0** Open **3** Percutaneous **4** Percutaneous Endoscopic **X** External	**0** Drainage Device **M** Bone Growth Stimulator	**Z** No Qualifier

Non-OR 0PP[C,D,F,G,H,J,K,L,M,N,P,Q,R,S,T,V]X[4,5]Z
Non-OR 0PPY30Z
Non-OR 0PPYX[0,M]Z

ICD-10-PCS 2025 — Upper Bones — 0PQ–0PQ

0 Medical and Surgical
P Upper Bones
Q Repair Definition: Restoring, to the extent possible, a body part to its normal anatomic structure and function
Explanation: Used only when the method to accomplish the repair is not one of the other root operations

Body Part Character 4	Approach Character 5	Device Character 6	Qualifier Character 7
0 Sternum Manubrium; Suprasternal notch; Xiphoid process **1 Ribs, 1 to 2** **2 Ribs, 3 or More** **3 Cervical Vertebra** Dens; Odontoid process; Spinous process; Transverse foramen; Transverse process; Vertebral arch; Vertebral body; Vertebral foramen; Vertebral lamina; Vertebral pedicle **4 Thoracic Vertebra** Spinous process; Transverse process; Vertebral arch; Vertebral body; Vertebral foramen; Vertebral lamina; Vertebral pedicle **5 Scapula, Right** Acromion (process); Coracoid process **6 Scapula, Left** *See 5 Scapula, Right* **7 Glenoid Cavity, Right** Glenoid fossa (of scapula) **8 Glenoid Cavity, Left** *See 7 Glenoid Cavity, Right* **9 Clavicle, Right** **B Clavicle, Left** **C Humeral Head, Right** Greater tuberosity; Lesser tuberosity; Neck of humerus (anatomical)(surgical) **D Humeral Head, Left** *See C Humeral Head, Right* **F Humeral Shaft, Right** Distal humerus; Humerus, distal; Lateral epicondyle of humerus; Medial epicondyle of humerus **G Humeral Shaft, Left** *See F Humeral Shaft, Right* **H Radius, Right** Ulnar notch **J Radius, Left** *See H Radius, Right* **K Ulna, Right** Olecranon process; Radial notch **L Ulna, Left** *See K Ulna, Right* **M Carpal, Right** Capitate bone; Hamate bone; Lunate bone; Pisiform bone; Scaphoid bone; Trapezium bone; Trapezoid bone; Triquetral bone **N Carpal, Left** *See M Carpal, Right* **P Metacarpal, Right** **Q Metacarpal, Left** **R Thumb Phalanx, Right** **S Thumb Phalanx, Left** **T Finger Phalanx, Right** **V Finger Phalanx, Left**	**0** Open **3** Percutaneous **4** Percutaneous Endoscopic **X** External	**Z** No Device	**Z** No Qualifier

Non-OR 0PQ[0,1,2,3,4,5,6,7,8,9,B,C,D,F,G,H,J,K,L,M,N,P,Q,R,S,T,V]XZZ

Upper Bones

ØPR–ØPR — ICD-10-PCS 2025

Ø Medical and Surgical
P Upper Bones
R Replacement

Definition: Putting in or on biological or synthetic material that physically takes the place and/or function of all or a portion of a body part
Explanation: The body part may have been taken out or replaced, or may be taken out, physically eradicated, or rendered nonfunctional during the REPLACEMENT procedure. A REMOVAL procedure is coded for taking out the device used in a previous replacement procedure.

Body Part Character 4	Approach Character 5	Device Character 6	Qualifier Character 7

Ø Sternum
  Manubrium
  Suprasternal notch
  Xiphoid process
1 Ribs, 1 to 2
2 Ribs, 3 or More
3 Cervical Vertebra
  Dens
  Odontoid process
  Spinous process
  Transverse foramen
  Transverse process
  Vertebral arch
  Vertebral body
  Vertebral foramen
  Vertebral lamina
  Vertebral pedicle
4 Thoracic Vertebra
  Spinous process
  Transverse process
  Vertebral arch
  Vertebral body
  Vertebral foramen
  Vertebral lamina
  Vertebral pedicle
5 Scapula, Right
  Acromion (process)
  Coracoid process
6 Scapula, Left
  See 5 Scapula, Right
7 Glenoid Cavity, Right
  Glenoid fossa (of scapula)
8 Glenoid Cavity, Left
  See 7 Glenoid Cavity, Right
9 Clavicle, Right
B Clavicle, Left
C Humeral Head, Right
  Greater tuberosity
  Lesser tuberosity
  Neck of humerus (anatomical)(surgical)
D Humeral Head, Left
  See C Humeral Head, Right
F Humeral Shaft, Right
  Distal humerus
  Humerus, distal
  Lateral epicondyle of humerus
  Medial epicondyle of humerus
G Humeral Shaft, Left
  See F Humeral Shaft, Right
H Radius, Right
  Ulnar notch
J Radius, Left
  See H Radius, Right
K Ulna, Right
  Olecranon process
  Radial notch
L Ulna, Left
  See K Ulna, Right
M Carpal, Right
  Capitate bone
  Hamate bone
  Lunate bone
  Pisiform bone
  Scaphoid bone
  Trapezium bone
  Trapezoid bone
  Triquetral bone
N Carpal, Left
  See M Carpal, Right
P Metacarpal, Right
Q Metacarpal, Left
R Thumb Phalanx, Right
S Thumb Phalanx, Left
T Finger Phalanx, Right
V Finger Phalanx, Left
	Ø Open
	3 Percutaneous
	4 Percutaneous Endoscopic
		7 Autologous Tissue Substitute
		J Synthetic Substitute
		K Nonautologous Tissue Substitute
			Z No Qualifier

ICD-10-PCS 2025 — Upper Bones — 0PS–0PS

- **0** Medical and Surgical
- **P** Upper Bones
- **S** Reposition

Definition: Moving to its normal location, or other suitable location, all or a portion of a body part
Explanation: The body part is moved to a new location from an abnormal location, or from a normal location where it is not functioning correctly. The body part may or may not be cut out or off to be moved to the new location.

Body Part Character 4	Approach Character 5	Device Character 6	Qualifier Character 7
0 Sternum Manubrium Suprasternal notch Xiphoid process	**0** Open **3** Percutaneous **4** Percutaneous Endoscopic	**0** Internal Fixation Device, Rigid Plate **4** Internal Fixation Device **Z** No Device	**Z** No Qualifier
0 Sternum Manubrium Suprasternal notch Xiphoid process	**X** External	**Z** No Device	**Z** No Qualifier
1 Ribs, 1 to 2 **2 Ribs, 3 or More** **3 Cervical Vertebra** ✚ Dens Odontoid process Spinous process Transverse foramen Transverse process Vertebral arch Vertebral body Vertebral foramen Vertebral lamina Vertebral pedicle **5 Scapula, Right** Acromion (process) Coracoid process **6 Scapula, Left** *See 5 Scapula, Right* **7 Glenoid Cavity, Right** Glenoid fossa (of scapula) **8 Glenoid Cavity, Left** *See 7 Glenoid Cavity, Right* **9 Clavicle, Right** **B Clavicle, Left**	**0** Open **3** Percutaneous **4** Percutaneous Endoscopic	**4** Internal Fixation Device **Z** No Device	**Z** No Qualifier
1 Ribs, 1 to 2 **2 Ribs, 3 or More** **3 Cervical Vertebra** Dens Odontoid process Spinous process Transverse foramen Transverse process Vertebral arch Vertebral body Vertebral foramen Vertebral lamina Vertebral pedicle **5 Scapula, Right** Acromion (process) Coracoid process **6 Scapula, Left** *See 5 Scapula, Right* **7 Glenoid Cavity, Right** Glenoid fossa (of scapula) **8 Glenoid Cavity, Left** *See 7 Glenoid Cavity, Right* **9 Clavicle, Right** **B Clavicle, Left**	**X** External	**Z** No Device	**Z** No Qualifier
4 Thoracic Vertebra Spinous process Transverse process Vertebral arch Vertebral body Vertebral foramen Vertebral lamina Vertebral pedicle	**0** Open **4** Percutaneous Endoscopic	**3** Spinal Stabilization Device, Vertebral Body Tether **4** Internal Fixation Device **Z** No Device	**Z** No Qualifier
4 Thoracic Vertebra ✚ Spinous process Transverse process Vertebral arch Vertebral body Vertebral foramen Vertebral lamina Vertebral pedicle	**3** Percutaneous	**4** Internal Fixation Device **Z** No Device	**Z** No Qualifier
4 Thoracic Vertebra Spinous process Transverse process Vertebral arch Vertebral body Vertebral foramen Vertebral lamina Vertebral pedicle	**X** External	**Z** No Device	**Z** No Qualifier
C Humeral Head, Right Greater tuberosity Lesser tuberosity Neck of humerus (anatomical)(surgical) **D Humeral Head, Left** *See C Humeral Head, Right* **F Humeral Shaft, Right** Distal humerus Humerus, distal Lateral epicondyle of humerus Medial epicondyle of humerus **G Humeral Shaft, Left** *See F Humeral Shaft, Right* **H Radius, Right** Ulnar notch **J Radius, Left** *See H Radius, Right* **K Ulna, Right** Olecranon process Radial notch **L Ulna, Left** *See K Ulna, Right*	**0** Open **3** Percutaneous **4** Percutaneous Endoscopic	**4** Internal Fixation Device **5** External Fixation Device **6** Internal Fixation Device, Intramedullary **B** External Fixation Device, Monoplanar **C** External Fixation Device, Ring **D** External Fixation Device, Hybrid **Z** No Device	**Z** No Qualifier

Non-OR 0PS0[3,4]ZZ
Non-OR 0PS0XZZ
Non-OR 0PS[1,2,5,6,7,8,9,B][3,4]ZZ
Non-OR 0PS[1,2,3,5,6,7,8,9,B]XZZ
Non-OR 0PS4XZZ
Non-OR 0PS[C,D,F,G,H,J,K,L][3,4]ZZ

See Appendix L for Procedure Combinations
✚ 0PS33ZZ
✚ 0PS43ZZ

0PS Continued on next page

Upper Bones

ØPS–ØPT   Upper Bones   ICD-10-PCS 2025

ØPS Continued

Ø Medical and Surgical
P Upper Bones
S Reposition

Definition: Moving to its normal location, or other suitable location, all or a portion of a body part
Explanation: The body part is moved to a new location from an abnormal location, or from a normal location where it is not functioning correctly. The body part may or may not be cut out or off to be moved to the new location.

Body Part Character 4	Approach Character 5	Device Character 6	Qualifier Character 7

C Humeral Head, Right
  Greater tuberosity
  Lesser tuberosity
  Neck of humerus
    (anatomical)(surgical)
D Humeral Head, Left
  See C Humeral Head, Right
F Humeral Shaft, Right
  Distal humerus
  Humerus, distal
  Lateral epicondyle of humerus
  Medial epicondyle of humerus
G Humeral Shaft, Left
  See F Humeral Shaft, Right
H Radius, Right
  Ulnar notch
J Radius, Left
  See H Radius, Right
K Ulna, Right
  Olecranon process
  Radial notch
L Ulna, Left
  See K Ulna, Right
	X External	Z No Device	Z No Qualifier

M Carpal, Right
  Capitate bone
  Hamate bone
  Lunate bone
  Pisiform bone
  Scaphoid bone
  Trapezium bone
  Trapezoid bone
  Triquetral bone
N Carpal, Left
  See M Carpal, Right
P Metacarpal, Right
Q Metacarpal, Left
R Thumb Phalanx, Right
S Thumb Phalanx, Left
T Finger Phalanx, Right
V Finger Phalanx, Left
	Ø Open
	3 Percutaneous
	4 Percutaneous Endoscopic
		4 Internal Fixation Device
		5 External Fixation Device
		Z No Device
			Z No Qualifier

M Carpal, Right
  Capitate bone
  Hamate bone
  Lunate bone
  Pisiform bone
  Scaphoid bone
  Trapezium bone
  Trapezoid bone
  Triquetral bone
N Carpal, Left
  See M Carpal, Right
P Metacarpal, Right
Q Metacarpal, Left
R Thumb Phalanx, Right
S Thumb Phalanx, Left
T Finger Phalanx, Right
V Finger Phalanx, Left
	X External	Z No Device	Z No Qualifier

Non-OR   ØPS[C,D,F,G,H,J,K,L]XZZ
Non-OR   ØPS[M,N,P,Q,R,S,T,V][3,4]ZZ
Non-OR   ØPS[M,N,P,Q,R,S,T,V]XZZ

Ø Medical and Surgical
P Upper Bones
T Resection

Definition: Cutting out or off, without replacement, all of a body part
Explanation: None

Body Part Character 4	Approach Character 5	Device Character 6	Qualifier Character 7

Ø Sternum
  Manubrium
  Suprasternal notch
  Xiphoid process
1 Ribs, 1 to 2
2 Ribs, 3 or More
5 Scapula, Right
  Acromion (process)
  Coracoid process
6 Scapula, Left
  See 5 Scapula, Right
7 Glenoid Cavity, Right
  Glenoid fossa (of scapula)
8 Glenoid Cavity, Left
  See 7 Glenoid Cavity, Right
9 Clavicle, Right
B Clavicle, Left
C Humeral Head, Right
  Greater tuberosity
  Lesser tuberosity
  Neck of humerus
    (anatomical) (surgical)
D Humeral Head, Left
  See C Humeral Head, Right
F Humeral Shaft, Right
  Distal humerus
  Humerus, distal
  Lateral epicondyle of humerus
  Medial epicondyle of humerus
G Humeral Shaft, Left
  See F Humeral Shaft, Right
H Radius, Right
  Ulnar notch
J Radius, Left
  See H Radius, Right
K Ulna, Right
  Olecranon process
  Radial notch
L Ulna, Left
  See K Ulna, Right
M Carpal, Right
  Capitate bone
  Hamate bone
  Lunate bone
  Pisiform bone
  Scaphoid bone
  Trapezium bone
  Trapezoid bone
  Triquetral bone
N Carpal, Left
  See M Carpal, Right
P Metacarpal, Right
Q Metacarpal, Left
R Thumb Phalanx, Right
S Thumb Phalanx, Left
T Finger Phalanx, Right
V Finger Phalanx, Left
	Ø Open	Z No Device	Z No Qualifier

ICD-10-PCS 2025 — Upper Bones — 0PU–0PU

0 **Medical and Surgical**
P **Upper Bones**
U **Supplement** Definition: Putting in or on biological or synthetic material that physically reinforces and/or augments the function of a portion of a body part
Explanation: The biological material is non-living, or is living and from the same individual. The body part may have been previously replaced, and the SUPPLEMENT procedure is performed to physically reinforce and/or augment the function of the replaced body part.

Body Part Character 4	Approach Character 5	Device Character 6	Qualifier Character 7

0 Sternum
   Manubrium
   Suprasternal notch
   Xiphoid process
1 Ribs, 1 to 2
2 Ribs, 3 or More
3 Cervical Vertebra ✚
   Dens
   Odontoid process
   Spinous process
   Transverse foramen
   Transverse process
   Vertebral arch
   Vertebral body
   Vertebral foramen
   Vertebral lamina
   Vertebral pedicle
4 Thoracic Vertebra ✚
   Spinous process
   Transverse process
   Vertebral arch
   Vertebral body
   Vertebral foramen
   Vertebral lamina
   Vertebral pedicle
5 Scapula, Right
   Acromion (process)
   Coracoid process
6 Scapula, Left
   See 5 Scapula, Right
7 Glenoid Cavity, Right
   Glenoid fossa (of scapula)
8 Glenoid Cavity, Left
   See 7 Glenoid Cavity, Right
9 Clavicle, Right
B Clavicle, Left
C Humeral Head, Right
   Greater tuberosity
   Lesser tuberosity
   Neck of humerus
      (anatomical) (surgical)
D Humeral Head, Left
   See C Humeral Head, Right
F Humeral Shaft, Right
   Distal humerus
   Humerus, distal
   Lateral epicondyle of humerus
   Medial epicondyle of humerus
G Humeral Shaft, Left
   See F Humeral Shaft, Right
H Radius, Right
   Ulnar notch
J Radius, Left
   See H Radius, Right
K Ulna, Right
   Olecranon process
   Radial notch
L Ulna, Left
   See K Ulna, Right
M Carpal, Right
   Capitate bone
   Hamate bone
   Lunate bone
   Pisiform bone
   Scaphoid bone
   Trapezium bone
   Trapezoid bone
   Triquetral bone
N Carpal, Left
   See M Carpal, Right
P Metacarpal, Right
Q Metacarpal, Left
R Thumb Phalanx, Right
S Thumb Phalanx, Left
T Finger Phalanx, Right
V Finger Phalanx, Left
	0 Open
	3 Percutaneous
	4 Percutaneous Endoscopic
		7 Autologous Tissue Substitute
		J Synthetic Substitute
		K Nonautologous Tissue Substitute
			Z No Qualifier

See Appendix L for Procedure Combinations
✚ 0PU[3,4]3JZ

0 Medical and Surgical
P Upper Bones
W Revision

Definition: Correcting, to the extent possible, a portion of a malfunctioning device or the position of a displaced device
Explanation: Revision can include correcting a malfunctioning or displaced device by taking out or putting in components of the device such as a screw or pin

Body Part Character 4	Approach Character 5	Device Character 6	Qualifier Character 7
0 Sternum Manubrium Suprasternal notch Xiphoid process **1 Ribs, 1 to 2** **2 Ribs, 3 or More** **3 Cervical Vertebra** Dens Odontoid process Spinous process Transverse foramen Transverse process Vertebral arch Vertebral body Vertebral foramen Vertebral lamina Vertebral pedicle **4 Thoracic Vertebra** Spinous process Transverse process Vertebral arch Vertebral body Vertebral foramen Vertebral lamina Vertebral pedicle **5 Scapula, Right** Acromion (process) Coracoid process **6 Scapula, Left** See 5 Scapula, Right **7 Glenoid Cavity, Right** Glenoid fossa (of scapula) **8 Glenoid Cavity, Left** See 7 Glenoid Cavity, Right **9 Clavicle, Right** **B Clavicle, Left**	0 Open 3 Percutaneous 4 Percutaneous Endoscopic X External	4 Internal Fixation Device 7 Autologous Tissue Substitute J Synthetic Substitute K Nonautologous Tissue Substitute	Z No Qualifier
C Humeral Head, Right Greater tuberosity Lesser tuberosity Neck of humerus (anatomical)(surgical) **D Humeral Head, Left** See C Humeral Head, Right **F Humeral Shaft, Right** Distal humerus Humerus, distal Lateral epicondyle of humerus Medial epicondyle of humerus **G Humeral Shaft, Left** See F Humeral Shaft, Right **H Radius, Right** Ulnar notch **J Radius, Left** See H Radius, Right **K Ulna, Right** Olecranon process Radial notch **L Ulna, Left** See K Ulna, Right **M Carpal, Right** Capitate bone Hamate bone Lunate bone Pisiform bone Scaphoid bone Trapezium bone Trapezoid bone Triquetral bone **N Carpal, Left** See M Carpal, Right **P Metacarpal, Right** **Q Metacarpal, Left** **R Thumb Phalanx, Right** **S Thumb Phalanx, Left** **T Finger Phalanx, Right** **V Finger Phalanx, Left**	0 Open 3 Percutaneous 4 Percutaneous Endoscopic X External	4 Internal Fixation Device 5 External Fixation Device 7 Autologous Tissue Substitute J Synthetic Substitute K Nonautologous Tissue Substitute	Z No Qualifier
Y Upper Bone	0 Open 3 Percutaneous 4 Percutaneous Endoscopic X External	0 Drainage Device M Bone Growth Stimulator	Z No Qualifier

Non-OR 0PW[0,1,2,3,4,5,6,7,8,9,B]X[4,7,J,K]Z
Non-OR 0PW[C,D,F,G,H,J,K,L,M,N,P,Q,R,S,T,V]X[4,5,7,J,K]Z
Non-OR 0PWYX[0,M]Z

Lower Bones ØQ2–ØQW

Character Meanings

This Character Meaning table is provided as a guide to assist the user in the identification of character members that may be found in this section of code tables. It **SHOULD NOT** be used to build a PCS code.

Operation–Character 3	Body Part–Character 4	Approach–Character 5	Device–Character 6	Qualifier–Character 7
2 Change	Ø Lumbar Vertebra	Ø Open	Ø Drainage Device	2 Sesamoid Bone(s) 1st Toe
5 Destruction	1 Sacrum	3 Percutaneous	3 Spinal Stabilization Device, Vertebral Body Tether	3 Laser Interstitial Thermal Therapy
8 Division	2 Pelvic Bone, Right	4 Percutaneous Endoscopic	4 Internal Fixation Device	X Diagnostic
9 Drainage	3 Pelvic Bone, Left	X External	5 External Fixation Device	Z No Qualifier
B Excision	4 Acetabulum, Right		6 Internal Fixation Device, Intramedullary	
C Extirpation	5 Acetabulum, Left		7 Autologous Tissue Substitute OR Internal Fixation Device, Intramedullary Limb Lengthening	
D Extraction	6 Upper Femur, Right		8 External Fixation Device, Limb Lengthening	
H Insertion	7 Upper Femur, Left		B External Fixation Device, Monoplanar	
J Inspection	8 Femoral Shaft, Right		C External Fixation Device, Ring	
N Release	9 Femoral Shaft, Left		D External Fixation Device, Hybrid	
P Removal	B Lower Femur, Right		J Synthetic Substitute	
Q Repair	C Lower Femur, Left		K Nonautologous Tissue Substitute	
R Replacement	D Patella, Right		M Bone Growth Stimulator	
S Reposition	F Patella, Left		Y Other Device	
T Resection	G Tibia, Right		Z No Device	
U Supplement	H Tibia, Left			
W Revision	J Fibula, Right			
	K Fibula, Left			
	L Tarsal, Right			
	M Tarsal, Left			
	N Metatarsal, Right			
	P Metatarsal, Left			
	Q Toe Phalanx, Right			
	R Toe Phalanx, Left			
	S Coccyx			
	Y Lower Bone			

Lower Bones

AHA Coding Clinic for table 0Q5
2023, 1Q, 10 — Laser interstitial thermal therapy

AHA Coding Clinic for table 0Q8
2018, 1Q, 25 — Periacetabular osteotomy for repair of congenital hip dysplasia
2016, 2Q, 31 — Periacetabular osteotomy for repair of congenital hip dysplasia

AHA Coding Clinic for table 0Q9
2022, 1Q, 31 — Septic arthritis/osteomyelitis of pubic symphysis and aspiration biopsy

AHA Coding Clinic for table 0QB
2023, 2Q, 30 — Excisional debridement and non-excisional debridement at deeper layer same site
2021, 4Q, 52-53 — Sesamoidectomy of great toe
2021, 2Q, 18 — Excision of tibial sesamoid
2020, 2Q, 26 — Sacral pressure ulcer with excisional and nonexcisional debridement of same site
2019, 2Q, 19 — Cervical spinal fusion, decompression and placement of interfacet stabilization device
2018, 3Q, 17 — Excisional debridement of periosteum
2017, 1Q, 23 — Reconstruction of mandible using titanium and bone
2016, 3Q, 30 — Resection of femur with interposition arthroplasty
2015, 3Q, 3-8 — Excisional and nonexcisional debridement
2015, 3Q, 26 — Femoral head resection
2015, 2Q, 34 — Decompressive laminectomy
2014, 4Q, 25 — Femoroacetabular impingement and labral tear with repair
2014, 2Q, 6 — Posterior lumbar fusion with discectomy
2013, 4Q, 116 — Spinal decompression
2013, 2Q, 39 — Ankle fusion, osteotomy, and removal of hardware
2012, 2Q, 19 — Multiple decompressive cervical laminectomies

AHA Coding Clinic for table 0QD
2023, 2Q, 30 — Excisional debridement and non-excisional debridement at deeper layer same site
2017, 4Q, 41 — Extraction procedures

AHA Coding Clinic for table 0QH
2022, 2Q, 19 — Limb lengthening surgery
2019, 4Q, 34 — Intramedullary limb lengthening internal fixation device
2017, 1Q, 21 — Staged scoliosis surgery with iliac fixation and spinal fusion
2016, 3Q, 34 — Tibial/fibula epiphysiodesis

AHA Coding Clinic for table 0QP
2023, 1Q, 33 — Removal of S2-Alar-Iliac screws
2020, 4Q, 56 — Removal of external fixation device
2017, 4Q, 74-75 — Magnetic growth rods
2015, 2Q, 6 — Planned implant break

AHA Coding Clinic for table 0QQ
2018, 1Q, 15 — Pubic symphysis fusion
2014, 3Q, 24 — Repair of lipomyelomeningocele and tethered cord

AHA Coding Clinic for table 0QR
2017, 1Q, 22 — Total knee replacement and patellar component
2016, 3Q, 30 — Resection of femur with interposition arthroplasty

AHA Coding Clinic for table 0QS
2023, 3Q, 23 — Aspiration and injection of bone marrow at fracture site
2022, 2Q, 19 — Limb lengthening surgery
2021, 4Q, 51-52 — Vertebral body tethering
2020, 1Q, 33 — Spinal fusion without use of bone graft
2019, 3Q, 26 — Open reduction with internal fixation and placement of strut allograft
2018, 1Q, 13 — Bilateral cuboid osteotomy for repair of congenital talipes equinovarus
2018, 1Q, 25 — Periacetabular osteotomy for repair of congenital hip dysplasia
2016, 3Q, 34 — Tibial/fibula epiphysiodesis
2014, 4Q, 29 — Rotational osteosynthesis
2014, 4Q, 31 — Reposition of femur for correction of valgus and recurvatum deformities

AHA Coding Clinic for table 0QT
2017, 1Q, 22 — Chopart amputation of foot
2016, 3Q, 30 — Resection of femur with interposition arthroplasty
2015, 3Q, 26 — Femoral head resection
2014, 4Q, 29 — Rotational osteosynthesis

AHA Coding Clinic for table 0QU
2023, 3Q, 22 — Patella resurfacing and tibial liner exchange
2019, 3Q, 26 — Open reduction with internal fixation and placement of strut allograft
2019, 2Q, 35 — Kiva® kyphoplasty
2015, 3Q, 18 — Total hip replacement with acetabular reconstruction
2014, 4Q, 31 — Reposition of femur for correction of valgus and recurvatum deformities
2014, 2Q, 12 — Percutaneous vertebroplasty using cement
2013, 2Q, 35 — Use of bone void filler in grafting

AHA Coding Clinic for table 0QW
2017, 4Q, 74-75 — Magnetic growth rods

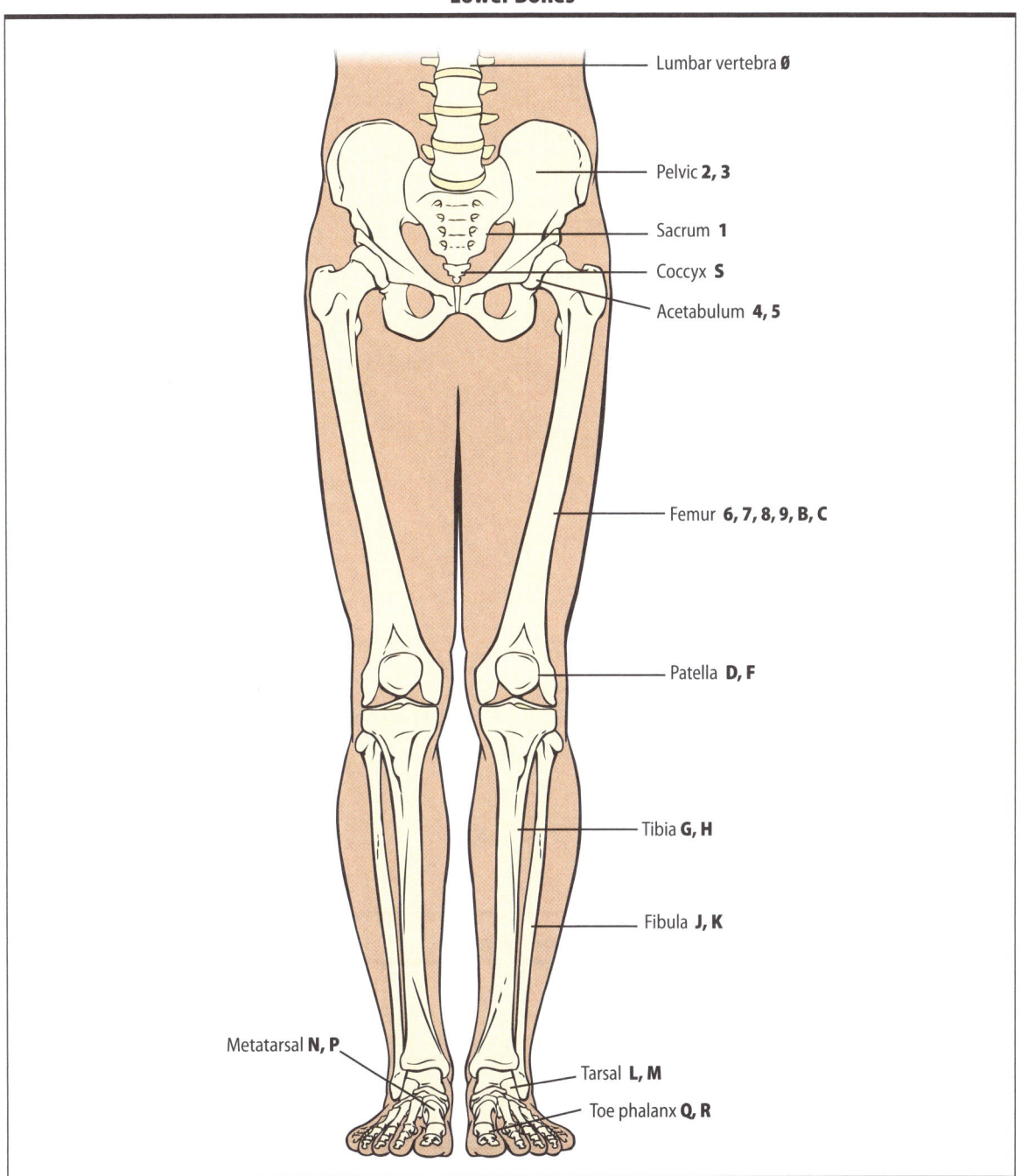

Lower Bones

- Lumbar vertebra **0**
- Pelvic **2, 3**
- Sacrum **1**
- Coccyx **S**
- Acetabulum **4, 5**
- Femur **6, 7, 8, 9, B, C**
- Patella **D, F**
- Tibia **G, H**
- Fibula **J, K**
- Metatarsal **N, P**
- Tarsal **L, M**
- Toe phalanx **Q, R**

Lower Bones

ICD-10-PCS 2025

Hip Bone Anatomy

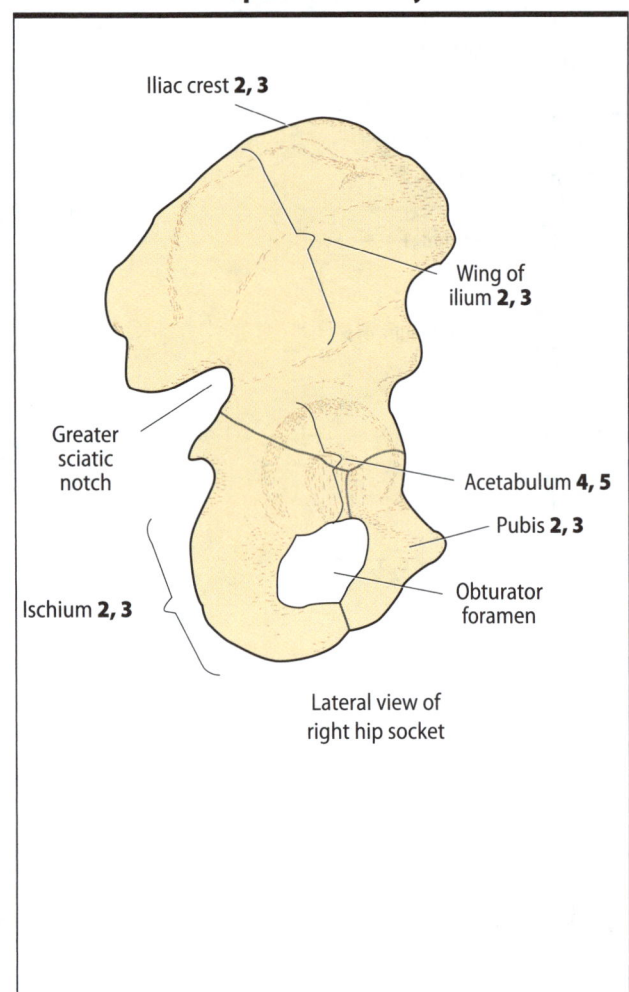

- Iliac crest **2, 3**
- Wing of ilium **2, 3**
- Greater sciatic notch
- Acetabulum **4, 5**
- Pubis **2, 3**
- Obturator foramen
- Ischium **2, 3**

Lateral view of right hip socket

Pelvic and Lower Extremity Bones

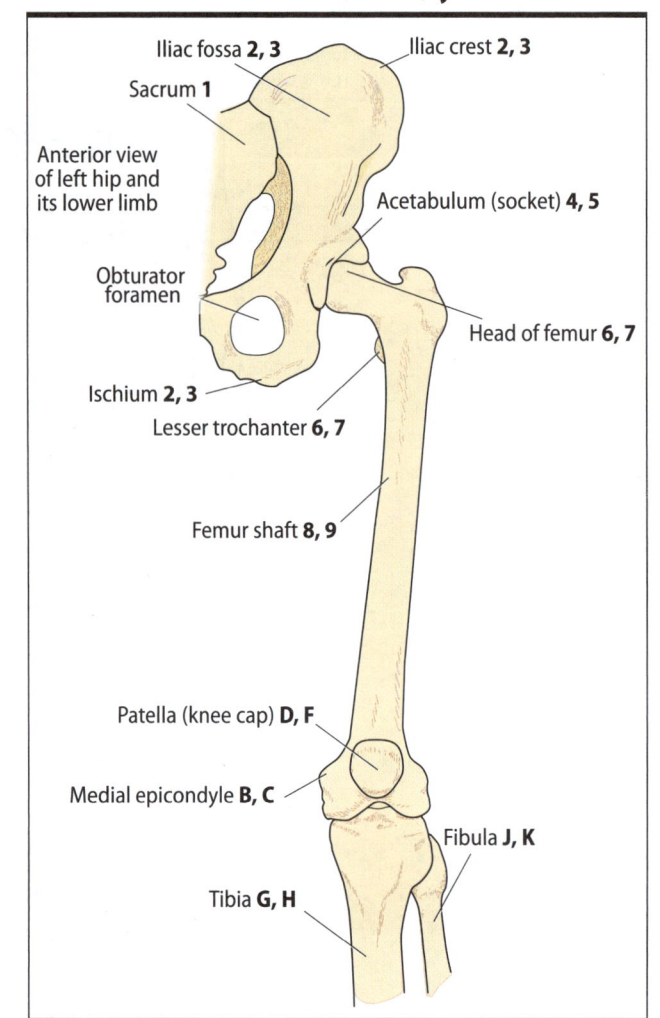

- Iliac fossa **2, 3**
- Iliac crest **2, 3**
- Sacrum **1**
- Acetabulum (socket) **4, 5**
- Obturator foramen
- Head of femur **6, 7**
- Ischium **2, 3**
- Lesser trochanter **6, 7**
- Femur shaft **8, 9**
- Patella (knee cap) **D, F**
- Medial epicondyle **B, C**
- Fibula **J, K**
- Tibia **G, H**

Anterior view of left hip and its lower limb

Foot Bones

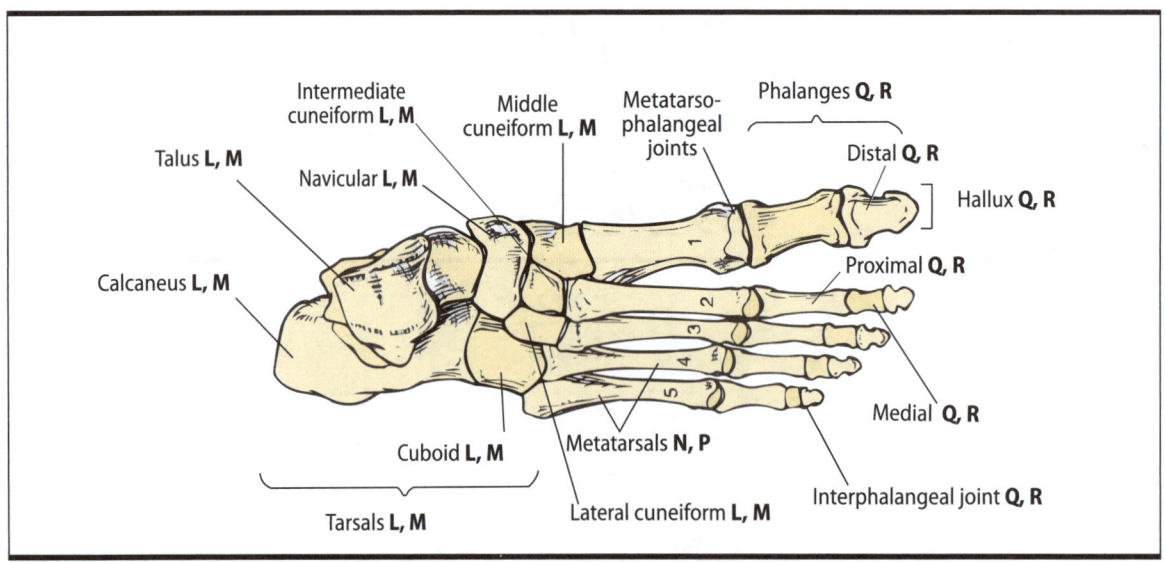

- Intermediate cuneiform **L, M**
- Middle cuneiform **L, M**
- Metatarsophalangeal joints
- Phalanges **Q, R**
- Talus **L, M**
- Navicular **L, M**
- Distal **Q, R**
- Hallux **Q, R**
- Calcaneus **L, M**
- Proximal **Q, R**
- Medial **Q, R**
- Cuboid **L, M**
- Metatarsals **N, P**
- Interphalangeal joint **Q, R**
- Tarsals **L, M**
- Lateral cuneiform **L, M**

Lower Bones

0 Medical and Surgical
Q Lower Bones
2 Change — Definition: Taking out or off a device from a body part and putting back an identical or similar device in or on the same body part without cutting or puncturing the skin or a mucous membrane
Explanation: All CHANGE procedures are coded using the approach EXTERNAL

Body Part Character 4	Approach Character 5	Device Character 6	Qualifier Character 7
Y Lower Bone	X External	0 Drainage Device Y Other Device	Z No Qualifier

Non-OR All body part, approach, device, and qualifier values

---

0 Medical and Surgical
Q Lower Bones
5 Destruction — Definition: Physical eradication of all or a portion of a body part by the direct use of energy, force, or a destructive agent
Explanation: None of the body part is physically taken out

Body Part Character 4	Approach Character 5	Device Character 6	Qualifier Character 7

0 Lumbar Vertebra
  Spinous process
  Transverse process
  Vertebral arch
  Vertebral body
  Vertebral foramen
  Vertebral lamina
  Vertebral pedicle
1 Sacrum
	0 Open
	3 Percutaneous
	4 Percutaneous Endoscopic
		Z No Device	3 Laser Interstitial Thermal Therapy
			Z No Qualifier

2 Pelvic Bone, Right
  Iliac crest
  Ilium
  Ischium
  Pubis
3 Pelvic Bone, Left
  See 2 Pelvic Bone, Right
4 Acetabulum, Right
5 Acetabulum, Left
6 Upper Femur, Right
  Femoral head
  Greater trochanter
  Lesser trochanter
  Neck of femur
7 Upper Femur, Left
  See 6 Upper Femur, Right
8 Femoral Shaft, Right
  Body of femur
9 Femoral Shaft, Left
  See 8 Femoral Shaft, Right
B Lower Femur, Right
  Lateral condyle of femur
  Lateral epicondyle of femur
  Medial condyle of femur
  Medial epicondyle of femur
C Lower Femur, Left
  See B Lower Femur, Right
D Patella, Right
F Patella, Left
G Tibia, Right
  Lateral condyle of tibia
  Medial condyle of tibia
  Medial malleolus
H Tibia, Left
  See G Tibia, Right
J Fibula, Right
  Body of fibula
  Head of fibula
  Lateral malleolus
K Fibula, Left
  See J Fibula, Right
L Tarsal, Right
  Calcaneus
  Cuboid bone
  Intermediate cuneiform bone
  Lateral cuneiform bone
  Medial cuneiform bone
  Navicular bone
  Talus bone
M Tarsal, Left
  See L Tarsal, Right
N Metatarsal, Right
  Fibular sesamoid
  Tibial sesamoid
P Metatarsal, Left
  See N Metatarsal, Right
Q Toe Phalanx, Right
R Toe Phalanx, Left
S Coccyx
	0 Open
	3 Percutaneous
	4 Percutaneous Endoscopic
		Z No Device	Z No Qualifier

0 Medical and Surgical
Q Lower Bones
8 Division Definition: Cutting into a body part, without draining fluids and/or gases from the body part, in order to separate or transect a body part
Explanation: All or a portion of the body part is separated into two or more portions

Body Part Character 4	Approach Character 5	Device Character 6	Qualifier Character 7

0 Lumbar Vertebra
    Spinous process
    Transverse process
    Vertebral arch
    Vertebral body
    Vertebral foramen
    Vertebral lamina
    Vertebral pedicle
1 Sacrum
2 Pelvic Bone, Right
    Iliac crest
    Ilium
    Ischium
    Pubis
3 Pelvic Bone, Left
    See 2 Pelvic Bone, Right
4 Acetabulum, Right
5 Acetabulum, Left
6 Upper Femur, Right
    Femoral head
    Greater trochanter
    Lesser trochanter
    Neck of femur
7 Upper Femur, Left
    See 6 Upper Femur, Right
8 Femoral Shaft, Right
    Body of femur
9 Femoral Shaft, Left
    See 8 Femoral Shaft, Right
B Lower Femur, Right
    Lateral condyle of femur
    Lateral epicondyle of femur
    Medial condyle of femur
    Medial epicondyle of femur
C Lower Femur, Left
    See B Lower Femur, Right
D Patella, Right
F Patella, Left
G Tibia, Right
    Lateral condyle of tibia
    Medial condyle of tibia
    Medial malleolus
H Tibia, Left
    See G Tibia, Right
J Fibula, Right
    Body of fibula
    Head of fibula
    Lateral malleolus
K Fibula, Left
    See J Fibula, Right
L Tarsal, Right
    Calcaneus
    Cuboid bone
    Intermediate cuneiform bone
    Lateral cuneiform bone
    Medial cuneiform bone
    Navicular bone
    Talus bone
M Tarsal, Left
    See L Tarsal, Right
N Metatarsal, Right
    Fibular sesamoid
    Tibial sesamoid
P Metatarsal, Left
    See N Metatarsal, Right
Q Toe Phalanx, Right
R Toe Phalanx, Left
S Coccyx
	0 Open
	3 Percutaneous
	4 Percutaneous Endoscopic
		Z No Device	**Z** No Qualifier

0 Medical and Surgical
Q Lower Bones
9 Drainage Definition: Taking or letting out fluids and/or gases from a body part
Explanation: The qualifier DIAGNOSTIC is used to identify drainage procedures that are biopsies

Body Part Character 4	Approach Character 5	Device Character 6	Qualifier Character 7
0 Lumbar Vertebra Spinous process, Transverse process, Vertebral arch, Vertebral body, Vertebral foramen, Vertebral lamina, Vertebral pedicle **1 Sacrum** **2 Pelvic Bone, Right** Iliac crest, Ilium, Ischium, Pubis **3 Pelvic Bone, Left** See 2 Pelvic Bone, Right **4 Acetabulum, Right** **5 Acetabulum, Left** **6 Upper Femur, Right** Femoral head, Greater trochanter, Lesser trochanter, Neck of femur **7 Upper Femur, Left** See 6 Upper Femur, Right **8 Femoral Shaft, Right** Body of femur **9 Femoral Shaft, Left** See 8 Femoral Shaft, Right **B Lower Femur, Right** Lateral condyle of femur, Lateral epicondyle of femur, Medial condyle of femur, Medial epicondyle of femur **C Lower Femur, Left** See B Lower Femur, Right **D Patella, Right** **F Patella, Left** **G Tibia, Right** Lateral condyle of tibia, Medial condyle of tibia, Medial malleolus **H Tibia, Left** See G Tibia, Right **J Fibula, Right** Body of fibula, Head of fibula, Lateral malleolus **K Fibula, Left** See J Fibula, Right **L Tarsal, Right** Calcaneus, Cuboid bone, Intermediate cuneiform bone, Lateral cuneiform bone, Medial cuneiform bone, Navicular bone, Talus bone **M Tarsal, Left** See L Tarsal, Right **N Metatarsal, Right** Fibular sesamoid, Tibial sesamoid **P Metatarsal, Left** See N Metatarsal, Right **Q Toe Phalanx, Right** **R Toe Phalanx, Left** **S Coccyx**	**0** Open **3** Percutaneous **4** Percutaneous Endoscopic	**0** Drainage Device	**Z** No Qualifier
0 Lumbar Vertebra Spinous process, Transverse process, Vertebral arch, Vertebral body, Vertebral foramen, Vertebral lamina, Vertebral pedicle **1 Sacrum** **2 Pelvic Bone, Right** Iliac crest, Ilium, Ischium, Pubis **3 Pelvic Bone, Left** See 2 Pelvic Bone, Right **4 Acetabulum, Right** **5 Acetabulum, Left** **6 Upper Femur, Right** Femoral head, Greater trochanter, Lesser trochanter, Neck of femur **7 Upper Femur, Left** See 6 Upper Femur, Right **8 Femoral Shaft, Right** Body of femur **9 Femoral Shaft, Left** See 8 Femoral Shaft, Right **B Lower Femur, Right** Lateral condyle of femur, Lateral epicondyle of femur, Medial condyle of femur, Medial epicondyle of femur **C Lower Femur, Left** See B Lower Femur, Right **D Patella, Right** **F Patella, Left** **G Tibia, Right** Lateral condyle of tibia, Medial condyle of tibia, Medial malleolus **H Tibia, Left** See G Tibia, Right **J Fibula, Right** Body of fibula, Head of fibula, Lateral malleolus **K Fibula, Left** See J Fibula, Right **L Tarsal, Right** Calcaneus, Cuboid bone, Intermediate cuneiform bone, Lateral cuneiform bone, Medial cuneiform bone, Navicular bone, Talus bone **M Tarsal, Left** See L Tarsal, Right **N Metatarsal, Right** Fibular sesamoid, Tibial sesamoid **P Metatarsal, Left** See N Metatarsal, Right **Q Toe Phalanx, Right** **R Toe Phalanx, Left** **S Coccyx**	**0** Open **3** Percutaneous **4** Percutaneous Endoscopic	**Z** No Device	**X** Diagnostic **Z** No Qualifier

Non-OR 0Q9[0,1,2,3,4,5,6,7,8,9,B,C,D,F,G,H,J,K,L,M,P,Q,R,S]30Z
Non-OR 0Q9[0,1,2,3,4,5,6,7,8,9,B,C,D,F,G,H,J,K,L,M,P,Q,R,S]3ZZ

0QB–0QB Lower Bones

0 Medical and Surgical
Q Lower Bones
B Excision Definition: Cutting out or off, without replacement, a portion of a body part
Explanation: The qualifier DIAGNOSTIC is used to identify excision procedures that are biopsies

Body Part Character 4	Approach Character 5	Device Character 6	Qualifier Character 7

0 Lumbar Vertebra
  Spinous process
  Transverse process
  Vertebral arch
  Vertebral body
  Vertebral foramen
  Vertebral lamina
  Vertebral pedicle
1 Sacrum
2 Pelvic Bone, Right
  Iliac crest
  Ilium
  Ischium
  Pubis
3 Pelvic Bone, Left
  See 2 Pelvic Bone, Right
4 Acetabulum, Right
5 Acetabulum, Left
6 Upper Femur, Right
  Femoral head
  Greater trochanter
  Lesser trochanter
  Neck of femur
7 Upper Femur, Left
  See 6 Upper Femur, Right
8 Femoral Shaft, Right
  Body of femur
9 Femoral Shaft, Left
  See 8 Femoral Shaft, Right
B Lower Femur, Right
  Lateral condyle of femur
  Lateral epicondyle of femur
  Medial condyle of femur
  Medial epicondyle of femur
C Lower Femur, Left
  See B Lower Femur, Right
D Patella, Right
F Patella, Left
G Tibia, Right
  Lateral condyle of tibia
  Medial condyle of tibia
  Medial malleolus
H Tibia, Left
  See G Tibia, Right
J Fibula, Right
  Body of fibula
  Head of fibula
  Lateral malleolus
K Fibula, Left
  See J Fibula, Right
L Tarsal, Right
  Calcaneus
  Cuboid bone
  Intermediate cuneiform bone
  Lateral cuneiform bone
  Medial cuneiform bone
  Navicular bone
  Talus bone
M Tarsal, Left
  See L Tarsal, Right
Q Toe Phalanx, Right
R Toe Phalanx, Left
S Coccyx
	0 Open
	3 Percutaneous
	4 Percutaneous Endoscopic
		Z No Device	**X** Diagnostic
			Z No Qualifier

N Metatarsal, Right
  Fibular sesamoid
  Tibial sesamoid
P Metatarsal, Left
  See N Metatarsal, Right
	0 Open
	3 Percutaneous
	4 Percutaneous Endoscopic
		Z No Device	**2** Sesamoid Bone(s) 1st Toe
			X Diagnostic
			Z No Qualifier

Non-OR Procedure   DRG Non-OR Procedure   Valid OR Procedure   HAC Associated Procedure   Combination Only   New/Revised April   New/Revised October

ICD-10-PCS 2025 — Lower Bones — 0QC–0QC

- **0 Medical and Surgical**
- **Q Lower Bones**
- **C Extirpation** Definition: Taking or cutting out solid matter from a body part
  Explanation: The solid matter may be an abnormal byproduct of a biological function or a foreign body; it may be imbedded in a body part or in the lumen of a tubular body part. The solid matter may or may not have been previously broken into pieces.

Body Part Character 4	Approach Character 5	Device Character 6	Qualifier Character 7
0 Lumbar Vertebra Spinous process Transverse process Vertebral arch Vertebral body Vertebral foramen Vertebral lamina Vertebral pedicle **1 Sacrum** **2 Pelvic Bone, Right** Iliac crest Ilium Ischium Pubis **3 Pelvic Bone, Left** See 2 Pelvic Bone, Right **4 Acetabulum, Right** **5 Acetabulum, Left** **6 Upper Femur, Right** Femoral head Greater trochanter Lesser trochanter Neck of femur **7 Upper Femur, Left** See 6 Upper Femur, Right **8 Femoral Shaft, Right** Body of femur **9 Femoral Shaft, Left** See 8 Femoral Shaft, Right **B Lower Femur, Right** Lateral condyle of femur Lateral epicondyle of femur Medial condyle of femur Medial epicondyle of femur **C Lower Femur, Left** See B Lower Femur, Right **D Patella, Right** **F Patella, Left** **G Tibia, Right** Lateral condyle of tibia Medial condyle of tibia Medial malleolus **H Tibia, Left** See G Tibia, Right **J Fibula, Right** Body of fibula Head of fibula Lateral malleolus **K Fibula, Left** See J Fibula, Right **L Tarsal, Right** Calcaneus Cuboid bone Intermediate cuneiform bone Lateral cuneiform bone Medial cuneiform bone Navicular bone Talus bone **M Tarsal, Left** See L Tarsal, Right **N Metatarsal, Right** Fibular sesamoid Tibial sesamoid **P Metatarsal, Left** See N Metatarsal, Right **Q Toe Phalanx, Right** **R Toe Phalanx, Left** **S Coccyx**	**0** Open **3** Percutaneous **4** Percutaneous Endoscopic	**Z** No Device	**Z** No Qualifier

0 Medical and Surgical
Q Lower Bones
D Extraction

Definition: Pulling or stripping out or off all or a portion of a body part by the use of force
Explanation: The qualifier DIAGNOSTIC is used to identify extraction procedures that are biopsies

Body Part Character 4	Approach Character 5	Device Character 6	Qualifier Character 7

0 Lumbar Vertebra
    Spinous process
    Transverse process
    Vertebral arch
    Vertebral body
    Vertebral foramen
    Vertebral lamina
    Vertebral pedicle
1 Sacrum
2 Pelvic Bone, Right
    Iliac crest
    Ilium
    Ischium
    Pubis
3 Pelvic Bone, Left
    See 2 Pelvic Bone, Right
4 Acetabulum, Right
5 Acetabulum, Left
6 Upper Femur, Right
    Femoral head
    Greater trochanter
    Lesser trochanter
    Neck of femur
7 Upper Femur, Left
    See 6 Upper Femur, Right
8 Femoral Shaft, Right
    Body of femur
9 Femoral Shaft, Left
    See 8 Femoral Shaft, Right
B Lower Femur, Right
    Lateral condyle of femur
    Lateral epicondyle of femur
    Medial condyle of femur
    Medial epicondyle of femur
C Lower Femur, Left
    See B Lower Femur, Right
D Patella, Right
F Patella, Left
G Tibia, Right
    Lateral condyle of tibia
    Medial condyle of tibia
    Medial malleolus
H Tibia, Left
    See G Tibia, Right
J Fibula, Right
    Body of fibula
    Head of fibula
    Lateral malleolus
K Fibula, Left
    See J Fibula, Right
L Tarsal, Right
    Calcaneus
    Cuboid bone
    Intermediate cuneiform bone
    Lateral cuneiform bone
    Medial cuneiform bone
    Navicular bone
    Talus bone
M Tarsal, Left
    See L Tarsal, Right
N Metatarsal, Right
    Fibular sesamoid
    Tibial sesamoid
P Metatarsal, Left
    See N Metatarsal, Right
Q Toe Phalanx, Right
R Toe Phalanx, Left
S Coccyx
	0 Open	**Z** No Device	**Z** No Qualifier

Lower Bones

0 Medical and Surgical
Q Lower Bones
H Insertion

Definition: Putting in a nonbiological appliance that monitors, assists, performs, or prevents a physiological function but does not physically take the place of a body part
Explanation: None

Body Part Character 4	Approach Character 5	Device Character 6	Qualifier Character 7

0 Lumbar Vertebra
  Spinous process
  Transverse process
  Vertebral arch
  Vertebral body
  Vertebral foramen
  Vertebral lamina
  Vertebral pedicle
1 Sacrum
2 Pelvic Bone, Right
  Iliac crest
  Ilium
  Ischium
  Pubis
3 Pelvic Bone, Left
  See 2 Pelvic Bone, Right
4 Acetabulum, Right
5 Acetabulum, Left
	D Patella, Right
	F Patella, Left
	L Tarsal, Right
	  Calcaneus
	  Cuboid bone
	  Intermediate cuneiform bone
	  Lateral cuneiform bone
	  Medial cuneiform bone
	  Navicular bone
	  Talus bone
	M Tarsal, Left
	  See L Tarsal, Right
	N Metatarsal, Right
	  Fibular sesamoid
	  Tibial sesamoid
	P Metatarsal, Left
	  See N Metatarsal, Right
	Q Toe Phalanx, Right
	R Toe Phalanx, Left
	S Coccyx
		0 Open
		3 Percutaneous
		4 Percutaneous Endoscopic
			4 Internal Fixation Device
			5 External Fixation Device
				Z No Qualifier

6 Upper Femur, Right
  Femoral head
  Greater trochanter
  Lesser trochanter
  Neck of femur
7 Upper Femur, Left
  See 6 Upper Femur, Right
B Lower Femur, Right
  Lateral condyle of femur
  Lateral epicondyle of femur
  Medial condyle of femur
  Medial epicondyle of femur
	C Lower Femur, Left
	  See B Lower Femur, Right
	J Fibula, Right
	  Body of fibula
	  Head of fibula
	  Lateral malleolus
	K Fibula, Left
	  See J Fibula, Right
		0 Open
		3 Percutaneous
		4 Percutaneous Endoscopic
			4 Internal Fixation Device
			5 External Fixation Device
			6 Internal Fixation Device, Intramedullary
			8 External Fixation Device, Limb Lengthening
			B External Fixation Device, Monoplanar
			C External Fixation Device, Ring
			D External Fixation Device, Hybrid
				Z No Qualifier

8 Femoral Shaft, Right
  Body of femur
9 Femoral Shaft, Left
  See 8 Femoral Shaft, Right
	G Tibia, Right
	  Lateral condyle of tibia
	  Medial condyle of tibia
	  Medial malleolus
	H Tibia, Left
	  See G Tibia, Right
		0 Open
		3 Percutaneous
		4 Percutaneous Endoscopic
			4 Internal Fixation Device
			5 External Fixation Device
			6 Internal Fixation Device, Intramedullary
			7 Internal Fixation Device, Intramedullary Limb Lengthening
			8 External Fixation Device, Limb Lengthening
			B External Fixation Device, Monoplanar
			C External Fixation Device, Ring
			D External Fixation Device, Hybrid
				Z No Qualifier

Y Lower Bone	**0** Open **3** Percutaneous **4** Percutaneous Endoscopic	**M** Bone Growth Stimulator	**Z** No Qualifier

Non-OR 0QH[6,7,B,C,J,K][0,3,4]8Z
Non-OR 0QH[8,9,G,H][0,3,4]8Z

0 Medical and Surgical
Q Lower Bones
J Inspection

Definition: Visually and/or manually exploring a body part
Explanation: Visual exploration may be performed with or without optical instrumentation. Manual exploration may be performed directly or through intervening body layers.

Body Part Character 4	Approach Character 5	Device Character 6	Qualifier Character 7
Y Lower Bone	**0** Open **3** Percutaneous **4** Percutaneous Endoscopic **X** External	**Z** No Device	**Z** No Qualifier

Non-OR 0QJY[3,X]ZZ

0 **Medical and Surgical**
Q **Lower Bones**
N **Release** Definition: Freeing a body part from an abnormal physical constraint by cutting or by the use of force
Explanation: Some of the restraining tissue may be taken out but none of the body part is taken out

Body Part Character 4	Approach Character 5	Device Character 6	Qualifier Character 7

0 Lumbar Vertebra
   Spinous process
   Transverse process
   Vertebral arch
   Vertebral body
   Vertebral foramen
   Vertebral lamina
   Vertebral pedicle
1 Sacrum
2 Pelvic Bone, Right
   Iliac crest
   Ilium
   Ischium
   Pubis
3 Pelvic Bone, Left
   See 2 Pelvic Bone, Right
4 Acetabulum, Right
5 Acetabulum, Left
6 Upper Femur, Right
   Femoral head
   Greater trochanter
   Lesser trochanter
   Neck of femur
7 Upper Femur, Left
   See 6 Upper Femur, Right
8 Femoral Shaft, Right
   Body of femur
9 Femoral Shaft, Left
   See 8 Femoral Shaft, Right
B Lower Femur, Right
   Lateral condyle of femur
   Lateral epicondyle of femur
   Medial condyle of femur
   Medial epicondyle of femur
C Lower Femur, Left
   See B Lower Femur, Right
D Patella, Right
F Patella, Left
G Tibia, Right
   Lateral condyle of tibia
   Medial condyle of tibia
   Medial malleolus
H Tibia, Left
   See G Tibia, Right
J Fibula, Right
   Body of fibula
   Head of fibula
   Lateral malleolus
K Fibula, Left
   See J Fibula, Right
L Tarsal, Right
   Calcaneus
   Cuboid bone
   Intermediate cuneiform bone
   Lateral cuneiform bone
   Medial cuneiform bone
   Navicular bone
   Talus bone
M Tarsal, Left
   See L Tarsal, Right
N Metatarsal, Right
   Fibular sesamoid
   Tibial sesamoid
P Metatarsal, Left
   See N Metatarsal, Right
Q Toe Phalanx, Right
R Toe Phalanx, Left
S Coccyx
	0 Open
	3 Percutaneous
	4 Percutaneous Endoscopic
		Z No Device	Z No Qualifier

ICD-10-PCS 2025 — Lower Bones — 0QP–0QP

- **0** Medical and Surgical
- **Q** Lower Bones
- **P** Removal

Definition: Taking out or off a device from a body part

Explanation: If a device is taken out and a similar device put in without cutting or puncturing the skin or mucous membrane, the procedure is coded to the root operation CHANGE. Otherwise, the procedure for taking out a device is coded to the root operation REMOVAL.

Body Part — Character 4	Approach — Character 5	Device — Character 6	Qualifier — Character 7
0 Lumbar Vertebra 　Spinous process 　Transverse process 　Vertebral arch 　Vertebral body 　Vertebral foramen 　Vertebral lamina 　Vertebral pedicle **1** Sacrum **2** Pelvic Bone, Right 　Iliac crest 　Ilium 　Ischium 　Pubis **3** Pelvic Bone, Left 　*See 2 Pelvic Bone, Right* **4** Acetabulum, Right **5** Acetabulum, Left **6** Upper Femur, Right 　Femoral head 　Greater trochanter 　Lesser trochanter 　Neck of femur **7** Upper Femur, Left 　*See 6 Upper Femur, Right* **8** Femoral Shaft, Right 　Body of femur **9** Femoral Shaft, Left 　*See 8 Femoral Shaft, Right* **B** Lower Femur, Right 　Lateral condyle of femur 　Lateral epicondyle of femur 　Medial condyle of femur 　Medial epicondyle of femur **C** Lower Femur, Left 　*See B Lower Femur, Right* **D** Patella, Right **F** Patella, Left **G** Tibia, Right 　Lateral condyle of tibia 　Medial condyle of tibia 　Medial malleolus **H** Tibia, Left 　*See G Tibia, Right* **J** Fibula, Right 　Body of fibula 　Head of fibula 　Lateral malleolus **K** Fibula, Left 　*See J Fibula, Right* **L** Tarsal, Right 　Calcaneus 　Cuboid bone 　Intermediate cuneiform bone 　Lateral cuneiform bone 　Medial cuneiform bone 　Navicular bone 　Talus bone **M** Tarsal, Left 　*See L Tarsal, Right* **N** Metatarsal, Right 　Fibular sesamoid 　Tibial sesamoid **P** Metatarsal, Left 　*See N Metatarsal, Right* **Q** Toe Phalanx, Right **R** Toe Phalanx, Left **S** Coccyx	**0** Open **3** Percutaneous **4** Percutaneous Endoscopic	**4** Internal Fixation Device **5** External Fixation Device **7** Autologous Tissue Substitute **J** Synthetic Substitute **K** Nonautologous Tissue Substitute	**Z** No Qualifier
0 Lumbar Vertebra 　Spinous process 　Transverse process 　Vertebral arch 　Vertebral body 　Vertebral foramen 　Vertebral lamina 　Vertebral pedicle **1** Sacrum **2** Pelvic Bone, Right 　Iliac crest 　Ilium 　Ischium 　Pubis **3** Pelvic Bone, Left 　*See 2 Pelvic Bone, Right* **4** Acetabulum, Right **5** Acetabulum, Left **6** Upper Femur, Right 　Femoral head 　Greater trochanter 　Lesser trochanter 　Neck of femur **7** Upper Femur, Left 　*See 6 Upper Femur, Right* **8** Femoral Shaft, Right 　Body of femur **9** Femoral Shaft, Left 　*See 8 Femoral Shaft, Right* **B** Lower Femur, Right 　Lateral condyle of femur 　Lateral epicondyle of femur 　Medial condyle of femur 　Medial epicondyle of femur **C** Lower Femur, Left 　*See B Lower Femur, Right* **D** Patella, Right **F** Patella, Left **G** Tibia, Right 　Lateral condyle of tibia 　Medial condyle of tibia 　Medial malleolus **H** Tibia, Left 　*See G Tibia, Right* **J** Fibula, Right 　Body of fibula 　Head of fibula 　Lateral malleolus **K** Fibula, Left 　*See J Fibula, Right* **L** Tarsal, Right 　Calcaneus 　Cuboid bone 　Intermediate cuneiform bone 　Lateral cuneiform bone 　Medial cuneiform bone 　Navicular bone 　Talus bone **M** Tarsal, Left 　*See L Tarsal, Right* **N** Metatarsal, Right 　Fibular sesamoid 　Tibial sesamoid **P** Metatarsal, Left 　*See N Metatarsal, Right* **Q** Toe Phalanx, Right **R** Toe Phalanx, Left **S** Coccyx	**X** External	**4** Internal Fixation Device **5** External Fixation Device	**Z** No Qualifier
Y Lower Bone	**0** Open **3** Percutaneous **4** Percutaneous Endoscopic **X** External	**0** Drainage Device **M** Bone Growth Stimulator	**Z** No Qualifier

Non-OR 0QPYX[0,M]Z
Non-OR 0QPY30Z
Non-OR 0QP[0,1,2,3,4,5,6,7,8,9,B,C,D,F,G,H,J,K,L,M,N,P,Q,R,S]X[4,5]Z

NC Noncovered Procedure　**LC** Limited Coverage　**QA** Questionable OB Admit　**NT** New Tech Add-on　✚ Combination Member　♂ Male　♀ Female

Lower Bones

0 Medical and Surgical
Q Lower Bones
Q Repair Definition: Restoring, to the extent possible, a body part to its normal anatomic structure and function
Explanation: Used only when the method to accomplish the repair is not one of the other root operations

Body Part Character 4	Approach Character 5	Device Character 6	Qualifier Character 7

0 Lumbar Vertebra
  Spinous process
  Transverse process
  Vertebral arch
  Vertebral body
  Vertebral foramen
  Vertebral lamina
  Vertebral pedicle
1 Sacrum
2 Pelvic Bone, Right
  Iliac crest
  Ilium
  Ischium
  Pubis
3 Pelvic Bone, Left
  See 2 Pelvic Bone, Right
4 Acetabulum, Right
5 Acetabulum, Left
6 Upper Femur, Right
  Femoral head
  Greater trochanter
  Lesser trochanter
  Neck of femur
7 Upper Femur, Left
  See 6 Upper Femur, Right
8 Femoral Shaft, Right
  Body of femur
9 Femoral Shaft, Left
  See 8 Femoral Shaft, Right
B Lower Femur, Right
  Lateral condyle of femur
  Lateral epicondyle of femur
  Medial condyle of femur
  Medial epicondyle of femur
C Lower Femur, Left
  See B Lower Femur, Right
D Patella, Right
F Patella, Left
G Tibia, Right
  Lateral condyle of tibia
  Medial condyle of tibia
  Medial malleolus
H Tibia, Left
  See G Tibia, Right
J Fibula, Right
  Body of fibula
  Head of fibula
  Lateral malleolus
K Fibula, Left
  See J Fibula, Right
L Tarsal, Right
  Calcaneus
  Cuboid bone
  Intermediate cuneiform bone
  Lateral cuneiform bone
  Medial cuneiform bone
  Navicular bone
  Talus bone
M Tarsal, Left
  See L Tarsal, Right
N Metatarsal, Right
  Fibular sesamoid
  Tibial sesamoid
P Metatarsal, Left
  See N Metatarsal, Right
Q Toe Phalanx, Right
R Toe Phalanx, Left
S Coccyx
	0 Open
	3 Percutaneous
	4 Percutaneous Endoscopic
	X External
		Z No Device	**Z** No Qualifier

Non-OR 0QQ[0,1,2,3,4,5,6,7,8,9,B,C,D,F,G,H,J,K,L,M,N,P,Q,R,S]XZZ

ICD-10-PCS 2025 — Lower Bones — 0QR–0QR

0 Medical and Surgical
Q Lower Bones
R Replacement

Definition: Putting in or on biological or synthetic material that physically takes the place and/or function of all or a portion of a body part
Explanation: The body part may have been taken out or replaced, or may be taken out, physically eradicated, or rendered nonfunctional during the REPLACEMENT procedure. A REMOVAL procedure is coded for taking out the device used in a previous replacement procedure.

Body Part Character 4	Approach Character 5	Device Character 6	Qualifier Character 7

0 Lumbar Vertebra
   Spinous process
   Transverse process
   Vertebral arch
   Vertebral body
   Vertebral foramen
   Vertebral lamina
   Vertebral pedicle
1 Sacrum
2 Pelvic Bone, Right
   Iliac crest
   Ilium
   Ischium
   Pubis
3 Pelvic Bone, Left
   See 2 Pelvic Bone, Right
4 Acetabulum, Right
5 Acetabulum, Left
6 Upper Femur, Right
   Femoral head
   Greater trochanter
   Lesser trochanter
   Neck of femur
7 Upper Femur, Left
   See 6 Upper Femur, Right
8 Femoral Shaft, Right
   Body of femur
9 Femoral Shaft, Left
   See 8 Femoral Shaft, Right
B Lower Femur, Right
   Lateral condyle of femur
   Lateral epicondyle of femur
   Medial condyle of femur
   Medial epicondyle of femur
C Lower Femur, Left
   See B Lower Femur, Right
D Patella, Right
F Patella, Left
G Tibia, Right
   Lateral condyle of tibia
   Medial condyle of tibia
   Medial malleolus
H Tibia, Left
   See G Tibia, Right
J Fibula, Right
   Body of fibula
   Head of fibula
   Lateral malleolus
K Fibula, Left
   See J Fibula, Right
L Tarsal, Right
   Calcaneus
   Cuboid bone
   Intermediate cuneiform bone
   Lateral cuneiform bone
   Medial cuneiform bone
   Navicular bone
   Talus bone
M Tarsal, Left
   See L Tarsal, Right
N Metatarsal, Right
   Fibular sesamoid
   Tibial sesamoid
P Metatarsal, Left
   See N Metatarsal, Right
Q Toe Phalanx, Right
R Toe Phalanx, Left
S Coccyx
	0 Open
	3 Percutaneous
	4 Percutaneous Endoscopic
		7 Autologous Tissue Substitute
		J Synthetic Substitute
		K Nonautologous Tissue Substitute
			Z No Qualifier

NC Noncovered Procedure   **LC** Limited Coverage   **QA** Questionable OB Admit   **NT** New Tech Add-on   ✚ Combination Member   ♂ Male   ♀ Female

Lower Bones

0 Medical and Surgical
Q Lower Bones
S Reposition Definition: Moving to its normal location, or other suitable location, all or a portion of a body part
Explanation: The body part is moved to a new location from an abnormal location, or from a normal location where it is not functioning correctly. The body part may or may not be cut out or off to be moved to the new location.

Body Part Character 4	Approach Character 5	Device Character 6	Qualifier Character 7
0 Lumbar Vertebra Spinous process Transverse process Vertebral arch Vertebral body Vertebral foramen Vertebral lamina Vertebral pedicle	**0** Open **4** Percutaneous Endoscopic	**3** Spinal Stabilization Device, Vertebral Body Tether **4** Internal Fixation Device **Z** No Device	**Z** No Qualifier
0 Lumbar Vertebra ⊕ Spinous process Transverse process Vertebral arch Vertebral body Vertebral foramen Vertebral lamina Vertebral pedicle	**3** Percutaneous	**4** Internal Fixation Device **Z** No Device	**Z** No Qualifier
0 Lumbar Vertebra Spinous process Transverse process Vertebral arch Vertebral body Vertebral foramen Vertebral lamina Vertebral pedicle	**X** External	**Z** No Device	**Z** No Qualifier
1 Sacrum ⊕ **4** Acetabulum, Right **5** Acetabulum, Left **S** Coccyx ⊕	**0** Open **3** Percutaneous **4** Percutaneous Endoscopic	**4** Internal Fixation Device **Z** No Device	**Z** No Qualifier
1 Sacrum **4** Acetabulum, Right **5** Acetabulum, Left **S** Coccyx	**X** External	**Z** No Device	**Z** No Qualifier
2 Pelvic Bone, Right Iliac crest Ilium Ischium Pubis **3** Pelvic Bone, Left *See 2 Pelvic Bone, Right* **D** Patella, Right **F** Patella, Left **L** Tarsal, Right Calcaneus Cuboid bone Intermediate cuneiform bone Lateral cuneiform bone Medial cuneiform bone Navicular bone Talus bone	**M** Tarsal, Left *See L Tarsal, Right* **Q** Toe Phalanx, Right **R** Toe Phalanx, Left	**0** Open **3** Percutaneous **4** Percutaneous Endoscopic	**4** Internal Fixation Device **5** External Fixation Device **Z** No Device	**Z** No Qualifier
2 Pelvic Bone, Right Iliac crest Ilium Ischium Pubis **3** Pelvic Bone, Left *See 2 Pelvic Bone, Right* **D** Patella, Right **F** Patella, Left **L** Tarsal, Right Calcaneus Cuboid bone Intermediate cuneiform bone Lateral cuneiform bone Medial cuneiform bone Navicular bone Talus bone	**M** Tarsal, Left *See L Tarsal, Right* **Q** Toe Phalanx, Right **R** Toe Phalanx, Left	**X** External	**Z** No Device	**Z** No Qualifier

Non-OR 0QS0XZZ
Non-OR 0QS[4,5][3,4]ZZ
Non-OR 0QS[1,4,5]XZZ
Non-OR 0QS[2,3,D,F,L,M,Q,R][3,4]ZZ
Non-OR 0QS[2,3,D,F,L,M,Q,R]XZZ

See Appendix L for Procedure Combinations
⊕ 0QS03ZZ
⊕ 0QS[1,S]3ZZ

0QS Continued on next page

ICD-10-PCS 2025 — Lower Bones — 0QS–0QS

0QS Continued

- **0** Medical and Surgical
- **Q** Lower Bones
- **S** Reposition

Definition: Moving to its normal location, or other suitable location, all or a portion of a body part

Explanation: The body part is moved to a new location from an abnormal location, or from a normal location where it is not functioning correctly. The body part may or may not be cut out or off to be moved to the new location.

Body Part — Character 4	Approach — Character 5	Device — Character 6	Qualifier — Character 7

6 Upper Femur, Right
   Femoral head
   Greater trochanter
   Lesser trochanter
   Neck of femur
7 Upper Femur, Left
   See 6 Upper Femur, Right
8 Femoral Shaft, Right
   Body of femur
9 Femoral Shaft, Left
   See 8 Femoral Shaft, Right
B Lower Femur, Right
   Lateral condyle of femur
   Lateral epicondyle of femur
   Medial condyle of femur
   Medial epicondyle of femur
C Lower Femur, Left
   See B Lower Femur, Right
G Tibia, Right
   Lateral condyle of tibia
   Medial condyle of tibia
   Medial malleolus
H Tibia, Left
   See G Tibia, Right
J Fibula, Right
   Body of fibula
   Head of fibula
   Lateral malleolus
K Fibula, Left
   See J Fibula, Right
	0 Open
	3 Percutaneous
	4 Percutaneous Endoscopic
		4 Internal Fixation Device
		5 External Fixation Device
		6 Internal Fixation Device, Intramedullary
		B External Fixation Device, Monoplanar
		C External Fixation Device, Ring
		D External Fixation Device, Hybrid
		Z No Device
			Z No Qualifier

6 Upper Femur, Right
   Femoral head
   Greater trochanter
   Lesser trochanter
   Neck of femur
7 Upper Femur, Left
   See 6 Upper Femur, Right
8 Femoral Shaft, Right
   Body of femur
9 Femoral Shaft, Left
   See 8 Femoral Shaft, Right
B Lower Femur, Right
   Lateral condyle of femur
   Lateral epicondyle of femur
   Medial condyle of femur
   Medial epicondyle of femur
C Lower Femur, Left
   See B Lower Femur, Right
G Tibia, Right
   Lateral condyle of tibia
   Medial condyle of tibia
   Medial malleolus
H Tibia, Left
   See G Tibia, Right
J Fibula, Right
   Body of fibula
   Head of fibula
   Lateral malleolus
K Fibula, Left
   See J Fibula, Right
	X External	**Z** No Device	**Z** No Qualifier

N Metatarsal, Right
   Fibular sesamoid
   Tibial sesamoid
P Metatarsal, Left
   See N Metatarsal, Right
	0 Open
	3 Percutaneous
	4 Percutaneous Endoscopic
		4 Internal Fixation Device
		5 External Fixation Device
		Z No Device
			2 Sesamoid Bone(s) 1st Toe
			Z No Qualifier

N Metatarsal, Right
   Fibular sesamoid
   Tibial sesamoid
P Metatarsal, Left
   See N Metatarsal, Right
	X External	**Z** No Device	**2** Sesamoid Bone(s) 1st Toe
			Z No Qualifier

Non-OR 0QS[6,7,8,9,B,C,G,H,J,K][3,4]ZZ
Non-OR 0QS[6,7,8,9,B,C,G,H,J,K]XZZ
Non-OR 0QS[N,P][3,4]Z[2,Z]
Non-OR 0QS[N,P]XZ[2,Z]

0QT–0QU — Lower Bones

0 Medical and Surgical
Q Lower Bones
T Resection

Definition: Cutting out or off, without replacement, all of a body part
Explanation: None

Body Part — Character 4	Approach — Character 5	Device — Character 6	Qualifier — Character 7

2 Pelvic Bone, Right
  Iliac crest
  Ilium
  Ischium
  Pubis
3 Pelvic Bone, Left
  See 2 Pelvic Bone, Right
4 Acetabulum, Right
5 Acetabulum, Left
6 Upper Femur, Right
  Femoral head
  Greater trochanter
  Lesser trochanter
  Neck of femur
7 Upper Femur, Left
  See 6 Upper Femur, Right
8 Femoral Shaft, Right
  Body of femur
9 Femoral Shaft, Left
  See 8 Femoral Shaft, Right
B Lower Femur, Right
  Lateral condyle of femur
  Lateral epicondyle of femur
  Medial condyle of femur
  Medial epicondyle of femur
C Lower Femur, Left
  See B Lower Femur, Right
D Patella, Right
F Patella, Left
G Tibia, Right
  Lateral condyle of tibia
  Medial condyle of tibia
  Medial malleolus
H Tibia, Left
  See G Tibia, Right
J Fibula, Right
  Body of fibula
  Head of fibula
  Lateral malleolus
K Fibula, Left
  See J Fibula, Right
L Tarsal, Right
  Calcaneus
  Cuboid bone
  Intermediate cuneiform bone
  Lateral cuneiform bone
  Medial cuneiform bone
  Navicular bone
  Talus bone
M Tarsal, Left
  See L Tarsal, Right
N Metatarsal, Right
  Fibular sesamoid
  Tibial sesamoid
P Metatarsal, Left
  See N Metatarsal, Right
Q Toe Phalanx, Right
R Toe Phalanx, Left
S Coccyx
	0 Open	**Z** No Device	**Z** No Qualifier

---

0 Medical and Surgical
Q Lower Bones
U Supplement

Definition: Putting in or on biological or synthetic material that physically reinforces and/or augments the function of a portion of a body part
Explanation: The biological material is non-living, or is living and from the same individual. The body part may have been previously replaced, and the SUPPLEMENT procedure is performed to physically reinforce and/or augment the function of the replaced body part.

Body Part — Character 4	Approach — Character 5	Device — Character 6	Qualifier — Character 7

0 Lumbar Vertebra ✚
  Spinous process
  Transverse process
  Vertebral arch
  Vertebral body
  Vertebral foramen
  Vertebral lamina
  Vertebral pedicle
1 Sacrum ✚
2 Pelvic Bone, Right
  Iliac crest
  Ilium
  Ischium
  Pubis
3 Pelvic Bone, Left
  See 2 Pelvic Bone, Right
4 Acetabulum, Right
5 Acetabulum, Left
6 Upper Femur, Right
  Femoral head
  Greater trochanter
  Lesser trochanter
  Neck of femur
7 Upper Femur, Left
  See 6 Upper Femur, Right
8 Femoral Shaft, Right
  Body of femur
9 Femoral Shaft, Left
  See 8 Femoral Shaft, Right
B Lower Femur, Right
  Lateral condyle of femur
  Lateral epicondyle of femur
  Medial condyle of femur
  Medial epicondyle of femur
C Lower Femur, Left
  See B Lower Femur, Right
D Patella, Right
F Patella, Left
G Tibia, Right
  Lateral condyle of tibia
  Medial condyle of tibia
  Medial malleolus
H Tibia, Left
  See G Tibia, Right
J Fibula, Right
  Body of fibula
  Head of fibula
  Lateral malleolus
K Fibula, Left
  See J Fibula, Right
L Tarsal, Right
  Calcaneus
  Cuboid bone
  Intermediate cuneiform bone
  Lateral cuneiform bone
  Medial cuneiform bone
  Navicular bone
  Talus bone
M Tarsal, Left
  See L Tarsal, Right
N Metatarsal, Right
  Fibular sesamoid
  Tibial sesamoid
P Metatarsal, Left
  See N Metatarsal, Right
Q Toe Phalanx, Right
R Toe Phalanx, Left
S Coccyx ✚
	0 Open
	3 Percutaneous
	4 Percutaneous Endoscopic
		7 Autologous Tissue Substitute
		J Synthetic Substitute
		K Nonautologous Tissue Substitute
			Z No Qualifier

See Appendix L for Procedure Combinations
  ✚ 0QU[0,1,S]3JZ

Non-OR Procedure | DRG Non-OR Procedure | Valid OR Procedure | HAC Associated Procedure | Combination Only | New/Revised April | New/Revised October

ICD-10-PCS 2025 — Lower Bones — 0QW–0QW

- **0 Medical and Surgical**
- **Q Lower Bones**
- **W Revision**

Definition: Correcting, to the extent possible, a portion of a malfunctioning device or the position of a displaced device

Explanation: Revision can include correcting a malfunctioning or displaced device by taking out or putting in components of the device such as a screw or pin

Body Part Character 4	Approach Character 5	Device Character 6	Qualifier Character 7

0 Lumbar Vertebra
  Spinous process
  Transverse process
  Vertebral arch
  Vertebral body
  Vertebral foramen
  Vertebral lamina
  Vertebral pedicle
1 Sacrum
4 Acetabulum, Right
5 Acetabulum, Left
S Coccyx
	0 Open
	3 Percutaneous
	4 Percutaneous Endoscopic
	X External
		4 Internal Fixation Device
		7 Autologous Tissue Substitute
		J Synthetic Substitute
		K Nonautologous Tissue Substitute
			Z No Qualifier

2 Pelvic Bone, Right
  Iliac crest
  Ilium
  Ischium
  Pubis
3 Pelvic Bone, Left
  See 2 Pelvic Bone, Right
6 Upper Femur, Right
  Femoral head
  Greater trochanter
  Lesser trochanter
  Neck of femur
7 Upper Femur, Left
  See 6 Upper Femur, Right
8 Femoral Shaft, Right
  Body of femur
9 Femoral Shaft, Left
  See 8 Femoral Shaft, Right
B Lower Femur, Right
  Lateral condyle of femur
  Lateral epicondyle of femur
  Medial condyle of femur
  Medial epicondyle of femur
C Lower Femur, Left
  See B Lower Femur, Right
D Patella, Right
F Patella, Left
G Tibia, Right
  Lateral condyle of tibia
  Medial condyle of tibia
  Medial malleolus
H Tibia, Left
  See G Tibia, Right
J Fibula, Right
  Body of fibula
  Head of fibula
  Lateral malleolus
K Fibula, Left
  See J Fibula, Right
L Tarsal, Right
  Calcaneus
  Cuboid bone
  Intermediate cuneiform bone
  Lateral cuneiform bone
  Medial cuneiform bone
  Navicular bone
  Talus bone
M Tarsal, Left
  See L Tarsal, Right
N Metatarsal, Right
  Fibular sesamoid
  Tibial sesamoid
P Metatarsal, Left
  See N Metatarsal, Right
Q Toe Phalanx, Right
R Toe Phalanx, Left
	0 Open
	3 Percutaneous
	4 Percutaneous Endoscopic
	X External
		4 Internal Fixation Device
		5 External Fixation Device
		7 Autologous Tissue Substitute
		J Synthetic Substitute
		K Nonautologous Tissue Substitute
			Z No Qualifier

Y Lower Bone	**0** Open **3** Percutaneous **4** Percutaneous Endoscopic **X** External	**0** Drainage Device **M** Bone Growth Stimulator	**Z** No Qualifier

Non-OR 0QW[0,1,4,5,S]X[4,7,J,K]Z
Non-OR 0QW[2,3,6,7,8,9,B,C,D,F,G,H,J,K,L,M,N,P,Q,R]X[4,5,7,J,K]Z
Non-OR 0QWYX[0,M]Z

Upper Joints 0R2–0RW

Character Meanings*

This Character Meaning table is provided as a guide to assist the user in the identification of character members that may be found in this section of code tables. It **SHOULD NOT** be used to build a PCS code.

Operation–Character 3	Body Part–Character 4	Approach–Character 5	Device–Character 6	Qualifier–Character 7
2 Change	0 Occipital-cervical Joint	0 Open	0 Drainage Device OR Synthetic Substitute, Reverse Ball and Socket	0 Anterior Approach, Anterior Column
5 Destruction	1 Cervical Vertebral Joint	3 Percutaneous	3 Infusion Device OR Internal Fixation Device, Sustained Compression	1 Posterior Approach, Posterior Column
9 Drainage	2 Cervical Vertebral Joint, 2 or more	4 Percutaneous Endoscopic	4 Internal Fixation Device	6 Humeral Surface
B Excision	3 Cervical Vertebral Disc	X External	5 External Fixation Device	7 Glenoid Surface
C Extirpation	4 Cervicothoracic Vertebral Joint		7 Autologous Tissue Substitute	J Posterior Approach, Anterior Column
G Fusion	5 Cervicothoracic Vertebral Disc		8 Spacer	X Diagnostic
H Insertion	6 Thoracic Vertebral Joint		A Interbody Fusion Device	Z No Qualifier
J Inspection	7 Thoracic Vertebral Joint, 2 to 7		B Spinal Stabilization Device, Interspinous Process	
N Release	8 Thoracic Vertebral Joint, 8 or more		C Spinal Stabilization Device, Pedicle-Based	
P Removal	9 Thoracic Vertebral Disc		D Spinal Stabilization Device, Facet Replacement	
Q Repair	A Thoracolumbar Vertebral Joint		J Synthetic Substitute	
R Replacement	B Thoracolumbar Vertebral Disc		K Nonautologous Tissue Substitute	
S Reposition	C Temporomandibular Joint, Right		Y Other Device	
T Resection	D Temporomandibular Joint, Left		Z No Device	
U Supplement	E Sternoclavicular Joint, Right			
W Revision	F Sternoclavicular Joint, Left			
	G Acromioclavicular Joint, Right			
	H Acromioclavicular Joint, Left			
	J Shoulder Joint, Right			
	K Shoulder Joint, Left			
	L Elbow Joint, Right			
	M Elbow Joint, Left			
	N Wrist Joint, Right			
	P Wrist Joint, Left			
	Q Carpal Joint, Right			
	R Carpal Joint, Left			
	S Carpometacarpal Joint, Right			
	T Carpometacarpal Joint, Left			
	U Metacarpophalangeal Joint, Right			
	V Metacarpophalangeal Joint, Left			
	W Finger Phalangeal Joint, Right			
	X Finger Phalangeal Joint, Left			
	Y Upper Joint			

* Includes synovial membrane.

Upper Joints

AHA Coding Clinic for table ØRB
2019, 3Q, 26	Acromioclavicular joint reconstruction using allograft

AHA Coding Clinic for table ØRG
2024, 2Q, 27	Stimulan® rapid cure antibiotic bead placement
2023, 2Q, 25	Spinal fusion using allograft bone graft and bone marrow aspirate
2022, 3Q, 21	Breakage of intervertebral cage during surgery
2021, 4Q, 67	Posterior dynamic distraction
2021, 1Q, 18	Placement of interspinous distraction device (spacer) for decompression
2021, 1Q, 53	Official guidelines for coding and reporting for interbody fusion device B3.10c
2020, 4Q, 56-58	Intramedullary sustained compression joint fusion
2020, 2Q, 27	Spinal fusion with NuVasive® VersaTie®
2020, 1Q, 33	Spinal fusion without use of bone graft
2019, 3Q, 28	Use of VERTE-STACK™ implant with fusion
2019, 3Q, 35	Fusion procedures of the spine (guideline B3.10c)
2019, 2Q, 19	Cervical spinal fusion, decompression and placement of interfacet stabilization device
2019, 1Q, 30	Spinal fusion performed at same level as decompressive laminectomy
2018, 4Q, 43	Joint fusion device value
2018, 1Q, 22	Spinal fusion procedures without bone graft
2017, 4Q, 62	Added and revised device values - Nerve substitutes
2017, 4Q, 76	Radiolucent porous interbody fusion device
2017, 2Q, 23	Decompression of spinal cord and placement of instrumentation
2014, 3Q, 30	Spinal fusion and fixation instrumentation
2014, 2Q, 7	Anterior cervical thoracic fusion with total discectomy
2013, 1Q, 21-23	Spinal fusion of thoracic and lumbar vertebrae
2013, 1Q, 29	Cervical and thoracic spinal fusion

AHA Coding Clinic for table ØRH
2021, 1Q, 18	Placement of interspinous distraction device (spacer) for decompression
2019, 2Q, 40	Decompression of spinal cord and placement of instrumentation
2018, 3Q, 26	Anterior vertebral tethering using Dynesys Tethering System
2017, 2Q, 23	Decompression of spinal cord and placement of instrumentation
2016, 3Q, 32	Rotator cuff repair, tenodesis, decompression, acromioplasty and coracoplasty

AHA Coding Clinic for table ØRN
2019, 1Q, 30	Spinal fusion performed at same level as decompressive laminectomy
2016, 3Q, 32	Rotator cuff repair, tenodesis, decompression, acromioplasty and coracoplasty
2015, 2Q, 22	Arthroscopic subacromial decompression
2015, 2Q, 23	Arthroscopic release of shoulder joint

AHA Coding Clinic for table ØRP
2022, 3Q, 21	Breakage of intervertebral cage during surgery
2021, 4Q, 53	Shoulder hemiarthroplasty
2017, 4Q, 107	Total ankle replacement versus revision

AHA Coding Clinic for table ØRQ
2016, 1Q, 30	Thermal capsulorrhaphy of shoulder

AHA Coding Clinic for table ØRR
2018, 4Q, 92	Radial head arthroplasty
2017, 4Q, 107	Total ankle replacement versus revision
2015, 3Q, 14	Endoprosthetic replacement of humerus and tendon reattachment
2015, 1Q, 27	Reverse total shoulder arthroplasty

AHA Coding Clinic for table ØRS
2019, 3Q, 26	Acromioclavicular joint reconstruction using allograft
2018, 3Q, 26	Anterior vertebral tethering using Dynesys Tethering System
2015, 2Q, 35	Application of tongs to reduce and stabilize cervical fracture
2014, 4Q, 32	Open reduction internal fixation of fracture with debridement
2014, 3Q, 33	Radial fracture treatment with open reduction internal fixation, and release of carpal ligament
2013, 2Q, 39	Application of cervical tongs for reduction of cervical fracture

AHA Coding Clinic for table ØRT
2019, 3Q, 26	Acromioclavicular joint reconstruction using allograft
2014, 2Q, 7	Anterior cervical thoracic fusion with total discectomy

AHA Coding Clinic for table ØRU
2019, 3Q, 26	Acromioclavicular joint reconstruction using allograft
2015, 3Q, 26	Thumb arthroplasty with resection of trapezium

AHA Coding Clinic for table ØRW
2021, 4Q, 53	Shoulder hemiarthroplasty
2017, 4Q, 107	Total ankle replacement versus revision

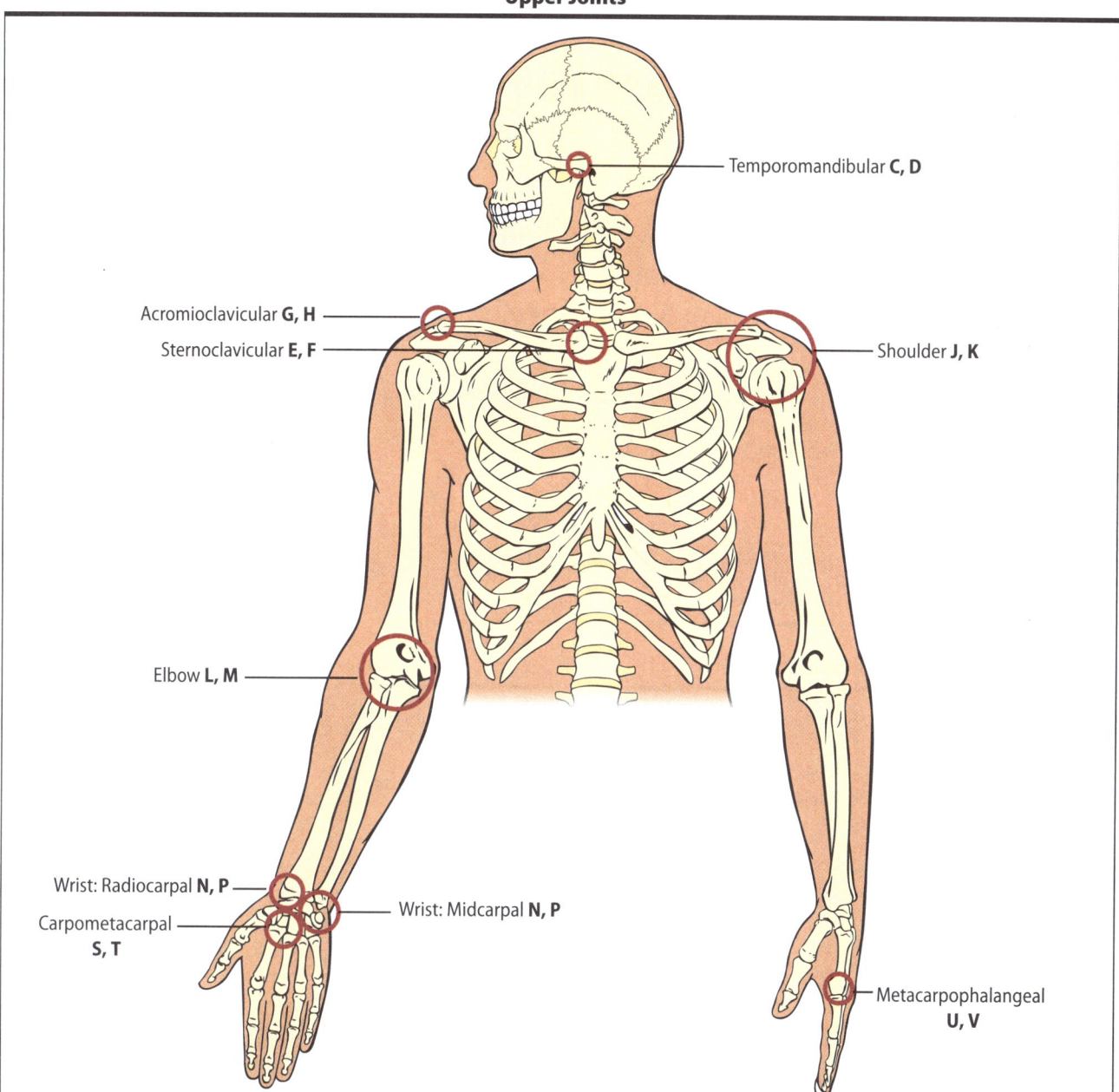

Upper Joints

- Temporomandibular **C, D**
- Acromioclavicular **G, H**
- Sternoclavicular **E, F**
- Shoulder **J, K**
- Elbow **L, M**
- Wrist: Radiocarpal **N, P**
- Wrist: Midcarpal **N, P**
- Carpometacarpal **S, T**
- Metacarpophalangeal **U, V**

Upper Joints

Hand Joints

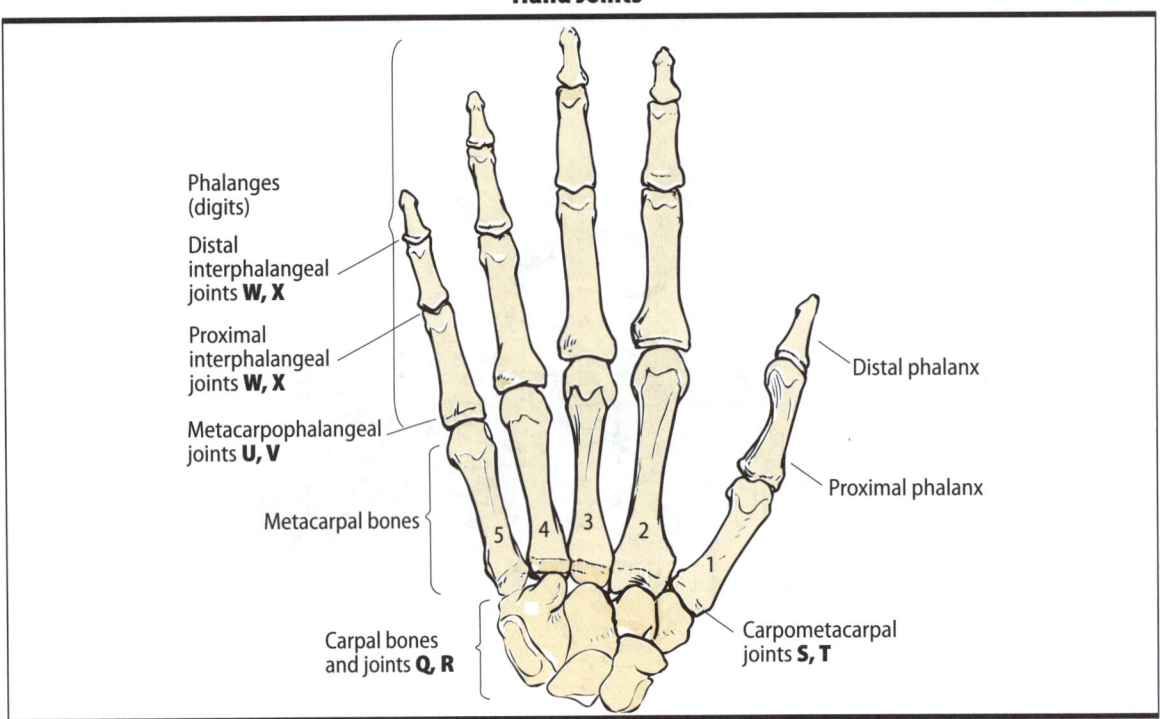

- Phalanges (digits)
- Distal interphalangeal joints **W, X**
- Proximal interphalangeal joints **W, X**
- Metacarpophalangeal joints **U, V**
- Metacarpal bones
- Carpal bones and joints **Q, R**
- Carpometacarpal joints **S, T**
- Distal phalanx
- Proximal phalanx

Shoulder Joints

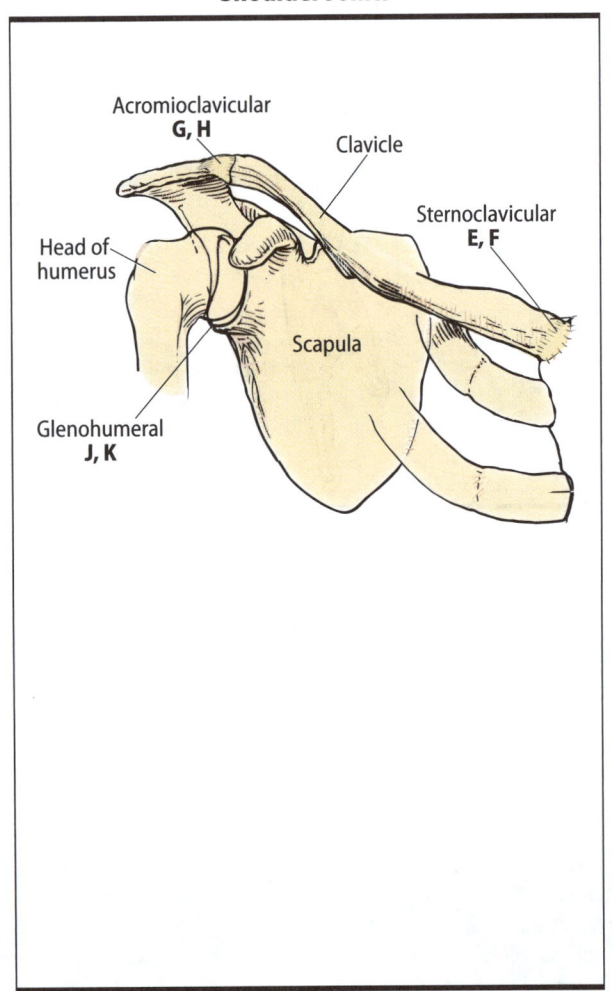

- Acromioclavicular **G, H**
- Clavicle
- Sternoclavicular **E, F**
- Head of humerus
- Scapula
- Glenohumeral **J, K**

Upper Vertebral Joints

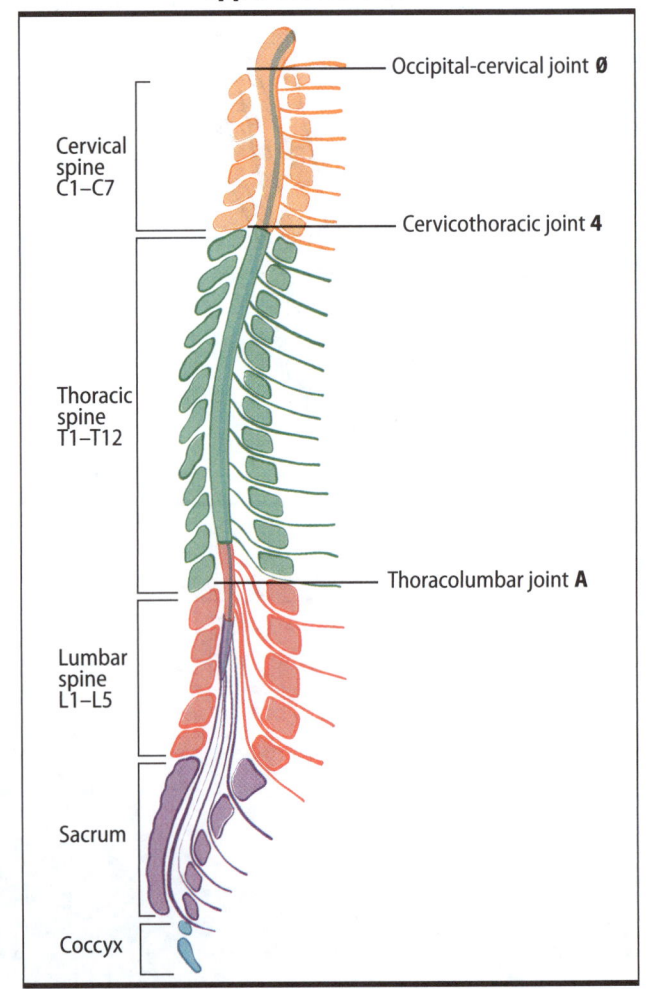

- Occipital-cervical joint **Ø**
- Cervical spine C1–C7
- Cervicothoracic joint **4**
- Thoracic spine T1–T12
- Thoracolumbar joint **A**
- Lumbar spine L1–L5
- Sacrum
- Coccyx

ICD-10-PCS 2025 — Upper Joints — 0R2–0R5

0 Medical and Surgical
R Upper Joints
2 Change — Definition: Taking out or off a device from a body part and putting back an identical or similar device in or on the same body part without cutting or puncturing the skin or a mucous membrane
Explanation: All CHANGE procedures are coded using the approach EXTERNAL

Body Part Character 4	Approach Character 5	Device Character 6	Qualifier Character 7
Y Upper Joint	X External	0 Drainage Device Y Other Device	Z No Qualifier

Non-OR All body part, approach, device, and qualifier values

---

0 Medical and Surgical
R Upper Joints
5 Destruction — Definition: Physical eradication of all or a portion of a body part by the direct use of energy, force, or a destructive agent
Explanation: None of the body part is physically taken out

Body Part Character 4	Approach Character 5	Device Character 6	Qualifier Character 7

0 Occipital-cervical Joint
1 Cervical Vertebral Joint
   Atlantoaxial joint
   Cervical facet joint
3 Cervical Vertebral Disc
4 Cervicothoracic Vertebral Joint
   Cervicothoracic facet joint
5 Cervicothoracic Vertebral Disc
6 Thoracic Vertebral Joint
   Costotransverse joint
   Costovertebral joint
   Thoracic facet joint
9 Thoracic Vertebral Disc
A Thoracolumbar Vertebral Joint
   Thoracolumbar facet joint
B Thoracolumbar Vertebral Disc
C Temporomandibular Joint, Right
D Temporomandibular Joint, Left
E Sternoclavicular Joint, Right
F Sternoclavicular Joint, Left
G Acromioclavicular Joint, Right
H Acromioclavicular Joint, Left
J Shoulder Joint, Right
   Glenohumeral joint
   Glenoid ligament (labrum)
K Shoulder Joint, Left
   See J Shoulder Joint, Right
L Elbow Joint, Right
   Distal humerus, involving joint
   Humeroradial joint
   Humeroulnar joint
   Proximal radioulnar joint
M Elbow Joint, Left
   See L Elbow Joint, Right
N Wrist Joint, Right
   Distal radioulnar joint
   Radiocarpal joint
P Wrist Joint, Left
   See N Wrist Joint, Right
Q Carpal Joint, Right
   Intercarpal joint
   Midcarpal joint
R Carpal Joint, Left
   See Q Carpal Joint, Right
S Carpometacarpal Joint, Right
T Carpometacarpal Joint, Left
U Metacarpophalangeal Joint, Right
V Metacarpophalangeal Joint, Left
W Finger Phalangeal Joint, Right
   Interphalangeal (IP) joint
X Finger Phalangeal Joint, Left
   See W Finger Phalangeal Joint, Right
	0 Open
	3 Percutaneous
	4 Percutaneous Endoscopic
		Z No Device	Z No Qualifier

Non-OR 0R5[3,5,9,B][3,4]ZZ

ØR9–ØR9 Upper Joints ICD-10-PCS 2025

Ø Medical and Surgical
R Upper Joints
9 Drainage

Definition: Taking or letting out fluids and/or gases from a body part
Explanation: The qualifier DIAGNOSTIC is used to identify drainage procedures that are biopsies

Body Part Character 4	Approach Character 5	Device Character 6	Qualifier Character 7

Ø Occipital-cervical Joint
1 Cervical Vertebral Joint
   Atlantoaxial joint
   Cervical facet joint
3 Cervical Vertebral Disc
4 Cervicothoracic Vertebral Joint
   Cervicothoracic facet joint
5 Cervicothoracic Vertebral Disc
6 Thoracic Vertebral Joint
   Costotransverse joint
   Costovertebral joint
   Thoracic facet joint
9 Thoracic Vertebral Disc
A Thoracolumbar Vertebral Joint
   Thoracolumbar facet joint
B Thoracolumbar Vertebral Disc
C Temporomandibular Joint, Right
D Temporomandibular Joint, Left
E Sternoclavicular Joint, Right
F Sternoclavicular Joint, Left
G Acromioclavicular Joint, Right
H Acromioclavicular Joint, Left
J Shoulder Joint, Right
   Glenohumeral joint
   Glenoid ligament (labrum)
K Shoulder Joint, Left
   See J Shoulder Joint, Right
	L Elbow Joint, Right
	   Distal humerus, involving joint
	   Humeroradial joint
	   Humeroulnar joint
	   Proximal radioulnar joint
	M Elbow Joint, Left
	   See L Elbow Joint, Right
	N Wrist Joint, Right
	   Distal radioulnar joint
	   Radiocarpal joint
	P Wrist Joint, Left
	   See N Wrist Joint, Right
	Q Carpal Joint, Right
	   Intercarpal joint
	   Midcarpal joint
	R Carpal Joint, Left
	   See Q Carpal Joint, Right
	S Carpometacarpal Joint, Right
	T Carpometacarpal Joint, Left
	U Metacarpophalangeal Joint, Right
	V Metacarpophalangeal Joint, Left
	W Finger Phalangeal Joint, Right
	   Interphalangeal (IP) joint
	X Finger Phalangeal Joint, Left
	   See W Finger Phalangeal Joint, Right
		Ø Open
		3 Percutaneous
		4 Percutaneous Endoscopic
			Ø Drainage Device	**Z** No Qualifier

Ø Occipital-cervical Joint
1 Cervical Vertebral Joint
   Atlantoaxial joint
   Cervical facet joint
3 Cervical Vertebral Disc
4 Cervicothoracic Vertebral Joint
   Cervicothoracic facet joint
5 Cervicothoracic Vertebral Disc
6 Thoracic Vertebral Joint
   Costotransverse joint
   Costovertebral joint
   Thoracic facet joint
9 Thoracic Vertebral Disc
A Thoracolumbar Vertebral Joint
   Thoracolumbar facet joint
B Thoracolumbar Vertebral Disc
C Temporomandibular Joint, Right
D Temporomandibular Joint, Left
E Sternoclavicular Joint, Right
F Sternoclavicular Joint, Left
G Acromioclavicular Joint, Right
H Acromioclavicular Joint, Left
J Shoulder Joint, Right
   Glenohumeral joint
   Glenoid ligament (labrum)
K Shoulder Joint, Left
   See J Shoulder Joint, Right
	L Elbow Joint, Right
	   Distal humerus, involving joint
	   Humeroradial joint
	   Humeroulnar joint
	   Proximal radioulnar joint
	M Elbow Joint, Left
	   See L Elbow Joint, Right
	N Wrist Joint, Right
	   Distal radioulnar joint
	   Radiocarpal joint
	P Wrist Joint, Left
	   See N Wrist Joint, Right
	Q Carpal Joint, Right
	   Intercarpal joint
	   Midcarpal joint
	R Carpal Joint, Left
	   See Q Carpal Joint, Right
	S Carpometacarpal Joint, Right
	T Carpometacarpal Joint, Left
	U Metacarpophalangeal Joint, Right
	V Metacarpophalangeal Joint, Left
	W Finger Phalangeal Joint, Right
	   Interphalangeal (IP) joint
	X Finger Phalangeal Joint, Left
	   See W Finger Phalangeal Joint, Right
		Ø Open
		3 Percutaneous
		4 Percutaneous Endoscopic
			Z No Device	**X** Diagnostic
				Z No Qualifier

Non-OR   ØR9[Ø,1,3,4,5,6,9,A,B,E,F,G,H,J,K,L,M,N,P,Q,R,S,T,U,V,W,X][3,4]ØZ
Non-OR   ØR9[C,D]3ØZ
Non-OR   ØR9[Ø,1,3,4,5,6,9,A,B,E,F,G,H,J,K,L,M,N,P,Q,R,S,T,U,V,W,X][Ø,3,4]ZX
Non-OR   ØR9[Ø,1,3,4,5,6,9,A,B,E,F,G,H,J,K,L,M,N,P,Q,R,S,T,U,V,W,X][3,4]ZZ
Non-OR   ØR9[C,D]3ZZ

Non-OR Procedure   DRG Non-OR Procedure   Valid OR Procedure   HAC Associated Procedure   Combination Only   New/Revised April   New/Revised October

ICD-10-PCS 2025   Upper Joints   0RB–0RB

- **0** Medical and Surgical
- **R** Upper Joints
- **B** Excision   Definition: Cutting out or off, without replacement, a portion of a body part
  Explanation: The qualifier DIAGNOSTIC is used to identify excision procedures that are biopsies

Body Part Character 4	Approach Character 5	Device Character 6	Qualifier Character 7

0 Occipital-cervical Joint
1 Cervical Vertebral Joint
   Atlantoaxial joint
   Cervical facet joint
3 Cervical Vertebral Disc
4 Cervicothoracic Vertebral Joint
   Cervicothoracic facet joint
5 Cervicothoracic Vertebral Disc
6 Thoracic Vertebral Joint
   Costotransverse joint
   Costovertebral joint
   Thoracic facet joint
9 Thoracic Vertebral Disc
A Thoracolumbar Vertebral Joint
   Thoracolumbar facet joint
B Thoracolumbar Vertebral Disc
C Temporomandibular Joint, Right
D Temporomandibular Joint, Left
E Sternoclavicular Joint, Right
F Sternoclavicular Joint, Left
G Acromioclavicular Joint, Right
H Acromioclavicular Joint, Left
J Shoulder Joint, Right
   Glenohumeral joint
   Glenoid ligament (labrum)
K Shoulder Joint, Left
   See J Shoulder Joint, Right
L Elbow Joint, Right
   Distal humerus, involving joint
   Humeroradial joint
   Humeroulnar joint
   Proximal radioulnar joint
M Elbow Joint, Left
   See L Elbow Joint, Right
N Wrist Joint, Right
   Distal radioulnar joint
   Radiocarpal joint
P Wrist Joint, Left
   See N Wrist Joint, Right
Q Carpal Joint, Right
   Intercarpal joint
   Midcarpal joint
R Carpal Joint, Left
   See Q Carpal Joint, Right
S Carpometacarpal Joint, Right
T Carpometacarpal Joint, Left
U Metacarpophalangeal Joint, Right
V Metacarpophalangeal Joint, Left
W Finger Phalangeal Joint, Right
   Interphalangeal (IP) joint
X Finger Phalangeal Joint, Left
   See W Finger Phalangeal Joint, Right
	0 Open
	3 Percutaneous
	4 Percutaneous Endoscopic
		Z No Device	**X** Diagnostic
			Z No Qualifier

Non-OR   0RB[0,1,3,4,5,6,9,A,B,E,F,G,H,J,K,L,M,N,P,Q,R,S,T,U,V,W,X][0,3,4]ZX

0RC–0RC Upper Joints ICD-10-PCS 2025

0 Medical and Surgical
R Upper Joints
C Extirpation Definition: Taking or cutting out solid matter from a body part
Explanation: The solid matter may be an abnormal byproduct of a biological function or a foreign body; it may be imbedded in a body part or in the lumen of a tubular body part. The solid matter may or may not have been previously broken into pieces.

Body Part Character 4	Approach Character 5	Device Character 6	Qualifier Character 7
0 Occipital-cervical Joint **1** Cervical Vertebral Joint 　Atlantoaxial joint 　Cervical facet joint **3** Cervical Vertebral Disc **4** Cervicothoracic Vertebral Joint 　Cervicothoracic facet joint **5** Cervicothoracic Vertebral Disc **6** Thoracic Vertebral Joint 　Costotransverse joint 　Costovertebral joint 　Thoracic facet joint **9** Thoracic Vertebral Disc **A** Thoracolumbar Vertebral Joint 　Thoracolumbar facet joint **B** Thoracolumbar Vertebral Disc **C** Temporomandibular Joint, Right **D** Temporomandibular Joint, Left **E** Sternoclavicular Joint, Right **F** Sternoclavicular Joint, Left **G** Acromioclavicular Joint, Right **H** Acromioclavicular Joint, Left **J** Shoulder Joint, Right 　Glenohumeral joint 　Glenoid ligament (labrum) **K** Shoulder Joint, Left 　*See J Shoulder Joint, Right* **L** Elbow Joint, Right 　Distal humerus, involving joint 　Humeroradial joint 　Humeroulnar joint 　Proximal radioulnar joint **M** Elbow Joint, Left 　*See L Elbow Joint, Right* **N** Wrist Joint, Right 　Distal radioulnar joint 　Radiocarpal joint **P** Wrist Joint, Left 　*See N Wrist Joint, Right* **Q** Carpal Joint, Right 　Intercarpal joint 　Midcarpal joint **R** Carpal Joint, Left 　*See Q Carpal Joint, Right* **S** Carpometacarpal Joint, Right **T** Carpometacarpal Joint, Left **U** Metacarpophalangeal Joint, Right **V** Metacarpophalangeal Joint, Left **W** Finger Phalangeal Joint, Right 　Interphalangeal (IP) joint **X** Finger Phalangeal Joint, Left 　*See W Finger Phalangeal Joint, Right*	**0** Open **3** Percutaneous **4** Percutaneous Endoscopic	**Z** No Device	**Z** No Qualifier

ICD-10-PCS 2025 — Upper Joints — 0RG–0RG

- **0** Medical and Surgical
- **R** Upper Joints
- **G** Fusion

Definition: Joining together portions of an articular body part rendering the articular body part immobile
Explanation: The body part is joined together by fixation device, bone graft, or other means

Body Part — Character 4	Approach — Character 5	Device — Character 6	Qualifier — Character 7

0 **Occipital-cervical Joint**
1 **Cervical Vertebral Joint**
   Atlantoaxial joint
   Cervical facet joint
2 **Cervical Vertebral Joints, 2 or more**
   Cervical facet joint
4 **Cervicothoracic Vertebral Joint**
   Cervicothoracic facet joint
6 **Thoracic Vertebral Joint**
   Costotransverse joint
   Costovertebral joint
   Thoracic facet joint
7 **Thoracic Vertebral Joints, 2 to 7** ✚
8 **Thoracic Vertebral Joints, 8 or more**
A **Thoracolumbar Vertebral Joint**
   Thoracolumbar facet joint
	0 Open
	3 Percutaneous
	4 Percutaneous Endoscopic
		7 Autologous Tissue Substitute
		J Synthetic Substitute
		K Nonautologous Tissue Substitute
			0 Anterior Approach, Anterior Column
			1 Posterior Approach, Posterior Column
			J Posterior Approach, Anterior Column

0 **Occipital-cervical Joint**
1 **Cervical Vertebral Joint**
   Atlantoaxial joint
   Cervical facet joint
2 **Cervical Vertebral Joints, 2 or more**
   Cervical facet joint
4 **Cervicothoracic Vertebral Joint**
   Cervicothoracic facet joint
6 **Thoracic Vertebral Joint**
   Costotransverse joint
   Costovertebral joint
   Thoracic facet joint
7 **Thoracic Vertebral Joints, 2 to 7** ✚
8 **Thoracic Vertebral Joints, 8 or more**
A **Thoracolumbar Vertebral Joint**
   Thoracolumbar facet joint
	0 Open
	3 Percutaneous
	4 Percutaneous Endoscopic
		A Interbody Fusion Device	**0** Anterior Approach, Anterior Column
			J Posterior Approach, Anterior Column

C Temporomandibular Joint, Right
D Temporomandibular Joint, Left
E **Sternoclavicular Joint, Right**
F **Sternoclavicular Joint, Left**
G **Acromioclavicular Joint, Right**
H **Acromioclavicular Joint, Left**
J **Shoulder Joint, Right**
   Glenohumeral joint
   Glenoid ligament (labrum)
K **Shoulder Joint, Left**
   See J Shoulder Joint, Right
	0 Open
	3 Percutaneous
	4 Percutaneous Endoscopic
		4 Internal Fixation Device
		7 Autologous Tissue Substitute
		J Synthetic Substitute
		K Nonautologous Tissue Substitute
			Z No Qualifier

L **Elbow Joint, Right**
   Distal humerus, involving joint
   Humeroradial joint
   Humeroulnar joint
   Proximal radioulnar joint
M **Elbow Joint, Left**
   See L Elbow Joint, Right
N Wrist Joint, Right
   Distal radioulnar joint
   Radiocarpal joint
P Wrist Joint, Left
   See N Wrist Joint, Right
Q Carpal Joint, Right
   Intercarpal joint
   Midcarpal joint
R Carpal Joint, Left
   See Q Carpal Joint, Right
S Carpometacarpal Joint, Right
T Carpometacarpal Joint, Left
U Metacarpophalangeal Joint, Right
V Metacarpophalangeal Joint, Left
W Finger Phalangeal Joint, Right
   Interphalangeal (IP) joint
X Finger Phalangeal Joint, Left
   See W Finger Phalangeal Joint, Right
	0 Open
	3 Percutaneous
	4 Percutaneous Endoscopic
		3 Internal Fixation Device, Sustained Compression
		4 Internal Fixation Device
		5 External Fixation Device
		7 Autologous Tissue Substitute
		J Synthetic Substitute
		K Nonautologous Tissue Substitute
			Z No Qualifier

HAC 0RG[0,1,2,4,6,7,8,A][0,3,4][7,J,K][0,1,J] when reported with SDx K68.11 or T81.40–T81.49, T84.60-T84.619, T84.63-T84.7 with 7th character A

HAC 0RG[0,1,2,4,6,7,8,A][0,3,4]A[0,J] when reported with SDx K68.11 or T81.40–T81.49, T84.60-T84.619, T84.63-T84.7 with 7th character A

HAC 0RG[E,F,G,H,J,K][0,3,4][4,7,J,K]Z when reported with SDx K68.11 or T81.40–T81.49, T84.60-T84.619, T84.63-T84.7 with 7th character A

HAC 0RG[L,M][0,3,4][3,4,5,7,J,K]Z when reported with SDx K68.11 or T81.40–T81.49, T84.60-T84.619, T84.63-T84.7 with 7th character A

See Appendix L for Procedure Combinations
✚ 0RG7[0,3,4][7,J,K][0,1,J]
✚ 0RG7[0,3,4]A[0,J]

Upper Joints

0RH–0RH   Upper Joints   ICD-10-PCS 2025

0 Medical and Surgical
R Upper Joints
H Insertion

Definition: Putting in a nonbiological appliance that monitors, assists, performs, or prevents a physiological function but does not physically take the place of a body part
Explanation: None

Body Part Character 4	Approach Character 5	Device Character 6	Qualifier Character 7

0 Occipital-cervical Joint
1 Cervical Vertebral Joint
   Atlantoaxial joint
   Cervical facet joint
4 Cervicothoracic Vertebral Joint
   Cervicothoracic facet joint
6 Thoracic Vertebral Joint
   Costotransverse joint
   Costovertebral joint
   Thoracic facet joint
A Thoracolumbar Vertebral Joint
   Thoracolumbar facet joint
	0 Open
	3 Percutaneous
	4 Percutaneous Endoscopic
		3 Infusion Device
		4 Internal Fixation Device
		8 Spacer
		B Spinal Stabilization Device, Interspinous Process
		C Spinal Stabilization Device, Pedicle-Based
		D Spinal Stabilization Device, Facet Replacement
			Z No Qualifier

3 Cervical Vertebral Disc 5 Cervicothoracic Vertebral Disc 9 Thoracic Vertebral Disc B Thoracolumbar Vertebral Disc	0 Open 3 Percutaneous 4 Percutaneous Endoscopic	3 Infusion Device	Z No Qualifier

C Temporomandibular Joint, Right
D Temporomandibular Joint, Left
E Sternoclavicular Joint, Right
F Sternoclavicular Joint, Left
G Acromioclavicular Joint, Right
H Acromioclavicular Joint, Left
J Shoulder Joint, Right
   Glenohumeral joint
   Glenoid ligament (labrum)
K Shoulder Joint, Left
   See J Shoulder Joint, Right
	0 Open
	3 Percutaneous
	4 Percutaneous Endoscopic
		3 Infusion Device
		4 Internal Fixation Device
		8 Spacer
			Z No Qualifier

L Elbow Joint, Right
   Distal humerus, involving joint
   Humeroradial joint
   Humeroulnar joint
   Proximal radioulnar joint
M Elbow Joint, Left
   See L Elbow Joint, Right
N Wrist Joint, Right
   Distal radioulnar joint
   Radiocarpal joint
P Wrist Joint, Left
   See N Wrist Joint, Right
Q Carpal Joint, Right
   Intercarpal joint
   Midcarpal joint
R Carpal Joint, Left
   See Q Carpal Joint, Right
S Carpometacarpal Joint, Right
T Carpometacarpal Joint, Left
U Metacarpophalangeal Joint, Right
V Metacarpophalangeal Joint, Left
W Finger Phalangeal Joint, Right
   Interphalangeal (IP) joint
X Finger Phalangeal Joint, Left
   See W Finger Phalangeal Joint, Right
	0 Open
	3 Percutaneous
	4 Percutaneous Endoscopic
		3 Infusion Device
		4 Internal Fixation Device
		5 External Fixation Device
		8 Spacer
			Z No Qualifier

Non-OR   0RH[0,1,4,6,A][0,3,4][3,8]Z
Non-OR   0RH[3,5,9,B][0,3,4]3Z
Non-OR   0RH[C,D][0,4]8Z
Non-OR   0RH[C,D]3[3,8]Z
Non-OR   0RH[E,F,G,H][0,3,4][3,8]Z
Non-OR   0RH[J,K][0,3,4]3Z
Non-OR   0RH[J,K]38Z
Non-OR   0RH[L,M,N,P,Q,R,S,T,U,V,W,X][0,3,4][3,8]Z

ICD-10-PCS 2025 — Upper Joints — ØRJ–ØRJ

- **Ø** Medical and Surgical
- **R** Upper Joints
- **J** Inspection

Definition: Visually and/or manually exploring a body part

Explanation: Visual exploration may be performed with or without optical instrumentation. Manual exploration may be performed directly or through intervening body layers.

Body Part Character 4	Approach Character 5	Device Character 6	Qualifier Character 7

Ø Occipital-cervical Joint
1 Cervical Vertebral Joint
   Atlantoaxial joint
   Cervical facet joint
3 Cervical Vertebral Disc
4 Cervicothoracic Vertebral Joint
   Cervicothoracic facet joint
5 Cervicothoracic Vertebral Disc
6 Thoracic Vertebral Joint
   Costotransverse joint
   Costovertebral joint
   Thoracic facet joint
9 Thoracic Vertebral Disc
A Thoracolumbar Vertebral Joint
   Thoracolumbar facet joint
B Thoracolumbar Vertebral Disc
C Temporomandibular Joint, Right
D Temporomandibular Joint, Left
E Sternoclavicular Joint, Right
F Sternoclavicular Joint, Left
G Acromioclavicular Joint, Right
H Acromioclavicular Joint, Left
J Shoulder Joint, Right
   Glenohumeral joint
   Glenoid ligament (labrum)
K Shoulder Joint, Left
   See J Shoulder Joint, Right
L Elbow Joint, Right
   Distal humerus, involving joint
   Humeroradial joint
   Humeroulnar joint
   Proximal radioulnar joint
M Elbow Joint, Left
   See L Elbow Joint, Right
N Wrist Joint, Right
   Distal radioulnar joint
   Radiocarpal joint
P Wrist Joint, Left
   See N Wrist Joint, Right
Q Carpal Joint, Right
   Intercarpal joint
   Midcarpal joint
R Carpal Joint, Left
   See Q Carpal Joint, Right
S Carpometacarpal Joint, Right
T Carpometacarpal Joint, Left
U Metacarpophalangeal Joint, Right
V Metacarpophalangeal Joint, Left
W Finger Phalangeal Joint, Right
   Interphalangeal (IP) joint
X Finger Phalangeal Joint, Left
   See W Finger Phalangeal Joint, Right
	Ø Open
	3 Percutaneous
	4 Percutaneous Endoscopic
	X External
		Z No Device	**Z** No Qualifier

Non-OR ØRJ[Ø,1,3,4,5,6,9,A,B,C,D,E,F,G,H,J,K,L,M,N,P,Q,R,S,T,U,V,W,X][3,X]ZZ

Upper Joints

0 Medical and Surgical
R Upper Joints
N Release

Definition: Freeing a body part from an abnormal physical constraint by cutting or by the use of force
Explanation: Some of the restraining tissue may be taken out but none of the body part is taken out

Body Part Character 4	Approach Character 5	Device Character 6	Qualifier Character 7

0 Occipital-cervical Joint
1 Cervical Vertebral Joint
   Atlantoaxial joint
   Cervical facet joint
3 Cervical Vertebral Disc
4 Cervicothoracic Vertebral Joint
   Cervicothoracic facet joint
5 Cervicothoracic Vertebral Disc
6 Thoracic Vertebral Joint
   Costotransverse joint
   Costovertebral joint
   Thoracic facet joint
9 Thoracic Vertebral Disc
A Thoracolumbar Vertebral Joint
   Thoracolumbar facet joint
B Thoracolumbar Vertebral Disc
C Temporomandibular Joint, Right
D Temporomandibular Joint, Left
E Sternoclavicular Joint, Right
F Sternoclavicular Joint, Left
G Acromioclavicular Joint, Right
H Acromioclavicular Joint, Left
J Shoulder Joint, Right
   Glenohumeral joint
   Glenoid ligament (labrum)
K Shoulder Joint, Left
   See J Shoulder Joint, Right
L Elbow Joint, Right
   Distal humerus, involving joint
   Humeroradial joint
   Humeroulnar joint
   Proximal radioulnar joint
M Elbow Joint, Left
   See L Elbow Joint, Right
N Wrist Joint, Right
   Distal radioulnar joint
   Radiocarpal joint
P Wrist Joint, Left
   See N Wrist Joint, Right
Q Carpal Joint, Right
   Intercarpal joint
   Midcarpal joint
R Carpal Joint, Left
   See Q Carpal Joint, Right
S Carpometacarpal Joint, Right
T Carpometacarpal Joint, Left
U Metacarpophalangeal Joint, Right
V Metacarpophalangeal Joint, Left
W Finger Phalangeal Joint, Right
   Interphalangeal (IP) joint
X Finger Phalangeal Joint, Left
   See W Finger Phalangeal Joint, Right
	0 Open
	3 Percutaneous
	4 Percutaneous Endoscopic
	X External
		Z No Device	**Z** No Qualifier

Non-OR 0RN[0,1,3,4,5,6,9,A,B,C,D,E,F,G,H,J,K,L,M,N,P,Q,R,S,T,U,V,W,X]XZZ

ICD-10-PCS 2025 Upper Joints ØRP–ØRP

- **Ø** Medical and Surgical
- **R** Upper Joints
- **P** Removal

Definition: Taking out or off a device from a body part

Explanation: If a device is taken out and a similar device put in without cutting or puncturing the skin or mucous membrane, the procedure is coded to the root operation CHANGE. Otherwise, the procedure for taking out the device is coded to the root operation REMOVAL.

Body Part Character 4	Approach Character 5	Device Character 6	Qualifier Character 7

Ø Occipital-cervical Joint
1 Cervical Vertebral Joint
   Atlantoaxial joint
   Cervical facet joint
4 Cervicothoracic Vertebral Joint
   Cervicothoracic facet joint
6 Thoracic Vertebral Joint
   Costotransverse joint
   Costovertebral joint
   Thoracic facet joint
A Thoracolumbar Vertebral Joint
   Thoracolumbar facet joint
	Ø Open
	3 Percutaneous
	4 Percutaneous Endoscopic
		Ø Drainage Device
		3 Infusion Device
		4 Internal Fixation Device
		7 Autologous Tissue Substitute
		8 Spacer
		A Interbody Fusion Device
		J Synthetic Substitute
		K Nonautologous Tissue Substitute
			Z No Qualifier

Ø Occipital-cervical Joint
1 Cervical Vertebral Joint
   Atlantoaxial joint
   Cervical facet joint
4 Cervicothoracic Vertebral Joint
   Cervicothoracic facet joint
6 Thoracic Vertebral Joint
   Costotransverse joint
   Costovertebral joint
   Thoracic facet joint
A Thoracolumbar Vertebral Joint
   Thoracolumbar facet joint
	X External	**Ø** Drainage Device
		3 Infusion Device
		4 Internal Fixation Device
			Z No Qualifier

3 Cervical Vertebral Disc **5** Cervicothoracic Vertebral Disc **9** Thoracic Vertebral Disc **B** Thoracolumbar Vertebral Disc	**Ø** Open **3** Percutaneous **4** Percutaneous Endoscopic	**Ø** Drainage Device **3** Infusion Device **7** Autologous Tissue Substitute **J** Synthetic Substitute **K** Nonautologous Tissue Substitute	**Z** No Qualifier
3 Cervical Vertebral Disc **5** Cervicothoracic Vertebral Disc **9** Thoracic Vertebral Disc **B** Thoracolumbar Vertebral Disc	**X** External	**Ø** Drainage Device **3** Infusion Device	**Z** No Qualifier
C Temporomandibular Joint, Right **D** Temporomandibular Joint, Left **E** Sternoclavicular Joint, Right **F** Sternoclavicular Joint, Left **G** Acromioclavicular Joint, Right **H** Acromioclavicular Joint, Left	**Ø** Open **3** Percutaneous **4** Percutaneous Endoscopic	**Ø** Drainage Device **3** Infusion Device **4** Internal Fixation Device **7** Autologous Tissue Substitute **8** Spacer **J** Synthetic Substitute **K** Nonautologous Tissue Substitute	**Z** No Qualifier
C Temporomandibular Joint, Right **D** Temporomandibular Joint, Left **E** Sternoclavicular Joint, Right **F** Sternoclavicular Joint, Left **G** Acromioclavicular Joint, Right **H** Acromioclavicular Joint, Left	**X** External	**Ø** Drainage Device **3** Infusion Device **4** Internal Fixation Device	**Z** No Qualifier

J Shoulder Joint, Right
   Glenohumeral joint
   Glenoid ligament (labrum)
K Shoulder Joint, Left
   See J Shoulder Joint, Right
	Ø Open
	3 Percutaneous
	4 Percutaneous Endoscopic
		Ø Drainage Device
		3 Infusion Device
		4 Internal Fixation Device
		7 Autologous Tissue Substitute
		8 Spacer
		K Nonautologous Tissue Substitute
			Z No Qualifier

J Shoulder Joint, Right
   Glenohumeral joint
   Glenoid ligament (labrum)
K Shoulder Joint, Left
   See J Shoulder Joint, Right
	Ø Open
	3 Percutaneous
	4 Percutaneous Endoscopic
		J Synthetic Substitute	**6** Humeral Surface
			7 Glenoid Surface
			Z No Qualifier

J Shoulder Joint, Right
   Glenohumeral joint
   Glenoid ligament (labrum)
K Shoulder Joint, Left
   See J Shoulder Joint, Right
	X External	**Ø** Drainage Device
		3 Infusion Device
		4 Internal Fixation Device
			Z No Qualifier

Non-OR ØRP[Ø,1,4,6,A]3[Ø,3,8]Z
Non-OR ØRP[Ø,1,4,6,A][Ø,4]8Z
Non-OR ØRP[Ø,1,4,6,A]X[Ø,3,4]Z
Non-OR ØRP[3,5,9,B]3[Ø,3]Z
Non-OR ØRP[3,5,9,B]X[Ø,3]Z
Non-OR ØRP[C,D,E,F,G,H]3[Ø,3,8]Z
Non-OR ØRP[C,D,E,F,G,H][Ø,4]8Z
Non-OR ØRP[C,D]X[Ø,3]Z
Non-OR ØRP[E,F,G,H,J,K]X[Ø,3,4]Z
Non-OR ØRP[J,K]3[Ø,3,8]Z
Non-OR ØRP[J,K]X[Ø,3,4]Z

ØRP Continued on next page

ØRP–ØRP Upper Joints ICD-10-PCS 2025

ØRP Continued

Ø Medical and Surgical
R Upper Joints
P Removal

Definition: Taking out or off a device from a body part
Explanation: If a device is taken out and a similar device put in without cutting or puncturing the skin or mucous membrane, the procedure is coded to the root operation CHANGE. Otherwise, the procedure for taking out the device is coded to the root operation REMOVAL.

Body Part Character 4	Approach Character 5	Device Character 6	Qualifier Character 7

L Elbow Joint, Right
  Distal humerus, involving joint
  Humeroradial joint
  Humeroulnar joint
  Proximal radioulnar joint
M Elbow Joint, Left
  See L Elbow Joint, Right
N Wrist Joint, Right
  Distal radioulnar joint
  Radiocarpal joint
P Wrist Joint, Left
  See N Wrist Joint, Right
Q Carpal Joint, Right
  Intercarpal joint
  Midcarpal joint
R Carpal Joint, Left
  See Q Carpal Joint, Right
S Carpometacarpal Joint, Right
T Carpometacarpal Joint, Left
U Metacarpophalangeal Joint, Right
V Metacarpophalangeal Joint, Left
W Finger Phalangeal Joint, Right
  Interphalangeal (IP) joint
X Finger Phalangeal Joint, Left
  See W Finger Phalangeal Joint, Right
	Ø Open
	3 Percutaneous
	4 Percutaneous Endoscopic
		Ø Drainage Device
		3 Infusion Device
		4 Internal Fixation Device
		5 External Fixation Device
		7 Autologous Tissue Substitute
		8 Spacer
		J Synthetic Substitute
		K Nonautologous Tissue Substitute
			Z No Qualifier

L Elbow Joint, Right
  Distal humerus, involving joint
  Humeroradial joint
  Humeroulnar joint
  Proximal radioulnar joint
M Elbow Joint, Left
  See L Elbow Joint, Right
N Wrist Joint, Right
  Distal radioulnar joint
  Radiocarpal joint
P Wrist Joint, Left
  See N Wrist Joint, Right
Q Carpal Joint, Right
  Intercarpal joint
  Midcarpal joint
R Carpal Joint, Left
  See Q Carpal Joint, Right
S Carpometacarpal Joint, Right
T Carpometacarpal Joint, Left
U Metacarpophalangeal Joint, Right
V Metacarpophalangeal Joint, Left
W Finger Phalangeal Joint, Right
  Interphalangeal (IP) joint
X Finger Phalangeal Joint, Left
  See W Finger Phalangeal Joint, Right
	X External	**Ø** Drainage Device
		3 Infusion Device
		4 Internal Fixation Device
		5 External Fixation Device
			Z No Qualifier

Non-OR   ØRP[L,M,N,P,Q,R,S,T,U,V,W,X]3[Ø,3,8]Z
Non-OR   ØRP[L,M,N,P,Q,R,S,T,U,V,W,X][Ø,4]8Z
Non-OR   ØRP[L,M,N,P,Q,R,S,T,U,V,W,X]X[Ø,3,4,5]Z

ICD-10-PCS 2025 Upper Joints ØRQ–ØRQ

Ø Medical and Surgical
R Upper Joints
Q Repair Definition: Restoring, to the extent possible, a body part to its normal anatomic structure and function
Explanation: Used only when the method to accomplish the repair is not one of the other root operations

Body Part Character 4	Approach Character 5	Device Character 6	Qualifier Character 7

Ø **Occipital-cervical Joint**
1 **Cervical Vertebral Joint**
  Atlantoaxial joint
  Cervical facet joint
3 **Cervical Vertebral Disc**
4 **Cervicothoracic Vertebral Joint**
  Cervicothoracic facet joint
5 **Cervicothoracic Vertebral Disc**
6 **Thoracic Vertebral Joint**
  Costotransverse joint
  Costovertebral joint
  Thoracic facet joint
9 **Thoracic Vertebral Disc**
A **Thoracolumbar Vertebral Joint**
  Thoracolumbar facet joint
B **Thoracolumbar Vertebral Disc**
C **Temporomandibular Joint, Right**
D **Temporomandibular Joint, Left**
E **Sternoclavicular Joint, Right**
F **Sternoclavicular Joint, Left**
G **Acromioclavicular Joint, Right**
H **Acromioclavicular Joint, Left**
J **Shoulder Joint, Right**
  Glenohumeral joint
  Glenoid ligament (labrum)
K **Shoulder Joint, Left**
  See J Shoulder Joint, Right
L **Elbow Joint, Right**
  Distal humerus, involving joint
  Humeroradial joint
  Humeroulnar joint
  Proximal radioulnar joint
M **Elbow Joint, Left**
  See L Elbow Joint, Right
N **Wrist Joint, Right**
  Distal radioulnar joint
  Radiocarpal joint
P **Wrist Joint, Left**
  See N Wrist Joint, Right
Q **Carpal Joint, Right**
  Intercarpal joint
  Midcarpal joint
R **Carpal Joint, Left**
  See Q Carpal Joint, Right
S **Carpometacarpal Joint, Right**
T **Carpometacarpal Joint, Left**
U **Metacarpophalangeal Joint, Right**
V **Metacarpophalangeal Joint, Left**
W **Finger Phalangeal Joint, Right**
  Interphalangeal (IP) joint
X **Finger Phalangeal Joint, Left**
  See W Finger Phalangeal Joint, Right
	Ø Open
	3 Percutaneous
	4 Percutaneous Endoscopic
	X External
		Z No Device	Z No Qualifier

Non-OR ØRQ[Ø,1,3,4,5,6,9,A,B,C,D,E,F,G,H,J,K,L,M,N,P,Q,R,S,T,U,V,W,X]XZZ
HAC ØRQ[E,F,G,H,J,K,L,M][Ø,3,4]ZZ when reported with SDx K68.11 or T81.4Ø–T81.49, T84.6Ø-T84.619, T84.63-T84.7 with 7th character A

0 **Medical and Surgical**
R **Upper Joints**
R **Replacement** Definition: Putting in or on biological or synthetic material that physically takes the place and/or function of all or a portion of a body part
Explanation: The body part may have been taken out or replaced, or may be taken out, physically eradicated, or rendered nonfunctional during the REPLACEMENT procedure. A REMOVAL procedure is coded for taking out the device used in a previous replacement procedure.

Body Part Character 4	Approach Character 5	Device Character 6	Qualifier Character 7

0 Occipital-cervical Joint
1 Cervical Vertebral Joint
   Atlantoaxial joint
   Cervical facet joint
3 Cervical Vertebral Disc
4 Cervicothoracic Vertebral Joint
   Cervicothoracic facet joint
5 Cervicothoracic Vertebral Disc
6 Thoracic Vertebral Joint
   Costotransverse joint
   Costovertebral joint
   Thoracic facet joint
9 Thoracic Vertebral Disc
A Thoracolumbar Vertebral Joint
   Thoracolumbar facet joint
B Thoracolumbar Vertebral Disc
C Temporomandibular Joint, Right
D Temporomandibular Joint, Left
E Sternoclavicular Joint, Right
F Sternoclavicular Joint, Left
G Acromioclavicular Joint, Right
H Acromioclavicular Joint, Left
L Elbow Joint, Right
   Distal humerus, involving joint
   Humeroradial joint
   Humeroulnar joint
   Proximal radioulnar joint
M Elbow Joint, Left
   See L Elbow Joint, Right
N Wrist Joint, Right
   Distal radioulnar joint
   Radiocarpal joint
P Wrist Joint, Left
   See N Wrist Joint, Right
Q Carpal Joint, Right
   Intercarpal joint
   Midcarpal joint
R Carpal Joint, Left
   See Q Carpal Joint, Right
S Carpometacarpal Joint, Right
T Carpometacarpal Joint, Left
U Metacarpophalangeal Joint, Right
V Metacarpophalangeal Joint, Left
W Finger Phalangeal Joint, Right
   Interphalangeal (IP) joint
X Finger Phalangeal Joint, Left
   See W Finger Phalangeal Joint, Right
	0 Open	7 Autologous Tissue Substitute
		J Synthetic Substitute
		K Nonautologous Tissue Substitute
			Z No Qualifier

J Shoulder Joint, Right
   Glenohumeral joint
   Glenoid ligament (labrum)
K Shoulder Joint, Left
   See J Shoulder Joint, Right
	0 Open	0 Synthetic Substitute, Reverse Ball and Socket
		7 Autologous Tissue Substitute
		K Nonautologous Tissue Substitute
			Z No Qualifier

J Shoulder Joint, Right
   Glenohumeral joint
   Glenoid ligament (labrum)
K Shoulder Joint, Left
   See J Shoulder Joint, Right
	0 Open	J Synthetic Substitute	6 Humeral Surface
			7 Glenoid Surface
			Z No Qualifier

ICD-10-PCS 2025 — Upper Joints — ØRS–ØRS

- **Ø** Medical and Surgical
- **R** Upper Joints
- **S** Reposition   Definition: Moving to its normal location, or other suitable location, all or a portion of a body part
  Explanation: The body part is moved to a new location from an abnormal location, or from a normal location where it is not functioning correctly. The body part may or may not be cut out or off to be moved to the new location.

Body Part Character 4	Approach Character 5	Device Character 6	Qualifier Character 7

Ø **Occipital-cervical Joint**
1 **Cervical Vertebral Joint**
  Atlantoaxial joint
  Cervical facet joint
4 **Cervicothoracic Vertebral Joint**
  Cervicothoracic facet joint
6 **Thoracic Vertebral Joint**
  Costotransverse joint
  Costovertebral joint
  Thoracic facet joint
A **Thoracolumbar Vertebral Joint**
  Thoracolumbar facet joint
C **Temporomandibular Joint, Right**
D **Temporomandibular Joint, Left**
E **Sternoclavicular Joint, Right**
F **Sternoclavicular Joint, Left**
G **Acromioclavicular Joint, Right**
H **Acromioclavicular Joint, Left**
J **Shoulder Joint, Right**
  Glenohumeral joint
  Glenoid ligament (labrum)
K **Shoulder Joint, Left**
  See J Shoulder Joint, Right
	Ø Open
	3 Percutaneous
	4 Percutaneous Endoscopic
	X External
		4 Internal Fixation Device
		Z No Device
			Z No Qualifier

L **Elbow Joint, Right**
  Distal humerus, involving joint
  Humeroradial joint
  Humeroulnar joint
  Proximal radioulnar joint
M **Elbow Joint, Left**
  See L Elbow Joint, Right
N **Wrist Joint, Right**
  Distal radioulnar joint
  Radiocarpal joint
P **Wrist Joint, Left**
  See N Wrist Joint, Right
Q **Carpal Joint, Right**
  Intercarpal joint
  Midcarpal joint
R **Carpal Joint, Left**
  See Q Carpal Joint, Right
S **Carpometacarpal Joint, Right**
T **Carpometacarpal Joint, Left**
U **Metacarpophalangeal Joint, Right**
V **Metacarpophalangeal Joint, Left**
W **Finger Phalangeal Joint, Right**
  Interphalangeal (IP) joint
X **Finger Phalangeal Joint, Left**
  See W Finger Phalangeal Joint, Right
	Ø Open
	3 Percutaneous
	4 Percutaneous Endoscopic
	X External
		4 Internal Fixation Device
		5 External Fixation Device
		Z No Device
			Z No Qualifier

Non-OR   ØRS[Ø,1,4,6,A,C,D,E,F,G,H,J,K][3,4,X][4,Z]Z
Non-OR   ØRS[L,M,N,P,Q,R,S,T,U,V,W,X][3,4,X][4,5,Z]Z

Upper Joints

0 Medical and Surgical
R Upper Joints
T Resection — Definition: Cutting out or off, without replacement, all of a body part
Explanation: None

Body Part Character 4	Approach Character 5	Device Character 6	Qualifier Character 7

3 Cervical Vertebral Disc
4 Cervicothoracic Vertebral Joint
  Cervicothoracic facet joint
5 Cervicothoracic Vertebral Disc
9 Thoracic Vertebral Disc
B Thoracolumbar Vertebral Disc
C Temporomandibular Joint, Right
D Temporomandibular Joint, Left
E Sternoclavicular Joint, Right
F Sternoclavicular Joint, Left
G Acromioclavicular Joint, Right
H Acromioclavicular Joint, Left
J Shoulder Joint, Right
  Glenohumeral joint
  Glenoid ligament (labrum)
K Shoulder Joint, Left
  See J Shoulder Joint, Right
L Elbow Joint, Right
  Distal humerus, involving joint
  Humeroradial joint
  Humeroulnar joint
  Proximal radioulnar joint
M Elbow Joint, Left
  See L Elbow Joint, Right
N Wrist Joint, Right
  Distal radioulnar joint
  Radiocarpal joint
P Wrist Joint, Left
  See N Wrist Joint, Right
Q Carpal Joint, Right
  Intercarpal joint
  Midcarpal joint
R Carpal Joint, Left
  See Q Carpal Joint, Right
S Carpometacarpal Joint, Right
T Carpometacarpal Joint, Left
U Metacarpophalangeal Joint, Right
V Metacarpophalangeal Joint, Left
W Finger Phalangeal Joint, Right
  Interphalangeal (IP) joint
X Finger Phalangeal Joint, Left
  See W Finger Phalangeal Joint, Right
	0 Open	**Z** No Device	**Z** No Qualifier

0 Medical and Surgical
R Upper Joints
U Supplement Definition: Putting in or on biological or synthetic material that physically reinforces and/or augments the function of a portion of a body part
Explanation: The biological material is non-living, or is living and from the same individual. The body part may have been previously replaced, and the SUPPLEMENT procedure is performed to physically reinforce and/or augment the function of the replaced body part.

Body Part Character 4	Approach Character 5	Device Character 6	Qualifier Character 7

0 Occipital-cervical Joint
1 Cervical Vertebral Joint
  Atlantoaxial joint
  Cervical facet joint
3 Cervical Vertebral Disc
4 Cervicothoracic Vertebral Joint
  Cervicothoracic facet joint
5 Cervicothoracic Vertebral Disc
6 Thoracic Vertebral Joint
  Costotransverse joint
  Costovertebral joint
  Thoracic facet joint
9 Thoracic Vertebral Disc
A Thoracolumbar Vertebral Joint
  Thoracolumbar facet joint
B Thoracolumbar Vertebral Disc
C Temporomandibular Joint, Right
D Temporomandibular Joint, Left
E Sternoclavicular Joint, Right
F Sternoclavicular Joint, Left
G Acromioclavicular Joint, Right
H Acromioclavicular Joint, Left
J Shoulder Joint, Right
  Glenohumeral joint
  Glenoid ligament (labrum)
K Shoulder Joint, Left
  See J Shoulder Joint, Right
L Elbow Joint, Right
  Distal humerus, involving joint
  Humeroradial joint
  Humeroulnar joint
  Proximal radioulnar joint
M Elbow Joint, Left
  See L Elbow Joint, Right
N Wrist Joint, Right
  Distal radioulnar joint
  Radiocarpal joint
P Wrist Joint, Left
  See N Wrist Joint, Right
Q Carpal Joint, Right
  Intercarpal joint
  Midcarpal joint
R Carpal Joint, Left
  See Q Carpal Joint, Right
S Carpometacarpal Joint, Right
T Carpometacarpal Joint, Left
U Metacarpophalangeal Joint, Right
V Metacarpophalangeal Joint, Left
W Finger Phalangeal Joint, Right
  Interphalangeal (IP) joint
X Finger Phalangeal Joint, Left
  See W Finger Phalangeal Joint, Right
	0 Open
	3 Percutaneous
	4 Percutaneous Endoscopic
		7 Autologous Tissue Substitute
		J Synthetic Substitute
		K Nonautologous Tissue Substitute
			Z No Qualifier

HAC 0RU[E,F,G,H,J,K,L,M][0,3,4][7,J,K]Z when reported with SDx K68.11 or T81.40–T81.49, T84.60-T84.619, T84.63-T84.7 with 7th character A

Upper Joints

0 Medical and Surgical
R Upper Joints
W Revision

Definition: Correcting, to the extent possible, a portion of a malfunctioning device or the position of a displaced device

Explanation: Revision can include correcting a malfunctioning or displaced device by taking out or putting in components of the device such as a screw or pin

Body Part Character 4	Approach Character 5	Device Character 6	Qualifier Character 7

0 Occipital-cervical Joint
1 Cervical Vertebral Joint
   Atlantoaxial joint
   Cervical facet joint
4 Cervicothoracic Vertebral Joint
   Cervicothoracic facet joint
6 Thoracic Vertebral Joint
   Costotransverse joint
   Costovertebral joint
   Thoracic facet joint
A Thoracolumbar Vertebral Joint
   Thoracolumbar facet joint
	0 Open
	3 Percutaneous
	4 Percutaneous Endoscopic
	X External
		0 Drainage Device
		3 Infusion Device
		4 Internal Fixation Device
		7 Autologous Tissue Substitute
		8 Spacer
		A Interbody Fusion Device
		J Synthetic Substitute
		K Nonautologous Tissue Substitute
			Z No Qualifier

3 Cervical Vertebral Disc 5 Cervicothoracic Vertebral Disc 9 Thoracic Vertebral Disc B Thoracolumbar Vertebral Disc	0 Open 3 Percutaneous 4 Percutaneous Endoscopic X External	0 Drainage Device 3 Infusion Device 7 Autologous Tissue Substitute J Synthetic Substitute K Nonautologous Tissue Substitute	Z No Qualifier
C Temporomandibular Joint, Right D Temporomandibular Joint, Left E Sternoclavicular Joint, Right F Sternoclavicular Joint, Left G Acromioclavicular Joint, Right H Acromioclavicular Joint, Left	0 Open 3 Percutaneous 4 Percutaneous Endoscopic X External	0 Drainage Device 3 Infusion Device 4 Internal Fixation Device 7 Autologous Tissue Substitute 8 Spacer J Synthetic Substitute K Nonautologous Tissue Substitute	Z No Qualifier

J Shoulder Joint, Right
   Glenohumeral joint
   Glenoid ligament (labrum)
K Shoulder Joint, Left
   See J Shoulder Joint, Right
	0 Open
	3 Percutaneous
	4 Percutaneous Endoscopic
	X External
		0 Drainage Device
		3 Infusion Device
		4 Internal Fixation Device
		7 Autologous Tissue Substitute
		8 Spacer
		J Synthetic Substitute
		K Nonautologous Tissue Substitute
			Z No Qualifier

J Shoulder Joint, Right
   Glenohumeral joint
   Glenoid ligament (labrum)
K Shoulder Joint, Left
   See J Shoulder Joint, Right
	0 Open
	3 Percutaneous
	4 Percutaneous Endoscopic
	X External
		J Synthetic Substitute	6 Humeral Surface
			7 Glenoid Surface
			Z No Qualifier

L Elbow Joint, Right
   Distal humerus, involving joint
   Humeroradial joint
   Humeroulnar joint
   Proximal radioulnar joint
M Elbow Joint, Left
   See L Elbow Joint, Right
N Wrist Joint, Right
   Distal radioulnar joint
   Radiocarpal joint
P Wrist Joint, Left
   See N Wrist Joint, Right
Q Carpal Joint, Right
   Intercarpal joint
   Midcarpal joint
R Carpal Joint, Left
   See Q Carpal Joint, Right
S Carpometacarpal Joint, Right
T Carpometacarpal Joint, Left
U Metacarpophalangeal Joint, Right
V Metacarpophalangeal Joint, Left
W Finger Phalangeal Joint, Right
   Interphalangeal (IP) joint
X Finger Phalangeal Joint, Left
   See W Finger Phalangeal Joint, Right
	0 Open
	3 Percutaneous
	4 Percutaneous Endoscopic
	X External
		0 Drainage Device
		3 Infusion Device
		4 Internal Fixation Device
		5 External Fixation Device
		7 Autologous Tissue Substitute
		8 Spacer
		J Synthetic Substitute
		K Nonautologous Tissue Substitute
			Z No Qualifier

Non-OR 0RW[0,1,4,6,A]X[0,3,4,7,8,A,J,K]Z
Non-OR 0RW[3,5,9,B]X[0,3,7,J,K]Z
Non-OR 0RW[C,D,E,F,G,H]X[0,3,4,7,8,J,K]Z
Non-OR 0RW[J,K]X[0,3,4,7,8,J,K]Z
Non-OR 0RW[J,K]XJ[6,7,Z]
Non-OR 0RW[L,M,N,P,Q,R,S,T,U,V,W,X]X[0,3,4,5,7,8,J,K]Z

Lower Joints ØS2–ØSW

Character Meanings*

This Character Meaning table is provided as a guide to assist the user in the identification of character members that may be found in this section of code tables. It **SHOULD NOT** be used to build a PCS code.

Operation–Character 3	Body Part–Character 4	Approach–Character 5	Device–Character 6	Qualifier–Character 7
2 Change	Ø Lumbar Vertebral Joint	Ø Open	Ø Drainage Device OR Synthetic Substitute, Polyethylene	Ø Anterior Approach, Anterior Column
5 Destruction	1 Lumbar Vertebral Joint, 2 or more	3 Percutaneous	1 Synthetic Substitute, Metal	1 Posterior Approach, Posterior Column
9 Drainage	2 Lumbar Vertebral Disc	4 Percutaneous Endoscopic	2 Synthetic Substitute, Metal on Polyethylene	9 Cemented
B Excision	3 Lumbosacral Joint	X External	3 Infusion Device OR Internal Fixation Device, Sustained Compression OR Synthetic Substitute, Ceramic	A Uncemented
C Extirpation	4 Lumbosacral Disc		4 Internal Fixation Device OR Synthetic Substitute, Ceramic on Polyethylene	C Patellar Surface
G Fusion	5 Sacrococcygeal Joint		5 External Fixation Device	J Posterior Approach, Anterior Column
H Insertion	6 Coccygeal Joint		6 Synthetic Substitute, Oxidized Zirconium on Polyethylene	X Diagnostic
J Inspection	7 Sacroiliac Joint, Right		7 Autologous Tissue Substitute	Z No Qualifier
N Release	8 Sacroiliac Joint, Left		8 Spacer	
P Removal	9 Hip Joint, Right		9 Liner	
Q Repair	A Hip Joint, Acetabular Surface, Right		A Interbody Fusion Device	
R Replacement	B Hip Joint, Left		B Resurfacing Device OR Spinal Stabilization Device, Interspinous Process	
S Reposition	C Knee Joint, Right		C Spinal Stabilization Device, Pedicle-Based	
T Resection	D Knee Joint, Left		D Spinal Stabilization Device, Facet Replacement	
U Supplement	E Hip Joint, Acetabular Surface, Left		E Articulating Spacer	
W Revision	F Ankle Joint, Right		J Synthetic Substitute	
	G Ankle Joint, Left		K Nonautologous Tissue Substitute	
	H Tarsal Joint, Right		L Synthetic Substitute, Unicondylar Medial	
	J Tarsal Joint, Left		M Synthetic Substitute, Unicondylar Lateral	
	K Tarsometatarsal Joint, Right		N Synthetic Substitute, Patellofemoral	
	L Tarsometatarsal Joint, Left		Y Other Device	
	M Metatarsal-Phalangeal Joint, Right		Z No Device	
	N Metatarsal-Phalangeal Joint, Left			
	P Toe Phalangeal Joint, Right			
	Q Toe Phalangeal Joint, Left			
	R Hip Joint, Femoral Surface, Right			
	S Hip Joint, Femoral Surface, Left			
	T Knee Joint, Femoral Surface, Right			
	U Knee Joint, Femoral Surface, Left			
	V Knee Joint, Tibial Surface, Right			
	W Knee Joint, Tibial Surface, Left			
	Y Lower Joint			

* Includes synovial membrane.

Lower Joints

AHA Coding Clinic for table 0S9
2018, 2Q, 17	Arthroscopic drainage of knee and nonexcisional debridement
2017, 1Q, 50	Dry aspiration of ankle joint

AHA Coding Clinic for table 0SB
2017, 4Q, 76	Radiolucent porous interbody fusion device
2016, 2Q, 16	Decompressive laminectomy/foraminotomy and lumbar discectomy
2016, 1Q, 20	Metatarsophalangeal joint resection arthroplasty
2015, 1Q, 34	Arthroscopic meniscectomy with debridement and abrasion chondroplasty
2014, 2Q, 6	Posterior lumbar fusion with discectomy

AHA Coding Clinic for table 0SG
2024, 2Q, 27	Stimulan® rapid cure antibiotic bead placement
2023, 2Q, 25	Spinal fusion using allograft bone graft and bone marrow aspirate
2022, 3Q, 21	Breakage of intervertebral cage during surgery
2022, 2Q, 23	Sacroiliac joint fusion
2021, 4Q, 67	Posterior dynamic distraction
2021, 3Q, 24	Mid-foot fusion with bone graft
2021, 3Q, 25	Placement of X-Spine Axle Cage
2021, 1Q, 18	Placement of interspinous distraction device (spacer) for decompression
2021, 1Q, 53	Official guidelines for coding and reporting for interbody fusion device B3.10c
2020, 4Q, 56-58	Intramedullary sustained compression joint fusion
2020, 2Q, 27	Spinal fusion with NuVasive® VersaTie®
2020, 1Q, 33	Spinal fusion without use of bone graft
2019, 3Q, 35	Fusion procedures of the spine (guideline B3.10c)
2019, 1Q, 30	Spinal fusion performed at same level as decompressive laminectomy
2018, 4Q, 43	Joint fusion device value
2018, 1Q, 22	Spinal fusion procedures without bone graft
2017, 4Q, 76	Radiolucent porous interbody fusion device
2017, 2Q, 23	Decompression of spinal cord and placement of instrumentation
2014, 3Q, 30	Spinal fusion and fixation instrumentation
2014, 3Q, 36	Lumbar interbody fusion of two vertebral levels
2014, 2Q, 6	Posterior lumbar fusion with discectomy
2013, 3Q, 25	360-degree spinal fusion
2013, 2Q, 39	Ankle fusion, osteotomy, and removal of hardware
2013, 1Q, 21-23	Spinal fusion of thoracic and lumbar vertebrae

AHA Coding Clinic for table 0SH
2021, 3Q, 25	Placement of X-Spine Axle Cage
2021, 1Q, 18	Placement of interspinous distraction device (spacer) for decompression
2017, 2Q, 23	Decompression of spinal cord and placement of instrumentation

AHA Coding Clinic for table 0SJ
2017, 1Q, 50	Dry aspiration of ankle joint

AHA Coding Clinic for table 0SN
2020, 2Q, 26	Arthroscopic manipulation and nonexcisional debridement of knee joint
2019, 1Q, 30	Spinal fusion performed at same level as decompressive laminectomy

AHA Coding Clinic for table 0SP
2023, 3Q, 22	Patella resurfacing and tibial liner exchange
2022, 3Q, 21	Breakage of intervertebral cage during surgery
2021, 3Q, 25	Revision total knee arthroplasty
2021, 1Q, 17	Revision of ankle arthroplasty with placement of tibial insert
2018, 4Q, 43	Articulating spacer for hip and knee joint
2018, 2Q, 16	Exchange of tibial polyethylene component with stabilizing insert (tibial tray)
2017, 4Q, 107	Total ankle replacement versus revision
2016, 4Q, 110-112	Removal and revision of hip and knee devices
2015, 2Q, 18	Total knee revision
2015, 2Q, 19	Revision of femoral head and acetabular liner
2013, 2Q, 39	Ankle fusion, osteotomy, and removal of hardware

AHA Coding Clinic for table 0SQ
2014, 4Q, 25	Femoroacetabular impingement and labral tear with repair

AHA Coding Clinic for table 0SR
2022, 1Q, 39	Provisional total hip arthroplasty
2021, 3Q, 25	Revision total knee arthroplasty
2021, 1Q, 17	Revision of ankle arthroplasty with placement of tibial insert
2020, 3Q, 33	Total hip arthroplasty using dual mobility components
2018, 4Q, 43	Articulating spacer for hip and knee joint
2018, 2Q, 16	Exchange of tibial polyethylene component with stabilizing insert (tibial tray)
2017, 4Q, 38-39	Oxidized zirconium on polyethylene bearing surface
2017, 4Q, 107	Total ankle replacement versus revision
2017, 1Q, 22	Total knee replacement and patellar component
2016, 4Q, 110-111	Partial (unicondylar) knee replacement
2016, 4Q, 111-112	Removal and revision of hip and knee devices
2016, 3Q, 35	Use of cemented versus uncemented qualifier for joint replacement
2015, 3Q, 18	Total hip replacement with acetabular reconstruction
2015, 2Q, 18	Total knee revision
2015, 2Q, 19	Revision of femoral head and acetabular liner

AHA Coding Clinic for table 0SS
2022, 3Q, 27	Ankle and tarsal joint distraction
2022, 2Q, 22	Ankle distraction procedure
2016, 2Q, 31	Periacetabular osteotomy for repair of congenital hip dysplasia

AHA Coding Clinic for table 0ST
2016, 1Q, 20	Metatarsophalangeal joint resection arthroplasty
2014, 4Q, 29	Rotational osteosynthesis

AHA Coding Clinic for table 0SU
2023, 3Q, 22	Patella resurfacing and tibial liner exchange
2022, 1Q, 47	Matrix-induced autologous chondrocyte implantation
2021, 1Q, 17	Revision of ankle arthroplasty with placement of tibial insert
2018, 2Q, 16	Exchange of tibial polyethylene component with stabilizing insert (tibial tray)
2016, 4Q, 111	Removal and revision of hip and knee devices
2015, 2Q, 19	Revision of femoral head and acetabular liner

AHA Coding Clinic for table 0SW
2017, 4Q, 107	Total ankle replacement versus revision
2016, 4Q, 110-112	Removal and revision of hip and knee devices
2015, 2Q, 18	Total knee revision
2015, 2Q, 19	Revision of femoral head and acetabular liner

Lower Joints

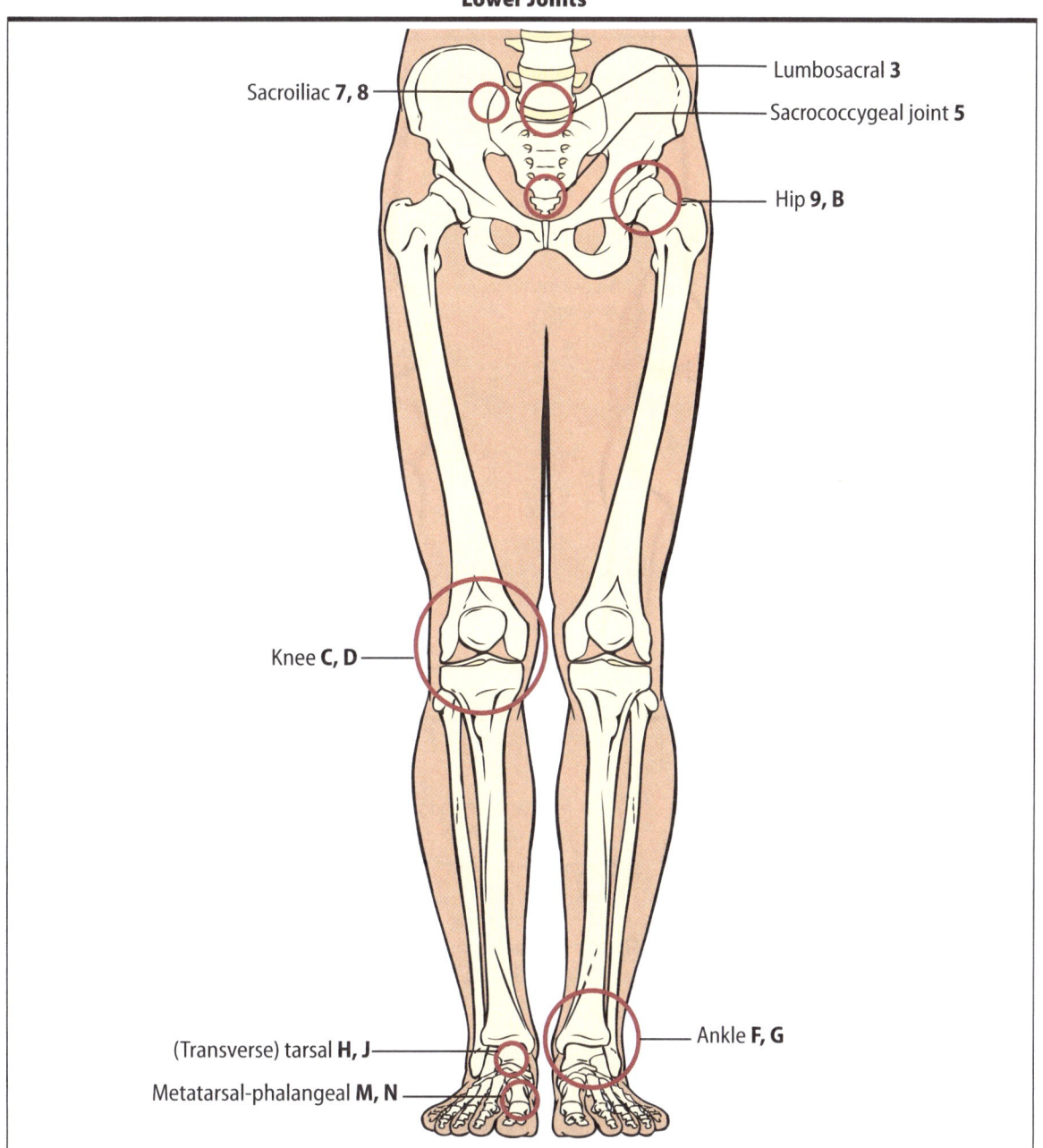

- Lumbosacral **3**
- Sacroiliac **7, 8**
- Sacrococcygeal joint **5**
- Hip **9, B**
- Knee **C, D**
- (Transverse) tarsal **H, J**
- Metatarsal-phalangeal **M, N**
- Ankle **F, G**

Hip Joint

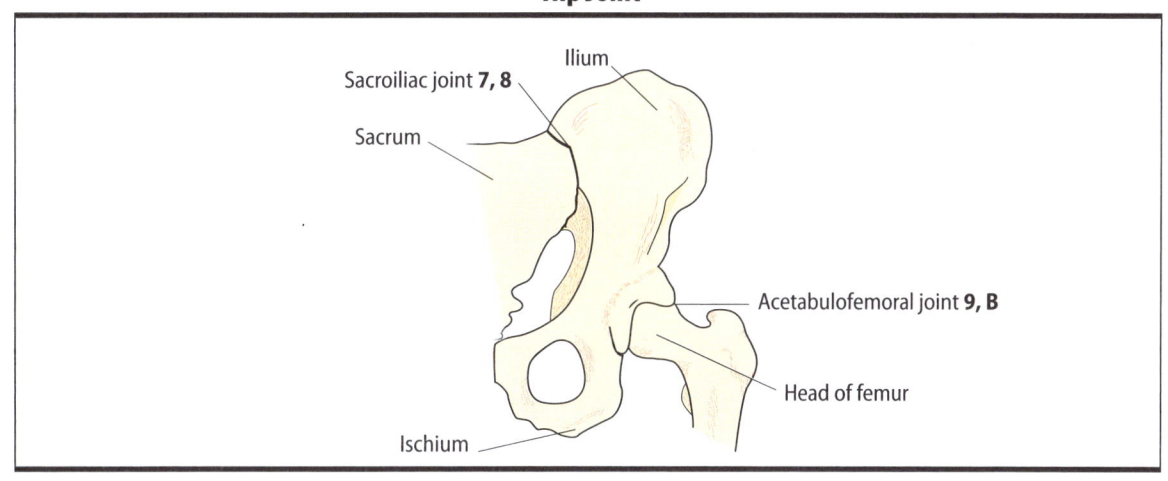

- Ilium
- Sacroiliac joint **7, 8**
- Sacrum
- Acetabulofemoral joint **9, B**
- Head of femur
- Ischium

Lower Joints

Knee Joint

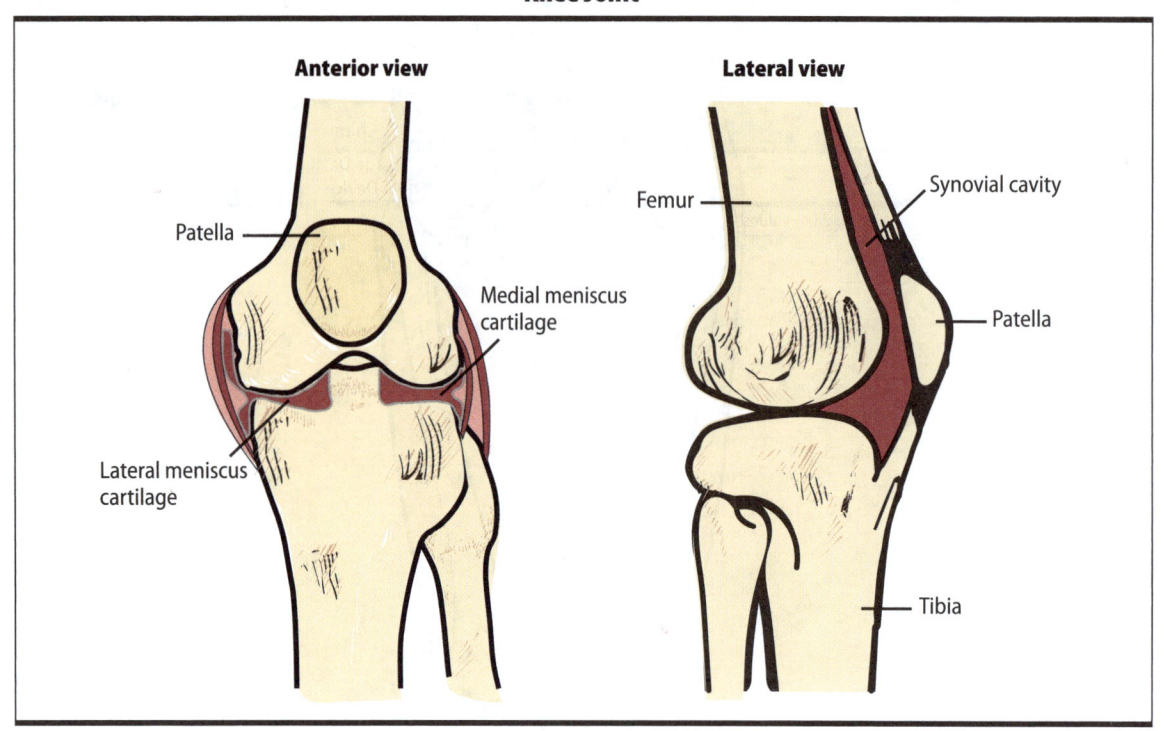

Anterior view
- Patella
- Medial meniscus cartilage
- Lateral meniscus cartilage

Lateral view
- Femur
- Synovial cavity
- Patella
- Tibia

Foot Joints

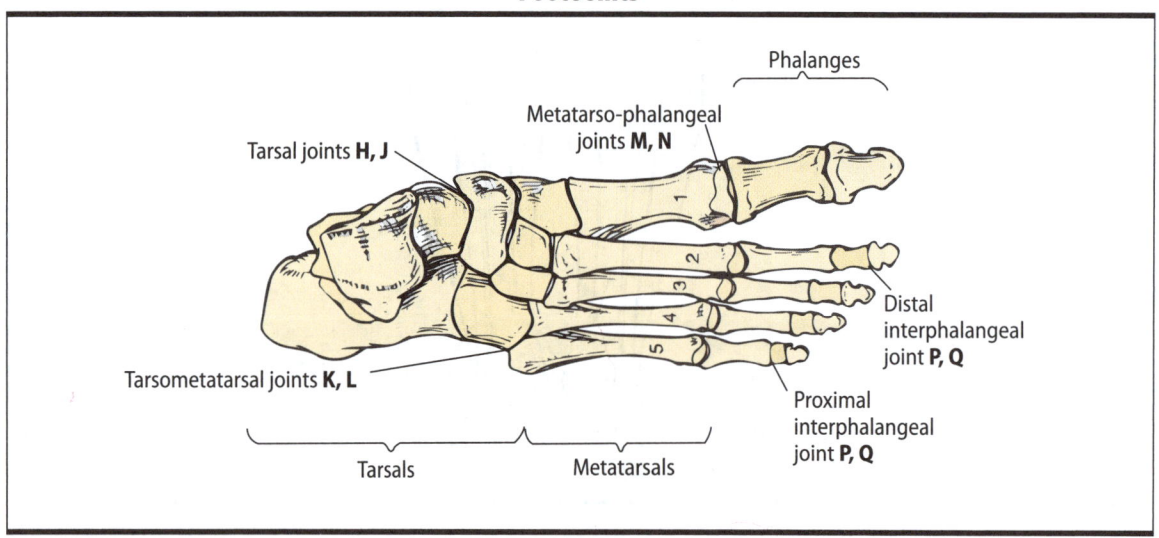

- Tarsal joints **H, J**
- Metatarso-phalangeal joints **M, N**
- Phalanges
- Distal interphalangeal joint **P, Q**
- Proximal interphalangeal joint **P, Q**
- Tarsometatarsal joints **K, L**
- Tarsals
- Metatarsals

0	**Medical and Surgical**	
S	**Lower Joints**	
2	**Change**	Definition: Taking out or off a device from a body part and putting back an identical or similar device in or on the same body part without cutting or puncturing the skin or a mucous membrane
		Explanation: ALL CHANGE procedures are coded using the approach EXTERNAL

Body Part Character 4	Approach Character 5	Device Character 6	Qualifier Character 7
Y Lower Joint	X External	0 Drainage Device Y Other Device	Z No Qualifier

Non-OR All body part, approach, device, and qualifier values

0	**Medical and Surgical**	
S	**Lower Joints**	
5	**Destruction**	Definition: Physical eradication of all or a portion of a body part by the direct use of energy, force, or a destructive agent
		Explanation: None of the body part is physically taken out

Body Part Character 4	Approach Character 5	Device Character 6	Qualifier Character 7

0 **Lumbar Vertebral Joint**
   Lumbar facet joint
2 **Lumbar Vertebral Disc**
3 **Lumbosacral Joint**
   Lumbosacral facet joint
4 **Lumbosacral Disc**
5 **Sacrococcygeal Joint**
   Sacrococcygeal symphysis
6 **Coccygeal Joint**
7 **Sacroiliac Joint, Right**
8 **Sacroiliac Joint, Left**
9 **Hip Joint, Right**
   Acetabulofemoral joint
B **Hip Joint, Left**
   See 9 Hip Joint, Right
C **Knee Joint, Right**
   Femoropatellar joint
   Femorotibial joint
   Lateral meniscus
   Medial meniscus
   Patellofemoral joint
   Tibiofemoral joint
D **Knee Joint, Left**
   See C Knee Joint, Right
F **Ankle Joint, Right**
   Inferior tibiofibular joint
   Talocrural joint
G **Ankle Joint, Left**
   See F Ankle Joint, Right
H **Tarsal Joint, Right**
   Calcaneocuboid joint
   Cuboideonavicular joint
   Cuneonavicular joint
   Intercuneiform joint
   Subtalar (talocalcaneal) joint
   Talocalcaneal (subtalar) joint
   Talocalcaneonavicular joint
J **Tarsal Joint, Left**
   See H Tarsal Joint, Right
K **Tarsometatarsal Joint, Right**
L **Tarsometatarsal Joint, Left**
M **Metatarsal-Phalangeal Joint, Right**
   Metatarsophalangeal (MTP) joint
N **Metatarsal-Phalangeal Joint, Left**
   See M Metatarsal-Phalangeal Joint, Right
P **Toe Phalangeal Joint, Right**
   Interphalangeal (IP) joint
Q **Toe Phalangeal Joint, Left**
   See P Toe Phalangeal Joint, Right
	0 Open
	3 Percutaneous
	4 Percutaneous Endoscopic
		Z No Device	Z No Qualifier

Lower Joints

0 Medical and Surgical
S Lower Joints
9 Drainage

Definition: Taking or letting out fluids and/or gases from a body part
Explanation: The qualifier DIAGNOSTIC is used to identify drainage procedures that are biopsies

Body Part Character 4	Approach Character 5	Device Character 6	Qualifier Character 7

0 Lumbar Vertebral Joint
   Lumbar facet joint
2 Lumbar Vertebral Disc
3 Lumbosacral Joint
   Lumbosacral facet joint
4 Lumbosacral Disc
5 Sacrococcygeal Joint
   Sacrococcygeal symphysis
6 Coccygeal Joint
7 Sacroiliac Joint, Right
8 Sacroiliac Joint, Left
9 Hip Joint, Right
   Acetabulofemoral joint
B Hip Joint, Left
   See 9 Hip Joint, Right
C Knee Joint, Right
   Femoropatellar joint
   Femorotibial joint
   Lateral meniscus
   Medial meniscus
   Patellofemoral joint
   Tibiofemoral joint
D Knee Joint, Left
   See C Knee Joint, Right
F Ankle Joint, Right
   Inferior tibiofibular joint
   Talocrural joint
G Ankle Joint, Left
   See F Ankle Joint, Right
	H Tarsal Joint, Right
	   Calcaneocuboid joint
	   Cuboideonavicular joint
	   Cuneonavicular joint
	   Intercuneiform joint
	   Subtalar (talocalcaneal) joint
	   Talocalcaneal (subtalar) joint
	   Talocalcaneonavicular joint
	J Tarsal Joint, Left
	   See H Tarsal Joint, Right
	K Tarsometatarsal Joint, Right
	L Tarsometatarsal Joint, Left
	M Metatarsal-Phalangeal Joint, Right
	   Metatarsophalangeal (MTP) joint
	N Metatarsal-Phalangeal Joint, Left
	   See M Metatarsal-Phalangeal Joint, Right
	P Toe Phalangeal Joint, Right
	   Interphalangeal (IP) joint
	Q Toe Phalangeal Joint, Left
	   See P Toe Phalangeal Joint, Right
		0 Open
		3 Percutaneous
		4 Percutaneous Endoscopic
			0 Drainage Device	**Z** No Qualifier

0 Lumbar Vertebral Joint
   Lumbar facet joint
2 Lumbar Vertebral Disc
3 Lumbosacral Joint
   Lumbosacral facet joint
4 Lumbosacral Disc
5 Sacrococcygeal Joint
   Sacrococcygeal symphysis
6 Coccygeal Joint
7 Sacroiliac Joint, Right
8 Sacroiliac Joint, Left
9 Hip Joint, Right
   Acetabulofemoral joint
B Hip Joint, Left
   See 9 Hip Joint, Right
C Knee Joint, Right
   Femoropatellar joint
   Femorotibial joint
   Lateral meniscus
   Medial meniscus
   Patellofemoral joint
   Tibiofemoral joint
D Knee Joint, Left
   See C Knee Joint, Right
F Ankle Joint, Right
   Inferior tibiofibular joint
   Talocrural joint
G Ankle Joint, Left
   See F Ankle Joint, Right
	H Tarsal Joint, Right
	   Calcaneocuboid joint
	   Cuboideonavicular joint
	   Cuneonavicular joint
	   Intercuneiform joint
	   Subtalar (talocalcaneal) joint
	   Talocalcaneal (subtalar) joint
	   Talocalcaneonavicular joint
	J Tarsal Joint, Left
	   See H Tarsal Joint, Right
	K Tarsometatarsal Joint, Right
	L Tarsometatarsal Joint, Left
	M Metatarsal-Phalangeal Joint, Right
	   Metatarsophalangeal (MTP) joint
	N Metatarsal-Phalangeal Joint, Left
	   See M Metatarsal-Phalangeal Joint, Right
	P Toe Phalangeal Joint, Right
	   Interphalangeal (IP) joint
	Q Toe Phalangeal Joint, Left
	   See P Toe Phalangeal Joint, Right
		0 Open
		3 Percutaneous
		4 Percutaneous Endoscopic
			Z No Device	**X** Diagnostic
				Z No Qualifier

Non-OR   0S9[0,2,3,4,5,6,7,8,9,B,C,D,F,G,H,J,K,L,M,N,P,Q][3,4]0Z
Non-OR   0S9[0,2,3,4,5,6,7,8,9,B,C,D,F,G,H,J,K,L,M,N,P,Q][0,3,4]ZX
Non-OR   0S9[0,2,3,4,5,6,7,8,9,B,C,D,F,G,H,J,K,L,M,N,P,Q][3,4]ZZ

Non-OR Procedure   DRG Non-OR Procedure   Valid OR Procedure   HAC Associated Procedure   Combination Only   New/Revised April   New/Revised October

ICD-10-PCS 2025 — Lower Joints — 0SB–0SB

- **0** Medical and Surgical
- **S** Lower Joints
- **B** Excision

Definition: Cutting out or off, without replacement, a portion of a body part
Explanation: The qualifier DIAGNOSTIC is used to identify excision procedures that are biopsies

Body Part Character 4	Approach Character 5	Device Character 6	Qualifier Character 7
0 Lumbar Vertebral Joint Lumbar facet joint **2 Lumbar Vertebral Disc** **3 Lumbosacral Joint** Lumbosacral facet joint **4 Lumbosacral Disc** **5 Sacrococcygeal Joint** Sacrococcygeal symphysis **6 Coccygeal Joint** **7 Sacroiliac Joint, Right** **8 Sacroiliac Joint, Left** **9 Hip Joint, Right** Acetabulofemoral joint **B Hip Joint, Left** See 9 Hip Joint, Right **C Knee Joint, Right** Femoropatellar joint Femorotibial joint Lateral meniscus Medial meniscus Patellofemoral joint Tibiofemoral joint **D Knee Joint, Left** See C Knee Joint, Right **F Ankle Joint, Right** Inferior tibiofibular joint Talocrural joint **G Ankle Joint, Left** See F Ankle Joint, Right **H Tarsal Joint, Right** Calcaneocuboid joint Cuboideonavicular joint Cuneonavicular joint Intercuneiform joint Subtalar (talocalcaneal) joint Talocalcaneal (subtalar) joint Talocalcaneonavicular joint **J Tarsal Joint, Left** See H Tarsal Joint, Right **K Tarsometatarsal Joint, Right** **L Tarsometatarsal Joint, Left** **M Metatarsal-Phalangeal Joint, Right** Metatarsophalangeal (MTP) joint **N Metatarsal-Phalangeal Joint, Left** See M Metatarsal-Phalangeal Joint, Right **P Toe Phalangeal Joint, Right** Interphalangeal (IP) joint **Q Toe Phalangeal Joint, Left** See P Toe Phalangeal Joint, Right	**0** Open **3** Percutaneous **4** Percutaneous Endoscopic	**Z** No Device	**X** Diagnostic **Z** No Qualifier

Non-OR 0SB[0,2,3,4,5,6,7,8,9,B,C,D,F,G,H,J,K,L,M,N,P,Q][0,3,4]ZX

0 Medical and Surgical
S Lower Joints
C Extirpation Definition: Taking or cutting out solid matter from a body part
Explanation: The solid matter may be an abnormal byproduct of a biological function or a foreign body; it may be imbedded in a body part or in the lumen of a tubular body part. The solid matter may or may not have been previously broken into pieces.

Body Part Character 4	Approach Character 5	Device Character 6	Qualifier Character 7
0 Lumbar Vertebral Joint Lumbar facet joint **2 Lumbar Vertebral Disc** **3 Lumbosacral Joint** Lumbosacral facet joint **4 Lumbosacral Disc** **5 Sacrococcygeal Joint** Sacrococcygeal symphysis **6 Coccygeal Joint** **7 Sacroiliac Joint, Right** **8 Sacroiliac Joint, Left** **9 Hip Joint, Right** Acetabulofemoral joint **B Hip Joint, Left** See 9 Hip Joint, Right **C Knee Joint, Right** Femoropatellar joint Femorotibial joint Lateral meniscus Medial meniscus Patellofemoral joint Tibiofemoral joint **D Knee Joint, Left** See C Knee Joint, Right **F Ankle Joint, Right** Inferior tibiofibular joint Talocrural joint **G Ankle Joint, Left** See F Ankle Joint, Right **H Tarsal Joint, Right** Calcaneocuboid joint Cuboideonavicular joint Cuneonavicular joint Intercuneiform joint Subtalar (talocalcaneal) joint Talocalcaneal (subtalar) joint Talocalcaneonavicular joint **J Tarsal Joint, Left** See H Tarsal Joint, Right **K Tarsometatarsal Joint, Right** **L Tarsometatarsal Joint, Left** **M Metatarsal-Phalangeal Joint, Right** Metatarsophalangeal (MTP) joint **N Metatarsal-Phalangeal Joint, Left** See M Metatarsal-Phalangeal Joint, Right **P Toe Phalangeal Joint, Right** Interphalangeal (IP) joint **Q Toe Phalangeal Joint, Left** See P Toe Phalangeal Joint, Right	**0** Open **3** Percutaneous **4** Percutaneous Endoscopic	**Z** No Device	**Z** No Qualifier

ICD-10-PCS 2025 — Lower Joints — 0SG–0SG

0 Medical and Surgical
S Lower Joints
G Fusion Definition: Joining together portions of an articular body part rendering the articular body part immobile
Explanation: The body part is joined together by fixation device, bone graft, or other means

Body Part Character 4	Approach Character 5	Device Character 6	Qualifier Character 7
0 Lumbar Vertebral Joint Lumbar facet joint **1** Lumbar Vertebral Joints, 2 or more ✚ **3** Lumbosacral Joint Lumbosacral facet joint	**0** Open **3** Percutaneous **4** Percutaneous Endoscopic	**7** Autologous Tissue Substitute **J** Synthetic Substitute **K** Nonautologous Tissue Substitute	**0** Anterior Approach, Anterior Column **1** Posterior Approach, Posterior Column **J** Posterior Approach, Anterior Column
0 Lumbar Vertebral Joint Lumbar facet joint **1** Lumbar Vertebral Joints, 2 or more ✚ **3** Lumbosacral Joint Lumbosacral facet joint	**0** Open **3** Percutaneous **4** Percutaneous Endoscopic	**A** Interbody Fusion Device	**0** Anterior Approach, Anterior Column **J** Posterior Approach, Anterior Column
5 Sacrococcygeal Joint Sacrococcygeal symphysis **6** Coccygeal Joint **7** Sacroiliac Joint, Right **8** Sacroiliac Joint, Left	**0** Open **3** Percutaneous **4** Percutaneous Endoscopic	**4** Internal Fixation Device **7** Autologous Tissue Substitute **J** Synthetic Substitute **K** Nonautologous Tissue Substitute	**Z** No Qualifier
9 Hip Joint, Right Acetabulofemoral joint **B** Hip Joint, Left *See 9 Hip Joint, Right* **C** Knee Joint, Right Femoropatellar joint Femorotibial joint Lateral meniscus Medial meniscus Patellofemoral joint Tibiofemoral joint **D** Knee Joint, Left *See C Knee Joint, Right* **F** Ankle Joint, Right Inferior tibiofibular joint Talocrural joint **G** Ankle Joint, Left *See F Ankle Joint, Right* **H** Tarsal Joint, Right Calcaneocuboid joint Cuboideonavicular joint Cuneonavicular joint Intercuneiform joint Subtalar (talocalcaneal) joint Talocalcaneal (subtalar) joint Talocalcaneonavicular joint **J** Tarsal Joint, Left *See H Tarsal Joint, Right* **K** Tarsometatarsal Joint, Right **L** Tarsometatarsal Joint, Left **M** Metatarsal-Phalangeal Joint, Right Metatarsophalangeal (MTP) joint **N** Metatarsal-Phalangeal Joint, Left *See M Metatarsal-Phalangeal Joint, Right* **P** Toe Phalangeal Joint, Right Interphalangeal (IP) joint **Q** Toe Phalangeal Joint, Left *See P Toe Phalangeal Joint, Right*	**0** Open **3** Percutaneous **4** Percutaneous Endoscopic	**3** Internal Fixation Device, Sustained Compression **4** Internal Fixation Device **5** External Fixation Device **7** Autologous Tissue Substitute **J** Synthetic Substitute **K** Nonautologous Tissue Substitute	**Z** No Qualifier

HAC 0SG[0,1,3][0,3,4][7,J,K][0,1,J] when reported with SDx K68.11 or T81.40–T81.49, T84.60-T84.619, T84.63-T84.7 with 7th character A
HAC 0SG[0,1,3][0,3,4]A[0,J] when reported with SDx K68.11 or T81.40–T81.49, T84.60-T84.619, T84.63-T84.7 with 7th character A
HAC 0SG[7,8][0,3,4][4,7,J,K]Z when reported with SDx K68.11 or T81.40–T81.49, T84.60-T84.619, T84.63-T84.7 with 7th character A

See Appendix L for Procedure Combinations
✚ 0SG1[0,3,4][7,J,K][0,1,J]
✚ 0SG1[0,3,4]A[0,J]

NC Noncovered Procedure **LC** Limited Coverage **QA** Questionable OB Admit **NT** New Tech Add-on ✚ Combination Member ♂ Male ♀ Female

0SH–0SH Lower Joints ICD-10-PCS 2025

0 Medical and Surgical
S Lower Joints
H Insertion Definition: Putting in a nonbiological appliance that monitors, assists, performs, or prevents a physiological function but does not physically take the place of a body part
Explanation: None

Body Part Character 4	Approach Character 5	Device Character 6	Qualifier Character 7
0 Lumbar Vertebral Joint Lumbar facet joint **3 Lumbosacral Joint** Lumbosacral facet joint	**0** Open **3** Percutaneous **4** Percutaneous Endoscopic	**3** Infusion Device **4** Internal Fixation Device **8** Spacer **B** Spinal Stabilization Device, Interspinous Process **C** Spinal Stabilization Device, Pedicle-Based **D** Spinal Stabilization Device, Facet Replacement	**Z** No Qualifier
2 Lumbar Vertebral Disc **4 Lumbosacral Disc**	**0** Open **3** Percutaneous **4** Percutaneous Endoscopic	**3** Infusion Device **8** Spacer	**Z** No Qualifier
5 Sacrococcygeal Joint Sacrococcygeal symphysis **6 Coccygeal Joint** **7 Sacroiliac Joint, Right** **8 Sacroiliac Joint, Left**	**0** Open **3** Percutaneous **4** Percutaneous Endoscopic	**3** Infusion Device **4** Internal Fixation Device **8** Spacer	**Z** No Qualifier
9 Hip Joint, Right Acetabulofemoral joint **B Hip Joint, Left** See 9 Hip Joint, Right **C Knee Joint, Right** Femoropatellar joint Femorotibial joint Lateral meniscus Medial meniscus Patellofemoral joint Tibiofemoral joint **D Knee Joint, Left** See C Knee Joint, Right **F Ankle Joint, Right** Inferior tibiofibular joint Talocrural joint **G Ankle Joint, Left** See F Ankle Joint, Right **H Tarsal Joint, Right** Calcaneocuboid joint Cuboideonavicular joint Cuneonavicular joint Intercuneiform joint Subtalar (talocalcaneal) joint Talocalcaneal (subtalar) joint Talocalcaneonavicular joint **J Tarsal Joint, Left** See H Tarsal Joint, Right **K Tarsometatarsal Joint, Right** **L Tarsometatarsal Joint, Left** **M Metatarsal-Phalangeal Joint, Right** Metatarsophalangeal (MTP) joint **N Metatarsal-Phalangeal Joint, Left** See M Metatarsal-Phalangeal Joint, Right **P Toe Phalangeal Joint, Right** Interphalangeal (IP) joint **Q Toe Phalangeal Joint, Left** See P Toe Phalangeal Joint, Right	**0** Open **3** Percutaneous **4** Percutaneous Endoscopic	**3** Infusion Device **4** Internal Fixation Device **5** External Fixation Device **8** Spacer	**Z** No Qualifier

Non-OR 0SH[0,3][0,3,4][3,8]Z
Non-OR 0SH[2,4][0,3,4][3,8]Z
Non-OR 0SH[5,6,7,8][0,3,4][3,8]Z
Non-OR 0SH[9,B,C,D][0,3,4]3Z
Non-OR 0SH[9,B,C,D][3,4]8Z
Non-OR 0SH[F,G,H,J,K,L,M,N,P,Q][0,3,4][3,8]Z

ICD-10-PCS 2025 — Lower Joints — 0SJ–0SN

- **0** Medical and Surgical
- **S** Lower Joints
- **J** Inspection

Definition: Visually and/or manually exploring a body part

Explanation: Visual exploration may be performed with or without optical instrumentation. Manual exploration may be performed directly or through intervening body layers.

Body Part — Character 4	Approach — Character 5	Device — Character 6	Qualifier — Character 7
0 Lumbar Vertebral Joint — Lumbar facet joint **2 Lumbar Vertebral Disc** **3 Lumbosacral Joint** — Lumbosacral facet joint **4 Lumbosacral Disc** **5 Sacrococcygeal Joint** — Sacrococcygeal symphysis **6 Coccygeal Joint** **7 Sacroiliac Joint, Right** **8 Sacroiliac Joint, Left** **9 Hip Joint, Right** — Acetabulofemoral joint **B Hip Joint, Left** — See 9 Hip Joint, Right **C Knee Joint, Right** — Femoropatellar joint, Femorotibial joint, Lateral meniscus, Medial meniscus, Patellofemoral joint, Tibiofemoral joint **D Knee Joint, Left** — See C Knee Joint, Right **F Ankle Joint, Right** — Inferior tibiofibular joint, Talocrural joint **G Ankle Joint, Left** — See F Ankle Joint, Right **H Tarsal Joint, Right** — Calcaneocuboid joint, Cuboideonavicular joint, Cuneonavicular joint, Intercuneiform joint, Subtalar (talocalcaneal) joint, Talocalcaneal (subtalar) joint, Talocalcaneonavicular joint **J Tarsal Joint, Left** — See H Tarsal Joint, Right **K Tarsometatarsal Joint, Right** **L Tarsometatarsal Joint, Left** **M Metatarsal-Phalangeal Joint, Right** — Metatarsophalangeal (MTP) joint **N Metatarsal-Phalangeal Joint, Left** — See M Metatarsal-Phalangeal Joint, Right **P Toe Phalangeal Joint, Right** — Interphalangeal (IP) joint **Q Toe Phalangeal Joint, Left** — See P Toe Phalangeal Joint, Right	**0** Open **3** Percutaneous **4** Percutaneous Endoscopic **X** External	**Z** No Device	**Z** No Qualifier

Non-OR 0SJ[0,2,3,4,5,6,7,8,9,B,C,D,F,G,H,J,K,L,M,N,P,Q][3,X]ZZ

- **0** Medical and Surgical
- **S** Lower Joints
- **N** Release

Definition: Freeing a body part from an abnormal physical constraint by cutting or by the use of force

Explanation: Some of the restraining tissue may be taken out but none of the body part is taken out

Body Part — Character 4	Approach — Character 5	Device — Character 6	Qualifier — Character 7
0 Lumbar Vertebral Joint — Lumbar facet joint **2 Lumbar Vertebral Disc** **3 Lumbosacral Joint** — Lumbosacral facet joint **4 Lumbosacral Disc** **5 Sacrococcygeal Joint** — Sacrococcygeal symphysis **6 Coccygeal Joint** **7 Sacroiliac Joint, Right** **8 Sacroiliac Joint, Left** **9 Hip Joint, Right** — Acetabulofemoral joint **B Hip Joint, Left** — See 9 Hip Joint, Right **C Knee Joint, Right** — Femoropatellar joint, Femorotibial joint, Lateral meniscus, Medial meniscus, Patellofemoral joint, Tibiofemoral joint **D Knee Joint, Left** — See C Knee Joint, Right **F Ankle Joint, Right** — Inferior tibiofibular joint, Talocrural joint **G Ankle Joint, Left** — See F Ankle Joint, Right **H Tarsal Joint, Right** — Calcaneocuboid joint, Cuboideonavicular joint, Cuneonavicular joint, Intercuneiform joint, Subtalar (talocalcaneal) joint, Talocalcaneal (subtalar) joint, Talocalcaneonavicular joint **J Tarsal Joint, Left** — See H Tarsal Joint, Right **K Tarsometatarsal Joint, Right** **L Tarsometatarsal Joint, Left** **M Metatarsal-Phalangeal Joint, Right** — Metatarsophalangeal (MTP) joint **N Metatarsal-Phalangeal Joint, Left** — See M Metatarsal-Phalangeal Joint, Right **P Toe Phalangeal Joint, Right** — Interphalangeal (IP) joint **Q Toe Phalangeal Joint, Left** — See P Toe Phalangeal Joint, Right	**0** Open **3** Percutaneous **4** Percutaneous Endoscopic **X** External	**Z** No Device	**Z** No Qualifier

Non-OR 0SN[0,2,3,4,5,6,7,8,9,B,C,D,F,G,H,J,K,L,M,N,P,Q]XZZ

Lower Joints

0 Medical and Surgical
S Lower Joints
P Removal

Definition: Taking out or off a device from a body part

Explanation: If a device is taken out and a similar device put in without cutting or puncturing the skin or mucous membrane, the procedure is coded to the root operation CHANGE. Otherwise, the procedure for taking out the device is coded to the root operation REMOVAL.

Body Part Character 4	Approach Character 5	Device Character 6	Qualifier Character 7

0 Lumbar Vertebral Joint
   Lumbar facet joint
3 Lumbosacral Joint
   Lumbosacral facet joint
	0 Open
	3 Percutaneous
	4 Percutaneous Endoscopic
		0 Drainage Device
		3 Infusion Device
		4 Internal Fixation Device
		7 Autologous Tissue Substitute
		8 Spacer
		A Interbody Fusion Device
		J Synthetic Substitute
		K Nonautologous Tissue Substitute
			Z No Qualifier

0 Lumbar Vertebral Joint
   Lumbar facet joint
3 Lumbosacral Joint
   Lumbosacral facet joint
	X External	0 Drainage Device
		3 Infusion Device
		4 Internal Fixation Device
			Z No Qualifier

2 Lumbar Vertebral Disc 4 Lumbosacral Disc	0 Open 3 Percutaneous 4 Percutaneous Endoscopic	0 Drainage Device 3 Infusion Device 7 Autologous Tissue Substitute J Synthetic Substitute K Nonautologous Tissue Substitute	Z No Qualifier
2 Lumbar Vertebral Disc 4 Lumbosacral Disc	X External	0 Drainage Device 3 Infusion Device	Z No Qualifier
5 Sacrococcygeal Joint Sacrococcygeal symphysis 6 Coccygeal Joint 7 Sacroiliac Joint, Right 8 Sacroiliac Joint, Left	0 Open 3 Percutaneous 4 Percutaneous Endoscopic	0 Drainage Device 3 Infusion Device 4 Internal Fixation Device 7 Autologous Tissue Substitute 8 Spacer J Synthetic Substitute K Nonautologous Tissue Substitute	Z No Qualifier
5 Sacrococcygeal Joint Sacrococcygeal symphysis 6 Coccygeal Joint 7 Sacroiliac Joint, Right 8 Sacroiliac Joint, Left	X External	0 Drainage Device 3 Infusion Device 4 Internal Fixation Device	Z No Qualifier

9 Hip Joint, Right
   Acetabulofemoral joint
B Hip Joint, Left
   See 9 Hip Joint, Right
	0 Open	0 Drainage Device
		3 Infusion Device
		4 Internal Fixation Device
		5 External Fixation Device
		7 Autologous Tissue Substitute
		8 Spacer
		9 Liner
		B Resurfacing Device
		E Articulating Spacer
		J Synthetic Substitute
		K Nonautologous Tissue Substitute
			Z No Qualifier

9 Hip Joint, Right
   Acetabulofemoral joint
B Hip Joint, Left
   See 9 Hip Joint, Right
	3 Percutaneous
	4 Percutaneous Endoscopic
		0 Drainage Device
		3 Infusion Device
		4 Internal Fixation Device
		5 External Fixation Device
		7 Autologous Tissue Substitute
		8 Spacer
		J Synthetic Substitute
		K Nonautologous Tissue Substitute
			Z No Qualifier

9 Hip Joint, Right
   Acetabulofemoral joint
B Hip Joint, Left
   See 9 Hip Joint, Right
	X External	0 Drainage Device
		3 Infusion Device
		4 Internal Fixation Device
		5 External Fixation Device
			Z No Qualifier

Non-OR 0SP[0,3][0,3,4]8Z
Non-OR 0SP[0,3]3[0,3]Z
Non-OR 0SP[0,3]X[0,3,4]Z
Non-OR 0SP[2,4]3[0,3]Z
Non-OR 0SP[2,4]X[0,3]Z
Non-OR 0SP[5,6,7,8][0,3,4]8Z
Non-OR 0SP[5,6,7,8]3[0,3]Z
Non-OR 0SP[5,6,7,8]X[0,3,4]Z
Non-OR 0SP[9,B]3[0,3,8]Z
Non-OR 0SP[9,B]X[0,3,4,5]Z

See Appendix L for Procedure Combinations
Combo-only 0SP[9,B]48Z
0SP[9,B]0[8,9,B,E,J]Z
0SP[9,B]4JZ

0SP Continued on next page

Non-OR Procedure | DRG Non-OR Procedure | Valid OR Procedure | HAC Associated Procedure | Combination Only | New/Revised April | New/Revised October

ICD-10-PCS 2025 — Lower Joints — ØSP–ØSP

ØSP Continued

- **Ø** Medical and Surgical
- **S** Lower Joints
- **P** Removal

Definition: Taking out or off a device from a body part

Explanation: If a device is taken out and a similar device put in without cutting or puncturing the skin or mucous membrane, the procedure is coded to the root operation CHANGE. Otherwise, the procedure for taking out the device is coded to the root operation REMOVAL.

Body Part Character 4	Approach Character 5	Device Character 6	Qualifier Character 7

A Hip Joint, Acetabular Surface, Right
E Hip Joint, Acetabular Surface, Left
R Hip Joint, Femoral Surface, Right
S Hip Joint, Femoral Surface, Left
T Knee Joint, Femoral Surface, Right
   Femoropatellar joint
   Patellofemoral joint
U Knee Joint, Femoral Surface, Left
   See T Knee Joint, Femoral Surface, Right
V Knee Joint, Tibial Surface, Right
   Femorotibial joint
   Tibiofemoral joint
W Knee Joint, Tibial Surface, Left
   See V Knee Joint, Tibial Surface, Right
	Ø Open
	3 Percutaneous
	4 Percutaneous Endoscopic
		J Synthetic Substitute	**Z** No Qualifier

C Knee Joint, Right
   Femoropatellar joint
   Femorotibial joint
   Lateral meniscus
   Medial meniscus
   Patellofemoral joint
   Tibiofemoral joint
D Knee Joint, Left
   See C Knee Joint, Right
	Ø Open	**Ø** Drainage Device
		3 Infusion Device
		4 Internal Fixation Device
		5 External Fixation Device
		7 Autologous Tissue Substitute
		8 Spacer
		9 Liner
		E Articulating Spacer
		K Nonautologous Tissue Substitute
		L Synthetic Substitute, Unicondylar Medial
		M Synthetic Substitute, Unicondylar Lateral
		N Synthetic Substitute, Patellofemoral
			Z No Qualifier

C Knee Joint, Right
   Femoropatellar joint
   Femorotibial joint
   Lateral meniscus
   Medial meniscus
   Patellofemoral joint
   Tibiofemoral joint
D Knee Joint, Left
   See C Knee Joint, Right
	Ø Open	**J** Synthetic Substitute	**C** Patellar Surface
			Z No Qualifier

C Knee Joint, Right
   Femoropatellar joint
   Femorotibial joint
   Lateral meniscus
   Medial meniscus
   Patellofemoral joint
   Tibiofemoral joint
D Knee Joint, Left
   See C Knee Joint, Right
	3 Percutaneous
	4 Percutaneous Endoscopic
		Ø Drainage Device
		3 Infusion Device
		4 Internal Fixation Device
		5 External Fixation Device
		7 Autologous Tissue Substitute
		8 Spacer
		K Nonautologous Tissue Substitute
		L Synthetic Substitute, Unicondylar Medial
		M Synthetic Substitute, Unicondylar Lateral
		N Synthetic Substitute, Patellofemoral
			Z No Qualifier

C Knee Joint, Right
   Femoropatellar joint
   Femorotibial joint
   Lateral meniscus
   Medial meniscus
   Patellofemoral joint
   Tibiofemoral joint
D Knee Joint, Left
   See C Knee Joint, Right
	3 Percutaneous
	4 Percutaneous Endoscopic
		J Synthetic Substitute	**C** Patellar Surface
			Z No Qualifier

Non-OR ØSP[C,D]3[Ø,3]Z

See Appendix L for Procedure Combinations
Combo-only
ØSP[C,D][3,4]8Z
ØSP[A,E,R,S,T,U,V,W][Ø,4]JZ
ØSP[C,D]Ø[8,9,E,L,M,N]Z
ØSP[C,D]ØJ[C,Z]
ØSP[C,D]4[L,M,N]Z
ØSP[C,D]4J[C,Z]

ØSP Continued on next page

NC Noncovered Procedure   **LC** Limited Coverage   **QA** Questionable OB Admit   **NT** New Tech Add-on   ➕ Combination Member   ♂ Male   ♀ Female

ØSP–ØSP Lower Joints ICD-10-PCS 2025

ØSP Continued

0	Medical and Surgical
S	Lower Joints
P	Removal

Definition: Taking out or off a device from a body part
Explanation: If a device is taken out and a similar device put in without cutting or puncturing the skin or mucous membrane, the procedure is coded to the root operation CHANGE. Otherwise, the procedure for taking out the device is coded to the root operation REMOVAL.

Body Part Character 4	Approach Character 5	Device Character 6	Qualifier Character 7
C Knee Joint, Right Femoropatellar joint Femorotibial joint Lateral meniscus Medial meniscus Patellofemoral joint Tibiofemoral joint **D Knee Joint, Left** See C Knee Joint, Right	X External	0 Drainage Device 3 Infusion Device 4 Internal Fixation Device 5 External Fixation Device	Z No Qualifier
F Ankle Joint, Right Inferior tibiofibular joint Talocrural joint **G Ankle Joint, Left** See F Ankle Joint, Right **H Tarsal Joint, Right** Calcaneocuboid joint Cuboideonavicular joint Cuneonavicular joint Intercuneiform joint Subtalar (talocalcaneal) joint Talocalcaneal (subtalar) joint Talocalcaneonavicular joint **J Tarsal Joint, Left** See H Tarsal Joint, Right **K Tarsometatarsal Joint, Right** **L Tarsometatarsal Joint, Left** **M Metatarsal-Phalangeal Joint, Right** Metatarsophalangeal (MTP) joint **N Metatarsal-Phalangeal Joint, Left** See M Metatarsal-Phalangeal Joint, Right **P Toe Phalangeal Joint, Right** Interphalangeal (IP) joint **Q Toe Phalangeal Joint, Left** See P Toe Phalangeal Joint, Right	0 Open 3 Percutaneous 4 Percutaneous Endoscopic	0 Drainage Device 3 Infusion Device 4 Internal Fixation Device 5 External Fixation Device 7 Autologous Tissue Substitute 8 Spacer J Synthetic Substitute K Nonautologous Tissue Substitute	Z No Qualifier
F Ankle Joint, Right Inferior tibiofibular joint Talocrural joint **G Ankle Joint, Left** See F Ankle Joint, Right **H Tarsal Joint, Right** Calcaneocuboid joint Cuboideonavicular joint Cuneonavicular joint Intercuneiform joint Subtalar (talocalcaneal) joint Talocalcaneal (subtalar) joint Talocalcaneonavicular joint **J Tarsal Joint, Left** See H Tarsal Joint, Right **K Tarsometatarsal Joint, Right** **L Tarsometatarsal Joint, Left** **M Metatarsal-Phalangeal Joint, Right** Metatarsophalangeal (MTP) joint **N Metatarsal-Phalangeal Joint, Left** See M Metatarsal-Phalangeal Joint, Right **P Toe Phalangeal Joint, Right** Interphalangeal (IP) joint **Q Toe Phalangeal Joint, Left** See P Toe Phalangeal Joint, Right	X External	0 Drainage Device 3 Infusion Device 4 Internal Fixation Device 5 External Fixation Device	Z No Qualifier

Non-OR ØSP[C,D]X[0,3,4,5]Z
Non-OR ØSP[F,G,H,J,K,L,M,N,P,Q]3[0,3,8]Z
Non-OR ØSP[F,G,H,J,K,L,M,N,P,Q][0,4]8Z
Non-OR ØSP[F,G,H,J,K,L,M,N,P,Q]X[0,3,4,5]Z

Non-OR Procedure   DRG Non-OR Procedure   Valid OR Procedure   HAC Associated Procedure   Combination Only   New/Revised April   New/Revised October

0 Medical and Surgical
S Lower Joints
Q Repair

Definition: Restoring, to the extent possible, a body part to its normal anatomic structure and function
Explanation: Used only when the method to accomplish the repair is not one of the other root operations

Body Part Character 4	Approach Character 5	Device Character 6	Qualifier Character 7

0 Lumbar Vertebral Joint
   Lumbar facet joint
2 Lumbar Vertebral Disc
3 Lumbosacral Joint
   Lumbosacral facet joint
4 Lumbosacral Disc
5 Sacrococcygeal Joint
   Sacrococcygeal symphysis
6 Coccygeal Joint
7 Sacroiliac Joint, Right
8 Sacroiliac Joint, Left
9 Hip Joint, Right
   Acetabulofemoral joint
B Hip Joint, Left
   See 9 Hip Joint, Right
C Knee Joint, Right
   Femoropatellar joint
   Femorotibial joint
   Lateral meniscus
   Medial meniscus
   Patellofemoral joint
   Tibiofemoral joint
D Knee Joint, Left
   See C Knee Joint, Right
F Ankle Joint, Right
   Inferior tibiofibular joint
   Talocrural joint
G Ankle Joint, Left
   See F Ankle Joint, Right
H Tarsal Joint, Right
   Calcaneocuboid joint
   Cuboideonavicular joint
   Cuneonavicular joint
   Intercuneiform joint
   Subtalar (talocalcaneal) joint
   Talocalcaneal (subtalar) joint
   Talocalcaneonavicular joint
J Tarsal Joint, Left
   See H Tarsal Joint, Right
K Tarsometatarsal Joint, Right
L Tarsometatarsal Joint, Left
M Metatarsal-Phalangeal Joint, Right
   Metatarsophalangeal (MTP) joint
N Metatarsal-Phalangeal Joint, Left
   See M Metatarsal-Phalangeal Joint, Right
P Toe Phalangeal Joint, Right
   Interphalangeal (IP) joint
Q Toe Phalangeal Joint, Left
   See P Toe Phalangeal Joint, Right
	0 Open
	3 Percutaneous
	4 Percutaneous Endoscopic
	X External
		Z No Device	**Z** No Qualifier

Non-OR   0SQ[0,2,3,4,5,6,7,8,9,B,C,D,F,G,H,J,K,L,M,N,P,Q]XZZ

Lower Joints

0 Medical and Surgical
S Lower Joints
R Replacement

Definition: Putting in or on biological or synthetic material that physically takes the place and/or function of all or a portion of a body part

Explanation: The body part may have been taken out or replaced, or may be taken out, physically eradicated, or rendered nonfunctional during the REPLACEMENT procedure. A REMOVAL procedure is coded for taking out the device used in a previous replacement procedure.

Body Part Character 4	Approach Character 5	Device Character 6	Qualifier Character 7

0 Lumbar Vertebral Joint
   Lumbar facet joint
2 Lumbar Vertebral Disc [NC]
3 Lumbosacral Joint
   Lumbosacral facet joint
4 Lumbosacral Disc [NC]
5 Sacrococcygeal Joint
   Sacrococcygeal symphysis
6 Coccygeal Joint
7 Sacroiliac Joint, Right
8 Sacroiliac Joint, Left
H Tarsal Joint, Right
   Calcaneocuboid joint
   Cuboideonavicular joint
   Cuneonavicular joint
   Intercuneiform joint
   Subtalar (talocalcaneal) joint
   Talocalcaneal (subtalar) joint
   Talocalcaneonavicular joint
J Tarsal Joint, Left
   See H Tarsal Joint, Right
K Tarsometatarsal Joint, Right
L Tarsometatarsal Joint, Left
M Metatarsal-Phalangeal Joint, Right
   Metatarsophalangeal (MTP) joint
N Metatarsal-Phalangeal Joint, Left
   See M Metatarsal-Phalangeal Joint, Right
P Toe Phalangeal Joint, Right
   Interphalangeal (IP) joint
Q Toe Phalangeal Joint, Left
   See P Toe Phalangeal Joint, Right
	0 Open	**7** Autologous Tissue Substitute
		J Synthetic Substitute
		K Nonautologous Tissue Substitute
			Z No Qualifier

9 Hip Joint, Right
   Acetabulofemoral joint
B Hip Joint, Left
   See 9 Hip Joint, Right
	0 Open	**1** Synthetic Substitute, Metal
		2 Synthetic Substitute, Metal on Polyethylene
		3 Synthetic Substitute, Ceramic
		4 Synthetic Substitute, Ceramic on Polyethylene
		6 Synthetic Substitute, Oxidized Zirconium on Polyethylene
		J Synthetic Substitute
			9 Cemented
			A Uncemented
			Z No Qualifier

9 Hip Joint, Right
   Acetabulofemoral joint
B Hip Joint, Left
   See 9 Hip Joint, Right
	0 Open	**7** Autologous Tissue Substitute
		E Articulating Spacer
		K Nonautologous Tissue Substitute
			Z No Qualifier

A Hip Joint, Acetabular Surface, Right **E** Hip Joint, Acetabular Surface, Left	**0** Open	**0** Synthetic Substitute, Polyethylene **1** Synthetic Substitute, Metal **3** Synthetic Substitute, Ceramic **J** Synthetic Substitute	**9** Cemented **A** Uncemented **Z** No Qualifier
A Hip Joint, Acetabular Surface, Right **E** Hip Joint, Acetabular Surface, Left	**0** Open	**7** Autologous Tissue Substitute **K** Nonautologous Tissue Substitute	**Z** No Qualifier

HAC 0SR[9,B]0[1,2,3,4,6,J][9,A,Z] when reported with SDx of I26.02-I26.09, I26.92-I26.99, or I82.401-I82.4Z9

HAC 0SR[9,B]0[7,E,K]Z when reported with SDx of I26.02-I26.09, I26.92-I26.99, or I82.401-I82.4Z9

HAC 0SR[A,E]0[0,1,3,J][9,A,Z] when reported with SDx of I26.02-I26.09, I26.92-I26.99, or I82.401-I82.4Z9

HAC 0SR[A,E]0[7,K]Z when reported with SDx of I26.02-I26.09, I26.92-I26.99, or I82.401-I82.4Z9

NC 0SR[2,4]0JZ when beneficiary age is over 60

See Appendix L for Procedure Combinations
- 0SR[9,B]0[1,2,3,4,6,J][9,A,Z]
- 0SR[9,B]0EZ
- 0SR[A,E]0[0,1,3,J][9,A,Z]

0SR Continued on next page

ICD-10-PCS 2025 — Lower Joints — ØSR–ØSR

Ø Medical and Surgical
S Lower Joints
R Replacement

ØSR Continued

Definition: Putting in or on biological or synthetic material that physically takes the place and/or function of all or a portion of a body part
Explanation: The body part may have been taken out or replaced, or may be taken out, physically eradicated, or rendered nonfunctional during the REPLACEMENT procedure. A REMOVAL procedure is coded for taking out the device used in a previous replacement procedure.

Body Part Character 4	Approach Character 5	Device Character 6	Qualifier Character 7

C Knee Joint, Right ➕
   Femoropatellar joint
   Femorotibial joint
   Lateral meniscus
   Medial meniscus
   Patellofemoral joint
   Tibiofemoral joint
D Knee Joint, Left ➕
   See C Knee Joint, Right
	Ø Open	6 Synthetic Substitute, Oxidized Zirconium on Polyethylene
		J Synthetic Substitute
		L Synthetic Substitute, Unicondylar Medial
		M Synthetic Substitute, Unicondylar Lateral
		N Synthetic Substitute, Patellofemoral
			9 Cemented
			A Uncemented
			Z No Qualifier

C Knee Joint, Right ➕
   Femoropatellar joint
   Femorotibial joint
   Lateral meniscus
   Medial meniscus
   Patellofemoral joint
   Tibiofemoral joint
D Knee Joint, Left ➕
   See C Knee Joint, Right
	Ø Open	7 Autologous Tissue Substitute
		E Articulating Spacer
		K Nonautologous Tissue Substitute
			Z No Qualifier

F Ankle Joint, Right
   Inferior tibiofibular joint
   Talocrural joint
G Ankle Joint, Left
   See F Ankle Joint, Right
T Knee Joint, Femoral Surface, Right
   Femoropatellar joint
   Patellofemoral joint
U Knee Joint, Femoral Surface, Left
   See T Knee Joint, Femoral Surface, Right
V Knee Joint, Tibial Surface, Right
   Femorotibial joint
   Tibiofemoral joint
W Knee Joint, Tibial Surface, Left
   See V Knee Joint, Tibial Surface, Right
	Ø Open	7 Autologous Tissue Substitute
		K Nonautologous Tissue Substitute
			Z No Qualifier

F Ankle Joint, Right
   Inferior tibiofibular joint
   Talocrural joint
G Ankle Joint, Left
   See F Ankle Joint, Right
T Knee Joint, Femoral Surface, Right ➕
   Femoropatellar joint
   Patellofemoral joint
U Knee Joint, Femoral Surface, Left ➕
   See T Knee Joint, Femoral Surface, Right
V Knee Joint, Tibial Surface, Right ➕
   Femorotibial joint
   Tibiofemoral joint
W Knee Joint, Tibial Surface, Left ➕
   See V Knee Joint, Tibial Surface, Right
	Ø Open	J Synthetic Substitute	9 Cemented
			A Uncemented
			Z No Qualifier

R Hip Joint, Femoral Surface, Right ➕ **S Hip Joint, Femoral Surface, Left** ➕	Ø Open	1 Synthetic Substitute, Metal 3 Synthetic Substitute, Ceramic J Synthetic Substitute	9 Cemented A Uncemented Z No Qualifier
R Hip Joint, Femoral Surface, Right **S Hip Joint, Femoral Surface, Left**	Ø Open	7 Autologous Tissue Substitute K Nonautologous Tissue Substitute	Z No Qualifier

HAC ØSR[C,D]Ø[6,J,L,M,N][9,A,Z] when reported with SDx of I26.02-I26.09, I26.92-I26.99 or I82.401-I82.4Z9
HAC ØSR[C,D]Ø[7,E,K]Z when reported with SDx of I26.02-I26.09, I26.92-I26.99 or I82.401-I82.4Z9
HAC ØSR[T,U,V,W]Ø[7,K]Z when reported with SDx of I26.02-I26.09, I26.92-I26.99 or I82.401-I82.4Z9
HAC ØSR[T,U,V,W]ØJ[9,A,Z] when reported with SDx of I26.02-I26.09, I26.92-I26.99 or I82.401-I82.4Z9
HAC ØSR[R,S]Ø[1,3,J][9,A,Z] when reported with SDx of I26.02-I26.09, I26.92-I26.99, or I82.401-I82.4Z9
HAC ØSR[R,S]Ø[7,K]Z when reported with SDx of I26.02-I26.09, I26.92-I26.99, or I82.401-I82.4Z9

See Appendix L for Procedure Combinations
➕ ØSR[C,D]Ø[6,J,L,M,N][9,A,Z]
➕ ØSR[C,D]ØEZ
➕ ØSR[T,U,V,W]ØJ[9,A,Z]
➕ ØSR[R,S]Ø[1,3,J][9,A,Z]

0 Medical and Surgical
S Lower Joints
S Reposition

Definition: Moving to its normal location, or other suitable location, all or a portion of a body part
Explanation: The body part is moved to a new location from an abnormal location, or from a normal location where it is not functioning correctly. The body part may or may not be cut out or off to be moved to the new location.

Body Part Character 4	Approach Character 5	Device Character 6	Qualifier Character 7
0 Lumbar Vertebral Joint Lumbar facet joint **3 Lumbosacral Joint** Lumbosacral facet joint **5 Sacrococcygeal Joint** Sacrococcygeal symphysis **6 Coccygeal Joint** **7 Sacroiliac Joint, Right** **8 Sacroiliac Joint, Left**	**0** Open **3** Percutaneous **4** Percutaneous Endoscopic **X** External	**4** Internal Fixation Device **Z** No Device	**Z** No Qualifier
9 Hip Joint, Right Acetabulofemoral joint **B Hip Joint, Left** See 9 Hip Joint, Right **C Knee Joint, Right** Femoropatellar joint Femorotibial joint Lateral meniscus Medial meniscus Patellofemoral joint Tibiofemoral joint **D Knee Joint, Left** See C Knee Joint, Right **F Ankle Joint, Right** Inferior tibiofibular joint Talocrural joint **G Ankle Joint, Left** See F Ankle Joint, Right **H Tarsal Joint, Right** Calcaneocuboid joint Cuboideonavicular joint Cuneonavicular joint Intercuneiform joint Subtalar (talocalcaneal) joint Talocalcaneal (subtalar) joint Talocalcaneonavicular joint **J Tarsal Joint, Left** See H Tarsal Joint, Right **K Tarsometatarsal Joint, Right** **L Tarsometatarsal Joint, Left** **M Metatarsal-Phalangeal Joint, Right** Metatarsophalangeal (MTP) joint **N Metatarsal-Phalangeal Joint, Left** See M Metatarsal-Phalangeal Joint, Right **P Toe Phalangeal Joint, Right** Interphalangeal (IP) joint **Q Toe Phalangeal Joint, Left** See P Toe Phalangeal Joint, Right	**0** Open **3** Percutaneous **4** Percutaneous Endoscopic **X** External	**4** Internal Fixation Device **5** External Fixation Device **Z** No Device	**Z** No Qualifier

Non-OR 0SS[0,3,5,6,][3,4,X][4,Z]Z
Non-OR 0SS[7,8]3ZZ
Non-OR 0SS[7,8][4,X][4,Z]Z
Non-OR 0SS[9,B]3ZZ
Non-OR 0SS[9,B][3,4,X]5Z
Non-OR 0SS[9,B][4,X][4,Z]Z
Non-OR 0SS[C,D,F,G,H,J,K,L,M,N,P,Q][3,4,X][4,5,Z]Z

ICD-10-PCS 2025 — Lower Joints — 0ST–0ST

- **0** Medical and Surgical
- **S** Lower Joints
- **T** Resection
  Definition: Cutting out or off, without replacement, all of a body part
  Explanation: None

Body Part Character 4	Approach Character 5	Device Character 6	Qualifier Character 7

2 Lumbar Vertebral Disc
4 Lumbosacral Disc
5 Sacrococcygeal Joint
    Sacrococcygeal symphysis
6 Coccygeal Joint
7 Sacroiliac Joint, Right
8 Sacroiliac Joint, Left
9 Hip Joint, Right
    Acetabulofemoral joint
B Hip Joint, Left
    See 9 Hip Joint, Right
C Knee Joint, Right
    Femoropatellar joint
    Femorotibial joint
    Lateral meniscus
    Medial meniscus
    Patellofemoral joint
    Tibiofemoral joint
D Knee Joint, Left
    See C Knee Joint, Right
F Ankle Joint, Right
    Inferior tibiofibular joint
    Talocrural joint
G Ankle Joint, Left
    See F Ankle Joint, Right
H Tarsal Joint, Right
    Calcaneocuboid joint
    Cuboideonavicular joint
    Cuneonavicular joint
    Intercuneiform joint
    Subtalar (talocalcaneal) joint
    Talocalcaneal (subtalar) joint
    Talocalcaneonavicular joint
J Tarsal Joint, Left
    See H Tarsal Joint, Right
K Tarsometatarsal Joint, Right
L Tarsometatarsal Joint, Left
M Metatarsal-Phalangeal Joint, Right
    Metatarsophalangeal (MTP) joint
N Metatarsal-Phalangeal Joint, Left
    See M Metatarsal-Phalangeal Joint, Right
P Toe Phalangeal Joint, Right
    Interphalangeal (IP) joint
Q Toe Phalangeal Joint, Left
    See P Toe Phalangeal Joint, Right
	0 Open	**Z** No Device	**Z** No Qualifier

0 Medical and Surgical
S Lower Joints
U Supplement: Putting in or on biological or synthetic material that physically reinforces and/or augments the function of a portion of a body part

Explanation: The biological material is non-living, or is living and from the same individual. The body part may have been previously replaced, and the SUPPLEMENT procedure is performed to physically reinforce and/or augment the function of the replaced body part.

Body Part Character 4	Approach Character 5	Device Character 6	Qualifier Character 7

0 Lumbar Vertebral Joint
   Lumbar facet joint
2 Lumbar Vertebral Disc
3 Lumbosacral Joint
   Lumbosacral facet joint
4 Lumbosacral Disc
5 Sacrococcygeal Joint
   Sacrococcygeal symphysis
6 Coccygeal Joint
7 Sacroiliac Joint, Right
8 Sacroiliac Joint, Left
F Ankle Joint, Right
   Inferior tibiofibular joint
   Talocrural joint
G Ankle Joint, Left
   See F Ankle Joint, Right
H Tarsal Joint, Right
   Calcaneocuboid joint
   Cuboideonavicular joint
   Cuneonavicular joint
   Intercuneiform joint
   Subtalar (talocalcaneal) joint
   Talocalcaneal (subtalar) joint
   Talocalcaneonavicular joint
J Tarsal Joint, Left
   See H Tarsal Joint, Right
K Tarsometatarsal Joint, Right
L Tarsometatarsal Joint, Left
M Metatarsal-Phalangeal Joint, Right
   Metatarsophalangeal (MTP) joint
N Metatarsal-Phalangeal Joint, Left
   See M Metatarsal-Phalangeal Joint, Right
P Toe Phalangeal Joint, Right
   Interphalangeal (IP) joint
Q Toe Phalangeal Joint, Left
   See P Toe Phalangeal Joint, Right
	0 Open
	3 Percutaneous
	4 Percutaneous Endoscopic
		7 Autologous Tissue Substitute
		J Synthetic Substitute
		K Nonautologous Tissue Substitute
			Z No Qualifier

9 Hip Joint, Right
   Acetabulofemoral joint
B Hip Joint, Left
   See 9 Hip Joint, Right
	0 Open	7 Autologous Tissue Substitute
		9 Liner
		B Resurfacing Device
		J Synthetic Substitute
		K Nonautologous Tissue Substitute
			Z No Qualifier

9 Hip Joint, Right
   Acetabulofemoral joint
B Hip Joint, Left
   See 9 Hip Joint, Right
	3 Percutaneous
	4 Percutaneous Endoscopic
		7 Autologous Tissue Substitute
		J Synthetic Substitute
		K Nonautologous Tissue Substitute
			Z No Qualifier

A Hip Joint, Acetabular Surface, Right E Hip Joint, Acetabular Surface, Left R Hip Joint, Femoral Surface, Right S Hip Joint, Femoral Surface, Left	0 Open	9 Liner B Resurfacing Device	Z No Qualifier

C Knee Joint, Right
   Femoropatellar joint
   Femorotibial joint
   Lateral meniscus
   Medial meniscus
   Patellofemoral joint
   Tibiofemoral joint
D Knee Joint, Left
   See C Knee Joint, Right
	0 Open	7 Autologous Tissue Substitute
		J Synthetic Substitute
		K Nonautologous Tissue Substitute
			Z No Qualifier

C Knee Joint, Right
   Femoropatellar joint
   Femorotibial joint
   Lateral meniscus
   Medial meniscus
   Patellofemoral joint
   Tibiofemoral joint
D Knee Joint, Left
   See C Knee Joint, Right
	0 Open	9 Liner	C Patellar Surface
			Z No Qualifier

HAC   0SU[9,B]0BZ when reported with SDx of I26.02-I26.09, I26.92-I26.99, or I82.401-I82.4Z9
HAC   0SU[A,E,R,S]0BZ when reported with SDx of I26.02-I26.09, I26.92-I26.99, or I82.401-I82.4Z9

See Appendix L for Procedure Combinations
- 0SU[9,B]09Z
- 0SU[A,E,R,S]09Z

0SU Continued on next page

ICD-10-PCS 2025 — Lower Joints — ØSU–ØSU

ØSU Continued

- **Ø** Medical and Surgical
- **S** Lower Joints
- **U** Supplement

Definition: Putting in or on biological or synthetic material that physically reinforces and/or augments the function of a portion of a body part

Explanation: The biological material is non-living, or is living and from the same individual. The body part may have been previously replaced, and the SUPPLEMENT procedure is performed to physically reinforce and/or augment the function of the replaced body part.

Body Part Character 4	Approach Character 5	Device Character 6	Qualifier Character 7
C Knee Joint, Right Femoropatellar joint Femorotibial joint Lateral meniscus Medial meniscus Patellofemoral joint Tibiofemoral joint **D** Knee Joint, Left *See C Knee Joint, Right*	**3** Percutaneous **4** Percutaneous Endoscopic	**7** Autologous Tissue Substitute **J** Synthetic Substitute **K** Nonautologous Tissue Substitute	**Z** No Qualifier
T Knee Joint, Femoral Surface, Right Femoropatellar joint Patellofemoral joint **U** Knee Joint, Femoral Surface, Left *See T Knee Joint, Femoral Surface, Right* **V** Knee Joint, Tibial Surface, Right ✚ Femorotibial joint Tibiofemoral joint **W** Knee Joint, Tibial Surface, Left ✚ *See V Knee Joint, Tibial Surface, Right*	**Ø** Open	**9** Liner	**Z** No Qualifier

See Appendix L for Procedure Combinations
✚ ØSU[V,W]09Z

0 Medical and Surgical
S Lower Joints
W Revision   Definition: Correcting, to the extent possible, a portion of a malfunctioning device or the position of a displaced device
Explanation: Revision can include correcting a malfunctioning or displaced device by taking out or putting in components of the device such as a screw or pin

Body Part Character 4	Approach Character 5	Device Character 6	Qualifier Character 7

0 Lumbar Vertebral Joint
   Lumbar facet joint
3 Lumbosacral Joint
   Lumbosacral facet joint
	0 Open
	3 Percutaneous
	4 Percutaneous Endoscopic
	X External
		0 Drainage Device
		3 Infusion Device
		4 Internal Fixation Device
		7 Autologous Tissue Substitute
		8 Spacer
		A Interbody Fusion Device
		J Synthetic Substitute
		K Nonautologous Tissue Substitute
			Z No Qualifier

2 Lumbar Vertebral Disc 4 Lumbosacral Disc	0 Open 3 Percutaneous 4 Percutaneous Endoscopic X External	0 Drainage Device 3 Infusion Device 7 Autologous Tissue Substitute J Synthetic Substitute K Nonautologous Tissue Substitute	Z No Qualifier
5 Sacrococcygeal Joint Sacrococcygeal symphysis 6 Coccygeal Joint 7 Sacroiliac Joint, Right 8 Sacroiliac Joint, Left	0 Open 3 Percutaneous 4 Percutaneous Endoscopic X External	0 Drainage Device 3 Infusion Device 4 Internal Fixation Device 7 Autologous Tissue Substitute 8 Spacer J Synthetic Substitute K Nonautologous Tissue Substitute	Z No Qualifier

9 Hip Joint, Right
   Acetabulofemoral joint
B Hip Joint, Left
   See 9 Hip Joint, Right
	0 Open	0 Drainage Device
		3 Infusion Device
		4 Internal Fixation Device
		5 External Fixation Device
		7 Autologous Tissue Substitute
		8 Spacer
		9 Liner
		B Resurfacing Device
		J Synthetic Substitute
		K Nonautologous Tissue Substitute
			Z No Qualifier

9 Hip Joint, Right
   Acetabulofemoral joint
B Hip Joint, Left
   See 9 Hip Joint, Right
	3 Percutaneous
	4 Percutaneous Endoscopic
	X External
		0 Drainage Device
		3 Infusion Device
		4 Internal Fixation Device
		5 External Fixation Device
		7 Autologous Tissue Substitute
		8 Spacer
		J Synthetic Substitute
		K Nonautologous Tissue Substitute
			Z No Qualifier

A Hip Joint, Acetabular Surface, Right
E Hip Joint, Acetabular Surface, Left
R Hip Joint, Femoral Surface, Right
S Hip Joint, Femoral Surface, Left
T Knee Joint, Femoral Surface, Right
   Femoropatellar joint
   Patellofemoral joint
U Knee Joint, Femoral Surface, Left
   See T Knee Joint, Femoral Surface, Right
V Knee Joint, Tibial Surface, Right
   Femorotibial joint
   Tibiofemoral joint
W Knee Joint, Tibial Surface, Left
   See V Knee Joint, Tibial Surface, Right
	0 Open
	3 Percutaneous
	4 Percutaneous Endoscopic
	X External
		J Synthetic Substitute	Z No Qualifier

C Knee Joint, Right
   Femoropatellar joint
   Femorotibial joint
   Lateral meniscus
   Medial meniscus
   Patellofemoral joint
   Tibiofemoral joint
D Knee Joint, Left
   See C Knee Joint, Right
	0 Open	0 Drainage Device
		3 Infusion Device
		4 Internal Fixation Device
		5 External Fixation Device
		7 Autologous Tissue Substitute
		8 Spacer
		9 Liner
		K Nonautologous Tissue Substitute
			Z No Qualifier

Non-OR 0SW[0,3]X[0,3,4,7,8,A,J,K]Z
Non-OR 0SW[2,4]X[0,3,7,J,K]Z
Non-OR 0SW[5,6,7,8]X[0,3,4,7,8,J,K]Z
Non-OR 0SW[9,B]X[0,3,4,5,7,8,J,K]Z
Non-OR 0SW[A,E,R,S,T,U,V,W]XJZ

0SW Continued on next page

ICD-10-PCS 2025 — Lower Joints — 0SW–0SW

0 Medical and Surgical
S Lower Joints
W Revision

0SW Continued

Definition: Correcting, to the extent possible, a portion of a malfunctioning device or the position of a displaced device
Explanation: Revision can include correcting a malfunctioning or displaced device by taking out or putting in components of the device such as a screw or pin

Body Part Character 4	Approach Character 5	Device Character 6	Qualifier Character 7
C Knee Joint, Right Femoropatellar joint Femorotibial joint Lateral meniscus Medial meniscus Patellofemoral joint Tibiofemoral joint **D Knee Joint, Left** *See C Knee Joint, Right*	0 Open	J Synthetic Substitute	C Patellar Surface Z No Qualifier
C Knee Joint, Right Femoropatellar joint Femorotibial joint Lateral meniscus Medial meniscus Patellofemoral joint Tibiofemoral joint **D Knee Joint, Left** *See C Knee Joint, Right*	3 Percutaneous 4 Percutaneous Endoscopic X External	0 Drainage Device 3 Infusion Device 4 Internal Fixation Device 5 External Fixation Device 7 Autologous Tissue Substitute 8 Spacer K Nonautologous Tissue Substitute	Z No Qualifier
C Knee Joint, Right Femoropatellar joint Femorotibial joint Lateral meniscus Medial meniscus Patellofemoral joint Tibiofemoral joint **D Knee Joint, Left** *See C Knee Joint, Right*	3 Percutaneous 4 Percutaneous Endoscopic X External	J Synthetic Substitute	C Patellar Surface Z No Qualifier
F Ankle Joint, Right Inferior tibiofibular joint Talocrural joint **G Ankle Joint, Left** *See F Ankle Joint, Right* **H Tarsal Joint, Right** Calcaneocuboid joint Cuboideonavicular joint Cuneonavicular joint Intercuneiform joint Subtalar (talocalcaneal) joint Talocalcaneal (subtalar) joint Talocalcaneonavicular joint **J Tarsal Joint, Left** *See H Tarsal Joint, Right* **K Tarsometatarsal Joint, Right** **L Tarsometatarsal Joint, Left** **M Metatarsal-Phalangeal Joint, Right** Metatarsophalangeal (MTP) joint **N Metatarsal-Phalangeal Joint, Left** *See M Metatarsal-Phalangeal Joint, Right* **P Toe Phalangeal Joint, Right** Interphalangeal (IP) joint **Q Toe Phalangeal Joint, Left** *See P Toe Phalangeal Joint, Right*	0 Open 3 Percutaneous 4 Percutaneous Endoscopic X External	0 Drainage Device 3 Infusion Device 4 Internal Fixation Device 5 External Fixation Device 7 Autologous Tissue Substitute 8 Spacer J Synthetic Substitute K Nonautologous Tissue Substitute	Z No Qualifier

Non-OR 0SW[C,D]X[0,3,4,5,7,8,K]Z
Non-OR 0SW[C,D]XJ[C,Z]
Non-OR 0SW[F,G,H,J,K,L,M,N,P,Q]X[0,3,4,5,7,8,J,K]Z

Urinary System ØT1–ØTY

Character Meanings

This Character Meaning table is provided as a guide to assist the user in the identification of character members that may be found in this section of code tables. It **SHOULD NOT** be used to build a PCS code.

	Operation–Character 3		Body Part–Character 4		Approach–Character 5		Device–Character 6		Qualifier–Character 7
1	Bypass	Ø	Kidney, Right	Ø	Open	Ø	Drainage Device	Ø	Allogeneic
2	Change	1	Kidney, Left	3	Percutaneous	1	Radioactive Element	1	Syngeneic
5	Destruction	2	Kidneys, Bilateral	4	Percutaneous Endoscopic	2	Monitoring Device	2	Zooplastic
7	Dilation	3	Kidney Pelvis, Right	7	Via Natural or Artificial Opening	3	Infusion Device	3	Kidney Pelvis, Right
8	Division	4	Kidney Pelvis, Left	8	Via Natural or Artificial Opening Endoscopic	7	Autologous Tissue Substitute	4	Kidney Pelvis, Left
9	Drainage	5	Kidney	X	External	C	Extraluminal Device	6	Ureter, Right
B	Excision	6	Ureter, Right			D	Intraluminal Device	7	Ureter, Left
C	Extirpation	7	Ureter, Left			J	Synthetic Substitute	8	Colon
D	Extraction	8	Ureters, Bilateral			K	Nonautologous Tissue Substitute	9	Colocutaneous
F	Fragmentation	9	Ureter			L	Artificial Sphincter	A	Ileum
H	Insertion	B	Bladder			M	Stimulator Lead	B	Bladder
J	Inspection	C	Bladder Neck			Y	Other Device	C	Ileocutaneous
L	Occlusion	D	Urethra			Z	No Device	D	Cutaneous
M	Reattachment							G	Hand-Assisted
N	Release							X	Diagnostic
P	Removal							Z	No Qualifier
Q	Repair								
R	Replacement								
S	Reposition								
T	Resection								
U	Supplement								
V	Restriction								
W	Revision								
Y	Transplantation								

AHA Coding Clinic for table ØT1
- 2017, 3Q, 20 — Creation of Indiana pouch
- 2017, 3Q, 21 — Augmentation cystoplasty with Indiana pouch and continent urinary diversion
- 2017, 1Q, 37 — Perineal urethrostomy
- 2015, 3Q, 34 — Redo urinary diversion surgery via left ureteral reimplantation

AHA Coding Clinic for table ØT7
- 2019, 2Q, 16 — Reimplantation of ureters with insertion of tubes
- 2017, 4Q, 111 — Exchange of ureteral stent
- 2016, 2Q, 27 — Exchange of ureteral stents
- 2015, 2Q, 8 — Urinary calculi fragmentation and evacuation
- 2013, 4Q, 123 — Urolift® procedure

AHA Coding Clinic for table ØT9
- 2017, 3Q, 19 — Ureteral stent placement for urinary leakage
- 2017, 3Q, 20 — Creation of Indiana pouch
- 2017, 3Q, 21 — Augmentation cystoplasty with Indiana pouch and continent urinary diversion

AHA Coding Clinic for table ØTB
- 2016, 1Q, 19 — Biopsy of neobladder malignancy
- 2015, 3Q, 34 — Excision of Mitrofanoff polyp
- 2014, 2Q, 8 — Ileoscopy with excision of polyp of Ileal loop urinary diversion

AHA Coding Clinic for table ØTC
- 2019, 3Q, 4 — Evacuation of clots from bladder dome
- 2016, 3Q, 23 — Ureteral stone migrating into bladder
- 2015, 2Q, 7 — Urinary calculi fragmentation and evacuation
- 2015, 2Q, 8 — Urinary calculi fragmentation and evacuation
- 2013, 4Q, 122 — Laser lithotripsy with removal of fragments

AHA Coding Clinic for table ØTF
- 2015, 2Q, 7 — Urinary calculi fragmentation and evacuation
- 2013, 4Q, 122 — Extracorporeal shock wave lithotripsy
- 2013, 4Q, 122 — Laser lithotripsy with removal of fragments

AHA Coding Clinic for table ØTH
- 2020, 4Q, 43-44 — Insertion of radioactive element
- 2019, 2Q, 16 — Reimplantation of ureters with insertion of tubes

AHA Coding Clinic for table ØTP
- 2017, 4Q, 111 — Exchange of ureteral stent
- 2016, 2Q, 27 — Exchange of ureteral stents

AHA Coding Clinic for table ØTQ
- 2018, 2Q, 27 — Dismembered pyeloplasty
- 2017, 1Q, 37 — Perineal urethrostomy

AHA Coding Clinic for table ØTR
- 2017, 3Q, 20 — Creation of Indiana pouch

AHA Coding Clinic for table ØTS
- 2019, 1Q, 29 — Young-Dees-Leadbetter bladder neck reconstruction
- 2018, 2Q, 27 — Dismembered pyeloplasty
- 2017, 1Q, 36 — Dismembered pyeloplasty
- 2016, 1Q, 15 — Pubovaginal sling placement

AHA Coding Clinic for table ØTT
- 2024, 1Q, 7 — Percutaneous endoscopic hand-assisted approach
- 2014, 3Q, 16 — Hand-assisted laparoscopy nephroureterectomy

AHA Coding Clinic for table ØTU
- 2019, 1Q, 29 — Young-Dees-Leadbetter bladder neck reconstruction
- 2017, 3Q, 21 — Augmentation cystoplasty with Indiana pouch and continent urinary diversion

AHA Coding Clinic for table ØTV
- 2015, 2Q, 11 — Cystourethroscopic Deflux® injection

AHA Coding Clinic for table ØTY
- 2023, 2Q, 32 — Preparation of donor organ before transplantation

Urinary System

Urinary System

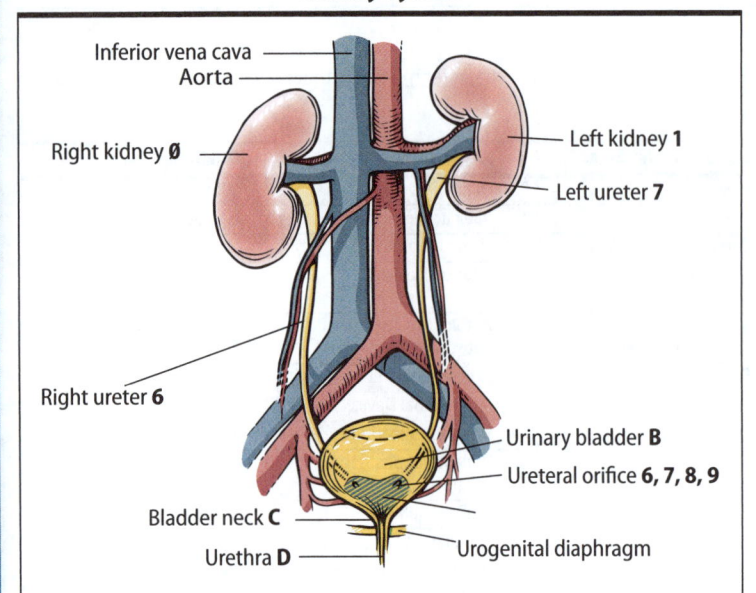

- Inferior vena cava
- Aorta
- Right kidney Ø
- Left kidney 1
- Left ureter 7
- Right ureter 6
- Urinary bladder B
- Ureteral orifice 6, 7, 8, 9
- Bladder neck C
- Urethra D
- Urogenital diaphragm

Kidney

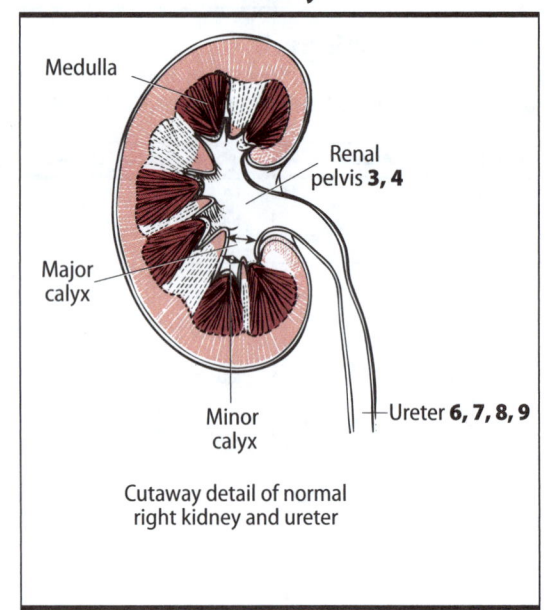

- Medulla
- Renal pelvis 3, 4
- Major calyx
- Minor calyx
- Ureter 6, 7, 8, 9

Cutaway detail of normal right kidney and ureter

Bladder

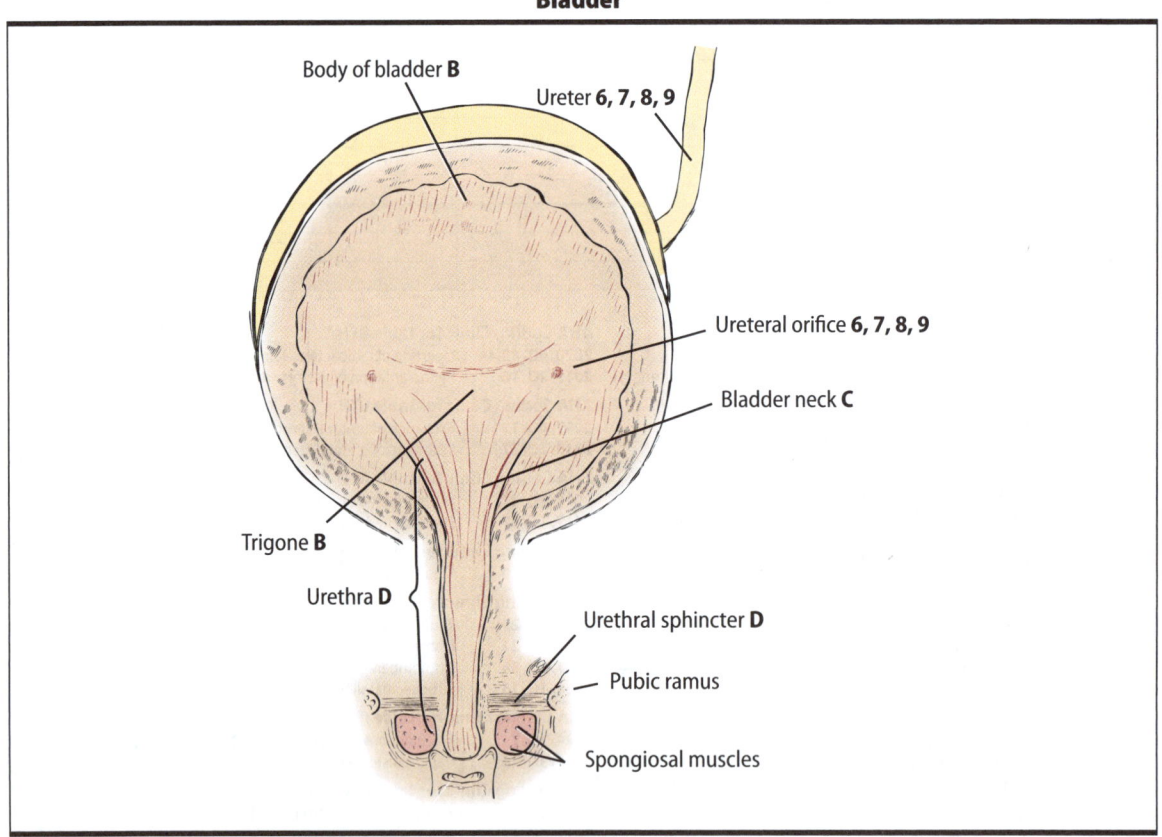

- Body of bladder B
- Ureter 6, 7, 8, 9
- Ureteral orifice 6, 7, 8, 9
- Bladder neck C
- Trigone B
- Urethra D
- Urethral sphincter D
- Pubic ramus
- Spongiosal muscles

ICD-10-PCS 2025 — Urinary System — 0T1–0T2

0 Medical and Surgical
T Urinary System
1 Bypass
Definition: Altering the route of passage of the contents of a tubular body part
Explanation: Rerouting contents of a body part to a downstream area of the normal route, to a similar route and body part, or to an abnormal route and dissimilar body part. Includes one or more anastomoses, with or without the use of a device.

Body Part Character 4	Approach Character 5	Device Character 6	Qualifier Character 7
3 Kidney Pelvis, Right Ureteropelvic junction (UPJ) 4 Kidney Pelvis, Left See 3 Kidney Pelvis, Right	0 Open 4 Percutaneous Endoscopic	7 Autologous Tissue Substitute J Synthetic Substitute K Nonautologous Tissue Substitute Z No Device	3 Kidney Pelvis, Right 4 Kidney Pelvis, Left 6 Ureter, Right 7 Ureter, Left 8 Colon 9 Colocutaneous A Ileum B Bladder C Ileocutaneous D Cutaneous
3 Kidney Pelvis, Right Ureteropelvic junction (UPJ) 4 Kidney Pelvis, Left See 3 Kidney Pelvis, Right	3 Percutaneous	J Synthetic Substitute	D Cutaneous
6 Ureter, Right Ureteral orifice Ureterovesical orifice 7 Ureter, Left See 6 Ureter, Right 8 Ureters, Bilateral See 6 Ureter, Right	0 Open 4 Percutaneous Endoscopic	7 Autologous Tissue Substitute J Synthetic Substitute K Nonautologous Tissue Substitute Z No Device	6 Ureter, Right 7 Ureter, Left 8 Colon 9 Colocutaneous A Ileum B Bladder C Ileocutaneous D Cutaneous
6 Ureter, Right Ureteral orifice Ureterovesical orifice 7 Ureter, Left See 6 Ureter, Right 8 Ureters, Bilateral See 6 Ureter, Right	3 Percutaneous	J Synthetic Substitute	D Cutaneous
B Bladder Trigone of bladder	0 Open 4 Percutaneous Endoscopic	7 Autologous Tissue Substitute J Synthetic Substitute K Nonautologous Tissue Substitute Z No Device	9 Colocutaneous C Ileocutaneous D Cutaneous
B Bladder Trigone of bladder	3 Percutaneous	J Synthetic Substitute	D Cutaneous

0 Medical and Surgical
T Urinary System
2 Change
Definition: Taking out or off a device from a body part and putting back an identical or similar device in or on the same body part without cutting or puncturing the skin or a mucous membrane
Explanation: All CHANGE procedures are coded using the approach EXTERNAL

Body Part Character 4	Approach Character 5	Device Character 6	Qualifier Character 7
5 Kidney Renal calyx Renal capsule Renal cortex Renal segment 9 Ureter Ureteral orifice Ureterovesical orifice B Bladder Trigone of bladder D Urethra Bulbourethral (Cowper's) gland Cowper's (bulbourethral) gland External urethral sphincter Internal urethral sphincter Membranous urethra Penile urethra Prostatic urethra	X External	0 Drainage Device Y Other Device	Z No Qualifier

Non-OR All body part, approach, device, and qualifier values

Urinary System

ØT5–ØT8 — ICD-10-PCS 2025

Ø Medical and Surgical
T Urinary System
5 Destruction

Definition: Physical eradication of all or a portion of a body part by the direct use of energy, force, or a destructive agent
Explanation: None of the body part is physically taken out

Body Part — Character 4	Approach — Character 5	Device — Character 6	Qualifier — Character 7
Ø Kidney, Right 　Renal calyx 　Renal capsule 　Renal cortex 　Renal segment **1** Kidney, Left 　*See Ø Kidney, Right* **3** Kidney Pelvis, Right 　Ureteropelvic junction (UPJ) **4** Kidney Pelvis, Left 　*See 3 Kidney Pelvis, Right* **6** Ureter, Right 　Ureteral orifice 　Ureterovesical orifice **7** Ureter, Left 　*See 6 Ureter, Right* **B** Bladder 　Trigone of bladder **C** Bladder Neck	**Ø** Open **3** Percutaneous **4** Percutaneous Endoscopic **7** Via Natural or Artificial Opening **8** Via Natural or Artificial Opening Endoscopic	**Z** No Device	**Z** No Qualifier
D Urethra 　Bulbourethral (Cowper's) gland 　Cowper's (bulbourethral) gland 　External urethral sphincter 　Internal urethral sphincter 　Membranous urethra 　Penile urethra 　Prostatic urethra	**Ø** Open **3** Percutaneous **4** Percutaneous Endoscopic **7** Via Natural or Artificial Opening **8** Via Natural or Artificial Opening Endoscopic **X** External	**Z** No Device	**Z** No Qualifier

Non-OR ØT5D[Ø,3,4,7,8,X]ZZ

Ø Medical and Surgical
T Urinary System
7 Dilation

Definition: Expanding an orifice or the lumen of a tubular body part
Explanation: The orifice can be a natural orifice or an artificially created orifice. Accomplished by stretching a tubular body part using intraluminal pressure or by cutting part of the orifice or wall of the tubular body part.

Body Part — Character 4	Approach — Character 5	Device — Character 6	Qualifier — Character 7
3 Kidney Pelvis, Right 　Ureteropelvic junction (UPJ) **4** Kidney Pelvis, Left 　*See 3 Kidney Pelvis, Right* **6** Ureter, Right 　Ureteral orifice 　Ureterovesical orifice **7** Ureter, Left 　*See 6 Ureter, Right* **8** Ureters, Bilateral 　*See 6 Ureter, Right* **B** Bladder 　Trigone of bladder **C** Bladder Neck **D** Urethra 　Bulbourethral (Cowper's) gland 　Cowper's (bulbourethral) gland 　External urethral sphincter 　Internal urethral sphincter 　Membranous urethra 　Penile urethra 　Prostatic urethra	**Ø** Open **3** Percutaneous **4** Percutaneous Endoscopic **7** Via Natural or Artificial Opening **8** Via Natural or Artificial Opening Endoscopic	**D** Intraluminal Device **Z** No Device	**Z** No Qualifier

Non-OR ØT7[6,7,8][Ø,3,4,7]DZ
Non-OR ØT7[6,7,8]7ZZ
Non-OR ØT788ZZ
Non-OR ØT7B7[D,Z]Z
Non-OR ØT7C[Ø,3,4]ZZ
Non-OR ØT7[C,D][Ø,3,4]DZ
Non-OR ØT7[C,D][7,8][D,Z]Z

Ø Medical and Surgical
T Urinary System
8 Division

Definition: Cutting into a body part, without draining fluids and/or gases from the body part, in order to separate or transect a body part
Explanation: All or a portion of the body part is separated into two or more portions

Body Part — Character 4	Approach — Character 5	Device — Character 6	Qualifier — Character 7
2 Kidneys, Bilateral 　Renal calyx 　Renal capsule 　Renal cortex 　Renal segment **C** Bladder Neck	**Ø** Open **3** Percutaneous **4** Percutaneous Endoscopic	**Z** No Device	**Z** No Qualifier

Non-OR Procedure　DRG Non-OR Procedure　Valid OR Procedure　HAC Associated Procedure　Combination Only　New/Revised April　New/Revised October

ICD-10-PCS 2025 — Urinary System — 0T9–0T9

- **0** Medical and Surgical
- **T** Urinary System
- **9** Drainage

Definition: Taking or letting out fluids and/or gases from a body part
Explanation: The qualifier DIAGNOSTIC is used to identify drainage procedures that are biopsies

Body Part Character 4	Approach Character 5	Device Character 6	Qualifier Character 7
0 Kidney, Right Renal calyx Renal capsule Renal cortex Renal segment **1** Kidney, Left *See 0 Kidney, Right* **3** Kidney Pelvis, Right Ureteropelvic junction (UPJ) **4** Kidney Pelvis, Left *See 3 Kidney Pelvis, Right* **6** Ureter, Right Ureteral orifice Ureterovesical orifice **7** Ureter, Left *See 6 Ureter, Right* **8** Ureters, Bilateral *See 6 Ureter, Right* **B** Bladder Trigone of bladder **C** Bladder Neck	**0** Open **3** Percutaneous **4** Percutaneous Endoscopic **7** Via Natural or Artificial Opening **8** Via Natural or Artificial Opening Endoscopic	**0** Drainage Device	**Z** No Qualifier
0 Kidney, Right Renal calyx Renal capsule Renal cortex Renal segment **1** Kidney, Left *See 0 Kidney, Right* **3** Kidney Pelvis, Right Ureteropelvic junction (UPJ) **4** Kidney Pelvis, Left *See 3 Kidney Pelvis, Right* **6** Ureter, Right Ureteral orifice Ureterovesical orifice **7** Ureter, Left *See 6 Ureter, Right* **8** Ureters, Bilateral *See 6 Ureter, Right* **B** Bladder Trigone of bladder **C** Bladder Neck	**0** Open **3** Percutaneous **4** Percutaneous Endoscopic **7** Via Natural or Artificial Opening **8** Via Natural or Artificial Opening Endoscopic	**Z** No Device	**X** Diagnostic **Z** No Qualifier
D Urethra Bulbourethral (Cowper's) gland Cowper's (bulbourethral) gland External urethral sphincter Internal urethral sphincter Membranous urethra Penile urethra Prostatic urethra	**0** Open **3** Percutaneous **4** Percutaneous Endoscopic **7** Via Natural or Artificial Opening **8** Via Natural or Artificial Opening Endoscopic **X** External	**0** Drainage Device	**Z** No Qualifier
D Urethra Bulbourethral (Cowper's) gland Cowper's (bulbourethral) gland External urethral sphincter Internal urethral sphincter Membranous urethra Penile urethra Prostatic urethra	**0** Open **3** Percutaneous **4** Percutaneous Endoscopic **7** Via Natural or Artificial Opening **8** Via Natural or Artificial Opening Endoscopic **X** External	**Z** No Device	**X** Diagnostic **Z** No Qualifier

Non-OR   0T9[0,1,3,4]30Z
Non-OR   0T9[6,7,8][0,3,4,7,8]0Z
Non-OR   0T9[B,C][3,4,7,8]0Z
Non-OR   0T9[0,1,3,4,6,7,8][3,4,7,8]ZX
Non-OR   0T9[0,1,3,4][3,4]ZZ
Non-OR   0T9[6,7,8]3ZZ
Non-OR   0T9[B,C][3,4,7,8]ZZ
Non-OR   0T9D30Z
Non-OR   0T9D[0,3,4,7,8,X]ZX
Non-OR   0T9D3ZZ

ØTB–ØTC — Urinary System — ICD-10-PCS 2025

Ø Medical and Surgical
T Urinary System
B Excision

Definition: Cutting out or off, without replacement, a portion of a body part
Explanation: The qualifier DIAGNOSTIC is used to identify excision procedures that are biopsies

Body Part Character 4	Approach Character 5	Device Character 6	Qualifier Character 7
Ø Kidney, Right Renal calyx Renal capsule Renal cortex Renal segment **1 Kidney, Left** *See Ø Kidney, Right* **3 Kidney Pelvis, Right** Ureteropelvic junction (UPJ) **4 Kidney Pelvis, Left** *See 3 Kidney Pelvis, Right* **6 Ureter, Right** Ureteral orifice Ureterovesical orifice **7 Ureter, Left** *See 6 Ureter, Right* **B Bladder** Trigone of bladder **C Bladder Neck**	**Ø** Open **3** Percutaneous **4** Percutaneous Endoscopic **7** Via Natural or Artificial Opening **8** Via Natural or Artificial Opening Endoscopic	**Z** No Device	**X** Diagnostic **Z** No Qualifier
D Urethra Bulbourethral (Cowper's) gland Cowper's (bulbourethral) gland External urethral sphincter Internal urethral sphincter Membranous urethra Penile urethra Prostatic urethra	**Ø** Open **3** Percutaneous **4** Percutaneous Endoscopic **7** Via Natural or Artificial Opening **8** Via Natural or Artificial Opening Endoscopic **X** External	**Z** No Device	**X** Diagnostic **Z** No Qualifier

Non-OR ØTB[Ø,1,3,4,6,7][3,4,7,8]ZX
Non-OR ØTBD[Ø,3,4,7,8,X]ZX

Ø Medical and Surgical
T Urinary System
C Extirpation

Definition: Taking or cutting out solid matter from a body part
Explanation: The solid matter may be an abnormal byproduct of a biological function or a foreign body; it may be imbedded in a body part or in the lumen of a tubular body part. The solid matter may or may not have been previously broken into pieces.

Body Part Character 4	Approach Character 5	Device Character 6	Qualifier Character 7
Ø Kidney, Right Renal calyx Renal capsule Renal cortex Renal segment **1 Kidney, Left** *See Ø Kidney, Right* **3 Kidney Pelvis, Right** Ureteropelvic junction (UPJ) **4 Kidney Pelvis, Left** *See 3 Kidney Pelvis, Right* **6 Ureter, Right** Ureteral orifice Ureterovesical orifice **7 Ureter, Left** *See 6 Ureter, Right* **B Bladder** Trigone of bladder **C Bladder Neck**	**Ø** Open **3** Percutaneous **4** Percutaneous Endoscopic **7** Via Natural or Artificial Opening **8** Via Natural or Artificial Opening Endoscopic	**Z** No Device	**Z** No Qualifier
D Urethra Bulbourethral (Cowper's) gland Cowper's (bulbourethral) gland External urethral sphincter Internal urethral sphincter Membranous urethra Penile urethra Prostatic urethra	**Ø** Open **3** Percutaneous **4** Percutaneous Endoscopic **7** Via Natural or Artificial Opening **8** Via Natural or Artificial Opening Endoscopic **X** External	**Z** No Device	**Z** No Qualifier

Non-OR ØTC[Ø,1,3,4,6,7]8ZZ
Non-OR ØTC[B,C][7,8]ZZ
Non-OR ØTCD[7,8,X]ZZ

ICD-10-PCS 2025 — Urinary System — 0TD–0TF

0 Medical and Surgical
T Urinary System
D Extraction Definition: Pulling or stripping out or off all or a portion of a body part by the use of force
Explanation: The qualifier DIAGNOSTIC is used to identify extraction procedures that are biopsies

Body Part Character 4	Approach Character 5	Device Character 6	Qualifier Character 7

0 Kidney, Right
  Renal calyx
  Renal capsule
  Renal cortex
  Renal segment
1 Kidney, Left
  See 0 Kidney, Right
	0 Open
	3 Percutaneous
	4 Percutaneous Endoscopic
		Z No Device	**Z** No Qualifier

0 Medical and Surgical
T Urinary System
F Fragmentation Definition: Breaking solid matter in a body part into pieces
Explanation: Physical force (e.g., manual, ultrasonic) applied directly or indirectly is used to break the solid matter into pieces. The solid matter may be an abnormal byproduct of a biological function or a foreign body. The pieces of solid matter are not taken out.

Body Part Character 4	Approach Character 5	Device Character 6	Qualifier Character 7

3 Kidney Pelvis, Right
  Ureteropelvic junction (UPJ)
4 Kidney Pelvis, Left
  See 3 Kidney Pelvis, Right
6 Ureter, Right
  Ureteral orifice
  Ureterovesical orifice
7 Ureter, Left
  See 6 Ureter, Right
B Bladder
  Trigone of bladder
C Bladder Neck
D Urethra **NC**
  Bulbourethral (Cowper's) gland
  Cowper's (bulbourethral) gland
  External urethral sphincter
  Internal urethral sphincter
  Membranous urethra
  Penile urethra
  Prostatic urethra
	0 Open
	3 Percutaneous
	4 Percutaneous Endoscopic
	7 Via Natural or Artificial Opening
	8 Via Natural or Artificial Opening Endoscopic
	X External
		Z No Device	**Z** No Qualifier

Non-OR 0TF[3,4][0,7,8]ZZ
Non-OR 0TF[6,7,B,C,D][0,3,4,7,8]ZZ
Non-OR 0TF[3,4,6,7,B,C,D]XZZ
NC 0TFDXZZ

ØTH–ØTH Urinary System ICD-10-PCS 2025

Ø Medical and Surgical
T Urinary System
H Insertion — Definition: Putting in a nonbiological appliance that monitors, assists, performs, or prevents a physiological function but does not physically take the place of a body part
Explanation: None

Body Part Character 4	Approach Character 5	Device Character 6	Qualifier Character 7
5 Kidney Renal calyx Renal capsule Renal cortex Renal segment	Ø Open 3 Percutaneous 4 Percutaneous Endoscopic 7 Via Natural or Artificial Opening 8 Via Natural or Artificial Opening Endoscopic	1 Radioactive Element 2 Monitoring Device 3 Infusion Device Y Other Device	Z No Qualifier
9 Ureter Ureteral orifice Ureterovesical orifice	Ø Open 3 Percutaneous 4 Percutaneous Endoscopic 7 Via Natural or Artificial Opening 8 Via Natural or Artificial Opening Endoscopic	1 Radioactive Element 2 Monitoring Device 3 Infusion Device M Stimulator Lead Y Other Device	Z No Qualifier
B Bladder NC Trigone of bladder	Ø Open 3 Percutaneous 4 Percutaneous Endoscopic 7 Via Natural or Artificial Opening 8 Via Natural or Artificial Opening Endoscopic	1 Radioactive Element 2 Monitoring Device 3 Infusion Device L Artificial Sphincter M Stimulator Lead Y Other Device	Z No Qualifier
C Bladder Neck	Ø Open 3 Percutaneous 4 Percutaneous Endoscopic 7 Via Natural or Artificial Opening 8 Via Natural or Artificial Opening Endoscopic	L Artificial Sphincter	Z No Qualifier
D Urethra Bulbourethral (Cowper's) gland Cowper's (bulbourethral) gland External urethral sphincter Internal urethral sphincter Membranous urethra Penile urethra Prostatic urethra	Ø Open 3 Percutaneous 4 Percutaneous Endoscopic 7 Via Natural or Artificial Opening 8 Via Natural or Artificial Opening Endoscopic	1 Radioactive Element 2 Monitoring Device 3 Infusion Device L Artificial Sphincter Y Other Device	Z No Qualifier
D Urethra Bulbourethral (Cowper's) gland Cowper's (bulbourethral) gland External urethral sphincter Internal urethral sphincter Membranous urethra Penile urethra Prostatic urethra	X External	2 Monitoring Device 3 Infusion Device L Artificial Sphincter	Z No Qualifier

Non-OR ØTH5Ø3Z
Non-OR ØTH53[1,3,Y]Z
Non-OR ØTH54[3,Y]Z
Non-OR ØTH57[1,2,3,Y]Z
Non-OR ØTH58[2,3]Z
Non-OR ØTH9Ø3Z
Non-OR ØTH93[1,3,Y]Z
Non-OR ØTH94[3,Y]Z
Non-OR ØTH97[1,2,3,Y]Z
Non-OR ØTH98[2,3]Z
Non-OR ØTHBØ3Z

Non-OR ØTHB3[1,3,Y]Z
Non-OR ØTHB4[3,Y]Z
Non-OR ØTHB7[1,2,3,Y]Z
Non-OR ØTHB8[2,3]Z
Non-OR ØTHDØ3Z
Non-OR ØTHD3[1,3,Y]Z
Non-OR ØTHD4[3,Y]Z
Non-OR ØTHD7[1,2,3,Y]Z
Non-OR ØTHD8[2,3]Z
Non-OR ØTHDX3Z
NC ØTHB[Ø,3,4,7,8]MZ

ICD-10-PCS 2025 — Urinary System — 0TJ–0TL

0 Medical and Surgical
T Urinary System
J Inspection   Definition: Visually and/or manually exploring a body part
Explanation: Visual exploration may be performed with or without optical instrumentation. Manual exploration may be performed directly or through intervening body layers.

Body Part Character 4	Approach Character 5	Device Character 6	Qualifier Character 7
5 Kidney Renal calyx Renal capsule Renal cortex Renal segment **9 Ureter** Ureteral orifice Ureterovesical orifice **B Bladder** Trigone of bladder **D Urethra** Bulbourethral (Cowper's) gland Cowper's (bulbourethral) gland External urethral sphincter Internal urethral sphincter Membranous urethra Penile urethra Prostatic urethra	0 Open 3 Percutaneous 4 Percutaneous Endoscopic 7 Via Natural or Artificial Opening 8 Via Natural or Artificial Opening Endoscopic X External	Z No Device	Z No Qualifier

Non-OR   0TJ[5,9,D][3,4,7,8,X]ZZ
Non-OR   0TJB[3,7,8,X]ZZ

0 Medical and Surgical
T Urinary System
L Occlusion   Definition: Completely closing an orifice or the lumen of a tubular body part
Explanation: The orifice can be a natural orifice or an artificially created orifice

Body Part Character 4	Approach Character 5	Device Character 6	Qualifier Character 7
3 Kidney Pelvis, Right Ureteropelvic junction (UPJ) **4 Kidney Pelvis, Left** See 3 Kidney Pelvis, Right **6 Ureter, Right** Ureteral orifice Ureterovesical orifice **7 Ureter, Left** See 6 Ureter, Right **B Bladder** Trigone of bladder **C Bladder Neck**	0 Open 3 Percutaneous 4 Percutaneous Endoscopic	C Extraluminal Device D Intraluminal Device Z No Device	Z No Qualifier
3 Kidney Pelvis, Right Ureteropelvic junction (UPJ) **4 Kidney Pelvis, Left** See 3 Kidney Pelvis, Right **6 Ureter, Right** Ureteral orifice Ureterovesical orifice **7 Ureter, Left** See 6 Ureter, Right **B Bladder** Trigone of bladder **C Bladder Neck**	7 Via Natural or Artificial Opening 8 Via Natural or Artificial Opening Endoscopic	D Intraluminal Device Z No Device	Z No Qualifier
D Urethra Bulbourethral (Cowper's) gland Cowper's (bulbourethral) gland External urethral sphincter Internal urethral sphincter Membranous urethra Penile urethra Prostatic urethra	0 Open 3 Percutaneous 4 Percutaneous Endoscopic X External	C Extraluminal Device D Intraluminal Device Z No Device	Z No Qualifier
D Urethra Bulbourethral (Cowper's) gland Cowper's (bulbourethral) gland External urethral sphincter Internal urethral sphincter Membranous urethra Penile urethra Prostatic urethra	7 Via Natural or Artificial Opening 8 Via Natural or Artificial Opening Endoscopic	D Intraluminal Device Z No Device	Z No Qualifier

NC Noncovered Procedure   LC Limited Coverage   QA Questionable OB Admit   NT New Tech Add-on   ✚ Combination Member   ♂ Male   ♀ Female

0TM–0TN Urinary System ICD-10-PCS 2025

0 Medical and Surgical
T Urinary System
M Reattachment   Definition: Putting back in or on all or a portion of a separated body part to its normal location or other suitable location
Explanation: Vascular circulation and nervous pathways may or may not be reestablished

Body Part Character 4	Approach Character 5	Device Character 6	Qualifier Character 7

0 Kidney, Right
   Renal calyx
   Renal capsule
   Renal cortex
   Renal segment
1 Kidney, Left
   See 0 Kidney, Right
2 Kidneys, Bilateral
   See 0 Kidney, Right
3 Kidney Pelvis, Right
   Ureteropelvic junction (UPJ)
4 Kidney Pelvis, Left
   See 3 Kidney Pelvis, Right
6 Ureter, Right
   Ureteral orifice
   Ureterovesical orifice
7 Ureter, Left
   See 6 Ureter, Right
8 Ureters, Bilateral
   See 6 Ureter, Right
B Bladder
   Trigone of bladder
C Bladder Neck
D Urethra
   Bulbourethral (Cowper's) gland
   Cowper's (bulbourethral) gland
   External urethral sphincter
   Internal urethral sphincter
   Membranous urethra
   Penile urethra
   Prostatic urethra
	0 Open
	4 Percutaneous Endoscopic
		Z No Device	**Z** No Qualifier

0 Medical and Surgical
T Urinary System
N Release   Definition: Freeing a body part from an abnormal physical constraint by cutting or by the use of force
Explanation: Some of the restraining tissue may be taken out but none of the body part is taken out

Body Part Character 4	Approach Character 5	Device Character 6	Qualifier Character 7

0 Kidney, Right
   Renal calyx
   Renal capsule
   Renal cortex
   Renal segment
1 Kidney, Left
   See 0 Kidney, Right
3 Kidney Pelvis, Right
   Ureteropelvic junction (UPJ)
4 Kidney Pelvis, Left
   See 3 Kidney Pelvis, Right
6 Ureter, Right
   Ureteral orifice
   Ureterovesical orifice
7 Ureter, Left
   See 6 Ureter, Right
B Bladder
   Trigone of bladder
C Bladder Neck
	0 Open
	3 Percutaneous
	4 Percutaneous Endoscopic
	7 Via Natural or Artificial Opening
	8 Via Natural or Artificial Opening Endoscopic
		Z No Device	**Z** No Qualifier

D Urethra
   Bulbourethral (Cowper's) gland
   Cowper's (bulbourethral) gland
   External urethral sphincter
   Internal urethral sphincter
   Membranous urethra
   Penile urethra
   Prostatic urethra
	0 Open
	3 Percutaneous
	4 Percutaneous Endoscopic
	7 Via Natural or Artificial Opening
	8 Via Natural or Artificial Opening Endoscopic
	X External
		Z No Device	**Z** No Qualifier

Non-OR Procedure   DRG Non-OR Procedure   Valid OR Procedure   HAC Associated Procedure   Combination Only   New/Revised April   New/Revised October

ICD-10-PCS 2025 — Urinary System — 0TP–0TP

0 Medical and Surgical
T Urinary System
P Removal   Definition: Taking out or off a device from a body part
Explanation: If a device is taken out and a similar device put in without cutting or puncturing the skin or mucous membrane, the procedure is coded to the root operation CHANGE. Otherwise, the procedure for taking out the device is coded to the root operation REMOVAL.

Body Part Character 4	Approach Character 5	Device Character 6	Qualifier Character 7
5 Kidney Renal calyx Renal capsule Renal cortex Renal segment	0 Open 3 Percutaneous 4 Percutaneous Endoscopic 7 Via Natural or Artificial Opening 8 Via Natural or Artificial Opening Endoscopic	0 Drainage Device 2 Monitoring Device 3 Infusion Device 7 Autologous Tissue Substitute C Extraluminal Device D Intraluminal Device J Synthetic Substitute K Nonautologous Tissue Substitute Y Other Device	Z No Qualifier
5 Kidney Renal calyx Renal capsule Renal cortex Renal segment	X External	0 Drainage Device 2 Monitoring Device 3 Infusion Device D Intraluminal Device	Z No Qualifier
9 Ureter Ureteral orifice Ureterovesical orifice	0 Open 3 Percutaneous 4 Percutaneous Endoscopic 7 Via Natural or Artificial Opening 8 Via Natural or Artificial Opening Endoscopic	0 Drainage Device 2 Monitoring Device 3 Infusion Device 7 Autologous Tissue Substitute C Extraluminal Device D Intraluminal Device J Synthetic Substitute K Nonautologous Tissue Substitute M Stimulator Lead Y Other Device	Z No Qualifier
9 Ureter Ureteral orifice Ureterovesical orifice	X External	0 Drainage Device 2 Monitoring Device 3 Infusion Device D Intraluminal Device M Stimulator Lead	Z No Qualifier
B Bladder NC Trigone of bladder	0 Open 3 Percutaneous 4 Percutaneous Endoscopic 7 Via Natural or Artificial Opening 8 Via Natural or Artificial Opening Endoscopic	0 Drainage Device 2 Monitoring Device 3 Infusion Device 7 Autologous Tissue Substitute C Extraluminal Device D Intraluminal Device J Synthetic Substitute K Nonautologous Tissue Substitute L Artificial Sphincter M Stimulator Lead Y Other Device	Z No Qualifier
B Bladder Trigone of bladder	X External	0 Drainage Device 2 Monitoring Device 3 Infusion Device D Intraluminal Device L Artificial Sphincter M Stimulator Lead	Z No Qualifier
D Urethra Bulbourethral (Cowper's) gland Cowper's (bulbourethral) gland External urethral sphincter Internal urethral sphincter Membranous urethra Penile urethra Prostatic urethra	0 Open 3 Percutaneous 4 Percutaneous Endoscopic 7 Via Natural or Artificial Opening 8 Via Natural or Artificial Opening Endoscopic	0 Drainage Device 2 Monitoring Device 3 Infusion Device 7 Autologous Tissue Substitute C Extraluminal Device D Intraluminal Device J Synthetic Substitute K Nonautologous Tissue Substitute L Artificial Sphincter Y Other Device	Z No Qualifier
D Urethra Bulbourethral (Cowper's) gland Cowper's (bulbourethral) gland External urethral sphincter Internal urethral sphincter Membranous urethra Penile urethra Prostatic urethra	X External	0 Drainage Device 2 Monitoring Device 3 Infusion Device D Intraluminal Device L Artificial Sphincter	Z No Qualifier

Non-OR 0TP5[3,4,7]YZ
Non-OR 0TP5[7,8][0,2,3,D]Z
Non-OR 0TP5X[0,2,3,D]Z
Non-OR 0TP9[3,4,7]YZ
Non-OR 0TP9[7,8][0,2,3,D]Z
Non-OR 0TP9X[0,2,3,D]Z
Non-OR 0TPB[3,4,7]YZ
Non-OR 0TPB[7,8][0,2,3,D]Z
Non-OR 0TPBX[0,2,3,D,L]Z
Non-OR 0TPD[3,4]YZ
Non-OR 0TPD[7,8][0,2,3,D,Y]Z
Non-OR 0TPDX[0,2,3,D]Z
NC 0TPB[0,3,4,7,8]MZ

NC Noncovered Procedure   **LC** Limited Coverage   **QA** Questionable OB Admit   **NT** New Tech Add-on   ✚ Combination Member   ♂ Male   ♀ Female

0 Medical and Surgical
T Urinary System
Q Repair

Definition: Restoring, to the extent possible, a body part to its normal anatomic structure and function

Explanation: Used only when the method to accomplish the repair is not one of the other root operations

Body Part Character 4	Approach Character 5	Device Character 6	Qualifier Character 7

0 Kidney, Right
   Renal calyx
   Renal capsule
   Renal cortex
   Renal segment
1 Kidney, Left
   See 0 Kidney, Right
3 Kidney Pelvis, Right
   Ureteropelvic junction (UPJ)
4 Kidney Pelvis, Left
   See 3 Kidney Pelvis, Right
6 Ureter, Right
   Ureteral orifice
   Ureterovesical orifice
7 Ureter, Left
   See 6 Ureter, Right
B Bladder ✚
   Trigone of bladder
C Bladder Neck
	0 Open
	3 Percutaneous
	4 Percutaneous Endoscopic
	7 Via Natural or Artificial Opening
	8 Via Natural or Artificial Opening Endoscopic
		Z No Device	Z No Qualifier

D Urethra
   Bulbourethral (Cowper's) gland
   Cowper's (bulbourethral) gland
   External urethral sphincter
   Internal urethral sphincter
   Membranous urethra
   Penile urethra
   Prostatic urethra
	0 Open
	3 Percutaneous
	4 Percutaneous Endoscopic
	7 Via Natural or Artificial Opening
	8 Via Natural or Artificial Opening Endoscopic
	X External
		Z No Device	Z No Qualifier

See Appendix L for Procedure Combinations
✚ 0TQB[0,3,4]ZZ

0 Medical and Surgical
T Urinary System
R Replacement

Definition: Putting in or on biological or synthetic material that physically takes the place and/or function of all or a portion of a body part

Explanation: The body part may have been taken out or replaced, or may be taken out, physically eradicated, or rendered nonfunctional during the REPLACEMENT procedure. A REMOVAL procedure is coded for taking out the device used in a previous replacement procedure.

Body Part Character 4	Approach Character 5	Device Character 6	Qualifier Character 7

3 Kidney Pelvis, Right
   Ureteropelvic junction (UPJ)
4 Kidney Pelvis, Left
   See 3 Kidney Pelvis, Right
6 Ureter, Right
   Ureteral orifice
   Ureterovesical orifice
7 Ureter, Left
   See 6 Ureter, Right
B Bladder
   Trigone of bladder
C Bladder Neck
	0 Open
	4 Percutaneous Endoscopic
	7 Via Natural or Artificial Opening
	8 Via Natural or Artificial Opening Endoscopic
		7 Autologous Tissue Substitute
		J Synthetic Substitute
		K Nonautologous Tissue Substitute
			Z No Qualifier

D Urethra
   Bulbourethral (Cowper's) gland
   Cowper's (bulbourethral) gland
   External urethral sphincter
   Internal urethral sphincter
   Membranous urethra
   Penile urethra
   Prostatic urethra
	0 Open
	4 Percutaneous Endoscopic
	7 Via Natural or Artificial Opening
	8 Via Natural or Artificial Opening Endoscopic
	X External
		7 Autologous Tissue Substitute
		J Synthetic Substitute
		K Nonautologous Tissue Substitute
			Z No Qualifier

ICD-10-PCS 2025 — Urinary System — 0TS–0TT

0 Medical and Surgical
T Urinary System
S Reposition

Definition: Moving to its normal location, or other suitable location, all or a portion of a body part

Explanation: The body part is moved to a new location from an abnormal location, or from a normal location where it is not functioning correctly. The body part may or may not be cut out or off to be moved to the new location.

Body Part Character 4	Approach Character 5	Device Character 6	Qualifier Character 7
0 Kidney, Right Renal calyx Renal capsule Renal cortex Renal segment **1 Kidney, Left** See 0 Kidney, Right **2 Kidneys, Bilateral** See 0 Kidney, Right **3 Kidney Pelvis, Right** Ureteropelvic junction (UPJ) **4 Kidney Pelvis, Left** See 3 Kidney Pelvis, Right **6 Ureter, Right** Ureteral orifice Ureterovesical orifice **7 Ureter, Left** See 6 Ureter, Right **8 Ureters, Bilateral** See 6 Ureter, Right **B Bladder** Trigone of bladder **C Bladder Neck** **D Urethra** Bulbourethral (Cowper's) gland Cowper's (bulbourethral) gland External urethral sphincter Internal urethral sphincter Membranous urethra Penile urethra Prostatic urethra	**0** Open **4** Percutaneous Endoscopic	**Z** No Device	**Z** No Qualifier

0 Medical and Surgical
T Urinary System
T Resection

Definition: Cutting out or off, without replacement, all of a body part

Explanation: None

Body Part Character 4	Approach Character 5	Device Character 6	Qualifier Character 7
0 Kidney, Right Renal calyx Renal capsule Renal cortex Renal segment	**1 Kidney, Left** See 0 Kidney, Right **2 Kidneys, Bilateral** See 0 Kidney, Right 	**0** Open	**Z** No Device	**Z** No Qualifier

Body Part Character 4	Approach Character 5	Device Character 6	Qualifier Character 7
0 Kidney, Right Renal calyx Renal capsule Renal cortex Renal segment **1 Kidney, Left** See 0 Kidney, Right **2 Kidneys, Bilateral** See 0 Kidney, Right	**0** Open	**Z** No Device	**Z** No Qualifier
0 Kidney, Right Renal calyx Renal capsule Renal cortex Renal segment **1 Kidney, Left** See 0 Kidney, Right **2 Kidneys, Bilateral** See 0 Kidney, Right	**4** Percutaneous Endoscopic	**Z** No Device	**G** Hand-assisted **Z** No Qualifier
3 Kidney Pelvis, Right Ureteropelvic junction (UPJ) **4 Kidney Pelvis, Left** See 3 Kidney Pelvis, Right **6 Ureter, Right** Ureteral orifice Ureterovesical orifice **7 Ureter, Left** See 6 Ureter, Right **B Bladder** ➕ Trigone of bladder **C Bladder Neck** **D Urethra** Bulbourethral (Cowper's) gland Cowper's (bulbourethral) gland External urethral sphincter Internal urethral sphincter Membranous urethra Penile urethra Prostatic urethra	**0** Open **4** Percutaneous Endoscopic **7** Via Natural or Artificial Opening **8** Via Natural or Artificial Opening Endoscopic	**Z** No Device	**Z** No Qualifier

Non-OR 0TTD[4,7,8]ZZ

See Appendix L for Procedure Combinations
Combo-only 0TTD0ZZ
➕ 0TTB0ZZ

0 Medical and Surgical
T Urinary System
U Supplement

Definition: Putting in or on biological or synthetic material that physically reinforces and/or augments the function of a portion of a body part

Explanation: The biological material is non-living, or is living and from the same individual. The body part may have been previously replaced, and the SUPPLEMENT procedure is performed to physically reinforce and/or augment the function of the replaced body part.

Body Part Character 4	Approach Character 5	Device Character 6	Qualifier Character 7

3 Kidney Pelvis, Right
   Ureteropelvic junction (UPJ)
4 Kidney Pelvis, Left
   See 3 Kidney Pelvis, Right
6 Ureter, Right
   Ureteral orifice
   Ureterovesical orifice
7 Ureter, Left
   See 6 Ureter, Right
B Bladder
   Trigone of bladder
C Bladder Neck
	0 Open
	4 Percutaneous Endoscopic
	7 Via Natural or Artificial Opening
	8 Via Natural or Artificial Opening Endoscopic
		7 Autologous Tissue Substitute
		J Synthetic Substitute
		K Nonautologous Tissue Substitute
			Z No Qualifier

D Urethra
   Bulbourethral (Cowper's) gland
   Cowper's (bulbourethral) gland
   External urethral sphincter
   Internal urethral sphincter
   Membranous urethra
   Penile urethra
   Prostatic urethra
	0 Open
	4 Percutaneous Endoscopic
	7 Via Natural or Artificial Opening
	8 Via Natural or Artificial Opening Endoscopic
	X External
		7 Autologous Tissue Substitute
		J Synthetic Substitute
		K Nonautologous Tissue Substitute
			Z No Qualifier

0 Medical and Surgical
T Urinary System
V Restriction

Definition: Partially closing an orifice or the lumen of a tubular body part

Explanation: The orifice can be a natural orifice or an artificially created orifice

Body Part Character 4	Approach Character 5	Device Character 6	Qualifier Character 7

3 Kidney Pelvis, Right
   Ureteropelvic junction (UPJ)
4 Kidney Pelvis, Left
   See 3 Kidney Pelvis, Right
6 Ureter, Right
   Ureteral orifice
   Ureterovesical orifice
7 Ureter, Left
   See 6 Ureter, Right
B Bladder
   Trigone of bladder
C Bladder Neck
	0 Open
	3 Percutaneous
	4 Percutaneous Endoscopic
		C Extraluminal Device
		D Intraluminal Device
		Z No Device
			Z No Qualifier

3 Kidney Pelvis, Right
   Ureteropelvic junction (UPJ)
4 Kidney Pelvis, Left
   See 3 Kidney Pelvis, Right
6 Ureter, Right
   Ureteral orifice
   Ureterovesical orifice
7 Ureter, Left
   See 6 Ureter, Right
B Bladder
   Trigone of bladder
C Bladder Neck
	7 Via Natural or Artificial Opening
	8 Via Natural or Artificial Opening Endoscopic
		D Intraluminal Device
		Z No Device
			Z No Qualifier

D Urethra
   Bulbourethral (Cowper's) gland
   Cowper's (bulbourethral) gland
   External urethral sphincter
   Internal urethral sphincter
   Membranous urethra
   Penile urethra
   Prostatic urethra
	0 Open
	3 Percutaneous
	4 Percutaneous Endoscopic
		C Extraluminal Device
		D Intraluminal Device
		Z No Device
			Z No Qualifier

D Urethra
   Bulbourethral (Cowper's) gland
   Cowper's (bulbourethral) gland
   External urethral sphincter
   Internal urethral sphincter
   Membranous urethra
   Penile urethra
   Prostatic urethra
	7 Via Natural or Artificial Opening
	8 Via Natural or Artificial Opening Endoscopic
		D Intraluminal Device
		Z No Device
			Z No Qualifier

D Urethra
   Bulbourethral (Cowper's) gland
   Cowper's (bulbourethral) gland
   External urethral sphincter
   Internal urethral sphincter
   Membranous urethra
   Penile urethra
   Prostatic urethra
	X External	Z No Device	Z No Qualifier

ICD-10-PCS 2025 Urinary System ØTW–ØTW

- Ø Medical and Surgical
- T Urinary System
- W Revision

Definition: Correcting, to the extent possible, a portion of a malfunctioning device or the position of a displaced device

Explanation: Revision can include correcting a malfunctioning or displaced device by taking out or putting in components of the device such as a screw or pin

Body Part Character 4	Approach Character 5	Device Character 6	Qualifier Character 7
5 Kidney Renal calyx Renal capsule Renal cortex Renal segment	Ø Open 3 Percutaneous 4 Percutaneous Endoscopic 7 Via Natural or Artificial Opening 8 Via Natural or Artificial Opening Endoscopic	Ø Drainage Device 2 Monitoring Device 3 Infusion Device 7 Autologous Tissue Substitute C Extraluminal Device D Intraluminal Device J Synthetic Substitute K Nonautologous Tissue Substitute Y Other Device	Z No Qualifier
5 Kidney Renal calyx Renal capsule Renal cortex Renal segment	X External	Ø Drainage Device 2 Monitoring Device 3 Infusion Device 7 Autologous Tissue Substitute C Extraluminal Device D Intraluminal Device J Synthetic Substitute K Nonautologous Tissue Substitute	Z No Qualifier
9 Ureter Ureteral orifice Ureterovesical orifice	Ø Open 3 Percutaneous 4 Percutaneous Endoscopic 7 Via Natural or Artificial Opening 8 Via Natural or Artificial Opening Endoscopic	Ø Drainage Device 2 Monitoring Device 3 Infusion Device 7 Autologous Tissue Substitute C Extraluminal Device D Intraluminal Device J Synthetic Substitute K Nonautologous Tissue Substitute M Stimulator Lead Y Other Device	Z No Qualifier
9 Ureter Ureteral orifice Ureterovesical orifice	X External	Ø Drainage Device 2 Monitoring Device 3 Infusion Device 7 Autologous Tissue Substitute C Extraluminal Device D Intraluminal Device J Synthetic Substitute K Nonautologous Tissue Substitute M Stimulator Lead	Z No Qualifier
B Bladder Trigone of bladder	Ø Open 3 Percutaneous 4 Percutaneous Endoscopic 7 Via Natural or Artificial Opening 8 Via Natural or Artificial Opening Endoscopic	Ø Drainage Device 2 Monitoring Device 3 Infusion Device 7 Autologous Tissue Substitute C Extraluminal Device D Intraluminal Device J Synthetic Substitute K Nonautologous Tissue Substitute L Artificial Sphincter M Stimulator Lead Y Other Device	Z No Qualifier
B Bladder Trigone of bladder	X External	Ø Drainage Device 2 Monitoring Device 3 Infusion Device 7 Autologous Tissue Substitute C Extraluminal Device D Intraluminal Device J Synthetic Substitute K Nonautologous Tissue Substitute L Artificial Sphincter M Stimulator Lead	Z No Qualifier

Non-OR ØTW5[3,4,7]YZ
Non-OR ØTW5X[Ø,2,3,7,C,D,J,K]Z
Non-OR ØTW9[3,4,7]YZ
Non-OR ØTW9X[Ø,2,3,7,C,D,J,K,M]Z
Non-OR ØTWB[3,4,7]YZ
Non-OR ØTWBX[Ø,2,3,7,C,D,J,K,L,M]Z

ØTW Continued on next page

Urinary System

0 Medical and Surgical
T Urinary System
W Revision — Definition: Correcting, to the extent possible, a portion of a malfunctioning device or the position of a displaced device
Explanation: Revision can include correcting a malfunctioning or displaced device by taking out or putting in components of the device such as a screw or pin

Body Part Character 4	Approach Character 5	Device Character 6	Qualifier Character 7
D Urethra Bulbourethral (Cowper's) gland Cowper's (bulbourethral) gland External urethral sphincter Internal urethral sphincter Membranous urethra Penile urethra Prostatic urethra	0 Open 3 Percutaneous 4 Percutaneous Endoscopic 7 Via Natural or Artificial Opening 8 Via Natural or Artificial Opening Endoscopic	0 Drainage Device 2 Monitoring Device 3 Infusion Device 7 Autologous Tissue Substitute C Extraluminal Device D Intraluminal Device J Synthetic Substitute K Nonautologous Tissue Substitute L Artificial Sphincter Y Other Device	Z No Qualifier
D Urethra Bulbourethral (Cowper's) gland Cowper's (bulbourethral) gland External urethral sphincter Internal urethral sphincter Membranous urethra Penile urethra Prostatic urethra	X External	0 Drainage Device 2 Monitoring Device 3 Infusion Device 7 Autologous Tissue Substitute C Extraluminal Device D Intraluminal Device J Synthetic Substitute K Nonautologous Tissue Substitute L Artificial Sphincter	Z No Qualifier

Non-OR 0TWD[3,4,7,8]YZ
Non-OR 0TWDX[0,2,3,7,C,D,J,K,L]Z

0 Medical and Surgical
T Urinary System
Y Transplantation — Definition: Putting in or on all or a portion of a living body part taken from another individual or animal to physically take the place and/or function of all or a portion of a similar body part
Explanation: The native body part may or may not be taken out, and the transplanted body part may take over all or a portion of its function

Body Part Character 4	Approach Character 5	Device Character 6	Qualifier Character 7
0 Kidney, Right LC + Renal calyx Renal capsule Renal cortex Renal segment **1 Kidney, Left** LC + See 0 Kidney, Right	0 Open	Z No Device	0 Allogeneic 1 Syngeneic 2 Zooplastic

LC 0TY[0,1]0Z[0,1,2]

See Appendix L for Procedure Combinations
+ 0TY[0,1]0Z[0,1,2]

Female Reproductive System 0U1–0UY

Character Meanings
This Character Meaning table is provided as a guide to assist the user in the identification of character members that may be found in this section of code tables. It **SHOULD NOT** be used to build a PCS code.

Operation–Character 3	Body Part–Character 4	Approach–Character 5	Device–Character 6	Qualifier–Character 7
1 Bypass	0 Ovary, Right	0 Open	0 Drainage Device	0 Allogeneic
2 Change	1 Ovary, Left	3 Percutaneous	1 Radioactive Element	1 Syngeneic
5 Destruction	2 Ovaries, Bilateral	4 Percutaneous Endoscopic	3 Infusion Device	2 Zooplastic
7 Dilation	3 Ovary	7 Via Natural or Artificial Opening	7 Autologous Tissue Substitute	5 Fallopian Tube, Right
8 Division	4 Uterine Supporting Structure	8 Via Natural or Artificial Opening Endoscopic	C Extraluminal Device	6 Fallopian Tube, Left
9 Drainage	5 Fallopian Tube, Right	F Via Natural or Artificial Opening With Percutaneous Endoscopic Assistance	D Intraluminal Device	9 Uterus
B Excision	6 Fallopian Tube, Left	X External	G Intraluminal Device, Pessary	L Supracervical
C Extirpation	7 Fallopian Tubes, Bilateral		H Contraceptive Device	X Diagnostic
D Extraction	8 Fallopian Tube		J Synthetic Substitute	Z No Qualifier
F Fragmentation	9 Uterus		K Nonautologous Tissue Substitute	
H Insertion	B Endometrium		Y Other Device	
J Inspection	C Cervix		Z No Device	
L Occlusion	D Uterus and Cervix			
M Reattachment	F Cul-de-sac			
N Release	G Vagina			
P Removal	H Vagina and Cul-de-sac			
Q Repair	J Clitoris			
S Reposition	K Hymen			
T Resection	L Vestibular Gland			
U Supplement	M Vulva			
V Restriction	N Ova			
W Revision				
Y Transplantation				

AHA Coding Clinic for table 0U5
2015, 3Q, 31 — Tubal ligation for sterilization

AHA Coding Clinic for table 0U7
2020, 2Q, 30 — Duhrssen cervical incision

AHA Coding Clinic for table 0U9
2016, 4Q, 58 — Longitudinal vaginal septum

AHA Coding Clinic for table 0UB
2018, 1Q, 23 — Tubal ligation procedure
2015, 3Q, 31 — Laparoscopic partial salpingectomy for ectopic pregnancy
2015, 3Q, 31 — Tubal ligation for sterilization
2014, 4Q, 16 — Excision of multiple uterine fibroids
2014, 3Q, 12 — Excision of skin tag from labia majora

AHA Coding Clinic for table 0UC
2015, 3Q, 30 — Removal of cervical cerclage
2013, 2Q, 38 — Evacuation of clot post-partum

AHA Coding Clinic for table 0UH
2020, 4Q, 43-44 — Insertion of radioactive element
2018, 1Q, 25 — Intrauterine brachytherapy & placement of tandems & ovoids
2013, 2Q, 34 — Placement of intrauterine device via open approach

AHA Coding Clinic for table 0UJ
2015, 1Q, 33 — Robotic-assisted laparoscopic hysterectomy converted to open procedure

AHA Coding Clinic for table 0UL
2018, 1Q, 23 — Tubal ligation procedure
2015, 3Q, 31 — Tubal ligation for sterilization

AHA Coding Clinic for table 0UP
2022, 3Q, 13 — Repair of prolapsed neovaginal graft

AHA Coding Clinic for table 0UQ
2020, 4Q, 59-60 — Extraction of ectopic products of conception
2014, 4Q, 18 — Obstetrical periurethral laceration
2013, 4Q, 120 — Repair of clitoral obstetric laceration

AHA Coding Clinic for table 0US
2016, 1Q, 9 — Anteversion of retroverted pregnant uterus

AHA Coding Clinic for table 0UT
2022, 1Q, 21 — Gravid hysterectomy due to placenta increta
2017, 4Q, 68 — New qualifier values - Supracervical hysterectomy
2015, 1Q, 33 — Robotic-assisted laparoscopic hysterectomy converted to open procedure
2013, 3Q, 28 — Total hysterectomy
2013, 1Q, 24 — Excision versus Resection of remaining ovarian remnant following previous excision

AHA Coding Clinic for table 0UV
2015, 3Q, 30 — Insertion of cervical cerclage

AHA Coding Clinic for table 0UY
2023, 2Q, 32 — Preparation of donor organ before transplantation
2018, 4Q, 40 — Uterus transplant

Female Reproductive System

Female Reproductive System

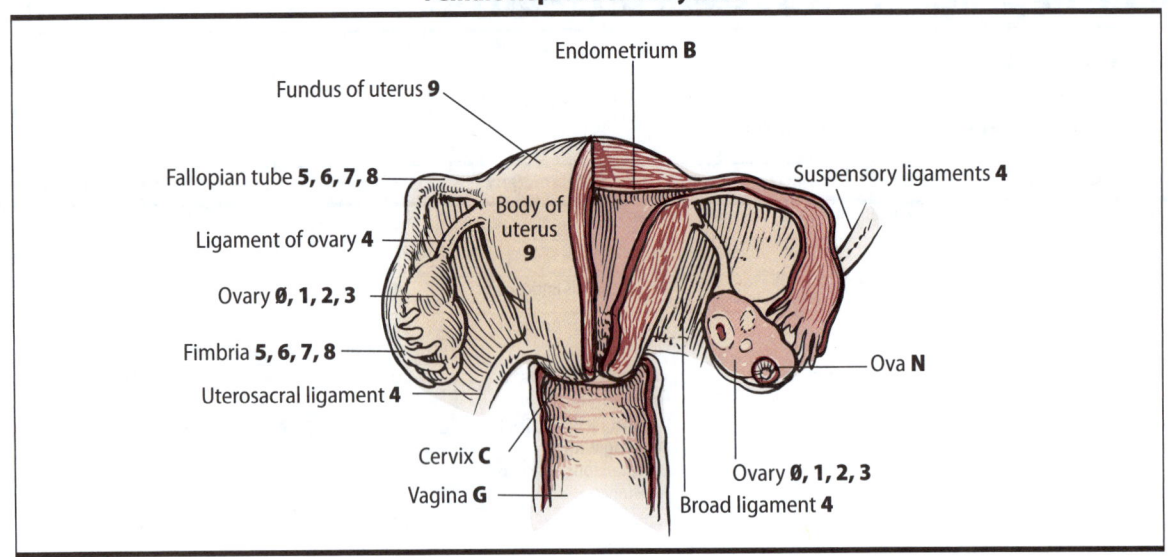

- Endometrium **B**
- Fundus of uterus **9**
- Fallopian tube **5, 6, 7, 8**
- Body of uterus **9**
- Suspensory ligaments **4**
- Ligament of ovary **4**
- Ovary **0, 1, 2, 3**
- Fimbria **5, 6, 7, 8**
- Ova **N**
- Uterosacral ligament **4**
- Cervix **C**
- Vagina **G**
- Ovary **0, 1, 2, 3**
- Broad ligament **4**

Female Internal/External Structures

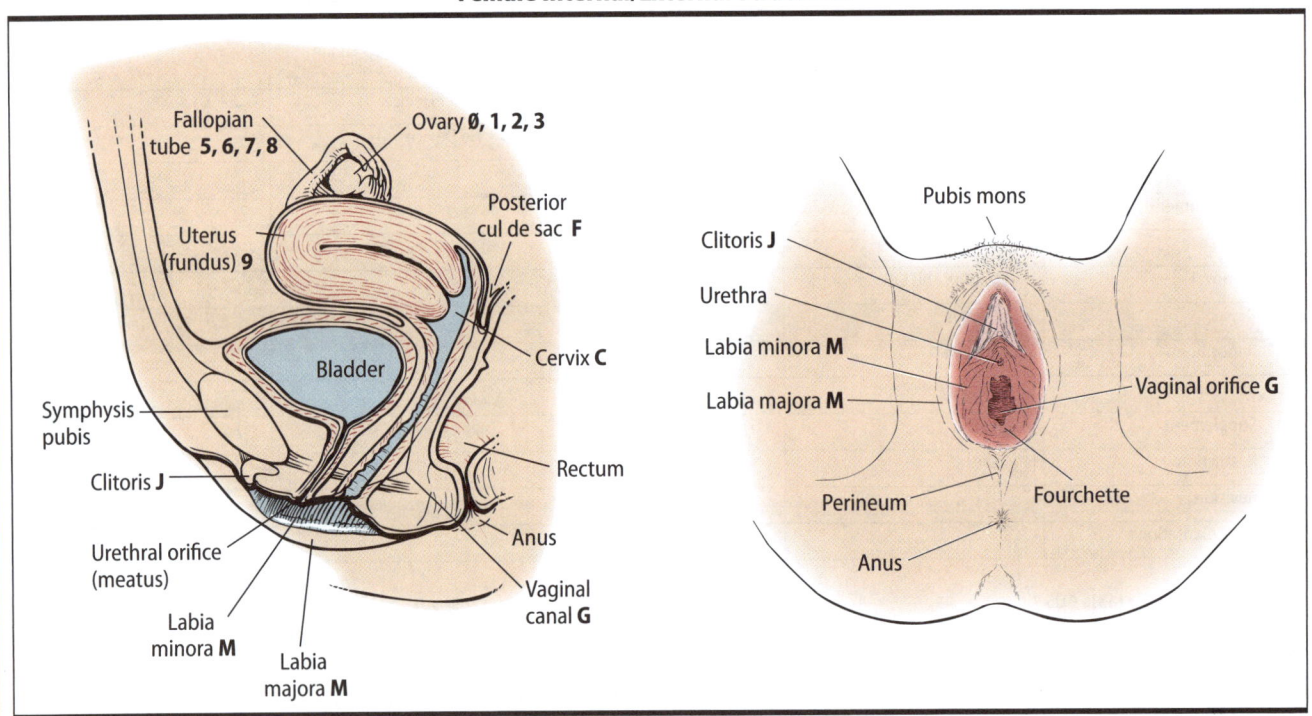

- Fallopian tube **5, 6, 7, 8**
- Ovary **0, 1, 2, 3**
- Uterus (fundus) **9**
- Posterior cul de sac **F**
- Bladder
- Cervix **C**
- Symphysis pubis
- Clitoris **J**
- Rectum
- Urethral orifice (meatus)
- Anus
- Labia minora **M**
- Vaginal canal **G**
- Labia majora **M**

- Pubis mons
- Clitoris **J**
- Urethra
- Labia minora **M**
- Labia majora **M**
- Vaginal orifice **G**
- Perineum
- Fourchette
- Anus

ICD-10-PCS 2025 — Female Reproductive System — 0U1–0U2

0 Medical and Surgical
U Female Reproductive System
1 Bypass   Definition: Altering the route of passage of the contents of a tubular body part

Explanation: Rerouting contents of a body part to a downstream area of the normal route, to a similar route and body part, or to an abnormal route and dissimilar body part. Includes one or more anastomoses, with or without the use of a device.

Body Part Character 4	Approach Character 5	Device Character 6	Qualifier Character 7

5 Fallopian Tube, Right
  Oviduct
  Salpinx
  Uterine tube
6 Fallopian Tube, Left
  See 5 Fallopian Tube, Right
	0 Open
	4 Percutaneous Endoscopic
		7 Autologous Tissue Substitute
		J Synthetic Substitute
		K Nonautologous Tissue Substitute
		Z No Device
			5 Fallopian Tube, Right
			6 Fallopian Tube, Left
			9 Uterus

0 Medical and Surgical
U Female Reproductive System
2 Change   Definition: Taking out or off a device from a body part and putting back an identical or similar device in or on the same body part without cutting or puncturing the skin or a mucous membrane

Explanation: All CHANGE procedures are coded using the approach EXTERNAL

Body Part Character 4	Approach Character 5	Device Character 6	Qualifier Character 7

3 Ovary
8 Fallopian Tube
M Vulva
  Labia majora
  Labia minora
	X External	0 Drainage Device
		Y Other Device
			Z No Qualifier

D Uterus and Cervix	X External	0 Drainage Device H Contraceptive Device Y Other Device	Z No Qualifier
H Vagina and Cul-de-sac	X External	0 Drainage Device G Intraluminal Device, Pessary Y Other Device	Z No Qualifier

Non-OR All body part, approach, device, and qualifier values

0 Medical and Surgical
U Female Reproductive System
5 Destruction   Definition: Physical eradication of all or a portion of a body part by the direct use of energy, force, or a destructive agent
   Explanation: None of the body part is physically taken out

Body Part Character 4	Approach Character 5	Device Character 6	Qualifier Character 7

0 Ovary, Right
1 Ovary, Left
2 Ovaries, Bilateral
4 Uterine Supporting Structure
    Broad ligament
    Infundibulopelvic ligament
    Ovarian ligament
    Round ligament of uterus
	0 Open
	3 Percutaneous
	4 Percutaneous Endoscopic
	8 Via Natural or Artificial Opening Endoscopic
		Z No Device	**Z** No Qualifier

5 Fallopian Tube, Right
    Oviduct
    Salpinx
    Uterine tube
6 Fallopian Tube, Left
    See 5 Fallopian Tube, Right
7 Fallopian Tubes, Bilateral `NC`
9 Uterus
    Fundus uteri
    Myometrium
    Perimetrium
    Uterine cornu
B Endometrium
C Cervix
F Cul-de-sac
	0 Open
	3 Percutaneous
	4 Percutaneous Endoscopic
	7 Via Natural or Artificial Opening
	8 Via Natural or Artificial Opening Endoscopic
		Z No Device	**Z** No Qualifier

G Vagina **K** Hymen	**0** Open **3** Percutaneous **4** Percutaneous Endoscopic **7** Via Natural or Artificial Opening **8** Via Natural or Artificial Opening Endoscopic **X** External	**Z** No Device	**Z** No Qualifier

J Clitoris
L Vestibular Gland
    Bartholin's (greater vestibular) gland
    Greater vestibular (Bartholin's) gland
    Paraurethral (Skene's) gland
    Skene's (paraurethral) gland
M Vulva
    Labia majora
    Labia minora
	0 Open
	X External
		Z No Device	**Z** No Qualifier

`NC` 0U57[0,3,4,7,8]ZZ with principal or secondary diagnosis of Z30.2

ICD-10-PCS 2025 — Female Reproductive System — 0U7–0U8

0 Medical and Surgical
U Female Reproductive System
7 Dilation Definition: Expanding an orifice or the lumen of a tubular body part
Explanation: The orifice can be a natural orifice or an artificially created orifice. Accomplished by stretching a tubular body part using intraluminal pressure or by cutting part of the orifice or wall of the tubular body part.

Body Part Character 4	Approach Character 5	Device Character 6	Qualifier Character 7

5 Fallopian Tube, Right
   Oviduct
   Salpinx
   Uterine tube
6 Fallopian Tube, Left
   See 5 Fallopian Tube, Right
7 Fallopian Tubes, Bilateral
9 Uterus
   Fundus uteri
   Myometrium
   Perimetrium
   Uterine cornu
C Cervix
G Vagina
	0 Open
	3 Percutaneous
	4 Percutaneous Endoscopic
	7 Via Natural or Artificial Opening
	8 Via Natural or Artificial Opening Endoscopic
		D Intraluminal Device
		Z No Device
			Z No Qualifier

K Hymen	0 Open 3 Percutaneous 4 Percutaneous Endoscopic 7 Via Natural or Artificial Opening 8 Via Natural or Artificial Opening Endoscopic X External	D Intraluminal Device Z No Device	Z No Qualifier

Non-OR 0U7C[0,3,4,7,8][D,Z]Z
Non-OR 0U7G[7,8][D,Z]Z

0 Medical and Surgical
U Female Reproductive System
8 Division Definition: Cutting into a body part, without draining fluids and/or gases from the body part, in order to separate or transect a body part
Explanation: All or a portion of the body part is separated into two or more portions

Body Part Character 4	Approach Character 5	Device Character 6	Qualifier Character 7

0 Ovary, Right
1 Ovary, Left
2 Ovaries, Bilateral
4 Uterine Supporting Structure
   Broad ligament
   Infundibulopelvic ligament
   Ovarian ligament
   Round ligament of uterus
	0 Open
	3 Percutaneous
	4 Percutaneous Endoscopic
		Z No Device	Z No Qualifier

K Hymen	7 Via Natural or Artificial Opening 8 Via Natural or Artificial Opening Endoscopic X External	Z No Device	Z No Qualifier

Non-OR 0U8K[7,8,X]ZZ

0 Medical and Surgical
U Female Reproductive System
9 Drainage — Definition: Taking or letting out fluids and/or gases from a body part
Explanation: The qualifier DIAGNOSTIC is used to identify drainage procedures that are biopsies

Body Part Character 4	Approach Character 5	Device Character 6	Qualifier Character 7
0 Ovary, Right 1 Ovary, Left 2 Ovaries, Bilateral	0 Open 3 Percutaneous 4 Percutaneous Endoscopic 8 Via Natural or Artificial Opening Endoscopic	0 Drainage Device	Z No Qualifier
0 Ovary, Right 1 Ovary, Left 2 Ovaries, Bilateral	0 Open 3 Percutaneous 4 Percutaneous Endoscopic 8 Via Natural or Artificial Opening Endoscopic	Z No Device	X Diagnostic Z No Qualifier
0 Ovary, Right 1 Ovary, Left 2 Ovaries, Bilateral	X External	Z No Device	Z No Qualifier

4 Uterine Supporting Structure
  Broad ligament
  Infundibulopelvic ligament
  Ovarian ligament
  Round ligament of uterus
	0 Open
	3 Percutaneous
	4 Percutaneous Endoscopic
	8 Via Natural or Artificial Opening Endoscopic
		0 Drainage Device	Z No Qualifier

4 Uterine Supporting Structure
  Broad ligament
  Infundibulopelvic ligament
  Ovarian ligament
  Round ligament of uterus
	0 Open
	3 Percutaneous
	4 Percutaneous Endoscopic
	8 Via Natural or Artificial Opening Endoscopic
		Z No Device	X Diagnostic
			Z No Qualifier

5 Fallopian Tube, Right
  Oviduct
  Salpinx
  Uterine tube
6 Fallopian Tube, Left
  See 5 Fallopian Tube, Right
7 Fallopian Tubes, Bilateral
9 Uterus
  Fundus uteri
  Myometrium
  Perimetrium
  Uterine cornu
C Cervix
F Cul-de-sac
	0 Open
	3 Percutaneous
	4 Percutaneous Endoscopic
	7 Via Natural or Artificial Opening
	8 Via Natural or Artificial Opening Endoscopic
		0 Drainage Device	Z No Qualifier

5 Fallopian Tube, Right
  Oviduct
  Salpinx
  Uterine tube
6 Fallopian Tube, Left
  See 5 Fallopian Tube, Right
7 Fallopian Tubes, Bilateral
9 Uterus
  Fundus uteri
  Myometrium
  Perimetrium
  Uterine cornu
C Cervix
F Cul-de-sac
	0 Open
	3 Percutaneous
	4 Percutaneous Endoscopic
	7 Via Natural or Artificial Opening
	8 Via Natural or Artificial Opening Endoscopic
		Z No Device	X Diagnostic
			Z No Qualifier

Non-OR 0U9[0,1,2][3,8]0Z
Non-OR 0U9[0,1,2][3,8]ZZ
Non-OR 0U9[0,1,2]8ZX
Non-OR 0U94[3,8]0Z
Non-OR 0U94[3,8]ZZ
Non-OR 0U948ZX
Non-OR 0U9[5,6,7,9,C]30Z
Non-OR 0U9F[3,4]0Z
Non-OR 0U9[5,6,7][3,4,7,8]ZZ
Non-OR 0U9[9,C]3ZZ
Non-OR 0U9F[3,4]ZZ

0U9 Continued on next page

ICD-10-PCS 2025 — Female Reproductive System — 0U9–0U9

0U9 Continued

- **0** Medical and Surgical
- **U** Female Reproductive System
- **9** Drainage   Definition: Taking or letting out fluids and/or gases from a body part
  Explanation: The qualifier DIAGNOSTIC is used to identify drainage procedures that are biopsies

Body Part Character 4	Approach Character 5	Device Character 6	Qualifier Character 7
G Vagina **K** Hymen	**0** Open **3** Percutaneous **4** Percutaneous Endoscopic **7** Via Natural or Artificial Opening **8** Via Natural or Artificial Opening Endoscopic **X** External	**0** Drainage Device	**Z** No Qualifier
G Vagina **K** Hymen	**0** Open **3** Percutaneous **4** Percutaneous Endoscopic **7** Via Natural or Artificial Opening **8** Via Natural or Artificial Opening Endoscopic **X** External	**Z** No Device	**X** Diagnostic **Z** No Qualifier

J Clitoris
L Vestibular Gland
   Bartholin's (greater vestibular) gland
   Greater vestibular (Bartholin's) gland
   Paraurethral (Skene's) gland
   Skene's (paraurethral) gland
M Vulva
   Labia majora
   Labia minora
	0 Open
	X External
		0 Drainage Device	**Z** No Qualifier

J Clitoris
L Vestibular Gland
   Bartholin's (greater vestibular) gland
   Greater vestibular (Bartholin's) gland
   Paraurethral (Skene's) gland
   Skene's (paraurethral) gland
M Vulva
   Labia majora
   Labia minora
	0 Open
	X External
		Z No Device	**X** Diagnostic
			Z No Qualifier

Non-OR   0U9G30Z
Non-OR   0U9K[0,3,4,7,8,X]0Z
Non-OR   0U9G3ZZ
Non-OR   0U9K[0,3,4,7,8,X]ZZ

Non-OR   0U9L[0,X]0Z
Non-OR   0U9L[0,X]Z[X,Z]

Female Reproductive System

0 Medical and Surgical
U Female Reproductive System
B Excision Definition: Cutting out or off, without replacement, a portion of a body part
Explanation: The qualifier DIAGNOSTIC is used to identify excision procedures that are biopsies

Body Part Character 4	Approach Character 5	Device Character 6	Qualifier Character 7
0 Ovary, Right **1** Ovary, Left **2** Ovaries, Bilateral **4** Uterine Supporting Structure 　Broad ligament 　Infundibulopelvic ligament 　Ovarian ligament 　Round ligament of uterus **5** Fallopian Tube, Right 　Oviduct 　Salpinx 　Uterine tube **6** Fallopian Tube, Left 　*See* 5 Fallopian Tube, Right **7** Fallopian Tubes, Bilateral **9** Uterus 　Fundus uteri 　Myometrium 　Perimetrium 　Uterine cornu **C** Cervix **F** Cul-de-sac	**0** Open **3** Percutaneous **4** Percutaneous Endoscopic **7** Via Natural or Artificial Opening **8** Via Natural or Artificial Opening Endoscopic	**Z** No Device	**X** Diagnostic **Z** No Qualifier
G Vagina **K** Hymen	**0** Open **3** Percutaneous **4** Percutaneous Endoscopic **7** Via Natural or Artificial Opening **8** Via Natural or Artificial Opening Endoscopic **X** External	**Z** No Device	**X** Diagnostic **Z** No Qualifier
J Clitoris **L** Vestibular Gland 　Bartholin's (greater vestibular) gland 　Greater vestibular (Bartholin's) gland 　Paraurethral (Skene's) gland 　Skene's (paraurethral) gland **M** Vulva 　Labia majora 　Labia minora	**0** Open **X** External	**Z** No Device	**X** Diagnostic **Z** No Qualifier

0 Medical and Surgical
U Female Reproductive System
C Extirpation   Definition: Taking or cutting out solid matter from a body part
Explanation: The solid matter may be an abnormal byproduct of a biological function or a foreign body; it may be imbedded in a body part or in the lumen of a tubular body part. The solid matter may or may not have been previously broken into pieces.

Body Part Character 4	Approach Character 5	Device Character 6	Qualifier Character 7

0 Ovary, Right
1 Ovary, Left
2 Ovaries, Bilateral
4 Uterine Supporting Structure
   Broad ligament
   Infundibulopelvic ligament
   Ovarian ligament
   Round ligament of uterus
	0 Open
	3 Percutaneous
	4 Percutaneous Endoscopic
	8 Via Natural or Artificial Opening Endoscopic
		Z No Device	**Z** No Qualifier

5 Fallopian Tube, Right
   Oviduct
   Salpinx
   Uterine tube
6 Fallopian Tube, Left
   See 5 Fallopian Tube, Right
7 Fallopian Tubes, Bilateral
9 Uterus
   Fundus uteri
   Myometrium
   Perimetrium
   Uterine cornu
B Endometrium
C Cervix
F Cul-de-sac
	0 Open
	3 Percutaneous
	4 Percutaneous Endoscopic
	7 Via Natural or Artificial Opening
	8 Via Natural or Artificial Opening Endoscopic
		Z No Device	**Z** No Qualifier

G Vagina **K** Hymen	**0** Open **3** Percutaneous **4** Percutaneous Endoscopic **7** Via Natural or Artificial Opening **8** Via Natural or Artificial Opening Endoscopic **X** External	**Z** No Device	**Z** No Qualifier

J Clitoris
L Vestibular Gland
   Bartholin's (greater vestibular) gland
   Greater vestibular (Bartholin's) gland
   Paraurethral (Skene's) gland
   Skene's (paraurethral) gland
M Vulva
   Labia majora
   Labia minora
	0 Open
	X External
		Z No Device	**Z** No Qualifier

Non-OR 0UC9[7,8]ZZ
Non-OR 0UCG[7,8,X]ZZ
Non-OR 0UCK[0,3,4,7,8,X]ZZ
Non-OR 0UCMXZZ

---

0 Medical and Surgical
U Female Reproductive System
D Extraction   Definition: Pulling or stripping out or off all or a portion of a body part by the use of force
Explanation: The qualifier DIAGNOSTIC is used to identify extraction procedures that are biopsies

Body Part Character 4	Approach Character 5	Device Character 6	Qualifier Character 7
B Endometrium	**7** Via Natural or Artificial Opening **8** Via Natural or Artificial Opening Endoscopic	**Z** No Device	**X** Diagnostic **Z** No Qualifier
N Ova	**0** Open **3** Percutaneous **4** Percutaneous Endoscopic	**Z** No Device	**Z** No Qualifier

Ø Medical and Surgical
U Female Reproductive System
F Fragmentation

Definition: Breaking solid matter in a body part into pieces

Explanation: Physical force (e.g., manual, ultrasonic) applied directly or indirectly is used to break the solid matter into pieces. The solid matter may be an abnormal byproduct of a biological function or a foreign body. The pieces of solid matter are not taken out.

Body Part Character 4	Approach Character 5	Device Character 6	Qualifier Character 7

5 Fallopian Tube, Right [NC]
   Oviduct
   Salpinx
   Uterine tube
6 Fallopian Tube, Left [NC]
   See 5 Fallopian Tube, Right
7 Fallopian Tubes, Bilateral [NC]
9 Uterus [NC]
   Fundus uteri
   Myometrium
   Perimetrium
   Uterine cornu
	Ø Open
	3 Percutaneous
	4 Percutaneous Endoscopic
	7 Via Natural or Artificial Opening
	8 Via Natural or Artificial Opening Endoscopic
	X External
		Z No Device	Z No Qualifier

Non-OR   ØUF[5,6,7,9]XZZ
[NC]   ØUF[5,6,7,9]XZZ

Ø Medical and Surgical
U Female Reproductive System
H Insertion

Definition: Putting in a nonbiological appliance that monitors, assists, performs, or prevents a physiological function but does not physically take the place of a body part

Explanation: None

Body Part Character 4	Approach Character 5	Device Character 6	Qualifier Character 7
3 Ovary	Ø Open 3 Percutaneous 4 Percutaneous Endoscopic	1 Radioactive Element 3 Infusion Device Y Other Device	Z No Qualifier
3 Ovary	7 Via Natural or Artificial Opening 8 Via Natural or Artificial Opening Endoscopic	1 Radioactive Element Y Other Device	Z No Qualifier
8 Fallopian Tube D Uterus and Cervix H Vagina and Cul-de-sac	Ø Open 3 Percutaneous 4 Percutaneous Endoscopic 7 Via Natural or Artificial Opening 8 Via Natural or Artificial Opening Endoscopic	3 Infusion Device Y Other Device	Z No Qualifier

9 Uterus
   Fundus uteri
   Myometrium
   Perimetrium
   Uterine cornu
	Ø Open
	7 Via Natural or Artificial Opening
	8 Via Natural or Artificial Opening Endoscopic
		1 Radioactive Element
		H Contraceptive Device
			Z No Qualifier

C Cervix	Ø Open 3 Percutaneous 4 Percutaneous Endoscopic	1 Radioactive Element	Z No Qualifier
C Cervix	7 Via Natural or Artificial Opening 8 Via Natural or Artificial Opening Endoscopic	1 Radioactive Element H Contraceptive Device	Z No Qualifier
F Cul-de-sac	7 Via Natural or Artificial Opening 8 Via Natural or Artificial Opening Endoscopic	G Intraluminal Device, Pessary	Z No Qualifier
G Vagina	Ø Open 3 Percutaneous 4 Percutaneous Endoscopic X External	1 Radioactive Element	Z No Qualifier
G Vagina	7 Via Natural or Artificial Opening 8 Via Natural or Artificial Opening Endoscopic	1 Radioactive Element G Intraluminal Device, Pessary	Z No Qualifier

Non-OR   ØUH3[Ø,4][3,Y]Z
Non-OR   ØUH33[1,3,Y]Z
Non-OR   ØUH3[7,8][1,Y]Z
Non-OR   ØUH[8,D][Ø,3,4,7,8][3,Y]Z
Non-OR   ØUHH[3,4]YZ
Non-OR   ØUHH[7,8][3,Y]Z
Non-OR   ØUH9[Ø,7,8][1,H]Z
Non-OR   ØUHC[7,8]HZ
Non-OR   ØUHF[7,8]HZ
Non-OR   ØUHG[7,8]HZ

Female Reproductive System

0 Medical and Surgical
U Female Reproductive System
J Inspection   Definition: Visually and/or manually exploring a body part
Explanation: Visual exploration may be performed with or without optical instrumentation. Manual exploration may be performed directly or through intervening body layers.

Body Part Character 4	Approach Character 5	Device Character 6	Qualifier Character 7
3 Ovary	**0** Open **3** Percutaneous **4** Percutaneous Endoscopic **8** Via Natural or Artificial Opening Endoscopic **X** External	**Z** No Device	**Z** No Qualifier
8 Fallopian Tube **D** Uterus and Cervix **H** Vagina and Cul-de-sac	**0** Open **3** Percutaneous **4** Percutaneous Endoscopic **7** Via Natural or Artificial Opening **8** Via Natural or Artificial Opening Endoscopic **X** External	**Z** No Device	**Z** No Qualifier
M Vulva Labia majora Labia minora	**0** Open **X** External	**Z** No Device	**Z** No Qualifier

Non-OR 0UJ3[3,8,X]ZZ
Non-OR 0UJ[8,D,H][3,7,8,X]ZZ
Non-OR 0UJMXZZ

---

0 Medical and Surgical
U Female Reproductive System
L Occlusion   Definition: Completely closing an orifice or the lumen of a tubular body part
Explanation: The orifice can be a natural orifice or an artificially created orifice

Body Part Character 4	Approach Character 5	Device Character 6	Qualifier Character 7
5 Fallopian Tube, Right Oviduct Salpinx Uterine tube **6** Fallopian Tube, Left *See 5 Fallopian Tube, Right* **7** Fallopian Tubes, Bilateral NC	**0** Open **3** Percutaneous **4** Percutaneous Endoscopic	**C** Extraluminal Device **D** Intraluminal Device **Z** No Device	**Z** No Qualifier
5 Fallopian Tube, Right Oviduct Salpinx Uterine tube **6** Fallopian Tube, Left *See 5 Fallopian Tube, Right* **7** Fallopian Tubes, Bilateral NC	**7** Via Natural or Artificial Opening **8** Via Natural or Artificial Opening Endoscopic	**D** Intraluminal Device **Z** No Device	**Z** No Qualifier
F Cul-de-sac **G** Vagina	**7** Via Natural or Artificial Opening **8** Via Natural or Artificial Opening Endoscopic	**D** Intraluminal Device **Z** No Device	**Z** No Qualifier

NC 0UL7[0,3,4][C,D,Z]Z with principal or secondary diagnosis of Z30.2
NC 0UL7[7,8][D,Z]Z with principal or secondary diagnosis of Z30.2

0 **Medical and Surgical**
U **Female Reproductive System**
M **Reattachment**   Definition: Putting back in or on all or a portion of a separated body part to its normal location or other suitable location
                      Explanation: Vascular circulation and nervous pathways may or may not be reestablished

Body Part Character 4	Approach Character 5	Device Character 6	Qualifier Character 7

0 Ovary, Right
1 Ovary, Left
2 Ovaries, Bilateral
4 Uterine Supporting Structure
   Broad ligament
   Infundibulopelvic ligament
   Ovarian ligament
   Round ligament of uterus
5 Fallopian Tube, Right
   Oviduct
   Salpinx
   Uterine tube
6 Fallopian Tube, Left
   See 5 Fallopian Tube, Right
7 Fallopian Tubes, Bilateral
9 Uterus
   Fundus uteri
   Myometrium
   Perimetrium
   Uterine cornu
C Cervix
F Cul-de-sac
G Vagina
	0 Open
	4 Percutaneous Endoscopic
		Z No Device	Z No Qualifier

J Clitoris
M Vulva
   Labia majora
   Labia minora
	X External	Z No Device	Z No Qualifier

K Hymen	0 Open 4 Percutaneous Endoscopic X External	Z No Device	Z No Qualifier

0 Medical and Surgical
U Female Reproductive System
N Release Definition: Freeing a body part from an abnormal physical constraint by cutting or by the use of force
Explanation: Some of the restraining tissue may be taken out but none of the body part is taken out

Body Part Character 4	Approach Character 5	Device Character 6	Qualifier Character 7
0 Ovary, Right **1** Ovary, Left **2** Ovaries, Bilateral **4** Uterine Supporting Structure 　Broad ligament 　Infundibulopelvic ligament 　Ovarian ligament 　Round ligament of uterus	**0** Open **3** Percutaneous **4** Percutaneous Endoscopic **8** Via Natural or Artificial Opening Endoscopic	**Z** No Device	**Z** No Qualifier
5 Fallopian Tube, Right 　Oviduct 　Salpinx 　Uterine tube **6** Fallopian Tube, Left 　See 5 Fallopian Tube, Right **7** Fallopian Tubes, Bilateral **9** Uterus 　Fundus uteri 　Myometrium 　Perimetrium 　Uterine cornu **C** Cervix **F** Cul-de-sac	**0** Open **3** Percutaneous **4** Percutaneous Endoscopic **7** Via Natural or Artificial Opening **8** Via Natural or Artificial Opening Endoscopic	**Z** No Device	**Z** No Qualifier
G Vagina **K** Hymen	**0** Open **3** Percutaneous **4** Percutaneous Endoscopic **7** Via Natural or Artificial Opening **8** Via Natural or Artificial Opening Endoscopic **X** External	**Z** No Device	**Z** No Qualifier
J Clitoris **L** Vestibular Gland 　Bartholin's (greater vestibular) gland 　Greater vestibular (Bartholin's) gland 　Paraurethral (Skene's) gland 　Skene's (paraurethral) gland **M** Vulva 　Labia majora 　Labia minora	**0** Open **X** External	**Z** No Device	**Z** No Qualifier

Female Reproductive System

0 **Medical and Surgical**
U **Female Reproductive System**
P **Removal** Definition: Taking out or off a device from a body part
Explanation: If a device is taken out and a similar device put in without cutting or puncturing the skin or mucous membrane, the procedure is coded to the root operation CHANGE. Otherwise, the procedure for taking out the device is coded to the root operation REMOVAL.

Body Part Character 4	Approach Character 5	Device Character 6	Qualifier Character 7
3 Ovary	0 Open 3 Percutaneous 4 Percutaneous Endoscopic	0 Drainage Device 3 Infusion Device Y Other Device	Z No Qualifier
3 Ovary	7 Via Natural or Artificial Opening 8 Via Natural or Artificial Opening Endoscopic	Y Other Device	Z No Qualifier
3 Ovary	X External	0 Drainage Device 3 Infusion Device	Z No Qualifier
8 Fallopian Tube	0 Open 3 Percutaneous 4 Percutaneous Endoscopic 7 Via Natural or Artificial Opening 8 Via Natural or Artificial Opening Endoscopic	0 Drainage Device 3 Infusion Device 7 Autologous Tissue Substitute C Extraluminal Device D Intraluminal Device J Synthetic Substitute K Nonautologous Tissue Substitute Y Other Device	Z No Qualifier
8 Fallopian Tube	X External	0 Drainage Device 3 Infusion Device D Intraluminal Device	Z No Qualifier
D Uterus and Cervix	0 Open 3 Percutaneous 4 Percutaneous Endoscopic 7 Via Natural or Artificial Opening 8 Via Natural or Artificial Opening Endoscopic	0 Drainage Device 1 Radioactive Element 3 Infusion Device 7 Autologous Tissue Substitute C Extraluminal Device D Intraluminal Device H Contraceptive Device J Synthetic Substitute K Nonautologous Tissue Substitute Y Other Device	Z No Qualifier
D Uterus and Cervix	X External	0 Drainage Device 3 Infusion Device D Intraluminal Device H Contraceptive Device	Z No Qualifier
H Vagina and Cul-de-sac	0 Open 3 Percutaneous 4 Percutaneous Endoscopic 7 Via Natural or Artificial Opening 8 Via Natural or Artificial Opening Endoscopic	0 Drainage Device 1 Radioactive Element 3 Infusion Device 7 Autologous Tissue Substitute D Intraluminal Device J Synthetic Substitute K Nonautologous Tissue Substitute Y Other Device	Z No Qualifier
H Vagina and Cul-de-sac	X External	0 Drainage Device 1 Radioactive Element 3 Infusion Device D Intraluminal Device	Z No Qualifier
M Vulva Labia majora Labia minora	0 Open	0 Drainage Device 7 Autologous Tissue Substitute J Synthetic Substitute K Nonautologous Tissue Substitute	Z No Qualifier
M Vulva Labia majora Labia minora	X External	0 Drainage Device	Z No Qualifier

Non-OR 0UP3[3,4]YZ
Non-OR 0UP3[7,8]YZ
Non-OR 0UP3X[0,3]Z
Non-OR 0UP8[3,4]YZ
Non-OR 0UP8[7,8][0,3,D,Y]Z
Non-OR 0UP8X[0,3,D]Z
Non-OR 0UPD[3,4][C,Y]Z
Non-OR 0UPD[7,8][0,3,C,D,H,Y]Z
Non-OR 0UPDX[0,3,D,H]Z
Non-OR 0UPH[3,4]YZ
Non-OR 0UPH[7,8][0,3,D,Y]Z
Non-OR 0UPHX[0,1,3,D]Z
Non-OR 0UPMX0Z

ICD-10-PCS 2025 — Female Reproductive System — ØUQ–ØUS

Ø Medical and Surgical
U Female Reproductive System
Q Repair — Definition: Restoring, to the extent possible, a body part to its normal anatomic structure and function
Explanation: Used only when the method to accomplish the repair is not one of the other root operations

Body Part Character 4	Approach Character 5	Device Character 6	Qualifier Character 7

Ø Ovary, Right
1 Ovary, Left
2 Ovaries, Bilateral
4 Uterine Supporting Structure
   Broad ligament
   Infundibulopelvic ligament
   Ovarian ligament
   Round ligament of uterus
	Ø Open
	3 Percutaneous
	4 Percutaneous Endoscopic
	8 Via Natural or Artificial Opening Endoscopic
		Z No Device	**Z** No Qualifier

5 Fallopian Tube, Right
   Oviduct
   Salpinx
   Uterine tube
6 Fallopian Tube, Left
   See 5 Fallopian Tube, Right
7 Fallopian Tubes, Bilateral
9 Uterus
   Fundus uteri
   Myometrium
   Perimetrium
   Uterine cornu
C Cervix
F Cul-de-sac
	Ø Open
	3 Percutaneous
	4 Percutaneous Endoscopic
	7 Via Natural or Artificial Opening
	8 Via Natural or Artificial Opening Endoscopic
		Z No Device	**Z** No Qualifier

G Vagina **K** Hymen	**Ø** Open **3** Percutaneous **4** Percutaneous Endoscopic **7** Via Natural or Artificial Opening **8** Via Natural or Artificial Opening Endoscopic **X** External	**Z** No Device	**Z** No Qualifier

J Clitoris
L Vestibular Gland
   Bartholin's (greater vestibular) gland
   Greater vestibular (Bartholin's) gland
   Paraurethral (Skene's) gland
   Skene's (paraurethral) gland
M Vulva
   Labia majora
   Labia minora
	Ø Open
	X External
		Z No Device	**Z** No Qualifier

Non-OR ØUQG[7,X]ZZ
Non-OR ØUQKXZZ
Non-OR ØUQMXZZ

Ø Medical and Surgical
U Female Reproductive System
S Reposition — Definition: Moving to its normal location, or other suitable location, all or a portion of a body part
Explanation: The body part is moved to a new location from an abnormal location, or from a normal location where it is not functioning correctly. The body part may or may not be cut out or off to be moved to the new location.

Body Part Character 4	Approach Character 5	Device Character 6	Qualifier Character 7

Ø Ovary, Right
1 Ovary, Left
2 Ovaries, Bilateral
4 Uterine Supporting Structure
   Broad ligament
   Infundibulopelvic ligament
   Ovarian ligament
   Round ligament of uterus
5 Fallopian Tube, Right
   Oviduct
   Salpinx
   Uterine tube
6 Fallopian Tube, Left
   See 5 Fallopian Tube, Right
7 Fallopian Tubes, Bilateral
C Cervix
F Cul-de-sac
	Ø Open
	4 Percutaneous Endoscopic
	8 Via Natural or Artificial Opening Endoscopic
		Z No Device	**Z** No Qualifier

9 Uterus
   Fundus uteri
   Myometrium
   Perimetrium
   Uterine cornu
G Vagina
	Ø Open
	4 Percutaneous Endoscopic
	7 Via Natural or Artificial Opening
	8 Via Natural or Artificial Opening Endoscopic
	X External
		Z No Device	**Z** No Qualifier

Non-OR ØUS9XZZ

Female Reproductive System

0 Medical and Surgical
U Female Reproductive System
T Resection   Definition: Cutting out or off, without replacement, all of a body part
            Explanation: None

Body Part Character 4	Approach Character 5	Device Character 6	Qualifier Character 7

0 Ovary, Right
1 Ovary, Left
2 Ovaries, Bilateral ✚
5 Fallopian Tube, Right
   Oviduct
   Salpinx
   Uterine tube
6 Fallopian Tube, Left
   See 5 Fallopian Tube, Right
7 Fallopian Tubes, Bilateral ✚
	0 Open
	4 Percutaneous Endoscopic
	7 Via Natural or Artificial Opening
	8 Via Natural or Artificial Opening Endoscopic
	F Via Natural or Artificial Opening With Percutaneous Endoscopic Assistance
		Z No Device	Z No Qualifier

4 Uterine Supporting Structure ✚
   Broad ligament
   Infundibulopelvic ligament
   Ovarian ligament
   Round ligament of uterus
C Cervix ✚
F Cul-de-sac
G Vagina ✚
	0 Open
	4 Percutaneous Endoscopic
	7 Via Natural or Artificial Opening
	8 Via Natural or Artificial Opening Endoscopic
		Z No Device	Z No Qualifier

9 Uterus ✚
   Fundus uteri
   Myometrium
   Perimetrium
   Uterine cornu
	0 Open
	4 Percutaneous Endoscopic
	7 Via Natural or Artificial Opening
	8 Via Natural or Artificial Opening Endoscopic
	F Via Natural or Artificial Opening With Percutaneous Endoscopic Assistance
		Z No Device	L Supracervical
			Z No Qualifier

J Clitoris
L Vestibular Gland
   Bartholin's (greater vestibular) gland
   Greater vestibular (Bartholin's) gland
   Paraurethral (Skene's) gland
   Skene's (paraurethral) gland
M Vulva ✚
   Labia majora
   Labia minora
	0 Open
	X External
		Z No Device	Z No Qualifier

K Hymen	0 Open 4 Percutaneous Endoscopic 7 Via Natural or Artificial Opening 8 Via Natural or Artificial Opening Endoscopic X External	Z No Device	Z No Device

See Appendix L for Procedure Combinations
   ✚ 0UT[2,7]0ZZ
   ✚ 0UT[4,C][0,4,7,8]ZZ
   ✚ 0UTG0ZZ
   ✚ 0UT9[0,4,7,8,F]ZZ
   ✚ 0UTM[0,X]ZZ

ICD-10-PCS 2025 — Female Reproductive System — 0UU–0UV

0 Medical and Surgical
U Female Reproductive System
U Supplement Definition: Putting in or on biological or synthetic material that physically reinforces and/or augments the function of a portion of a body part
Explanation: The biological material is non-living, or is living and from the same individual. The body part may have been previously replaced, and the SUPPLEMENT procedure is performed to physically reinforce and/or augment the function of the replaced body part.

Body Part Character 4	Approach Character 5	Device Character 6	Qualifier Character 7
4 Uterine Supporting Structure Broad ligament Infundibulopelvic ligament Ovarian ligament Round ligament of uterus	**0** Open **4** Percutaneous Endoscopic	**7** Autologous Tissue Substitute **J** Synthetic Substitute **K** Nonautologous Tissue Substitute	**Z** No Qualifier
5 Fallopian Tube, Right Oviduct Salpinx Uterine tube **6** Fallopian Tube, Left See 5 Fallopian Tube, Right **7** Fallopian Tubes, Bilateral **F** Cul-de-sac	**0** Open **4** Percutaneous Endoscopic **7** Via Natural or Artificial Opening **8** Via Natural or Artificial Opening Endoscopic	**7** Autologous Tissue Substitute **J** Synthetic Substitute **K** Nonautologous Tissue Substitute	**Z** No Qualifier
G Vagina **K** Hymen	**0** Open **4** Percutaneous Endoscopic **7** Via Natural or Artificial Opening **8** Via Natural or Artificial Opening Endoscopic **X** External	**7** Autologous Tissue Substitute **J** Synthetic Substitute **K** Nonautologous Tissue Substitute	**Z** No Qualifier
J Clitoris **M** Vulva Labia majora Labia minora	**0** Open **X** External	**7** Autologous Tissue Substitute **J** Synthetic Substitute **K** Nonautologous Tissue Substitute	**Z** No Qualifier

0 Medical and Surgical
U Female Reproductive System
V Restriction Definition: Partially closing an orifice or the lumen of a tubular body part
Explanation: The orifice can be a natural orifice or an artificially created orifice

Body Part Character 4	Approach Character 5	Device Character 6	Qualifier Character 7
C Cervix	**0** Open **3** Percutaneous **4** Percutaneous Endoscopic	**C** Extraluminal Device **D** Intraluminal Device **Z** No Device	**Z** No Qualifier
C Cervix	**7** Via Natural or Artificial Opening **8** Via Natural or Artificial Opening Endoscopic	**D** Intraluminal Device **Z** No Device	**Z** No Qualifier

NC Noncovered Procedure   LC Limited Coverage   QA Questionable OB Admit   NT New Tech Add-on   ✚ Combination Member   ♂ Male   ♀ Female

Female Reproductive System

0 Medical and Surgical
U Female Reproductive System
W Revision Definition: Correcting, to the extent possible, a portion of a malfunctioning device or the position of a displaced device
Explanation: Revision can include correcting a malfunctioning or displaced device by taking out or putting in components of the device such as a screw or pin

Body Part Character 4	Approach Character 5	Device Character 6	Qualifier Character 7
3 Ovary	0 Open 3 Percutaneous 4 Percutaneous Endoscopic	0 Drainage Device 3 Infusion Device Y Other Device	Z No Qualifier
3 Ovary	7 Via Natural or Artificial Opening 8 Via Natural or Artificial Opening Endoscopic	Y Other Device	Z No Qualifier
3 Ovary	X External	0 Drainage Device 3 Infusion Device	Z No Qualifier
8 Fallopian Tube	0 Open 3 Percutaneous 4 Percutaneous Endoscopic 7 Via Natural or Artificial Opening 8 Via Natural or Artificial Opening Endoscopic	0 Drainage Device 3 Infusion Device 7 Autologous Tissue Substitute C Extraluminal Device D Intraluminal Device J Synthetic Substitute K Nonautologous Tissue Substitute Y Other Device	Z No Qualifier
8 Fallopian Tube	X External	0 Drainage Device 3 Infusion Device 7 Autologous Tissue Substitute C Extraluminal Device D Intraluminal Device J Synthetic Substitute K Nonautologous Tissue Substitute	Z No Qualifier
D Uterus and Cervix	0 Open 3 Percutaneous 4 Percutaneous Endoscopic 7 Via Natural or Artificial Opening 8 Via Natural or Artificial Opening Endoscopic	0 Drainage Device 1 Radioactive Element 3 Infusion Device 7 Autologous Tissue Substitute C Extraluminal Device D Intraluminal Device H Contraceptive Device J Synthetic Substitute K Nonautologous Tissue Substitute Y Other Device	Z No Qualifier
D Uterus and Cervix	X External	0 Drainage Device 3 Infusion Device 7 Autologous Tissue Substitute C Extraluminal Device D Intraluminal Device H Contraceptive Device J Synthetic Substitute K Nonautologous Tissue Substitute	Z No Qualifier
H Vagina and Cul-de-sac	0 Open 3 Percutaneous 4 Percutaneous Endoscopic 7 Via Natural or Artificial Opening 8 Via Natural or Artificial Opening Endoscopic	0 Drainage Device 1 Radioactive Element 3 Infusion Device 7 Autologous Tissue Substitute D Intraluminal Device J Synthetic Substitute K Nonautologous Tissue Substitute Y Other Device	Z No Qualifier
H Vagina and Cul-de-sac	X External	0 Drainage Device 3 Infusion Device 7 Autologous Tissue Substitute D Intraluminal Device J Synthetic Substitute K Nonautologous Tissue Substitute	Z No Qualifier

M Vulva
  Labia majora
  Labia minora
	0 Open
	X External
		0 Drainage Device
		7 Autologous Tissue Substitute
		J Synthetic Substitute
		K Nonautologous Tissue Substitute
			Z No Qualifier

Non-OR 0UW3[3,4]YZ
Non-OR 0UW3[7,8]YZ
Non-OR 0UW3X[0,3]Z
Non-OR 0UW8[3,4,7,8]YZ
Non-OR 0UW8X[0,3,7,C,D,J,K]Z
Non-OR 0UWD[3,4,7,8]YZ
Non-OR 0UWDX[0,3,7,C,D,H,J,K]Z
Non-OR 0UWH[3,4,7,8]YZ
Non-OR 0UWHX[0,3,7,D,J,K]Z
Non-OR 0UWMX[0,7,J,K]Z

Non-OR Procedure   DRG Non-OR Procedure   Valid OR Procedure   HAC Associated Procedure   Combination Only   New/Revised April   New/Revised October

0 **Medical and Surgical**
U **Female Reproductive System**
Y **Transplantation** Definition: Putting in or on all or a portion of a living body part taken from another individual or animal to physically take the place and/or function of all or a portion of a similar body part

Explanation: The native body part may or may not be taken out, and the transplanted body part may take over all or a portion of its function

Body Part Character 4	Approach Character 5	Device Character 6	Qualifier Character 7
0 Ovary, Right 1 Ovary, Left 9 Uterus	0 Open	Z No Device	0 Allogeneic 1 Syngeneic 2 Zooplastic

Male Reproductive System ØV1–ØVY

Character Meanings

This Character Meaning table is provided as a guide to assist the user in the identification of character members that may be found in this section of code tables. It **SHOULD NOT** be used to build a PCS code.

Operation–Character 3		Body Part–Character 4		Approach–Character 5		Device–Character 6		Qualifier–Character 7	
1	Bypass	Ø	Prostate	Ø	Open	Ø	Drainage Device	Ø	Allogeneic
2	Change	1	Seminal Vesicle, Right	3	Percutaneous	1	Radioactive Element	1	Syngeneic
5	Destruction	2	Seminal Vesicle, Left	4	Percutaneous Endoscopic	3	Infusion Device	2	Zooplastic
7	Dilation	3	Seminal Vesicles, Bilateral	7	Via Natural or Artificial Opening	7	Autologous Tissue Substitute	3	Laser Interstitial Thermal Therapy
9	Drainage	4	Prostate and Seminal Vesicles	8	Via Natural or Artificial Opening Endoscopic	C	Extraluminal Device	D	Urethra
B	Excision	5	Scrotum	X	External	D	Intraluminal Device	J	Epididymis, Right
C	Extirpation	6	Tunica Vaginalis, Right			J	Synthetic Substitute	K	Epididymis, Left
H	Insertion	7	Tunica Vaginalis, Left			K	Nonautologous Tissue Substitute	N	Vas Deferens, Right
J	Inspection	8	Scrotum and Tunica Vaginalis			Y	Other Device	P	Vas Deferens, Left
L	Occlusion	9	Testis, Right			Z	No Device	S	Penis
M	Reattachment	B	Testis, Left					X	Diagnostic
N	Release	C	Testes, Bilateral					Z	No Qualifier
P	Removal	D	Testis						
Q	Repair	F	Spermatic Cord, Right						
R	Replacement	G	Spermatic Cord, Left						
S	Reposition	H	Spermatic Cords, Bilateral						
T	Resection	J	Epididymis, Right						
U	Supplement	K	Epididymis, Left						
W	Revision	L	Epididymis, Bilateral						
X	Transfer	M	Epididymis and Spermatic Cord						
Y	Transplantation	N	Vas Deferens, Right						
		P	Vas Deferens, Left						
		Q	Vas Deferens, Bilateral						
		R	Vas Deferens						
		S	Penis						
		T	Prepuce						

AHA Coding Clinic for table ØV1
2018, 3Q, 12   Al-Ghorab distal penile shunt surgery

AHA Coding Clinic for table ØV5
2022, 4Q, 53-54   Laser interstitial thermal therapy

AHA Coding Clinic for table ØV9
2018, 3Q, 12   Al-Ghorab distal penile shunt surgery

AHA Coding Clinic for table ØVB
2020, 1Q, 31   Repair of buried penis
2019, 3Q, 18   Radical prostatectomy and lymph node dissection with biopsy of neurovascular bundle
2016, 1Q, 23   Transurethral resection of ejaculatory ducts
2014, 4Q, 33   Radical prostatectomy

AHA Coding Clinic for table ØVH
2020, 4Q, 43-44   Insertion of radioactive element

AHA Coding Clinic for table ØVP
2016, 2Q, 28   Removal of multi-component inflatable penile prosthesis with placement of new malleable device

AHA Coding Clinic for table ØVQ
2018, 3Q, 12   Al-Ghorab distal penile shunt surgery

AHA Coding Clinic for table ØVT
2020, 4Q, 99   Robotic-assisted prostatectomy with extension of incision for specimen removal
2019, 3Q, 18   Radical prostatectomy and lymph node dissection with biopsy of neurovascular bundle
2014, 4Q, 33   Radical prostatectomy

AHA Coding Clinic for table ØVU
2020, 1Q, 31   Repair of buried penis
2016, 2Q, 28   Removal of multi-component inflatable penile prosthesis with placement of new malleable device
2015, 3Q, 25   Placement of inflatable penile prosthesis

AHA Coding Clinic for table ØVX
2018, 4Q, 40   Transfer of prepuce

AHA Coding Clinic for table ØVY
2023, 2Q, 32   Preparation of donor organ before transplantation
2020, 4Q, 58   Male reproductive organ transplant

Male Reproductive System

Male Reproductive System

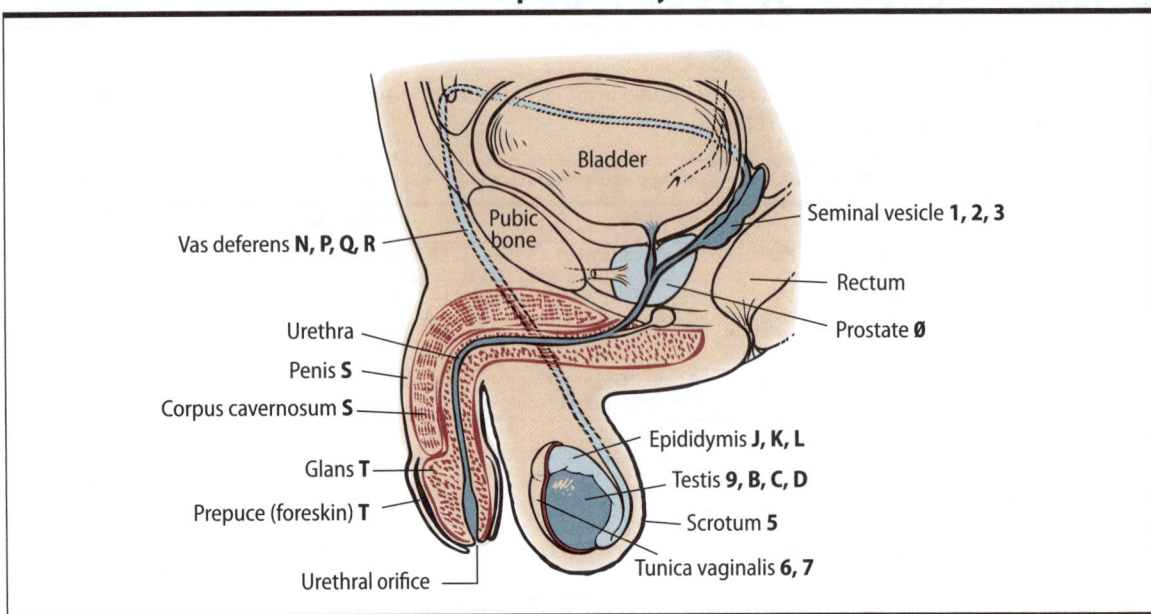

- Vas deferens **N, P, Q, R**
- Seminal vesicle **1, 2, 3**
- Rectum
- Prostate **Ø**
- Bladder
- Pubic bone
- Urethra
- Penis **S**
- Corpus cavernosum **S**
- Glans **T**
- Prepuce (foreskin) **T**
- Urethral orifice
- Epididymis **J, K, L**
- Testis **9, B, C, D**
- Scrotum **5**
- Tunica vaginalis **6, 7**

Penis

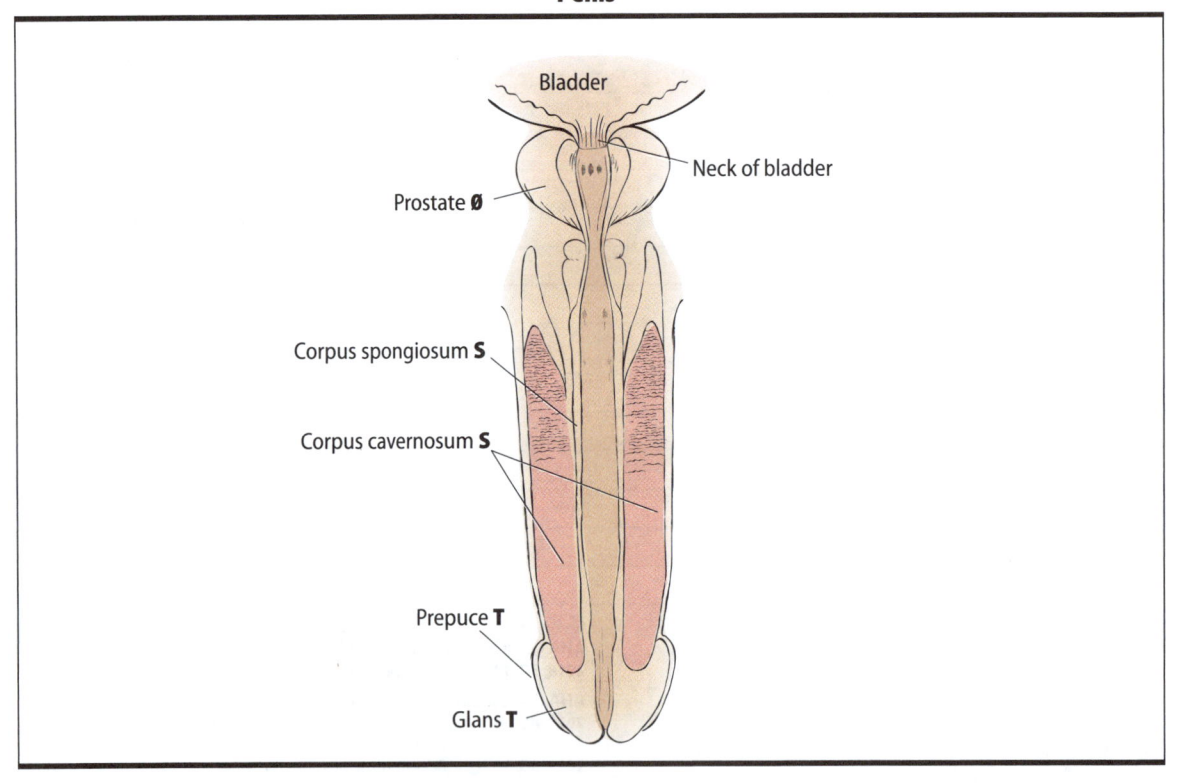

- Bladder
- Neck of bladder
- Prostate **Ø**
- Corpus spongiosum **S**
- Corpus cavernosum **S**
- Prepuce **T**
- Glans **T**

ICD-10-PCS 2025 — Male Reproductive System — 0V1–0V5

0 Medical and Surgical
V Male Reproductive System
1 Bypass   Definition: Altering the route of passage of the contents of a tubular body part
Explanation: Rerouting contents of a body part to a downstream area of the normal route, to a similar route and body part, or to an abnormal route and dissimilar body part. Includes one or more anastomoses, with or without the use of a device.

Body Part Character 4	Approach Character 5	Device Character 6	Qualifier Character 7

N Vas Deferens, Right
  Ductus deferens
  Ejaculatory duct
P Vas Deferens, Left
  See N Vas Deferens, Right
Q Vas Deferens, Bilateral
  See N Vas Deferens, Right
	0 Open
	4 Percutaneous Endoscopic
		7 Autologous Tissue Substitute
		J Synthetic Substitute
		K Nonautologous Tissue Substitute
		Z No Device
			J Epididymis, Right
			K Epididymis, Left
			N Vas Deferens, Right
			P Vas Deferens, Left

0 Medical and Surgical
V Male Reproductive System
2 Change   Definition: Taking out or off a device from a body part and putting back an identical or similar device in or on the same body part without cutting or puncturing the skin or a mucous membrane
Explanation: All CHANGE procedures are coded using the approach EXTERNAL

Body Part Character 4	Approach Character 5	Device Character 6	Qualifier Character 7

4 Prostate and Seminal Vesicles
8 Scrotum and Tunica Vaginalis
D Testis
M Epididymis and Spermatic Cord
R Vas Deferens
  Ductus deferens
  Ejaculatory duct
S Penis
  Corpus cavernosum
  Corpus spongiosum
	X External	**0** Drainage Device
		Y Other Device
			Z No Qualifier

Non-OR All body part, approach, device, and qualifier values

0 Medical and Surgical
V Male Reproductive System
5 Destruction   Definition: Physical eradication of all or a portion of a body part by the direct use of energy, force, or a destructive agent
Explanation: None of the body part is physically taken out

Body Part Character 4	Approach Character 5	Device Character 6	Qualifier Character 7
0 Prostate	**0** Open **3** Percutaneous **4** Percutaneous Endoscopic	**Z** No Device	**3** Laser Interstitial Thermal Therapy **Z** No Qualifier
0 Prostate	**7** Via Natural or Artificial Opening **8** Via Natural or Artificial Opening Endoscopic	**Z** No Device	**Z** No Qualifier
1 Seminal Vesicle, Right **2** Seminal Vesicle, Left **3** Seminal Vesicles, Bilateral **6** Tunica Vaginalis, Right **7** Tunica Vaginalis, Left **9** Testis, Right **B** Testis, Left **C** Testes, Bilateral	**0** Open **3** Percutaneous **4** Percutaneous Endoscopic	**Z** No Device	**Z** No Qualifier

5 Scrotum
S Penis
  Corpus cavernosum
  Corpus spongiosum
T Prepuce
  Foreskin
  Glans penis
	0 Open
	3 Percutaneous
	4 Percutaneous Endoscopic
	X External
		Z No Device	**Z** No Qualifier

F Spermatic Cord, Right
G Spermatic Cord, Left
H Spermatic Cords, Bilateral
J Epididymis, Right
K Epididymis, Left
L Epididymis, Bilateral
N Vas Deferens, Right [NC]
  Ductus deferens
  Ejaculatory duct
P Vas Deferens, Left [NC]
  See N Vas Deferens, Right
Q Vas Deferens, Bilateral [NC]
  See N Vas Deferens, Right
	0 Open
	3 Percutaneous
	4 Percutaneous Endoscopic
	8 Via Natural or Artificial Opening Endoscopic
		Z No Device	**Z** No Qualifier

Non-OR 0V55[0,3,4,X]ZZ
Non-OR 0V5[N,P,Q][0,3,4,8]ZZ
NC 0V5[N,P,Q][0,3,4]ZZ with principal or secondary diagnosis of Z30.2

NC Noncovered Procedure   **LC** Limited Coverage   **QA** Questionable OB Admit   **NT** New Tech Add-on   ✚ Combination Member   ♂ Male   ♀ Female

0V7–0V9 — Male Reproductive System — ICD-10-PCS 2025

0 Medical and Surgical
V Male Reproductive System
7 Dilation

Definition: Expanding an orifice or the lumen of a tubular body part

Explanation: The orifice can be a natural orifice or an artificially created orifice. Accomplished by stretching a tubular body part using intraluminal pressure or by cutting part of the orifice or wall of the tubular body part.

Body Part Character 4	Approach Character 5	Device Character 6	Qualifier Character 7

N Vas Deferens, Right
   Ductus deferens
   Ejaculatory duct
P Vas Deferens, Left
   See N Vas Deferens, Right
Q Vas Deferens, Bilateral
   See N Vas Deferens, Right
	0 Open
	3 Percutaneous
	4 Percutaneous Endoscopic
		D Intraluminal Device
		Z No Device
			Z No Qualifier

0 Medical and Surgical
V Male Reproductive System
9 Drainage

Definition: Taking or letting out fluids and/or gases from a body part

Explanation: The qualifier DIAGNOSTIC is used to identify drainage procedures that are biopsies

Body Part Character 4	Approach Character 5	Device Character 6	Qualifier Character 7
0 Prostate	0 Open 3 Percutaneous 4 Percutaneous Endoscopic 7 Via Natural or Artificial Opening 8 Via Natural or Artificial Opening Endoscopic	0 Drainage Device	Z No Qualifier
0 Prostate	0 Open 3 Percutaneous 4 Percutaneous Endoscopic 7 Via Natural or Artificial Opening 8 Via Natural or Artificial Opening Endoscopic	Z No Device	X Diagnostic Z No Qualifier

1 Seminal Vesicle, Right
2 Seminal Vesicle, Left
3 Seminal Vesicles, Bilateral
6 Tunica Vaginalis, Right
7 Tunica Vaginalis, Left
9 Testis, Right
B Testis, Left
C Testes, Bilateral
F Spermatic Cord, Right
G Spermatic Cord, Left
H Spermatic Cords, Bilateral
J Epididymis, Right
K Epididymis, Left
L Epididymis, Bilateral
N Vas Deferens, Right
   Ductus deferens
   Ejaculatory duct
P Vas Deferens, Left
   See N Vas Deferens, Right
Q Vas Deferens, Bilateral
   See N Vas Deferens, Right
	0 Open
	3 Percutaneous
	4 Percutaneous Endoscopic
		0 Drainage Device	Z No Qualifier

Non-OR 0V90[3,4]0Z
Non-OR 0V90[3,4]Z[X,Z]
Non-OR 0V90[7,8]ZX
Non-OR 0V9[1,2,3,9,B,C][3,4]0Z
Non-OR 0V9[6,7,F,G,H,N,P,Q][0,3,4]0Z
Non-OR 0V9[J,K,L]30Z

0V9 Continued on next page

Male Reproductive System

0 Medical and Surgical
V Male Reproductive System
9 Drainage — Definition: Taking or letting out fluids and/or gases from a body part
Explanation: The qualifier DIAGNOSTIC is used to identify drainage procedures that are biopsies

0V9 Continued

Body Part Character 4	Approach Character 5	Device Character 6	Qualifier Character 7

1 Seminal Vesicle, Right
2 Seminal Vesicle, Left
3 Seminal Vesicles, Bilateral
6 Tunica Vaginalis, Right
7 Tunica Vaginalis, Left
9 Testis, Right
B Testis, Left
C Testes, Bilateral
F Spermatic Cord, Right
G Spermatic Cord, Left
H Spermatic Cords, Bilateral
J Epididymis, Right
K Epididymis, Left
L Epididymis, Bilateral
N Vas Deferens, Right
   Ductus deferens
   Ejaculatory duct
P Vas Deferens, Left
   See N Vas Deferens, Right
Q Vas Deferens, Bilateral
   See N Vas Deferens, Right
	0 Open
	3 Percutaneous
	4 Percutaneous Endoscopic
		Z No Device	X Diagnostic
			Z No Qualifier

5 Scrotum
S Penis
   Corpus cavernosum
   Corpus spongiosum
T Prepuce
   Foreskin
   Glans penis
	0 Open
	3 Percutaneous
	4 Percutaneous Endoscopic
	X External
		0 Drainage Device	Z No Qualifier

5 Scrotum
S Penis
   Corpus cavernosum
   Corpus spongiosum
T Prepuce
   Foreskin
   Glans penis
	0 Open
	3 Percutaneous
	4 Percutaneous Endoscopic
	X External
		Z No Device	X Diagnostic
			Z No Qualifier

Non-OR 0V9[1,2,3,9,B,C][3,4]Z[X,Z]
Non-OR 0V9[6,7,F,G,H,J,K,L,N,P,Q][0,3,4]ZX
Non-OR 0V9[6,7,F,G,H,N,P,Q][0,3,4]ZZ
Non-OR 0V9[J,K,L]3ZZ
Non-OR 0V95[0,3,4,X]0Z
Non-OR 0V9[S,T]30Z
Non-OR 0V950ZX
Non-OR 0V95[3,4,X]Z[X,Z]
Non-OR 0V9[S,T]3ZZ

Male Reproductive System

0 Medical and Surgical
V Male Reproductive System
B Excision   Definition: Cutting out or off, without replacement, a portion of a body part
Explanation: The qualifier DIAGNOSTIC is used to identify excision procedures that are biopsies

Body Part Character 4	Approach Character 5	Device Character 6	Qualifier Character 7
0 Prostate	**0** Open **3** Percutaneous **4** Percutaneous Endoscopic **7** Via Natural or Artificial Opening **8** Via Natural or Artificial Opening Endoscopic	**Z** No Device	**X** Diagnostic **Z** No Qualifier
1 Seminal Vesicle, Right **2** Seminal Vesicle, Left **3** Seminal Vesicles, Bilateral **6** Tunica Vaginalis, Right **7** Tunica Vaginalis, Left **9** Testis, Right **B** Testis, Left **C** Testes, Bilateral	**0** Open **3** Percutaneous **4** Percutaneous Endoscopic	**Z** No Device	**X** Diagnostic **Z** No Qualifier

5 Scrotum
S Penis
   Corpus cavernosum
   Corpus spongiosum
T Prepuce
   Foreskin
   Glans penis
	0 Open
	3 Percutaneous
	4 Percutaneous Endoscopic
	X External
		Z No Device	**X** Diagnostic
			Z No Qualifier

F Spermatic Cord, Right
G Spermatic Cord, Left
H Spermatic Cords, Bilateral
J Epididymis, Right
K Epididymis, Left
L Epididymis, Bilateral
N Vas Deferens, Right [NC]
   Ductus deferens
   Ejaculatory duct
P Vas Deferens, Left [NC]
   See N Vas Deferens, Right
Q Vas Deferens, Bilateral [NC]
   See N Vas Deferens, Right
	0 Open
	3 Percutaneous
	4 Percutaneous Endoscopic
	8 Via Natural or Artificial Opening Endoscopic
		Z No Device	**X** Diagnostic
			Z No Qualifier

Non-OR   0VB0[3,4,7,8]ZX
Non-OR   0VB[1,2,3,9,B,C][3,4]ZX
Non-OR   0VB[6,7][0,3,4]ZX
Non-OR   0VB50ZX
Non-OR   0VB5[3,4,X]Z[X,Z]

Non-OR   0VB[F,G,H,J,K,L][0,3,4,8]ZX
Non-OR   0VB[N,P,Q][0,3,4,8]Z[X,Z]
[NC]   0VB[N,P,Q][0,3,4]ZZ with principal or secondary diagnosis of Z30.2

ICD-10-PCS 2025 Male Reproductive System 0VC–0VC

- **0** Medical and Surgical
- **V** Male Reproductive System
- **C** Extirpation Definition: Taking or cutting out solid matter from a body part
  Explanation: The solid matter may be an abnormal byproduct of a biological function or a foreign body; it may be imbedded in a body part or in the lumen of a tubular body part. The solid matter may or may not have been previously broken into pieces.

Body Part Character 4	Approach Character 5	Device Character 6	Qualifier Character 7
0 Prostate	**0** Open **3** Percutaneous **4** Percutaneous Endoscopic **7** Via Natural or Artificial Opening **8** Via Natural or Artificial Opening Endoscopic	**Z** No Device	**Z** No Qualifier

1 Seminal Vesicle, Right
2 Seminal Vesicle, Left
3 Seminal Vesicles, Bilateral
6 Tunica Vaginalis, Right
7 Tunica Vaginalis, Left
9 Testis, Right
B Testis, Left
C Testes, Bilateral
F Spermatic Cord, Right
G Spermatic Cord, Left
H Spermatic Cords, Bilateral
J Epididymis, Right
K Epididymis, Left
L Epididymis, Bilateral
N Vas Deferens, Right
  Ductus deferens
  Ejaculatory duct
P Vas Deferens, Left
  See N Vas Deferens, Right
Q Vas Deferens, Bilateral
  See N Vas Deferens, Right
	0 Open
	3 Percutaneous
	4 Percutaneous Endoscopic
		Z No Device	**Z** No Qualifier

5 Scrotum
S Penis
  Corpus cavernosum
  Corpus spongiosum
T Prepuce
  Foreskin
  Glans penis
	0 Open
	3 Percutaneous
	4 Percutaneous Endoscopic
	X External
		Z No Device	**Z** No Qualifier

Non-OR 0VC[6,7,N,P,Q][0,3,4]ZZ
Non-OR 0VC5[3,4,X]ZZ
Non-OR 0VCSXZZ

Male Reproductive System

ØVH–ØVJ — ICD-10-PCS 2025

Ø Medical and Surgical
V Male Reproductive System
H Insertion Definition: Putting in a nonbiological appliance that monitors, assists, performs, or prevents a physiological function but does not physically take the place of a body part
Explanation: None

Body Part Character 4	Approach Character 5	Device Character 6	Qualifier Character 7
Ø Prostate	**Ø** Open **3** Percutaneous **4** Percutaneous Endoscopic **7** Via Natural or Artificial Opening **8** Via Natural or Artificial Opening Endoscopic	**1** Radioactive Element	**Z** No Qualifier

4 Prostate and Seminal Vesicles
8 Scrotum and Tunica Vaginalis
M Epididymis and Spermatic Cord
R Vas Deferens
  Ductus deferens
  Ejaculatory duct
	Ø Open
	3 Percutaneous
	4 Percutaneous Endoscopic
	7 Via Natural or Artificial Opening
	8 Via Natural or Artificial Opening Endoscopic
		3 Infusion Device
		Y Other Device
			Z No Qualifier

D Testis	**Ø** Open **3** Percutaneous **4** Percutaneous Endoscopic **7** Via Natural or Artificial Opening **8** Via Natural or Artificial Opening Endoscopic	**1** Radioactive Element **3** Infusion Device **Y** Other Device	**Z** No Qualifier

S Penis
  Corpus cavernosum
  Corpus spongiosum
	Ø Open
	3 Percutaneous
	4 Percutaneous Endoscopic
		3 Infusion Device
		Y Other Device
			Z No Qualifier

S Penis
  Corpus cavernosum
  Corpus spongiosum
	7 Via Natural or Artificial Opening
	8 Via Natural or Artificial Opening Endoscopic
		Y Other Device	**Z** No Qualifier

S Penis
  Corpus cavernosum
  Corpus spongiosum
	X External	**3** Infusion Device	**Z** No Qualifier

Non-OR ØVH[4,8,M,R][Ø,3,4,7,8][3,Y]Z
Non-OR ØVHD[Ø,3,4,7,8][1,3,Y]Z
Non-OR ØVHS[Ø,3,4][3,Y]Z
Non-OR ØVHS[7,8]YZ

Non-OR ØVHSX3Z

Ø Medical and Surgical
V Male Reproductive System
J Inspection Definition: Visually and/or manually exploring a body part
Explanation: Visual exploration may be performed with or without optical instrumentation. Manual exploration may be performed directly or through intervening body layers.

Body Part Character 4	Approach Character 5	Device Character 6	Qualifier Character 7

4 Prostate and Seminal Vesicles
8 Scrotum and Tunica Vaginalis
D Testis
M Epididymis and Spermatic Cord
R Vas Deferens
  Ductus deferens
  Ejaculatory duct
S Penis
  Corpus cavernosum
  Corpus spongiosum
	Ø Open
	3 Percutaneous
	4 Percutaneous Endoscopic
	X External
		Z No Device	**Z** No Qualifier

Non-OR ØVJ[4,D,M,R][3,X]ZZ
Non-OR ØVJ8[Ø,3,4,X]ZZ
Non-OR ØVJS[3,4,X]ZZ

ICD-10-PCS 2025 — Male Reproductive System — ØVL–ØVM

Ø Medical and Surgical
V Male Reproductive System
L Occlusion Definition: Completely closing an orifice or the lumen of a tubular body part
Explanation: The orifice can be a natural orifice or an artificially created orifice

Body Part Character 4	Approach Character 5	Device Character 6	Qualifier Character 7
F Spermatic Cord, Right [NC] G Spermatic Cord, Left [NC] H Spermatic Cords, Bilateral [NC] N Vas Deferens, Right [NC] 　Ductus deferens 　Ejaculatory duct P Vas Deferens, Left [NC] 　See N Vas Deferens, Right Q Vas Deferens, Bilateral [NC] 　See N Vas Deferens, Right	Ø Open 3 Percutaneous 4 Percutaneous Endoscopic 8 Via Natural or Artificial Opening Endoscopic	C Extraluminal Device D Intraluminal Device Z No Device	Z No Qualifier

Non-OR ØVL[F,G,H][Ø,3,4,8][C,D,Z]Z
Non-OR ØVL[N,P,Q][Ø,3,4,8][C,Z]Z
[NC] ØVL[F,G,H][Ø,3,4][C,D,Z]Z with principal or secondary diagnosis of Z30.2
[NC] ØVL[N,P,Q][Ø,3,4][C,Z]Z with principal or secondary diagnosis of Z30.2

Ø Medical and Surgical
V Male Reproductive System
M Reattachment Definition: Putting back in or on all or a portion of a separated body part to its normal location or other suitable location
Explanation: Vascular circulation and nervous pathways may or may not be reestablished

Body Part Character 4	Approach Character 5	Device Character 6	Qualifier Character 7
5 Scrotum S Penis 　Corpus cavernosum 　Corpus spongiosum	X External	Z No Device	Z No Qualifier
6 Tunica Vaginalis, Right 7 Tunica Vaginalis, Left 9 Testis, Right B Testis, Left C Testes, Bilateral F Spermatic Cord, Right G Spermatic Cord, Left H Spermatic Cords, Bilateral	Ø Open 4 Percutaneous Endoscopic	Z No Device	Z No Qualifier

Male Reproductive System

0VN–0VN   Male Reproductive System   ICD-10-PCS 2025

0 Medical and Surgical
V Male Reproductive System
N Release   Definition: Freeing a body part from an abnormal physical constraint by cutting or by the use of force
Explanation: Some of the restraining tissue may be taken out but none of the body part is taken out

Body Part Character 4	Approach Character 5	Device Character 6	Qualifier Character 7
0 Prostate	**0** Open **3** Percutaneous **4** Percutaneous Endoscopic **7** Via Natural or Artificial Opening **8** Via Natural or Artificial Opening Endoscopic	**Z** No Device	**Z** No Qualifier
1 Seminal Vesicle, Right **2** Seminal Vesicle, Left **3** Seminal Vesicles, Bilateral **6** Tunica Vaginalis, Right **7** Tunica Vaginalis, Left **9** Testis, Right **B** Testis, Left **C** Testes, Bilateral	**0** Open **3** Percutaneous **4** Percutaneous Endoscopic	**Z** No Device	**Z** No Qualifier

5 Scrotum
S Penis
   Corpus cavernosum
   Corpus spongiosum
T Prepuce
   Foreskin
   Glans penis
	0 Open
	3 Percutaneous
	4 Percutaneous Endoscopic
	X External
		Z No Device	**Z** No Qualifier

F Spermatic Cord, Right
G Spermatic Cord, Left
H Spermatic Cords, Bilateral
J Epididymis, Right
K Epididymis, Left
L Epididymis, Bilateral
N Vas Deferens, Right
   Ductus deferens
   Ejaculatory duct
P Vas Deferens, Left
   See N Vas Deferens, Right
Q Vas Deferens, Bilateral
   See N Vas Deferens, Right
	0 Open
	3 Percutaneous
	4 Percutaneous Endoscopic
	8 Via Natural or Artificial Opening Endoscopic
		Z No Device	**Z** No Qualifier

Non-OR 0VN[9,B,C][0,3,4]ZZ
Non-OR 0VNT[0,3,4,X]ZZ

Non-OR Procedure   DRG Non-OR Procedure   Valid OR Procedure   HAC Associated Procedure   Combination Only   New/Revised April   New/Revised October

ICD-10-PCS 2025 — Male Reproductive System — 0VP–0VP

0 Medical and Surgical
V Male Reproductive System
P Removal   Definition: Taking out or off a device from a body part
Explanation: If a device is taken out and a similar device put in without cutting or puncturing the skin or mucous membrane, the procedure is coded to the root operation CHANGE. Otherwise, the procedure for taking out the device is coded to the root operation REMOVAL.

Body Part Character 4	Approach Character 5	Device Character 6	Qualifier Character 7
4 Prostate and Seminal Vesicles	**0** Open **3** Percutaneous **4** Percutaneous Endoscopic **7** Via Natural or Artificial Opening **8** Via Natural or Artificial Opening Endoscopic	**0** Drainage Device **1** Radioactive Element **3** Infusion Device **7** Autologous Tissue Substitute **J** Synthetic Substitute **K** Nonautologous Tissue Substitute **Y** Other Device	**Z** No Qualifier
4 Prostate and Seminal Vesicles	**X** External	**0** Drainage Device **1** Radioactive Element **3** Infusion Device	**Z** No Qualifier

8 Scrotum and Tunica Vaginalis
D Testis
S Penis
   Corpus cavernosum
   Corpus spongiosum
	0 Open
	3 Percutaneous
	4 Percutaneous Endoscopic
	7 Via Natural or Artificial Opening
	8 Via Natural or Artificial Opening Endoscopic
		0 Drainage Device
		3 Infusion Device
		7 Autologous Tissue Substitute
		J Synthetic Substitute
		K Nonautologous Tissue Substitute
		Y Other Device
			Z No Qualifier

8 Scrotum and Tunica Vaginalis
D Testis
S Penis
   Corpus cavernosum
   Corpus spongiosum
	X External	**0** Drainage Device
		3 Infusion Device
			Z No Qualifier

M Epididymis and Spermatic Cord	**0** Open **3** Percutaneous **4** Percutaneous Endoscopic **7** Via Natural or Artificial Opening **8** Via Natural or Artificial Opening Endoscopic	**0** Drainage Device **3** Infusion Device **7** Autologous Tissue Substitute **C** Extraluminal Device **J** Synthetic Substitute **K** Nonautologous Tissue Substitute **Y** Other Device	**Z** No Qualifier
M Epididymis and Spermatic Cord	**X** External	**0** Drainage Device **3** Infusion Device	**Z** No Qualifier

R Vas Deferens
   Ductus deferens
   Ejaculatory duct
	0 Open
	3 Percutaneous
	4 Percutaneous Endoscopic
	7 Via Natural or Artificial Opening
	8 Via Natural or Artificial Opening Endoscopic
		0 Drainage Device
		3 Infusion Device
		7 Autologous Tissue Substitute
		C Extraluminal Device
		D Intraluminal Device
		J Synthetic Substitute
		K Nonautologous Tissue Substitute
		Y Other Device
			Z No Qualifier

R Vas Deferens
   Ductus deferens
   Ejaculatory duct
	X External	**0** Drainage Device
		3 Infusion Device
		D Intraluminal Device
			Z No Qualifier

Non-OR 0VP4[3,4]YZ
Non-OR 0VP4[7,8][0,3,Y]Z
Non-OR 0VP4X[0,1,3]Z
Non-OR 0VP8[0,3,4,7,8][0,3,7,J,K,Y]Z
Non-OR 0VP[D,S][3,4]YZ
Non-OR 0VP[D,S][7,8][0,3,Y]Z
Non-OR 0VP[8,D,S]X[0,3]Z
Non-OR 0VPM[3,4]YZ
Non-OR 0VPM[7,8][0,3,Y]Z
Non-OR 0VPMX[0,3]Z
Non-OR 0VPR[0,3,4][0,3,7,C,J,K,Y]Z
Non-OR 0VPR[7,8][0,3,7,C,D,J,K,Y]Z
Non-OR 0VPRX[0,3,D]Z

Male Reproductive System

0 Medical and Surgical
V Male Reproductive System
Q Repair   Definition: Restoring, to the extent possible, a body part to its normal anatomic structure and function
   Explanation: Used only when the method to accomplish the repair is not one of the other root operations

Body Part Character 4	Approach Character 5	Device Character 6	Qualifier Character 7
0 Prostate	**0** Open **3** Percutaneous **4** Percutaneous Endoscopic **7** Via Natural or Artificial Opening **8** Via Natural or Artificial Opening Endoscopic	**Z** No Device	**Z** No Qualifier
1 Seminal Vesicle, Right **2** Seminal Vesicle, Left **3** Seminal Vesicles, Bilateral **6** Tunica Vaginalis, Right **7** Tunica Vaginalis, Left **9** Testis, Right **B** Testis, Left **C** Testes, Bilateral	**0** Open **3** Percutaneous **4** Percutaneous Endoscopic	**Z** No Device	**Z** No Qualifier

5 Scrotum
S Penis
   Corpus cavernosum
   Corpus spongiosum
T Prepuce
   Foreskin
   Glans penis
	0 Open
	3 Percutaneous
	4 Percutaneous Endoscopic
	X External
		Z No Device	**Z** No Qualifier

F Spermatic Cord, Right
G Spermatic Cord, Left
H Spermatic Cords, Bilateral
J Epididymis, Right
K Epididymis, Left
L Epididymis, Bilateral
N Vas Deferens, Right
   Ductus deferens
   Ejaculatory duct
P Vas Deferens, Left
   See N Vas Deferens, Right
Q Vas Deferens, Bilateral
   See N Vas Deferens, Right
	0 Open
	3 Percutaneous
	4 Percutaneous Endoscopic
	8 Via Natural or Artificial Opening Endoscopic
		Z No Device	**Z** No Qualifier

Non-OR   0VQ[6,7][0,3,4]ZZ
Non-OR   0VQ5[0,3,4,X]ZZ

---

0 Medical and Surgical
V Male Reproductive System
R Replacement   Definition: Putting in or on biological or synthetic material that physically takes the place and/or function of all or a portion of a body part
   Explanation: The body part may have been taken out or replaced, or may be taken out, physically eradicated, or rendered nonfunctional during the REPLACEMENT procedure. A REMOVAL procedure is coded for taking out the device used in a previous replacement procedure.

Body Part Character 4	Approach Character 5	Device Character 6	Qualifier Character 7
9 Testis, Right **B** Testis, Left **C** Testes, Bilateral	**0** Open	**J** Synthetic Substitute	**Z** No Qualifier

---

0 Medical and Surgical
V Male Reproductive System
S Reposition   Definition: Moving to its normal location, or other suitable location, all or a portion of a body part
   Explanation: The body part is moved to a new location from an abnormal location, or from a normal location where it is not functioning correctly. The body part may or may not be cut out or off to be moved to the new location.

Body Part Character 4	Approach Character 5	Device Character 6	Qualifier Character 7
9 Testis, Right **B** Testis, Left **C** Testes, Bilateral **F** Spermatic Cord, Right **G** Spermatic Cord, Left **H** Spermatic Cords, Bilateral	**0** Open **3** Percutaneous **4** Percutaneous Endoscopic **8** Via Natural or Artificial Opening Endoscopic	**Z** No Device	**Z** No Qualifier

ICD-10-PCS 2025 — Male Reproductive System — ØVT–ØVT

0 Medical and Surgical
V Male Reproductive System
T Resection Definition: Cutting out or off, without replacement, all of a body part
Explanation: None

Body Part Character 4	Approach Character 5	Device Character 6	Qualifier Character 7
0 Prostate	**0** Open **4** Percutaneous Endoscopic **7** Via Natural or Artificial Opening **8** Via Natural or Artificial Opening Endoscopic	**Z** No Device	**Z** No Qualifier

1 Seminal Vesicle, Right
2 Seminal Vesicle, Left
3 Seminal Vesicles, Bilateral ✚
6 Tunica Vaginalis, Right
7 Tunica Vaginalis, Left
9 Testis, Right
B Testis, Left
C Testes, Bilateral
F Spermatic Cord, Right
G Spermatic Cord, Left
H Spermatic Cords, Bilateral
J Epididymis, Right
K Epididymis, Left
L Epididymis, Bilateral
N Vas Deferens, Right [NC]
  Ductus deferens
  Ejaculatory duct
P Vas Deferens, Left [NC]
  See N Vas Deferens, Right
Q Vas Deferens, Bilateral [NC]
  See N Vas Deferens, Right
	0 Open
	4 Percutaneous Endoscopic
		Z No Device	**Z** No Qualifier

5 Scrotum
S Penis
  Corpus cavernosum
  Corpus spongiosum
T Prepuce
  Foreskin
  Glans penis
	0 Open
	4 Percutaneous Endoscopic
	X External
		Z No Device	**Z** No Qualifier

Non-OR ØVT[N,P,Q][0,4]ZZ
Non-OR ØVT[5,T][0,4,X]ZZ
[NC] ØVT[N,P,Q][0,4]ZZ with principal or secondary diagnosis of Z30.2

See Appendix L for Procedure Combinations
✚ ØVT0[0,4,7,8]ZZ
✚ ØVT3[0,4]ZZ

0 Medical and Surgical
V Male Reproductive System
U Supplement

Definition: Putting in or on biological or synthetic material that physically reinforces and/or augments the function of a portion of a body part

Explanation: The biological material is non-living, or is living and from the same individual. The body part may have been previously replaced, and the SUPPLEMENT procedure is performed to physically reinforce and/or augment the function of the replaced body part.

Body Part Character 4	Approach Character 5	Device Character 6	Qualifier Character 7

1 Seminal Vesicle, Right
2 Seminal Vesicle, Left
3 Seminal Vesicles, Bilateral
6 Tunica Vaginalis, Right
7 Tunica Vaginalis, Left
F Spermatic Cord, Right
G Spermatic Cord, Left
H Spermatic Cords, Bilateral
J Epididymis, Right
K Epididymis, Left
L Epididymis, Bilateral
N Vas Deferens, Right
   Ductus deferens
   Ejaculatory duct
P Vas Deferens, Left
   See N Vas Deferens, Right
Q Vas Deferens, Bilateral
   See N Vas Deferens, Right
	0 Open
	4 Percutaneous Endoscopic
	8 Via Natural or Artificial Opening Endoscopic
		7 Autologous Tissue Substitute
		J Synthetic Substitute
		K Nonautologous Tissue Substitute
			Z No Qualifier

5 Scrotum
S Penis
   Corpus cavernosum
   Corpus spongiosum
T Prepuce
   Foreskin
   Glans penis
	0 Open
	4 Percutaneous Endoscopic
	X External
		7 Autologous Tissue Substitute
		J Synthetic Substitute
		K Nonautologous Tissue Substitute
			Z No Qualifier

9 Testis, Right B Testis, Left C Testes, Bilateral	0 Open	7 Autologous Tissue Substitute J Synthetic Substitute K Nonautologous Tissue Substitute	Z No Qualifier

Non-OR 0VUSX[7,J,K]Z

ICD-10-PCS 2025 — Male Reproductive System — 0VW–0VW

0 Medical and Surgical
V Male Reproductive System
W Revision   Definition: Correcting, to the extent possible, a portion of a malfunctioning device or the position of a displaced device
Explanation: Revision can include correcting a malfunctioning or displaced device by taking out or putting in components of the device such as a screw or pin

Body Part Character 4	Approach Character 5	Device Character 6	Qualifier Character 7

4 Prostate and Seminal Vesicles
8 Scrotum and Tunica Vaginalis
D Testis
S Penis
   Corpus cavernosum
   Corpus spongiosum
	0 Open
	3 Percutaneous
	4 Percutaneous Endoscopic
	7 Via Natural or Artificial Opening
	8 Via Natural or Artificial Opening Endoscopic
		0 Drainage Device
		3 Infusion Device
		7 Autologous Tissue Substitute
		J Synthetic Substitute
		K Nonautologous Tissue Substitute
		Y Other Device
			Z No Qualifier

4 Prostate and Seminal Vesicles
8 Scrotum and Tunica Vaginalis
D Testis
S Penis
   Corpus cavernosum
   Corpus spongiosum
	X External	0 Drainage Device
		3 Infusion Device
		7 Autologous Tissue Substitute
		J Synthetic Substitute
		K Nonautologous Tissue Substitute
			Z No Qualifier

M Epididymis and Spermatic Cord	0 Open 3 Percutaneous 4 Percutaneous Endoscopic 7 Via Natural or Artificial Opening 8 Via Natural or Artificial Opening Endoscopic	0 Drainage Device 3 Infusion Device 7 Autologous Tissue Substitute C Extraluminal Device J Synthetic Substitute K Nonautologous Tissue Substitute Y Other Device	Z No Qualifier
M Epididymis and Spermatic Cord	X External	0 Drainage Device 3 Infusion Device 7 Autologous Tissue Substitute C Extraluminal Device J Synthetic Substitute K Nonautologous Tissue Substitute	Z No Qualifier

R Vas Deferens
   Ductus deferens
   Ejaculatory duct
	0 Open
	3 Percutaneous
	4 Percutaneous Endoscopic
	7 Via Natural or Artificial Opening
	8 Via Natural or Artificial Opening Endoscopic
		0 Drainage Device
		3 Infusion Device
		7 Autologous Tissue Substitute
		C Extraluminal Device
		D Intraluminal Device
		J Synthetic Substitute
		K Nonautologous Tissue Substitute
		Y Other Device
			Z No Qualifier

R Vas Deferens
   Ductus deferens
   Ejaculatory duct
	X External	0 Drainage Device
		3 Infusion Device
		7 Autologous Tissue Substitute
		C Extraluminal Device
		D Intraluminal Device
		J Synthetic Substitute
		K Nonautologous Tissue Substitute
			Z No Qualifier

Non-OR 0VW[4,D,S][3,4,7,8]YZ
Non-OR 0VW8[0,3,4,7,8][0,3,7,J,K,Y]Z
Non-OR 0VW[4,8,D,S]X[0,3,7,J,K]Z
Non-OR 0VWM[3,4,7,8]YZ
Non-OR 0VWMX[0,3,7,C,J,K]Z
Non-OR 0VWR[0,3,4,7,8][0,3,7,C,D,J,K,Y]Z
Non-OR 0VWRX[0,3,7,C,D,J,K]Z

Male Reproductive System

0 Medical and Surgical
V Male Reproductive System
X Transfer Definition: Moving, without taking out, all or a portion of a body part to another location to take over the function of all or a portion of a body part
Explanation: The body part transferred remains connected to its vascular and nervous supply

Body Part Character 4	Approach Character 5	Device Character 6	Qualifier Character 7

T Prepuce
  Foreskin
  Glans penis
	0 Open
	X External
		Z No Device	D Urethra
			S Penis

0 Medical and Surgical
V Male Reproductive System
Y Transplantation Definition: Putting in or on all or a portion of a living body part taken from another individual or animal to physically take the place and/or function of all or a portion of a similar body part
Explanation: The native body part may or may not be taken out, and the transplanted body part may take over all or a portion of its function

Body Part Character 4	Approach Character 5	Device Character 6	Qualifier Character 7

5 Scrotum
S Penis
  Corpus cavernosum
  Corpus spongiosum
	0 Open	Z No Device	0 Allogeneic
			1 Syngeneic
			2 Zooplastic

Anatomical Regions, General ØWØ–ØWY

Character Meanings

This Character Meaning table is provided as a guide to assist the user in the identification of character members that may be found in this section of code tables. It **SHOULD NOT** be used to build a PCS code.

Operation–Character 3	Body Region–Character 4	Approach–Character 5	Device–Character 6	Qualifier–Character 7
Ø Alteration	Ø Head	Ø Open	Ø Drainage Device	Ø Vagina OR Allogeneic
1 Bypass	1 Cranial Cavity	3 Percutaneous	1 Radioactive Element	1 Penis OR Syngeneic
2 Change	2 Face	4 Percutaneous Endoscopic	3 Infusion Device	2 Stoma
3 Control	3 Oral Cavity and Throat	7 Via Natural or Artificial Opening	7 Autologous Tissue Substitute	4 Cutaneous
4 Creation	4 Upper Jaw	8 Via Natural or Artificial Opening Endoscopic	G Defibrillator Lead	6 Bladder
8 Division	5 Lower Jaw	X External	J Synthetic Substitute	9 Pleural Cavity, Right
9 Drainage	6 Neck		K Nonautologous Tissue Substitute	B Pleural Cavity, Left
B Excision	8 Chest Wall		Y Other Device	G Peritoneal Cavity
C Extirpation	9 Pleural Cavity, Right		Z No Device	J Pelvic Cavity
F Fragmentation	B Pleural Cavity, Left			W Upper Vein
H Insertion	C Mediastinum			X Diagnostic
J Inspection	D Pericardial Cavity			Y Lower Vein
M Reattachment	F Abdominal Wall			Z No Qualifier
P Removal	G Peritoneal Cavity			
Q Repair	H Retroperitoneum			
U Supplement	J Pelvic Cavity			
W Revision	K Upper Back			
Y Transplantation	L Lower Back			
	M Perineum, Male			
	N Perineum, Female			
	P Gastrointestinal Tract			
	Q Respiratory Tract			
	R Genitourinary Tract			

AHA Coding Clinic for table ØWØ
2015, 1Q, 31 Bilateral browpexy

AHA Coding Clinic for table ØW1
2020, 4Q, 55 Insertion of subcutaneous pump system for ascites drainage
2018, 4Q, 41-42 Anatomical regions bypass qualifiers
2015, 2Q, 36 Insertion of infusion device into peritoneal cavity
2013, 4Q, 126-127 Creation of percutaneous cutaneoperitoneal fistula

AHA Coding Clinic for table ØW3
2023, 3Q, 5 Control postpartum hemorrhage with Jada® system
2023, 3Q, 7 Control of bleeding with hemostatic clip and Hemospray®
2023, 2Q, 26 Control of bleeding with Hemospray®
2021, 3Q, 26 Cavoatrial junction tear with repair and relief of cardiac tamponade
2019, 3Q, 4 Evacuation of subdural hematoma and control of bleeding artery
2018, 4Q, 38 Control of epistaxis
2018, 1Q, 19 Argon plasma coagulation of duodenal arteriovenous malformation
2018, 1Q, 19 Control of epistaxis via silver nitrate cauterization
2017, 4Q, 57-58 Added approach values - Transorifice esophageal vein banding
2017, 4Q, 105 Control of gastrointestinal bleeding
2017, 4Q, 106 Control of bleeding of external naris using suture
2017, 4Q, 106 Nasal packing for epistaxis
2016, 4Q, 99-100 Root operation Control
2014, 4Q, 44 Bakri balloon for control of postpartum hemorrhage
2013, 3Q, 23 Control of intraoperative bleeding

AHA Coding Clinic for table ØW4
2019, 4Q, 30 Transfer large intestine to vagina
2016, 4Q, 101 Root operation Creation

AHA Coding Clinic for table ØW9
2022, 4Q, 59-60 Drainage of the parapharyngeal space and retropharyngeal space
2021, 3Q, 17 Incision and drainage of retropharyngeal space abscess
2021, 3Q, 21 Drainage of midline neck abscess
2021, 3Q, 26 Cavoatrial junction tear with repair and relief of cardiac tamponade
2020, 4Q, 56 Transvaginal drainage of pelvis
2017, 3Q, 12 Therapeutic and diagnostic paracentesis
2017, 2Q, 16 Incision and drainage of floor of mouth

AHA Coding Clinic for table ØWB
2021, 3Q, 21 Excision of thyroglossal duct cyst
2019, 1Q, 27 Excision of pelvic sidewall mass
2017, 2Q, 16 Excision of floor of mouth
2016, 1Q, 21 Excision of urachal mass
2013, 4Q, 119 Excision of inclusion cyst of perineum

AHA Coding Clinic for table ØWC
2022, 1Q, 42 Removal of fat necrosis from retroperitoneum and space of Retzius
2019, 4Q, 35 Extirpation of jaw
2017, 2Q, 16 Excision of floor of mouth

AHA Coding Clinic for table ØWH
2023, 4Q, 54-55 Implantable defibrillator lead into mediastinum
2021, 2Q, 14 Peritoneal dialysis catheter placement
2019, 4Q, 43 Unidirectional source brachytherapy
2018, 1Q, 25 Intrauterine brachytherapy & placement of tandems & ovoids
2017, 4Q, 104 Intrauterine brachytherapy & placement of tandems & ovoids
2016, 2Q, 14 Insertion of peritoneal totally implantable venous access device
2015, 2Q, 36 Insertion of infusion device into peritoneal cavity

AHA Coding Clinic for table ØWJ
2022, 3Q, 19 Aortic cross-clamping and exploratory thoracotomy
2021, 2Q, 19 Electromagnetic stealth guided ventriculoperitoneal shunt insertion with endoscopy
2019, 1Q, 3-8 Whipple procedure
2019, 1Q, 25 Laparoscopic appendectomy converted to open procedure
2018, 3Q, 29 Decommissioning of left ventricular assist device with exploration of mediastinum
2016, 4Q, 58 Longitudinal vaginal septum
2013, 2Q, 36 Insertion of ventriculoperitoneal shunt with laparoscopic assistance

AHA Coding Clinic for table ØWP
2023, 4Q, 54-55 Implantable defibrillator lead into mediastinum
2021, 2Q, 14 Removal of peritoneal dialysis catheter

AHA Coding Clinic for table ØWQ
2017, 4Q, 106 Control of bleeding of external naris using suture
2017, 3Q, 8 Removal of silo and closure of gastroschisis
2016, 3Q, 3-7 Stoma creation & takedown procedures
2014, 4Q, 38 Abdominoplasty and abdominal wall plication for hernia repair
2014, 3Q, 28 Ileostomy takedown and parastomal hernia repair

AHA Coding Clinic for table ØWU
2017, 3Q, 8 First stage of gastroschisis repair with silo placement
2016, 3Q, 40 Omentoplasty
2015, 2Q, 29 Placement of Ioban™ antimicrobial drape over surgical wound
2014, 4Q, 39 Abdominal component release with placement of mesh for hernia repair
2012, 4Q, 101 Rib resection with reconstruction of anterior chest wall

AHA Coding Clinic for table ØWW
2023, 4Q, 54-55 Implantable defibrillator lead into mediastinum
2015, 2Q, 9 Revision of ventriculoperitoneal (VP) shunt

AHA Coding Clinic for table ØWY
2016, 4Q, 112-113 Transplantation

Anatomical Regions, General

0 Medical and Surgical
W Anatomical Regions, General
0 Alteration   Definition: Modifying the anatomic structure of a body part without affecting the function of the body part
                    Explanation: Principal purpose is to improve appearance

Body Part Character 4	Approach Character 5	Device Character 6	Qualifier Character 7

0 Head
2 Face
4 Upper Jaw
5 Lower Jaw
6 Neck
   Parapharyngeal space
   Retropharyngeal space
8 Chest Wall
F Abdominal Wall
K Upper Back
L Lower Back
M Perineum, Male
N Perineum, Female
	0 Open
	3 Percutaneous
	4 Percutaneous Endoscopic
		7 Autologous Tissue Substitute
		J Synthetic Substitute
		K Nonautologous Tissue Substitute
		Z No Device
			Z No Qualifier

0 Medical and Surgical
W Anatomical Regions, General
1 Bypass   Definition: Altering the route of passage of the contents of a tubular body part
                 Explanation: Rerouting contents of a body part to a downstream area of the normal route, to a similar route and body part, or to an abnormal route and dissimilar body part. Includes one or more anastomoses, with or without the use of a device.

Body Part Character 4	Approach Character 5	Device Character 6	Qualifier Character 7
1 Cranial Cavity	0 Open	J Synthetic Substitute	9 Pleural Cavity, Right B Pleural Cavity, Left G Peritoneal Cavity J Pelvic Cavity

9 Pleural Cavity, Right
B Pleural Cavity, Left
J Pelvic Cavity
   Prevesical space
   Retropubic space
   Space of Retzius
	0 Open
	3 Percutaneous
	4 Percutaneous Endoscopic
		J Synthetic Substitute	4 Cutaneous
			9 Pleural Cavity, Right
			B Pleural Cavity, Left
			G Peritoneal Cavity
			J Pelvic Cavity
			W Upper Vein
			Y Lower Vein

G Peritoneal Cavity Abdominal cavity	0 Open 3 Percutaneous 4 Percutaneous Endoscopic	J Synthetic Substitute	4 Cutaneous 6 Bladder 9 Pleural Cavity, Right B Pleural Cavity, Left G Peritoneal Cavity J Pelvic Cavity W Upper Vein Y Lower Vein

Non-OR   0W1[9,B][0,3,4]J[4,G,W,Y]
Non-OR   0W1J[0,3,4]J[4,W,Y]
Non-OR   0W1G[0,3,4]J[9,B,G,J]

Anatomical Regions, General

0 Medical and Surgical
W Anatomical Regions, General
2 Change: Definition: Taking out or off a device from a body part and putting back an identical or similar device in or on the same body part without cutting or puncturing the skin or a mucous membrane
Explanation: All CHANGE procedures are coded using the approach EXTERNAL

Body Part Character 4	Approach Character 5	Device Character 6	Qualifier Character 7

0 Head
1 Cranial Cavity
2 Face
4 Upper Jaw
5 Lower Jaw
6 Neck
    Parapharyngeal space
    Retropharyngeal space
8 Chest Wall
9 Pleural Cavity, Right
B Pleural Cavity, Left
C Mediastinum
    Mediastinal cavity
    Mediastinal space
D Pericardial Cavity
F Abdominal Wall
G Peritoneal Cavity
    Abdominal cavity
H Retroperitoneum
    Retroperitoneal cavity
    Retroperitoneal space
J Pelvic Cavity
    Prevesical space
    Retropubic space
    Space of Retzius
K Upper Back
L Lower Back
M Perineum, Male
N Perineum, Female
	X External	**0** Drainage Device
		Y Other Device
			Z No Qualifier

Non-OR All body part, approach, device, and qualifier values

0 Medical and Surgical
W Anatomical Regions, General
3 Control

Definition: Stopping, or attempting to stop, postprocedural or other acute bleeding
Explanation: None

Body Part Character 4	Approach Character 5	Device Character 6	Qualifier Character 7

0 Head
1 Cranial Cavity
2 Face
4 Upper Jaw
5 Lower Jaw
6 Neck
   Parapharyngeal space
   Retropharyngeal space
8 Chest Wall
9 Pleural Cavity, Right
B Pleural Cavity, Left
C Mediastinum
   Mediastinal cavity
   Mediastinal space
D Pericardial Cavity
F Abdominal Wall
G Peritoneal Cavity
   Abdominal cavity
H Retroperitoneum
   Retroperitoneal cavity
   Retroperitoneal space
J Pelvic Cavity
   Prevesical space
   Retropubic space
   Space of Retzius
K Upper Back
L Lower Back
M Perineum, Male
N Perineum, Female
	0 Open
	3 Percutaneous
	4 Percutaneous Endoscopic
		Z No Device	Z No Qualifier

3 Oral Cavity and Throat	0 Open 3 Percutaneous 4 Percutaneous Endoscopic 7 Via Natural or Artificial Opening 8 Via Natural or Artificial Opening Endoscopic X External	Z No Device	Z No Qualifier
P Gastrointestinal Tract Q Respiratory Tract R Genitourinary Tract	0 Open 3 Percutaneous 4 Percutaneous Endoscopic 7 Via Natural or Artificial Opening 8 Via Natural or Artificial Opening Endoscopic	Z No Device	Z No Qualifier

Non-OR 0W3P8ZZ

0 Medical and Surgical
W Anatomical Regions, General
4 Creation

Definition: Putting in or on biological or synthetic material to form a new body part that to the extent possible replicates the anatomic structure or function of an absent body part
Explanation: Used for gender reassignment surgery and corrective procedures in individuals with congenital anomalies

Body Part Character 4	Approach Character 5	Device Character 6	Qualifier Character 7
M Perineum, Male	0 Open	7 Autologous Tissue Substitute J Synthetic Substitute K Nonautologous Tissue Substitute	0 Vagina
N Perineum, Female	0 Open	7 Autologous Tissue Substitute J Synthetic Substitute K Nonautologous Tissue Substitute	1 Penis

0 Medical and Surgical
W Anatomical Regions, General
8 Division

Definition: Cutting into a body part, without draining fluids and/or gases from the body part, in order to separate or transect a body part
Explanation: All or a portion of the body part is separated into two or more portions

Body Part Character 4	Approach Character 5	Device Character 6	Qualifier Character 7
N Perineum, Female	X External	Z No Device	Z No Qualifier

Non-OR 0W8NXZZ

ICD-10-PCS 2025 — Anatomical Regions, General — 0W9–0W9

0 Medical and Surgical
W Anatomical Regions, General
9 Drainage Definition: Taking or letting out fluids and/or gases from a body part
Explanation: The qualifier DIAGNOSTIC is used to identify drainage procedures that are biopsies

Body Part Character 4	Approach Character 5	Device Character 6	Qualifier Character 7

0 Head
1 Cranial Cavity
2 Face
3 Oral Cavity and Throat
4 Upper Jaw
5 Lower Jaw
8 Chest Wall
9 Pleural Cavity, Right
B Pleural Cavity, Left
C Mediastinum
  Mediastinal cavity
  Mediastinal space
D Pericardial Cavity
F Abdominal Wall
G Peritoneal Cavity
  Abdominal cavity
H Retroperitoneum
  Retroperitoneal cavity
  Retroperitoneal space
K Upper Back
L Lower Back
M Perineum, Male
N Perineum, Female
	0 Open
	3 Percutaneous
	4 Percutaneous Endoscopic
		0 Drainage Device	**Z** No Qualifier

0 Head
1 Cranial Cavity
2 Face
3 Oral Cavity and Throat
4 Upper Jaw
5 Lower Jaw
8 Chest Wall
9 Pleural Cavity, Right
B Pleural Cavity, Left
C Mediastinum
  Mediastinal cavity
  Mediastinal space
D Pericardial Cavity
F Abdominal Wall
G Peritoneal Cavity
  Abdominal cavity
H Retroperitoneum
  Retroperitoneal cavity
  Retroperitoneal space
K Upper Back
L Lower Back
M Perineum, Male
N Perineum, Female
	0 Open
	3 Percutaneous
	4 Percutaneous Endoscopic
		Z No Device	**X** Diagnostic
			Z No Qualifier

6 Neck
  Parapharyngeal space
  Retropharyngeal space
J Pelvic Cavity
  Prevesical space
  Retropubic space
  Space of Retzius
	0 Open
	3 Percutaneous
	4 Percutaneous Endoscopic
	7 Via Natural or Artificial Opening
	8 Via Natural or Artificial Opening Endoscopic
		0 Drainage Device	**Z** No Qualifier

6 Neck
  Parapharyngeal space
  Retropharyngeal space
J Pelvic Cavity
  Prevesical space
  Retropubic space
  Space of Retzius
	0 Open
	3 Percutaneous
	4 Percutaneous Endoscopic
	7 Via Natural or Artificial Opening
	8 Via Natural or Artificial Opening Endoscopic
		Z No Device	**X** Diagnostic
			Z No Qualifier

Non-OR 0W9[0,8,9,B,K,L,M]00Z
Non-OR 0W9[0,1,2,3,4,5,8,9,B,C,D,F,G,H,K,L,M,N]3 0Z
Non-OR 0W9[0,1,8,F,K,L,M]40Z
Non-OR 0W9[0,2,3,4,5,8,9,B,K,L,M,N]0ZX
Non-OR 0W9[0,1,2,3,4,5,8,9,B,C,D,G,K,L,M,N]3ZX
Non-OR 0W9[0,1,2,3,4,5,8,C,K,L,M,N]4ZX
Non-OR 0W9[0,8,9,B,K,L,M]0ZZ
Non-OR 0W9[0,1,2,3,4,5,8,9,B,C,D,F,G,H,K,L,M,N]3ZZ
Non-OR 0W9[0,1,8,F,K,L,M]4ZZ
Non-OR 0W9[6,J][3,7,8]0Z
Non-OR 0W96[0,4]ZX
Non-OR 0W9[6,J][3,7,8]Z[X,Z]

NC Noncovered Procedure   LC Limited Coverage   QA Questionable OB Admit   NT New Tech Add-on   ⊞ Combination Member   ♂ Male   ♀ Female

0 Medical and Surgical
W Anatomical Regions, General
B Excision

Definition: Cutting out or off, without replacement, a portion of a body part

Explanation: The qualifier DIAGNOSTIC is used to identify excision procedures that are biopsies

Body Part Character 4	Approach Character 5	Device Character 6	Qualifier Character 7
0 Head 2 Face 3 Oral Cavity and Throat 4 Upper Jaw 5 Lower Jaw 8 Chest Wall K Upper Back L Lower Back M Perineum, Male N Perineum, Female	0 Open 3 Percutaneous 4 Percutaneous Endoscopic X External	Z No Device	X Diagnostic Z No Qualifier

6 Neck
  Parapharyngeal space
  Retropharyngeal space
F Abdominal Wall
	0 Open
	3 Percutaneous
	4 Percutaneous Endoscopic
		Z No Device	X Diagnostic
			Z No Qualifier

6 Neck
  Parapharyngeal space
  Retropharyngeal space
F Abdominal Wall
	X External	Z No Device	2 Stoma
			X Diagnostic
			Z No Qualifier

C Mediastinum
  Mediastinal cavity
  Mediastinal space
H Retroperitoneum
  Retroperitoneal cavity
  Retroperitoneal space
	0 Open
	3 Percutaneous
	4 Percutaneous Endoscopic
		Z No Device	X Diagnostic
			Z No Qualifier

Non-OR   0WB[0,2,4,5,8,K,L,M][0,3,4,X]ZX
Non-OR   0WB6[0,3,4]ZX
Non-OR   0WB6XZX
Non-OR   0WBH[3,4]ZX

0 Medical and Surgical
W Anatomical Regions, General
C Extirpation

Definition: Taking or cutting out solid matter from a body part

Explanation: The solid matter may be an abnormal byproduct of a biological function or a foreign body; it may be imbedded in a body part or in the lumen of a tubular body part. The solid matter may or may not have been previously broken into pieces.

Body Part Character 4	Approach Character 5	Device Character 6	Qualifier Character 7

1 Cranial Cavity
3 Oral Cavity and Throat
9 Pleural Cavity, Right
B Pleural Cavity, Left
C Mediastinum
  Mediastinal cavity
  Mediastinal space
D Pericardial Cavity
G Peritoneal Cavity
  Abdominal cavity
H Retroperitoneum
  Retroperitoneal cavity
  Retroperitoneal space
J Pelvic Cavity
  Prevesical space
  Retropubic space
  Space of Retzius
	0 Open
	3 Percutaneous
	4 Percutaneous Endoscopic
	X External
		Z No Device	Z No Qualifier

4 Upper Jaw 5 Lower Jaw	0 Open 3 Percutaneous 4 Percutaneous Endoscopic	Z No Device	Z No Qualifier
P Gastrointestinal Tract Q Respiratory Tract R Genitourinary Tract	0 Open 3 Percutaneous 4 Percutaneous Endoscopic 7 Via Natural or Artificial Opening 8 Via Natural or Artificial Opening Endoscopic X External	Z No Device	Z No Qualifier

Non-OR   0WC[1,3]XZZ
Non-OR   0WC[9,B][0,3,4,X]ZZ
Non-OR   0WC[C,D,G,H,J]XZZ
Non-OR   0WC[4,5]3ZZ
Non-OR   0WC[P,R][7,8,X]ZZ
Non-OR   0WCQ[0,3,4,X]ZZ

0 Medical and Surgical
W Anatomical Regions, General
F Fragmentation Definition: Breaking solid matter in a body part into pieces
Explanation: Physical force (e.g., manual, ultrasonic) applied directly or indirectly is used to break the solid matter into pieces. The solid matter may be an abnormal byproduct of a biological function or a foreign body. The pieces of solid matter are not taken out.

Body Part Character 4	Approach Character 5	Device Character 6	Qualifier Character 7

1 Cranial Cavity NC
3 Oral Cavity and Throat NC
9 Pleural Cavity, Right NC
B Pleural Cavity, Left NC
C Mediastinum NC
   Mediastinal cavity
   Mediastinal space
D Pericardial Cavity
G Peritoneal Cavity NC
   Abdominal cavity
J Pelvic Cavity NC
   Prevesical space
   Retropubic space
   Space of Retzius
	0 Open
	3 Percutaneous
	4 Percutaneous Endoscopic
	X External
		Z No Device	Z No Qualifier

P Gastrointestinal Tract NC Q Respiratory Tract NC R Genitourinary Tract	0 Open 3 Percutaneous 4 Percutaneous Endoscopic 7 Via Natural or Artificial Opening 8 Via Natural or Artificial Opening Endoscopic X External	Z No Device	Z No Qualifier

Non-OR 0WF[1,3,9,B,C,G]XZZ
Non-OR 0WFJ[0,3,4,X]ZZ
Non-OR 0WFP[0,3,4,7,8,X]ZZ
Non-OR 0WFQXZZ
Non-OR 0WFR[0,3,4,7,8,X]ZZ

NC 0WF[1,3,9,B,C,G,J]XZZ
NC 0WF[P,Q]XZZ

Anatomical Regions, General

0 Medical and Surgical
W Anatomical Regions, General
H Insertion Definition: Putting in a nonbiological appliance that monitors, assists, performs, or prevents a physiological function but does not physically take the place of a body part
  Explanation: None

Body Part Character 4	Approach Character 5	Device Character 6	Qualifier Character 7

0 Head
1 Cranial Cavity
2 Face
3 Oral Cavity and Throat
4 Upper Jaw
5 Lower Jaw
6 Neck
   Parapharyngeal space
   Retropharyngeal space
8 Chest Wall
9 Pleural Cavity, Right
B Pleural Cavity, Left
D Pericardial Cavity
F Abdominal Wall
G Peritoneal Cavity
   Abdominal cavity
H Retroperitoneum
   Retroperitoneal cavity
   Retroperitoneal space
J Pelvic Cavity
   Prevesical space
   Retropubic space
   Space of Retzius
K Upper Back
L Lower Back
M Perineum, Male
N Perineum, Female
	0 Open
	3 Percutaneous
	4 Percutaneous Endoscopic
		1 Radioactive Element
		3 Infusion Device
		Y Other Device
			Z No Qualifier

C Mediastinum
   Mediastinal cavity
   Mediastinal space
	0 Open
	3 Percutaneous
	4 Percutaneous Endoscopic
		1 Radioactive Element
		3 Infusion Device
		G Defibrillator Lead
		Y Other Device
			Z No Qualifier

P Gastrointestinal Tract Q Respiratory Tract R Genitourinary Tract	0 Open 3 Percutaneous 4 Percutaneous Endoscopic 7 Via Natural or Artificial Opening 8 Via Natural or Artificial Opening Endoscopic	1 Radioactive Element 3 Infusion Device Y Other Device	Z No Qualifier

DRG Non-OR 0WH[0,2,4,5,6,K,L,M][0,3,4][3,Y]Z
Non-OR 0WH1[0,3,4]3Z
Non-OR 0WH[8,9,B][0,3,4][3,Y]Z
Non-OR 0WHP0YZ
Non-OR 0WHP[3,4,7,8][3,Y]Z
Non-OR 0WHQ[0,7,8][3,Y]Z
Non-OR 0WHR[0,3,4,7,8][3,Y]Z

See Appendix L for Procedure Combinations
  0WHC[0,3,4]GZ

ICD-10-PCS 2025 — Anatomical Regions, General — 0WJ–0WM

0 Medical and Surgical
W Anatomical Regions, General
J Inspection   Definition: Visually and/or manually exploring a body part
Explanation: Visual exploration may be performed with or without optical instrumentation. Manual exploration may be performed directly or through intervening body layers.

Body Part Character 4	Approach Character 5	Device Character 6	Qualifier Character 7

0 Head
2 Face
3 Oral Cavity and Throat
4 Upper Jaw
5 Lower Jaw
6 Neck
  Parapharyngeal space
  Retropharyngeal space
8 Chest Wall
F Abdominal Wall
K Upper Back
L Lower Back
M Perineum, Male
N Perineum, Female
	0 Open
	3 Percutaneous
	4 Percutaneous Endoscopic
	X External
		Z No Device	Z No Qualifier

1 Cranial Cavity
9 Pleural Cavity, Right
B Pleural Cavity, Left
C Mediastinum
  Mediastinal cavity
  Mediastinal space
D Pericardial Cavity
G Peritoneal Cavity
  Abdominal cavity
H Retroperitoneum
  Retroperitoneal cavity
  Retroperitoneal space
J Pelvic Cavity
  Prevesical space
  Retropubic space
  Space of Retzius
	0 Open
	3 Percutaneous
	4 Percutaneous Endoscopic
		Z No Device	Z No Qualifier

P Gastrointestinal Tract Q Respiratory Tract R Genitourinary Tract	0 Open 3 Percutaneous 4 Percutaneous Endoscopic 7 Via Natural or Artificial Opening 8 Via Natural or Artificial Opening Endoscopic	Z No Device	Z No Qualifier

DRG Non-OR   0WJ[0,2,4,5,K,L]0ZZ
DRG Non-OR   0WJM[0,4]ZZ
Non-OR   0WJ30ZZ
Non-OR   0WJ[0,2,3,4,5,6,8,F,K,L,M,N][3,X]ZZ
Non-OR   0WJ[0,2,3,4,5,K,L]4ZZ
Non-OR   0WJD0ZZ
Non-OR   0WJ[1,9,B,C,D,G,H,J]3ZZ
Non-OR   0WJ[P,Q,R][3,7,8]ZZ

0 Medical and Surgical
W Anatomical Regions, General
M Reattachment   Definition: Putting back in or on all or a portion of a separated body part to its normal location or other suitable location
Explanation: Vascular circulation and nervous pathways may or may not be reestablished

Body Part Character 4	Approach Character 5	Device Character 6	Qualifier Character 7

2 Face
4 Upper Jaw
5 Lower Jaw
6 Neck
  Parapharyngeal space
  Retropharyngeal space
8 Chest Wall
F Abdominal Wall
K Upper Back
L Lower Back
M Perineum, Male
N Perineum, Female
	0 Open	Z No Device	Z No Qualifier

0 Medical and Surgical
W Anatomical Regions, General
P Removal

Definition: Taking out or off a device from a body part

Explanation: If a device is taken out and a similar device put in without cutting or puncturing the skin or mucous membrane, the procedure is coded to the root operation CHANGE. Otherwise, the procedure for taking out the device is coded to the root operation REMOVAL.

Body Part Character 4	Approach Character 5	Device Character 6	Qualifier Character 7

0 Head
2 Face
4 Upper Jaw
5 Lower Jaw
6 Neck
  Parapharyngeal space
  Retropharyngeal space
8 Chest Wall
F Abdominal Wall
K Upper Back
L Lower Back
M Perineum, Male
N Perineum, Female
	0 Open
	3 Percutaneous
	4 Percutaneous Endoscopic
	X External
		0 Drainage Device
		1 Radioactive Element
		3 Infusion Device
		7 Autologous Tissue Substitute
		J Synthetic Substitute
		K Nonautologous Tissue Substitute
		Y Other Device
			Z No Qualifier

1 Cranial Cavity
9 Pleural Cavity, Right
B Pleural Cavity, Left
G Peritoneal Cavity
  Abdominal cavity
J Pelvic Cavity
  Prevesical space
  Retropubic space
  Space of Retzius
	0 Open
	3 Percutaneous
	4 Percutaneous Endoscopic
		0 Drainage Device
		1 Radioactive Element
		3 Infusion Device
		J Synthetic Substitute
		Y Other Device
			Z No Qualifier

1 Cranial Cavity
9 Pleural Cavity, Right
B Pleural Cavity, Left
G Peritoneal Cavity
  Abdominal cavity
J Pelvic Cavity
  Prevesical space
  Retropubic space
  Space of Retzius
	X External	0 Drainage Device
		1 Radioactive Element
		3 Infusion Device
			Z No Qualifier

C Mediastinum
  Mediastinal cavity
  Mediastinal space
	0 Open
	3 Percutaneous
	4 Percutaneous Endoscopic
	X External
		0 Drainage Device
		1 Radioactive Element
		3 Infusion Device
		7 Autologous Tissue Substitute
		G Defibrillator Lead
		J Synthetic Substitute
		K Nonautologous Tissue Substitute
		Y Other Device
			Z No Qualifier

D Pericardial Cavity
H Retroperitoneum
  Retroperitoneal cavity
  Retroperitoneal space
	0 Open
	3 Percutaneous
	4 Percutaneous Endoscopic
		0 Drainage Device
		1 Radioactive Element
		3 Infusion Device
		Y Other Device
			Z No Qualifier

D Pericardial Cavity
H Retroperitoneum
  Retroperitoneal cavity
  Retroperitoneal space
	X External	0 Drainage Device
		1 Radioactive Element
		3 Infusion Device
			Z No Qualifier

P Gastrointestinal Tract Q Respiratory Tract R Genitourinary Tract	0 Open 3 Percutaneous 4 Percutaneous Endoscopic 7 Via Natural or Artificial Opening 8 Via Natural or Artificial Opening Endoscopic X External	1 Radioactive Element 3 Infusion Device Y Other Device	Z No Qualifier

Non-OR 0WP[0,2,4,5,6,8][0,3,4,X][0,1,3,7,J,K,Y]Z
Non-OR 0WPFX[0,1,3,7,J,K,Y]Z
Non-OR 0WP[K,L][0,3,4,X][0,1,3,7,J,K,Y]Z
Non-OR 0WPM[0,3,4][0,1,3,J,Y]Z
Non-OR 0WPMX[0,1,3,Y]Z
Non-OR 0WPNX[0,1,3,7,J,K,Y]Z
Non-OR 0WP1[0,3,4]3Z
Non-OR 0WP[9,B,J][0,3,4][0,1,3,J,Y]Z
Non-OR 0WP[1,9,B,G,J]X[0,1,3]Z
Non-OR 0WPCX[0,1,3,7,G,J,K,Y]Z
Non-OR 0WP[D,H]X[0,1,3]Z
Non-OR 0WPP[3,4,7,8,X][1,3,Y]Z
Non-OR 0WPQ73Z
Non-OR 0WPQ8[3,Y]Z
Non-OR 0WPQ[0,X][1,3,Y]Z
Non-OR 0WPR[0,3,4,7,8,X][1,3,Y]Z

ICD-10-PCS 2025 — Anatomical Regions, General — 0WQ–0WU

0 Medical and Surgical
W Anatomical Regions, General
Q Repair Definition: Restoring, to the extent possible, a body part to its normal anatomic structure and function
  Explanation: Used only when the method to accomplish the repair is not one of the other root operations

Body Part Character 4	Approach Character 5	Device Character 6	Qualifier Character 7
0 Head 2 Face 3 Oral Cavity and Throat 4 Upper Jaw 5 Lower Jaw 8 Chest Wall K Upper Back L Lower Back M Perineum, Male N Perineum, Female	0 Open 3 Percutaneous 4 Percutaneous Endoscopic X External	Z No Device	Z No Qualifier

6 Neck
  Parapharyngeal space
  Retropharyngeal space
F Abdominal Wall
	0 Open
	3 Percutaneous
	4 Percutaneous Endoscopic
		Z No Device	Z No Qualifier

6 Neck
  Parapharyngeal space
  Retropharyngeal space
F Abdominal Wall ✚
	X External	Z No Device	2 Stoma
			Z No Qualifier

C Mediastinum
  Mediastinal cavity
  Mediastinal space
	0 Open
	3 Percutaneous
	4 Percutaneous Endoscopic
		Z No Device	Z No Qualifier

Non-OR 0WQNXZZ

See Appendix L for Procedure Combinations
✚ 0WQFXZ[2,Z]

0 Medical and Surgical
W Anatomical Regions, General
U Supplement Definition: Putting in or on biological or synthetic material that physically reinforces and/or augments the function of a portion of a body part
  Explanation: The biological material is non-living, or is living and from the same individual. The body part may have been previously replaced, and the SUPPLEMENT procedure is performed to physically reinforce and/or augment the function of the replaced body part.

Body Part Character 4	Approach Character 5	Device Character 6	Qualifier Character 7

0 Head
2 Face
4 Upper Jaw
5 Lower Jaw
6 Neck
  Parapharyngeal space
  Retropharyngeal space
8 Chest Wall
C Mediastinum
  Mediastinal cavity
  Mediastinal space
F Abdominal Wall
K Upper Back
L Lower Back
M Perineum, Male
N Perineum, Female
	0 Open
	4 Percutaneous Endoscopic
		7 Autologous Tissue Substitute
		J Synthetic Substitute
		K Nonautologous Tissue Substitute
			Z No Qualifier

0 Medical and Surgical
W Anatomical Regions, General
W Revision   Definition: Correcting, to the extent possible, a portion of a malfunctioning device or the position of a displaced device
Explanation: Revision can include correcting a malfunctioning or displaced device by taking out or putting in components of the device such as a screw or pin

Body Part Character 4	Approach Character 5	Device Character 6	Qualifier Character 7

0 Head
2 Face
4 Upper Jaw
5 Lower Jaw
6 Neck
    Parapharyngeal space
    Retropharyngeal space
8 Chest Wall
F Abdominal Wall
K Upper Back
L Lower Back
M Perineum, Male
N Perineum, Female
	0 Open
	3 Percutaneous
	4 Percutaneous Endoscopic
	X External
		0 Drainage Device
		1 Radioactive Element
		3 Infusion Device
		7 Autologous Tissue Substitute
		J Synthetic Substitute
		K Nonautologous Tissue Substitute
		Y Other Device
			Z No Qualifier

1 Cranial Cavity
9 Pleural Cavity, Right
B Pleural Cavity, Left
G Peritoneal Cavity
    Abdominal cavity
J Pelvic Cavity
    Prevesical space
    Retropubic space
    Space of Retzius
	0 Open
	3 Percutaneous
	4 Percutaneous Endoscopic
	X External
		0 Drainage Device
		1 Radioactive Element
		3 Infusion Device
		J Synthetic Substitute
		Y Other Device
			Z No Qualifier

C Mediastinum
    Mediastinal cavity
    Mediastinal space
	0 Open
	3 Percutaneous
	4 Percutaneous Endoscopic
	X External
		0 Drainage Device
		1 Radioactive Element
		3 Infusion Device
		7 Autologous Tissue Substitute
		G Defibrillator Lead
		J Synthetic Substitute
		K Nonautologous Tissue Substitute
		Y Other Device
			Z No Qualifier

D Pericardial Cavity
H Retroperitoneum
    Retroperitoneal cavity
    Retroperitoneal space
	0 Open
	3 Percutaneous
	4 Percutaneous Endoscopic
	X External
		0 Drainage Device
		1 Radioactive Element
		3 Infusion Device
		Y Other Device
			Z No Qualifier

P Gastrointestinal Tract **Q** Respiratory Tract **R** Genitourinary Tract	**0** Open **3** Percutaneous **4** Percutaneous Endoscopic **7** Via Natural or Artificial Opening **8** Via Natural or Artificial Opening Endoscopic **X** External	**1** Radioactive Element **3** Infusion Device **Y** Other Device	**Z** No Qualifier

DRG Non-OR   0WW[0,2,4,5,6,K,L][0,3,4][0,1,3,7,J,K,Y]Z
DRG Non-OR   0WWM[0,3,4][0,1,3,J,Y]Z
Non-OR   0WW[0,2,4,5,6,F,K,L,M,N]X[0,1,3,7,J,K,Y]Z
Non-OR   0WW8[0,3,4,X][0,1,3,7,J,K,Y]Z
Non-OR   0WW[1,G,J]X[0,1,3,J,Y]Z
Non-OR   0WW[9,B][0,3,4,X][0,1,3,J,Y]Z
Non-OR   0WWCX[0,1,3,7,G,J,K,Y]Z
Non-OR   0WW[D,H]X[0,1,3,Y]Z
Non-OR   0WWP[3,4,7,8,X][1,3,Y]Z
Non-OR   0WWQ[0,X][1,3,Y]Z
Non-OR   0WWR[0,3,4,7,8,X][1,3,Y]Z

0 Medical and Surgical
W Anatomical Regions, General
Y Transplantation   Definition: Putting in or on all or a portion of a living body part taken from another individual or animal to physically take the place and/or function of all or a portion of a similar body part
Explanation: The native body part may or may not be taken out, and the transplanted body part may take over all or a portion of its function

Body Part Character 4	Approach Character 5	Device Character 6	Qualifier Character 7
2 Face	**0** Open	**Z** No Device	**0** Allogeneic **1** Syngeneic

Anatomical Regions, Upper Extremities 0X0–0XY

Character Meanings

This Character Meaning table is provided as a guide to assist the user in the identification of character members that may be found in this section of code tables. It **SHOULD NOT** be used to build a PCS code.

Operation–Character 3	Body Part–Character 4	Approach–Character 5	Device–Character 6	Qualifier–Character 7
0 Alteration	0 Forequarter, Right	0 Open	0 Drainage Device	0 Complete OR Allogeneic
2 Change	1 Forequarter, Left	3 Percutaneous	1 Radioactive Element	1 High OR Syngeneic
3 Control	2 Shoulder Region, Right	4 Percutaneous Endoscopic	3 Infusion Device	2 Mid
6 Detachment	3 Shoulder Region, Left	X External	7 Autologous Tissue Substitute	3 Low
9 Drainage	4 Axilla, Right		J Synthetic Substitute	4 Complete 1st Ray
B Excision	5 Axilla, Left		K Nonautologous Tissue Substitute	5 Complete 2nd Ray
H Insertion	6 Upper Extremity, Right		Y Other Device	6 Complete 3rd Ray
J Inspection	7 Upper Extremity, Left		Z No Device	7 Complete 4th Ray
M Reattachment	8 Upper Arm, Right			8 Complete 5th Ray
P Removal	9 Upper Arm, Left			9 Partial 1st Ray
Q Repair	B Elbow Region, Right			B Partial 2nd Ray
R Replacement	C Elbow Region, Left			C Partial 3rd Ray
U Supplement	D Lower Arm, Right			D Partial 4th Ray
W Revision	F Lower Arm, Left			F Partial 5th Ray
X Transfer	G Wrist Region, Right			L Thumb, Right
Y Transplantation	H Wrist Region, Left			M Thumb, Left
	J Hand, Right			N Toe, Right
	K Hand, Left			P Toe, Left
	L Thumb, Right			X Diagnostic
	M Thumb, Left			Z No Qualifier
	N Index Finger, Right			
	P Index Finger, Left			
	Q Middle Finger, Right			
	R Middle Finger, Left			
	S Ring Finger, Right			
	T Ring Finger, Left			
	V Little Finger, Right			
	W Little Finger, Left			

AHA Coding Clinic for table 0X3
2016, 4Q, 99 Root operation Control
2015, 1Q, 35 Evacuation of hematoma for control of postprocedural bleeding
2013, 3Q, 23 Control of intraoperative bleeding

AHA Coding Clinic for table 0X6
2017, 2Q, 3-4 Qualifiers for the root operation detachment
2017, 2Q, 18 Removal of polydactyl digits
2017, 1Q, 52 Further distal phalangeal amputation
2016, 3Q, 33 Traumatic amputation of fingers with further revision amputation

AHA Coding Clinic for table 0XH
2017, 2Q, 20 Exchange of intramedullary antibiotic impregnated spacer

AHA Coding Clinic for table 0XP
2017, 2Q, 20 Exchange of intramedullary antibiotic impregnated spacer

AHA Coding Clinic for table 0XY
2016, 4Q, 112-113 Transplantation

Anatomical Regions, Upper Extremities

Detachment Qualifier Descriptions

	Qualifier Definition	Upper Arm	Lower Arm
1	**High:** Amputation at the proximal portion of the shaft of the:	Humerus	Radius/Ulna
2	**Mid:** Amputation at the middle portion of the shaft of the:	Humerus	Radius/Ulna
3	**Low:** Amputation at the distal portion of the shaft of the:	Humerus	Radius/Ulna

	Qualifier Definition	Hand
0	Complete 1st through 5th Rays Ray: digit of hand or foot with corresponding metacarpus or metatarsus	Through carpo-metacarpal joint, **Wrist**
4	Complete 1st Ray	Through carpo-metacarpal joint, **Thumb**
5	Complete 2nd Ray	Through carpo-metacarpal joint, **Index Finger**
6	Complete 3rd Ray	Through carpo-metacarpal joint, **Middle Finger**
7	Complete 4th Ray	Through carpo-metacarpal joint, **Ring Finger**
8	Complete 5th Ray	Through carpo-metacarpal joint, **Little Finger**
9	Partial 1st Ray	Anywhere along shaft or head of metacarpal bone, **Thumb**
B	Partial 2nd Ray	Anywhere along shaft or head of metacarpal bone, **Index Finger**
C	Partial 3rd Ray	Anywhere along shaft or head of metacarpal bone, **Middle Finger**
D	Partial 4th Ray	Anywhere along shaft or head of metacarpal bone, **Ring Finger**
F	Partial 5th Ray	Anywhere along shaft or head of metacarpal bone, **Little Finger**

	Qualifier Definition	Thumb/Finger
0	Complete	At the metacarpophalangeal joint
1	High	Anywhere along the proximal phalanx
2	Mid	Through the proximal interphalangeal joint or anywhere along the middle phalanx
3	Low	Through the distal interphalangeal joint or anywhere along the distal phalanx

Anatomical Regions, Upper Extremities

0 Medical and Surgical
X Anatomical Regions, Upper Extremities
0 Alteration   Definition: Modifying the anatomic structure of a body part without affecting the function of the body part
        Explanation: Principal purpose is to improve appearance

Body Part Character 4	Approach Character 5	Device Character 6	Qualifier Character 7
2 Shoulder Region, Right 3 Shoulder Region, Left 4 Axilla, Right 5 Axilla, Left 6 Upper Extremity, Right 7 Upper Extremity, Left 8 Upper Arm, Right 9 Upper Arm, Left B Elbow Region, Right C Elbow Region, Left D Lower Arm, Right F Lower Arm, Left G Wrist Region, Right H Wrist Region, Left	0 Open 3 Percutaneous 4 Percutaneous Endoscopic	7 Autologous Tissue Substitute J Synthetic Substitute K Nonautologous Tissue Substitute Z No Device	Z No Qualifier

0 Medical and Surgical
X Anatomical Regions, Upper Extremities
2 Change   Definition: Taking out or off a device from a body part and putting back an identical or similar device in or on the same body part without cutting or puncturing the skin or a mucous membrane
        Explanation: All CHANGE procedures are coded using the approach EXTERNAL

Body Part Character 4	Approach Character 5	Device Character 6	Qualifier Character 7
6 Upper Extremity, Right 7 Upper Extremity, Left	X External	0 Drainage Device Y Other Device	Z No Qualifier

Non-OR All body part, approach, device, and qualifier values

0 Medical and Surgical
X Anatomical Regions, Upper Extremities
3 Control   Definition: Stopping, or attempting to stop, postprocedural or other acute bleeding
        Explanation: None

Body Part Character 4	Approach Character 5	Device Character 6	Qualifier Character 7
2 Shoulder Region, Right 3 Shoulder Region, Left 4 Axilla, Right 5 Axilla, Left 6 Upper Extremity, Right 7 Upper Extremity, Left 8 Upper Arm, Right 9 Upper Arm, Left B Elbow Region, Right C Elbow Region, Left D Lower Arm, Right F Lower Arm, Left G Wrist Region, Right H Wrist Region, Left J Hand, Right K Hand, Left	0 Open 3 Percutaneous 4 Percutaneous Endoscopic	Z No Device	Z No Qualifier

0 Medical and Surgical
X Anatomical Regions, Upper Extremities
6 Detachment Definition: Cutting off all or a portion of the upper or lower extremities
Explanation: The body part value is the site of the detachment, with a qualifier if applicable to further specify the level where the extremity was detached

Body Part Character 4	Approach Character 5	Device Character 6	Qualifier Character 7
0 Forequarter, Right 1 Forequarter, Left 2 Shoulder Region, Right 3 Shoulder Region, Left B Elbow Region, Right C Elbow Region, Left	0 Open	Z No Device	Z No Qualifier
8 Upper Arm, Right 9 Upper Arm, Left D Lower Arm, Right F Lower Arm, Left	0 Open	Z No Device	1 High 2 Mid 3 Low
J Hand, Right K Hand, Left	0 Open	Z No Device	0 Complete 4 Complete 1st Ray 5 Complete 2nd Ray 6 Complete 3rd Ray 7 Complete 4th Ray 8 Complete 5th Ray 9 Partial 1st Ray B Partial 2nd Ray C Partial 3rd Ray D Partial 4th Ray F Partial 5th Ray
L Thumb, Right M Thumb, Left	0 Open	Z No Device	0 Complete 1 High 3 Low
N Index Finger, Right P Index Finger, Left Q Middle Finger, Right R Middle Finger, Left S Ring Finger, Right T Ring Finger, Left V Little Finger, Right W Little Finger, Left	0 Open	Z No Device	0 Complete 1 High 2 Mid 3 Low

ICD-10-PCS 2025 — Anatomical Regions, Upper Extremities — 0X9–0XB

- **0** Medical and Surgical
- **X** Anatomical Regions, Upper Extremities
- **9** Drainage — Definition: Taking or letting out fluids and/or gases from a body part
  Explanation: The qualifier DIAGNOSTIC is used to identify drainage procedures that are biopsies

Body Part Character 4	Approach Character 5	Device Character 6	Qualifier Character 7
2 Shoulder Region, Right 3 Shoulder Region, Left 4 Axilla, Right 5 Axilla, Left 6 Upper Extremity, Right 7 Upper Extremity, Left 8 Upper Arm, Right 9 Upper Arm, Left B Elbow Region, Right C Elbow Region, Left D Lower Arm, Right F Lower Arm, Left G Wrist Region, Right H Wrist Region, Left J Hand, Right K Hand, Left	0 Open 3 Percutaneous 4 Percutaneous Endoscopic	0 Drainage Device	Z No Qualifier
2 Shoulder Region, Right 3 Shoulder Region, Left 4 Axilla, Right 5 Axilla, Left 6 Upper Extremity, Right 7 Upper Extremity, Left 8 Upper Arm, Right 9 Upper Arm, Left B Elbow Region, Right C Elbow Region, Left D Lower Arm, Right F Lower Arm, Left G Wrist Region, Right H Wrist Region, Left J Hand, Right K Hand, Left	0 Open 3 Percutaneous 4 Percutaneous Endoscopic	Z No Device	X Diagnostic Z No Qualifier

Non-OR All body part, approach, device, and qualifier values

- **0** Medical and Surgical
- **X** Anatomical Regions, Upper Extremities
- **B** Excision — Definition: Cutting out or off, without replacement, a portion of a body part
  Explanation: The qualifier DIAGNOSTIC is used to identify excision procedures that are biopsies

Body Part Character 4	Approach Character 5	Device Character 6	Qualifier Character 7
2 Shoulder Region, Right 3 Shoulder Region, Left 4 Axilla, Right 5 Axilla, Left 6 Upper Extremity, Right 7 Upper Extremity, Left 8 Upper Arm, Right 9 Upper Arm, Left B Elbow Region, Right C Elbow Region, Left D Lower Arm, Right F Lower Arm, Left G Wrist Region, Right H Wrist Region, Left J Hand, Right K Hand, Left	0 Open 3 Percutaneous 4 Percutaneous Endoscopic	Z No Device	X Diagnostic Z No Qualifier

Non-OR 0XB[2,3,4,5,6,7,8,9,B,C,D,F,G,H,J,K][0,3,4]ZX

0XH–0XJ Anatomical Regions, Upper Extremities ICD-10-PCS 2025

0 Medical and Surgical
X Anatomical Regions, Upper Extremities
H Insertion Definition: Putting in a nonbiological appliance that monitors, assists, performs, or prevents a physiological function but does not physically take the place of a body part
Explanation: None

Body Part Character 4	Approach Character 5	Device Character 6	Qualifier Character 7
2 Shoulder Region, Right 3 Shoulder Region, Left 4 Axilla, Right 5 Axilla, Left 6 Upper Extremity, Right 7 Upper Extremity, Left 8 Upper Arm, Right 9 Upper Arm, Left B Elbow Region, Right C Elbow Region, Left D Lower Arm, Right F Lower Arm, Left G Wrist Region, Right H Wrist Region, Left J Hand, Right K Hand, Left	0 Open 3 Percutaneous 4 Percutaneous Endoscopic	1 Radioactive Element 3 Infusion Device Y Other Device	Z No Qualifier

DRG Non-OR 0XH[2,3,4,5,6,7,8,9,B,C,D,F,G,H,J,K][0,3,4][3,Y]Z

0 Medical and Surgical
X Anatomical Regions, Upper Extremities
J Inspection Definition: Visually and/or manually exploring a body part
Explanation: Visual exploration may be performed with or without optical instrumentation. Manual exploration may be performed directly or through intervening body layers.

Body Part Character 4	Approach Character 5	Device Character 6	Qualifier Character 7
2 Shoulder Region, Right 3 Shoulder Region, Left 4 Axilla, Right 5 Axilla, Left 6 Upper Extremity, Right 7 Upper Extremity, Left 8 Upper Arm, Right 9 Upper Arm, Left B Elbow Region, Right C Elbow Region, Left D Lower Arm, Right F Lower Arm, Left G Wrist Region, Right H Wrist Region, Left J Hand, Right K Hand, Left	0 Open 3 Percutaneous 4 Percutaneous Endoscopic X External	Z No Device	Z No Qualifier

DRG Non-OR 0XJ[2,3,4,5,6,7,8,9,B,C,D,F,G,H,J,K]0ZZ
Non-OR 0XJ[2,3,4,5,6,7,8,9,B,C,D,F,G,H][3,4,X]ZZ
Non-OR 0XJ[J,K][3,X]ZZ

0 Medical and Surgical
X Anatomical Regions, Upper Extremities
M Reattachment   Definition: Putting back in or on all or a portion of a separated body part to its normal location or other suitable location
                  Explanation: Vascular circulation and nervous pathways may or may not be reestablished

Body Part Character 4	Approach Character 5	Device Character 6	Qualifier Character 7
0 Forequarter, Right 1 Forequarter, Left 2 Shoulder Region, Right 3 Shoulder Region, Left 4 Axilla, Right 5 Axilla, Left 6 Upper Extremity, Right 7 Upper Extremity, Left 8 Upper Arm, Right 9 Upper Arm, Left B Elbow Region, Right C Elbow Region, Left D Lower Arm, Right F Lower Arm, Left G Wrist Region, Right H Wrist Region, Left J Hand, Right K Hand, Left L Thumb, Right M Thumb, Left N Index Finger, Right P Index Finger, Left Q Middle Finger, Right R Middle Finger, Left S Ring Finger, Right T Ring Finger, Left V Little Finger, Right W Little Finger, Left	0 Open	Z No Device	Z No Qualifier

0 Medical and Surgical
X Anatomical Regions, Upper Extremities
P Removal   Definition: Taking out or off a device from a body part
              Explanation: If a device is taken out and a similar device put in without cutting or puncturing the skin or mucous membrane, the procedure is coded to the root operation CHANGE. Otherwise, the procedure for taking out the device is coded to the root operation REMOVAL.

Body Part Character 4	Approach Character 5	Device Character 6	Qualifier Character 7
6 Upper Extremity, Right 7 Upper Extremity, Left	0 Open 3 Percutaneous 4 Percutaneous Endoscopic X External	0 Drainage Device 1 Radioactive Element 3 Infusion Device 7 Autologous Tissue Substitute J Synthetic Substitute K Nonautologous Tissue Substitute Y Other Device	Z No Qualifier

Non-OR   All body part, approach, device, and qualifier values

ØXQ–ØXR — Anatomical Regions, Upper Extremities

Ø Medical and Surgical
X Anatomical Regions, Upper Extremities
Q Repair — **Definition:** Restoring, to the extent possible, a body part to its normal anatomic structure and function
    Explanation: Used only when the method to accomplish the repair is not one of the other root operations

Body Part — Character 4	Approach — Character 5	Device — Character 6	Qualifier — Character 7
2 Shoulder Region, Right 3 Shoulder Region, Left 4 Axilla, Right 5 Axilla, Left 6 Upper Extremity, Right 7 Upper Extremity, Left 8 Upper Arm, Right 9 Upper Arm, Left B Elbow Region, Right C Elbow Region, Left D Lower Arm, Right F Lower Arm, Left G Wrist Region, Right H Wrist Region, Left J Hand, Right K Hand, Left L Thumb, Right M Thumb, Left N Index Finger, Right P Index Finger, Left Q Middle Finger, Right R Middle Finger, Left S Ring Finger, Right T Ring Finger, Left V Little Finger, Right W Little Finger, Left	Ø Open 3 Percutaneous 4 Percutaneous Endoscopic X External	Z No Device	Z No Qualifier

Ø Medical and Surgical
X Anatomical Regions, Upper Extremities
R Replacement — **Definition:** Putting in or on biological or synthetic material that physically takes the place and/or function of all or a portion of a body part
    Explanation: The body part may have been taken out or replaced, or may be taken out, physically eradicated, or rendered nonfunctional during the REPLACEMENT procedure. A REMOVAL procedure is coded for taking out the device used in a previous replacement procedure.

Body Part — Character 4	Approach — Character 5	Device — Character 6	Qualifier — Character 7
L Thumb, Right M Thumb, Left	Ø Open 4 Percutaneous Endoscopic	7 Autologous Tissue Substitute	N Toe, Right P Toe, Left

Non-OR Procedure   DRG Non-OR Procedure   Valid OR Procedure   HAC Associated Procedure   Combination Only   New/Revised April   New/Revised October

ICD-10-PCS 2025 — Anatomical Regions, Upper Extremities — ØXU–ØXY

Ø Medical and Surgical
X Anatomical Regions, Upper Extremities
U Supplement Definition: Putting in or on biological or synthetic material that physically reinforces and/or augments the function of a portion of a body part
Explanation: The biological material is non-living, or is living and from the same individual. The body part may have been previously replaced, and the SUPPLEMENT procedure is performed to physically reinforce and/or augment the function of the replaced body part.

Body Part Character 4	Approach Character 5	Device Character 6	Qualifier Character 7
2 Shoulder Region, Right 3 Shoulder Region, Left 4 Axilla, Right 5 Axilla, Left 6 Upper Extremity, Right 7 Upper Extremity, Left 8 Upper Arm, Right 9 Upper Arm, Left B Elbow Region, Right C Elbow Region, Left D Lower Arm, Right F Lower Arm, Left G Wrist Region, Right H Wrist Region, Left J Hand, Right K Hand, Left L Thumb, Right M Thumb, Left N Index Finger, Right P Index Finger, Left Q Middle Finger, Right R Middle Finger, Left S Ring Finger, Right T Ring Finger, Left V Little Finger, Right W Little Finger, Left	Ø Open 4 Percutaneous Endoscopic	7 Autologous Tissue Substitute J Synthetic Substitute K Nonautologous Tissue Substitute	Z No Qualifier

Ø Medical and Surgical
X Anatomical Regions, Upper Extremities
W Revision Definition: Correcting, to the extent possible, a portion of a malfunctioning device or the position of a displaced device
Explanation: Revision can include correcting a malfunctioning or displaced device by taking out or putting in components of the device such as a screw or pin

Body Part Character 4	Approach Character 5	Device Character 6	Qualifier Character 7
6 Upper Extremity, Right 7 Upper Extremity, Left	Ø Open 3 Percutaneous 4 Percutaneous Endoscopic X External	Ø Drainage Device 3 Infusion Device 7 Autologous Tissue Substitute J Synthetic Substitute K Nonautologous Tissue Substitute Y Other Device	Z No Qualifier

DRG Non-OR ØXW[6,7][Ø,3,4][Ø,3,7,J,K,Y]Z
Non-OR ØXW[6,7]X[Ø,3,7,J,K,Y]Z

Ø Medical and Surgical
X Anatomical Regions, Upper Extremities
X Transfer Definition: Moving, without taking out, all or a portion of a body part to another location to take over the function of all or a portion of a body part
Explanation: The body part transferred remains connected to its vascular and nervous supply

Body Part Character 4	Approach Character 5	Device Character 6	Qualifier Character 7
N Index Finger, Right	Ø Open	Z No Device	L Thumb, Right
P Index Finger, Left	Ø Open	Z No Device	M Thumb, Left

Ø Medical and Surgical
X Anatomical Regions, Upper Extremities
Y Transplantation Definition: Putting in or on all or a portion of a living body part taken from another individual or animal to physically take the place and/or function of all or a portion of a similar body part
Explanation: The native body part may or may not be taken out, and the transplanted body part may take over all or a portion of its function

Body Part Character 4	Approach Character 5	Device Character 6	Qualifier Character 7
J Hand, Right K Hand, Left	Ø Open	Z No Device	Ø Allogeneic 1 Syngeneic

Anatomical Regions, Lower Extremities ØYØ–ØYW

Character Meanings

This Character Meaning table is provided as a guide to assist the user in the identification of character members that may be found in this section of code tables. It **SHOULD NOT** be used to build a PCS code.

Operation–Character 3		Body Part–Character 4		Approach–Character 5		Device–Character 6		Qualifier–Character 7	
Ø	Alteration	Ø	Buttock, Right	Ø	Open	Ø	Drainage Device	Ø	Complete
2	Change	1	Buttock, Left	3	Percutaneous	1	Radioactive Element	1	High
3	Control	2	Hindquarter, Right	4	Percutaneous Endoscopic	3	Infusion Device	2	Mid
6	Detachment	3	Hindquarter, Left	X	External	7	Autologous Tissue Substitute	3	Low
9	Drainage	4	Hindquarter, Bilateral			J	Synthetic Substitute	4	Complete 1st Ray
B	Excision	5	Inguinal Region, Right			K	Nonautologous Tissue Substitute	5	Complete 2nd Ray
H	Insertion	6	Inguinal Region, Left			Y	Other Device	6	Complete 3rd Ray
J	Inspection	7	Femoral Region, Right			Z	No Device	7	Complete 4th Ray
M	Reattachment	8	Femoral Region, Left					8	Complete 5th Ray
P	Removal	9	Lower Extremity, Right					9	Partial 1st Ray
Q	Repair	A	Inguinal Region, Bilateral					B	Partial 2nd Ray
U	Supplement	B	Lower Extremity, Left					C	Partial 3rd Ray
W	Revision	C	Upper Leg, Right					D	Partial 4th Ray
		D	Upper Leg, Left					F	Partial 5th Ray
		E	Femoral Region, Bilateral					X	Diagnostic
		F	Knee Region, Right					Z	No Qualifier
		G	Knee Region, Left						
		H	Lower Leg, Right						
		J	Lower Leg, Left						
		K	Ankle Region, Right						
		L	Ankle Region, Left						
		M	Foot, Right						
		N	Foot, Left						
		P	1st Toe, Right						
		Q	1st Toe, Left						
		R	2nd Toe, Right						
		S	2nd Toe, Left						
		T	3rd Toe, Right						
		U	3rd Toe, Left						
		V	4th Toe, Right						
		W	4th Toe, Left						
		X	5th Toe, Right						
		Y	5th Toe, Left						

AHA Coding Clinic for table ØY3
2016, 4Q, 99   Root operation Control
2013, 3Q, 23   Control of intraoperative bleeding

AHA Coding Clinic for table ØY6
2019, 2Q, 17   Cryoamputation of lower leg
2017, 2Q, 3-4   Qualifiers for the root operation detachment
2017, 1Q, 22   Chopart amputation of foot
2015, 2Q, 28   Partial amputation of hallux at interphalangeal Joint
2015, 1Q, 28   Mid-foot amputation

AHA Coding Clinic for table ØY9
2015, 1Q, 22   Incision and drainage of abscess of femoropopliteal bypass site
2015, 1Q, 22   Incision and drainage of groin abscess

AHA Coding Clinic for table ØYH
2023, 1Q, 27   Bilateral traumatic amputation with Stage 1 placement of OPRA device
2023, 1Q, 29   Stage 2 placement of OPRA device

AHA Coding Clinic for table ØYW
2023, 1Q, 29   Stage 2 placement of OPRA device

Anatomical Regions, Lower Extremities

Detachment Qualifier Descriptions

	Qualifier Definition	Upper Leg	Lower Leg
1	**High:** Amputation at the proximal portion of the shaft of the:	Femur	Tibia/Fibula
2	**Mid:** Amputation at the middle portion of the shaft of the:	Femur	Tibia/Fibula
3	**Low:** Amputation at the distal portion of the shaft of the:	Femur	Tibia/Fibula

	Qualifier Definition	Foot
0	Complete 1st through 5th Rays Ray: digit of hand or foot with corresponding metacarpus or metatarsus	Through tarso-metatarsal Joint, **Ankle**
4	Complete 1st Ray	Through tarso-metatarsal joint, **Great Toe**
5	Complete 2nd Ray	Through tarso-metatarsal joint, **2nd Toe**
6	Complete 3rd Ray	Through tarso-metatarsal joint, **3rd Toe**
7	Complete 4th Ray	Through tarso-metatarsal joint, **4th Toe**
8	Complete 5th Ray	Through tarso-metatarsal joint, **Little Toe**
9	Partial 1st Ray	Anywhere along shaft or head of metatarsal bone, **Great Toe**
B	Partial 2nd Ray	Anywhere along shaft or head of metatarsal bone, **2nd Toe**
C	Partial 3rd Ray	Anywhere along shaft or head of metatarsal bone, **3rd Toe**
D	Partial 4th Ray	Anywhere along shaft or head of metatarsal bone, **4th Toe**
F	Partial 5th Ray	Anywhere along shaft or head of metatarsal bone, **Little Toe**

	Qualifier Definition	Toe
0	Complete	At the metatarsal-phalangeal joint
1	High	Anywhere along the proximal phalanx
2	Mid	Through the proximal interphalangeal joint or anywhere along the middle phalanx
3	Low	Through the distal interphalangeal joint or anywhere along the distal phalanx

ICD-10-PCS 2025 — Anatomical Regions, Lower Extremities — ØYØ–ØY3

Ø   Medical and Surgical
Y   Anatomical Regions, Lower Extremities
Ø   Alteration   Definition: Modifying the anatomic structure of a body part without affecting the function of the body part
Explanation: Principal purpose is to improve appearance

Body Part Character 4	Approach Character 5	Device Character 6	Qualifier Character 7

Ø Buttock, Right
1 Buttock, Left
9 Lower Extremity, Right
B Lower Extremity, Left
C Upper Leg, Right
D Upper Leg, Left
F Knee Region, Right
    Popliteal fossa
G Knee Region, Left
    See Knee Region, Right
H Lower Leg, Right
J Lower Leg, Left
K Ankle Region, Right
L Ankle Region, Left
	Ø Open
	3 Percutaneous
	4 Percutaneous Endoscopic
		7 Autologous Tissue Substitute
		J Synthetic Substitute
		K Nonautologous Tissue Substitute
		Z No Device
			Z No Qualifier

Ø   Medical and Surgical
Y   Anatomical Regions, Lower Extremities
2   Change   Definition: Taking out or off a device from a body part and putting back an identical or similar device in or on the same body part without cutting or puncturing the skin or a mucous membrane
Explanation: All CHANGE procedures are coded using the approach EXTERNAL

Body Part Character 4	Approach Character 5	Device Character 6	Qualifier Character 7
9 Lower Extremity, Right B Lower Extremity, Left	X External	Ø Drainage Device Y Other Device	Z No Qualifier

Non-OR All body part, approach, device, and qualifier values

Ø   Medical and Surgical
Y   Anatomical Regions, Lower Extremities
3   Control   Definition: Stopping, or attempting to stop, postprocedural or other acute bleeding
Explanation: None

Body Part Character 4	Approach Character 5	Device Character 6	Qualifier Character 7

Ø Buttock, Right
1 Buttock, Left
5 Inguinal Region, Right
    Inguinal canal
    Inguinal triangle
6 Inguinal Region, Left
    See 5 Inguinal Region, Right
7 Femoral Region, Right
8 Femoral Region, Left
9 Lower Extremity, Right
B Lower Extremity, Left
C Upper Leg, Right
D Upper Leg, Left
F Knee Region, Right
    Popliteal fossa
G Knee Region, Left
    See Knee Region, Right
H Lower Leg, Right
J Lower Leg, Left
K Ankle Region, Right
L Ankle Region, Left
M Foot, Right
N Foot, Left
	Ø Open
	3 Percutaneous
	4 Percutaneous Endoscopic
		Z No Device	Z No Qualifier

NC Noncovered Procedure   **LC** Limited Coverage   **QA** Questionable OB Admit   **NT** New Tech Add-on   ✚ Combination Member   ♂ Male   ♀ Female

Anatomical Regions, Lower Extremities

0 Medical and Surgical
Y Anatomical Regions, Lower Extremities
6 Detachment

Definition: Cutting off all or a portion of the upper or lower extremities
Explanation: The body part value is the site of the detachment, with a qualifier if applicable to further specify the level where the extremity was detached

Body Part Character 4	Approach Character 5	Device Character 6	Qualifier Character 7

2 Hindquarter, Right
3 Hindquarter, Left
4 Hindquarter, Bilateral
7 Femoral Region, Right
8 Femoral Region, Left
F Knee Region, Right
   Popliteal fossa
G Knee Region, Left
   See Knee Region, Right
	0 Open	Z No Device	Z No Qualifier

C Upper Leg, Right D Upper Leg, Left H Lower Leg, Right J Lower Leg, Left	0 Open	Z No Device	1 High 2 Mid 3 Low
M Foot, Right N Foot, Left	0 Open	Z No Device	0 Complete 4 Complete 1st Ray 5 Complete 2nd Ray 6 Complete 3rd Ray 7 Complete 4th Ray 8 Complete 5th Ray 9 Partial 1st Ray B Partial 2nd Ray C Partial 3rd Ray D Partial 4th Ray F Partial 5th Ray

P 1st Toe, Right
   Hallux
Q 1st Toe, Left
   See 1st Toe, Right
	0 Open	Z No Device	0 Complete
			1 High
			3 Low

R 2nd Toe, Right S 2nd Toe, Left T 3rd Toe, Right U 3rd Toe, Left V 4th Toe, Right W 4th Toe, Left X 5th Toe, Right Y 5th Toe, Left	0 Open	Z No Device	0 Complete 1 High 2 Mid 3 Low

0 Medical and Surgical
Y Anatomical Regions, Lower Extremities
9 Drainage   Definition: Taking or letting out fluids and/or gases from a body part
                     Explanation: The qualifier DIAGNOSTIC is used to identify drainage procedures that are biopsies

Body Part Character 4	Approach Character 5	Device Character 6	Qualifier Character 7

0 Buttock, Right
1 Buttock, Left
5 Inguinal Region, Right
    Inguinal canal
    Inguinal triangle
6 Inguinal Region, Left
    See 5 Inguinal Region, Right
7 Femoral Region, Right
8 Femoral Region, Left
9 Lower Extremity, Right
B Lower Extremity, Left
C Upper Leg, Right
D Upper Leg, Left
F Knee Region, Right
    Popliteal fossa
G Knee Region, Left
    See Knee Region, Right
H Lower Leg, Right
J Lower Leg, Left
K Ankle Region, Right
L Ankle Region, Left
M Foot, Right
N Foot, Left
	0 Open
	3 Percutaneous
	4 Percutaneous Endoscopic
		0 Drainage Device	**Z** No Qualifier

0 Buttock, Right
1 Buttock, Left
5 Inguinal Region, Right
    Inguinal canal
    Inguinal triangle
6 Inguinal Region, Left
    See 5 Inguinal Region, Right
7 Femoral Region, Right
8 Femoral Region, Left
9 Lower Extremity, Right
B Lower Extremity, Left
C Upper Leg, Right
D Upper Leg, Left
F Knee Region, Right
    Popliteal fossa
G Knee Region, Left
    See Knee Region, Right
H Lower Leg, Right
J Lower Leg, Left
K Ankle Region, Right
L Ankle Region, Left
M Foot, Right
N Foot, Left
	0 Open
	3 Percutaneous
	4 Percutaneous Endoscopic
		Z No Device	**X** Diagnostic
			Z No Qualifier

Non-OR   0Y9[0,1,7,8,9,B,C,D,F,G,H,J,K,L,M,N][0,3,4]0Z
Non-OR   0Y9[5,6]30Z
Non-OR   0Y9[0,1,7,8,9,B,C,D,F,G,H,J,K,L,M,N][0,3,4]Z[X,Z]
Non-OR   0Y9[5,6]3ZZ

ØYB–ØYH Anatomical Regions, Lower Extremities ICD-10-PCS 2025

Ø Medical and Surgical
Y Anatomical Regions, Lower Extremities
B Excision Definition: Cutting out or off, without replacement, a portion of a body part
Explanation: The qualifier DIAGNOSTIC is used to identify excision procedures that are biopsies

Body Part Character 4	Approach Character 5	Device Character 6	Qualifier Character 7

Ø Buttock, Right
1 Buttock, Left
5 Inguinal Region, Right
  Inguinal canal
  Inguinal triangle
6 Inguinal Region, Left
  See 5 Inguinal Region, Right
7 Femoral Region, Right
8 Femoral Region, Left
9 Lower Extremity, Right
B Lower Extremity, Left
C Upper Leg, Right
D Upper Leg, Left
F Knee Region, Right
  Popliteal fossa
G Knee Region, Left
  See Knee Region, Right
H Lower Leg, Right
J Lower Leg, Left
K Ankle Region, Right
L Ankle Region, Left
M Foot, Right
N Foot, Left
	Ø Open
	3 Percutaneous
	4 Percutaneous Endoscopic
		Z No Device	X Diagnostic
			Z No Qualifier

Non-OR ØYB[Ø,1,9,B,C,D,F,G,H,J,K,L,M,N][Ø,3,4]ZX

Ø Medical and Surgical
Y Anatomical Regions, Lower Extremities
H Insertion Definition: Putting in a nonbiological appliance that monitors, assists, performs, or prevents a physiological function but does not physically take the place of a body part
Explanation: None

Body Part Character 4	Approach Character 5	Device Character 6	Qualifier Character 7

Ø Buttock, Right
1 Buttock, Left
5 Inguinal Region, Right
  Inguinal canal
  Inguinal triangle
6 Inguinal Region, Left
  See 5 Inguinal Region, Right
7 Femoral Region, Right
8 Femoral Region, Left
9 Lower Extremity, Right
B Lower Extremity, Left
C Upper Leg, Right
D Upper Leg, Left
F Knee Region, Right
  Popliteal fossa
G Knee Region, Left
  See Knee Region, Right
H Lower Leg, Right
J Lower Leg, Left
K Ankle Region, Right
L Ankle Region, Left
M Foot, Right
N Foot, Left
	Ø Open
	3 Percutaneous
	4 Percutaneous Endoscopic
		1 Radioactive Element
		3 Infusion Device
		Y Other Device
			Z No Qualifier

DRG Non-OR ØYH[Ø,1,5,6,7,8,9,B,C,D,F,G,H,J,K,L,M,N][Ø,3,4][3,Y]Z

Non-OR Procedure DRG Non-OR Procedure Valid OR Procedure HAC Associated Procedure Combination Only New/Revised April New/Revised October

0 Medical and Surgical
Y Anatomical Regions, Lower Extremities
J Inspection Definition: Visually and/or manually exploring a body part
Explanation: Visual exploration may be performed with or without optical instrumentation. Manual exploration may be performed directly or through intervening body layers.

Body Part Character 4	Approach Character 5	Device Character 6	Qualifier Character 7

0 Buttock, Right
1 Buttock, Left
5 Inguinal Region, Right
   Inguinal canal
   Inguinal triangle
6 Inguinal Region, Left
   See 5 Inguinal Region, Right
7 Femoral Region, Right
8 Femoral Region, Left
9 Lower Extremity, Right
A Inguinal Region, Bilateral
   See 5 Inguinal Region, Right
B Lower Extremity, Left
C Upper Leg, Right
D Upper Leg, Left
E Femoral Region, Bilateral
F Knee Region, Right
   Popliteal fossa
G Knee Region, Left
   See Knee Region, Right
H Lower Leg, Right
J Lower Leg, Left
K Ankle Region, Right
L Ankle Region, Left
M Foot, Right
N Foot, Left
	0 Open
	3 Percutaneous
	4 Percutaneous Endoscopic
	X External
		Z No Device	Z No Qualifier

DRG Non-OR   0YJ[0,1,8,9,B,C,D,E,F,G,H,J,K,L,M,N]0ZZ
Non-OR   0YJ[0,1,9,B,C,D,F,G,H,J,K,L,M,N][3,4,X]ZZ
Non-OR   0YJ[5,6,7,8,A,E][3,X]ZZ

0YM–0YP Anatomical Regions, Lower Extremities

0 Medical and Surgical
Y Anatomical Regions, Lower Extremities
M Reattachment   **Definition:** Putting back in or on all or a portion of a separated body part to its normal location or other suitable location
      Explanation: Vascular circulation and nervous pathways may or may not be reestablished

Body Part Character 4	Approach Character 5	Device Character 6	Qualifier Character 7

0 Buttock, Right
1 Buttock, Left
2 Hindquarter, Right
3 Hindquarter, Left
4 Hindquarter, Bilateral
5 Inguinal Region, Right
    Inguinal canal
    Inguinal triangle
6 Inguinal Region, Left
    See 5 Inguinal Region, Right
7 Femoral Region, Right
8 Femoral Region, Left
9 Lower Extremity, Right
B Lower Extremity, Left
C Upper Leg, Right
D Upper Leg, Left
F Knee Region, Right
    Popliteal fossa
G Knee Region, Left
    See Knee Region, Right
H Lower Leg, Right
J Lower Leg, Left
K Ankle Region, Right
L Ankle Region, Left
M Foot, Right
N Foot, Left
P 1st Toe, Right
    Hallux
Q 1st Toe, Left
    See 1st Toe, Right
R 2nd Toe, Right
S 2nd Toe, Left
T 3rd Toe, Right
U 3rd Toe, Left
V 4th Toe, Right
W 4th Toe, Left
X 5th Toe, Right
Y 5th Toe, Left
	0 Open	**Z** No Device	**Z** No Qualifier

0 Medical and Surgical
Y Anatomical Regions, Lower Extremities
P Removal   **Definition:** Taking out or off a device from a body part
      Explanation: If a device is taken out and a similar device put in without cutting or puncturing the skin or mucous membrane, the procedure is coded to the root operation CHANGE. Otherwise, the procedure for taking out the device is coded to the root operation REMOVAL.

Body Part Character 4	Approach Character 5	Device Character 6	Qualifier Character 7
9 Lower Extremity, Right **B** Lower Extremity, Left	**0** Open **3** Percutaneous **4** Percutaneous Endoscopic **X** External	**0** Drainage Device **1** Radioactive Element **3** Infusion Device **7** Autologous Tissue Substitute **J** Synthetic Substitute **K** Nonautologous Tissue Substitute **Y** Other Device	**Z** No Qualifier

Non-OR All body part, approach, device, and qualifier values

0 Medical and Surgical
Y Anatomical Regions, Lower Extremities
Q Repair   Definition: Restoring, to the extent possible, a body part to its normal anatomic structure and function
                Explanation: Used only when the method to accomplish the repair is not one of the other root operations

Body Part Character 4	Approach Character 5	Device Character 6	Qualifier Character 7

0 Buttock, Right
1 Buttock, Left
5 Inguinal Region, Right
    Inguinal canal
    Inguinal triangle
6 Inguinal Region, Left
    See 5 Inguinal Region, Right
7 Femoral Region, Right
8 Femoral Region, Left
9 Lower Extremity, Right
A Inguinal Region, Bilateral
    See 5 Inguinal Region, Right
B Lower Extremity, Left
C Upper Leg, Right
D Upper Leg, Left
E Femoral Region, Bilateral
F Knee Region, Right
    Popliteal fossa
G Knee Region, Left
    See Knee Region, Right
H Lower Leg, Right
J Lower Leg, Left
K Ankle Region, Right
L Ankle Region, Left
M Foot, Right
N Foot, Left
P 1st Toe, Right
    Hallux
Q 1st Toe, Left
    See 1st Toe, Right
R 2nd Toe, Right
S 2nd Toe, Left
T 3rd Toe, Right
U 3rd Toe, Left
V 4th Toe, Right
W 4th Toe, Left
X 5th Toe, Right
Y 5th Toe, Left
	0 Open
	3 Percutaneous
	4 Percutaneous Endoscopic
	X External
		Z No Device	**Z** No Qualifier

Non-OR   0YQ[5,6,7,8,A,E]XZZ

0 Medical and Surgical
Y Anatomical Regions, Lower Extremities
U Supplement

Definition: Putting in or on biological or synthetic material that physically reinforces and/or augments the function of a portion of a body part

Explanation: The biological material is non-living, or is living and from the same individual. The body part may have been previously replaced, and the SUPPLEMENT procedure is performed to physically reinforce and/or augment the function of the replaced body part.

Body Part Character 4	Approach Character 5	Device Character 6	Qualifier Character 7

0 Buttock, Right
1 Buttock, Left
5 Inguinal Region, Right
    Inguinal canal
    Inguinal triangle
6 Inguinal Region, Left
    See 5 Inguinal Region, Right
7 Femoral Region, Right
8 Femoral Region, Left
9 Lower Extremity, Right
A Inguinal Region, Bilateral
    See 5 Inguinal Region, Right
B Lower Extremity, Left
C Upper Leg, Right
D Upper Leg, Left
E Femoral Region, Bilateral
F Knee Region, Right
    Popliteal fossa
G Knee Region, Left
    See Knee Region, Right
H Lower Leg, Right
J Lower Leg, Left
K Ankle Region, Right
L Ankle Region, Left
M Foot, Right
N Foot, Left
P 1st Toe, Right
    Hallux
Q 1st Toe, Left
    See 1st Toe, Right
R 2nd Toe, Right
S 2nd Toe, Left
T 3rd Toe, Right
U 3rd Toe, Left
V 4th Toe, Right
W 4th Toe, Left
X 5th Toe, Right
Y 5th Toe, Left
	0 Open
	4 Percutaneous Endoscopic
		7 Autologous Tissue Substitute
		J Synthetic Substitute
		K Nonautologous Tissue Substitute
			Z No Qualifier

0 Medical and Surgical
Y Anatomical Regions, Lower Extremities
W Revision

Definition: Correcting, to the extent possible, a portion of a malfunctioning device or the position of a displaced device

Explanation: Revision can include correcting a malfunctioning or displaced device by taking out or putting in components of the device such as a screw or pin

Body Part Character 4	Approach Character 5	Device Character 6	Qualifier Character 7
9 Lower Extremity, Right **B** Lower Extremity, Left	**0** Open **3** Percutaneous **4** Percutaneous Endoscopic **X** External	**0** Drainage Device **3** Infusion Device **7** Autologous Tissue Substitute **J** Synthetic Substitute **K** Nonautologous Tissue Substitute **Y** Other Device	**Z** No Qualifier

DRG Non-OR 0YW[9,B][0,3,4][0,3,7,J,K,Y]Z
Non-OR 0YW[9,B]X[0,3,7,J,K,Y]Z

Obstetrics 1Ø2–1ØY

Character Meanings
This Character Meaning table is provided as a guide to assist the user in the identification of character members that may be found in this section of code tables. It **SHOULD NOT** be used to build a PCS code.

Ø: Pregnancy

Operation–Character 3		Body Part–Character 4		Approach–Character 5		Device–Character 6		Qualifier–Character 7	
2	Change	Ø	Products of Conception	Ø	Open	3	Monitoring Electrode	Ø	High
9	Drainage	1	Products of Conception, Retained	3	Percutaneous	Y	Other Device	1	Low
A	Abortion	2	Products of Conception, Ectopic	4	Percutaneous Endoscopic	Z	No Device	2	Extraperitoneal
D	Extraction			7	Via Natural or Artificial Opening			3	Low Forceps
E	Delivery			8	Via Natural or Artificial Opening Endoscopic			4	Mid Forceps
H	Insertion			X	External			5	High Forceps
J	Inspection							6	Vacuum
P	Removal							7	Internal Version
Q	Repair							8	Other
S	Reposition							9	Fetal Blood OR Manual
T	Resection							A	Fetal Cerebrospinal Fluid
Y	Transplantation							B	Fetal Fluid, Other
								C	Amniotic Fluid, Therapeutic
								D	Fluid, Other
								E	Nervous System
								F	Cardiovascular System
								G	Lymphatics & Hemic
								H	Eye
								J	Ear, Nose & Sinus
								K	Respiratory System
								L	Mouth & Throat
								M	Gastrointestinal System
								N	Hepatobiliary & Pancreas
								P	Endocrine System
								Q	Skin
								R	Musculoskeletal System
								S	Urinary System
								T	Female Reproductive System
								U	Amniotic Fluid, Diagnostic
								V	Male Reproductive System
								W	Laminaria
								X	Abortifacient
								Y	Other Body System
								Z	No Qualifier

AHA Coding Clinic for table 1Ø9
2014, 3Q, 12   Fetoscopic laser photocoagulation and laser microseptostomy for twin-twin transfusion syndrome
2014, 2Q, 9   Pitocin administration to augment labor

AHA Coding Clinic for table 1ØA
2022, 1Q, 21   Gravid hysterectomy due to placenta increta
2022, 1Q, 41   Intrauterine Cook balloon placement for ectopic pregnancy

AHA Coding Clinic for table 1ØD
2022, 1Q, 19   Spontaneous abortion with retained placenta of Twin B
2021, 1Q, 52   Removal of ectopic pregnancy via laparotomy
2020, 4Q, 59-60   Extraction of ectopic products of conception
2018, 4Q, 49-51   Revised qualifier values for root operation "extraction" (cesarean delivery)
2018, 2Q, 17   High transverse cesarean section
2016, 1Q, 9   Vaginal delivery assisted by vacuum and low forceps extraction
2014, 4Q, 43   Cesarean delivery assisted by vacuum extraction
2014, 4Q, 43   Vacuum dilation and curettage for blighted ovum

AHA Coding Clinic for table 1ØE
2017, 3Q, 5   Delivery of placenta
2016, 2Q, 34   Assisted vaginal delivery
2014, 4Q, 17   RH (D) alloimmunization (sensitization)
2014, 2Q, 9   Pitocin administration to augment labor

AHA Coding Clinic for table 1ØH
2013, 2Q, 36   Intrauterine pressure monitor

AHA Coding Clinic for table 1ØQ
2021, 2Q, 21   Ex Utero intrapartum treatment procedure
2014, 3Q, 12   Fetoscopic laser photocoagulation and laser microseptostomy for twin-twin transfusion syndrome

AHA Coding Clinic for table 1ØT
2020, 3Q, 47   Removal of ectopic cornual pregnancy
2015, 3Q, 31   Laparoscopic partial salpingectomy for ectopic pregnancy

1 Obstetrics
0 Pregnancy
2 Change

Definition: Taking out or off a device from a body part and putting back an identical or similar device in or on the same body part without cutting or puncturing the skin or a mucous membrane

Explanation: None

Body Part Character 4	Approach Character 5	Device Character 6	Qualifier Character 7
0 Products of Conception	7 Via Natural or Artificial Opening	3 Monitoring Electrode Y Other Device	Z No Qualifier

Non-OR All body part, approach, device, and qualifier values

1 Obstetrics
0 Pregnancy
9 Drainage

Definition: Taking or letting out fluids and/or gases from a body part

Explanation: None

Body Part Character 4	Approach Character 5	Device Character 6	Qualifier Character 7
0 Products of Conception	0 Open 3 Percutaneous 4 Percutaneous Endoscopic 7 Via Natural or Artificial Opening 8 Via Natural or Artificial Opening Endoscopic	Z No Device	9 Fetal Blood A Fetal Cerebrospinal Fluid B Fetal Fluid, Other C Amniotic Fluid, Therapeutic D Fluid, Other U Amniotic Fluid, Diagnostic

Non-OR All body part, approach, device, and qualifier values

1 Obstetrics
0 Pregnancy
A Abortion

Definition: Artificially terminating a pregnancy

Explanation: None

Body Part Character 4	Approach Character 5	Device Character 6	Qualifier Character 7
0 Products of Conception	0 Open 3 Percutaneous 4 Percutaneous Endoscopic 8 Via Natural or Artificial Opening Endoscopic	Z No Device	Z No Qualifier
0 Products of Conception	7 Via Natural or Artificial Opening	Z No Device	6 Vacuum W Laminaria X Abortifacient Z No Qualifier

Non-OR 10A07Z[6,W,X]

1 Obstetrics
0 Pregnancy
D Extraction

Definition: Pulling or stripping out or off all or a portion of a body part by the use of force

Explanation: None

Body Part Character 4	Approach Character 5	Device Character 6	Qualifier Character 7
0 Products of Conception ᴼᴬ	0 Open	Z No Device	0 High 1 Low 2 Extraperitoneal
0 Products of Conception ᴼᴬ	7 Via Natural or Artificial Opening	Z No Device	3 Low Forceps 4 Mid Forceps 5 High Forceps 6 Vacuum 7 Internal Version 8 Other
1 Products of Conception, Retained	7 Via Natural or Artificial Opening 8 Via Natural or Artificial Opening Endoscopic	Z No Device	9 Manual Z No Qualifier
2 Products of Conception, Ectopic	0 Open 4 Percutaneous Endoscopic 7 Via Natural or Artificial Opening 8 Via Natural or Artificial Opening Endoscopic	Z No Device	Z No Qualifier

DRG Non-OR 10D07Z[3,4,5,6,7,8]
QA 10D00Z[0,1,2] except when a corresponding SDX of Z37.0-Z37.9 is also reported
QA 10D07Z[3,4,5,7] except when a corresponding SDX of Z37.0-Z37.9 is also reported

1 Obstetrics
0 Pregnancy
E Delivery

Definition: Assisting the passage of the products of conception from the genital canal
Explanation: None

Body Part Character 4	Approach Character 5	Device Character 6	Qualifier Character 7
0 Products of Conception	QA X External	Z No Device	Z No Qualifier

DRG Non-OR 10E0XZZ
QA 10E0XZZ except when a corresponding SDX of Z37.0-Z37.9 is also reported

1 Obstetrics
0 Pregnancy
H Insertion

Definition: Putting in a nonbiological appliance that monitors, assists, performs, or prevents a physiological function but does not physically take the place of a body part
Explanation: None

Body Part Character 4	Approach Character 5	Device Character 6	Qualifier Character 7
0 Products of Conception	0 Open 7 Via Natural or Artificial Opening	3 Monitoring Electrode Y Other Device	Z No Qualifier

Non-OR All body part, approach, device, and qualifier values

1 Obstetrics
0 Pregnancy
J Inspection

Definition: Visually and/or manually exploring a body part
Explanation: Visual exploration may be performed with or without optical instrumentation. Manual exploration may be performed directly or through intervening body layers.

Body Part Character 4	Approach Character 5	Device Character 6	Qualifier Character 7
0 Products of Conception 1 Products of Conception, Retained 2 Products of Conception, Ectopic	0 Open 3 Percutaneous 4 Percutaneous Endoscopic 7 Via Natural or Artificial Opening 8 Via Natural or Artificial Opening Endoscopic X External	Z No Device	Z No Qualifier

Non-OR All body part, approach, device, and qualifier values

1 Obstetrics
0 Pregnancy
P Removal

Definition: Taking out or off a device from a body part, region or orifice
Explanation: If a device is taken out and a similar device put in without cutting or puncturing the skin or mucous membrane, the procedure is coded to the root operation CHANGE. Otherwise, the procedure for taking out a device is coded to the root operation REMOVAL.

Body Part Character 4	Approach Character 5	Device Character 6	Qualifier Character 7
0 Products of Conception	0 Open 7 Via Natural or Artificial Opening	3 Monitoring Electrode Y Other Device	Z No Qualifier

Non-OR All body part, approach, device, and qualifier values

1 Obstetrics
0 Pregnancy
Q Repair

Definition: Restoring, to the extent possible, a body part to its normal anatomic structure and function
Explanation: Used only when the method to accomplish the repair is not one of the other root operations

Body Part Character 4	Approach Character 5	Device Character 6	Qualifier Character 7
0 Products of Conception	0 Open 3 Percutaneous 4 Percutaneous Endoscopic 7 Via Natural or Artificial Opening 8 Via Natural or Artificial Opening Endoscopic	Y Other Device Z No Device	E Nervous System F Cardiovascular System G Lymphatics and Hemic H Eye J Ear, Nose and Sinus K Respiratory System L Mouth and Throat M Gastrointestinal System N Hepatobiliary and Pancreas P Endocrine System Q Skin R Musculoskeletal System S Urinary System T Female Reproductive System V Male Reproductive System Y Other Body System

Non-OR All body part, approach, device, and qualifier values

1 Obstetrics
0 Pregnancy
S Reposition

Definition: Moving to its normal location, or other suitable location, all or a portion of a body part

Explanation: The body part is moved to a new location from an abnormal location, or from a normal location where it is not functioning correctly. The body part may or may not be cut out or off to be moved to the new location.

Body Part Character 4	Approach Character 5	Device Character 6	Qualifier Character 7
0 Products of Conception	7 Via Natural or Artificial Opening X External	Z No Device	Z No Qualifier
2 Products of Conception, Ectopic	0 Open 3 Percutaneous 4 Percutaneous Endoscopic 7 Via Natural or Artificial Opening 8 Via Natural or Artificial Opening Endoscopic	Z No Device	Z No Qualifier

Non-OR 10S0[7,X]ZZ

1 Obstetrics
0 Pregnancy
T Resection

Definition: Cutting out or off, without replacement, all of a body part

Explanation: None

Body Part Character 4	Approach Character 5	Device Character 6	Qualifier Character 7
2 Products of Conception, Ectopic	0 Open 3 Percutaneous 4 Percutaneous Endoscopic 7 Via Natural or Artificial Opening 8 Via Natural or Artificial Opening Endoscopic	Z No Device	Z No Qualifier

1 Obstetrics
0 Pregnancy
Y Transplantation

Definition: Putting in or on all or a portion of a living body part taken from another individual or animal to physically take the place and/or function of all or a portion of a similar body part

Explanation: The native body part may or may not be taken out, and the transplanted body part may take over all or a portion of its function

Body Part Character 4	Approach Character 5	Device Character 6	Qualifier Character 7
0 Products of Conception	3 Percutaneous 4 Percutaneous Endoscopic 7 Via Natural or Artificial Opening	Z No Device	E Nervous System F Cardiovascular System G Lymphatics and Hemic H Eye J Ear, Nose and Sinus K Respiratory System L Mouth and Throat M Gastrointestinal System N Hepatobiliary and Pancreas P Endocrine System Q Skin R Musculoskeletal System S Urinary System T Female Reproductive System V Male Reproductive System Y Other Body System

Non-OR All body part, approach, device, and qualifier values

Placement 2W0–2Y5

AHA Coding Clinic for table 2W6
- 2015, 2Q, 35 — Application of tongs to reduce and stabilize cervical fracture
- 2013, 2Q, 39 — Application of cervical tongs for reduction of cervical fracture

AHA Coding Clinic for table 2Y4
- 2018, 4Q, 38 — Control of epistaxis
- 2017, 4Q, 106 — Nasal packing for epistaxis

2 Placement
W Anatomical Regions
0 Change — Definition: Taking out or off a device from a body part and putting back an identical or similar device in or on the same body part without cutting or puncturing the skin or a mucous membrane

Body Region Character 4	Approach Character 5	Device Character 6	Qualifier Character 7
0 Head 2 Neck 3 Abdominal Wall 4 Chest Wall 5 Back 6 Inguinal Region, Right 7 Inguinal Region, Left 8 Upper Extremity, Right 9 Upper Extremity, Left A Upper Arm, Right B Upper Arm, Left C Lower Arm, Right D Lower Arm, Left E Hand, Right F Hand, Left G Thumb, Right H Thumb, Left J Finger, Right K Finger, Left L Lower Extremity, Right M Lower Extremity, Left N Upper Leg, Right P Upper Leg, Left Q Lower Leg, Right R Lower Leg, Left S Foot, Right T Foot, Left U Toe, Right V Toe, Left	X External	0 Traction Apparatus 1 Splint 2 Cast 3 Brace 4 Bandage 5 Packing Material 6 Pressure Dressing 7 Intermittent Pressure Device Y Other Device	Z No Qualifier
1 Face	X External	0 Traction Apparatus 1 Splint 2 Cast 3 Brace 4 Bandage 5 Packing Material 6 Pressure Dressing 7 Intermittent Pressure Device 9 Wire Y Other Device	Z No Qualifier

2 Placement
W Anatomical Regions
1 Compression
Definition: Putting pressure on a body region

Body Region Character 4	Approach Character 5	Device Character 6	Qualifier Character 7
0 Head 1 Face 2 Neck 3 Abdominal Wall 4 Chest Wall 5 Back 6 Inguinal Region, Right 7 Inguinal Region, Left 8 Upper Extremity, Right 9 Upper Extremity, Left A Upper Arm, Right B Upper Arm, Left C Lower Arm, Right D Lower Arm, Left E Hand, Right F Hand, Left G Thumb, Right H Thumb, Left J Finger, Right K Finger, Left L Lower Extremity, Right M Lower Extremity, Left N Upper Leg, Right P Upper Leg, Left Q Lower Leg, Right R Lower Leg, Left S Foot, Right T Foot, Left U Toe, Right V Toe, Left	X External	6 Pressure Dressing 7 Intermittent Pressure Device	Z No Qualifier

2 Placement
W Anatomical Regions
2 Dressing
Definition: Putting material on a body region for protection

Body Region Character 4	Approach Character 5	Device Character 6	Qualifier Character 7
0 Head 1 Face 2 Neck 3 Abdominal Wall 4 Chest Wall 5 Back 6 Inguinal Region, Right 7 Inguinal Region, Left 8 Upper Extremity, Right 9 Upper Extremity, Left A Upper Arm, Right B Upper Arm, Left C Lower Arm, Right D Lower Arm, Left E Hand, Right F Hand, Left G Thumb, Right H Thumb, Left J Finger, Right K Finger, Left L Lower Extremity, Right M Lower Extremity, Left N Upper Leg, Right P Upper Leg, Left Q Lower Leg, Right R Lower Leg, Left S Foot, Right T Foot, Left U Toe, Right V Toe, Left	X External	4 Bandage	Z No Qualifier

Non-OR Procedure DRG Non-OR Procedure Valid OR Procedure HAC Associated Procedure Combination Only New/Revised April New/Revised October

2 Placement
W Anatomical Regions
3 Immobilization   Definition: Limiting or preventing motion of a body region

Body Region Character 4	Approach Character 5	Device Character 6	Qualifier Character 7
0 Head 2 Neck 3 Abdominal Wall 4 Chest Wall 5 Back 6 Inguinal Region, Right 7 Inguinal Region, Left 8 Upper Extremity, Right 9 Upper Extremity, Left A Upper Arm, Right B Upper Arm, Left C Lower Arm, Right D Lower Arm, Left E Hand, Right F Hand, Left G Thumb, Right H Thumb, Left J Finger, Right K Finger, Left L Lower Extremity, Right M Lower Extremity, Left N Upper Leg, Right P Upper Leg, Left Q Lower Leg, Right R Lower Leg, Left S Foot, Right T Foot, Left U Toe, Right V Toe, Left	X External	1 Splint 2 Cast 3 Brace Y Other Device	Z No Qualifier
1 Face	X External	1 Splint 2 Cast 3 Brace 9 Wire Y Other Device	Z No Qualifier

2 Placement
W Anatomical Regions
4 Packing   Definition: Putting material in a body region or orifice

Body Region Character 4	Approach Character 5	Device Character 6	Qualifier Character 7
0 Head 1 Face 2 Neck 3 Abdominal Wall 4 Chest Wall 5 Back 6 Inguinal Region, Right 7 Inguinal Region, Left 8 Upper Extremity, Right 9 Upper Extremity, Left A Upper Arm, Right B Upper Arm, Left C Lower Arm, Right D Lower Arm, Left E Hand, Right F Hand, Left G Thumb, Right H Thumb, Left J Finger, Right K Finger, Left L Lower Extremity, Right M Lower Extremity, Left N Upper Leg, Right P Upper Leg, Left Q Lower Leg, Right R Lower Leg, Left S Foot, Right T Foot, Left U Toe, Right V Toe, Left	X External	5 Packing Material	Z No Qualifier

NC Noncovered Procedure   **LC** Limited Coverage   **QA** Questionable OB Admit   **NT** New Tech Add-on   ✚ Combination Member   ♂ Male   ♀ Female

2 Placement
W Anatomical Regions
5 Removal   Definition: Taking out or off a device from a body part

Body Region Character 4	Approach Character 5	Device Character 6	Qualifier Character 7
0 Head 2 Neck 3 Abdominal Wall 4 Chest Wall 5 Back 6 Inguinal Region, Right 7 Inguinal Region, Left 8 Upper Extremity, Right 9 Upper Extremity, Left A Upper Arm, Right B Upper Arm, Left C Lower Arm, Right D Lower Arm, Left E Hand, Right F Hand, Left G Thumb, Right H Thumb, Left J Finger, Right K Finger, Left L Lower Extremity, Right M Lower Extremity, Left N Upper Leg, Right P Upper Leg, Left Q Lower Leg, Right R Lower Leg, Left S Foot, Right T Foot, Left U Toe, Right V Toe, Left	X External	0 Traction Apparatus 1 Splint 2 Cast 3 Brace 4 Bandage 5 Packing Material 6 Pressure Dressing 7 Intermittent Pressure Device Y Other Device	Z No Qualifier
1 Face	X External	0 Traction Apparatus 1 Splint 2 Cast 3 Brace 4 Bandage 5 Packing Material 6 Pressure Dressing 7 Intermittent Pressure Device 9 Wire Y Other Device	Z No Qualifier

2 Placement
W Anatomical Regions
6 Traction
Definition: Exerting a pulling force on a body region in a distal direction

Body Region Character 4	Approach Character 5	Device Character 6	Qualifier Character 7
0 Head 1 Face 2 Neck 3 Abdominal Wall 4 Chest Wall 5 Back 6 Inguinal Region, Right 7 Inguinal Region, Left 8 Upper Extremity, Right 9 Upper Extremity, Left A Upper Arm, Right B Upper Arm, Left C Lower Arm, Right D Lower Arm, Left E Hand, Right F Hand, Left G Thumb, Right H Thumb, Left J Finger, Right K Finger, Left L Lower Extremity, Right M Lower Extremity, Left N Upper Leg, Right P Upper Leg, Left Q Lower Leg, Right R Lower Leg, Left S Foot, Right T Foot, Left U Toe, Right V Toe, Left	X External	0 Traction Apparatus Z No Device	Z No Qualifier

2 Placement
Y Anatomical Orifices
0 Change
Definition: Taking out or off a device from a body part and putting back an identical or similar device in or on the same body part without cutting or puncturing the skin or a mucous membrane

Body Region Character 4	Approach Character 5	Device Character 6	Qualifier Character 7
0 Mouth and Pharynx 1 Nasal 2 Ear 3 Anorectal 4 Female Genital Tract 5 Urethra	X External	5 Packing Material	Z No Qualifier

2 Placement
Y Anatomical Orifices
4 Packing
Definition: Putting material in a body region or orifice

Body Region Character 4	Approach Character 5	Device Character 6	Qualifier Character 7
0 Mouth and Pharynx 1 Nasal 2 Ear 3 Anorectal 4 Female Genital Tract 5 Urethra	X External	5 Packing Material	Z No Qualifier

2 Placement
Y Anatomical Orifices
5 Removal
Definition: Taking out or off a device from a body part

Body Region Character 4	Approach Character 5	Device Character 6	Qualifier Character 7
0 Mouth and Pharynx 1 Nasal 2 Ear 3 Anorectal 4 Female Genital Tract 5 Urethra	X External	5 Packing Material	Z No Qualifier

Administration 3Ø2–3E1

AHA Coding Clinic for table 3Ø2
2023, 1Q, 10-11	Intraosseous administration of blood products
2021, 4Q, 54	Nonautologous pathogen reduced cryoprecipitated fibrinogen complex
2020, 4Q, 60-61	Transfusion stem cell progenitor cells
2019, 4Q, 35	Transfusion of blood products
2019, 4Q, 36	T-cell depleted hematopoietic stem cells for transplantation
2016, 4Q, 113	Bone marrow and stem cell transfusion (Transplantation)

AHA Coding Clinic for table 3EØ
2024, 1Q, 9	Introduction of other therapeutic monoclonal antibody
2023, 2Q, 33	Testing of premature rupture of membranes via indigo carmine injection
2022, 4Q, 60-61	Introduction of other therapeutic monoclonal antibody
2022, 4Q, 61	Introduction of bone-substitute material
2022, 3Q, 26	Tumor-infiltrating lymphocyte therapy
2022, 1Q, 8	Other monoclonal antibody
2021, 4Q, 54-55	Antineoplastic monoclonal antibody
2021, 4Q, 110	New/revised frequently asked questions regarding ICD-10-CM/PCS coding for COVID-19
2021, 1Q, 49	Frequently asked questions regarding ICD-10-CM and ICD-10-PCS coding for COVID-19
2020, 4Q, 49-50	Intravascular ultrasound assisted thrombolysis
2020, 4Q, 95	Frequently asked questions regarding ICD-10-PCS coding for COVID-19
2020, 3Q, 17-21	New procedure codes for introduction or infusion of therapeutics
2019, 4Q, 36-37	Hyperthermic antineoplastic chemotherapy
2018, 3Q, 7	Coronary brachytherapy with angioplasty
2018, 1Q, 8	Placement of bone morphogenetic protein & spinal fusion surgery
2017, 2Q, 14	Infusion of tPA into pleural cavity
2017, 1Q, 37	Injection of glue into enteric fistula tract
2016, 4Q, 113-114	Substances applied to cranial cavity and brain
2016, 3Q, 29	Closure of bilateral alveolar clefts
2016, 1Q, 20	Metatarsophalangeal joint resection arthroplasty

AHA Coding Clinic for table 3EØ (Continued)
2015, 3Q, 24	Esophagogastroduodenoscopy with epinephrine injection for control of bleeding
2015, 3Q, 29	Placement of adhesion barrier
2015, 2Q, 29	Insertion of nasogastric tube for drainage and feeding
2015, 2Q, 31	Thoracoscopic talc pleurodesis
2015, 1Q, 31	Intrathecal chemotherapy
2015, 1Q, 38	Chemoembolization of the hepatic artery
2014, 4Q, 16	Administration of RH (D) immunoglobulin
2014, 4Q, 17	RH (D) alloimmunization (sensitization)
2014, 4Q, 19	Ultrasound accelerated thrombolysis
2014, 4Q, 34	Resection of brain malignancy with implantation of chemotherapeutic wafer
2014, 4Q, 38	Placement of saline and Seprafilm solution into abdominal cavity
2014, 3Q, 26	Coil embolization of gastroduodenal artery with chemoembolization of hepatic artery
2014, 2Q, 8	Medical induction of labor with Cervidil tampon insertion
2014, 2Q, 10	Prophylactic Neulasta injection for infection prevention
2013, 4Q, 124	Administration of tPA for stroke treatment prior to transfer
2013, 1Q, 27	Injection of sclerosing agent into an esophageal varix

AHA Coding Clinic for table 3E1
2021, 4Q, 55	Laparoscopic irrigation of peritoneal cavity
2019, 4Q, 38	Irrigation of joint using irrigating substance
2017, 3Q, 14	Bronchoscopy with suctioning and washings for removal of mucus plug

3 Administration
0 Circulatory
2 Transfusion
Definition: Putting in blood or blood products

Body System/Region Character 4	Approach Character 5	Substance Character 6	Qualifier Character 7
3 Peripheral Vein [NC] 4 Central Vein [NC]	3 Percutaneous	A Stem Cells, Embryonic	Z No Qualifier
3 Peripheral Vein 4 Central Vein	3 Percutaneous	C Hematopoietic Stem/Progenitor Cells, Genetically Modified	0 Autologous
3 Peripheral Vein 4 Central Vein	3 Percutaneous	D Pathogen Reduced Cryoprecipitated Fibrinogen Complex	1 Nonautologous
3 Peripheral Vein [NC] 4 Central Vein [NC]	3 Percutaneous	G Bone Marrow X Stem Cells, Cord Blood Y Stem Cells, Hematopoietic	0 Autologous 2 Allogeneic, Related 3 Allogeneic, Unrelated 4 Allogeneic, Unspecified
3 Peripheral Vein 4 Central Vein	3 Percutaneous	H Whole Blood J Serum Albumin K Frozen Plasma L Fresh Plasma M Plasma Cryoprecipitate N Red Blood Cells P Frozen Red Cells Q White Cells R Platelets S Globulin T Fibrinogen V Antihemophilic Factors W Factor IX	0 Autologous 1 Nonautologous
3 Peripheral Vein 4 Central Vein	3 Percutaneous	U Stem Cells, T-cell Depleted Hematopoietic	2 Allogeneic, Related 3 Allogeneic, Unrelated 4 Allogeneic, Unspecified
7 Products of Conception, Circulatory	3 Percutaneous 7 Via Natural or Artificial Opening	H Whole Blood J Serum Albumin K Frozen Plasma L Fresh Plasma M Plasma Cryoprecipitate N Red Blood Cells P Frozen Red Cells Q White Cells R Platelets S Globulin T Fibrinogen V Antihemophilic Factors W Factor IX	1 Nonautologous
8 Vein	3 Percutaneous	B 4-Factor Prothrombin Complex Concentrate	1 Nonautologous
A Bone Marrow	3 Percutaneous	H Whole Blood J Serum Albumin K Frozen Plasma L Fresh Plasma N Red Blood Cells P Frozen Red Cells R Platelets	0 Autologous 1 Nonautologous

DRG Non-OR	302[3,4]3AZ
DRG Non-OR	302[3,4]3C0
DRG Non-OR	302[3,4]3[G,X,Y][0,2,3,4]
DRG Non-OR	302[3,4]3U[2,3,4]

[NC] 302[3,4]3AZ Only when reported with PDx or SDx of C91.00, C92.00, C92.10, C92.11, C92.40, C92.50, C92.60, C92.A0, C93.00, C94.00, C95.00
[NC] 302[3,4]3[G,Y]0 Only when reported with PDx or SDx of C91.00, C92.00, C92.10, C92.11, C92.40, C92.50, C92.60, C92.A0, C93.00, C94.00, C95.00

3 Administration
C Indwelling Device
1 Irrigation
Definition: Putting in or on a cleansing substance

Body System/Region Character 4	Approach Character 5	Substance Character 6	Qualifier Character 7
Z None	X External	8 Irrigating Substance	Z No Qualifier

3 Administration
E Physiological Systems and Anatomical Regions
0 Introduction

Definition: Putting in or on a therapeutic, diagnostic, nutritional, physiological, or prophylactic substance except blood or blood products

Body System/Region Character 4	Approach Character 5	Substance Character 6	Qualifier Character 7
0 Skin and Mucous Membranes	X External	0 Antineoplastic	5 Other Antineoplastic M Monoclonal Antibody
0 Skin and Mucous Membranes	X External	2 Anti-infective	8 Oxazolidinones 9 Other Anti-infective
0 Skin and Mucous Membranes	X External	3 Anti-inflammatory 4 Serum, Toxoid and Vaccine B Anesthetic Agent K Other Diagnostic Substance M Pigment N Analgesics, Hypnotics, Sedatives T Destructive Agent	Z No Qualifier
0 Skin and Mucous Membranes	X External	G Other Therapeutic Substance	C Other Substance
1 Subcutaneous Tissue	0 Open	2 Anti-infective	A Anti-Infective Envelope
1 Subcutaneous Tissue	3 Percutaneous	0 Antineoplastic	5 Other Antineoplastic M Monoclonal Antibody
1 Subcutaneous Tissue	3 Percutaneous	2 Anti-infective	8 Oxazolidinones 9 Other Anti-infective A Anti-Infective Envelope
1 Subcutaneous Tissue	3 Percutaneous	3 Anti-inflammatory 6 Nutritional Substance 7 Electrolytic and Water Balance Substance B Anesthetic Agent H Radioactive Substance K Other Diagnostic Substance N Analgesics, Hypnotics, Sedatives T Destructive Agent	Z No Qualifier
1 Subcutaneous Tissue	3 Percutaneous	4 Serum, Toxoid and Vaccine	0 Influenza Vaccine Z No Qualifier
1 Subcutaneous Tissue	3 Percutaneous	G Other Therapeutic Substance	C Other Substance
1 Subcutaneous Tissue	3 Percutaneous	V Hormone	G Insulin J Other Hormone
2 Muscle	3 Percutaneous	0 Antineoplastic	5 Other Antineoplastic M Monoclonal Antibody
2 Muscle	3 Percutaneous	2 Anti-infective	8 Oxazolidinones 9 Other Anti-infective
2 Muscle	3 Percutaneous	3 Anti-inflammatory 6 Nutritional Substance 7 Electrolytic and Water Balance Substance B Anesthetic Agent H Radioactive Substance K Other Diagnostic Substance N Analgesics, Hypnotics, Sedatives T Destructive Agent	Z No Qualifier
2 Muscle	3 Percutaneous	4 Serum, Toxoid and Vaccine	0 Influenza Vaccine Z No Qualifier
2 Muscle	3 Percutaneous	G Other Therapeutic Substance	C Other Substance
3 Peripheral Vein	0 Open	0 Antineoplastic	2 High-dose Interleukin-2 3 Low-dose Interleukin-2 5 Other Antineoplastic M Monoclonal Antibody P Clofarabine
3 Peripheral Vein	0 Open	1 Thrombolytic	6 Recombinant Human-activated Protein C 7 Other Thrombolytic
3 Peripheral Vein	0 Open	2 Anti-infective	8 Oxazolidinones 9 Other Anti-infective

DRG Non-OR 3E03002
DRG Non-OR 3E03017

3E0 Continued on next page

Administration

3E0–3E0 Administration — ICD-10-PCS 2025

3E0 Continued

3 Administration
E Physiological Systems and Anatomical Regions
0 Introduction   Definition: Putting in or on a therapeutic, diagnostic, nutritional, physiological, or prophylactic substance except blood or blood products

Body System/Region Character 4	Approach Character 5	Substance Character 6	Qualifier Character 7
3 Peripheral Vein	0 Open	3 Anti-inflammatory 4 Serum, Toxoid and Vaccine 6 Nutritional Substance 7 Electrolytic and Water Balance Substance F Intracirculatory Anesthetic H Radioactive Substance K Other Diagnostic Substance N Analgesics, Hypnotics, Sedatives P Platelet Inhibitor R Antiarrhythmic T Destructive Agent X Vasopressor	Z No Qualifier
3 Peripheral Vein	0 Open	G Other Therapeutic Substance	C Other Substance N Blood Brain Barrier Disruption
3 Peripheral Vein	0 Open	U Pancreatic Islet Cells	0 Autologous 1 Nonautologous
3 Peripheral Vein	0 Open	V Hormone	G Insulin H Human B-type Natriuretic Peptide J Other Hormone
3 Peripheral Vein	0 Open	W Immunotherapeutic	K Immunostimulator L Immunosuppressive
3 Peripheral Vein	3 Percutaneous	0 Antineoplastic	2 High-dose Interleukin-2 3 Low-dose Interleukin-2 5 Other Antineoplastic M Monoclonal Antibody P Clofarabine
3 Peripheral Vein	3 Percutaneous	1 Thrombolytic	6 Recombinant Human- activated Protein C 7 Other Thrombolytic
3 Peripheral Vein	3 Percutaneous	2 Anti-infective	8 Oxazolidinones 9 Other Anti-infective
3 Peripheral Vein	3 Percutaneous	3 Anti-inflammatory 4 Serum, Toxoid and Vaccine 6 Nutritional Substance 7 Electrolytic and Water Balance Substance F Intracirculatory Anesthetic H Radioactive Substance K Other Diagnostic Substance N Analgesics, Hypnotics, Sedatives P Platelet Inhibitor R Antiarrhythmic T Destructive Agent X Vasopressor	Z No Qualifier
3 Peripheral Vein	3 Percutaneous	G Other Therapeutic Substance	C Other Substance N Blood Brain Barrier Disruption Q Glucarpidase R Other Therapeutic Monoclonal Antibody
3 Peripheral Vein	3 Percutaneous	U Pancreatic Islet Cells	0 Autologous 1 Nonautologous
3 Peripheral Vein	3 Percutaneous	V Hormone	G Insulin H Human B-type Natriuretic Peptide J Other Hormone
3 Peripheral Vein	3 Percutaneous	W Immunotherapeutic	K Immunostimulator L Immunosuppressive
4 Central Vein	0 Open	0 Antineoplastic	2 High-dose Interleukin-2 3 Low-dose Interleukin-2 5 Other Antineoplastic M Monoclonal Antibody P Clofarabine
4 Central Vein	0 Open	1 Thrombolytic	6 Recombinant Human- activated Protein C 7 Other Thrombolytic

Valid OR   3E030TZ
DRG Non-OR   3E030U[0,1]
DRG Non-OR   3E03302
DRG Non-OR   3E03317
DRG Non-OR   3E033U[0,1]
DRG Non-OR   3E04002
DRG Non-OR   3E04017

3E0 Continued on next page

Non-OR Procedure   DRG Non-OR Procedure   Valid OR Procedure   HAC Associated Procedure   Combination Only   New/Revised April   New/Revised October

ICD-10-PCS 2025 — Administration — 3E0–3E0

3 Administration
E Physiological Systems and Anatomical Regions
0 Introduction — Definition: Putting in or on a therapeutic, diagnostic, nutritional, physiological, or prophylactic substance except blood or blood products

3E0 Continued

Body System/Region Character 4	Approach Character 5	Substance Character 6	Qualifier Character 7
4 Central Vein	0 Open	2 Anti-infective	8 Oxazolidinones 9 Other Anti-infective
4 Central Vein	0 Open	3 Anti-inflammatory 4 Serum, Toxoid and Vaccine 6 Nutritional Substance 7 Electrolytic and Water Balance Substance F Intracirculatory Anesthetic H Radioactive Substance K Other Diagnostic Substance N Analgesics, Hypnotics, Sedatives P Platelet Inhibitor R Antiarrhythmic T Destructive Agent X Vasopressor	Z No Qualifier
4 Central Vein	0 Open	G Other Therapeutic Substance	C Other Substance N Blood Brain Barrier Disruption
4 Central Vein	0 Open	V Hormone	G Insulin H Human B-type Natriuretic Peptide J Other Hormone
4 Central Vein	0 Open	W Immunotherapeutic	K Immunostimulator L Immunosuppressive
4 Central Vein	3 Percutaneous	0 Antineoplastic	2 High-dose Interleukin-2 3 Low-dose Interleukin-2 5 Other Antineoplastic M Monoclonal Antibody P Clofarabine
4 Central Vein	3 Percutaneous	1 Thrombolytic	6 Recombinant Human- activated Protein C 7 Other Thrombolytic
4 Central Vein	3 Percutaneous	2 Anti-infective	8 Oxazolidinones 9 Other Anti-infective
4 Central Vein	3 Percutaneous	3 Anti-inflammatory 4 Serum, Toxoid and Vaccine 6 Nutritional Substance 7 Electrolytic and Water Balance Substance F Intracirculatory Anesthetic H Radioactive Substance K Other Diagnostic Substance N Analgesics, Hypnotics, Sedatives P Platelet Inhibitor R Antiarrhythmic T Destructive Agent X Vasopressor	Z No Qualifier
4 Central Vein	3 Percutaneous	G Other Therapeutic Substance	C Other Substance N Blood Brain Barrier Disruption Q Glucarpidase R Other Therapeutic Monoclonal Antibody
4 Central Vein	3 Percutaneous	V Hormone	G Insulin H Human B-type Natriuretic Peptide J Other Hormone
4 Central Vein	3 Percutaneous	W Immunotherapeutic	K Immunostimulator L Immunosuppressive
5 Peripheral Artery 6 Central Artery	0 Open 3 Percutaneous	0 Antineoplastic	2 High-dose Interleukin-2 3 Low-dose Interleukin-2 5 Other Antineoplastic M Monoclonal Antibody P Clofarabine
5 Peripheral Artery 6 Central Artery	0 Open 3 Percutaneous	1 Thrombolytic	6 Recombinant Human- activated Protein C 7 Other Thrombolytic
5 Peripheral Artery 6 Central Artery	0 Open 3 Percutaneous	2 Anti-infective	8 Oxazolidinones 9 Other Anti-infective

Valid OR 3E040TZ
DRG Non-OR 3E04302
DRG Non-OR 3E04317
DRG Non-OR 3E0[5,6][0,3]02
DRG Non-OR 3E0[5,6][0,3]17

3E0 Continued on next page

NC Noncovered Procedure   LC Limited Coverage   QA Questionable OB Admit   NT New Tech Add-on   ✚ Combination Member   ♂ Male   ♀ Female

Administration

3EØ Continued

3 Administration
E Physiological Systems and Anatomical Regions
Ø Introduction — Definition: Putting in or on a therapeutic, diagnostic, nutritional, physiological, or prophylactic substance except blood or blood products

Body System/Region Character 4	Approach Character 5	Substance Character 6	Qualifier Character 7
5 Peripheral Artery 6 Central Artery	Ø Open 3 Percutaneous	3 Anti-inflammatory 4 Serum, Toxoid and Vaccine 6 Nutritional Substance 7 Electrolytic and Water Balance Substance F Intracirculatory Anesthetic H Radioactive Substance K Other Diagnostic Substance N Analgesics, Hypnotics, Sedatives P Platelet Inhibitor R Antiarrhythmic T Destructive Agent X Vasopressor	Z No Qualifier
5 Peripheral Artery 6 Central Artery	Ø Open 3 Percutaneous	G Other Therapeutic Substance	C Other Substance N Blood Brain Barrier Disruption
5 Peripheral Artery 6 Central Artery	Ø Open 3 Percutaneous	V Hormone	G Insulin H Human B-type Natriuretic Peptide J Other Hormone
5 Peripheral Artery 6 Central Artery	Ø Open 3 Percutaneous	W Immunotherapeutic	K Immunostimulator L Immunosuppressive
7 Coronary Artery 8 Heart	Ø Open 3 Percutaneous	1 Thrombolytic	6 Recombinant Human- activated Protein C 7 Other Thrombolytic
7 Coronary Artery 8 Heart	Ø Open 3 Percutaneous	G Other Therapeutic Substance	C Other Substance
7 Coronary Artery 8 Heart	Ø Open 3 Percutaneous	K Other Diagnostic Substance P Platelet Inhibitor	Z No Qualifier
7 Coronary Artery 8 Heart	4 Percutaneous Endoscopic	G Other Therapeutic Substance	C Other Substance
9 Nose	3 Percutaneous 7 Via Natural or Artificial Opening X External	Ø Antineoplastic	5 Other Antineoplastic M Monoclonal Antibody
9 Nose	3 Percutaneous 7 Via Natural or Artificial Opening X External	2 Anti-infective	8 Oxazolidinones 9 Other Anti-infective
9 Nose	3 Percutaneous 7 Via Natural or Artificial Opening X External	3 Anti-inflammatory 4 Serum, Toxoid and Vaccine B Anesthetic Agent H Radioactive Substance K Other Diagnostic Substance N Analgesics, Hypnotics, Sedatives T Destructive Agent	Z No Qualifier
9 Nose	3 Percutaneous 7 Via Natural or Artificial Opening X External	G Other Therapeutic Substance	C Other Substance
A Bone Marrow	3 Percutaneous	Ø Antineoplastic	5 Other Antineoplastic M Monoclonal Antibody
A Bone Marrow	3 Percutaneous	G Other Therapeutic Substance	C Other Substance
B Ear	3 Percutaneous 7 Via Natural or Artificial Opening X External	Ø Antineoplastic	4 Liquid Brachytherapy Radioisotope 5 Other Antineoplastic M Monoclonal Antibody
B Ear	3 Percutaneous 7 Via Natural or Artificial Opening X External	2 Anti-infective	8 Oxazolidinones 9 Other Anti-infective
B Ear	3 Percutaneous 7 Via Natural or Artificial Opening X External	3 Anti-inflammatory B Anesthetic Agent H Radioactive Substance K Other Diagnostic Substance N Analgesics, Hypnotics, Sedatives T Destructive Agent	Z No Qualifier
B Ear	3 Percutaneous 7 Via Natural or Artificial Opening X External	G Other Therapeutic Substance	C Other Substance

DRG Non-OR 3E08[Ø,3]17

3EØ Continued on next page

Administration

3 Administration
E Physiological Systems and Anatomical Regions
0 Introduction — Definition: Putting in or on a therapeutic, diagnostic, nutritional, physiological, or prophylactic substance except blood or blood products

3E0 Continued

Body System/Region Character 4	Approach Character 5	Substance Character 6	Qualifier Character 7
C Eye	3 Percutaneous 7 Via Natural or Artificial Opening X External	0 Antineoplastic	4 Liquid Brachytherapy Radioisotope 5 Other Antineoplastic M Monoclonal Antibody
C Eye	3 Percutaneous 7 Via Natural or Artificial Opening X External	2 Anti-infective	8 Oxazolidinones 9 Other Anti-infective
C Eye	3 Percutaneous 7 Via Natural or Artificial Opening X External	3 Anti-inflammatory B Anesthetic Agent H Radioactive Substance K Other Diagnostic Substance M Pigment N Analgesics, Hypnotics, Sedatives T Destructive Agent	Z No Qualifier
C Eye	3 Percutaneous 7 Via Natural or Artificial Opening X External	G Other Therapeutic Substance	C Other Substance
C Eye	3 Percutaneous 7 Via Natural or Artificial Opening X External	S Gas	F Other Gas
D Mouth and Pharynx	3 Percutaneous 7 Via Natural or Artificial Opening X External	0 Antineoplastic	4 Liquid Brachytherapy Radioisotope 5 Other Antineoplastic M Monoclonal Antibody
D Mouth and Pharynx	3 Percutaneous 7 Via Natural or Artificial Opening X External	2 Anti-infective	8 Oxazolidinones 9 Other Anti-infective
D Mouth and Pharynx	3 Percutaneous 7 Via Natural or Artificial Opening X External	3 Anti-inflammatory 4 Serum, Toxoid and Vaccine 6 Nutritional Substance 7 Electrolytic and Water Balance Substance B Anesthetic Agent H Radioactive Substance K Other Diagnostic Substance N Analgesics, Hypnotics, Sedatives R Antiarrhythmic T Destructive Agent	Z No Qualifier
D Mouth and Pharynx	3 Percutaneous 7 Via Natural or Artificial Opening X External	G Other Therapeutic Substance	C Other Substance
E Products of Conception G Upper GI H Lower GI K Genitourinary Tract N Male Reproductive	3 Percutaneous 7 Via Natural or Artificial Opening 8 Via Natural or Artificial Opening Endoscopic	0 Antineoplastic	4 Liquid Brachytherapy Radioisotope 5 Other Antineoplastic M Monoclonal Antibody
E Products of Conception G Upper GI H Lower GI K Genitourinary Tract N Male Reproductive	3 Percutaneous 7 Via Natural or Artificial Opening 8 Via Natural or Artificial Opening Endoscopic	2 Anti-infective	8 Oxazolidinones 9 Other Anti-infective
E Products of Conception G Upper GI H Lower GI K Genitourinary Tract N Male Reproductive	3 Percutaneous 7 Via Natural or Artificial Opening 8 Via Natural or Artificial Opening Endoscopic	3 Anti-inflammatory 6 Nutritional Substance 7 Electrolytic and Water Balance Substance B Anesthetic Agent H Radioactive Substance K Other Diagnostic Substance N Analgesics, Hypnotics, Sedatives T Destructive Agent	Z No Qualifier
E Products of Conception G Upper GI H Lower GI K Genitourinary Tract N Male Reproductive	3 Percutaneous 7 Via Natural or Artificial Opening 8 Via Natural or Artificial Opening Endoscopic	G Other Therapeutic Substance	C Other Substance

3E0 Continued on next page

3 Administration
E Physiological Systems and Anatomical Regions
Ø Introduction

Definition: Putting in or on a therapeutic, diagnostic, nutritional, physiological, or prophylactic substance except blood or blood products

3EØ Continued

Body System/Region Character 4	Approach Character 5	Substance Character 6	Qualifier Character 7
E Products of Conception G Upper GI H Lower GI K Genitourinary Tract N Male Reproductive	3 Percutaneous 7 Via Natural or Artificial Opening 8 Via Natural or Artificial Opening Endoscopic	S Gas	F Other Gas
E Products of Conception G Upper GI H Lower GI K Genitourinary Tract N Male Reproductive	4 Percutaneous Endoscopic	G Other Therapeutic Substance	C Other Substance
F Respiratory Tract	3 Percutaneous 7 Via Natural or Artificial Opening 8 Via Natural or Artificial Opening Endoscopic	Ø Antineoplastic	4 Liquid Brachytherapy Radioisotope 5 Other Antineoplastic M Monoclonal Antibody
F Respiratory Tract	3 Percutaneous 7 Via Natural or Artificial Opening 8 Via Natural or Artificial Opening Endoscopic	2 Anti-infective	8 Oxazolidinones 9 Other Anti-infective
F Respiratory Tract	3 Percutaneous 7 Via Natural or Artificial Opening 8 Via Natural or Artificial Opening Endoscopic	3 Anti-inflammatory 6 Nutritional Substance 7 Electrolytic and Water Balance Substance B Anesthetic Agent H Radioactive Substance K Other Diagnostic Substance N Analgesics, Hypnotics, Sedatives T Destructive Agent	Z No Qualifier
F Respiratory Tract	3 Percutaneous 7 Via Natural or Artificial Opening 8 Via Natural or Artificial Opening Endoscopic	G Other Therapeutic Substance	C Other Substance
F Respiratory Tract	3 Percutaneous 7 Via Natural or Artificial Opening 8 Via Natural or Artificial Opening Endoscopic	S Gas	D Nitric Oxide F Other Gas
F Respiratory Tract	4 Percutaneous Endoscopic	G Other Therapeutic Substance	C Other Substance
J Biliary and Pancreatic Tract	3 Percutaneous 7 Via Natural or Artificial Opening 8 Via Natural or Artificial Opening Endoscopic	Ø Antineoplastic	4 Liquid Brachytherapy Radioisotope 5 Other Antineoplastic M Monoclonal Antibody
J Biliary and Pancreatic Tract	3 Percutaneous 7 Via Natural or Artificial Opening 8 Via Natural or Artificial Opening Endoscopic	2 Anti-infective	8 Oxazolidinones 9 Other Anti-infective
J Biliary and Pancreatic Tract	3 Percutaneous 7 Via Natural or Artificial Opening 8 Via Natural or Artificial Opening Endoscopic	3 Anti-inflammatory 6 Nutritional Substance 7 Electrolytic and Water Balance Substance B Anesthetic Agent H Radioactive Substance K Other Diagnostic Substance N Analgesics, Hypnotics, Sedatives T Destructive Agent	Z No Qualifier
J Biliary and Pancreatic Tract	3 Percutaneous 7 Via Natural or Artificial Opening 8 Via Natural or Artificial Opening Endoscopic	G Other Therapeutic Substance	C Other Substance
J Biliary and Pancreatic Tract	3 Percutaneous 7 Via Natural or Artificial Opening 8 Via Natural or Artificial Opening Endoscopic	S Gas	F Other Gas

3EØ Continued on next page

ICD-10-PCS 2025 — Administration — 3E0–3E0

3 Administration
E Physiological Systems and Anatomical Regions
0 Introduction Definition: Putting in or on a therapeutic, diagnostic, nutritional, physiological, or prophylactic substance except blood or blood products

3E0 Continued

Body System/Region Character 4	Approach Character 5	Substance Character 6	Qualifier Character 7
J Biliary and Pancreatic Tract	3 Percutaneous 7 Via Natural or Artificial Opening 8 Via Natural or Artificial Opening Endoscopic	U Pancreatic Islet Cells	0 Autologous 1 Nonautologous
J Biliary and Pancreatic Tract	4 Percutaneous Endoscopic	G Other Therapeutic Substance	C Other Substance
L Pleural Cavity	0 Open	5 Adhesion Barrier	Z No Qualifier
L Pleural Cavity	3 Percutaneous	0 Antineoplastic	4 Liquid Brachytherapy Radioisotope 5 Other Antineoplastic M Monoclonal Antibody
L Pleural Cavity	3 Percutaneous	1 Thrombolytic	7 Other Thrombolytic
L Pleural Cavity	3 Percutaneous	2 Anti-infective	8 Oxazolidinones 9 Other Anti-infective
L Pleural Cavity	3 Percutaneous	3 Anti-inflammatory 5 Adhesion Barrier 6 Nutritional Substance 7 Electrolytic and Water Balance Substance B Anesthetic Agent H Radioactive Substance K Other Diagnostic Substance N Analgesics, Hypnotics, Sedatives T Destructive Agent	Z No Qualifier
L Pleural Cavity	3 Percutaneous	G Other Therapeutic Substance	C Other Substance
L Pleural Cavity	3 Percutaneous	S Gas	F Other Gas
L Pleural Cavity	4 Percutaneous Endoscopic	5 Adhesion Barrier	Z No Qualifier
L Pleural Cavity	4 Percutaneous Endoscopic	G Other Therapeutic Substance	C Other Substance
L Pleural Cavity	7 Via Natural or Artificial Opening	0 Antineoplastic	4 Liquid Brachytherapy Radioisotope 5 Other Antineoplastic M Monoclonal Antibody
L Pleural Cavity	7 Via Natural or Artificial Opening	S Gas	F Other Gas
M Peritoneal Cavity	0 Open	5 Adhesion Barrier	Z No Qualifier
M Peritoneal Cavity	3 Percutaneous	0 Antineoplastic	4 Liquid Brachytherapy Radioisotope 5 Other Antineoplastic M Monoclonal Antibody Y Hyperthermic
M Peritoneal Cavity	3 Percutaneous	2 Anti-infective	8 Oxazolidinones 9 Other Anti-infective
M Peritoneal Cavity	3 Percutaneous	3 Anti-inflammatory 5 Adhesion Barrier 6 Nutritional Substance 7 Electrolytic and Water Balance Substance B Anesthetic Agent H Radioactive Substance K Other Diagnostic Substance N Analgesics, Hypnotics, Sedatives T Destructive Agent	Z No Qualifier
M Peritoneal Cavity	3 Percutaneous	G Other Therapeutic Substance	C Other Substance
M Peritoneal Cavity	3 Percutaneous	S Gas	F Other Gas
M Peritoneal Cavity	4 Percutaneous Endoscopic	5 Adhesion Barrier	Z No Qualifier
M Peritoneal Cavity	4 Percutaneous Endoscopic	G Other Therapeutic Substance	C Other Substance
M Peritoneal Cavity	7 Via Natural or Artificial Opening	0 Antineoplastic	4 Liquid Brachytherapy Radioisotope 5 Other Antineoplastic M Monoclonal Antibody
M Peritoneal Cavity	7 Via Natural or Artificial Opening	S Gas	F Other Gas
P Female Reproductive	0 Open	5 Adhesion Barrier	Z No Qualifier
P Female Reproductive	3 Percutaneous	0 Antineoplastic	4 Liquid Brachytherapy Radioisotope 5 Other Antineoplastic M Monoclonal Antibody
P Female Reproductive	3 Percutaneous	2 Anti-infective	8 Oxazolidinones 9 Other Anti-infective

Valid OR 3E0L4GC
DRG Non-OR 3E0J[3,7,8]U[0,1]

3E0 Continued on next page

NC Noncovered Procedure · LC Limited Coverage · QA Questionable OB Admit · NT New Tech Add-on · ✚ Combination Member · ♂ Male · ♀ Female

ICD-10-PCS 2025 — 733

3E0 Continued

3 Administration
E Physiological Systems and Anatomical Regions
0 Introduction   Definition: Putting in or on a therapeutic, diagnostic, nutritional, physiological, or prophylactic substance except blood or blood products

Body System/Region Character 4	Approach Character 5	Substance Character 6	Qualifier Character 7
P Female Reproductive	3 Percutaneous	3 Anti-inflammatory 5 Adhesion Barrier 6 Nutritional Substance 7 Electrolytic and Water Balance Substance B Anesthetic Agent H Radioactive Substance K Other Diagnostic Substance L Sperm N Analgesics, Hypnotics, Sedatives T Destructive Agent V Hormone	Z No Qualifier
P Female Reproductive	3 Percutaneous	G Other Therapeutic Substance	C Other Substance
P Female Reproductive	3 Percutaneous	Q Fertilized Ovum	0 Autologous 1 Nonautologous
P Female Reproductive	3 Percutaneous	S Gas	F Other Gas
P Female Reproductive	4 Percutaneous Endoscopic	5 Adhesion Barrier	Z No Qualifier
P Female Reproductive	4 Percutaneous Endoscopic	G Other Therapeutic Substance	C Other Substance
P Female Reproductive	7 Via Natural or Artificial Opening	0 Antineoplastic	4 Liquid Brachytherapy Radioisotope 5 Other Antineoplastic M Monoclonal Antibody
P Female Reproductive	7 Via Natural or Artificial Opening	2 Anti-infective	8 Oxazolidinones 9 Other Anti-infective
P Female Reproductive	7 Via Natural or Artificial Opening	3 Anti-inflammatory 6 Nutritional Substance 7 Electrolytic and Water Balance Substance B Anesthetic Agent H Radioactive Substance K Other Diagnostic Substance L Sperm N Analgesics, Hypnotics, Sedatives T Destructive Agent V Hormone	Z No Qualifier
P Female Reproductive	7 Via Natural or Artificial Opening	G Other Therapeutic Substance	C Other Substance
P Female Reproductive	7 Via Natural or Artificial Opening	Q Fertilized Ovum	0 Autologous 1 Nonautologous
P Female Reproductive	7 Via Natural or Artificial Opening	S Gas	F Other Gas
P Female Reproductive	8 Via Natural or Artificial Opening Endoscopic	0 Antineoplastic	4 Liquid Brachytherapy Radioisotope 5 Other Antineoplastic M Monoclonal Antibody
P Female Reproductive	8 Via Natural or Artificial Opening Endoscopic	2 Anti-infective	8 Oxazolidinones 9 Other Anit-infective
P Female Reproductive	8 Via Natural or Artificial Opening Endoscopic	3 Anti-inflammatory 6 Nutritional Substance 7 Electrolytic and Water Balance Substance B Anesthetic Agent H Radioactive Substance K Other Diagnostic Substance N Analgesics, Hypnotics, Sedatives T Destructive Agent	Z No Qualifier
P Female Reproductive	8 Via Natural or Artificial Opening Endoscopic	G Other Therapeutic Substance	C Other Substance
P Female Reproductive	8 Via Natural or Artificial Opening Endoscopic	S Gas	F Other Gas
Q Cranial Cavity and Brain	0 Open 3 Percutaneous	0 Antineoplastic	4 Liquid Brachytherapy Radioisotope 5 Other Antineoplastic M Monoclonal Antibody
Q Cranial Cavity and Brain	0 Open 3 Percutaneous	2 Anti-infective	8 Oxazolidinones 9 Other Anti-infective

Valid OR   3E0P3Q[0,1]
Valid OR   3E0P7Q[0,1]
DRG Non-OR   3E0Q[0,3]05

3E0 Continued on next page

ICD-10-PCS 2025 — Administration — 3E0–3E0

3E0 Continued

3 Administration
E Physiological Systems and Anatomical Regions
0 Introduction — Definition: Putting in or on a therapeutic, diagnostic, nutritional, physiological, or prophylactic substance except blood or blood products

Body System/Region Character 4	Approach Character 5	Substance Character 6	Qualifier Character 7
Q Cranial Cavity and Brain	0 Open 3 Percutaneous	3 Anti-inflammatory 6 Nutritional Substance 7 Electrolytic and Water Balance Substance A Stem Cells, Embryonic B Anesthetic Agent H Radioactive Substance K Other Diagnostic Substance N Analgesics, Hypnotics, Sedatives T Destructive Agent	Z No Qualifier
Q Cranial Cavity and Brain	0 Open 3 Percutaneous	E Stem Cells, Somatic	0 Autologous 1 Nonautologous
Q Cranial Cavity and Brain	0 Open 3 Percutaneous	G Other Therapeutic Substance	C Other Substance
Q Cranial Cavity and Brain	0 Open 3 Percutaneous	S Gas	F Other Gas
Q Cranial Cavity and Brain	7 Via Natural or Artificial Opening	0 Antineoplastic	4 Liquid Brachytherapy Radioisotope 5 Other Antineoplastic M Monoclonal Antibody
Q Cranial Cavity and Brain	7 Via Natural or Artificial Opening	S Gas	F Other Gas
R Spinal Canal	0 Open	A Stem Cells, Embryonic	Z No Qualifier
R Spinal Canal	0 Open	E Stem Cells, Somatic	0 Autologous 1 Nonautologous
R Spinal Canal	3 Percutaneous	0 Antineoplastic	2 High-dose Interleukin-2 3 Low-dose Interleukin-2 4 Liquid Brachytherapy Radioisotope 5 Other Antineoplastic M Monoclonal Antibody
R Spinal Canal	3 Percutaneous	2 Anti-infective	8 Oxazolidinones 9 Other Anti-infective
R Spinal Canal	3 Percutaneous	3 Anti-inflammatory 6 Nutritional Substance 7 Electrolytic and Water Balance Substance A Stem Cells, Embryonic B Anesthetic Agent H Radioactive Substance K Other Diagnostic Substance N Analgesics, Hypnotics, Sedatives T Destructive Agent	Z No Qualifier
R Spinal Canal	3 Percutaneous	E Stem Cells, Somatic	0 Autologous 1 Nonautologous
R Spinal Canal	3 Percutaneous	G Other Therapeutic Substance	C Other Substance
R Spinal Canal	3 Percutaneous	S Gas	F Other Gas
R Spinal Canal	7 Via Natural or Artificial Opening	S Gas	F Other Gas
S Epidural Space	3 Percutaneous	0 Antineoplastic	2 High-dose Interleukin-2 3 Low-dose Interleukin-2 4 Liquid Brachytherapy Radioisotope 5 Other Antineoplastic M Monoclonal Antibody
S Epidural Space	3 Percutaneous	2 Anti-infective	8 Oxazolidinones 9 Other Anti-infective
S Epidural Space	3 Percutaneous	3 Anti-inflammatory 6 Nutritional Substance 7 Electrolytic and Water Balance Substance B Anesthetic Agent H Radioactive Substance K Other Diagnostic Substance N Analgesics, Hypnotics, Sedatives T Destructive Agent	Z No Qualifier

DRG Non-OR 3E0Q705
DRG Non-OR 3E0R302
DRG Non-OR 3E0S302

3E0 Continued on next page

Administration

3 Administration
E Physiological Systems and Anatomical Regions
0 Introduction Definition: Putting in or on a therapeutic, diagnostic, nutritional, physiological, or prophylactic substance except blood or blood products

3E0 Continued

Body System/Region Character 4	Approach Character 5	Substance Character 6	Qualifier Character 7
S Epidural Space	3 Percutaneous	G Other Therapeutic Substance	C Other Substance
S Epidural Space	3 Percutaneous	S Gas	F Other Gas
S Epidural Space	7 Via Natural or Artificial Opening	S Gas	F Other Gas
T Peripheral Nerves and Plexi X Cranial Nerves	3 Percutaneous	3 Anti-inflammatory B Anesthetic Agent T Destructive Agent	Z No Qualifier
T Peripheral Nerves and Plexi X Cranial Nerves	3 Percutaneous	G Other Therapeutic Substance	C Other Substance
U Joints	0 Open	2 Anti-infective	8 Oxazolidinones 9 Other Anti-infective
U Joints	0 Open	G Other Therapeutic Substance	B Recombinant Bone Morphogenetic Protein
U Joints	3 Percutaneous	0 Antineoplastic	4 Liquid Brachytherapy Radioisotope 5 Other Antineoplastic M Monoclonal Antibody
U Joints	3 Percutaneous	2 Anti-infective	8 Oxazolidinones 9 Other Anti-infective
U Joints	3 Percutaneous	3 Anti-inflammatory 6 Nutritional Substance 7 Electrolytic and Water Balance Substance B Anesthetic Agent H Radioactive Substance K Other Diagnostic Substance N Analgesics, Hypnotics, Sedatives T Destructive Agent	Z No Qualifier
U Joints	3 Percutaneous	G Other Therapeutic Substance	B Recombinant Bone Morphogenetic Protein C Other Substance
U Joints	3 Percutaneous	S Gas	F Other Gas
U Joints	4 Percutaneous Endoscopic	G Other Therapeutic Substance	C Other Substance
V Bones	0 Open	G Other Therapeutic Substance	B Recombinant Bone Morphogenetic Protein C Other Substance
V Bones	3 Percutaneous	0 Antineoplastic	5 Other Antineoplastic M Monoclonal Antibody
V Bones	3 Percutaneous	2 Anti-infective	8 Oxazolidinones 9 Other Anti-infective
V Bones	3 Percutaneous	3 Anti-inflammatory 6 Nutritional Substance 7 Electrolytic and Water Balance Substance B Anesthetic Agent H Radioactive Substance K Other Diagnostic Substance N Analgesics, Hypnotics, Sedatives T Destructive Agent	Z No Qualifier
V Bones	3 Percutaneous	G Other Therapeutic Substance	B Recombinant Bone Morphogenetic Protein C Other Substance
V Bones	4 Percutaneous Endoscopic	G Other Therapeutic Substance	C Other Substance
W Lymphatics	3 Percutaneous	0 Antineoplastic	5 Other Antineoplastic M Monoclonal Antibody
W Lymphatics	3 Percutaneous	2 Anti-infective	8 Oxazolidinones 9 Other Anti-infective
W Lymphatics	3 Percutaneous	3 Anti-inflammatory 6 Nutritional Substance 7 Electrolytic and Water Balance Substance B Anesthetic Agent H Radioactive Substance K Other Diagnostic Substance N Analgesics, Hypnotics, Sedatives T Destructive Agent	Z No Qualifier
W Lymphatics	3 Percutaneous	G Other Therapeutic Substance	C Other Substance

3E0 Continued on next page

ICD-10-PCS 2025 — Administration — 3E0–3E1

3 Administration
E Physiological Systems and Anatomical Regions
0 Introduction — Definition: Putting in or on a therapeutic, diagnostic, nutritional, physiological, or prophylactic substance except blood or blood products

3E0 Continued

Body System/Region Character 4	Approach Character 5	Substance Character 6	Qualifier Character 7
Y Pericardial Cavity	3 Percutaneous	0 Antineoplastic	4 Liquid Brachytherapy Radioisotope 5 Other Antineoplastic M Monoclonal Antibody
Y Pericardial Cavity	3 Percutaneous	2 Anti-infective	8 Oxazolidinones 9 Other Anti-infective
Y Pericardial Cavity	3 Percutaneous	3 Anti-inflammatory 6 Nutritional Substance 7 Electrolytic and Water Balance Substance B Anesthetic Agent H Radioactive Substance K Other Diagnostic Substance N Analgesics, Hypnotics, Sedatives T Destructive Agent	Z No Qualifier
Y Pericardial Cavity	3 Percutaneous	G Other Therapeutic Substance	C Other Substance
Y Pericardial Cavity	3 Percutaneous	S Gas	F Other Gas
Y Pericardial Cavity	4 Percutaneous Endoscopic	G Other Therapeutic Substance	C Other Substance
Y Pericardial Cavity	7 Via Natural or Artificial Opening	0 Antineoplastic	4 Liquid Brachytherapy Radioisotope 5 Other Antineoplastic M Monoclonal Antibody
Y Pericardial Cavity	7 Via Natural or Artificial Opening	S Gas	F Other Gas

3 Administration
E Physiological Systems and Anatomical Regions
1 Irrigation — Definition: Putting in or on a cleansing substance

Body System/Region Character 4	Approach Character 5	Substance Character 6	Qualifier Character 7
0 Skin and Mucous Membranes C Eye	3 Percutaneous X External	8 Irrigating Substance	X Diagnostic Z No Qualifier
9 Nose B Ear F Respiratory Tract G Upper GI H Lower GI J Biliary and Pancreatic Tract K Genitourinary Tract N Male Reproductive P Female Reproductive	3 Percutaneous 7 Via Natural or Artificial Opening 8 Via Natural or Artificial Opening Endoscopic	8 Irrigating Substance	X Diagnostic Z No Qualifier
L Pleural Cavity Q Cranial Cavity and Brain R Spinal Canal S Epidural Space Y Pericardial Cavity	3 Percutaneous	8 Irrigating Substance	X Diagnostic Z No Qualifier
M Peritoneal Cavity	3 Percutaneous	8 Irrigating Substance	X Diagnostic Z No Qualifier
M Peritoneal Cavity	3 Percutaneous	9 Dialysate	Z No Qualifier
M Peritoneal Cavity	4 Percutaneous Endoscopic	8 Irrigating Substance	X Diagnostic Z No Qualifier
U Joints	3 Percutaneous 4 Percutaneous Endoscopic	8 Irrigating Substance	X Diagnostic Z No Qualifier

NC Noncovered Procedure   LC Limited Coverage   QA Questionable OB Admit   NT New Tech Add-on   ➕ Combination Member   ♂ Male   ♀ Female

Measurement and Monitoring 4A0–4B0

AHA Coding Clinic for table 4A0
2022, 1Q, 46	Internal cardioversion
2020, 4Q, 62	Measurement of intracranial arterial flow
2020, 4Q, 62	Percutaneous endoscopic measurement of portal venous pressure
2020, 4Q, 63	Intercompartmental pressure measurement
2019, 3Q, 32	Endomyocardial biopsy and right heart catheterization
2018, 1Q, 12	Percutaneous balloon valvuloplasty & cardiac catheterization with ventriculogram
2016, 3Q, 37	Fractional flow reserve
2015, 3Q, 29	Approach value for esophageal electrophysiology study

AHA Coding Clinic for table 4B0
2021, 4Q, 55-56	Measurement of flow in a cerebral fluid shunt

AHA Coding Clinic for table 4A1
2019, 4Q, 38-39	Intraoperative fluorescence lymphatic mapping using Indocyanine green dye
2016, 4Q, 114	Fluorescence vascular angiography
2016, 2Q, 29	Decompressive craniectomy with cryopreservation and storage of bone flap
2016, 2Q, 33	Monitoring of arterial pressure & pulse
2015, 3Q, 35	Swan Ganz catheterization
2015, 2Q, 14	Intraoperative EMG monitoring via endotracheal tube
2015, 1Q, 26	Intraoperative monitoring using Sentio MMG®
2014, 4Q, 28	Removal and replacement of displaced growing rods

4 Measurement and Monitoring
A Physiological Systems
0 Measurement   Definition: Determining the level of a physiological or physical function at a point in time

Body System Character 4	Approach Character 5	Function/Device Character 6	Qualifier Character 7
0 Central Nervous	0 Open	2 Conductivity 4 Electrical Activity B Pressure	Z No Qualifier
0 Central Nervous	3 Percutaneous 7 Via Natural or Artificial Opening 8 Via Natural or Artificial Opening Endoscopic	4 Electrical Activity	Z No Qualifier
0 Central Nervous	3 Percutaneous 7 Via Natural or Artificial Opening 8 Via Natural or Artificial Opening Endoscopic	B Pressure K Temperature R Saturation	D Intracranial
0 Central Nervous	X External	2 Conductivity 4 Electrical Activity	Z No Qualifier
1 Peripheral Nervous	0 Open 3 Percutaneous 7 Via Natural or Artificial Opening 8 Via Natural or Artificial Opening Endoscopic X External	2 Conductivity	9 Sensory B Motor
1 Peripheral Nervous	0 Open 3 Percutaneous 7 Via Natural or Artificial Opening 8 Via Natural or Artificial Opening Endoscopic X External	4 Electrical Activity	Z No Qualifier
2 Cardiac	0 Open 3 Percutaneous 7 Via Natural or Artificial Opening 8 Via Natural or Artificial Opening Endoscopic	4 Electrical Activity 9 Output C Rate F Rhythm H Sound P Action Currents	Z No Qualifier
2 Cardiac	0 Open 3 Percutaneous 7 Via Natural or Artificial Opening 8 Via Natural or Artificial Opening Endoscopic	N Sampling and Pressure	6 Right Heart 7 Left Heart 8 Bilateral
2 Cardiac	X External	4 Electrical Activity	A Guidance Z No Qualifier
2 Cardiac	X External	9 Output C Rate F Rhythm H Sound P Action Currents	Z No Qualifier
2 Cardiac	X External	M Total Activity	4 Stress
3 Arterial	0 Open 3 Percutaneous	5 Flow J Pulse	1 Peripheral 3 Pulmonary C Coronary
3 Arterial	0 Open 3 Percutaneous	B Pressure	1 Peripheral 3 Pulmonary C Coronary F Other Thoracic

DRG Non-OR 4A02[3,7,8]FZ
DRG Non-OR 4A02[0,3,7,8]N[6,7,8]

4A0 Continued on next page

Measurement and Monitoring

4 Measurement and Monitoring
A Physiological Systems
0 Measurement   Definition: Determining the level of a physiological or physical function at a point in time

4A0 Continued

Body System Character 4	Approach Character 5	Function/Device Character 6	Qualifier Character 7
3 Arterial	0 Open 3 Percutaneous	H Sound R Saturation	1 Peripheral
3 Arterial	X External	5 Flow	1 Peripheral D Intracranial
3 Arterial	X External	B Pressure H Sound J Pulse R Saturation	1 Peripheral
4 Venous	0 Open 3 Percutaneous	5 Flow B Pressure J Pulse	0 Central 1 Peripheral 2 Portal 3 Pulmonary
4 Venous	0 Open 3 Percutaneous	R Saturation	1 Peripheral
4 Venous	4 Percutaneous Endoscopic	B Pressure	2 Portal
4 Venous	X External	5 Flow B Pressure J Pulse R Saturation	1 Peripheral
5 Circulatory	X External	L Volume	Z No Qualifier
6 Lymphatic	0 Open 3 Percutaneous 7 Via Natural or Artificial Opening 8 Via Natural or Artificial Opening Endoscopic	5 Flow B Pressure	Z No Qualifier
7 Visual	X External	0 Acuity 7 Mobility B Pressure	Z No Qualifier
8 Olfactory	X External	0 Acuity	Z No Qualifier
9 Respiratory	7 Via Natural or Artificial Opening 8 Via Natural or Artificial Opening Endoscopic X External	1 Capacity 5 Flow C Rate D Resistance L Volume M Total Activity	Z No Qualifier
B Gastrointestinal	7 Via Natural or Artificial Opening 8 Via Natural or Artificial Opening Endoscopic	8 Motility B Pressure G Secretion	Z No Qualifier
C Biliary	3 Percutaneous 4 Percutaneous Endoscopic 7 Via Natural or Artificial Opening 8 Via Natural or Artificial Opening Endoscopic	5 Flow B Pressure	Z No Qualifier
D Urinary	7 Via Natural or Artificial Opening 8 Via Natural or Artificial Opening Endoscopic	3 Contractility 5 Flow B Pressure D Resistance L Volume	Z No Qualifier
F Musculoskeletal	3 Percutaneous	3 Contractility	Z No Qualifier
F Musculoskeletal	3 Percutaneous	B Pressure	E Compartment
F Musculoskeletal	X External	3 Contractility	Z No Qualifier
H Products of Conception, Cardiac	7 Via Natural or Artificial Opening 8 Via Natural or Artificial Opening Endoscopic X External	4 Electrical Activity C Rate F Rhythm H Sound	Z No Qualifier
J Products of Conception, Nervous	7 Via Natural or Artificial Opening 8 Via Natural or Artificial Opening Endoscopic X External	2 Conductivity 4 Electrical Activity B Pressure	Z No Qualifier
Z None	7 Via Natural or Artificial Opening	6 Metabolism K Temperature	Z No Qualifier
Z None	X External	6 Metabolism K Temperature Q Sleep	Z No Qualifier

Valid OR   4A060[5,B]Z
Valid OR   4A0C4[5,B]Z

Measurement and Monitoring

4 Measurement and Monitoring
A Physiological Systems
1 Monitoring   Definition: Determining the level of a physiological or physical function repetitively over a period of time

Body System Character 4	Approach Character 5	Function/Device Character 6	Qualifier Character 7
Ø Central Nervous	Ø Open	2 Conductivity B Pressure	Z No Qualifier
Ø Central Nervous	Ø Open	4 Electrical Activity	G Intraoperative Z No Qualifier
Ø Central Nervous	3 Percutaneous 7 Via Natural or Artificial Opening 8 Via Natural or Artificial Opening Endoscopic	4 Electrical Activity	G Intraoperative Z No Qualifier
Ø Central Nervous	3 Percutaneous 7 Via Natural or Artificial Opening 8 Via Natural or Artificial Opening Endoscopic	B Pressure K Temperature R Saturation	D Intracranial
Ø Central Nervous	X External	2 Conductivity	Z No Qualifier
Ø Central Nervous	X External	4 Electrical Activity	G Intraoperative Z No Qualifier
1 Peripheral Nervous	Ø Open 3 Percutaneous 7 Via Natural or Artificial Opening 8 Via Natural or Artificial Opening Endoscopic X External	2 Conductivity	9 Sensory B Motor
1 Peripheral Nervous	Ø Open 3 Percutaneous 7 Via Natural or Artificial Opening 8 Via Natural or Artificial Opening Endoscopic X External	4 Electrical Activity	G Intraoperative Z No Qualifier
2 Cardiac	Ø Open 3 Percutaneous 7 Via Natural or Artificial Opening 8 Via Natural or Artificial Opening Endoscopic	4 Electrical Activity 9 Output C Rate F Rhythm H Sound	Z No Qualifier
2 Cardiac	X External	4 Electrical Activity	5 Ambulatory Z No Qualifier
2 Cardiac	X External	9 Output C Rate F Rhythm H Sound	Z No Qualifier
2 Cardiac	X External	M Total Activity	4 Stress
2 Cardiac	X External	S Vascular Perfusion	H Indocyanine Green Dye
3 Arterial	Ø Open 3 Percutaneous	5 Flow B Pressure J Pulse	1 Peripheral 3 Pulmonary C Coronary
3 Arterial	Ø Open 3 Percutaneous	H Sound R Saturation	1 Peripheral
3 Arterial	X External	5 Flow B Pressure H Sound J Pulse R Saturation	1 Peripheral
4 Venous	Ø Open 3 Percutaneous	5 Flow B Pressure J Pulse	Ø Central 1 Peripheral 2 Portal 3 Pulmonary
4 Venous	Ø Open 3 Percutaneous	R Saturation	Ø Central 2 Portal 3 Pulmonary
4 Venous	X External	5 Flow B Pressure J Pulse	1 Peripheral
6 Lymphatic	Ø Open 3 Percutaneous 7 Via Natural or Artificial Opening 8 Via Natural or Artificial Opening Endoscopic	5 Flow	H Indocyanine Green Dye Z No Qualifier

Valid OR 4A1ized

4A1 Continued on next page

4 Measurement and Monitoring
A Physiological Systems
1 Monitoring
Definition: Determining the level of a physiological or physical function repetitively over a period of time

Body System Character 4	Approach Character 5	Function/Device Character 6	Qualifier Character 7
6 Lymphatic	0 Open 3 Percutaneous 7 Via Natural or Artificial Opening 8 Via Natural or Artificial Opening Endoscopic	B Pressure	Z No Qualifier
9 Respiratory	7 Via Natural or Artificial Opening X External	1 Capacity 5 Flow C Rate D Resistance L Volume	Z No Qualifier
B Gastrointestinal	7 Via Natural or Artificial Opening 8 Via Natural or Artificial Opening Endoscopic	8 Motility B Pressure G Secretion	Z No Qualifier
B Gastrointestinal	X External	S Vascular Perfusion	H Indocyanine Green Dye
D Urinary	7 Via Natural or Artificial Opening 8 Via Natural or Artificial Opening Endoscopic	3 Contractility 5 Flow B Pressure D Resistance L Volume	Z No Qualifier
G Skin and Breast	X External	S Vascular Perfusion	H Indocyanine Green Dye
H Products of Conception, Cardiac	7 Via Natural or Artificial Opening 8 Via Natural or Artificial Opening Endoscopic X External	4 Electrical Activity C Rate F Rhythm H Sound	Z No Qualifier
J Products of Conception, Nervous	7 Via Natural or Artificial Opening 8 Via Natural or Artificial Opening Endoscopic X External	2 Conductivity 4 Electrical Activity B Pressure	Z No Qualifier
Z None	7 Via Natural or Artificial Opening	K Temperature	Z No Qualifier
Z None	X External	K Temperature Q Sleep	Z No Qualifier

Valid OR 4A160BZ

4 Measurement and Monitoring
B Physiological Devices
0 Measurement
Definition: Determining the level of a physiological or physical function at a point in time

Body System Character 4	Approach Character 5	Function/Device Character 6	Qualifier Character 7
0 Central Nervous	X External	V Stimulator	Z No Qualifier
0 Central Nervous	X External	W Cerebrospinal Fluid Shunt	0 Wireless Sensor
1 Peripheral Nervous F Musculoskeletal	X External	V Stimulator	Z No Qualifier
2 Cardiac	X External	S Pacemaker T Defibrillator	Z No Qualifier
9 Respiratory	X External	S Pacemaker	Z No Qualifier

Extracorporeal or Systemic Assistance and Performance 5A0–5A2

AHA Coding Clinic for table 5A0

2024, 1Q, 30	PROTEKDuo® cannula insertion with CentriMag®
2023, 4Q, 55-56	Intubated prone positioning
2023, 3Q, 9	Neurally-adjusted ventilatory assistance
2022, 4Q, 61-62	Cardiac perfusion with intra-arterial supersaturated oxygen
2022, 3Q, 23	Placement of preCARDIA device
2021, 2Q, 12	Repositioning of displaced intra-aortic balloon pump
2020, 4Q, 64-65	Ventilatory assistance by high flow or high velocity nasal cannula devices
2020, 1Q, 10	Intermittent use of continuous positive airway pressure
2018, 2Q, 3-5	Intra-aortic balloon pump
2017, 4Q, 43-44	Insertion of external heart assist devices
2017, 3Q, 18	Intra-aortic balloon pump removal
2017, 1Q, 10-11	External heart assist device
2017, 1Q, 29	Newborn resuscitation using positive pressure ventilation
2017, 1Q, 29	Newborn noninvasive ventilation
2016, 4Q, 137-139	Heart assist device systems
2014, 4Q, 9	Mechanical ventilation
2014, 3Q, 19	Ablation of ventricular tachycardia with Impella® support
2013, 3Q, 18	Heart transplant surgery

AHA Coding Clinic for table 5A1

2022, 2Q, 25	Temporary-permanent pacemaker placement
2021, 4Q, 56	Automated chest compression
2019, 4Q, 39-41	Intraoperative extracorporeal membrane oxygenation
2019, 3Q, 19	Insertion of left ventricular catheter
2019, 3Q, 20	Removal and revision of ECMO component
2019, 3Q, 21	Exchange of extracorporeal membrane oxygenation component (oxygenator)

AHA Coding Clinic for table 5A1 (Continued)

2019, 2Q, 36	Veno-arterial extracorporeal membrane oxygenation via sternotomy
2019, 3Q, 22	Extracorporeal membrane oxygenation and Centrimag™ pump
2019, 3Q, 22	Extracorporeal membrane oxygenation transfers
2018, 4Q, 52-54	Percutaneous extracorporeal membrane oxygenation
2018, 1Q, 13	Mechanical ventilation using patient's equipment
2017, 4Q, 71-73	Hemodialysis and renal replacement therapy
2017, 3Q, 7	Senning procedure (arterial switch)
2017, 1Q, 19	Norwood Sano procedure
2016, 1Q, 27	Aortocoronary bypass graft utilizing Y-graft
2016, 1Q, 28	Extracorporeal liver assist device
2016, 1Q, 29	Duration of hemodialysis
2015, 4Q, 22-24	Congenital heart corrective procedures
2014, 4Q, 3-10	Mechanical ventilation
2014, 4Q, 11-15	Sequencing of mechanical ventilation with other procedures
2014, 3Q, 16	Repair of Tetralogy of Fallot
2014, 3Q, 20	MAZE procedure performed with coronary artery bypass graft
2014, 1Q, 10	Repair of thoracic aortic aneurysm & coronary artery bypass graft
2013, 3Q, 18	Heart transplant surgery

AHA Coding Clinic for table 5A2

2022, 1Q, 46	Internal cardioversion

5 Extracorporeal or Systemic Assistance and Performance
A Physiological Systems
0 Assistance   Definition: Taking over a portion of a physiological function by extracorporeal means

Body System Character 4	Duration Character 5	Function Character 6	Qualifier Character 7
2 Cardiac	1 Intermittent	1 Output	0 Balloon Pump 5 Pulsatile Compression 6 Other Pump D Impeller Pump
2 Cardiac	2 Continuous	1 Output	0 Balloon Pump 5 Pulsatile Compression 6 Other Pump D Impeller Pump
2 Cardiac	2 Continuous	2 Oxygenation	C Supersaturated
5 Circulatory	1 Intermittent 2 Continuous	2 Oxygenation	1 Hyperbaric
5 Circulatory	A Intraoperative	0 Filtration	L Peripheral Veno-venous
9 Respiratory	2 Continuous	0 Filtration	Z No Qualifier
9 Respiratory	3 Less than 24 Consecutive Hours 4 24-96 Consecutive Hours 5 Greater than 96 Consecutive Hours	5 Ventilation	7 Continuous Positive Airway Pressure 8 Intermittent Positive Airway Pressure 9 Continuous Negative Airway Pressure A High Flow/Velocity Cannula B Intermittent Negative Airway Pressure Z No Qualifier
9 Respiratory	B Less than 8 Consecutive Hours C 8-24 Consecutive Hours D Greater than 24 Consecutive Hours	5 Ventilation	K Intubated Prone Positioning

Valid OR   5A0211[0,6,D]
Valid OR   5A0221[0,6,D]

5 Extracorporeal or Systemic Assistance and Performance
A Physiological Systems
1 Performance
Definition: Completely taking over a physiological function by extracorporeal means

Body System Character 4	Duration Character 5	Function Character 6	Qualifier Character 7
2 Cardiac	0 Single	1 Output	2 Manual
2 Cardiac	1 Intermittent	3 Pacing	Z No Qualifier
2 Cardiac	2 Continuous	1 Output	J Automated Z No Qualifier
2 Cardiac	2 Continuous	3 Pacing	Z No Qualifier
5 Circulatory	2 Continuous A Intraoperative	2 Oxygenation	F Membrane, Central G Membrane, Peripheral Veno-arterial H Membrane, Peripheral Veno-venous
9 Respiratory	0 Single	5 Ventilation	4 Nonmechanical
9 Respiratory	3 Less than 24 Consecutive Hours 4 24-96 Consecutive Hours 5 Greater than 96 Consecutive Hours	5 Ventilation	Z No Qualifier
C Biliary	0 Single 6 Multiple	0 Filtration	Z No Qualifier
D Urinary	7 Intermittent, Less than 6 Hours per day 8 Prolonged Intermittent, 6-18 Hours per day 9 Continuous, Greater than 18 Hours per day	0 Filtration	Z No Qualifier

Valid OR 5A1522F
DRG Non-OR 5A1522[G,H]
DRG Non-OR 5A19[3,4]5Z
DRG Non-OR 5A1955Z Length of stay must be > 4 consecutive days.
DRG Non-OR 5A1D[7,8,9]0Z

5 Extracorporeal or Systemic Assistance and Performance
A Physiological Systems
2 Restoration
Definition: Returning, or attempting to return, a physiological function to its original state by extracorporeal means.

Body System Character 4	Duration Character 5	Function Character 6	Qualifier Character 7
2 Cardiac	0 Single	4 Rhythm	Z No Qualifier

Extracorporeal or Systemic Therapies 6A0–6AB

AHA Coding Clinic for table 6A4
2019, 2Q, 17 — Cryoamputation of lower leg

AHA Coding Clinic for table 6A5
2022, 1Q, 48 — Umbilical cord blood sampling

AHA Coding Clinic for table 6A7
2014, 4Q, 19 — Ultrasound accelerated thrombolysis

AHA Coding Clinic for table 6AB
2023, 2Q, 32 — Preparation of donor organ before transplantation
2016, 4Q, 115 — Donor organ perfusion

6 Extracorporeal or Systemic Therapies
A Physiological Systems
0 Atmospheric Control   Definition: Extracorporeal control of atmospheric pressure and composition

Body System Character 4	Duration Character 5	Qualifier Character 6	Qualifier Character 7
Z None	0 Single 1 Multiple	Z No Qualifier	Z No Qualifier

6 Extracorporeal or Systemic Therapies
A Physiological Systems
1 Decompression   Definition: Extracorporeal elimination of undissolved gas from body fluids

Body System Character 4	Duration Character 5	Qualifier Character 6	Qualifier Character 7
5 Circulatory	0 Single 1 Multiple	Z No Qualifier	Z No Qualifier

6 Extracorporeal or Systemic Therapies
A Physiological Systems
2 Electromagnetic Therapy   Definition: Extracorporeal treatment by electromagnetic rays

Body System Character 4	Duration Character 5	Qualifier Character 6	Qualifier Character 7
1 Urinary 2 Central Nervous	0 Single 1 Multiple	Z No Qualifier	Z No Qualifier

6 Extracorporeal or Systemic Therapies
A Physiological Systems
3 Hyperthermia   Definition: Extracorporeal raising of body temperature

Body System Character 4	Duration Character 5	Qualifier Character 6	Qualifier Character 7
Z None	0 Single 1 Multiple	Z No Qualifier	Z No Qualifier

6 Extracorporeal or Systemic Therapies
A Physiological Systems
4 Hypothermia   Definition: Extracorporeal lowering of body temperature

Body System Character 4	Duration Character 5	Qualifier Character 6	Qualifier Character 7
Z None	0 Single 1 Multiple	Z No Qualifier	Z No Qualifier

6 Extracorporeal or Systemic Therapies
A Physiological Systems
5 Pheresis   Definition: Extracorporeal separation of blood products

Body System Character 4	Duration Character 5	Qualifier Character 6	Qualifier Character 7
5 Circulatory	0 Single 1 Multiple	Z No Qualifier	0 Erythrocytes 1 Leukocytes 2 Platelets 3 Plasma T Stem Cells, Cord Blood V Stem Cells, Hematopoietic

6 Extracorporeal or Systemic Therapies
A Physiological Systems
6 Phototherapy   Definition: Extracorporeal treatment by light rays

Body System Character 4	Duration Character 5	Qualifier Character 6	Qualifier Character 7
0 Skin 5 Circulatory	0 Single 1 Multiple	Z No Qualifier	Z No Qualifier

6 Extracorporeal or Systemic Therapies
A Physiological Systems
7 Ultrasound Therapy   Definition: Extracorporeal treatment by ultrasound

Body System Character 4	Duration Character 5	Qualifier Character 6	Qualifier Character 7
5 Circulatory	0 Single 1 Multiple	Z No Qualifier	4 Head and Neck Vessels 5 Heart 6 Peripheral Vessels 7 Other Vessels Z No Qualifier

6 Extracorporeal or Systemic Therapies
A Physiological Systems
8 Ultraviolet Light Therapy   Definition: Extracorporeal treatment by ultraviolet light

Body System Character 4	Duration Character 5	Qualifier Character 6	Qualifier Character 7
0 Skin	0 Single 1 Multiple	Z No Qualifier	Z No Qualifier

6 Extracorporeal or Systemic Therapies
A Physiological Systems
9 Shock Wave Therapy   Definition: Extracorporeal treatment by shock waves

Body System Character 4	Duration Character 5	Qualifier Character 6	Qualifier Character 7
3 Musculoskeletal	0 Single 1 Multiple	Z No Qualifier	Z No Qualifier

6 Extracorporeal or Systemic Therapies
A Physiological Systems
B Perfusion   Definition: Extracorporeal treatment by diffusion of therapeutic fluid

Body System Character 4	Duration Character 5	Qualifier Character 6	Qualifier Character 7
5 Circulatory B Respiratory System F Hepatobiliary System and Pancreas T Urinary System	0 Single	B Donor Organ	Z No Qualifier

Osteopathic 7W0

7 Osteopathic
W Anatomical Regions
0 Treatment — Definition: Manual treatment to eliminate or alleviate somatic dysfunction and related disorders

Body Region Character 4	Approach Character 5	Method Character 6	Qualifier Character 7
0 Head	X External	0 Articulatory-Raising	Z None
1 Cervical		1 Fascial Release	
2 Thoracic		2 General Mobilization	
3 Lumbar		3 High Velocity-Low Amplitude	
4 Sacrum		4 Indirect	
5 Pelvis		5 Low Velocity-High Amplitude	
6 Lower Extremities		6 Lymphatic Pump	
7 Upper Extremities		7 Muscle Energy-Isometric	
8 Rib Cage		8 Muscle Energy-Isotonic	
9 Abdomen		9 Other Method	

Other Procedures 8C0–8E0

AHA Coding Clinic for table 8E0

2023, 4Q, 56-57	Fluorescence-guided surgery using Pafolacianine
2021, 4Q, 49	Division of liver for staged hepatectomy
2021, 2Q, 19	Electromagnetic stealth guided ventriculoperitoneal shunt insertion with endoscopy
2020, 4Q, 53	Bypass pancreatic duct to stomach
2020, 4Q, 65-66	Near infrared spectroscopy for tissue viability assessment
2020, 4Q, 99	Robotic-assisted prostatectomy with extension of incision for specimen removal
2020, 4Q, 100	Robotic-assisted sigmoid colectomy with extension of incision for specimen removal
2019, 4Q, 41-42	Intraoperative fluorescence guidance
2019, 1Q, 30	Laparoscopic-assisted rectopexy with manual reduction of prolapse
2015, 1Q, 33	Robotic-assisted laparoscopic hysterectomy converted to open procedure
2014, 4Q, 33	Radical prostatectomy

8 Other Procedures
C Indwelling Device
0 Other Procedures Definition: Methodologies which attempt to remediate or cure a disorder or disease

Body Region Character 4	Approach Character 5	Method Character 6	Qualifier Character 7
1 Nervous System	X External	6 Collection	J Cerebrospinal Fluid L Other Fluid
2 Circulatory System	X External	6 Collection	K Blood L Other Fluid

8E0–8E0 — Other Procedures

8 Other Procedures
E Physiological Systems and Anatomical Regions
0 Other Procedures   Definition: Methodologies which attempt to remediate or cure a disorder or disease

Body Region Character 4	Approach Character 5	Method Character 6	Qualifier Character 7
1 Nervous System	X External	Y Other Method	7 Examination
2 Circulatory System	3 Percutaneous	D Near Infrared Spectroscopy F Fiber Optic 3D Guided Procedure	Z No Qualifier
2 Circulatory System	X External	D Near Infrared Spectroscopy	Z No Qualifier
9 Head and Neck Region	0 Open	C Robotic Assisted Procedure	Z No Qualifier
9 Head and Neck Region	0 Open	E Fluorescence Guided Procedure	M Aminolevulinic Acid Z No Qualifier
9 Head and Neck Region	3 Percutaneous 4 Percutaneous Endoscopic 7 Via Natural or Artificial Opening 8 Via Natural or Artificial Opening Endoscopic	C Robotic Assisted Procedure E Fluorescence Guided Procedure	Z No Qualifier
9 Head and Neck Region	X External	B Computer Assisted Procedure	F With Fluoroscopy G With Computerized Tomography H With Magnetic Resonance Imaging Z No Qualifier
9 Head and Neck Region	X External	C Robotic Assisted Procedure	Z No Qualifier
9 Head and Neck Region	X External	Y Other Method	8 Suture Removal
H Integumentary System and Breast	3 Percutaneous	0 Acupuncture	0 Anesthesia Z No Qualifier
H Integumentary System and Breast	X External	6 Collection	2 Breast Milk
H Integumentary System and Breast	X External	Y Other Method	9 Piercing
K Musculoskeletal System	X External	1 Therapeutic Massage	Z No Qualifier
K Musculoskeletal System	X External	Y Other Method	7 Examination
U Female Reproductive System	0 Open 3 Percutaneous 4 Percutaneous Endoscopic 7 Via Natural or Artificial Opening 8 Via Natural or Artificial Opening Endoscopic	E Fluorescence Guided Procedure [NT]	N Pafolacianine
U Female Reproductive System	X External	Y Other Method	7 Examination
V Male Reproductive System	X External	1 Therapeutic Massage	C Prostate D Rectum
V Male Reproductive System	X External	6 Collection	3 Sperm
W Trunk Region	0 Open 3 Percutaneous 4 Percutaneous Endoscopic 7 Via Natural or Artificial Opening 8 Via Natural or Artificial Opening Endoscopic	C Robotic Assisted Procedure	Z No Qualifier
W Trunk Region	0 Open 3 Percutaneous 4 Percutaneous Endoscopic 7 Via Natural or Artificial Opening 8 Via Natural or Artificial Opening Endoscopic	E Fluorescence Guided Procedure [NT]	N Pafolacianine Z No Qualifier
W Trunk Region	X External	B Computer Assisted Procedure	F With Fluoroscopy G With Computerized Tomography H With Magnetic Resonance Imaging Z No Qualifier
W Trunk Region	X External	C Robotic Assisted Procedure	Z No Qualifier
W Trunk Region	X External	Y Other Method	8 Suture Removal
X Upper Extremity Y Lower Extremity	0 Open 3 Percutaneous 4 Percutaneous Endoscopic	C Robotic Assisted Procedure E Fluorescence Guided Procedure	Z No Qualifier
X Upper Extremity Y Lower Extremity	X External	B Computer Assisted Procedure	F With Fluoroscopy G With Computerized Tomography H With Magnetic Resonance Imaging Z No Qualifier
X Upper Extremity Y Lower Extremity	X External	C Robotic Assisted Procedure	Z No Qualifier
X Upper Extremity Y Lower Extremity	X External	Y Other Method	8 Suture Removal
Z None	X External	Y Other Method	1 In Vitro Fertilization 4 Yoga Therapy 5 Meditation 6 Isolation

[NT] 8E0U[0,3,4,7,8]EN for CYTALUX® when used for ovarian indications
[NT] 8E0W[0,3,4,7,8]EN for CYTALUX® when used for lung indications

Non-OR Procedure   DRG Non-OR Procedure   Valid OR Procedure   HAC Associated Procedure   Combination Only   New/Revised April   New/Revised October

Chiropractic 9WB

9 Chiropractic
W Anatomical Regions
B Manipulation Definition: Manual procedure that involves a directed thrust to move a joint past the physiological range of motion, without exceeding the anatomical limit

Body Region Character 4	Approach Character 5	Method Character 6	Qualifier Character 7
0 Head 1 Cervical 2 Thoracic 3 Lumbar 4 Sacrum 5 Pelvis 6 Lower Extremities 7 Upper Extremities 8 Rib Cage 9 Abdomen	X External	B Non-Manual C Indirect Visceral D Extra-Articular F Direct Visceral G Long Lever Specific Contact H Short Lever Specific Contact J Long and Short Lever Specific Contact K Mechanically Assisted L Other Method	Z None

Imaging B00–BY4

AHA Coding Clinic for table B21
2018, 1Q, 12 — Percutaneous balloon valvuloplasty & cardiac catheterization with ventriculogram
2016, 3Q, 36 — Type of contrast medium for angiography (high osmolar, low osmolar, and other)

AHA Coding Clinic for table B41
2015, 3Q, 9 — Aborted endovascular stenting of superficial femoral artery

AHA Coding Clinic for table B51
2015, 4Q, 30 — Vascular access devices

AHA Coding Clinic for table BB3
2022, 4Q, 62 — Hyperpolarized Xenon-129 gas for imaging of lung function

AHA Coding Clinic for table BF1
2021, 4Q, 57 — Fluoroscopic guidance of hepatobiliary sites

AHA Coding Clinic for table BF4
2014, 3Q, 15 — Drainage of pancreatic pseudocyst
2020, 4Q, 66 — Other imaging type

AHA Coding Clinic for table BF5
2020, 4Q, 66 — Other imaging type
2020, 4Q, 66-67 — Fluorescence imaging of hepatobiliary system

AHA Coding Clinic for table BW5
2020, 4Q, 66 — Other imaging type
2020, 4Q, 68 — Bacterial autofluorescence detection

Contrast Agents

High Osmolar (0)	Low Osmolar (1)	Other Contrast (Y)
cholografin meglumine	hexabrix	iodixanol
conray	iohexol	iotrolan
cysto-conray II	iomeprol	isovist
cystografin	iomeron	visipaque
cystografin-dilute	iopamidol	
diatrizoate	iopromide	
gastrografin	ioversol	
hypaque	ioxaglate	
iothalamate	ioxilan	
isopaque	isovue	
md-76r	omnipaque	
metrizoate	optiray	
reno-dip	oxilan	
sinografin	ultravist	

B Imaging
0 Central Nervous System
0 Plain Radiography   Definition: Planar display of an image developed from the capture of external ionizing radiation on photographic or photoconductive plate

Body Part Character 4	Contrast Character 5	Qualifier Character 6	Qualifier Character 7
B Spinal Cord	0 High Osmolar 1 Low Osmolar Y Other Contrast Z None	Z None	Z None

B Imaging
0 Central Nervous System
1 Fluoroscopy   Definition: Single plane or bi-plane real time display of an image developed from the capture of external ionizing radiation on a fluorescent screen. The image may also be stored by either digital or analog means.

Body Part Character 4	Contrast Character 5	Qualifier Character 6	Qualifier Character 7
B Spinal Cord	0 High Osmolar 1 Low Osmolar Y Other Contrast Z None	Z None	Z None

B Imaging
0 Central Nervous System
2 Computerized Tomography (CT Scan)

Definition: Computer reformatted digital display of multiplanar images developed from the capture of multiple exposures of external ionizing radiation

Body Part Character 4	Contrast Character 5	Qualifier Character 6	Qualifier Character 7
0 Brain 7 Cisterna 8 Cerebral Ventricle(s) 9 Sella Turcica/Pituitary Gland B Spinal Cord	0 High Osmolar 1 Low Osmolar Y Other Contrast	0 Unenhanced and Enhanced Z None	Z None
0 Brain 7 Cisterna 8 Cerebral Ventricle(s) 9 Sella Turcica/Pituitary Gland B Spinal Cord	Z None	Z None	Z None

B Imaging
0 Central Nervous System
3 Magnetic Resonance Imaging (MRI)

Definition: Computer reformatted digital display of multiplanar images developed from the capture of radio-frequency signals emitted by nuclei in a body site excited within a magnetic field

Body Part Character 4	Contrast Character 5	Qualifier Character 6	Qualifier Character 7
0 Brain 9 Sella Turcica/Pituitary Gland B Spinal Cord C Acoustic Nerves	Y Other Contrast	0 Unenhanced and Enhanced Z None	Z None
0 Brain 9 Sella Turcica/Pituitary Gland B Spinal Cord C Acoustic Nerves	Z None	Z None	Z None

B Imaging
0 Central Nervous System
4 Ultrasonography

Definition: Real time display of images of anatomy or flow information developed from the capture of reflected and attenuated high frequency sound waves

Body Part Character 4	Contrast Character 5	Qualifier Character 6	Qualifier Character 7
0 Brain B Spinal Cord	Z None	Z None	Z None

B Imaging
2 Heart
0 Plain Radiography

Definition: Planar display of an image developed from the capture of external ionizing radiation on photographic or photoconductive plate

Body Part Character 4	Contrast Character 5	Qualifier Character 6	Qualifier Character 7
0 Coronary Artery, Single 1 Coronary Arteries, Multiple 2 Coronary Artery Bypass Graft, Single 3 Coronary Artery Bypass Grafts, Multiple 4 Heart, Right 5 Heart, Left 6 Heart, Right and Left 7 Internal Mammary Bypass Graft, Right 8 Internal Mammary Bypass Graft, Left F Bypass Graft, Other	0 High Osmolar 1 Low Osmolar Y Other Contrast	Z None	Z None

DRG Non-OR All body part, contrast, and qualifier values

ICD-10-PCS 2025 — Imaging — B21–B23

B Imaging
2 Heart
1 Fluoroscopy   Definition: Single plane or bi-plane real time display of an image developed from the capture of external ionizing radiation on a fluorescent screen. The image may also be stored by either digital or analog means.

Body Part Character 4	Contrast Character 5	Qualifier Character 6	Qualifier Character 7
0 Coronary Artery, Single 1 Coronary Arteries, Multiple 2 Coronary Artery Bypass Graft, Single 3 Coronary Artery Bypass Grafts, Multiple	0 High Osmolar 1 Low Osmolar Y Other Contrast	1 Laser	0 Intraoperative
0 Coronary Artery, Single 1 Coronary Arteries, Multiple 2 Coronary Artery Bypass Graft, Single 3 Coronary Artery Bypass Grafts, Multiple	0 High Osmolar 1 Low Osmolar Y Other Contrast	Z None	Z None
4 Heart, Right 5 Heart, Left 6 Heart, Right and Left 7 Internal Mammary Bypass Graft, Right 8 Internal Mammary Bypass Graft, Left F Bypass Graft, Other	0 High Osmolar 1 Low Osmolar Y Other Contrast	Z None	Z None

DRG Non-OR   B21[0,1,2,3][0,1,Y]ZZ
DRG Non-OR   B21[4,5,6,7,8,F][0,1,Y]ZZ

B Imaging
2 Heart
2 Computerized Tomography (CT Scan)   Definition: Computer reformatted digital display of multiplanar images developed from the capture of multiple exposures of external ionizing radiation

Body Part Character 4	Contrast Character 5	Qualifier Character 6	Qualifier Character 7
1 Coronary Arteries, Multiple 3 Coronary Artery Bypass Grafts, Multiple 6 Heart, Right and Left	0 High Osmolar 1 Low Osmolar Y Other Contrast	0 Unenhanced and Enhanced Z None	Z None
1 Coronary Arteries, Multiple 3 Coronary Artery Bypass Grafts, Multiple 6 Heart, Right and Left	Z None	2 Intravascular Optical Coherence Z None	Z None

B Imaging
2 Heart
3 Magnetic Resonance Imaging (MRI)   Definition: Computer reformatted digital display of multiplanar images developed from the capture of radio-frequency signals emitted by nuclei in a body site excited within a magnetic field

Body Part Character 4	Contrast Character 5	Qualifier Character 6	Qualifier Character 7
1 Coronary Arteries, Multiple 3 Coronary Artery Bypass Grafts, Multiple 6 Heart, Right and Left	Y Other Contrast	0 Unenhanced and Enhanced Z None	Z None
1 Coronary Arteries, Multiple 3 Coronary Artery Bypass Grafts, Multiple 6 Heart, Right and Left	Z None	Z None	Z None

NC Noncovered Procedure   LC Limited Coverage   QA Questionable OB Admit   NT New Tech Add-on   ✚ Combination Member   ♂ Male   ♀ Female

B Imaging
2 Heart
4 Ultrasonography

Definition: Real time display of images of anatomy or flow information developed from the capture of reflected and attenuated high frequency sound waves

Body Part Character 4	Contrast Character 5	Qualifier Character 6	Qualifier Character 7
0 Coronary Artery, Single 1 Coronary Arteries, Multiple 4 Heart, Right 5 Heart, Left 6 Heart, Right and Left B Heart with Aorta C Pericardium D Pediatric Heart	Y Other Contrast	Z None	Z None
0 Coronary Artery, Single 1 Coronary Arteries, Multiple 4 Heart, Right 5 Heart, Left 6 Heart, Right and Left B Heart with Aorta C Pericardium D Pediatric Heart	Z None	Z None	3 Intravascular 4 Transesophageal Z None

B Imaging
3 Upper Arteries
0 Plain Radiography

Definition: Planar display of an image developed from the capture of external ionizing radiation on photographic or photoconductive plate

Body Part Character 4	Contrast Character 5	Qualifier Character 6	Qualifier Character 7
0 Thoracic Aorta 1 Brachiocephalic-Subclavian Artery, Right 2 Subclavian Artery, Left 3 Common Carotid Artery, Right 4 Common Carotid Artery, Left 5 Common Carotid Arteries, Bilateral 6 Internal Carotid Artery, Right 7 Internal Carotid Artery, Left 8 Internal Carotid Arteries, Bilateral 9 External Carotid Artery, Right B External Carotid Artery, Left C External Carotid Arteries, Bilateral D Vertebral Artery, Right F Vertebral Artery, Left G Vertebral Arteries, Bilateral H Upper Extremity Arteries, Right J Upper Extremity Arteries, Left K Upper Extremity Arteries, Bilateral L Intercostal and Bronchial Arteries M Spinal Arteries N Upper Arteries, Other P Thoraco-Abdominal Aorta Q Cervico-Cerebral Arch R Intracranial Arteries S Pulmonary Artery, Right T Pulmonary Artery, Left	0 High Osmolar 1 Low Osmolar Y Other Contrast Z None	Z None	Z None

B	Imaging
3	Upper Arteries
1	Fluoroscopy

Definition: Single plane or bi-plane real time display of an image developed from the capture of external ionizing radiation on a fluorescent screen. The image may also be stored by either digital or analog means.

Body Part Character 4	Contrast Character 5	Qualifier Character 6	Qualifier Character 7
0 Thoracic Aorta 1 Brachiocephalic-Subclavian Artery, Right 2 Subclavian Artery, Left 3 Common Carotid Artery, Right 4 Common Carotid Artery, Left 5 Common Carotid Arteries, Bilateral 6 Internal Carotid Artery, Right 7 Internal Carotid Artery, Left 8 Internal Carotid Arteries, Bilateral 9 External Carotid Artery, Right B External Carotid Artery, Left C External Carotid Arteries, Bilateral D Vertebral Artery, Right F Vertebral Artery, Left G Vertebral Arteries, Bilateral H Upper Extremity Arteries, Right J Upper Extremity Arteries, Left K Upper Extremity Arteries, Bilateral L Intercostal and Bronchial Arteries M Spinal Arteries N Upper Arteries, Other P Thoraco-Abdominal Aorta Q Cervico-Cerebral Arch R Intracranial Arteries S Pulmonary Artery, Right T Pulmonary Artery, Left U Pulmonary Trunk	0 High Osmolar 1 Low Osmolar Y Other Contrast	1 Laser	0 Intraoperative
0 Thoracic Aorta 1 Brachiocephalic-Subclavian Artery, Right 2 Subclavian Artery, Left 3 Common Carotid Artery, Right 4 Common Carotid Artery, Left 5 Common Carotid Arteries, Bilateral 6 Internal Carotid Artery, Right 7 Internal Carotid Artery, Left 8 Internal Carotid Arteries, Bilateral 9 External Carotid Artery, Right B External Carotid Artery, Left C External Carotid Arteries, Bilateral D Vertebral Artery, Right F Vertebral Artery, Left G Vertebral Arteries, Bilateral H Upper Extremity Arteries, Right J Upper Extremity Arteries, Left K Upper Extremity Arteries, Bilateral L Intercostal and Bronchial Arteries M Spinal Arteries N Upper Arteries, Other P Thoraco-Abdominal Aorta Q Cervico-Cerebral Arch R Intracranial Arteries S Pulmonary Artery, Right T Pulmonary Artery, Left U Pulmonary Trunk	0 High Osmolar 1 Low Osmolar Y Other Contrast	Z None	Z None

B31 Continued on next page

B Imaging
3 Upper Arteries
1 Fluoroscopy

Definition: Single plane or bi-plane real time display of an image developed from the capture of external ionizing radiation on a fluorescent screen. The image may also be stored by either digital or analog means.

Body Part Character 4	Contrast Character 5	Qualifier Character 6	Qualifier Character 7
0 Thoracic Aorta 1 Brachiocephalic-Subclavian Artery, Right 2 Subclavian Artery, Left 3 Common Carotid Artery, Right 4 Common Carotid Artery, Left 5 Common Carotid Arteries, Bilateral 6 Internal Carotid Artery, Right 7 Internal Carotid Artery, Left 8 Internal Carotid Arteries, Bilateral 9 External Carotid Artery, Right B External Carotid Artery, Left C External Carotid Arteries, Bilateral D Vertebral Artery, Right F Vertebral Artery, Left G Vertebral Arteries, Bilateral H Upper Extremity Arteries, Right J Upper Extremity Arteries, Left K Upper Extremity Arteries, Bilateral L Intercostal and Bronchial Arteries M Spinal Arteries N Upper Arteries, Other P Thoraco-Abdominal Aorta Q Cervico-Cerebral Arch R Intracranial Arteries S Pulmonary Artery, Right T Pulmonary Artery, Left U Pulmonary Trunk	Z None	Z None	Z None

B Imaging
3 Upper Arteries
2 Computerized Tomography (CT Scan)

Definition: Computer reformatted digital display of multiplanar images developed from the capture of multiple exposures of external ionizing radiation

Body Part Character 4	Contrast Character 5	Qualifier Character 6	Qualifier Character 7
0 Thoracic Aorta 5 Common Carotid Arteries, Bilateral 8 Internal Carotid Arteries, Bilateral G Vertebral Arteries, Bilateral R Intracranial Arteries S Pulmonary Artery, Right T Pulmonary Artery, Left	0 High Osmolar 1 Low Osmolar Y Other Contrast	Z None	Z None
0 Thoracic Aorta 5 Common Carotid Arteries, Bilateral 8 Internal Carotid Arteries, Bilateral G Vertebral Arteries, Bilateral R Intracranial Arteries S Pulmonary Artery, Right T Pulmonary Artery, Left	Z None	2 Intravascular Optical Coherence Z None	Z None

ICD-10-PCS 2025   Imaging   B33–B40

B   Imaging
3   Upper Arteries
3   Magnetic Resonance Imaging (MRI)   **Definition:** Computer reformatted digital display of multiplanar images developed from the capture of radio-frequency signals emitted by nuclei in a body site excited within a magnetic field

Body Part Character 4	Contrast Character 5	Qualifier Character 6	Qualifier Character 7
0 Thoracic Aorta **5** Common Carotid Arteries, Bilateral **8** Internal Carotid Arteries, Bilateral **G** Vertebral Arteries, Bilateral **H** Upper Extremity Arteries, Right **J** Upper Extremity Arteries, Left **K** Upper Extremity Arteries, Bilateral **M** Spinal Arteries **Q** Cervico-Cerebral Arch **R** Intracranial Arteries	**Y** Other Contrast	**0** Unenhanced and Enhanced **Z** None	**Z** None
0 Thoracic Aorta **5** Common Carotid Arteries, Bilateral **8** Internal Carotid Arteries, Bilateral **G** Vertebral Arteries, Bilateral **H** Upper Extremity Arteries, Right **J** Upper Extremity Arteries, Left **K** Upper Extremity Arteries, Bilateral **M** Spinal Arteries **Q** Cervico-Cerebral Arch **R** Intracranial Arteries	**Z** None	**Z** None	**Z** None

B   Imaging
3   Upper Arteries
4   Ultrasonography   **Definition:** Real time display of images of anatomy or flow information developed from the capture of reflected and attenuated high frequency sound waves

Body Part Character 4	Contrast Character 5	Qualifier Character 6	Qualifier Character 7
0 Thoracic Aorta **1** Brachiocephalic-Subclavian Artery, Right **2** Subclavian Artery, Left **3** Common Carotid Artery, Right **4** Common Carotid Artery, Left **5** Common Carotid Arteries, Bilateral **6** Internal Carotid Artery, Right **7** Internal Carotid Artery, Left **8** Internal Carotid Arteries, Bilateral **H** Upper Extremity Arteries, Right **J** Upper Extremity Arteries, Left **K** Upper Extremity Arteries, Bilateral **R** Intracranial Arteries **S** Pulmonary Artery, Right **T** Pulmonary Artery, Left **V** Ophthalmic Arteries	**Z** None	**Z** None	**3** Intravascular **Z** None

B   Imaging
4   Lower Arteries
0   Plain Radiography   **Definition:** Planar display of an image developed from the capture of external ionizing radiation on photographic or photoconductive plate

Body Part Character 4	Contrast Character 5	Qualifier Character 6	Qualifier Character 7
0 Abdominal Aorta **2** Hepatic Artery **3** Splenic Arteries **4** Superior Mesenteric Artery **5** Inferior Mesenteric Artery **6** Renal Artery, Right **7** Renal Artery, Left **8** Renal Arteries, Bilateral **9** Lumbar Arteries **B** Intra-Abdominal Arteries, Other **C** Pelvic Arteries **D** Aorta and Bilateral Lower Extremity Arteries **F** Lower Extremity Arteries, Right **G** Lower Extremity Arteries, Left **J** Lower Arteries, Other **M** Renal Artery Transplant	**0** High Osmolar **1** Low Osmolar **Y** Other Contrast	**Z** None	**Z** None

NC Noncovered Procedure   **LC** Limited Coverage   **QA** Questionable OB Admit   **NT** New Tech Add-on   ✚ Combination Member   ♂ Male   ♀ Female

B Imaging
4 Lower Arteries
1 Fluoroscopy

Definition: Single plane or bi-plane real time display of an image developed from the capture of external ionizing radiation on a fluorescent screen. The image may also be stored by either digital or analog means.

Body Part Character 4	Contrast Character 5	Qualifier Character 6	Qualifier Character 7
0 Abdominal Aorta 2 Hepatic Artery 3 Splenic Arteries 4 Superior Mesenteric Artery 5 Inferior Mesenteric Artery 6 Renal Artery, Right 7 Renal Artery, Left 8 Renal Arteries, Bilateral 9 Lumbar Arteries B Intra-Abdominal Arteries, Other C Pelvic Arteries D Aorta and Bilateral Lower Extremity Arteries F Lower Extremity Arteries, Right G Lower Extremity Arteries, Left J Lower Arteries, Other	0 High Osmolar 1 Low Osmolar Y Other Contrast	1 Laser	0 Intraoperative
0 Abdominal Aorta 2 Hepatic Artery 3 Splenic Arteries 4 Superior Mesenteric Artery 5 Inferior Mesenteric Artery 6 Renal Artery, Right 7 Renal Artery, Left 8 Renal Arteries, Bilateral 9 Lumbar Arteries B Intra-Abdominal Arteries, Other C Pelvic Arteries D Aorta and Bilateral Lower Extremity Arteries F Lower Extremity Arteries, Right G Lower Extremity Arteries, Left J Lower Arteries, Other	0 High Osmolar 1 Low Osmolar Y Other Contrast	Z None	Z None
0 Abdominal Aorta 2 Hepatic Artery 3 Splenic Arteries 4 Superior Mesenteric Artery 5 Inferior Mesenteric Artery 6 Renal Artery, Right 7 Renal Artery, Left 8 Renal Arteries, Bilateral 9 Lumbar Arteries B Intra-Abdominal Arteries, Other C Pelvic Arteries D Aorta and Bilateral Lower Extremity Arteries F Lower Extremity Arteries, Right G Lower Extremity Arteries, Left J Lower Arteries, Other	Z None	Z None	Z None

ICD-10-PCS 2025 — Imaging — B42–B44

B Imaging
4 Lower Arteries
2 Computerized Tomography (CT Scan) — Definition: Computer reformatted digital display of multiplanar images developed from the capture of multiple exposures of external ionizing radiation

Body Part — Character 4	Contrast — Character 5	Qualifier — Character 6	Qualifier — Character 7
0 Abdominal Aorta 1 Celiac Artery 4 Superior Mesenteric Artery 8 Renal Arteries, Bilateral C Pelvic Arteries F Lower Extremity Arteries, Right G Lower Extremity Arteries, Left H Lower Extremity Arteries, Bilateral M Renal Artery Transplant	0 High Osmolar 1 Low Osmolar Y Other Contrast	Z None	Z None
0 Abdominal Aorta 1 Celiac Artery 4 Superior Mesenteric Artery 8 Renal Arteries, Bilateral C Pelvic Arteries F Lower Extremity Arteries, Right G Lower Extremity Arteries, Left H Lower Extremity Arteries, Bilateral M Renal Artery Transplant	Z None	2 Intravascular Optical Coherence Z None	Z None

B Imaging
4 Lower Arteries
3 Magnetic Resonance Imaging (MRI) — Definition: Computer reformatted digital display of multiplanar images developed from the capture of radio-frequency signals emitted by nuclei in a body site excited within a magnetic field

Body Part — Character 4	Contrast — Character 5	Qualifier — Character 6	Qualifier — Character 7
0 Abdominal Aorta 1 Celiac Artery 4 Superior Mesenteric Artery 8 Renal Arteries, Bilateral C Pelvic Arteries F Lower Extremity Arteries, Right G Lower Extremity Arteries, Left H Lower Extremity Arteries, Bilateral	Y Other Contrast	0 Unenhanced and Enhanced Z None	Z None
0 Abdominal Aorta 1 Celiac Artery 4 Superior Mesenteric Artery 8 Renal Arteries, Bilateral C Pelvic Arteries F Lower Extremity Arteries, Right G Lower Extremity Arteries, Left H Lower Extremity Arteries, Bilateral	Z None	Z None	Z None

B Imaging
4 Lower Arteries
4 Ultrasonography — Definition: Real time display of images of anatomy or flow information developed from the capture of reflected and attenuated high frequency sound waves

Body Part — Character 4	Contrast — Character 5	Qualifier — Character 6	Qualifier — Character 7
0 Abdominal Aorta 4 Superior Mesenteric Artery 5 Inferior Mesenteric Artery 6 Renal Artery, Right 7 Renal Artery, Left 8 Renal Arteries, Bilateral B Intra-Abdominal Arteries, Other F Lower Extremity Arteries, Right G Lower Extremity Arteries, Left H Lower Extremity Arteries, Bilateral K Celiac and Mesenteric Arteries L Femoral Artery N Penile Arteries	Z None	Z None	3 Intravascular Z None

NC Noncovered Procedure   LC Limited Coverage   QA Questionable OB Admit   NT New Tech Add-on   ✚ Combination Member   ♂ Male   ♀ Female

B	Imaging
5	Veins
0	**Plain Radiography** Definition: Planar display of an image developed from the capture of external ionizing radiation on photographic or photoconductive plate

Body Part Character 4	Contrast Character 5	Qualifier Character 6	Qualifier Character 7
0 Epidural Veins 1 Cerebral and Cerebellar Veins 2 Intracranial Sinuses 3 Jugular Veins, Right 4 Jugular Veins, Left 5 Jugular Veins, Bilateral 6 Subclavian Vein, Right 7 Subclavian Vein, Left 8 Superior Vena Cava 9 Inferior Vena Cava B Lower Extremity Veins, Right C Lower Extremity Veins, Left D Lower Extremity Veins, Bilateral F Pelvic (Iliac) Veins, Right G Pelvic (Iliac) Veins, Left H Pelvic (Iliac) Veins, Bilateral J Renal Vein, Right K Renal Vein, Left L Renal Veins, Bilateral M Upper Extremity Veins, Right N Upper Extremity Veins, Left P Upper Extremity Veins, Bilateral Q Pulmonary Vein, Right R Pulmonary Vein, Left S Pulmonary Veins, Bilateral T Portal and Splanchnic Veins V Veins, Other W Dialysis Shunt/Fistula	0 High Osmolar 1 Low Osmolar Y Other Contrast	Z None	Z None

B	Imaging
5	Veins
1	**Fluoroscopy** Definition: Single plane or bi-plane real time display of an image developed from the capture of external ionizing radiation on a fluorescent screen. The image may also be stored by either digital or analog means.

Body Part Character 4	Contrast Character 5	Qualifier Character 6	Qualifier Character 7
0 Epidural Veins 1 Cerebral and Cerebellar Veins 2 Intracranial Sinuses 3 Jugular Veins, Right 4 Jugular Veins, Left 5 Jugular Veins, Bilateral 6 Subclavian Vein, Right 7 Subclavian Vein, Left 8 Superior Vena Cava 9 Inferior Vena Cava B Lower Extremity Veins, Right C Lower Extremity Veins, Left D Lower Extremity Veins, Bilateral F Pelvic (Iliac) Veins, Right G Pelvic (Iliac) Veins, Left H Pelvic (Iliac) Veins, Bilateral J Renal Vein, Right K Renal Vein, Left L Renal Veins, Bilateral M Upper Extremity Veins, Right N Upper Extremity Veins, Left P Upper Extremity Veins, Bilateral Q Pulmonary Vein, Right R Pulmonary Vein, Left S Pulmonary Veins, Bilateral T Portal and Splanchnic Veins V Veins, Other W Dialysis Shunt/Fistula	0 High Osmolar 1 Low Osmolar Y Other Contrast Z None	Z None	A Guidance Z None

B	Imaging
5	Veins
2	**Computerized Tomography (CT Scan)** Definition: Computer reformatted digital display of multiplanar images developed from the capture of multiple exposures of external ionizing radiation

Body Part Character 4	Contrast Character 5	Qualifier Character 6	Qualifier Character 7
2 Intracranial Sinuses 8 Superior Vena Cava 9 Inferior Vena Cava F Pelvic (Iliac) Veins, Right G Pelvic (Iliac) Veins, Left H Pelvic (Iliac) Veins, Bilateral J Renal Vein, Right K Renal Vein, Left L Renal Veins, Bilateral Q Pulmonary Vein, Right R Pulmonary Vein, Left S Pulmonary Veins, Bilateral T Portal and Splanchnic Veins	0 High Osmolar 1 Low Osmolar Y Other Contrast	0 Unenhanced and Enhanced Z None	Z None
2 Intracranial Sinuses 8 Superior Vena Cava 9 Inferior Vena Cava F Pelvic (Iliac) Veins, Right G Pelvic (Iliac) Veins, Left H Pelvic (Iliac) Veins, Bilateral J Renal Vein, Right K Renal Vein, Left L Renal Veins, Bilateral Q Pulmonary Vein, Right R Pulmonary Vein, Left S Pulmonary Veins, Bilateral T Portal and Splanchnic Veins	Z None	2 Intravascular Optical Coherence Z None	Z None

B	Imaging
5	Veins
3	**Magnetic Resonance Imaging (MRI)** Definition: Computer reformatted digital display of multiplanar images developed from the capture of radio-frequency signals emitted by nuclei in a body site excited within a magnetic field

Body Part Character 4	Contrast Character 5	Qualifier Character 6	Qualifier Character 7
1 Cerebral and Cerebellar Veins 2 Intracranial Sinuses 5 Jugular Veins, Bilateral 8 Superior Vena Cava 9 Inferior Vena Cava B Lower Extremity Veins, Right C Lower Extremity Veins, Left D Lower Extremity Veins, Bilateral H Pelvic (Iliac) Veins, Bilateral L Renal Veins, Bilateral M Upper Extremity Veins, Right N Upper Extremity Veins, Left P Upper Extremity Veins, Bilateral S Pulmonary Veins, Bilateral T Portal and Splanchnic Veins V Veins, Other	Y Other Contrast	0 Unenhanced and Enhanced Z None	Z None
1 Cerebral and Cerebellar Veins 2 Intracranial Sinuses 5 Jugular Veins, Bilateral 8 Superior Vena Cava 9 Inferior Vena Cava B Lower Extremity Veins, Right C Lower Extremity Veins, Left D Lower Extremity Veins, Bilateral H Pelvic (Iliac) Veins, Bilateral L Renal Veins, Bilateral M Upper Extremity Veins, Right N Upper Extremity Veins, Left P Upper Extremity Veins, Bilateral S Pulmonary Veins, Bilateral T Portal and Splanchnic Veins V Veins, Other	Z None	Z None	Z None

B Imaging
5 Veins
4 Ultrasonography

Definition: Real time display of images of anatomy or flow information developed from the capture of reflected and attenuated high frequency sound waves

Body Part Character 4	Contrast Character 5	Qualifier Character 6	Qualifier Character 7
3 Jugular Veins, Right 4 Jugular Veins, Left 6 Subclavian Vein, Right 7 Subclavian Vein, Left 8 Superior Vena Cava 9 Inferior Vena Cava B Lower Extremity Veins, Right C Lower Extremity Veins, Left D Lower Extremity Veins, Bilateral J Renal Vein, Right K Renal Vein, Left L Renal Veins, Bilateral M Upper Extremity Veins, Right N Upper Extremity Veins, Left P Upper Extremity Veins, Bilateral T Portal and Splanchnic Veins	Z None	Z None	3 Intravascular A Guidance Z None

B Imaging
7 Lymphatic System
0 Plain Radiography

Definition: Planar display of an image developed from the capture of external ionizing radiation on photographic or photoconductive plate

Body Part Character 4	Contrast Character 5	Qualifier Character 6	Qualifier Character 7
0 Abdominal/Retroperitoneal Lymphatics, Unilateral 1 Abdominal/Retroperitoneal Lymphatics, Bilateral 4 Lymphatics, Head and Neck 5 Upper Extremity Lymphatics, Right 6 Upper Extremity Lymphatics, Left 7 Upper Extremity Lymphatics, Bilateral 8 Lower Extremity Lymphatics, Right 9 Lower Extremity Lymphatics, Left B Lower Extremity Lymphatics, Bilateral C Lymphatics, Pelvic	0 High Osmolar 1 Low Osmolar Y Other Contrast	Z None	Z None

B Imaging
8 Eye
0 Plain Radiography

Definition: Planar display of an image developed from the capture of external ionizing radiation on photographic or photoconductive plate

Body Part Character 4	Contrast Character 5	Qualifier Character 6	Qualifier Character 7
0 Lacrimal Duct, Right 1 Lacrimal Duct, Left 2 Lacrimal Ducts, Bilateral	0 High Osmolar 1 Low Osmolar Y Other Contrast	Z None	Z None
3 Optic Foramina, Right 4 Optic Foramina, Left 5 Eye, Right 6 Eye, Left 7 Eyes, Bilateral	Z None	Z None	Z None

B Imaging
8 Eye
2 Computerized Tomography (CT Scan)

Definition: Computer reformatted digital display of multiplanar images developed from the capture of multiple exposures of external ionizing radiation

Body Part Character 4	Contrast Character 5	Qualifier Character 6	Qualifier Character 7
5 Eye, Right 6 Eye, Left 7 Eyes, Bilateral	0 High Osmolar 1 Low Osmolar Y Other Contrast	0 Unenhanced and Enhanced Z None	Z None
5 Eye, Right 6 Eye, Left 7 Eyes, Bilateral	Z None	Z None	Z None

ICD-10-PCS 2025 — Imaging — B83–B92

B Imaging
8 Eye
3 Magnetic Resonance Imaging (MRI) Definition: Computer reformatted digital display of multiplanar images developed from the capture of radio-frequency signals emitted by nuclei in a body site excited within a magnetic field

Body Part Character 4	Contrast Character 5	Qualifier Character 6	Qualifier Character 7
5 Eye, Right 6 Eye, Left 7 Eyes, Bilateral	Y Other Contrast	0 Unenhanced and Enhanced Z None	Z None
5 Eye, Right 6 Eye, Left 7 Eyes, Bilateral	Z None	Z None	Z None

B Imaging
8 Eye
4 Ultrasonography Definition: Real time display of images of anatomy or flow information developed from the capture of reflected and attenuated high frequency sound waves

Body Part Character 4	Contrast Character 5	Qualifier Character 6	Qualifier Character 7
5 Eye, Right 6 Eye, Left 7 Eyes, Bilateral	Z None	Z None	Z None

B Imaging
9 Ear, Nose, Mouth and Throat
0 Plain Radiography Definition: Planar display of an image developed from the capture of external ionizing radiation on photographic or photoconductive plate

Body Part Character 4	Contrast Character 5	Qualifier Character 6	Qualifier Character 7
2 Paranasal Sinuses F Nasopharynx/Oropharynx H Mastoids	Z None	Z None	Z None
4 Parotid Gland, Right 5 Parotid Gland, Left 6 Parotid Glands, Bilateral 7 Submandibular Gland, Right 8 Submandibular Gland, Left 9 Submandibular Glands, Bilateral B Salivary Gland, Right C Salivary Gland, Left D Salivary Glands, Bilateral	0 High Osmolar 1 Low Osmolar Y Other Contrast	Z None	Z None

B Imaging
9 Ear, Nose, Mouth and Throat
1 Fluoroscopy Definition: Single plane or bi-plane real time display of an image developed from the capture of external ionizing radiation on a fluorescent screen. The image may also be stored by either digital or analog means.

Body Part Character 4	Contrast Character 5	Qualifier Character 6	Qualifier Character 7
G Pharynx and Epiglottis J Larynx	Y Other Contrast Z None	Z None	Z None

B Imaging
9 Ear, Nose, Mouth and Throat
2 Computerized Tomography (CT Scan) Definition: Computer reformatted digital display of multiplanar images developed from the capture of multiple exposures of external ionizing radiation

Body Part Character 4	Contrast Character 5	Qualifier Character 6	Qualifier Character 7
0 Ear 2 Paranasal Sinuses 6 Parotid Glands, Bilateral 9 Submandibular Glands, Bilateral D Salivary Glands, Bilateral F Nasopharynx/Oropharynx J Larynx	0 High Osmolar 1 Low Osmolar Y Other Contrast	0 Unenhanced and Enhanced Z None	Z None
0 Ear 2 Paranasal Sinuses 6 Parotid Glands, Bilateral 9 Submandibular Glands, Bilateral D Salivary Glands, Bilateral F Nasopharynx/Oropharynx J Larynx	Z None	Z None	Z None

NC Noncovered Procedure   LC Limited Coverage   QA Questionable OB Admit   NT New Tech Add-on   ✚ Combination Member   ♂ Male   ♀ Female

B Imaging
9 Ear, Nose, Mouth and Throat
3 Magnetic Resonance Imaging (MRI) Definition: Computer reformatted digital display of multiplanar images developed from the capture of radio-frequency signals emitted by nuclei in a body site excited within a magnetic field

Body Part Character 4	Contrast Character 5	Qualifier Character 6	Qualifier Character 7
0 Ear 2 Paranasal Sinuses 6 Parotid Glands, Bilateral 9 Submandibular Glands, Bilateral D Salivary Glands, Bilateral F Nasopharynx/Oropharynx J Larynx	Y Other Contrast	0 Unenhanced and Enhanced Z None	Z None
0 Ear 2 Paranasal Sinuses 6 Parotid Glands, Bilateral 9 Submandibular Glands, Bilateral D Salivary Glands, Bilateral F Nasopharynx/Oropharynx J Larynx	Z None	Z None	Z None

B Imaging
B Respiratory System
0 Plain Radiography Definition: Planar display of an image developed from the capture of external ionizing radiation on photographic or photoconductive plate

Body Part Character 4	Contrast Character 5	Qualifier Character 6	Qualifier Character 7
7 Tracheobronchial Tree, Right 8 Tracheobronchial Tree, Left 9 Tracheobronchial Trees, Bilateral	Y Other Contrast	Z None	Z None
D Upper Airways	Z None	Z None	Z None

B Imaging
B Respiratory System
1 Fluoroscopy Definition: Single plane or bi-plane real time display of an image developed from the capture of external ionizing radiation on a fluorescent screen. The image may also be stored by either digital or analog means.

Body Part Character 4	Contrast Character 5	Qualifier Character 6	Qualifier Character 7
2 Lung, Right 3 Lung, Left 4 Lungs, Bilateral 6 Diaphragm C Mediastinum D Upper Airways	Z None	Z None	Z None
7 Tracheobronchial Tree, Right 8 Tracheobronchial Tree, Left 9 Tracheobronchial Trees, Bilateral	Y Other Contrast	Z None	Z None

B Imaging
B Respiratory System
2 Computerized Tomography (CT Scan) Definition: Computer reformatted digital display of multiplanar images developed from the capture of multiple exposures of external ionizing radiation

Body Part Character 4	Contrast Character 5	Qualifier Character 6	Qualifier Character 7
4 Lungs, Bilateral 7 Tracheobronchial Tree, Right 8 Tracheobronchial Tree, Left 9 Tracheobronchial Trees, Bilateral F Trachea/Airways	0 High Osmolar 1 Low Osmolar Y Other Contrast	0 Unenhanced and Enhanced Z None	Z None
4 Lungs, Bilateral 7 Tracheobronchial Tree, Right 8 Tracheobronchial Tree, Left 9 Tracheobronchial Trees, Bilateral F Trachea/Airways	Z None	Z None	Z None

B Imaging
B Respiratory System
3 Magnetic Resonance Imaging (MRI)
Definition: Computer reformatted digital display of multiplanar images developed from the capture of radio-frequency signals emitted by nuclei in a body site excited within a magnetic field

Body Part Character 4	Contrast Character 5	Qualifier Character 6	Qualifier Character 7
4 Lungs, Bilateral	Z None	3 Hyperpolarized Xenon 129 (Xe-129)	Z None
G Lung Apices	Y Other Contrast	0 Unenhanced and Enhanced Z None	Z None
G Lung Apices	Z None	Z None	Z None

B Imaging
B Respiratory System
4 Ultrasonography
Definition: Real time display of images of anatomy or flow information developed from the capture of reflected and attenuated high frequency sound waves

Body Part Character 4	Contrast Character 5	Qualifier Character 6	Qualifier Character 7
B Pleura C Mediastinum	Z None	Z None	Z None

B Imaging
D Gastrointestinal System
1 Fluoroscopy
Definition: Single plane or bi-plane real time display of an image developed from the capture of external ionizing radiation on a fluorescent screen. The image may also be stored by either digital or analog means.

Body Part Character 4	Contrast Character 5	Qualifier Character 6	Qualifier Character 7
1 Esophagus 2 Stomach 3 Small Bowel 4 Colon 5 Upper GI 6 Upper GI and Small Bowel 9 Duodenum B Mouth/Oropharynx	Y Other Contrast Z None	Z None	Z None

B Imaging
D Gastrointestinal System
2 Computerized Tomography (CT Scan)
Definition: Computer reformatted digital display of multiplanar images developed from the capture of multiple exposures of external ionizing radiation

Body Part Character 4	Contrast Character 5	Qualifier Character 6	Qualifier Character 7
4 Colon	0 High Osmolar 1 Low Osmolar Y Other Contrast	0 Unenhanced and Enhanced Z None	Z None
4 Colon	Z None	Z None	Z None

B Imaging
D Gastrointestinal System
4 Ultrasonography
Definition: Real time display of images of anatomy or flow information developed from the capture of reflected and attenuated high frequency sound waves

Body Part Character 4	Contrast Character 5	Qualifier Character 6	Qualifier Character 7
1 Esophagus 2 Stomach 7 Gastrointestinal Tract 8 Appendix 9 Duodenum C Rectum	Z None	Z None	Z None

B Imaging
F Hepatobiliary System and Pancreas
0 Plain Radiography
Definition: Planar display of an image developed from the capture of external ionizing radiation on photographic or photoconductive plate

Body Part Character 4	Contrast Character 5	Qualifier Character 6	Qualifier Character 7
0 Bile Ducts 3 Gallbladder and Bile Ducts C Hepatobiliary System, All	0 High Osmolar 1 Low Osmolar Y Other Contrast	Z None	Z None

B Imaging
F Hepatobiliary System and Pancreas
1 Fluoroscopy
Definition: Single plane or bi-plane real time display of an image developed from the capture of external ionizing radiation on a fluorescent screen. The image may also be stored by either digital or analog means.

Body Part – Character 4	Contrast – Character 5	Qualifier – Character 6	Qualifier – Character 7
0 Bile Ducts 1 Biliary and Pancreatic Ducts 2 Gallbladder 3 Gallbladder and Bile Ducts 4 Gallbladder, Bile Ducts and Pancreatic Ducts 8 Pancreatic Ducts	0 High Osmolar 1 Low Osmolar Y Other Contrast	Z None	Z None
5 Liver	0 High Osmolar 1 Low Osmolar Y Other Contrast	Z None	Z None
5 Liver	Z None	Z None	A Guidance

B Imaging
F Hepatobiliary System and Pancreas
2 Computerized Tomography (CT Scan)
Definition: Computer reformatted digital display of multiplanar images developed from the capture of multiple exposures of external ionizing radiation

Body Part – Character 4	Contrast – Character 5	Qualifier – Character 6	Qualifier – Character 7
5 Liver 6 Liver and Spleen 7 Pancreas C Hepatobiliary System, All	0 High Osmolar 1 Low Osmolar Y Other Contrast	0 Unenhanced and Enhanced Z None	Z None
5 Liver 6 Liver and Spleen 7 Pancreas C Hepatobiliary System, All	Z None	Z None	Z None

B Imaging
F Hepatobiliary System and Pancreas
3 Magnetic Resonance Imaging (MRI)
Definition: Computer reformatted digital display of multiplanar images developed from the capture of radio-frequency signals emitted by nuclei in a body site excited within a magnetic field

Body Part – Character 4	Contrast – Character 5	Qualifier – Character 6	Qualifier – Character 7
5 Liver 6 Liver and Spleen 7 Pancreas	Y Other Contrast	0 Unenhanced and Enhanced Z None	Z None
5 Liver 6 Liver and Spleen 7 Pancreas	Z None	Z None	Z None

B Imaging
F Hepatobiliary System and Pancreas
4 Ultrasonography
Definition: Real time display of images of anatomy or flow information developed from the capture of reflected and attenuated high frequency sound waves

Body Part – Character 4	Contrast – Character 5	Qualifier – Character 6	Qualifier – Character 7
0 Bile Ducts 2 Gallbladder 3 Gallbladder and Bile Ducts 5 Liver 6 Liver and Spleen 7 Pancreas C Hepatobiliary System, All	Z None	Z None	Z None

B Imaging
F Hepatobiliary System and Pancreas
5 Other Imaging
Definition: Other specified modality for visualizing a body part

Body Part – Character 4	Contrast – Character 5	Qualifier – Character 6	Qualifier – Character 7
0 Bile Ducts 2 Gallbladder 3 Gallbladder and Bile Ducts 5 Liver 6 Liver and Spleen 7 Pancreas C Hepatobiliary System, All	2 Fluorescing Agent	0 Indocyanine Green Dye Z None	0 Intraoperative Z None

B Imaging
G Endocrine System
2 Computerized Tomography (CT Scan)
Definition: Computer reformatted digital display of multiplanar images developed from the capture of multiple exposures of external ionizing radiation

Body Part Character 4	Contrast Character 5	Qualifier Character 6	Qualifier Character 7
2 Adrenal Glands, Bilateral 3 Parathyroid Glands 4 Thyroid Gland	0 High Osmolar 1 Low Osmolar Y Other Contrast	0 Unenhanced and Enhanced Z None	Z None
2 Adrenal Glands, Bilateral 3 Parathyroid Glands 4 Thyroid Gland	Z None	Z None	Z None

B Imaging
G Endocrine System
3 Magnetic Resonance Imaging (MRI)
Definition: Computer reformatted digital display of multiplanar images developed from the capture of radio-frequency signals emitted by nuclei in a body site excited within a magnetic field

Body Part Character 4	Contrast Character 5	Qualifier Character 6	Qualifier Character 7
2 Adrenal Glands, Bilateral 3 Parathyroid Glands 4 Thyroid Gland	Y Other Contrast	0 Unenhanced and Enhanced Z None	Z None
2 Adrenal Glands, Bilateral 3 Parathyroid Glands 4 Thyroid Gland	Z None	Z None	Z None

B Imaging
G Endocrine System
4 Ultrasonography
Definition: Real time display of images of anatomy or flow information developed from the capture of reflected and attenuated high frequency sound waves

Body Part Character 4	Contrast Character 5	Qualifier Character 6	Qualifier Character 7
0 Adrenal Gland, Right 1 Adrenal Gland, Left 2 Adrenal Glands, Bilateral 3 Parathyroid Glands 4 Thyroid Gland	Z None	Z None	Z None

B Imaging
H Skin, Subcutaneous Tissue and Breast
0 Plain Radiography
Definition: Planar display of an image developed from the capture of external ionizing radiation on photographic or photoconductive plate

Body Part Character 4	Contrast Character 5	Qualifier Character 6	Qualifier Character 7
0 Breast, Right 1 Breast, Left 2 Breasts, Bilateral	Z None	Z None	Z None
3 Single Mammary Duct, Right 4 Single Mammary Duct, Left 5 Multiple Mammary Ducts, Right 6 Multiple Mammary Ducts, Left	0 High Osmolar 1 Low Osmolar Y Other Contrast Z None	Z None	Z None

B Imaging
H Skin, Subcutaneous Tissue and Breast
3 Magnetic Resonance Imaging (MRI)

Definition: Computer reformatted digital display of multiplanar images developed from the capture of radio-frequency signals emitted by nuclei in a body site excited within a magnetic field

Body Part Character 4	Contrast Character 5	Qualifier Character 6	Qualifier Character 7
0 Breast, Right 1 Breast, Left 2 Breasts, Bilateral D Subcutaneous Tissue, Head/Neck F Subcutaneous Tissue, Upper Extremity G Subcutaneous Tissue, Thorax H Subcutaneous Tissue, Abdomen and Pelvis J Subcutaneous Tissue, Lower Extremity	Y Other Contrast	0 Unenhanced and Enhanced Z None	Z None
0 Breast, Right 1 Breast, Left 2 Breasts, Bilateral D Subcutaneous Tissue, Head/Neck F Subcutaneous Tissue, Upper Extremity G Subcutaneous Tissue, Thorax H Subcutaneous Tissue, Abdomen and Pelvis J Subcutaneous Tissue, Lower Extremity	Z None	Z None	Z None

B Imaging
H Skin, Subcutaneous Tissue and Breast
4 Ultrasonography

Definition: Real time display of images of anatomy or flow information developed from the capture of reflected and attenuated high frequency sound waves

Body Part Character 4	Contrast Character 5	Qualifier Character 6	Qualifier Character 7
0 Breast, Right 1 Breast, Left 2 Breasts, Bilateral 7 Extremity, Upper 8 Extremity, Lower 9 Abdominal Wall B Chest Wall C Head and Neck	Z None	Z None	Z None

B Imaging
L Connective Tissue
3 Magnetic Resonance Imaging (MRI)

Definition: Computer reformatted digital display of multiplanar images developed from the capture of radio-frequency signals emitted by nuclei in a body site excited within a magnetic field

Body Part Character 4	Contrast Character 5	Qualifier Character 6	Qualifier Character 7
0 Connective Tissue, Upper Extremity 1 Connective Tissue, Lower Extremity 2 Tendons, Upper Extremity 3 Tendons, Lower Extremity	Y Other Contrast	0 Unenhanced and Enhanced Z None	Z None
0 Connective Tissue, Upper Extremity 1 Connective Tissue, Lower Extremity 2 Tendons, Upper Extremity 3 Tendons, Lower Extremity	Z None	Z None	Z None

B Imaging
L Connective Tissue
4 Ultrasonography

Definition: Real time display of images of anatomy or flow information developed from the capture of reflected and attenuated high frequency sound waves

Body Part Character 4	Contrast Character 5	Qualifier Character 6	Qualifier Character 7
0 Connective Tissue, Upper Extremity 1 Connective Tissue, Lower Extremity 2 Tendons, Upper Extremity 3 Tendons, Lower Extremity	Z None	Z None	Z None

B Imaging
N Skull and Facial Bones
0 Plain Radiography

Definition: Planar display of an image developed from the capture of external ionizing radiation on photographic or photoconductive plate

Body Part Character 4	Contrast Character 5	Qualifier Character 6	Qualifier Character 7
0 Skull 1 Orbit, Right 2 Orbit, Left 3 Orbits, Bilateral 4 Nasal Bones 5 Facial Bones 6 Mandible B Zygomatic Arch, Right C Zygomatic Arch, Left D Zygomatic Arches, Bilateral G Tooth, Single H Teeth, Multiple J Teeth, All	Z None	Z None	Z None
7 Temporomandibular Joint, Right 8 Temporomandibular Joint, Left 9 Temporomandibular Joints, Bilateral	0 High Osmolar 1 Low Osmolar Y Other Contrast Z None	Z None	Z None

B Imaging
N Skull and Facial Bones
1 Fluoroscopy

Definition: Single plane or bi-plane real time display of an image developed from the capture of external ionizing radiation on a fluorescent screen. The image may also be stored by either digital or analog means.

Body Part Character 4	Contrast Character 5	Qualifier Character 6	Qualifier Character 7
7 Temporomandibular Joint, Right 8 Temporomandibular Joint, Left 9 Temporomandibular Joints, Bilateral	0 High Osmolar 1 Low Osmolar Y Other Contrast Z None	Z None	Z None

B Imaging
N Skull and Facial Bones
2 Computerized Tomography (CT Scan)

Definition: Computer reformatted digital display of multiplanar images developed from the capture of multiple exposures of external ionizing radiation

Body Part Character 4	Contrast Character 5	Qualifier Character 6	Qualifier Character 7
0 Skull 3 Orbits, Bilateral 5 Facial Bones 6 Mandible 9 Temporomandibular Joints, Bilateral F Temporal Bones	0 High Osmolar 1 Low Osmolar Y Other Contrast Z None	Z None	Z None

B Imaging
N Skull and Facial Bones
3 Magnetic Resonance Imaging (MRI)

Definition: Computer reformatted digital display of multiplanar images developed from the capture of radio-frequency signals emitted by nuclei in a body site excited within a magnetic field

Body Part Character 4	Contrast Character 5	Qualifier Character 6	Qualifier Character 7
9 Temporomandibular Joints, Bilateral	Y Other Contrast Z None	Z None	Z None

B Imaging
P Non-Axial Upper Bones
0 Plain Radiography
Definition: Planar display of an image developed from the capture of external ionizing radiation on photographic or photoconductive plate

Body Part — Character 4	Contrast — Character 5	Qualifier — Character 6	Qualifier — Character 7
0 Sternoclavicular Joint, Right 1 Sternoclavicular Joint, Left 2 Sternoclavicular Joints, Bilateral 3 Acromioclavicular Joints, Bilateral 4 Clavicle, Right 5 Clavicle, Left 6 Scapula, Right 7 Scapula, Left A Humerus, Right B Humerus, Left E Upper Arm, Right F Upper Arm, Left J Forearm, Right K Forearm, Left N Hand, Right P Hand, Left R Finger(s), Right S Finger(s), Left X Ribs, Right Y Ribs, Left	Z None	Z None	Z None
8 Shoulder, Right 9 Shoulder, Left C Hand/Finger Joint, Right D Hand/Finger Joint, Left G Elbow, Right H Elbow, Left L Wrist, Right M Wrist, Left	0 High Osmolar 1 Low Osmolar Y Other Contrast Z None	Z None	Z None

B Imaging
P Non-Axial Upper Bones
1 Fluoroscopy
Definition: Single plane or bi-plane real time display of an image developed from the capture of external ionizing radiation on a fluorescent screen. The image may also be stored by either digital or analog means.

Body Part — Character 4	Contrast — Character 5	Qualifier — Character 6	Qualifier — Character 7
0 Sternoclavicular Joint, Right 1 Sternoclavicular Joint, Left 2 Sternoclavicular Joints, Bilateral 3 Acromioclavicular Joints, Bilateral 4 Clavicle, Right 5 Clavicle, Left 6 Scapula, Right 7 Scapula, Left A Humerus, Right B Humerus, Left E Upper Arm, Right F Upper Arm, Left J Forearm, Right K Forearm, Left N Hand, Right P Hand, Left R Finger(s), Right S Finger(s), Left X Ribs, Right Y Ribs, Left	Z None	Z None	Z None
8 Shoulder, Right 9 Shoulder, Left L Wrist, Right M Wrist, Left	0 High Osmolar 1 Low Osmolar Y Other Contrast Z None	Z None	Z None
C Hand/Finger Joint, Right D Hand/Finger Joint, Left G Elbow, Right H Elbow, Left	0 High Osmolar 1 Low Osmolar Y Other Contrast	Z None	Z None

Non-OR Procedure | DRG Non-OR Procedure | Valid OR Procedure | HAC Associated Procedure | Combination Only | New/Revised April | New/Revised October

B   Imaging
P   Non-Axial Upper Bones
2   Computerized Tomography (CT Scan) Definition: Computer reformatted digital display of multiplanar images developed from the capture of multiple exposures of external ionizing radiation

Body Part Character 4	Contrast Character 5	Qualifier Character 6	Qualifier Character 7
0 Sternoclavicular Joint, Right 1 Sternoclavicular Joint, Left W Thorax	0 High Osmolar 1 Low Osmolar Y Other Contrast	Z None	Z None
2 Sternoclavicular Joints, Bilateral 3 Acromioclavicular Joints, Bilateral 4 Clavicle, Right 5 Clavicle, Left 6 Scapula, Right 7 Scapula, Left 8 Shoulder, Right 9 Shoulder, Left A Humerus, Right B Humerus, Left E Upper Arm, Right F Upper Arm, Left G Elbow, Right H Elbow, Left J Forearm, Right K Forearm, Left L Wrist, Right M Wrist, Left N Hand, Right P Hand, Left Q Hands and Wrists, Bilateral R Finger(s), Right S Finger(s), Left T Upper Extremity, Right U Upper Extremity, Left V Upper Extremities, Bilateral X Ribs, Right Y Ribs, Left	0 High Osmolar 1 Low Osmolar Y Other Contrast Z None	Z None	Z None
C Hand/Finger Joint, Right D Hand/Finger Joint, Left	Z None	Z None	Z None

B   Imaging
P   Non-Axial Upper Bones
3   Magnetic Resonance Imaging (MRI) Definition: Computer reformatted digital display of multiplanar images developed from the capture of radio-frequency signals emitted by nuclei in a body site excited within a magnetic field

Body Part Character 4	Contrast Character 5	Qualifier Character 6	Qualifier Character 7
8 Shoulder, Right 9 Shoulder, Left C Hand/Finger Joint, Right D Hand/Finger Joint, Left E Upper Arm, Right F Upper Arm, Left G Elbow, Right H Elbow, Left J Forearm, Right K Forearm, Left L Wrist, Right M Wrist, Left	Y Other Contrast	0 Unenhanced and Enhanced Z None	Z None
8 Shoulder, Right 9 Shoulder, Left C Hand/Finger Joint, Right D Hand/Finger Joint, Left E Upper Arm, Right F Upper Arm, Left G Elbow, Right H Elbow, Left J Forearm, Right K Forearm, Left L Wrist, Right M Wrist, Left	Z None	Z None	Z None

B Imaging
P Non-Axial Upper Bones
4 Ultrasonography
Definition: Real time display of images of anatomy or flow information developed from the capture of reflected and attenuated high frequency sound waves

Body Part Character 4	Contrast Character 5	Qualifier Character 6	Qualifier Character 7
8 Shoulder, Right 9 Shoulder, Left G Elbow, Right H Elbow, Left L Wrist, Right M Wrist, Left N Hand, Right P Hand, Left	Z None	Z None	1 Densitometry Z None

B Imaging
Q Non-Axial Lower Bones
0 Plain Radiography
Definition: Planar display of an image developed from the capture of external ionizing radiation on photographic or photoconductive plate

Body Part Character 4	Contrast Character 5	Qualifier Character 6	Qualifier Character 7
0 Hip, Right 1 Hip, Left	0 High Osmolar 1 Low Osmolar Y Other Contrast	Z None	Z None
0 Hip, Right 1 Hip, Left	Z None	Z None	1 Densitometry Z None
3 Femur, Right 4 Femur, Left	Z None	Z None	1 Densitometry Z None
7 Knee, Right 8 Knee, Left G Ankle, Right H Ankle, Left	0 High Osmolar 1 Low Osmolar Y Other Contrast Z None	Z None	Z None
D Lower Leg, Right F Lower Leg, Left J Calcaneus, Right K Calcaneus, Left L Foot, Right M Foot, Left P Toe(s), Right Q Toe(s), Left V Patella, Right W Patella, Left	Z None	Z None	Z None
X Foot/Toe Joint, Right Y Foot/Toe Joint, Left	0 High Osmolar 1 Low Osmolar Y Other Contrast	Z None	Z None

B Imaging
Q Non-Axial Lower Bones
1 Fluoroscopy
Definition: Single plane or bi-plane real time display of an image developed from the capture of external ionizing radiation on a fluorescent screen. The image may also be stored by either digital or analog means.

Body Part Character 4	Contrast Character 5	Qualifier Character 6	Qualifier Character 7
0 Hip, Right 1 Hip, Left 7 Knee, Right 8 Knee, Left G Ankle, Right H Ankle, Left X Foot/Toe Joint, Right Y Foot/Toe Joint, Left	0 High Osmolar 1 Low Osmolar Y Other Contrast Z None	Z None	Z None
3 Femur, Right 4 Femur, Left D Lower Leg, Right F Lower Leg, Left J Calcaneus, Right K Calcaneus, Left L Foot, Right M Foot, Left P Toe(s), Right Q Toe(s), Left V Patella, Right W Patella, Left	Z None	Z None	Z None

ICD-10-PCS 2025 — Imaging — BQ2–BQ3

B Imaging
Q Non-Axial Lower Bones
2 Computerized Tomography (CT Scan) Definition: Computer reformatted digital display of multiplanar images developed from the capture of multiple exposures of external ionizing radiation

Body Part Character 4	Contrast Character 5	Qualifier Character 6	Qualifier Character 7
0 Hip, Right 1 Hip, Left 3 Femur, Right 4 Femur, Left 7 Knee, Right 8 Knee, Left D Lower Leg, Right F Lower Leg, Left G Ankle, Right H Ankle, Left J Calcaneus, Right K Calcaneus, Left L Foot, Right M Foot, Left P Toe(s), Right Q Toe(s), Left R Lower Extremity, Right S Lower Extremity, Left V Patella, Right W Patella, Left X Foot/Toe Joint, Right Y Foot/Toe Joint, Left	0 High Osmolar 1 Low Osmolar Y Other Contrast Z None	Z None	Z None
B Tibia/Fibula, Right C Tibia/Fibula, Left	0 High Osmolar 1 Low Osmolar Y Other Contrast	Z None	Z None

B Imaging
Q Non-Axial Lower Bones
3 Magnetic Resonance Imaging (MRI) Definition: Computer reformatted digital display of multiplanar images developed from the capture of radio-frequency signals emitted by nuclei in a body site excited within a magnetic field

Body Part Character 4	Contrast Character 5	Qualifier Character 6	Qualifier Character 7
0 Hip, Right 1 Hip, Left 3 Femur, Right 4 Femur, Left 7 Knee, Right 8 Knee, Left D Lower Leg, Right F Lower Leg, Left G Ankle, Right H Ankle, Left J Calcaneus, Right K Calcaneus, Left L Foot, Right M Foot, Left P Toe(s), Right Q Toe(s), Left V Patella, Right W Patella, Left	Y Other Contrast	0 Unenhanced and Enhanced Z None	Z None
0 Hip, Right 1 Hip, Left 3 Femur, Right 4 Femur, Left 7 Knee, Right 8 Knee, Left D Lower Leg, Right F Lower Leg, Left G Ankle, Right H Ankle, Left J Calcaneus, Right K Calcaneus, Left L Foot, Right M Foot, Left P Toe(s), Right Q Toe(s), Left V Patella, Right W Patella, Left	Z None	Z None	Z None

NC Noncovered Procedure   LC Limited Coverage   QA Questionable OB Admit   NT New Tech Add-on   ➕ Combination Member   ♂ Male   ♀ Female

B Imaging
Q Non-Axial Lower Bones
4 Ultrasonography   Definition: Real time display of images of anatomy or flow information developed from the capture of reflected and attenuated high frequency sound waves

Body Part Character 4	Contrast Character 5	Qualifier Character 6	Qualifier Character 7
0 Hip, Right 1 Hip, Left 2 Hips, Bilateral 7 Knee, Right 8 Knee, Left 9 Knees, Bilateral	Z None	Z None	Z None

B Imaging
R Axial Skeleton, Except Skull and Facial Bones
0 Plain Radiography   Definition: Planar display of an image developed from the capture of external ionizing radiation on photographic or photoconductive plate

Body Part Character 4	Contrast Character 5	Qualifier Character 6	Qualifier Character 7
0 Cervical Spine 7 Thoracic Spine 9 Lumbar Spine G Whole Spine	Z None	Z None	1 Densitometry Z None
1 Cervical Disc(s) 2 Thoracic Disc(s) 3 Lumbar Disc(s) 4 Cervical Facet Joint(s) 5 Thoracic Facet Joint(s) 6 Lumbar Facet Joint(s) D Sacroiliac Joints	0 High Osmolar 1 Low Osmolar Y Other Contrast Z None	Z None	Z None
8 Thoracolumbar Joint B Lumbosacral Joint C Pelvis F Sacrum and Coccyx H Sternum	Z None	Z None	Z None

B Imaging
R Axial Skeleton, Except Skull and Facial Bones
1 Fluoroscopy   Definition: Single plane or bi-plane real time display of an image developed from the capture of external ionizing radiation on a fluorescent screen. The image may also be stored by either digital or analog means.

Body Part Character 4	Contrast Character 5	Qualifier Character 6	Qualifier Character 7
0 Cervical Spine 1 Cervical Disc(s) 2 Thoracic Disc(s) 3 Lumbar Disc(s) 4 Cervical Facet Joint(s) 5 Thoracic Facet Joint(s) 6 Lumbar Facet Joint(s) 7 Thoracic Spine 8 Thoracolumbar Joint 9 Lumbar Spine B Lumbosacral Joint C Pelvis D Sacroiliac Joints F Sacrum and Coccyx G Whole Spine H Sternum	0 High Osmolar 1 Low Osmolar Y Other Contrast Z None	Z None	Z None

B Imaging
R Axial Skeleton, Except Skull and Facial Bones
2 Computerized Tomography (CT Scan)   Definition: Computer reformatted digital display of multiplanar images developed from the capture of multiple exposures of external ionizing radiation

Body Part Character 4	Contrast Character 5	Qualifier Character 6	Qualifier Character 7
0 Cervical Spine 7 Thoracic Spine 9 Lumbar Spine C Pelvis D Sacroiliac Joints F Sacrum and Coccyx	0 High Osmolar 1 Low Osmolar Y Other Contrast Z None	Z None	Z None

Imaging

B Imaging
R Axial Skeleton, Except Skull and Facial Bones
3 Magnetic Resonance Imaging (MRI)   Definition: Computer reformatted digital display of multiplanar images developed from the capture of radio-frequency signals emitted by nuclei in a body site excited within a magnetic field

Body Part Character 4	Contrast Character 5	Qualifier Character 6	Qualifier Character 7
0 Cervical Spine 1 Cervical Disc(s) 2 Thoracic Disc(s) 3 Lumbar Disc(s) 7 Thoracic Spine 9 Lumbar Spine C Pelvis F Sacrum and Coccyx	Y Other Contrast	0 Unenhanced and Enhanced Z None	Z None
0 Cervical Spine 1 Cervical Disc(s) 2 Thoracic Disc(s) 3 Lumbar Disc(s) 7 Thoracic Spine 9 Lumbar Spine C Pelvis F Sacrum and Coccyx	Z None	Z None	Z None

B Imaging
R Axial Skeleton, Except Skull and Facial Bones
4 Ultrasonography   Definition: Real time display of images of anatomy or flow information developed from the capture of reflected and attenuated high frequency sound waves

Body Part Character 4	Contrast Character 5	Qualifier Character 6	Qualifier Character 7
0 Cervical Spine 7 Thoracic Spine 9 Lumbar Spine F Sacrum and Coccyx	Z None	Z None	Z None

B Imaging
T Urinary System
0 Plain Radiography   Definition: Planar display of an image developed from the capture of external ionizing radiation on photographic or photoconductive plate

Body Part Character 4	Contrast Character 5	Qualifier Character 6	Qualifier Character 7
0 Bladder 1 Kidney, Right 2 Kidney, Left 3 Kidneys, Bilateral 4 Kidneys, Ureters and Bladder 5 Urethra 6 Ureter, Right 7 Ureter, Left 8 Ureters, Bilateral B Bladder and Urethra C Ileal Diversion Loop	0 High Osmolar 1 Low Osmolar Y Other Contrast Z None	Z None	Z None

B Imaging
T Urinary System
1 Fluoroscopy   Definition: Single plane or bi-plane real time display of an image developed from the capture of external ionizing radiation on a fluorescent screen. The image may also be stored by either digital or analog means.

Body Part Character 4	Contrast Character 5	Qualifier Character 6	Qualifier Character 7
0 Bladder 1 Kidney, Right 2 Kidney, Left 3 Kidneys, Bilateral 4 Kidneys, Ureters and Bladder 5 Urethra 6 Ureter, Right 7 Ureter, Left B Bladder and Urethra C Ileal Diversion Loop D Kidney, Ureter and Bladder, Right F Kidney, Ureter and Bladder, Left G Ileal Loop, Ureters and Kidneys	0 High Osmolar 1 Low Osmolar Y Other Contrast Z None	Z None	Z None

B Imaging
T Urinary System
2 Computerized Tomography (CT Scan)
Definition: Computer reformatted digital display of multiplanar images developed from the capture of multiple exposures of external ionizing radiation

Body Part Character 4	Contrast Character 5	Qualifier Character 6	Qualifier Character 7
0 Bladder 1 Kidney, Right 2 Kidney, Left 3 Kidneys, Bilateral 9 Kidney Transplant	0 High Osmolar 1 Low Osmolar Y Other Contrast	0 Unenhanced and Enhanced Z None	Z None
0 Bladder 1 Kidney, Right 2 Kidney, Left 3 Kidneys, Bilateral 9 Kidney Transplant	Z None	Z None	Z None

B Imaging
T Urinary System
3 Magnetic Resonance Imaging (MRI)
Definition: Computer reformatted digital display of multiplanar images developed from the capture of radio-frequency signals emitted by nuclei in a body site excited within a magnetic field

Body Part Character 4	Contrast Character 5	Qualifier Character 6	Qualifier Character 7
0 Bladder 1 Kidney, Right 2 Kidney, Left 3 Kidneys, Bilateral 9 Kidney Transplant	Y Other Contrast	0 Unenhanced and Enhanced Z None	Z None
0 Bladder 1 Kidney, Right 2 Kidney, Left 3 Kidneys, Bilateral 9 Kidney Transplant	Z None	Z None	Z None

B Imaging
T Urinary System
4 Ultrasonography
Definition: Real time display of images of anatomy or flow information developed from the capture of reflected and attenuated high frequency sound waves

Body Part Character 4	Contrast Character 5	Qualifier Character 6	Qualifier Character 7
0 Bladder 1 Kidney, Right 2 Kidney, Left 3 Kidneys, Bilateral 5 Urethra 6 Ureter, Right 7 Ureter, Left 8 Ureters, Bilateral 9 Kidney Transplant J Kidneys and Bladder	Z None	Z None	Z None

B Imaging
U Female Reproductive System
0 Plain Radiography
Definition: Planar display of an image developed from the capture of external ionizing radiation on photographic or photoconductive plate

Body Part Character 4	Contrast Character 5	Qualifier Character 6	Qualifier Character 7
0 Fallopian Tube, Right 1 Fallopian Tube, Left 2 Fallopian Tubes, Bilateral 6 Uterus 8 Uterus and Fallopian Tubes 9 Vagina	0 High Osmolar 1 Low Osmolar Y Other Contrast	Z None	Z None

B Imaging
U Female Reproductive System
1 Fluoroscopy
Definition: Single plane or bi-plane real time display of an image developed from the capture of external ionizing radiation on a fluorescent screen. The image may also be stored by either digital or analog means.

Body Part Character 4	Contrast Character 5	Qualifier Character 6	Qualifier Character 7
0 Fallopian Tube, Right 1 Fallopian Tube, Left 2 Fallopian Tubes, Bilateral 6 Uterus 8 Uterus and Fallopian Tubes 9 Vagina	0 High Osmolar 1 Low Osmolar Y Other Contrast Z None	Z None	Z None

B Imaging
U Female Reproductive System
3 Magnetic Resonance Imaging (MRI)
Definition: Computer reformatted digital display of multiplanar images developed from the capture of radio-frequency signals emitted by nuclei in a body site excited within a magnetic field

Body Part Character 4	Contrast Character 5	Qualifier Character 6	Qualifier Character 7
3 Ovary, Right 4 Ovary, Left 5 Ovaries, Bilateral 6 Uterus 9 Vagina B Pregnant Uterus C Uterus and Ovaries	Y Other Contrast	0 Unenhanced and Enhanced Z None	Z None
3 Ovary, Right 4 Ovary, Left 5 Ovaries, Bilateral 6 Uterus 9 Vagina B Pregnant Uterus C Uterus and Ovaries	Z None	Z None	Z None

B Imaging
U Female Reproductive System
4 Ultrasonography
Definition: Real time display of images of anatomy or flow information developed from the capture of reflected and attenuated high frequency sound waves

Body Part Character 4	Contrast Character 5	Qualifier Character 6	Qualifier Character 7
0 Fallopian Tube, Right 1 Fallopian Tube, Left 2 Fallopian Tubes, Bilateral 3 Ovary, Right 4 Ovary, Left 5 Ovaries, Bilateral 6 Uterus C Uterus and Ovaries	Y Other Contrast Z None	Z None	Z None

B Imaging
V Male Reproductive System
0 Plain Radiography
Definition: Planar display of an image developed from the capture of external ionizing radiation on photographic or photoconductive plate

Body Part Character 4	Contrast Character 5	Qualifier Character 6	Qualifier Character 7
0 Corpora Cavernosa 1 Epididymis, Right 2 Epididymis, Left 3 Prostate 5 Testicle, Right 6 Testicle, Left 8 Vasa Vasorum	0 High Osmolar 1 Low Osmolar Y Other Contrast	Z None	Z None

B Imaging
V Male Reproductive System
1 Fluoroscopy
Definition: Single plane or bi-plane real time display of an image developed from the capture of external ionizing radiation on a fluorescent screen. The image may also be stored by either digital or analog means.

Body Part Character 4	Contrast Character 5	Qualifier Character 6	Qualifier Character 7
0 Corpora Cavernosa 8 Vasa Vasorum	0 High Osmolar 1 Low Osmolar Y Other Contrast Z None	Z None	Z None

B Imaging
V Male Reproductive System
2 Computerized Tomography (CT Scan)

Definition: Computer reformatted digital display of multiplanar images developed from the capture of multiple exposures of external ionizing radiation

Body Part Character 4	Contrast Character 5	Qualifier Character 6	Qualifier Character 7
3 Prostate	0 High Osmolar 1 Low Osmolar Y Other Contrast	0 Unenhanced and Enhanced Z None	Z None
3 Prostate	Z None	Z None	Z None

B Imaging
V Male Reproductive System
3 Magnetic Resonance Imaging (MRI)

Definition: Computer reformatted digital display of multiplanar images developed from the capture of radio-frequency signals emitted by nuclei in a body site excited within a magnetic field

Body Part Character 4	Contrast Character 5	Qualifier Character 6	Qualifier Character 7
0 Corpora Cavernosa 3 Prostate 4 Scrotum 5 Testicle, Right 6 Testicle, Left 7 Testicles, Bilateral	Y Other Contrast	0 Unenhanced and Enhanced Z None	Z None
0 Corpora Cavernosa 3 Prostate 4 Scrotum 5 Testicle, Right 6 Testicle, Left 7 Testicles, Bilateral	Z None	Z None	Z None

B Imaging
V Male Reproductive System
4 Ultrasonography

Definition: Real time display of images of anatomy or flow information developed from the capture of reflected and attenuated high frequency sound waves

Body Part Character 4	Contrast Character 5	Qualifier Character 6	Qualifier Character 7
4 Scrotum 9 Prostate and Seminal Vesicles B Penis	Z None	Z None	Z None

B Imaging
W Anatomical Regions
0 Plain Radiography

Definition: Planar display of an image developed from the capture of external ionizing radiation on photographic or photoconductive plate

Body Part Character 4	Contrast Character 5	Qualifier Character 6	Qualifier Character 7
0 Abdomen 1 Abdomen and Pelvis 3 Chest B Long Bones, All C Lower Extremity J Upper Extremity K Whole Body L Whole Skeleton M Whole Body, Infant	Z None	Z None	Z None

B Imaging
W Anatomical Regions
1 Fluoroscopy

Definition: Single plane or bi-plane real time display of an image developed from the capture of external ionizing radiation on a fluorescent screen. The image may also be stored by either digital or analog means.

Body Part Character 4	Contrast Character 5	Qualifier Character 6	Qualifier Character 7
1 Abdomen and Pelvis 9 Head and Neck C Lower Extremity J Upper Extremity	0 High Osmolar 1 Low Osmolar Y Other Contrast Z None	Z None	Z None

Imaging

B Imaging
W Anatomical Regions
2 Computerized Tomography (CT Scan) Definition: Computer reformatted digital display of multiplanar images developed from the capture of multiple exposures of external ionizing radiation

Body Part Character 4	Contrast Character 5	Qualifier Character 6	Qualifier Character 7
0 Abdomen 1 Abdomen and Pelvis 4 Chest and Abdomen 5 Chest, Abdomen and Pelvis 8 Head 9 Head and Neck F Neck G Pelvic Region	0 High Osmolar 1 Low Osmolar Y Other Contrast	0 Unenhanced and Enhanced Z None	Z None
0 Abdomen 1 Abdomen and Pelvis 4 Chest and Abdomen 5 Chest, Abdomen and Pelvis 8 Head 9 Head and Neck F Neck G Pelvic Region	Z None	Z None	Z None

B Imaging
W Anatomical Regions
3 Magnetic Resonance Imaging (MRI) Definition: Computer reformatted digital display of multiplanar images developed from the capture of radio-frequency signals emitted by nuclei in a body site excited within a magnetic field

Body Part Character 4	Contrast Character 5	Qualifier Character 6	Qualifier Character 7
0 Abdomen 8 Head F Neck G Pelvic Region H Retroperitoneum P Brachial Plexus	Y Other Contrast	0 Unenhanced and Enhanced Z None	Z None
0 Abdomen 8 Head F Neck G Pelvic Region H Retroperitoneum P Brachial Plexus	Z None	Z None	Z None
3 Chest	Y Other Contrast	0 Unenhanced and Enhanced Z None	Z None

B Imaging
W Anatomical Regions
4 Ultrasonography Definition: Real time display of images of anatomy or flow information developed from the capture of reflected and attenuated high frequency sound waves

Body Part Character 4	Contrast Character 5	Qualifier Character 6	Qualifier Character 7
0 Abdomen 1 Abdomen and Pelvis F Neck G Pelvic Region	Z None	Z None	Z None

B Imaging
W Anatomical Regions
5 Other Imaging Definition: Other specified modality for visualizing a body part

Body Part Character 4	Contrast Character 5	Qualifier Character 6	Qualifier Character 7
2 Trunk 9 Head and Neck C Lower Extremity J Upper Extremity	Z None	1 Bacterial Autofluorescence	Z None

B Imaging
Y Fetus and Obstetrical
3 Magnetic Resonance Imaging (MRI)

Definition: Computer reformatted digital display of multiplanar images developed from the capture of radio-frequency signals emitted by nuclei in a body site excited within a magnetic field

Body Part Character 4	Contrast Character 5	Qualifier Character 6	Qualifier Character 7
0 Fetal Head 1 Fetal Heart 2 Fetal Thorax 3 Fetal Abdomen 4 Fetal Spine 5 Fetal Extremities 6 Whole Fetus	Y Other Contrast	0 Unenhanced and Enhanced Z None	Z None
0 Fetal Head 1 Fetal Heart 2 Fetal Thorax 3 Fetal Abdomen 4 Fetal Spine 5 Fetal Extremities 6 Whole Fetus	Z None	Z None	Z None

B Imaging
Y Fetus and Obstetrical
4 Ultrasonography

Definition: Real time display of images of anatomy or flow information developed from the capture of reflected and attenuated high frequency sound waves

Body Part Character 4	Contrast Character 5	Qualifier Character 6	Qualifier Character 7
7 Fetal Umbilical Cord 8 Placenta 9 First Trimester, Single Fetus B First Trimester, Multiple Gestation C Second Trimester, Single Fetus D Second Trimester, Multiple Gestation F Third Trimester, Single Fetus G Third Trimester, Multiple Gestation	Z None	Z None	Z None

Nuclear Medicine C01–CW7

- **C** Nuclear Medicine
- **0** Central Nervous System
- **1** Planar Nuclear Medicine Imaging   Definition: Introduction of radioactive materials into the body for single plane display of images developed from the capture of radioactive emissions

Body Part Character 4	Radionuclide Character 5	Qualifier Character 6	Qualifier Character 7
0 Brain	1 Technetium 99m (Tc-99m) Y Other Radionuclide	Z None	Z None
5 Cerebrospinal Fluid	D Indium 111 (In-111) Y Other Radionuclide	Z None	Z None
Y Central Nervous System	Y Other Radionuclide	Z None	Z None

- **C** Nuclear Medicine
- **0** Central Nervous System
- **2** Tomographic (Tomo) Nuclear Medicine Imaging   Definition: Introduction of radioactive materials into the body for three dimensional display of images developed from the capture of radioactive emissions

Body Part Character 4	Radionuclide Character 5	Qualifier Character 6	Qualifier Character 7
0 Brain	1 Technetium 99m (Tc-99m) F Iodine 123 (I-123) S Thallium 201 (Tl-201) Y Other Radionuclide	Z None	Z None
5 Cerebrospinal Fluid	D Indium 111 (In-111) Y Other Radionuclide	Z None	Z None
Y Central Nervous System	Y Other Radionuclide	Z None	Z None

- **C** Nuclear Medicine
- **0** Central Nervous System
- **3** Positron Emission Tomographic (PET) Imaging   Definition: Introduction of radioactive materials into the body for three dimensional display of images developed from the simultaneous capture, 180 degrees apart, of radioactive emissions

Body Part Character 4	Radionuclide Character 5	Qualifier Character 6	Qualifier Character 7
0 Brain	B Carbon 11 (C-11) K Fluorine 18 (F-18) M Oxygen 15 (O-15) Y Other Radionuclide	Z None	Z None
Y Central Nervous System	Y Other Radionuclide	Z None	Z None

- **C** Nuclear Medicine
- **0** Central Nervous System
- **5** Nonimaging Nuclear Medicine Probe   Definition: Introduction of radioactive materials into the body for the study of distribution and fate of certain substances by the detection of radioactive emissions; or, alternatively, measurement of absorption of radioactive emissions from an external source

Body Part Character 4	Radionuclide Character 5	Qualifier Character 6	Qualifier Character 7
0 Brain	V Xenon 133 (Xe-133) Y Other Radionuclide	Z None	Z None
Y Central Nervous System	Y Other Radionuclide	Z None	Z None

- **C** Nuclear Medicine
- **2** Heart
- **1** Planar Nuclear Medicine Imaging   Definition: Introduction of radioactive materials into the body for single plane display of images developed from the capture of radioactive emissions

Body Part Character 4	Radionuclide Character 5	Qualifier Character 6	Qualifier Character 7
6 Heart, Right and Left	1 Technetium 99m (Tc-99m) Y Other Radionuclide	Z None	Z None
G Myocardium	1 Technetium 99m (Tc-99m) D Indium 111 (In-111) S Thallium 201 (Tl-201) Y Other Radionuclide Z None	Z None	Z None
Y Heart	Y Other Radionuclide	Z None	Z None

C Nuclear Medicine
2 Heart
2 Tomographic (Tomo) Nuclear Medicine Imaging Definition: Introduction of radioactive materials into the body for three dimensional display of images developed from the capture of radioactive emissions

Body Part Character 4	Radionuclide Character 5	Qualifier Character 6	Qualifier Character 7
6 Heart, Right and Left	**1** Technetium 99m (Tc-99m) **Y** Other Radionuclide	**Z** None	**Z** None
G Myocardium	**1** Technetium 99m (Tc-99m) **D** Indium 111 (In-111) **K** Fluorine 18 (F-18) **S** Thallium 201 (Tl-201) **Y** Other Radionuclide **Z** None	**Z** None	**Z** None
Y Heart	**Y** Other Radionuclide	**Z** None	**Z** None

C Nuclear Medicine
2 Heart
3 Positron Emission Tomographic (PET) Imaging Definition: Introduction of radioactive materials into the body for three dimensional display of images developed from the simultaneous capture, 180 degrees apart, of radioactive emissions

Body Part Character 4	Radionuclide Character 5	Qualifier Character 6	Qualifier Character 7
G Myocardium	**K** Fluorine 18 (F-18) **M** Oxygen 15 (O-15) **Q** Rubidium 82 (Rb-82) **R** Nitrogen 13 (N-13) **Y** Other Radionuclide	**Z** None	**Z** None
Y Heart	**Y** Other Radionuclide	**Z** None	**Z** None

C Nuclear Medicine
2 Heart
5 Nonimaging Nuclear Medicine Probe Definition: Introduction of radioactive materials into the body for the study of distribution and fate of certain substances by the detection of radioactive emissions; or, alternatively, measurement of absorption of radioactive emissions from an external source

Body Part Character 4	Radionuclide Character 5	Qualifier Character 6	Qualifier Character 7
6 Heart, Right and Left	**1** Technetium 99m (Tc-99m) **Y** Other Radionuclide	**Z** None	**Z** None
Y Heart	**Y** Other Radionuclide	**Z** None	**Z** None

C Nuclear Medicine
5 Veins
1 Planar Nuclear Medicine Imaging Definition: Introduction of radioactive materials into the body for single plane display of images developed from the capture of radioactive emissions

Body Part Character 4	Radionuclide Character 5	Qualifier Character 6	Qualifier Character 7
B Lower Extremity Veins, Right **C** Lower Extremity Veins, Left **D** Lower Extremity Veins, Bilateral **N** Upper Extremity Veins, Right **P** Upper Extremity Veins, Left **Q** Upper Extremity Veins, Bilateral **R** Central Veins	**1** Technetium 99m (Tc-99m) **Y** Other Radionuclide	**Z** None	**Z** None
Y Veins	**Y** Other Radionuclide	**Z** None	**Z** None

C Nuclear Medicine
7 Lymphatic and Hematologic System
1 Planar Nuclear Medicine Imaging Definition: Introduction of radioactive materials into the body for single plane display of images developed from the capture of radioactive emissions

Body Part Character 4	Radionuclide Character 5	Qualifier Character 6	Qualifier Character 7
0 Bone Marrow	1 Technetium 99m (Tc-99m) D Indium 111 (In-111) Y Other Radionuclide	Z None	Z None
2 Spleen 5 Lymphatics, Head and Neck D Lymphatics, Pelvic J Lymphatics, Head K Lymphatics, Neck L Lymphatics, Upper Chest M Lymphatics, Trunk N Lymphatics, Upper Extremity P Lymphatics, Lower Extremity	1 Technetium 99m (Tc-99m) Y Other Radionuclide	Z None	Z None
3 Blood	D Indium 111 (In-111) Y Other Radionuclide	Z None	Z None
Y Lymphatic and Hematologic System	Y Other Radionuclide	Z None	Z None

C Nuclear Medicine
7 Lymphatic and Hematologic System
2 Tomographic (Tomo) Nuclear Medicine Imaging Definition: Introduction of radioactive materials into the body for three dimensional display of images developed from the capture of radioactive emissions

Body Part Character 4	Radionuclide Character 5	Qualifier Character 6	Qualifier Character 7
2 Spleen	1 Technetium 99m (Tc-99m) Y Other Radionuclide	Z None	Z None
Y Lymphatic and Hematologic System	Y Other Radionuclide	Z None	Z None

C Nuclear Medicine
7 Lymphatic and Hematologic System
5 Nonimaging Nuclear Medicine Probe Definition: Introduction of radioactive materials into the body for the study of distribution and fate of certain substances by the detection of radioactive emissions; or, alternatively, measurement of absorption of radioactive emissions from an external source

Body Part Character 4	Radionuclide Character 5	Qualifier Character 6	Qualifier Character 7
5 Lymphatics, Head and Neck D Lymphatics, Pelvic J Lymphatics, Head K Lymphatics, Neck L Lymphatics, Upper Chest M Lymphatics, Trunk N Lymphatics, Upper Extremity P Lymphatics, Lower Extremity	1 Technetium 99m (Tc-99m) Y Other Radionuclide	Z None	Z None
Y Lymphatic and Hematologic System	Y Other Radionuclide	Z None	Z None

C Nuclear Medicine
7 Lymphatic and Hematologic System
6 Nonimaging Nuclear Medicine Assay Definition: Introduction of radioactive materials into the body for the study of body fluids and blood elements, by the detection of radioactive emissions

Body Part Character 4	Radionuclide Character 5	Qualifier Character 6	Qualifier Character 7
3 Blood	1 Technetium 99m (Tc-99m) 7 Cobalt 58 (Co-58) C Cobalt 57 (Co-57) D Indium 111 (In-111) H Iodine 125 (I-125) W Chromium (Cr-51) Y Other Radionuclide	Z None	Z None
Y Lymphatic and Hematologic System	Y Other Radionuclide	Z None	Z None

Nuclear Medicine

C Nuclear Medicine
8 Eye
1 Planar Nuclear Medicine Imaging — Definition: Introduction of radioactive materials into the body for single plane display of images developed from the capture of radioactive emissions

Body Part Character 4	Radionuclide Character 5	Qualifier Character 6	Qualifier Character 7
9 Lacrimal Ducts, Bilateral	1 Technetium 99m (Tc-99m) Y Other Radionuclide	Z None	Z None
Y Eye	Y Other Radionuclide	Z None	Z None

C Nuclear Medicine
9 Ear, Nose, Mouth and Throat
1 Planar Nuclear Medicine Imaging — Definition: Introduction of radioactive materials into the body for single plane display of images developed from the capture of radioactive emissions

Body Part Character 4	Radionuclide Character 5	Qualifier Character 6	Qualifier Character 7
B Salivary Glands, Bilateral	1 Technetium 99m (Tc-99m) Y Other Radionuclide	Z None	Z None
Y Ear, Nose, Mouth and Throat	Y Other Radionuclide	Z None	Z None

C Nuclear Medicine
B Respiratory System
1 Planar Nuclear Medicine Imaging — Definition: Introduction of radioactive materials into the body for single plane display of images developed from the capture of radioactive emissions

Body Part Character 4	Radionuclide Character 5	Qualifier Character 6	Qualifier Character 7
2 Lungs and Bronchi	1 Technetium 99m (Tc-99m) 9 Krypton (Kr-81m) T Xenon 127 (Xe-127) V Xenon 133 (Xe-133) Y Other Radionuclide	Z None	Z None
Y Respiratory System	Y Other Radionuclide	Z None	Z None

C Nuclear Medicine
B Respiratory System
2 Tomographic (Tomo) Nuclear Medicine Imaging — Definition: Introduction of radioactive materials into the body for three dimensional display of images developed from the capture of radioactive emissions

Body Part Character 4	Radionuclide Character 5	Qualifier Character 6	Qualifier Character 7
2 Lungs and Bronchi	1 Technetium 99m (Tc-99m) 9 Krypton (Kr-81m) Y Other Radionuclide	Z None	Z None
Y Respiratory System	Y Other Radionuclide	Z None	Z None

C Nuclear Medicine
B Respiratory System
3 Positron Emission Tomographic (PET) Imaging — Definition: Introduction of radioactive materials into the body for three dimensional display of images developed from the simultaneous capture, 180 degrees apart, of radioactive emissions

Body Part Character 4	Radionuclide Character 5	Qualifier Character 6	Qualifier Character 7
2 Lungs and Bronchi	K Fluorine 18 (F-18) Y Other Radionuclide	Z None	Z None
Y Respiratory System	Y Other Radionuclide	Z None	Z None

C Nuclear Medicine
D Gastrointestinal System
1 Planar Nuclear Medicine Imaging — Definition: Introduction of radioactive materials into the body for single plane display of images developed from the capture of radioactive emissions

Body Part Character 4	Radionuclide Character 5	Qualifier Character 6	Qualifier Character 7
5 Upper Gastrointestinal Tract 7 Gastrointestinal Tract	1 Technetium 99m (Tc-99m) D Indium 111 (In-111) Y Other Radionuclide	Z None	Z None
Y Digestive System	Y Other Radionuclide	Z None	Z None

ICD-10-PCS 2025 — Nuclear Medicine — CD2–CG2

C Nuclear Medicine
D Gastrointestinal System
2 Tomographic (Tomo) Nuclear Medicine Imaging — Definition: Introduction of radioactive materials into the body for three dimensional display of images developed from the capture of radioactive emissions

Body Part Character 4	Radionuclide Character 5	Qualifier Character 6	Qualifier Character 7
7 Gastrointestinal Tract	1 Technetium 99m (Tc-99m) D Indium 111 (In-111) Y Other Radionuclide	Z None	Z None
Y Digestive System	Y Other Radionuclide	Z None	Z None

C Nuclear Medicine
F Hepatobiliary System and Pancreas
1 Planar Nuclear Medicine Imaging — Definition: Introduction of radioactive materials into the body for single plane display of images developed from the capture of radioactive emissions

Body Part Character 4	Radionuclide Character 5	Qualifier Character 6	Qualifier Character 7
4 Gallbladder 5 Liver 6 Liver and Spleen C Hepatobiliary System, All	1 Technetium 99m (Tc-99m) Y Other Radionuclide	Z None	Z None
Y Hepatobiliary System and Pancreas	Y Other Radionuclide	Z None	Z None

C Nuclear Medicine
F Hepatobiliary System and Pancreas
2 Tomographic (Tomo) Nuclear Medicine Imaging — Definition: Introduction of radioactive materials into the body for three dimensional display of images developed from the capture of radioactive emissions

Body Part Character 4	Radionuclide Character 5	Qualifier Character 6	Qualifier Character 7
4 Gallbladder 5 Liver 6 Liver and Spleen	1 Technetium 99m (Tc-99m) Y Other Radionuclide	Z None	Z None
Y Hepatobiliary System and Pancreas	Y Other Radionuclide	Z None	Z None

C Nuclear Medicine
G Endocrine System
1 Planar Nuclear Medicine Imaging — Definition: Introduction of radioactive materials into the body for single plane display of images developed from the capture of radioactive emissions

Body Part Character 4	Radionuclide Character 5	Qualifier Character 6	Qualifier Character 7
1 Parathyroid Glands	1 Technetium 99m (Tc-99m) S Thallium 201 (Tl-201) Y Other Radionuclide	Z None	Z None
2 Thyroid Gland	1 Technetium 99m (Tc-99m) F Iodine 123 (I-123) G Iodine 131 (I-131) Y Other Radionuclide	Z None	Z None
4 Adrenal Glands, Bilateral	G Iodine 131 (I-131) Y Other Radionuclide	Z None	Z None
Y Endocrine System	Y Other Radionuclide	Z None	Z None

C Nuclear Medicine
G Endocrine System
2 Tomographic (Tomo) Nuclear Medicine Imaging — Definition: Introduction of radioactive materials into the body for three dimensional display of images developed from the capture of radioactive emissions

Body Part Character 4	Radionuclide Character 5	Qualifier Character 6	Qualifier Character 7
1 Parathyroid Glands	1 Technetium 99m (Tc-99m) S Thallium 201 (Tl-201) Y Other Radionuclide	Z None	Z None
Y Endocrine System	Y Other Radionuclide	Z None	Z None

Nuclear Medicine

C Nuclear Medicine
G Endocrine System
4 Nonimaging Nuclear Medicine Uptake — Definition: Introduction of radioactive materials into the body for measurements of organ function, from the detection of radioactive emissions

Body Part Character 4	Radionuclide Character 5	Qualifier Character 6	Qualifier Character 7
2 Thyroid Gland	1 Technetium 99m (Tc-99m) F Iodine 123 (I-123) G Iodine 131 (I-131) Y Other Radionuclide	Z None	Z None
Y Endocrine System	Y Other Radionuclide	Z None	Z None

C Nuclear Medicine
H Skin, Subcutaneous Tissue and Breast
1 Planar Nuclear Medicine Imaging — Definition: Introduction of radioactive materials into the body for single plane display of images developed from the capture of radioactive emissions

Body Part Character 4	Radionuclide Character 5	Qualifier Character 6	Qualifier Character 7
0 Breast, Right 1 Breast, Left 2 Breasts, Bilateral	1 Technetium 99m (Tc-99m) S Thallium 201 (Tl-201) Y Other Radionuclide	Z None	Z None
Y Skin, Subcutaneous Tissue and Breast	Y Other Radionuclide	Z None	Z None

C Nuclear Medicine
H Skin, Subcutaneous Tissue and Breast
2 Tomographic (Tomo) Nuclear Medicine Imaging — Definition: Introduction of radioactive materials into the body for three dimensional display of images developed from the capture of radioactive emissions

Body Part Character 4	Radionuclide Character 5	Qualifier Character 6	Qualifier Character 7
0 Breast, Right 1 Breast, Left 2 Breasts, Bilateral	1 Technetium 99m (Tc-99m) S Thallium 201 (Tl-201) Y Other Radionuclide	Z None	Z None
Y Skin, Subcutaneous Tissue and Breast	Y Other Radionuclide	Z None	Z None

C Nuclear Medicine
P Musculoskeletal System
1 Planar Nuclear Medicine Imaging — Definition: Introduction of radioactive materials into the body for single plane display of images developed from the capture of radioactive emissions

Body Part Character 4	Radionuclide Character 5	Qualifier Character 6	Qualifier Character 7
1 Skull 4 Thorax 5 Spine 6 Pelvis 7 Spine and Pelvis 8 Upper Extremity, Right 9 Upper Extremity, Left B Upper Extremities, Bilateral C Lower Extremity, Right D Lower Extremity, Left F Lower Extremities, Bilateral Z Musculoskeletal System, All	1 Technetium 99m (Tc-99m) Y Other Radionuclide	Z None	Z None
Y Musculoskeletal System, Other	Y Other Radionuclide	Z None	Z None

Non-OR Procedure | DRG Non-OR Procedure | Valid OR Procedure | HAC Associated Procedure | Combination Only | New/Revised April | New/Revised October

ICD-10-PCS 2025 — Nuclear Medicine — CP2–CT6

C Nuclear Medicine
P Musculoskeletal System
2 Tomographic (Tomo) Nuclear Medicine Imaging — Definition: Introduction of radioactive materials into the body for three dimensional display of images developed from the capture of radioactive emissions

Body Part Character 4	Radionuclide Character 5	Qualifier Character 6	Qualifier Character 7
1 Skull 2 Cervical Spine 3 Skull and Cervical Spine 4 Thorax 6 Pelvis 7 Spine and Pelvis 8 Upper Extremity, Right 9 Upper Extremity, Left B Upper Extremities, Bilateral C Lower Extremity, Right D Lower Extremity, Left F Lower Extremities, Bilateral G Thoracic Spine H Lumbar Spine J Thoracolumbar Spine	1 Technetium 99m (Tc-99m) Y Other Radionuclide	Z None	Z None
Y Musculoskeletal System, Other	Y Other Radionuclide	Z None	Z None

C Nuclear Medicine
P Musculoskeletal System
5 Nonimaging Nuclear Medicine Probe — Definition: Introduction of radioactive materials into the body for the study of distribution and fate of certain substances by the detection of radioactive emissions; or, alternatively, measurement of absorption of radioactive emissions from an external source

Body Part Character 4	Radionuclide Character 5	Qualifier Character 6	Qualifier Character 7
5 Spine N Upper Extremities P Lower Extremities	Z None	Z None	Z None
Y Musculoskeletal System, Other	Y Other Radionuclide	Z None	Z None

C Nuclear Medicine
T Urinary System
1 Planar Nuclear Medicine Imaging — Definition: Introduction of radioactive materials into the body for single plane display of images developed from the capture of radioactive emissions

Body Part Character 4	Radionuclide Character 5	Qualifier Character 6	Qualifier Character 7
3 Kidneys, Ureters and Bladder	1 Technetium 99m (Tc-99m) F Iodine 123 (I-123) G Iodine 131 (I-131) Y Other Radionuclide	Z None	Z None
H Bladder and Ureters	1 Technetium 99m (Tc-99m) Y Other Radionuclide	Z None	Z None
Y Urinary System	Y Other Radionuclide	Z None	Z None

C Nuclear Medicine
T Urinary System
2 Tomographic (Tomo) Nuclear Medicine Imaging — Definition: Introduction of radioactive materials into the body for three dimensional display of images developed from the capture of radioactive emissions

Body Part Character 4	Radionuclide Character 5	Qualifier Character 6	Qualifier Character 7
3 Kidneys, Ureters and Bladder	1 Technetium 99m (Tc-99m) Y Other Radionuclide	Z None	Z None
Y Urinary System	Y Other Radionuclide	Z None	Z None

C Nuclear Medicine
T Urinary System
6 Nonimaging Nuclear Medicine Assay — Definition: Introduction of radioactive materials into the body for the study of body fluids and blood elements, by the detection of radioactive emissions

Body Part Character 4	Radionuclide Character 5	Qualifier Character 6	Qualifier Character 7
3 Kidneys, Ureters and Bladder	1 Technetium 99m (Tc-99m) F Iodine 123 (I-123) G Iodine 131 (I-131) H Iodine 125 (I-125) Y Other Radionuclide	Z None	Z None
Y Urinary System	Y Other Radionuclide	Z None	Z None

NC Noncovered Procedure LC Limited Coverage OA Questionable OB Admit NT New Tech Add-on ✚ Combination Member ♂ Male ♀ Female

Nuclear Medicine

C Nuclear Medicine
V Male Reproductive System
1 Planar Nuclear Medicine Imaging

Definition: Introduction of radioactive materials into the body for single plane display of images developed from the capture of radioactive emissions

Body Part Character 4	Radionuclide Character 5	Qualifier Character 6	Qualifier Character 7
9 Testicles, Bilateral	1 Technetium 99m (Tc-99m) Y Other Radionuclide	Z None	Z None
Y Male Reproductive System	Y Other Radionuclide	Z None	Z None

C Nuclear Medicine
W Anatomical Regions
1 Planar Nuclear Medicine Imaging

Definition: Introduction of radioactive materials into the body for single plane display of images developed from the capture of radioactive emissions

Body Part Character 4	Radionuclide Character 5	Qualifier Character 6	Qualifier Character 7
0 Abdomen 1 Abdomen and Pelvis 4 Chest and Abdomen 6 Chest and Neck B Head and Neck D Lower Extremity J Pelvic Region M Upper Extremity N Whole Body	1 Technetium 99m (Tc-99m) D Indium 111 (In-111) F Iodine 123 (I-123) G Iodine 131 (I-131) L Gallium 67 (Ga-67) S Thallium 201 (Tl-201) Y Other Radionuclide	Z None	Z None
3 Chest	1 Technetium 99m (Tc-99m) D Indium 111 (In-111) F Iodine 123 (I-123) G Iodine 131 (I-131) K Fluorine 18 (F-18) L Gallium 67 (Ga-67) S Thallium 201 (Tl-201) Y Other Radionuclide	Z None	Z None
Y Anatomical Regions, Multiple	Y Other Radionuclide	Z None	Z None
Z Anatomical Region, Other	Z None	Z None	Z None

C Nuclear Medicine
W Anatomical Regions
2 Tomographic (Tomo) Nuclear Medicine Imaging

Definition: Introduction of radioactive materials into the body for three dimensional display of images developed from the capture of radioactive emissions

Body Part Character 4	Radionuclide Character 5	Qualifier Character 6	Qualifier Character 7
0 Abdomen 1 Abdomen and Pelvis 3 Chest 4 Chest and Abdomen 6 Chest and Neck B Head and Neck D Lower Extremity J Pelvic Region M Upper Extremity	1 Technetium 99m (Tc-99m) D Indium 111 (In-111) F Iodine 123 (I-123) G Iodine 131 (I-131) K Fluorine 18 (F-18) L Gallium 67 (Ga-67) S Thallium 201 (Tl-201) Y Other Radionuclide	Z None	Z None
Y Anatomical Regions, Multiple	Y Other Radionuclide	Z None	Z None

C Nuclear Medicine
W Anatomical Regions
3 Positron Emission Tomographic (PET) Imaging

Definition: Introduction of radioactive materials into the body for three dimensional display of images developed from the simultaneous capture, 180 degrees apart, of radioactive emissions

Body Part Character 4	Radionuclide Character 5	Qualifier Character 6	Qualifier Character 7
N Whole Body	Y Other Radionuclide	Z None	Z None

C Nuclear Medicine
W Anatomical Regions
5 Nonimaging Nuclear Medicine Probe — Definition: Introduction of radioactive materials into the body for the study of distribution and fate of certain substances by the detection of radioactive emissions; or, alternatively, measurement of absorption of radioactive emissions from an external source

Body Part Character 4	Radionuclide Character 5	Qualifier Character 6	Qualifier Character 7
0 Abdomen 1 Abdomen and Pelvis 3 Chest 4 Chest and Abdomen 6 Chest and Neck B Head and Neck D Lower Extremity J Pelvic Region M Upper Extremity	1 Technetium 99m (Tc-99m) D Indium 111 (In-111) Y Other Radionuclide	Z None	Z None

C Nuclear Medicine
W Anatomical Regions
7 Systemic Nuclear Medicine Therapy — Definition: Introduction of unsealed radioactive materials into the body for treatment

Body Part Character 4	Radionuclide Character 5	Qualifier Character 6	Qualifier Character 7
0 Abdomen 3 Chest	N Phosphorus 32 (P-32) Y Other Radionuclide	Z None	Z None
G Thyroid	G Iodine 131 (I-131) Y Other Radionuclide	Z None	Z None
N Whole Body	8 Samarium 153 (Sm-153) G Iodine 131 (I-131) N Phosphorus 32 (P-32) P Strontium 89 (Sr-89) Y Other Radionuclide	Z None	Z None
Y Anatomical Regions, Multiple	Y Other Radionuclide	Z None	Z None

Radiation Therapy D00–DWY

AHA Coding Clinic for table D01
2020, 4Q, 43-44   Insertion of radioactive element
2020, 4Q, 69-70   Cesium 131 brachytherapy
2019, 4Q, 42-44   Unidirectional source brachytherapy

AHA Coding Clinic for table D0Y
2022, 4Q, 62   Deletion of qualifier value for laser interstitial thermal therapy
2020, 4Q, 70   Intraoperative radiation therapy

AHA Coding Clinic for table D71
2020, 4Q, 43-44   Insertion of radioactive element
2020, 4Q, 69-70   Cesium 131 brachytherapy
2019, 4Q, 42-44   Unidirectional source brachytherapy

AHA Coding Clinic for table D81
2020, 4Q, 43-44   Insertion of radioactive element
2020, 4Q, 69-70   Cesium 131 brachytherapy
2019, 4Q, 42-44   Unidirectional source brachytherapy

AHA Coding Clinic for table D91
2020, 4Q, 43-44   Insertion of radioactive element
2020, 4Q, 69-70   Cesium 131 brachytherapy
2019, 4Q, 42-44   Unidirectional source brachytherapy

AHA Coding Clinic for table DB1
2020, 4Q, 43-44   Insertion of radioactive element
2020, 4Q, 69-70   Cesium 131 brachytherapy
2019, 4Q, 42-44   Unidirectional source brachytherapy

AHA Coding Clinic for table DBY
2022, 4Q, 62   Deletion of qualifier value for laser interstitial thermal therapy

AHA Coding Clinic for table DD1
2020, 4Q, 43-44   Insertion of radioactive element
2020, 4Q, 69-70   Cesium 131 brachytherapy
2019, 4Q, 42-44   Unidirectional source brachytherapy

AHA Coding Clinic for table DDY
2022, 4Q, 62   Deletion of qualifier value for laser interstitial thermal therapy

AHA Coding Clinic for table DF1
2022, 2Q, 26   Radioembolization of right hepatic lobe
2020, 4Q, 43-44   Insertion of radioactive element
2020, 4Q, 69-70   Cesium 131 brachytherapy
2019, 4Q, 42-44   Unidirectional source brachytherapy

AHA Coding Clinic for table DFY
2022, 4Q, 62   Deletion of qualifier value for laser interstitial thermal therapy

AHA Coding Clinic for table DG1
2020, 4Q, 43-44   Insertion of radioactive element
2020, 4Q, 69-70   Cesium 131 brachytherapy
2019, 4Q, 42-44   Unidirectional source brachytherapy

AHA Coding Clinic for table DGY
2022, 4Q, 62   Deletion of qualifier value for laser interstitial thermal therapy

AHA Coding Clinic for table DM1
2020, 4Q, 43-44   Insertion of radioactive element
2020, 4Q, 69-70   Cesium 131 brachytherapy
2019, 4Q, 42-44   Unidirectional source brachytherapy

AHA Coding Clinic for table DMY
2022, 4Q, 62   Deletion of qualifier value for laser interstitial thermal therapy

AHA Coding Clinic for table DT1
2020, 4Q, 43-44   Insertion of radioactive element
2020, 4Q, 69-70   Cesium 131 brachytherapy
2019, 4Q, 42-44   Unidirectional source brachytherapy

AHA Coding Clinic for table DU1
2020, 4Q, 43-44   Insertion of radioactive element
2020, 4Q, 69-70   Cesium 131 brachytherapy
2019, 4Q, 42-44   Unidirectional source brachytherapy
2017, 4Q, 104   Intrauterine brachytherapy & placement of tandems & ovoids

AHA Coding Clinic for table DV1
2020, 4Q, 43-44   Insertion of radioactive element
2020, 4Q, 69-70   Cesium 131 brachytherapy
2019, 4Q, 42-44   Unidirectional source brachytherapy

AHA Coding Clinic for table DVY
2022, 4Q, 62   Deletion of qualifier value for laser interstitial thermal therapy

AHA Coding Clinic for table DW1
2020, 4Q, 43-44   Insertion of radioactive element
2020, 4Q, 69-70   Cesium 131 brachytherapy
2019, 4Q, 42-44   Unidirectional source brachytherapy

AHA Coding Clinic for table DWY
2019, 4Q, 37   Hyperthermic antineoplastic chemotherapy

D   Radiation Therapy
0   Central and Peripheral Nervous System
0   Beam Radiation

Treatment Site Character 4	Modality Qualifier Character 5	Isotope Character 6	Qualifier Character 7
0 Brain 1 Brain Stem 6 Spinal Cord 7 Peripheral Nerve	0 Photons <1 MeV 1 Photons 1- 10 MeV 2 Photons >10 MeV 4 Heavy Particles (Protons, Ions) 5 Neutrons 6 Neutron Capture	Z None	Z None
0 Brain 1 Brain Stem 6 Spinal Cord 7 Peripheral Nerve	3 Electrons	Z None	0 Intraoperative Z None

Radiation Therapy

D Radiation Therapy
0 Central and Peripheral Nervous System
1 Brachytherapy

Treatment Site Character 4	Modality Qualifier Character 5	Isotope Character 6	Qualifier Character 7
0 Brain 1 Brain Stem 6 Spinal Cord 7 Peripheral Nerve	9 High Dose Rate (HDR)	7 Cesium 137 (Cs-137) 8 Iridium 192 (Ir-192) 9 Iodine 125 (I-125) B Palladium 103 (Pd-103) C Californium 252 (Cf-252) Y Other Isotope	Z None
0 Brain 1 Brain Stem 6 Spinal Cord 7 Peripheral Nerve	B Low Dose Rate (LDR)	6 Cesium 131 (Cs-131) 7 Cesium 137 (Cs-137) 8 Iridium 192 (Ir-192) 9 Iodine 125 (I-125) C Californium 252 (Cf-252) Y Other Isotope	Z None
0 Brain 1 Brain Stem 6 Spinal Cord 7 Peripheral Nerve	B Low Dose Rate (LDR)	B Palladium 103 (Pd-103)	1 Unidirectional Source Z None

D Radiation Therapy
0 Central and Peripheral Nervous System
2 Stereotactic Radiosurgery

Treatment Site Character 4	Modality Qualifier Character 5	Isotope Character 6	Qualifier Character 7
0 Brain 1 Brain Stem 6 Spinal Cord 7 Peripheral Nerve	D Stereotactic Other Photon Radiosurgery H Stereotactic Particulate Radiosurgery J Stereotactic Gamma Beam Radiosurgery	Z None	Z None

DRG Non-OR All treatment site, modality, isotope, and qualifier values

D Radiation Therapy
0 Central and Peripheral Nervous System
Y Other Radiation

Treatment Site Character 4	Modality Qualifier Character 5	Isotope Character 6	Qualifier Character 7
0 Brain 1 Brain Stem 6 Spinal Cord 7 Peripheral Nerve	7 Contact Radiation 8 Hyperthermia C Intraoperative Radiation Therapy (IORT) F Plaque Radiation	Z None	Z None

D Radiation Therapy
7 Lymphatic and Hematologic System
0 Beam Radiation

Treatment Site Character 4	Modality Qualifier Character 5	Isotope Character 6	Qualifier Character 7
0 Bone Marrow 1 Thymus 2 Spleen 3 Lymphatics, Neck 4 Lymphatics, Axillary 5 Lymphatics, Thorax 6 Lymphatics, Abdomen 7 Lymphatics, Pelvis 8 Lymphatics, Inguinal	0 Photons <1 MeV 1 Photons 1- 10 MeV 2 Photons >10 MeV 4 Heavy Particles (Protons, Ions) 5 Neutrons 6 Neutron Capture	Z None	Z None
0 Bone Marrow 1 Thymus 2 Spleen 3 Lymphatics, Neck 4 Lymphatics, Axillary 5 Lymphatics, Thorax 6 Lymphatics, Abdomen 7 Lymphatics, Pelvis 8 Lymphatics, Inguinal	3 Electrons	Z None	0 Intraoperative Z None

D Radiation Therapy
7 Lymphatic and Hematologic System
1 Brachytherapy

Treatment Site Character 4	Modality Qualifier Character 5	Isotope Character 6	Qualifier Character 7
0 Bone Marrow 1 Thymus 2 Spleen 3 Lymphatics, Neck 4 Lymphatics, Axillary 5 Lymphatics, Thorax 6 Lymphatics, Abdomen 7 Lymphatics, Pelvis 8 Lymphatics, Inguinal	9 High Dose Rate (HDR)	7 Cesium 137 (Cs-137) 8 Iridium 192 (Ir-192) 9 Iodine 125 (I-125) B Palladium 103 (Pd-103) C Californium 252 (Cf-252) Y Other Isotope	Z None
0 Bone Marrow 1 Thymus 2 Spleen 3 Lymphatics, Neck 4 Lymphatics, Axillary 5 Lymphatics, Thorax 6 Lymphatics, Abdomen 7 Lymphatics, Pelvis 8 Lymphatics, Inguinal	B Low Dose Rate (LDR)	6 Cesium 131 (Cs-131) 7 Cesium 137 (Cs-137) 8 Iridium 192 (Ir-192) 9 Iodine 125 (I-125) C Californium 252 (Cf-252) Y Other Isotope	Z None
0 Bone Marrow 1 Thymus 2 Spleen 3 Lymphatics, Neck 4 Lymphatics, Axillary 5 Lymphatics, Thorax 6 Lymphatics, Abdomen 7 Lymphatics, Pelvis 8 Lymphatics, Inguinal	B Low Dose Rate (LDR)	B Palladium 103 (Pd-103)	1 Unidirectional Source Z None

D Radiation Therapy
7 Lymphatic and Hematologic System
2 Stereotactic Radiosurgery

Treatment Site Character 4	Modality Qualifier Character 5	Isotope Character 6	Qualifier Character 7
0 Bone Marrow 1 Thymus 2 Spleen 3 Lymphatics, Neck 4 Lymphatics, Axillary 5 Lymphatics, Thorax 6 Lymphatics, Abdomen 7 Lymphatics, Pelvis 8 Lymphatics, Inguinal	D Stereotactic Other Photon Radiosurgery H Stereotactic Particulate Radiosurgery J Stereotactic Gamma Beam Radiosurgery	Z None	Z None

DRG Non-OR All treatment site, modality, isotope, and qualifier values

D Radiation Therapy
7 Lymphatic and Hematologic System
Y Other Radiation

Treatment Site Character 4	Modality Qualifier Character 5	Isotope Character 6	Qualifier Character 7
0 Bone Marrow 1 Thymus 2 Spleen 3 Lymphatics, Neck 4 Lymphatics, Axillary 5 Lymphatics, Thorax 6 Lymphatics, Abdomen 7 Lymphatics, Pelvis 8 Lymphatics, Inguinal	8 Hyperthermia F Plaque Radiation	Z None	Z None

Radiation Therapy

D Radiation Therapy
8 Eye
0 Beam Radiation

Treatment Site Character 4	Modality Qualifier Character 5	Isotope Character 6	Qualifier Character 7
0 Eye	0 Photons <1 MeV 1 Photons 1- 10 MeV 2 Photons >10 MeV 4 Heavy Particles (Protons, Ions) 5 Neutrons 6 Neutron Capture	Z None	Z None
0 Eye	3 Electrons	Z None	0 Intraoperative Z None

D Radiation Therapy
8 Eye
1 Brachytherapy

Treatment Site Character 4	Modality Qualifier Character 5	Isotope Character 6	Qualifier Character 7
0 Eye	9 High Dose Rate (HDR)	7 Cesium 137 (Cs-137) 8 Iridium 192 (Ir-192) 9 Iodine 125 (I-125) B Palladium 103 (Pd-103) C Californium 252 (Cf-252) Y Other Isotope	Z None
0 Eye	B Low Dose Rate (LDR)	6 Cesium 131 (Cs-131) 7 Cesium 137 (Cs-137) 8 Iridium 192 (Ir-192) 9 Iodine 125 (I-125) C Californium 252 (Cf-252) Y Other Isotope	Z None
0 Eye	B Low Dose Rate (LDR)	B Palladium 103 (Pd-103)	1 Unidirectional Source Z None

D Radiation Therapy
8 Eye
2 Stereotactic Radiosurgery

Treatment Site Character 4	Modality Qualifier Character 5	Isotope Character 6	Qualifier Character 7
0 Eye	D Stereotactic Other Photon Radiosurgery H Stereotactic Particulate Radiosurgery J Stereotactic Gamma Beam Radiosurgery	Z None	Z None

DRG Non-OR All treatment site, modality, isotope, and qualifier values

D Radiation Therapy
8 Eye
Y Other Radiation

Treatment Site Character 4	Modality Qualifier Character 5	Isotope Character 6	Qualifier Character 7
0 Eye	7 Contact Radiation 8 Hyperthermia F Plaque Radiation	Z None	Z None

ICD-10-PCS 2025 — Radiation Therapy — D90–D91

D Radiation Therapy
9 Ear, Nose, Mouth and Throat
0 Beam Radiation

Treatment Site Character 4	Modality Qualifier Character 5	Isotope Character 6	Qualifier Character 7
0 Ear 1 Nose 3 Hypopharynx 4 Mouth 5 Tongue 6 Salivary Glands 7 Sinuses 8 Hard Palate 9 Soft Palate B Larynx D Nasopharynx F Oropharynx	0 Photons <1 MeV 1 Photons 1- 10 MeV 2 Photons >10 MeV 4 Heavy Particles (Protons, Ions) 5 Neutrons 6 Neutron Capture	Z None	Z None
0 Ear 1 Nose 3 Hypopharynx 4 Mouth 5 Tongue 6 Salivary Glands 7 Sinuses 8 Hard Palate 9 Soft Palate B Larynx D Nasopharynx F Oropharynx	3 Electrons	Z None	0 Intraoperative Z None

D Radiation Therapy
9 Ear, Nose, Mouth and Throat
1 Brachytherapy

Treatment Site Character 4	Modality Qualifier Character 5	Isotope Character 6	Qualifier Character 7
0 Ear 1 Nose 3 Hypopharynx 4 Mouth 5 Tongue 6 Salivary Glands 7 Sinuses 8 Hard Palate 9 Soft Palate B Larynx D Nasopharynx F Oropharynx	9 High Dose Rate (HDR)	7 Cesium 137 (Cs-137) 8 Iridium 192 (Ir-192) 9 Iodine 125 (I-125) B Palladium 103 (Pd-103) C Californium 252 (Cf-252) Y Other Isotope	Z None
0 Ear 1 Nose 3 Hypopharynx 4 Mouth 5 Tongue 6 Salivary Glands 7 Sinuses 8 Hard Palate 9 Soft Palate B Larynx D Nasopharynx F Oropharynx	B Low Dose Rate (LDR)	6 Cesium 131 (Cs-131) 7 Cesium 137 (Cs-137) 8 Iridium 192 (Ir-192) 9 Iodine 125 (I-125) C Californium 252 (Cf-252) Y Other Isotope	Z None
0 Ear 1 Nose 3 Hypopharynx 4 Mouth 5 Tongue 6 Salivary Glands 7 Sinuses 8 Hard Palate 9 Soft Palate B Larynx D Nasopharynx F Oropharynx	B Low Dose Rate (LDR)	B Palladium 103 (Pd-103)	1 Unidirectional Source Z None

NC Noncovered Procedure   **LC** Limited Coverage   **QA** Questionable OB Admit   **NT** New Tech Add-on   ✚ Combination Member   ♂ Male   ♀ Female

Radiation Therapy

D Radiation Therapy
9 Ear, Nose, Mouth and Throat
2 Stereotactic Radiosurgery

Treatment Site Character 4	Modality Qualifier Character 5	Isotope Character 6	Qualifier Character 7
0 Ear 1 Nose 4 Mouth 5 Tongue 6 Salivary Glands 7 Sinuses 8 Hard Palate 9 Soft Palate B Larynx C Pharynx D Nasopharynx	D Stereotactic Other Photon Radiosurgery H Stereotactic Particulate Radiosurgery J Stereotactic Gamma Beam Radiosurgery	Z None	Z None

DRG Non-OR All treatment site, modality, isotope, and qualifier values

---

D Radiation Therapy
9 Ear, Nose, Mouth and Throat
Y Other Radiation

Treatment Site Character 4	Modality Qualifier Character 5	Isotope Character 6	Qualifier Character 7
0 Ear 1 Nose 5 Tongue 6 Salivary Glands 7 Sinuses 8 Hard Palate 9 Soft Palate	7 Contact Radiation 8 Hyperthermia F Plaque Radiation	Z None	Z None
3 Hypopharynx F Oropharynx	7 Contact Radiation 8 Hyperthermia	Z None	Z None
4 Mouth B Larynx D Nasopharynx	7 Contact Radiation 8 Hyperthermia C Intraoperative Radiation Therapy (IORT) F Plaque Radiation	Z None	Z None
C Pharynx	C Intraoperative Radiation Therapy (IORT) F Plaque Radiation	Z None	Z None

---

D Radiation Therapy
B Respiratory System
0 Beam Radiation

Treatment Site Character 4	Modality Qualifier Character 5	Isotope Character 6	Qualifier Character 7
0 Trachea 1 Bronchus 2 Lung 5 Pleura 6 Mediastinum 7 Chest Wall 8 Diaphragm	0 Photons <1 MeV 1 Photons 1- 10 MeV 2 Photons >10 MeV 4 Heavy Particles (Protons, Ions) 5 Neutrons 6 Neutron Capture	Z None	Z None
0 Trachea 1 Bronchus 2 Lung 5 Pleura 6 Mediastinum 7 Chest Wall 8 Diaphragm	3 Electrons	Z None	0 Intraoperative Z None

ICD-10-PCS 2025 — Radiation Therapy — DB1–DBY

D Radiation Therapy
B Respiratory System
1 Brachytherapy

Treatment Site Character 4	Modality Qualifier Character 5	Isotope Character 6	Qualifier Character 7
0 Trachea 1 Bronchus 2 Lung 5 Pleura 6 Mediastinum 7 Chest Wall 8 Diaphragm	9 High Dose Rate (HDR)	7 Cesium 137 (Cs-137) 8 Iridium 192 (Ir-192) 9 Iodine 125 (I-125) B Palladium 103 (Pd-103) C Californium 252 (Cf-252) Y Other Isotope	Z None
0 Trachea 1 Bronchus 2 Lung 5 Pleura 6 Mediastinum 7 Chest Wall 8 Diaphragm	B Low Dose Rate (LDR)	6 Cesium 131 (Cs-131) 7 Cesium 137 (Cs-137) 8 Iridium 192 (Ir-192) 9 Iodine 125 (I-125) C Californium 252 (Cf-252) Y Other Isotope	Z None
0 Trachea 1 Bronchus 2 Lung 5 Pleura 6 Mediastinum 7 Chest Wall 8 Diaphragm	B Low Dose Rate (LDR)	B Palladium 103 (Pd-103)	1 Unidirectional Source Z None

D Radiation Therapy
B Respiratory System
2 Stereotactic Radiosurgery

Treatment Site Character 4	Modality Qualifier Character 5	Isotope Character 6	Qualifier Character 7
0 Trachea 1 Bronchus 2 Lung 5 Pleura 6 Mediastinum 7 Chest Wall 8 Diaphragm	D Stereotactic Other Photon Radiosurgery H Stereotactic Particulate Radiosurgery J Stereotactic Gamma Beam Radiosurgery	Z None	Z None

DRG Non-OR All treatment site, modality, isotope, and qualifier values

D Radiation Therapy
B Respiratory System
Y Other Radiation

Treatment Site Character 4	Modality Qualifier Character 5	Isotope Character 6	Qualifier Character 7
0 Trachea 1 Bronchus 2 Lung 5 Pleura 6 Mediastinum 7 Chest Wall 8 Diaphragm	7 Contact Radiation 8 Hyperthermia F Plaque Radiation	Z None	Z None

NC Noncovered Procedure   **LC** Limited Coverage   **QA** Questionable OB Admit   **NT** New Tech Add-on   ✚ Combination Member   ♂ Male   ♀ Female

Radiation Therapy

D Radiation Therapy
D Gastrointestinal System
0 Beam Radiation

Treatment Site Character 4	Modality Qualifier Character 5	Isotope Character 6	Qualifier Character 7
0 Esophagus 1 Stomach 2 Duodenum 3 Jejunum 4 Ileum 5 Colon 7 Rectum	0 Photons <1 MeV 1 Photons 1- 10 MeV 2 Photons >10 MeV 4 Heavy Particles (Protons, Ions) 5 Neutrons 6 Neutron Capture	Z None	Z None
0 Esophagus 1 Stomach 2 Duodenum 3 Jejunum 4 Ileum 5 Colon 7 Rectum	3 Electrons	Z None	0 Intraoperative Z None

D Radiation Therapy
D Gastrointestinal System
1 Brachytherapy

Treatment Site Character 4	Modality Qualifier Character 5	Isotope Character 6	Qualifier Character 7
0 Esophagus 1 Stomach 2 Duodenum 3 Jejunum 4 Ileum 5 Colon 7 Rectum	9 High Dose Rate (HDR)	7 Cesium 137 (Cs-137) 8 Iridium 192 (Ir-192) 9 Iodine 125 (I-125) B Palladium 103 (Pd-103) C Californium 252 (Cf-252) Y Other Isotope	Z None
0 Esophagus 1 Stomach 2 Duodenum 3 Jejunum 4 Ileum 5 Colon 7 Rectum	B Low Dose Rate (LDR)	6 Cesium 131 (Cs-131) 7 Cesium 137 (Cs-137) 8 Iridium 192 (Ir-192) 9 Iodine 125 (I-125) C Californium 252 (Cf-252) Y Other Isotope	Z None
0 Esophagus 1 Stomach 2 Duodenum 3 Jejunum 4 Ileum 5 Colon 7 Rectum	B Low Dose Rate (LDR)	B Palladium 103 (Pd-103)	1 Unidirectional Source Z None

D Radiation Therapy
D Gastrointestinal System
2 Stereotactic Radiosurgery

Treatment Site Character 4	Modality Qualifier Character 5	Isotope Character 6	Qualifier Character 7
0 Esophagus 1 Stomach 2 Duodenum 3 Jejunum 4 Ileum 5 Colon 7 Rectum	D Stereotactic Other Photon Radiosurgery H Stereotactic Particulate Radiosurgery J Stereotactic Gamma Beam Radiosurgery	Z None	Z None

DRG Non-OR All treatment site, modality, isotope, and qualifier values

D Radiation therapy
D Gastrointestinal System
Y Other Radiation

Treatment Site Character 4	Modality Qualifier Character 5	Isotope Character 6	Qualifier Character 7
0 Esophagus	7 Contact Radiation 8 Hyperthermia F Plaque Radiation	Z None	Z None
1 Stomach 2 Duodenum 3 Jejunum 4 Ileum 5 Colon 7 Rectum	7 Contact Radiation 8 Hyperthermia C Intraoperative Radiation Therapy (IORT) F Plaque Radiation	Z None	Z None
8 Anus	C Intraoperative Radiation Therapy (IORT) F Plaque Radiation	Z None	Z None

D Radiation Therapy
F Hepatobiliary System and Pancreas
0 Beam Radiation

Treatment Site Character 4	Modality Qualifier Character 5	Isotope Character 6	Qualifier Character 7
0 Liver 1 Gallbladder 2 Bile Ducts 3 Pancreas	0 Photons <1 MeV 1 Photons 1- 10 MeV 2 Photons >10 MeV 4 Heavy Particles (Protons, Ions) 5 Neutrons 6 Neutron Capture	Z None	Z None
0 Liver 1 Gallbladder 2 Bile Ducts 3 Pancreas	3 Electrons	Z None	0 Intraoperative Z None

D Radiation Therapy
F Hepatobiliary System and Pancreas
1 Brachytherapy

Treatment Site Character 4	Modality Qualifier Character 5	Isotope Character 6	Qualifier Character 7
0 Liver 1 Gallbladder 2 Bile Ducts 3 Pancreas	9 High Dose Rate (HDR)	7 Cesium 137 (Cs-137) 8 Iridium 192 (Ir-192) 9 Iodine 125 (I-125) B Palladium 103 (Pd-103) C Californium 252 (Cf-252) Y Other Isotope	Z None
0 Liver 1 Gallbladder 2 Bile Ducts 3 Pancreas	B Low Dose Rate (LDR)	6 Cesium 131 (Cs-131) 7 Cesium 137 (Cs-137) 8 Iridium 192 (Ir-192) 9 Iodine 125 (I-125) C Californium 252 (Cf-252) Y Other Isotope	Z None
0 Liver 1 Gallbladder 2 Bile Ducts 3 Pancreas	B Low Dose Rate (LDR)	B Palladium 103 (Pd-103)	1 Unidirectional Source Z None

D Radiation Therapy
F Hepatobiliary System and Pancreas
2 Stereotactic Radiosurgery

Treatment Site Character 4	Modality Qualifier Character 5	Isotope Character 6	Qualifier Character 7
0 Liver 1 Gallbladder 2 Bile Ducts 3 Pancreas	D Stereotactic Other Photon Radiosurgery H Stereotactic Particulate Radiosurgery J Stereotactic Gamma Beam Radiosurgery	Z None	Z None

DRG Non-OR All treatment site, modality, isotope, and qualifier values

Radiation Therapy

D Radiation Therapy
F Hepatobiliary System and Pancreas
Y Other Radiation

Treatment Site Character 4	Modality Qualifier Character 5	Isotope Character 6	Qualifier Character 7
0 Liver 1 Gallbladder 2 Bile Ducts 3 Pancreas	7 Contact Radiation 8 Hyperthermia C Intraoperative Radiation Therapy (IORT) F Plaque Radiation	Z None	Z None

D Radiation Therapy
G Endocrine System
0 Beam Radiation

Treatment Site Character 4	Modality Qualifier Character 5	Isotope Character 6	Qualifier Character 7
0 Pituitary Gland 1 Pineal Body 2 Adrenal Glands 4 Parathyroid Glands 5 Thyroid	0 Photons <1 MeV 1 Photons 1- 10 MeV 2 Photons >10 MeV 5 Neutrons 6 Neutron Capture	Z None	Z None
0 Pituitary Gland 1 Pineal Body 2 Adrenal Glands 4 Parathyroid Glands 5 Thyroid	3 Electrons	Z None	0 Intraoperative Z None

D Radiation Therapy
G Endocrine System
1 Brachytherapy

Treatment Site Character 4	Modality Qualifier Character 5	Isotope Character 6	Qualifier Character 7
0 Pituitary Gland 1 Pineal Body 2 Adrenal Glands 4 Parathyroid Glands 5 Thyroid	9 High Dose Rate (HDR)	7 Cesium 137 (Cs-137) 8 Iridium 192 (Ir-192) 9 Iodine 125 (I-125) B Palladium 103 (Pd-103) C Californium 252 (Cf-252) Y Other Isotope	Z None
0 Pituitary Gland 1 Pineal Body 2 Adrenal Glands 4 Parathyroid Glands 5 Thyroid	B Low Dose Rate (LDR)	6 Cesium 131 (Cs-131) 7 Cesium 137 (Cs-137) 8 Iridium 192 (Ir-192) 9 Iodine 125 (I-125) C Californium 252 (Cf-252) Y Other Isotope	Z None
0 Pituitary Gland 1 Pineal Body 2 Adrenal Glands 4 Parathyroid Glands 5 Thyroid	B Low Dose Rate (LDR)	B Palladium 103 (Pd-103)	1 Unidirectional Source Z None

D Radiation Therapy
G Endocrine System
2 Stereotactic Radiosurgery

Treatment Site Character 4	Modality Qualifier Character 5	Isotope Character 6	Qualifier Character 7
0 Pituitary Gland 1 Pineal Body 2 Adrenal Glands 4 Parathyroid Glands 5 Thyroid	D Stereotactic Other Photon Radiosurgery H Stereotactic Particulate Radiosurgery J Stereotactic Gamma Beam Radiosurgery	Z None	Z None

DRG Non-OR All treatment site, modality, isotope, and qualifier values

D Radiation therapy
G Endocrine System
Y Other Radiation

Treatment Site Character 4	Modality Qualifier Character 5	Isotope Character 6	Qualifier Character 7
0 Pituitary Gland 1 Pineal Body 2 Adrenal Glands 4 Parathyroid Glands 5 Thyroid	7 Contact Radiation 8 Hyperthermia F Plaque Radiation	Z None	Z None

D Radiation Therapy
H Skin
0 Beam Radiation

Treatment Site Character 4	Modality Qualifier Character 5	Isotope Character 6	Qualifier Character 7
2 Skin, Face 3 Skin, Neck 4 Skin, Arm 6 Skin, Chest 7 Skin, Back 8 Skin, Abdomen 9 Skin, Buttock B Skin, Leg	0 Photons <1 MeV 1 Photons 1-10 MeV 2 Photons >10 MeV 4 Heavy Particles (Protons, Ions) 5 Neutrons 6 Neutron Capture	Z None	Z None
2 Skin, Face 3 Skin, Neck 4 Skin, Arm 6 Skin, Chest 7 Skin, Back 8 Skin, Abdomen 9 Skin, Buttock B Skin, Leg	3 Electrons	Z None	0 Intraoperative Z None

D Radiation Therapy
H Skin
Y Other Radiation

Treatment Site Character 4	Modality Qualifier Character 5	Isotope Character 6	Qualifier Character 7
2 Skin, Face 3 Skin, Neck 4 Skin, Arm 6 Skin, Chest 7 Skin, Back 8 Skin, Abdomen 9 Skin, Buttock B Skin, Leg	7 Contact Radiation 8 Hyperthermia F Plaque Radiation	Z None	Z None
5 Skin, Hand C Skin, Foot	F Plaque Radiation	Z None	Z None

D Radiation Therapy
M Breast
0 Beam Radiation

Treatment Site Character 4	Modality Qualifier Character 5	Isotope Character 6	Qualifier Character 7
0 Breast, Left 1 Breast, Right	0 Photons <1 MeV 1 Photons 1-10 MeV 2 Photons >10 MeV 4 Heavy Particles (Protons, Ions) 5 Neutrons 6 Neutron Capture	Z None	Z None
0 Breast, Left 1 Breast, Right	3 Electrons	Z None	0 Intraoperative Z None

Radiation Therapy

D Radiation Therapy
M Breast
1 Brachytherapy

Treatment Site Character 4	Modality Qualifier Character 5	Isotope Character 6	Qualifier Character 7
0 Breast, Left 1 Breast, Right	9 High Dose Rate (HDR)	7 Cesium 137 (Cs-137) 8 Iridium 192 (Ir-192) 9 Iodine 125 (I-125) B Palladium 103 (Pd-103) C Californium 252 (Cf-252) Y Other Isotope	Z None
0 Breast, Left 1 Breast, Right	B Low Dose Rate (LDR)	6 Cesium 131 (Cs-131) 7 Cesium 137 (Cs-137) 8 Iridium 192 (Ir-192) 9 Iodine 125 (I-125) C Californium 252 (Cf-252) Y Other Isotope	Z None
0 Breast, Left 1 Breast, Right	B Low Dose Rate (LDR)	B Palladium 103 (Pd-103)	1 Unidirectional Source Z None

D Radiation Therapy
M Breast
2 Stereotactic Radiosurgery

Treatment Site Character 4	Modality Qualifier Character 5	Isotope Character 6	Qualifier Character 7
0 Breast, Left 1 Breast, Right	D Stereotactic Other Photon Radiosurgery H Stereotactic Particulate Radiosurgery J Stereotactic Gamma Beam Radiosurgery	Z None	Z None

DRG Non-OR All treatment site, modality, isotope, and qualifier values

D Radiation Therapy
M Breast
Y Other Radiation

Treatment Site Character 4	Modality Qualifier Character 5	Isotope Character 6	Qualifier Character 7
0 Breast, Left 1 Breast, Right	7 Contact Radiation 8 Hyperthermia F Plaque Radiation	Z None	Z None

D Radiation Therapy
P Musculoskeletal System
0 Beam Radiation

Treatment Site Character 4	Modality Qualifier Character 5	Isotope Character 6	Qualifier Character 7
0 Skull 2 Maxilla 3 Mandible 4 Sternum 5 Rib(s) 6 Humerus 7 Radius/Ulna 8 Pelvic Bones 9 Femur B Tibia/Fibula C Other Bone	0 Photons <1 MeV 1 Photons 1- 10 MeV 2 Photons >10 MeV 4 Heavy Particles (Protons, Ions) 5 Neutrons 6 Neutron Capture	Z None	Z None
0 Skull 2 Maxilla 3 Mandible 4 Sternum 5 Rib(s) 6 Humerus 7 Radius/Ulna 8 Pelvic Bones 9 Femur B Tibia/Fibula C Other Bone	3 Electrons	Z None	0 Intraoperative Z None

ICD-10-PCS 2025 — Radiation Therapy — DPY–DT2

D Radiation Therapy
P Musculoskeletal System
Y Other Radiation

Treatment Site Character 4	Modality Qualifier Character 5	Isotope Character 6	Qualifier Character 7
0 Skull 2 Maxilla 3 Mandible 4 Sternum 5 Rib(s) 6 Humerus 7 Radius/Ulna 8 Pelvic Bones 9 Femur B Tibia/Fibula C Other Bone	7 Contact Radiation 8 Hyperthermia F Plaque Radiation	Z None	Z None

D Radiation Therapy
T Urinary System
0 Beam Radiation

Treatment Site Character 4	Modality Qualifier Character 5	Isotope Character 6	Qualifier Character 7
0 Kidney 1 Ureter 2 Bladder 3 Urethra	0 Photons <1 MeV 1 Photons 1-10 MeV 2 Photons >10 MeV 4 Heavy Particles (Protons, Ions) 5 Neutrons 6 Neutron Capture	Z None	Z None
0 Kidney 1 Ureter 2 Bladder 3 Urethra	3 Electrons	Z None	0 Intraoperative Z None

D Radiation Therapy
T Urinary System
1 Brachytherapy

Treatment Site Character 4	Modality Qualifier Character 5	Isotope Character 6	Qualifier Character 7
0 Kidney 1 Ureter 2 Bladder 3 Urethra	9 High Dose Rate (HDR)	7 Cesium 137 (Cs-137) 8 Iridium 192 (Ir-192) 9 Iodine 125 (I-125) B Palladium 103 (Pd-103) C Californium 252 (Cf-252) Y Other Isotope	Z None
0 Kidney 1 Ureter 2 Bladder 3 Urethra	B Low Dose Rate (LDR)	6 Cesium 131 (Cs-131) 7 Cesium 137 (Cs-137) 8 Iridium 192 (Ir-192) 9 Iodine 125 (I-125) C Californium 252 (Cf-252) Y Other Isotope	Z None
0 Kidney 1 Ureter 2 Bladder 3 Urethra	B Low Dose Rate (LDR)	B Palladium 103 (Pd-103)	1 Unidirectional Source Z None

D Radiation Therapy
T Urinary System
2 Stereotactic Radiosurgery

Treatment Site Character 4	Modality Qualifier Character 5	Isotope Character 6	Qualifier Character 7
0 Kidney 1 Ureter 2 Bladder 3 Urethra	D Stereotactic Other Photon Radiosurgery H Stereotactic Particulate Radiosurgery J Stereotactic Gamma Beam Radiosurgery	Z None	Z None

DRG Non-OR All treatment site, modality, isotope, and qualifier values

Radiation Therapy

D Radiation Therapy
T Urinary System
Y Other Radiation

Treatment Site Character 4	Modality Qualifier Character 5	Isotope Character 6	Qualifier Character 7
0 Kidney 1 Ureter 2 Bladder 3 Urethra	7 Contact Radiation 8 Hyperthermia C Intraoperative Radiation Therapy (IORT) F Plaque Radiation	Z None	Z None

D Radiation Therapy
U Female Reproductive System
0 Beam Radiation

Treatment Site Character 4	Modality Qualifier Character 5	Isotope Character 6	Qualifier Character 7
0 Ovary 1 Cervix 2 Uterus	0 Photons <1 MeV 1 Photons 1- 10 MeV 2 Photons >10 MeV 4 Heavy Particles (Protons, Ions) 5 Neutrons 6 Neutron Capture	Z None	Z None
0 Ovary 1 Cervix 2 Uterus	3 Electrons	Z None	0 Intraoperative Z None

D Radiation Therapy
U Female Reproductive System
1 Brachytherapy

Treatment Site Character 4	Modality Qualifier Character 5	Isotope Character 6	Qualifier Character 7
0 Ovary 1 Cervix 2 Uterus	9 High Dose Rate (HDR)	7 Cesium 137 (Cs-137) 8 Iridium 192 (Ir-192) 9 Iodine 125 (I-125) B Palladium 103 (Pd-103) C Californium 252 (Cf-252) Y Other Isotope	Z None
0 Ovary 1 Cervix 2 Uterus	B Low Dose Rate (LDR)	6 Cesium 131 (Cs-131) 7 Cesium 137 (Cs-137) 8 Iridium 192 (Ir-192) 9 Iodine 125 (I-125) C Californium 252 (Cf-252) Y Other Isotope	Z None
0 Ovary 1 Cervix 2 Uterus	B Low Dose Rate (LDR)	B Palladium 103 (Pd-103)	1 Unidirectional Source Z None

D Radiation Therapy
U Female Reproductive System
2 Stereotactic Radiosurgery

Treatment Site Character 4	Modality Qualifier Character 5	Isotope Character 6	Qualifier Character 7
0 Ovary 1 Cervix 2 Uterus	D Stereotactic Other Photon Radiosurgery H Stereotactic Particulate Radiosurgery J Stereotactic Gamma Beam Radiosurgery	Z None	Z None

DRG Non-OR All treatment site, modality, isotope, and qualifier values

D Radiation Therapy
U Female Reproductive System
Y Other Radiation

Treatment Site Character 4	Modality Qualifier Character 5	Isotope Character 6	Qualifier Character 7
0 Ovary 1 Cervix 2 Uterus	7 Contact Radiation 8 Hyperthermia C Intraoperative Radiation Therapy (IORT) F Plaque Radiation	Z None	Z None

D Radiation Therapy
V Male Reproductive System
0 Beam Radiation

Treatment Site Character 4	Modality Qualifier Character 5	Isotope Character 6	Qualifier Character 7
0 Prostate 1 Testis	0 Photons <1 MeV 1 Photons 1- 10 MeV 2 Photons >10 MeV 4 Heavy Particles (Protons, Ions) 5 Neutrons 6 Neutron Capture	Z None	Z None
0 Prostate 1 Testis	3 Electrons	Z None	0 Intraoperative Z None

D Radiation Therapy
V Male Reproductive System
1 Brachytherapy

Treatment Site Character 4	Modality Qualifier Character 5	Isotope Character 6	Qualifier Character 7
0 Prostate 1 Testis	9 High Dose Rate (HDR)	7 Cesium 137 (Cs-137) 8 Iridium 192 (Ir-192) 9 Iodine 125 (I-125) B Palladium 103 (Pd-103) C Californium 252 (Cf-252) Y Other Isotope	Z None
0 Prostate 1 Testis	B Low Dose Rate (LDR)	6 Cesium 131 (Cs-131) 7 Cesium 137 (Cs-137) 8 Iridium 192 (Ir-192) 9 Iodine 125 (I-125) C Californium 252 (Cf-252) Y Other Isotope	Z None
0 Prostate 1 Testis	B Low Dose Rate (LDR)	B Palladium 103 (Pd-103)	1 Unidirectional Source Z None

D Radiation Therapy
V Male Reproductive System
2 Stereotactic Radiosurgery

Treatment Site Character 4	Modality Qualifier Character 5	Isotope Character 6	Qualifier Character 7
0 Prostate 1 Testis	D Stereotactic Other Photon Radiosurgery H Stereotactic Particulate Radiosurgery J Stereotactic Gamma Beam Radiosurgery	Z None	Z None

DRG Non-OR All treatment site, modality, isotope, and qualifier values

D Radiation Therapy
V Male Reproductive System
Y Other Radiation

Treatment Site Character 4	Modality Qualifier Character 5	Isotope Character 6	Qualifier Character 7
0 Prostate	7 Contact Radiation 8 Hyperthermia C Intraoperative Radiation Therapy (IORT) F Plaque Radiation	Z None	Z None
1 Testis	7 Contact Radiation 8 Hyperthermia F Plaque Radiation	Z None	Z None

Radiation Therapy

D Radiation Therapy
W Anatomical Regions
0 Beam Radiation

Treatment Site Character 4	Modality Qualifier Character 5	Isotope Character 6	Qualifier Character 7
1 Head and Neck 2 Chest 3 Abdomen 4 Hemibody 5 Whole Body 6 Pelvic Region	0 Photons <1 MeV 1 Photons 1- 10 MeV 2 Photons >10 MeV 4 Heavy Particles (Protons, Ions) 5 Neutrons 6 Neutron Capture	Z None	Z None
1 Head and Neck 2 Chest 3 Abdomen 4 Hemibody 5 Whole Body 6 Pelvic Region	3 Electrons	Z None	0 Intraoperative Z None

D Radiation Therapy
W Anatomical Regions
1 Brachytherapy

Treatment Site Character 4	Modality Qualifier Character 5	Isotope Character 6	Qualifier Character 7
0 Cranial Cavity K Upper Back L Lower Back P Gastrointestinal Tract Q Respiratory Tract R Genitourinary Tract X Upper Extremity Y Lower Extremity	B Low Dose Rate (LDR)	B Palladium 103 (Pd-103)	1 Unidirectional Source Z None
1 Head and Neck 2 Chest 3 Abdomen 6 Pelvic Region	9 High Dose Rate (HDR)	7 Cesium 137 (Cs-137) 8 Iridium 192 (Ir-192) 9 Iodine 125 (I-125) B Palladium 103 (Pd-103) C Californium 252 (Cf-252) Y Other Isotope	Z None
1 Head and Neck 2 Chest 3 Abdomen 6 Pelvic Region	B Low Dose Rate (LDR)	6 Cesium 131 (Cs-131) 7 Cesium 137 (Cs-137) 8 Iridium 192 (Ir-192) 9 Iodine 125 (I-125) C Californium 252 (Cf-252) Y Other Isotope	Z None
1 Head and Neck 2 Chest 3 Abdomen 6 Pelvic Region	B Low Dose Rate (LDR)	B Palladium 103 (Pd-103)	1 Unidirectional Source Z None

D Radiation Therapy
W Anatomical Regions
2 Stereotactic Radiosurgery

Treatment Site Character 4	Modality Qualifier Character 5	Isotope Character 6	Qualifier Character 7
1 Head and Neck 2 Chest 3 Abdomen 6 Pelvic Region	D Stereotactic Other Photon Radiosurgery H Stereotactic Particulate Radiosurgery J Stereotactic Gamma Beam Radiosurgery	Z None	Z None

DRG Non-OR All treatment site, modality, isotope, and qualifier values

D   Radiation Therapy
W   Anatomical Regions
Y   Other Radiation

Treatment Site Character 4	Modality Qualifier Character 5	Isotope Character 6	Qualifier Character 7
1 Head and Neck 2 Chest 3 Abdomen 4 Hemibody 6 Pelvic Region	7 Contact Radiation 8 Hyperthermia F Plaque Radiation	Z None	Z None
5 Whole Body	7 Contact Radiation 8 Hyperthermia F Plaque Radiation	Z None	Z None
5 Whole Body	G Isotope Administration	D Iodine 131 (I-131) F Phosphorus 32 (P-32) G Strontium 89 (Sr-89) H Strontium 90 (Sr-90) Y Other Isotope	Z None

Physical Rehabilitation and Diagnostic Audiology F00–F15

- **F** Physical Rehabilitation and Diagnostic Audiology
- **0** Rehabilitation
- **0** Speech Assessment   Definition: Measurement of speech and related functions

Body System/Region Character 4	Type Qualifier Character 5	Equipment Character 6	Qualifier Character 7
3 Neurological System - Whole Body	G Communicative/Cognitive Integration Skills	K Audiovisual M Augmentative / Alternative Communication P Computer Y Other Equipment Z None	Z None
Z None	0 Filtered Speech 3 Staggered Spondaic Word Q Performance Intensity Phonetically Balanced Speech Discrimination R Brief Tone Stimuli S Distorted Speech T Dichotic Stimuli V Temporal Ordering of Stimuli W Masking Patterns	1 Audiometer 2 Sound Field / Booth K Audiovisual Z None	Z None
Z None	1 Speech Threshold 2 Speech/Word Recognition	1 Audiometer 2 Sound Field / Booth 9 Cochlear Implant K Audiovisual Z None	Z None
Z None	4 Sensorineural Acuity Level	1 Audiometer 2 Sound Field / Booth Z None	Z None
Z None	5 Synthetic Sentence Identification	1 Audiometer 2 Sound Field / Booth 9 Cochlear Implant K Audiovisual	Z None
Z None	6 Speech and/or Language Screening 7 Nonspoken Language 8 Receptive/Expressive Language C Aphasia G Communicative/Cognitive Integration Skills L Augmentative/Alternative Communication System	K Audiovisual M Augmentative / Alternative Communication P Computer Y Other Equipment Z None	Z None
Z None	9 Articulation/Phonology	K Audiovisual P Computer Q Speech Analysis Y Other Equipment Z None	Z None
Z None	B Motor Speech	K Audiovisual N Biosensory Feedback P Computer Q Speech Analysis T Aerodynamic Function Y Other Equipment Z None	Z None
Z None	D Fluency	K Audiovisual N Biosensory Feedback P Computer Q Speech Analysis S Voice Analysis T Aerodynamic Function Y Other Equipment Z None	Z None
Z None	F Voice	K Audiovisual N Biosensory Feedback P Computer S Voice Analysis T Aerodynamic Function Y Other Equipment Z None	Z None

DRG Non-OR All body system/region, type qualifier, equipment, and qualifier values

F00 Continued on next page

F00–F01   Physical Rehabilitation and Diagnostic Audiology   ICD-10-PCS 2025

F00 Continued

F   Physical Rehabilitation and Diagnostic Audiology
0   Rehabilitation
0   Speech Assessment   Definition: Measurement of speech and related functions

Body System/Region Character 4	Type Qualifier Character 5	Equipment Character 6	Qualifier Character 7
Z None	H Bedside Swallowing and Oral Function P Oral Peripheral Mechanism	Y Other Equipment Z None	Z None
Z None	J Instrumental Swallowing and Oral Function	T Aerodynamic Function W Swallowing Y Other Equipment	Z None
Z None	K Orofacial Myofunctional	K Audiovisual P Computer Y Other Equipment Z None	Z None
Z None	M Voice Prosthetic	K Audiovisual P Computer S Voice Analysis V Speech Prosthesis Y Other Equipment Z None	Z None
Z None	N Non-invasive Instrumental Status	N Biosensory Feedback P Computer Q Speech Analysis S Voice Analysis T Aerodynamic Function Y Other Equipment	Z None
Z None	X Other Specified Central Auditory Processing	Z None	Z None

DRG Non-OR   All body system/region, type qualifier, equipment, and qualifier values

---

F   Physical Rehabilitation and Diagnostic Audiology
0   Rehabilitation
1   Motor and/or Nerve Function Assessment   Definition: Measurement of motor, nerve, and related functions

Body System/Region Character 4	Type Qualifier Character 5	Equipment Character 6	Qualifier Character 7
0 Neurological System - Head and Neck 1 Neurological System - Upper Back/ Upper Extremity 2 Neurological System - Lower Back/ Lower Extremity 3 Neurological System - Whole Body	0 Muscle Performance	E Orthosis F Assistive, Adaptive, Supportive or Protective U Prosthesis Y Other Equipment Z None	Z None
0 Neurological System - Head and Neck 1 Neurological System - Upper Back/ Upper Extremity 2 Neurological System - Lower Back/ Lower Extremity 3 Neurological System - Whole Body	1 Integumentary Integrity 3 Coordination/Dexterity 4 Motor Function G Reflex Integrity	Z None	Z None
0 Neurological System - Head and Neck 1 Neurological System - Upper Back/ Upper Extremity 2 Neurological System - Lower Back/ Lower Extremity 3 Neurological System - Whole Body	5 Range of Motion and Joint Integrity 6 Sensory Awareness/Processing/ Integrity	Y Other Equipment Z None	Z None
D Integumentary System - Head and Neck F Integumentary System - Upper Back/ Upper Extremity G Integumentary System - Lower Back/ Lower Extremity H Integumentary System - Whole Body J Musculoskeletal System - Head and Neck K Musculoskeletal System - Upper Back/ Upper Extremity L Musculoskeletal System - Lower Back/ Lower Extremity M Musculoskeletal System - Whole Body	0 Muscle Performance	E Orthosis F Assistive, Adaptive, Supportive or Protective U Prosthesis Y Other Equipment Z None	Z None

DRG Non-OR   All body system/region, type qualifier, equipment, and qualifier values

F01 Continued on next page

Non-OR Procedure   DRG Non-OR Procedure   Valid OR Procedure   HAC Associated Procedure   Combination Only   New/Revised April   New/Revised October

ICD-10-PCS 2025　　Physical Rehabilitation and Diagnostic Audiology　　F01–F01

F **Physical Rehabilitation and Diagnostic Audiology**
0 **Rehabilitation**
1 **Motor and/or Nerve Function Assessment**　Definition: Measurement of motor, nerve, and related functions

F01 Continued

Body System/Region Character 4	Type Qualifier Character 5	Equipment Character 6	Qualifier Character 7
D Integumentary System - Head and Neck F Integumentary System - Upper Back/ Upper Extremity G Integumentary System - Lower Back/ Lower Extremity H Integumentary System - Whole Body J Musculoskeletal System - Head and Neck K Musculoskeletal System - Upper Back/ Upper Extremity L Musculoskeletal System - Lower Back/ Lower Extremity M Musculoskeletal System - Whole Body	1 Integumentary Integrity	Z None	Z None
D Integumentary System - Head and Neck F Integumentary System - Upper Back/ Upper Extremity G Integumentary System - Lower Back/ Lower Extremity H Integumentary System - Whole Body J Musculoskeletal System - Head and Neck K Musculoskeletal System - Upper Back/ Upper Extremity L Musculoskeletal System - Lower Back/ Lower Extremity M Musculoskeletal System - Whole Body	5 Range of Motion and Joint Integrity 6 Sensory Awareness/Processing/ Integrity	Y Other Equipment Z None	Z None
N Genitourinary System	0 Muscle Performance	E Orthosis F Assistive, Adaptive, Supportive or Protective U Prosthesis Y Other Equipment Z None	Z None
Z None	2 Visual Motor Integration	K Audiovisual M Augmentative / Alternative Communication N Biosensory Feedback P Computer Q Speech Analysis S Voice Analysis Y Other Equipment Z None	Z None
Z None	7 Facial Nerve Function	7 Electrophysiologic	Z None
Z None	9 Somatosensory Evoked Potentials	J Somatosensory	Z None
Z None	B Bed Mobility C Transfer F Wheelchair Mobility	E Orthosis F Assistive, Adaptive, Supportive or Protective U Prosthesis Z None	Z None
Z None	D Gait and/or Balance	E Orthosis F Assistive, Adaptive, Supportive or Protective U Prosthesis Y Other Equipment Z None	Z None

DRG Non-OR All body system/region, type qualifier, equipment, and qualifier values

Physical Rehabilitation and Diagnostic Audiology

F Physical Rehabilitation and Diagnostic Audiology
0 Rehabilitation
2 Activities of Daily Living Assessment Definition: Measurement of functional level for activities of daily living

Body System/Region Character 4	Type Qualifier Character 5	Equipment Character 6	Qualifier Character 7
0 Neurological System - Head and Neck	**9** Cranial Nerve Integrity **D** Neuromotor Development	**Y** Other Equipment **Z** None	**Z** None
1 Neurological System - Upper Back/ Upper Extremity **2** Neurological System - Lower Back/ Lower Extremity **3** Neurological System - Whole Body	**D** Neuromotor Development	**Y** Other Equipment **Z** None	**Z** None
4 Circulatory System - Head and Neck **5** Circulatory System - Upper Back/ Upper Extremity **6** Circulatory System - Lower Back/ Lower Extremity **8** Respiratory System - Head and Neck **9** Respiratory System - Upper Back/ Upper Extremity **B** Respiratory System - Lower Back/ Lower Extremity	**G** Ventilation, Respiration and Circulation	**C** Mechanical **G** Aerobic Endurance and Conditioning **Y** Other Equipment **Z** None	**Z** None
7 Circulatory System - Whole Body **C** Respiratory System - Whole Body	**7** Aerobic Capacity and Endurance	**E** Orthosis **G** Aerobic Endurance and Conditioning **U** Prosthesis **Y** Other Equipment **Z** None	**Z** None
7 Circulatory System - Whole Body **C** Respiratory System - Whole Body	**G** Ventilation, Respiration and Circulation	**C** Mechanical **G** Aerobic Endurance and Conditioning **Y** Other Equipment **Z** None	**Z** None
Z None	**0** Bathing/Showering **1** Dressing **3** Grooming/Personal Hygiene **4** Home Management	**E** Orthosis **F** Assistive, Adaptive, Supportive or Protective **U** Prosthesis **Z** None	**Z** None
Z None	**2** Feeding/Eating **8** Anthropometric Characteristics **F** Pain	**Y** Other Equipment **Z** None	**Z** None
Z None	**5** Perceptual Processing	**K** Audiovisual **M** Augmentative / Alternative Communication **N** Biosensory Feedback **P** Computer **Q** Speech Analysis **S** Voice Analysis **Y** Other Equipment **Z** None	**Z** None
Z None	**6** Psychosocial Skills	**Z** None	**Z** None
Z None	**B** Environmental, Home and Work Barriers **C** Ergonomics and Body Mechanics	**E** Orthosis **F** Assistive, Adaptive, Supportive or Protective **U** Prosthesis **Y** Other Equipment **Z** None	**Z** None
Z None	**H** Vocational Activities and Functional Community or Work Reintegration Skills	**E** Orthosis **F** Assistive, Adaptive, Supportive or Protective **G** Aerobic Endurance and Conditioning **U** Prosthesis **Y** Other Equipment **Z** None	**Z** None

DRG Non-OR All body system/region, type qualifier, equipment, and qualifier values

F Physical Rehabilitation and Diagnostic Audiology
0 Rehabilitation
6 Speech Treatment   Definition: Application of techniques to improve, augment, or compensate for speech and related functional impairment

Body System/Region Character 4	Type Qualifier Character 5	Equipment Character 6	Qualifier Character 7
3 Neurological System - Whole Body	6 Communicative/Cognitive Integration Skills	K Audiovisual M Augmentative / Alternative Communication P Computer Y Other Equipment Z None	Z None
Z None	0 Nonspoken Language 3 Aphasia 6 Communicative/Cognitive Integration Skills	K Audiovisual M Augmentative / Alternative Communication P Computer Y Other Equipment Z None	Z None
Z None	1 Speech-Language Pathology and Related Disorders Counseling 2 Speech-Language Pathology and Related Disorders Prevention	K Audiovisual Z None	Z None
Z None	4 Articulation/Phonology	K Audiovisual P Computer Q Speech Analysis T Aerodynamic Function Y Other Equipment Z None	Z None
Z None	5 Aural Rehabilitation	K Audiovisual L Assistive Listening M Augmentative / Alternative Communication N Biosensory Feedback P Computer Q Speech Analysis S Voice Analysis Y Other Equipment Z None	Z None
Z None	7 Fluency	4 Electroacoustic Immitance / Acoustic Reflex K Audiovisual N Biosensory Feedback Q Speech Analysis S Voice Analysis T Aerodynamic Function Y Other Equipment Z None	Z None
Z None	8 Motor Speech	K Audiovisual N Biosensory Feedback P Computer Q Speech Analysis S Voice Analysis T Aerodynamic Function Y Other Equipment Z None	Z None
Z None	9 Orofacial Myofunctional	K Audiovisual P Computer Y Other Equipment Z None	Z None
Z None	B Receptive/Expressive Language	K Audiovisual L Assistive Listening M Augmentative / Alternative Communication P Computer Y Other Equipment Z None	Z None

DRG Non-OR All body system/region, type qualifier, equipment, and qualifier values

F06 Continued on next page

Physical Rehabilitation and Diagnostic Audiology

F Physical Rehabilitation and Diagnostic Audiology
0 Rehabilitation
6 Speech Treatment   Definition: Application of techniques to improve, augment, or compensate for speech and related functional impairment

F06 Continued

Body System/Region Character 4	Type Qualifier Character 5	Equipment Character 6	Qualifier Character 7
Z None	C Voice	K Audiovisual N Biosensory Feedback P Computer S Voice Analysis T Aerodynamic Function V Speech Prosthesis Y Other Equipment Z None	Z None
Z None	D Swallowing Dysfunction	M Augmentative / Alternative Communication T Aerodynamic Function V Speech Prosthesis Y Other Equipment Z None	Z None

DRG Non-OR All body system/region, type qualifier, equipment, and qualifier values

---

F Physical Rehabilitation and Diagnostic Audiology
0 Rehabilitation
7 Motor Treatment   Definition: Exercise or activities to increase or facilitate motor function

Body System/Region Character 4	Type Qualifier Character 5	Equipment Character 6	Qualifier Character 7
0 Neurological System - Head and Neck 1 Neurological System - Upper Back/Upper Extremity 2 Neurological System - Lower Back/Lower Extremity 3 Neurological System - Whole Body D Integumentary System - Head and Neck F Integumentary System - Upper Back/Upper Extremity G Integumentary System - Lower Back/Lower Extremity H Integumentary System - Whole Body J Musculoskeletal System - Head and Neck K Musculoskeletal System - Upper Back/Upper Extremity L Musculoskeletal System - Lower Back/Lower Extremity M Musculoskeletal System - Whole Body	0 Range of Motion and Joint Mobility 1 Muscle Performance 2 Coordination/Dexterity 3 Motor Function	E Orthosis F Assistive, Adaptive, Supportive or Protective U Prosthesis Y Other Equipment Z None	Z None
0 Neurological System - Head and Neck 1 Neurological System - Upper Back/Upper Extremity 2 Neurological System - Lower Back/Lower Extremity 3 Neurological System - Whole Body D Integumentary System - Head and Neck F Integumentary System - Upper Back/Upper Extremity G Integumentary System - Lower Back/Lower Extremity H Integumentary System - Whole Body J Musculoskeletal System - Head and Neck K Musculoskeletal System - Upper Back/Upper Extremity L Musculoskeletal System - Lower Back/Lower Extremity M Musculoskeletal System - Whole Body	6 Therapeutic Exercise	B Physical Agents C Mechanical D Electrotherapeutic E Orthosis F Assistive, Adaptive, Supportive or Protective G Aerobic Endurance and Conditioning H Mechanical or Electromechanical U Prosthesis Y Other Equipment Z None	Z None

DRG Non-OR All body system/region, type qualifier, equipment, and qualifier values

F07 Continued on next page

ICD-10-PCS 2025 — Physical Rehabilitation and Diagnostic Audiology — F07–F07

F07 Continued

- **F** Physical Rehabilitation and Diagnostic Audiology
- **0** Rehabilitation
- **7** Motor Treatment   Definition: Exercise or activities to increase or facilitate motor function

Body System/Region Character 4	Type Qualifier Character 5	Equipment Character 6	Qualifier Character 7
0 Neurological System - Head and Neck 1 Neurological System - Upper Back/Upper Extremity 2 Neurological System - Lower Back/Lower Extremity 3 Neurological System - Whole Body D Integumentary System - Head and Neck F Integumentary System - Upper Back/Upper Extremity G Integumentary System - Lower Back/Lower Extremity H Integumentary System - Whole Body J Musculoskeletal System - Head and Neck K Musculoskeletal System - Upper Back/Upper Extremity L Musculoskeletal System - Lower Back/Lower Extremity M Musculoskeletal System - Whole Body	7 Manual Therapy Techniques	Z None	Z None
4 Circulatory System - Head and Neck 5 Circulatory System - Upper Back / Upper Extremity 6 Circulatory System - Lower Back / Lower Extremity 7 Circulatory System - Whole Body 8 Respiratory System - Head and Neck 9 Respiratory System - Upper Back / Upper Extremity B Respiratory System - Lower Back / Lower Extremity C Respiratory System - Whole Body	6 Therapeutic Exercise	B Physical Agents C Mechanical D Electrotherapeutic E Orthosis F Assistive, Adaptive, Supportive or Protective G Aerobic Endurance and Conditioning H Mechanical or Electromechanical U Prosthesis Y Other Equipment Z None	Z None
N Genitourinary System	1 Muscle Performance	E Orthosis F Assistive, Adaptive, Supportive or Protective U Prosthesis Y Other Equipment Z None	Z None
N Genitourinary System	6 Therapeutic Exercise	B Physical Agents C Mechanical D Electrotherapeutic E Orthosis F Assistive, Adaptive, Supportive or Protective G Aerobic Endurance and Conditioning H Mechanical or Electromechanical U Prosthesis Y Other Equipment Z None	Z None
Z None	4 Wheelchair Mobility	D Electrotherapeutic E Orthosis F Assistive, Adaptive, Supportive or Protective U Prosthesis Y Other Equipment Z None	Z None
Z None	5 Bed Mobility	C Mechanical E Orthosis F Assistive, Adaptive, Supportive or Protective U Prosthesis Y Other Equipment Z None	Z None
Z None	8 Transfer Training	C Mechanical D Electrotherapeutic E Orthosis F Assistive, Adaptive, Supportive or Protective U Prosthesis Y Other Equipment Z None	Z None

DRG Non-OR All body system/region, type qualifier, equipment, and qualifier values

F07 Continued on next page

NC Noncovered Procedure   **LC** Limited Coverage   **QA** Questionable OB Admit   **NT** New Tech Add-on   ✚ Combination Member   ♂ Male   ♀ Female

F Physical Rehabilitation and Diagnostic Audiology
0 Rehabilitation
7 Motor Treatment
Definition: Exercise or activities to increase or facilitate motor function

Body System/Region Character 4	Type Qualifier Character 5	Equipment Character 6	Qualifier Character 7
Z None	9 Gait Training/Functional Ambulation	C Mechanical D Electrotherapeutic E Orthosis F Assistive, Adaptive, Supportive or Protective G Aerobic Endurance and Conditioning U Prosthesis Y Other Equipment Z None	Z None

DRG Non-OR All body system/region, type qualifier, equipment, and qualifier values

F Physical Rehabilitation and Diagnostic Audiology
0 Rehabilitation
8 Activities of Daily Living Treatment
Definition: Exercise or activities to facilitate functional competence for activities of daily living

Body System/Region Character 4	Type Qualifier Character 5	Equipment Character 6	Qualifier Character 7
D Integumentary System - Head and Neck F Integumentary System - Upper Back/Upper Extremity G Integumentary System - Lower Back/Lower Extremity H Integumentary System - Whole Body J Musculoskeletal System - Head and Neck K Musculoskeletal System - Upper Back/Upper Extremity L Musculoskeletal System - Lower Back/Lower Extremity M Musculoskeletal System - Whole Body	5 Wound Management	B Physical Agents C Mechanical D Electrotherapeutic E Orthosis F Assistive, Adaptive, Supportive or Protective U Prosthesis Y Other Equipment Z None	Z None
Z None	0 Bathing/Showering Techniques 1 Dressing Techniques 2 Grooming/Personal Hygiene	E Orthosis F Assistive, Adaptive, Supportive or Protective U Prosthesis Y Other Equipment Z None	Z None
Z None	3 Feeding/Eating	C Mechanical D Electrotherapeutic E Orthosis F Assistive, Adaptive, Supportive or Protective U Prosthesis Y Other Equipment Z None	Z None
Z None	4 Home Management	D Electrotherapeutic E Orthosis F Assistive, Adaptive, Supportive or Protective U Prosthesis Y Other Equipment Z None	Z None
Z None	6 Psychosocial Skills	Z None	Z None
Z None	7 Vocational Activities and Functional Community or Work Reintegration Skills	B Physical Agents C Mechanical D Electrotherapeutic E Orthosis F Assistive, Adaptive, Supportive or Protective G Aerobic Endurance and Conditioning U Prosthesis Y Other Equipment Z None	Z None

DRG Non-OR All body system/region, type qualifier, equipment, and qualifier values

F Physical Rehabilitation and Diagnostic Audiology
0 Rehabilitation
9 Hearing Treatment   Definition: Application of techniques to improve, augment, or compensate for hearing and related functional impairment

Body System/Region Character 4	Type Qualifier Character 5	Equipment Character 6	Qualifier Character 7
Z None	0 Hearing and Related Disorders Counseling 1 Hearing and Related Disorders Prevention	K Audiovisual Z None	Z None
Z None	2 Auditory Processing	K Audiovisual L Assistive Listening P Computer Y Other Equipment Z None	Z None
Z None	3 Cerumen Management	X Cerumen Management Z None	Z None

DRG Non-OR   All body system/region, type qualifier, equipment, and qualifier values

---

F Physical Rehabilitation and Diagnostic Audiology
0 Rehabilitation
B Cochlear Implant Treatment   Definition: Application of techniques to improve the communication abilities of individuals with cochlear implant

Body System/Region Character 4	Type Qualifier Character 5	Equipment Character 6	Qualifier Character 7
Z None	0 Cochlear Implant Rehabilitation	1 Audiometer 2 Sound Field / Booth 9 Cochlear Implant K Audiovisual P Computer Y Other Equipment	Z None

DRG Non-OR   All body system/region, type qualifier, equipment, and qualifier values

---

F Physical Rehabilitation and Diagnostic Audiology
0 Rehabilitation
C Vestibular Treatment   Definition: Application of techniques to improve, augment, or compensate for vestibular and related functional impairment

Body System/Region Character 4	Type Qualifier Character 5	Equipment Character 6	Qualifier Character 7
3 Neurological System - Whole Body H Integumentary System - Whole Body M Musculoskeletal System - Whole Body	3 Postural Control	E Orthosis F Assistive, Adaptive, Supportive or Protective U Prosthesis Y Other Equipment Z None	Z None
Z None	0 Vestibular	8 Vestibular / Balance Z None	Z None
Z None	1 Perceptual Processing 2 Visual Motor Integration	K Audiovisual L Assistive Listening N Biosensory Feedback P Computer Q Speech Analysis S Voice Analysis T Aerodynamic Function Y Other Equipment Z None	Z None

DRG Non-OR   All body system/region, type qualifier, equipment, and qualifier values

F Physical Rehabilitation and Diagnostic Audiology
0 Rehabilitation
D Device Fitting

Definition: Fitting of a device designed to facilitate or support achievement of a higher level of function

Body System/Region Character 4	Type Qualifier Character 5	Equipment Character 6	Qualifier Character 7
Z None	0 Tinnitus Masker	5 Hearing Aid Selection / Fitting / Test Z None	Z None
Z None	1 Monaural Hearing Aid 2 Binaural Hearing Aid 5 Assistive Listening Device	1 Audiometer 2 Sound Field / Booth 5 Hearing Aid Selection / Fitting / Test K Audiovisual L Assistive Listening Z None	Z None
Z None	3 Augmentative/Alternative Communication System	M Augmentative / Alternative Communication	Z None
Z None	4 Voice Prosthetic	S Voice Analysis V Speech Prosthesis	Z None
Z None	6 Dynamic Orthosis 7 Static Orthosis 8 Prosthesis 9 Assistive, Adaptive, Supportive or Protective Devices	E Orthosis F Assistive, Adaptive, Supportive or Protective U Prosthesis Z None	Z None

DRG Non-OR F0DZ0[5,Z]Z
DRG Non-OR F0DZ[1, 2,5][1,2,5, K,L,Z]Z
DRG Non-OR F0DZ3MZ
DRG Non-OR F0DZ4[S,V]Z
DRG Non-OR F0DZ[6,7][E,F,U,Z]Z
DRG Non-OR F0DZ8[E,F,U]Z

F Physical Rehabilitation and Diagnostic Audiology
0 Rehabilitation
F Caregiver Training

Definition: Training in activities to support patient's optimal level of function

Body System/Region Character 4	Type Qualifier Character 5	Equipment Character 6	Qualifier Character 7
Z None	0 Bathing/Showering Technique 1 Dressing 2 Feeding and Eating 3 Grooming/Personal Hygiene 4 Bed Mobility 5 Transfer 6 Wheelchair Mobility 7 Therapeutic Exercise 8 Airway Clearance Techniques 9 Wound Management B Vocational Activities and Functional Community or Work Reintegration Skills C Gait Training/Functional Ambulation D Application, Proper Use and Care of Devices F Application, Proper Use and Care of Orthoses G Application, Proper Use and Care of Prosthesis H Home Management	E Orthosis F Assistive, Adaptive, Supportive or Protective U Prosthesis Z None	Z None
Z None	J Communication Skills	K Audiovisual L Assistive Listening M Augmentative / Alternative Communication P Computer Z None	Z None

DRG Non-OR All body system/region, type qualifier, equipment, and qualifier values

ICD-10-PCS 2025 — Physical Rehabilitation and Diagnostic Audiology

F Physical Rehabilitation and Diagnostic Audiology
1 Diagnostic Audiology
3 Hearing Assessment Definition: Measurement of hearing and related functions

Body System/Region Character 4	Type Qualifier Character 5	Equipment Character 6	Qualifier Character 7
Z None	0 Hearing Screening	0 Occupational Hearing 1 Audiometer 2 Sound Field / Booth 3 Tympanometer 8 Vestibular / Balance 9 Cochlear Implant Z None	Z None
Z None	1 Pure Tone Audiometry, Air 2 Pure Tone Audiometry, Air and Bone	0 Occupational Hearing 1 Audiometer 2 Sound Field / Booth Z None	Z None
Z None	3 Bekesy Audiometry 6 Visual Reinforcement Audiometry 9 Short Increment Sensitivity Index B Stenger C Pure Tone Stenger	1 Audiometer 2 Sound Field / Booth Z None	Z None
Z None	4 Conditioned Play Audiometry 5 Select Picture Audiometry	1 Audiometer 2 Sound Field / Booth K Audiovisual Z None	Z None
Z None	7 Alternate Binaural or Monaural Loudness Balance	1 Audiometer K Audiovisual Z None	Z None
Z None	8 Tone Decay D Tympanometry F Eustachian Tube Function G Acoustic Reflex Patterns H Acoustic Reflex Threshold J Acoustic Reflex Decay	3 Tympanometer 4 Electroacoustic Immitance / Acoustic Reflex Z None	Z None
Z None	K Electrocochleography L Auditory Evoked Potentials	7 Electrophysiologic Z None	Z None
Z None	M Evoked Otoacoustic Emissions, Screening N Evoked Otoacoustic Emissions, Diagnostic	6 Otoacoustic Emission (OAE) Z None	Z None
Z None	P Aural Rehabilitation Status	1 Audiometer 2 Sound Field / Booth 4 Electroacoustic Immitance / Acoustic Reflex 9 Cochlear Implant K Audiovisual L Assistive Listening P Computer Z None	Z None
Z None	Q Auditory Processing	K Audiovisual P Computer Y Other Equipment Z None	Z None

F Physical Rehabilitation and Diagnostic Audiology
1 Diagnostic Audiology
4 Hearing Aid Assessment

Definition: Measurement of the appropriateness and/or effectiveness of a hearing device

Body System/Region Character 4	Type Qualifier Character 5	Equipment Character 6	Qualifier Character 7
Z None	0 Cochlear Implant	1 Audiometer 2 Sound Field / Booth 3 Tympanometer 4 Electroacoustic Immitance / Acoustic Reflex 5 Hearing Aid Selection / Fitting / Test 7 Electrophysiologic 9 Cochlear Implant K Audiovisual L Assistive Listening P Computer Y Other Equipment Z None	Z None
Z None	1 Ear Canal Probe Microphone 6 Binaural Electroacoustic Hearing Aid Check 8 Monaural Electroacoustic Hearing Aid Check	5 Hearing Aid Selection / Fitting / Test Z None	Z None
Z None	2 Monaural Hearing Aid 3 Binaural Hearing Aid	1 Audiometer 2 Sound Field / Booth 3 Tympanometer 4 Electroacoustic Immitance / Acoustic Reflex 5 Hearing Aid Selection / Fitting / Test K Audiovisual L Assistive Listening P Computer Z None	Z None
Z None	4 Assistive Listening System/Device Selection	1 Audiometer 2 Sound Field / Booth 3 Tympanometer 4 Electroacoustic Immitance / Acoustic Reflex K Audiovisual L Assistive Listening Z None	Z None
Z None	5 Sensory Aids	1 Audiometer 2 Sound Field / Booth 3 Tympanometer 4 Electroacoustic Immitance / Acoustic Reflex 5 Hearing Aid Selection / Fitting / Test K Audiovisual L Assistive Listening Z None	Z None
Z None	7 Ear Protector Attentuation	0 Occupational Hearing Z None	Z None

F Physical Rehabilitation and Diagnostic Audiology
1 Diagnostic Audiology
5 Vestibular Assessment

Definition: Measurement of the vestibular system and related functions

Body System/Region Character 4	Type Qualifier Character 5	Equipment Character 6	Qualifier Character 7
Z None	0 Bithermal, Binaural Caloric Irrigation 1 Bithermal, Monaural Caloric Irrigation 2 Unithermal Binaural Screen 3 Oscillating Tracking 4 Sinusoidal Vertical Axis Rotational 5 Dix-Hallpike Dynamic 6 Computerized Dynamic Posturography	8 Vestibular / Balance Z None	Z None
Z None	7 Tinnitus Masker	5 Hearing Aid Selection / Fitting / Test Z None	Z None

Mental Health GZ1–GZJ

G Mental Health
Z None
1 Psychological Tests — Definition: The administration and interpretation of standardized psychological tests and measurement instruments for the assessment of psychological function

Qualifier Character 4	Qualifier Character 5	Qualifier Character 6	Qualifier Character 7
0 Developmental 1 Personality and Behavioral 2 Intellectual and Psychoeducational 3 Neuropsychological 4 Neurobehavioral and Cognitive Status	Z None	Z None	Z None

G Mental Health
Z None
2 Crisis Intervention — Definition: Treatment of a traumatized, acutely disturbed or distressed individual for the purpose of short-term stabilization

Qualifier Character 4	Qualifier Character 5	Qualifier Character 6	Qualifier Character 7
Z None	Z None	Z None	Z None

G Mental Health
Z None
3 Medication Management — Definition: Monitoring and adjusting the use of medications for the treatment of a mental health disorder

Qualifier Character 4	Qualifier Character 5	Qualifier Character 6	Qualifier Character 7
Z None	Z None	Z None	Z None

G Mental Health
Z None
5 Individual Psychotherapy — Definition: Treatment of an individual with a mental health disorder by behavioral, cognitive, psychoanalytic, psychodynamic or psychophysiological means to improve functioning or well-being

Qualifier Character 4	Qualifier Character 5	Qualifier Character 6	Qualifier Character 7
0 Interactive 1 Behavioral 2 Cognitive 3 Interpersonal 4 Psychoanalysis 5 Psychodynamic 6 Supportive 8 Cognitive-Behavioral 9 Psychophysiological	Z None	Z None	Z None

G Mental Health
Z None
6 Counseling — Definition: The application of psychological methods to treat an individual with normal developmental issues and psychological problems in order to increase function, improve well-being, alleviate distress, maladjustment or resolve crises

Qualifier Character 4	Qualifier Character 5	Qualifier Character 6	Qualifier Character 7
0 Educational 1 Vocational 3 Other Counseling	Z None	Z None	Z None

G Mental Health
Z None
7 Family Psychotherapy — Definition: Treatment that includes one or more family members of an individual with a mental health disorder by behavioral, cognitive, psychoanalytic, psychodynamic or psychophysiological means to improve functioning or well-being
Explanation: Remediation of emotional or behavioral problems presented by one or more family members in cases where psychotherapy with more than one family member is indicated

Qualifier Character 4	Qualifier Character 5	Qualifier Character 6	Qualifier Character 7
2 Other Family Psychotherapy	Z None	Z None	Z None

Mental Health

G Mental Health
Z None
B Electroconvulsive Therapy   Definition: The application of controlled electrical voltages to treat a mental health disorder

Qualifier Character 4	Qualifier Character 5	Qualifier Character 6	Qualifier Character 7
0 Unilateral-Single Seizure 2 Bilateral-Single Seizure 4 Other Electroconvulsive Therapy	Z None	Z None	Z None

G Mental Health
Z None
C Biofeedback   Definition: Provision of information from the monitoring and regulating of physiological processes in conjunction with cognitive-behavioral techniques to improve patient functioning or well-being

Qualifier Character 4	Qualifier Character 5	Qualifier Character 6	Qualifier Character 7
9 Other Biofeedback	Z None	Z None	Z None

G Mental Health
Z None
F Hypnosis   Definition: Induction of a state of heightened suggestibility by auditory, visual and tactile techniques to elicit an emotional or behavioral response

Qualifier Character 4	Qualifier Character 5	Qualifier Character 6	Qualifier Character 7
Z None	Z None	Z None	Z None

G Mental Health
Z None
G Narcosynthesis   Definition: Administration of intravenous barbiturates in order to release suppressed or repressed thoughts

Qualifier Character 4	Qualifier Character 5	Qualifier Character 6	Qualifier Character 7
Z None	Z None	Z None	Z None

G Mental Health
Z None
H Group Psychotherapy   Definition: Treatment of two or more individuals with a mental health disorder by behavioral, cognitive, psychoanalytic, psychodynamic or psychophysiological means to improve functioning or well-being

Qualifier Character 4	Qualifier Character 5	Qualifier Character 6	Qualifier Character 7
Z None	Z None	Z None	Z None

G Mental Health
Z None
J Light Therapy   Definition: Application of specialized light treatments to improve functioning or well-being

Qualifier Character 4	Qualifier Character 5	Qualifier Character 6	Qualifier Character 7
Z None	Z None	Z None	Z None

Substance Abuse Treatment HZ2–HZ9

AHA Coding Clinic for table HZ2
2020, 1Q, 21 — Inpatient detoxification services

AHA Coding Clinic for table HZ9
2020, 1Q, 21 — Inpatient detoxification services

H Substance Abuse Treatment
Z None
2 Detoxification Services

Definition: Detoxification from alcohol and/or drugs

Explanation: Not a treatment modality, but helps the patient stabilize physically and psychologically until the body becomes free of drugs and the effects of alcohol

Qualifier Character 4	Qualifier Character 5	Qualifier Character 6	Qualifier Character 7
Z None	Z None	Z None	Z None

H Substance Abuse Treatment
Z None
3 Individual Counseling

Definition: The application of psychological methods to treat an individual with addictive behavior

Explanation: Comprised of several different techniques, which apply various strategies to address drug addiction

Qualifier Character 4	Qualifier Character 5	Qualifier Character 6	Qualifier Character 7
0 Cognitive 1 Behavioral 2 Cognitive-Behavioral 3 12-Step 4 Interpersonal 5 Vocational 6 Psychoeducation 7 Motivational Enhancement 8 Confrontational 9 Continuing Care B Spiritual C Pre/Post-Test Infectious Disease	Z None	Z None	Z None

DRG Non-OR HZ3[0,1,2,3,4,5,6,7,8,9,B]ZZZ

H Substance Abuse Treatment
Z None
4 Group Counseling

Definition: The application of psychological methods to treat two or more individuals with addictive behavior

Explanation: Provides structured group counseling sessions and healing power through the connection with others

Qualifier Character 4	Qualifier Character 5	Qualifier Character 6	Qualifier Character 7
0 Cognitive 1 Behavioral 2 Cognitive-Behavioral 3 12-Step 4 Interpersonal 5 Vocational 6 Psychoeducation 7 Motivational Enhancement 8 Confrontational 9 Continuing Care B Spiritual C Pre/Post-Test Infectious Disease	Z None	Z None	Z None

DRG Non-OR HZ4[0,1,2,3,4,5,6,7,8,9,B]ZZZ

Substance Abuse Treatment

H Substance Abuse Treatment
Z None
5 Individual Psychotherapy Definition: Treatment of an individual with addictive behavior by behavioral, cognitive, psychoanalytic, psychodynamic or psychophysiological means

Qualifier Character 4	Qualifier Character 5	Qualifier Character 6	Qualifier Character 7
0 Cognitive 1 Behavioral 2 Cognitive-Behavioral 3 12-Step 4 Interpersonal 5 Interactive 6 Psychoeducation 7 Motivational Enhancement 8 Confrontational 9 Supportive B Psychoanalysis C Psychodynamic D Psychophysiological	Z None	Z None	Z None

DRG Non-OR For all qualifier values

H Substance Abuse Treatment
Z None
6 Family Counseling Definition: The application of psychological methods that includes one or more family members to treat an individual with addictive behavior
  Explanation: Provides support and education for family members of addicted individuals. Family member participation is seen as a critical area of substance abuse treatment

Qualifier Character 4	Qualifier Character 5	Qualifier Character 6	Qualifier Character 7
3 Other Family Counseling	Z None	Z None	Z None

H Substance Abuse Treatment
Z None
8 Medication Management Definition: Monitoring or adjusting the use of replacement medications for the treatment of addiction

Qualifier Character 4	Qualifier Character 5	Qualifier Character 6	Qualifier Character 7
0 Nicotine Replacement 1 Methadone Maintenance 2 Levo-alpha-acetyl-methadol (LAAM) 3 Antabuse 4 Naltrexone 5 Naloxone 6 Clonidine 7 Bupropion 8 Psychiatric Medication 9 Other Replacement Medication	Z None	Z None	Z None

H Substance Abuse Treatment
Z None
9 Pharmacotherapy Definition: The use of replacement medications for the treatment of addiction

Qualifier Character 4	Qualifier Character 5	Qualifier Character 6	Qualifier Character 7
0 Nicotine Replacement 1 Methadone Maintenance 2 Levo-alpha-acetyl-methadol (LAAM) 3 Antabuse 4 Naltrexone 5 Naloxone 6 Clonidine 7 Bupropion 8 Psychiatric Medication 9 Other Replacement Medication	Z None	Z None	Z None

New Technology X05–XY0

AHA Coding Clinic for all tables in the New Technology Section
2015, 4Q, 8-11   New Section X codes - New Technology procedures

AHA Coding Clinic for table XKU
2022, 4Q, 67-68   Posterior vertebral body tethering
2015, 4Q, 8-11   New Section X codes - New Technology procedures

AHA Coding Clinic for table X05
2023, 4Q, 57-58   Ultrasound ablation of renal sympathetic nerves

AHA Coding Clinic for table X0H
2022, 4Q, 63-64   Implantation of sphenopalatine ganglion stimulator for ischemic stroke
2022, 4Q, 64-65   Implantation of paired vagus nerve stimulator using an external controller

AHA Coding Clinic for table X0Z
2022, 4Q, 65-66   Computer-assisted transcranial magnetic stimulation of the prefrontal cortex

AHA Coding Clinic for table X27
2019, 4Q, 45-46   Sustained released drug-eluting stent

AHA Coding Clinic for table X2A
2023, 3Q, 25   Placement of Emboshield embolic filter
2022, 4Q, 66   Pressure-controlled intermittent coronary sinus occlusion
2021, 1Q, 16   Placement of Sentinel™ embolic protection device with deployment of single filter
2020, 4Q, 70-71   Cerebral embolic filtration extracorporeal flow reversal circuit
2019, 4Q, 46   Cerebral embolic filtration
2016, 4Q, 115-116   Cerebral embolic filtration

AHA Coding Clinic for table X2C
2021, 4Q, 58-59   Computer-aided mechanical aspiration thrombectomy
2016, 4Q, 82-83   Coronary artery, number of arteries
2015, 4Q, 8-14   New Section X codes—New Technology procedures

AHA Coding Clinic for table X2H
2023, 4Q, 58-59   Transcatheter bicaval valves system
2023, 4Q, 59-60   Bioprosthetic femoral venous valves
2023, 4Q, 60-61   Dual-chamber leadless intracardiac pacemaker
2023, 4Q, 61-62   Short-term external heart assist system with axillary artery or ascending thoracic aorta conduit

AHA Coding Clinic for table X2J
2021, 4Q, 59   Transthoracic echocardiography with computer-aided image acquisition

AHA Coding Clinic for table X2K
2024, 1Q, 32   Percutaneous creation of arteriovenous fistula with Ellipsys® Vascular Access System
2023, 4Q, 62-63   Percutaneous femoral-popliteal artery bypass with conduit through femoral vein
2021, 4Q, 60   Percutaneous creation of arteriovenous fistula using thermal resistance energy

AHA Coding Clinic for table X2R
2022, 4Q, 54-55   Rapid deployment technique for replacement of aortic valve using zooplastic tissue
2021, 4Q, 61-62   Replacement combined with restriction of descending thoracic aorta
2016, 4Q, 116   Aortic valve rapid deployment
2015, 4Q, 8-12   New Section X codes—New Technology procedures

AHA Coding Clinic for table X2U
2023, 4Q, 63-64   Placement of extraluminal vein graft support device during coronary artery bypass graft surgery
2023, 4Q, 64-65   Implantation of extraluminal support device during creation of arteriovenous fistula

AHA Coding Clinic for table X2V
2021, 4Q, 61-62   Replacement combined with restriction of descending thoracic aorta
2021, 4Q, 63   Restriction of coronary sinus

AHA Coding Clinic for table XD2
2021, 4Q, 63-64   Monitoring of tissue oxygen saturation in gastrointestinal tract

AHA Coding Clinic for table XDP
2021, 4Q, 64-65   Colonic irrigation for colonoscopy

AHA Coding Clinic for table XF5
2022, 4Q, 67   Extracorporeal histotripsy of targeted liver tissue using ultrasound-guided cavitation

AHA Coding Clinic for table XFJ
2021, 4Q, 65-66   Single-use duodenoscope during endoscopic retrograde cholangiopancreatography

AHA Coding Clinic for table XHR
2021, 4Q, 66   Application of bioengineered allogeneic construct
2016, 4Q, 116   Application of wound matrix

AHA Coding Clinic for table XK0
2017, 4Q, 74   Intramuscular autologous bone marrow cell therapy

AHA Coding Clinic for table XNH
2023, 4Q, 65-66   Insertion of Canturio™ tibial extension implant with motion sensors during total knee arthroplasty
2022, 4Q, 69   Internal fixation device with Tulip connector

AHA Coding Clinic for table XNR
2023, 4Q, 66-67   Ultrasound penetrable cranioplasty Longeviti ClearFit® device
2023, 4Q, 67   Total talar prosthesis with total ankle replacement

AHA Coding Clinic for table XNS
2021, 4Q, 67   Posterior dynamic distraction
2017, 4Q, 74-75   Magnetic growth rods
2016, 4Q, 117   Placement of magnetic growth rods

AHA Coding Clinic for table XNU
2020, 4Q, 72   Implantation of vertebral mechanically expandable device

AHA Coding Clinic for table XRG
2023, 4Q, 68   Ankle fusion with open-truss device
2022, 4Q, 69   Internal fixation device with Tulip connector
2021, 4Q, 68   Customizable interbody fusion
2017, 4Q, 76   Radiolucent porous interbody fusion device

AHA Coding Clinic for table XRH
2022, 4Q, 70   Insertion of posterior spinal motion preservation device

AHA Coding Clinic for table XRR
2022, 4Q, 70-71   Replacement of synthetic substitute meniscus of knee

AHA Coding Clinic for table XT2
2019, 4Q, 46-47   Renal function monitoring

AHA Coding Clinic for table XV5
2018, 4Q, 55   Robotic waterjet ablation

AHA Coding Clinic for table XW0
2024, 1Q, 9-10   Talquetamab antineoplastic
2023, 4Q, 69   Quizartinib
2023, 4Q, 69   Sulbactam-durlobactam
2023, 4Q, 69   Elranatamab antineoplastic
2023, 4Q, 69-70   SER-109
2023, 4Q, 70   Glofitamab antineoplastic
2023, 4Q, 70   Posoleucel
2023, 4Q, 70   Rezafungin
2023, 4Q, 71   Epcoritamab monoclonal antibody
2023, 4Q, 71   Melphalan hydrochloride antineoplastic
2023, 3Q, 7   Control of bleeding with hemostatic clip and Hemospray®
2023, 2Q, 26   Control of bleeding with Hemospray®
2023, 1Q, 12   REGN-COV2 monoclonal antibody
2023, 1Q, 12   Sabizabulin
2022, 4Q, 60-61   Introduction of other therapeutic monoclonal antibody
2022, 4Q, 71-72   Spesolimab monoclonal antibody
2022, 4Q, 72   Daratumumab and hyaluronidase-fihj
2022, 4Q, 72   Maribavir anti-infective
2022, 4Q, 72   Teclistamab antineoplastic
2022, 4Q, 72-73   Mosunetuzumab antineoplatic
2022, 4Q, 73   Afamitresgene autoleucel immunotherapy
2022, 4Q, 73   Tabelecleucel immunotherapy
2022, 4Q, 74   Treosulfan
2022, 4Q, 74   Inebilizumab-cdon
2022, 4Q, 74   Engineered allogeneic thymus tissue
2022, 4Q, 74   Broad consortium microbiota-based live biotherapeutic suspension
2022, 3Q, 26   Tumor-infiltrating lymphocyte therapy
2022, 1Q, 5-6   COVID-19 vaccine administration
2022, 1Q, 7   Fostamatinib
2022, 1Q, 7-8   Tixagevimab and cilgavimab
2022, 1Q, 8   Other monoclonal antibody
2021, 4Q, 69-71   Introduction of new therapeutic substances
2021, 4Q, 71-74   Chimeric antigen receptor T-cell immunotherapy
2021, 4Q, 74-75   Antibiotic-eluting bone void filler
2021, 4Q, 110   New/revised frequently asked questions regarding ICD-10-CM/PCS coding for COVID-19
2021, 1Q, 49   Frequently asked questions regarding ICD-10-CM and ICD-10-PCS coding for COVID-19
2020, 4Q, 72-76   Introduction of new therapeutic substances
2020, 4Q, 95   Frequently asked questions regarding ICD-10-PCS coding for COVID-19
2020, 3Q, 17-21   New procedure codes for introduction or infusion of therapeutics
2019, 4Q, 47-50   New therapeutic substances
2018, 4Q, 56   New therapeutic substances
2015, 4Q, 8-15   New Section X codes—New Technology procedures

AHA Coding Clinic for table XW1
2023, 4Q, 71-72   Transfusion of lovotibeglogene autotemcel
2023, 1Q, 13   Exagamglogene autotemcel
2022, 4Q, 75   Betibeglogene autotemcel
2022, 4Q, 75   Omidubicel
2022, 4Q, 76   OTL-103
2022, 4Q, 76   OTL-200
2021, 4Q, 76   Transfusion of hyperimmune globulin and high-dose immune globulin
2020, 3Q, 17-21   New procedure codes for introduction or infusion of therapeutics

AHA Coding Clinic for table XWH
2021, 4Q, 76-77   Pharyngeal electrical stimulation

X05–Z28   New Technology   ICD-10-PCS 2025

AHA Coding Clinic for table XX2

2024, 1Q, 10	Electrical biocapacitance for assessment of pressure injuries
2023, 4Q, 72	Monitoring of brain electrical activity computer-aided detection and notification
2023, 4Q, 72-73	Monitoring of muscle compartment pressure

AHA Coding Clinic for table XXE

2023, 4Q, 73-74	Computer-aided assessment of cardiac output
2023, 4Q, 74	Rapid antimicrobial susceptibility testing system for blood and body fluid cultures using phenotypic susceptibility
2022, 4Q, 76	Computer-aided analysis for the detection and classification of epileptic events
2022, 4Q, 77	Quantitative flow rate for noninvasive analysis of coronary angiography
2022, 4Q, 77	Simulation for assessment of coronary obstruction risk
2022, 4Q, 78	Gene expression assay
2021, 4Q, 77	Computer-aided assessment of intracranial vascular activity

AHA Coding Clinic for table XXE (continued)

2021, 4Q, 77-78	Computer-aided triage and notification of pulmonary artery flow
2021, 4Q, 78-79	Mechanical initial specimen diversion of whole blood using active negative pressure
2021, 4Q, 79-80	Concurrent measurement of mRNA, PCR test and detection of antibodies
2020, 4Q, 78-79	Measurement of infection
2020, 4Q, 78-79	Positive blood culture fluorescence hybridization
2020, 4Q, 79	Nucleic acid-base microbial detection
2019, 4Q, 50-51	Whole blood nucleic acid-base microbial detection

AHA Coding Clinic for table XY0

2022, 4Q, 78	Extracorporeal antimicrobial administration during renal replacement therapy
2021, 4Q, 80	Regional anticoagulation for renal replacement therapy
2017, 4Q, 78	Intraoperative treatment of vascular grafts

X New Technology
0 Nervous System
5 Destruction

Definition: Physical eradication of all or a portion of a body part by the direct use of energy, force, or a destructive agent
Explanation: None of the body part is physically taken out

Body Part Character 4	Approach Character 5	Device/Substance/Technology Character 6	Qualifier Character 7
1 Renal Sympathetic Nerve(s)	3 Percutaneous	2 Ultrasound Ablation	9 New Technology Group 9
1 Renal Sympathetic Nerve(s)	3 Percutaneous	2 Radiofrequency Ablation	A New Technology Group 10

Valid OR X051329

X New Technology
0 Nervous System
H Insertion

Definition: Putting in a nonbiological appliance that monitors, assists, performs, or prevents a physiological function but does not physically take the place of a body part
Explanation: None

Body Part Character 4	Approach Character 5	Device/Substance/Technology Character 6	Qualifier Character 7
K Sphenopalatine Ganglion	3 Percutaneous	Q Neurostimulator Lead	8 New Technology Group 8
Q Vagus Nerve	3 Percutaneous	R Neurostimulator Lead with Paired Stimulation System	8 New Technology Group 8

Valid OR: All body part, approach, device/substance/technology, and qualifier values
NT X0HQ3R8 for ViviStim® Paired VNS System

See Appendix L for Procedure Combinations
X0HQ3R8

X New Technology
0 Nervous System
Z Other Procedures

Definition: Methodologies which attempt to remediate or cure a disorder or disease
Explanation: None

Body Part Character 4	Approach Character 5	Device/Substance/Technology Character 6	Qualifier Character 7
0 Prefrontal Cortex	X External	1 Computer-assisted Transcranial Magnetic Stimulation	8 New Technology Group 8

NT X0Z0X18 for SAINT Neuromodulation System

X New Technology
2 Cardiovascular System
7 Dilation

Definition: Expanding an orifice or the lumen of a tubular body part
Explanation: The orifice can be a natural orifice or an artificially created orifice. Accomplished by stretching a tubular body part using intraluminal pressure or by cutting part of the orifice or wall of the tubular body part.

Body Part Character 4	Approach Character 5	Device/Substance/Technology Character 6	Qualifier Character 7
P Anterior Tibial Artery, Right	3 Percutaneous	T Intraluminal Device, Everolimus-eluting Resorbable Scaffold(s)	A New Technology Group 10
Q Anterior Tibial Artery, Left			
R Posterior Tibial Artery, Right			
S Posterior Tibial Artery, Left			
T Peroneal Artery, Right			
U Peroneal Artery, Left			

X New Technology
2 Cardiovascular System
8 Division

Definition: Cutting into a body part, without draining fluids and/or gases from the body part, in order to separate or transect a body part
Explanation: All or a portion of the body part is separated into two or more portions

Body Part Character 4	Approach Character 5	Device/Substance/Technology Character 6	Qualifier Character 7
F Aortic Valve	3 Percutaneous	V Intraluminal Bioprosthetic Valve Leaflet Splitting Technology in Existing Valve	A New Technology Group 10

Non-OR Procedure   DRG Non-OR Procedure   Valid OR Procedure   HAC Associated Procedure   Combination Only   New/Revised April   New/Revised October

New Technology

X New Technology
2 Cardiovascular System
A Assistance Definition: Taking over a portion of a physiological function by extracorporeal means
  Explanation: None

Body Part Character 4	Approach Character 5	Device/Substance/Technology Character 6	Qualifier Character 7
5 Innominate Artery and Left Common Carotid Artery	3 Percutaneous	1 Cerebral Embolic Filtration, Dual Filter	2 New Technology Group 2
6 Aortic Arch	3 Percutaneous	2 Cerebral Embolic Filtration, Single Deflection Filter	5 New Technology Group 5
7 Coronary Sinus	3 Percutaneous	5 Intermittent Coronary Sinus Occlusion	8 New Technology Group 8
H Common Carotid Artery, Right J Common Carotid Artery, Left	3 Percutaneous	3 Cerebral Embolic Filtration, Extracorporeal Flow Reversal Circuit	6 New Technology Group 6

DRG Non-OR X2A7358

X New Technology
2 Cardiovascular System
C Extirpation Definition: Taking or cutting out solid matter from a body part
  Explanation: The solid matter may be an abnormal byproduct of a biological function or a foreign body; it may be imbedded in a body part or in the lumen of a tubular body part. The solid matter may or may not have been previously broken into pieces.

Body Part Character 4	Approach Character 5	Device/Substance/Technology Character 6	Qualifier Character 7
P Abdominal Aorta Q Upper Extremity Vein, Right R Upper Extremity Vein, Left S Lower Extremity Artery, Right T Lower Extremity Artery, Left U Lower Extremity Vein, Right V Lower Extremity Vein, Left Y Great Vessel	3 Percutaneous	T Computer-aided Mechanical Aspiration	7 New Technology Group 7

Valid OR All body part, approach, device/substance/technology, and qualifier values

X New Technology
2 Cardiovascular System
H Insertion Definition: Putting in a nonbiological appliance that monitors, assists, performs, or prevents a physiological function but does not physically take the place of a body part
  Explanation: None

Body Part Character 4	Approach Character 5	Device/Substance/Technology Character 6	Qualifier Character 7
0 Inferior Vena Cava 1 Superior Vena Cava	3 Percutaneous	R Intraluminal Device, Bioprosthetic Valve	9 New Technology Group 9
2 Femoral Vein, Right 3 Femoral Vein, Left	0 Open	R Intraluminal Device, Bioprosthetic Valve	9 New Technology Group 9
6 Atrium, Right K Ventricle, Right	3 Percutaneous	V Intracardiac Pacemaker, Dual-Chamber [NT]	9 New Technology Group 9
L Axillary Artery, Right M Axillary Artery, Left X Thoracic Aorta, Ascending	0 Open	F Conduit to Short-term External Heart Assist System	9 New Technology Group 9

Valid OR X2H13R9
Valid OR X2H[2,3]0R9
Valid OR X2H[6,K]3V9
Valid OR X2H[L,M,X]0F9
HAC X2H[6,K]3V9 when reported with SDx K68.11, or T81.40-T81.49, T82.7 with 7th character A
NT X2H63V9 for Aveir™ AR Leadless Pacemaker
NT X2H63V9 with X2HK3V9 for Aveir™ Leadless Pacemaker Dual-Chamber System

See Appendix L for Procedure Combinations
  X2H[L,M,X]0F9

X New Technology
2 Cardiovascular System
J Inspection Definition: Visually and/or manually exploring a body part
  Explanation: None

Body Part Character 4	Approach Character 5	Device/Substance/Technology Character 6	Qualifier Character 7
A Heart	X External	4 Transthoracic Echocardiography, Computer-aided Guidance	7 New Technology Group 7

NC Noncovered Procedure **LC** Limited Coverage **QA** Questionable OB Admit **NT** New Tech Add-on ✚ Combination Member ♂ Male ♀ Female

New Technology

X New Technology
2 Cardiovascular System
K Bypass Definition: Altering the route of passage of the contents of a tubular body part
  Explanation: None

Body Part Character 4	Approach Character 5	Device/Substance/Technology Character 6	Qualifier Character 7
B Radial Artery, Right **C** Radial Artery, Left	**3** Percutaneous	**1** Thermal Resistance Energy	**7** New Technology Group 7
H Femoral Artery, Right **J** Femoral Artery, Left	**3** Percutaneous	**D** Conduit through Femoral Vein to Superficial Femoral Artery [NT] **E** Conduit through Femoral Vein to Popliteal Artery [NT]	**9** New Technology Group 9

Valid OR All body part, approach, device/substance/technology, and qualifier values
[NT] X2K[H,J]3[D,E]9 for DETOUR System

X New Technology
2 Cardiovascular System
R Replacement Definition: Putting in or on biological or synthetic material that physically takes the place and/or function of all or a portion of a body part
  Explanation: None

Body Part Character 4	Approach Character 5	Device/Substance/Technology Character 6	Qualifier Character 7
5 Upper Extremity Artery, Right **6** Upper Extremity Artery, Left **7** Lower Extremity Artery, Right **8** Lower Extremity Artery, Left	**0** Open	**W** Bioengineered Human Acellular Vessel	**A** New Technology Group 10
J Tricuspid Valve	**3** Percutaneous	**R** Multi-plane Flex Technology Bioprosthetic Valve	**A** New Technology Group 10
X Thoracic Aorta, Arch	**0** Open	**N** Branched Synthetic Substitute with Intraluminal Device [NT]	**7** New Technology Group 7

Valid OR X2RX0N7
[NT] X2RX0N7 with X2VW0N7 for Thoraflex™ Hybrid System

X New Technology
2 Cardiovascular System
U Supplememt Definition: Putting in or on biological or synthetic material that physically reinforces and/or augments the function of a portion of a body part
  Explanation: None

Body Part Character 4	Approach Character 5	Device/Substance/Technology Character 6	Qualifier Character 7
4 Coronary Artery/Arteries	**0** Open	**7** Vein Graft Extraluminal Support Device(s)	**9** New Technology Group 9
Q Upper Extremity Vein, Right **R** Upper Extremity Vein, Left	**0** Open	**P** Synthetic Substitute, Extraluminal Support Device	**9** New Technology Group 9

Valid OR All body part, approach, device/substance/technology, and qualifier values

---

X New Technology
2 Cardiovascular System
V Restriction Definition: Partially closing an orifice or the lumen of a tubular body part
  Explanation: None

Body Part Character 4	Approach Character 5	Device/Substance/Technology Character 6	Qualifier Character 7
7 Coronary Sinus	**3** Percutaneous	**Q** Reduction Device	**7** New Technology Group 7
E Descending Thoracic Aorta and Abdominal Aorta	**3** Percutaneous	**S** Branched Intraluminal Device, Manufactured Integrated System, Four or More Arteries	**A** New Technology Group 10
W Thoracic Aorta, Descending	**0** Open	**N** Branched Synthetic Substitute with Intraluminal Device [NT]	**7** New Technology Group 7

Valid OR X2V73Q7
Valid OR X2VW0N7
[NT] X2VW0N7 with X2RX0N7 for Thoraflex™ Hybrid System

X New Technology
D Gastrointestinal System
2 Monitoring Definition: Determining the level of a physiological or physical function repetitively over a period of time
  Explanation: None

Body Part Character 4	Approach Character 5	Device/Substance/Technology Character 6	Qualifier Character 7
G Upper GI **H** Lower GI	**4** Percutaneous Endoscopic **8** Via Natural or Artificial Opening Endoscopic	**V** Oxygen Saturation	**7** New Technology Group 7

ICD-10-PCS 2025 — New Technology — XDP–XNH

- X New Technology
- D Gastrointestinal System
- P Irrigation   Definition: Putting in or on a cleansing substance
     Explanation: None

Body Part Character 4	Approach Character 5	Device/Substance/Technology Character 6	Qualifier Character 7
H Lower GI	8 Via Natural or Artificial Opening Endoscopic	K Intraoperative Single-use Oversleeve	7 New Technology Group 7

- X New Technology
- F Hepatobiliary System and Pancreas
- 5 Destruction   Definition: Physical eradication of all or a portion of a body part by the direct use of energy, force, or a destructive agent
     Explanation: None of the body part is physically taken out

Body Part Character 4	Approach Character 5	Device/Substance/Technology Character 6	Qualifier Character 7
0 Liver 1 Liver, Right Lobe 2 Liver, Left Lobe	X External	0 Ultrasound-guided Cavitation	8 New Technology Group 8

DRG Non-OR All body part, approach, device/substance/technology, and qualifier values

- X New Technology
- F Hepatobiliary System and Pancreas
- J Inspection   Definition: Visually and/or manually exploring a body part
     Explanation: None

Body Part Character 4	Approach Character 5	Device/Substance/Technology Character 6	Qualifier Character 7
B Hepatobiliary Duct D Pancreatic Duct	8 Via Natural or Artificial Opening Endoscopic	A Single-use Duodenoscope	7 New Technology Group 7

- X New Technology
- H Skin, Subcutaneous Tissue, Fascia and Breast
- R Replacement   Definition: Putting in or on biological or synthetic material that physically takes the place and/or function of all or a portion of a body part
     Explanation: None

Body Part Character 4	Approach Character 5	Device/Substance/Technology Character 6	Qualifier Character 7
0 Skin, Head and Neck 1 Skin, Chest 2 Skin, Abdomen 3 Skin, Back 4 Skin, Right Upper Extremity 5 Skin, Left Upper Extremity 6 Skin, Right Lower Extremity 7 Skin, Left Lower Extremity	X External	G Prademagene Zamikeracel, Genetically Engineered Autologous Cell Therapy	A New Technology Group 10
P Skin	X External	F Bioengineered Allogeneic Construct	7 New Technology Group 7

Valid OR XHRPXF7

- X New Technology
- K Muscles, Tendons, Bursae and Ligaments
- U Supplement   Definition: Putting in or on biological or synthetic material that physically reinforces and/or augments the function of a portion of a body part
     Explanation: None

Body Part Character 4	Approach Character 5	Device/Substance/Technology Character 6	Qualifier Character 7
C Upper Spine Bursa and Ligament D Lower Spine Bursa and Ligament	0 Open	6 Posterior Vertebral Tether	8 New Technology Group 8

Valid OR All body part, approach, device/substance/technology, and qualifier values

- X New Technology
- N Bones
- H Insertion   Definition: Putting in a nonbiological appliance that monitors, assists, performs, or prevents a physiological function but does not physically take the place of a body part
     Explanation: None

Body Part Character 4	Approach Character 5	Device/Substance/Technology Character 6	Qualifier Character 7
6 Pelvic Bone, Right 7 Pelvic Bone, Left	0 Open 3 Percutaneous	5 Internal Fixation Device with Tulip Connector [NT]	8 New Technology Group 8
G Tibia, Right H Tibia, Left	0 Open	F Tibial Extension with Motion Sensors	9 New Technology Group 9

Valid OR XNH[6,7][0,3]58
DRG Non-OR XNH[G,H]0F9
NT XNH[6,7][0,3]58 for iFuse Bedrock Granite Implant System

X New Technology
N Bones
R Replacement Definition: Putting in or on biological or synthetic material that physically takes the place and/or function of all or a portion of a body part
Explanation: None

Body Part Character 4	Approach Character 5	Device/Substance/Technology Character 6	Qualifier Character 7
8 Skull	Ø Open	D Synthetic Substitute, Ultrasound Penetrable	9 New Technology Group 9
L Tarsal, Right M Tarsal, Left	Ø Open	9 Synthetic Substitute, Talar Prosthesis	9 New Technology Group 9

Valid OR   All body part, approach, device/substance/technology, and qualifier values

X New Technology
N Bones
S Reposition Definition: Moving to its normal location, or other suitable location, all or a portion of a body part
Explanation: The body part is moved to a new location from an abnormal location, or from a normal location where it is not functioning correctly. The body part may or may not be cut out or off to be moved to the new location.

Body Part Character 4	Approach Character 5	Device/Substance/Technology Character 6	Qualifier Character 7
Ø Lumbar Vertebra	Ø Open	3 Magnetically Controlled Growth Rod(s)	2 New Technology Group 2
Ø Lumbar Vertebra	Ø Open	C Posterior (Dynamic) Distraction Device	7 New Technology Group 7
Ø Lumbar Vertebra	3 Percutaneous	3 Magnetically Controlled Growth Rod(s)	2 New Technology Group 2
Ø Lumbar Vertebra	3 Percutaneous	C Posterior (Dynamic) Distraction Device	7 New Technology Group 7
3 Cervical Vertebra	Ø Open 3 Percutaneous	3 Magnetically Controlled Growth Rod(s)	2 New Technology Group 2
4 Thoracic Vertebra	Ø Open	3 Magnetically Controlled Growth Rod(s)	2 New Technology Group 2
4 Thoracic Vertebra	Ø Open	C Posterior (Dynamic) Distraction Device	7 New Technology Group 7
4 Thoracic Vertebra	3 Percutaneous	3 Magnetically Controlled Growth Rod(s)	2 New Technology Group 2
4 Thoracic Vertebra	3 Percutaneous	C Posterior (Dynamic) Distraction Device	7 New Technology Group 7

Valid OR   All body part, approach, device/substance/technology, and qualifier values

X New Technology
N Bones
U Supplement Definition: Putting in or on biological or synthetic material that physically reinforces and/or augments the function of a portion of a body part
Explanation: None

Body Part Character 4	Approach Character 5	Device/Substance/Technology Character 6	Qualifier Character 7
Ø Lumbar Vertebra 4 Thoracic Vertebra	3 Percutaneous	5 Synthetic Substitute, Mechanically Expandable (Paired)	6 New Technology Group 6

Valid OR   All body part, approach, device/substance/technology, and qualifier values

ICD-10-PCS 2025 — New Technology — XRG–XRG

- **X** New Technology
- **R** Joints
- **G** Fusion

Definition: Joining together portions of an articular body part rendering the articular body part immobile
Explanation: None

Body Part Character 4	Approach Character 5	Device/Substance/Technology Character 6	Qualifier Character 7
A Thoracolumbar Vertebral Joint	0 Open	E Facet Joint Fusion Device, Paired Titanium Cages	A New Technology Group 10
A Thoracolumbar Vertebral Joint	0 Open 3 Percutaneous 4 Percutaneous Endoscopic	R Interbody Fusion Device, Custom-Made Anatomically Designed	7 New Technology Group 7
B Lumbar Vertebral Joint	0 Open	E Facet Joint Fusion Device, Paired Titanium Cages	A New Technology Group 10
B Lumbar Vertebral Joint	0 Open 3 Percutaneous 4 Percutaneous Endoscopic	R Interbody Fusion Device, Custom-Made Anatomically Designed	7 New Technology Group 7
C Lumbar Vertebral Joints, 2 or more	0 Open	E Facet Joint Fusion Device, Paired Titanium Cages	A New Technology Group 10
C Lumbar Vertebral Joints, 2 or more ✚	0 Open 3 Percutaneous 4 Percutaneous Endoscopic	R Interbody Fusion Device, Custom-Made Anatomically Designed	7 New Technology Group 7
D Lumbosacral Joint	0 Open	E Facet Joint Fusion Device, Paired Titanium Cages	A New Technology Group 10
D Lumbosacral Joint	0 Open 3 Percutaneous 4 Percutaneous Endoscopic	R Interbody Fusion Device, Custom-Made Anatomically Designed	7 New Technology Group 7
E Sacroiliac Joint, Right F Sacroiliac Joint, Left	0 Open 3 Percutaneous	5 Internal Fixation Device with Tulip Connector [NT]	8 New Technology Group 8
J Ankle Joint, Right	0 Open	B Internal Fixation Device, Open-truss Design	9 New Technology Group 9
J Ankle Joint, Right	0 Open	C Internal Fixation Device, Gyroid-Sheet Lattice Design	A New Technology Group 10
K Ankle Joint, Left	0 Open	B Internal Fixation Device, Open-truss Design	9 New Technology Group 9
K Ankle Joint, Left	0 Open	C Internal Fixation Device, Gyroid-Sheet Lattice Design	A New Technology Group 10
L Tarsal Joint, Right	0 Open	B Internal Fixation Device, Open-truss Design	9 New Technology Group 9
L Tarsal Joint, Right	0 Open	C Internal Fixation Device, Gyroid-Sheet Lattice Design	A New Technology Group 10
M Tarsal Joint, Left	0 Open	B Internal Fixation Device, Open-truss Design	9 New Technology Group 9
M Tarsal Joint, Left	0 Open	C Internal Fixation Device, Gyroid-Sheet Lattice Design	A New Technology Group 10

Valid OR XRGA[0,3,4]R7
Valid OR XRGB[0,3,4]R7
Valid OR XRGC[0,3,4]R7
Valid OR XRGD[0,3,4]R7
Valid OR XRG[E,F][0,3]58
Valid OR XRGJ0B9
Valid OR XRGK0B9
Valid OR XRGL0B9
Valid OR XRGM0B9

See Appendix L for Procedure Combinations
✚ XRGC[0,3,4]R7

HAC XRG[A,B,C,D][0,3,4]R7 when reported with SDx K68.11 or T81.40-T81.49, T84.60-T84.619, T84.63-T84.7 with 7th character A
HAC XRG[E,F][0,3]58 when reported with SDx K68.11 or T81.40-T81.49, T84.60-T84.619, T84.63-T84.7 with 7th character A
NT XRG[E,F][0,3]58 for iFuse Bedrock Granite Implant System

XRH–XT2   New Technology   ICD-10-PCS 2025

X New Technology
R Joints
H Insertion   **Definition:** Putting in a nonbiological appliance that monitors, assists, performs, or prevents a physiological function but does not physically take the place of a body part
    Explanation: None

Body Part Character 4	Approach Character 5	Device/Substance/Technology Character 6	Qualifier Character 7
6 Thoracic Vertebral Joint 7 Thoracic Vertebral Joints, 2 to 7 8 Thoracic Vertebral Joints, 8 or more A Thoracolumbar Vertebral Joint	0 Open 3 Percutaneous 4 Percutaneous Endoscopic	F Carbon/PEEK Spinal Stabilization Device, Pedicle Based	A New Technology Group 10
B Lumbar Vertebral Joint	0 Open	1 Posterior Spinal Motion Preservation Device **NT**	8 New Technology Group 8
B Lumbar Vertebral Joint C Lumbar Vertebral Joints, 2 or more	0 Open 3 Percutaneous 4 Percutaneous Endoscopic	F Carbon/PEEK Spinal Stabilization Device, Pedicle Based	A New Technology Group 10
D Lumbosacral Joint	0 Open	1 Posterior Spinal Motion Preservation Device **NT**	8 New Technology Group 8
D Lumbosacral Joint	0 Open 3 Percutaneous 4 Percutaneous Endoscopic	F Carbon/PEEK Spinal Stabilization Device, Pedicle Based	A New Technology Group 10

Valid OR   XRHB018
Valid OR   XRHD018
NT   XRHB018 for TOPS™ System in combination with dx code M48.062

X New Technology
R Joints
R Replacement   **Definition:** Putting in or on biological or synthetic material that physically takes the place and/or function of all or a portion of a body part
    Explanation: None

Body Part Character 4	Approach Character 5	Device/Substance/Technology Character 6	Qualifier Character 7
G Knee Joint, Right ⊕ H Knee Joint, Left ⊕	0 Open	L Synthetic Substitute, Lateral Meniscus M Synthetic Substitute, Medial Meniscus	8 New Technology Group 8

Valid OR   All body part, approach, device/substance/technology, and qualifier values
HAC   XRR[G,H]0[L,M]8 when reported with SDx of I26.02-I26.09, I26.92-I26.99, or I82.401-I82.4Z9

See Appendix L for Procedure Combinations
    ⊕ XRR[G,H]0[L,M]8

X New Technology
T Urinary System
2 Monitoring   **Definition:** Determining the level of a physiological or physical function repetitively over a period of time
    Explanation: None

Body Part Character 4	Approach Character 5	Device/Substance/Technology Character 6	Qualifier Character 7
5 Kidney	X External	E Fluorescent Pyrazine	5 New Technology Group 5

ICD-10-PCS 2025 — New Technology — XW0–XW0

X New Technology
W Anatomical Regions
0 Introduction Definition: Putting in or on a therapeutic, diagnostic, nutritional, physiological, or prophylactic substance except blood or blood products
Explanation: None

Body Part Character 4	Approach Character 5	Device/Substance/Technology Character 6	Qualifier Character 7
0 Skin	X External	2 Anacaulase-bcdb	7 New Technology Group 7
1 Subcutaneous Tissue	3 Percutaneous	1 Daratumumab and Hyaluronidase-fihj	8 New Technology Group 8
1 Subcutaneous Tissue	3 Percutaneous	2 Talquetamab Antineoplastic	9 New Technology Group 9
1 Subcutaneous Tissue	3 Percutaneous	4 Teclistamab Antineoplastic [NT]	8 New Technology Group 8
1 Subcutaneous Tissue	3 Percutaneous	6 Dasiglucagon	A New Technology Group 10
1 Subcutaneous Tissue	3 Percutaneous	9 Satralizumab-mwge	7 New Technology Group 7
1 Subcutaneous Tissue	3 Percutaneous	F Other New Technology Therapeutic Substance	5 New Technology Group 5
1 Subcutaneous Tissue	3 Percutaneous	G REGN-COV2 Monoclonal Antibody H Other New Technology Monoclonal Antibody K Leronlimab Monoclonal Antibody	6 New Technology Group 6
1 Subcutaneous Tissue	3 Percutaneous	L Elranatamab Antineoplastic	9 New Technology Group 9
1 Subcutaneous Tissue	3 Percutaneous	S COVID-19 Vaccine Dose 1	6 New Technology Group 6
1 Subcutaneous Tissue	3 Percutaneous	S Epcoritamab Monoclonal Antibody [NT]	9 New Technology Group 9
1 Subcutaneous Tissue	3 Percutaneous	T COVID-19 Vaccine Dose 2 U COVID-19 Vaccine	6 New Technology Group 6
1 Subcutaneous Tissue	3 Percutaneous	V COVID-19 Vaccine Dose 3	7 New Technology Group 7
1 Subcutaneous Tissue	3 Percutaneous	W Caplacizumab	5 New Technology Group 5
1 Subcutaneous Tissue	3 Percutaneous	W COVID-19 Vaccine Booster	7 New Technology Group 7
1 Subcutaneous Tissue	X External	2 Anacaulase-bcdb	7 New Technology Group 7
2 Muscle	0 Open	D Engineered Allogeneic Thymus Tissue	8 New Technology Group 8
2 Muscle	3 Percutaneous	S COVID-19 Vaccine Dose 1 T COVID-19 Vaccine Dose 2 U COVID-19 Vaccine	6 New Technology Group 6
2 Muscle	3 Percutaneous	V COVID-19 Vaccine Dose 3 W COVID-19 Vaccine Booster X Tixagevimab and Cilgavimab Monoclonal Antibody Y Other New Technology Monoclonal Antibody	7 New Technology Group 7
3 Peripheral Vein	3 Percutaneous	0 Brexanolone	6 New Technology Group 6
3 Peripheral Vein	3 Percutaneous	0 Spesolimab Monoclonal Antibody [NT]	8 New Technology Group 8
3 Peripheral Vein	3 Percutaneous	2 Nerinitide 3 Durvalumab Antineoplastic	6 New Technology Group 6
3 Peripheral Vein	3 Percutaneous	3 Bentracimab, Ticagrelor Reversal Agent 4 Cefepime-taniborbactam Anti-infective	A New Technology Group 10
3 Peripheral Vein	3 Percutaneous	5 Narsoplimab Monoclonal Antibody	7 New Technology Group 7
3 Peripheral Vein	3 Percutaneous	5 Mosunetuzumab Antineoplastic [NT]	8 New Technology Group 8
3 Peripheral Vein	3 Percutaneous	5 Ceftobiprole Medocaril Anti-infective	A New Technology Group 10
3 Peripheral Vein	3 Percutaneous	6 Lefamulin Anti-infective	6 New Technology Group 6
3 Peripheral Vein	3 Percutaneous	6 Terlipressin [NT]	7 New Technology Group 7
3 Peripheral Vein	3 Percutaneous	6 Afamitresgene Autoleucel Immunotherapy	8 New Technology Group 8
3 Peripheral Vein	3 Percutaneous	7 Coagulation Factor Xa, Inactivated	2 New Technology Group 2
3 Peripheral Vein	3 Percutaneous	7 Trilaciclib	7 New Technology Group 7
3 Peripheral Vein	3 Percutaneous	7 Tabelecleucel Immunotherapy	8 New Technology Group 8
0 Peripheral Vein	3 Percutaneous	8 Lurbinectedin	7 New Technology Group 7
3 Peripheral Vein	3 Percutaneous	8 Treosulfan	8 New Technology Group 8
3 Peripheral Vein	3 Percutaneous	8 Obecabtagene Autoleucel	A New Technology Group 10
3 Peripheral Vein	3 Percutaneous	9 Ceftolozane/Tazobactam Anti-infective	6 New Technology Group 6
3 Peripheral Vein	3 Percutaneous	9 Inebilizumab-cdon	8 New Technology Group 8
3 Peripheral Vein	3 Percutaneous	9 Odronextamab Antineoplastic	A New Technology Group 10
3 Peripheral Vein	3 Percutaneous	A Cefiderocol Anti-infective	6 New Technology Group 6
3 Peripheral Vein	3 Percutaneous	A Ciltacabtagene Autoleucel	7 New Technology Group 7
3 Peripheral Vein	3 Percutaneous	B Cytarabine and Daunorubicin Liposome Antineoplastic	3 New Technology Group 3
3 Peripheral Vein	3 Percutaneous	B Omadacycline Anti-infective	6 New Technology Group 6
3 Peripheral Vein	3 Percutaneous	B Amivantamab Monoclonal Antibody	7 New Technology Group 7
3 Peripheral Vein	3 Percutaneous	B Orca-T Allogeneic T-cell Immunotherapy	A New Technology Group 10
3 Peripheral Vein	3 Percutaneous	C Eculizumab	6 New Technology Group 6

Valid OR XW020D8
DRG Non-OR XW03368
DRG Non-OR XW03378
DRG Non-OR XW033A7

[NT] XW01348 for TECVAYLI™
[NT] XW013S9 for EPKINLY™
[NT] XW03308 for SPEVIGO®
[NT] XW03358 for Lunsumio™
[NT] XW03367 for TERLIVAZ®

XW0 Continued on next page

NC Noncovered Procedure   LC Limited Coverage   QA Questionable OB Admit   NT New Tech Add-on   ⊕ Combination Member   ♂ Male   ♀ Female

New Technology

X New Technology
W Anatomical Regions
0 Introduction   Definition: Putting in or on a therapeutic, diagnostic, nutritional, physiological, or prophylactic substance except blood or blood products
Explanation: None

Body Part Character 4	Approach Character 5	Device/Substance/Technology Character 6	Qualifier Character 7
3 Peripheral Vein	3 Percutaneous	C Engineered Chimeric Antigen Receptor T-cell Immunotherapy, Autologous	7 New Technology Group 7
3 Peripheral Vein	3 Percutaneous	C Zanidatamab Antineoplastic	A New Technology Group 10
3 Peripheral Vein	3 Percutaneous	D Atezolizumab Antineoplastic	6 New Technology Group 6
3 Peripheral Vein	3 Percutaneous	D Donislecel-jujn Allogeneic Pancreatic Islet Cellular Suspension	A New Technology Group 10
3 Peripheral Vein	3 Percutaneous	E Remdesivir Anti-infective	5 New Technology Group 5
3 Peripheral Vein	3 Percutaneous	E Etesevimab Monoclonal Antibody	6 New Technology Group 6
3 Peripheral Vein	3 Percutaneous	F Other New Technology Therapeutic Substance	3 New Technology Group 3
3 Peripheral Vein	3 Percutaneous	F Other New Technology Therapeutic Substance	5 New Technology Group 5
3 Peripheral Vein	3 Percutaneous	F Bamlanivimab Monoclonal Antibody	6 New Technology Group 6
3 Peripheral Vein	3 Percutaneous	F Non-Chimeric Antigen Receptor T-cell Immune Effector Cell Therapy	A New Technology Group 10
3 Peripheral Vein	3 Percutaneous	G Sarilumab	5 New Technology Group 5
3 Peripheral Vein	3 Percutaneous	G REGN-COV2 Monoclonal Antibody	6 New Technology Group 6
3 Peripheral Vein	3 Percutaneous	G Engineered Chimeric Antigen Receptor T-cell Immunotherapy, Allogeneic	7 New Technology Group 7
3 Peripheral Vein	3 Percutaneous	H Tocilizumab	5 New Technology Group 5
3 Peripheral Vein	3 Percutaneous	H Other New Technology Monoclonal Antibody	6 New Technology Group 6
3 Peripheral Vein	3 Percutaneous	H Axicabtagene Ciloleucel Immunotherapy J Tisagenlecleucel Immunotherapy K Idecabtagene Vicleucel Immunotherapy	7 New Technology Group 7
3 Peripheral Vein	3 Percutaneous	K Sulbactam-Durlobactam [NT]	9 New Technology Group 9
3 Peripheral Vein	3 Percutaneous	L CD24Fc Immunomodulator	6 New Technology Group 6
3 Peripheral Vein	3 Percutaneous	L Lifileucel Immunotherapy M Brexucabtagene Autoleucel Immunotherapy N Lisocabtagene Maraleucel Immunotherapy	7 New Technology Group 7
3 Peripheral Vein	3 Percutaneous	P Glofitamab Antineoplastic [NT]	9 New Technology Group 9
3 Peripheral Vein	3 Percutaneous	Q Tagraxofusp-erzs Antineoplastic	5 New Technology Group 5
3 Peripheral Vein	3 Percutaneous	Q Posoleucel R Rezafungin [NT]	9 New Technology Group 9
3 Peripheral Vein	3 Percutaneous	S Iobenguane I-131 Antineoplastic W Caplacizumab	5 New Technology Group 5
4 Central Vein	3 Percutaneous	0 Brexanolone	6 New Technology Group 6
4 Central Vein	3 Percutaneous	0 Spesolimab Monoclonal Antibody	8 New Technology Group 8
4 Central Vein	3 Percutaneous	2 Nerinitide 3 Durvalumab Antineoplastic	6 New Technology Group 6
4 Central Vein	3 Percutaneous	3 Bentracimab, Ticagrelor Reversal Agent 4 Cefepime-taniborbactam Anti-infective	A New Technology Group 10
4 Central Vein	3 Percutaneous	5 Narsoplimab Monoclonal Antibody	7 New Technology Group 7
4 Central Vein	3 Percutaneous	5 Mosunetuzumab Antineoplastic [NT]	8 New Technology Group 8
4 Central Vein	3 Percutaneous	5 Ceftobiprole Medocaril Anti-infective	A New Technology Group 10
4 Central Vein	3 Percutaneous	6 Lefamulin Anti-infective	6 New Technology Group 6
4 Central Vein	3 Percutaneous	6 Terlipressin [NT]	7 New Technology Group 7
4 Central Vein	3 Percutaneous	6 Afamitresgene Autoleucel Immunotherapy	8 New Technology Group 8
4 Central Vein	3 Percutaneous	7 Coagulation Factor Xa, Inactivated	2 New Technology Group 2
4 Central Vein	3 Percutaneous	7 Trilaciclib	7 New Technology Group 7
4 Central Vein	3 Percutaneous	7 Tabelecleucel Immunotherapy	8 New Technology Group 8
4 Central Vein	3 Percutaneous	8 Lurbinectedin	7 New Technology Group 7
4 Central Vein	3 Percutaneous	8 Treosulfan	8 New Technology Group 8
4 Central Vein	3 Percutaneous	8 Obecabtagene Autoleucel	A New Technology Group 10
4 Central Vein	3 Percutaneous	9 Ceftolozane/Tazobactam Anti-infective	6 New Technology Group 6
4 Central Vein	3 Percutaneous	9 Inebilizumab-cdon	8 New Technology Group 8
4 Central Vein	3 Percutaneous	9 Odronextamab Antineoplastic	A New Technology Group 10
4 Central Vein	3 Percutaneous	A Cefiderocol Anti-infective	6 New Technology Group 6
4 Central Vein	3 Percutaneous	A Ciltacabtagene Autoleucel	7 New Technology Group 7

DRG Non-OR XW033C7
DRG Non-OR XW033G7
DRG Non-OR XW033[H,J]7
DRG Non-OR XW033K7
DRG Non-OR XW033[L,M]7
DRG Non-OR XW04368
DRG Non-OR XW04378
DRG Non-OR XW043A7

[NT] XW033K9 for XACDURO® in combination with one of the following: J15.61 and Y95 or J95.851 and B96.83
[NT] XW033P9 for EPKINLY™
[NT] XW033R9 for REZZAYO™
[NT] XW04358 for Lunsumio™
[NT] XW04367 for TERLIVAZ®

XW0 Continued on next page

ICD-10-PCS 2025 — New Technology — XW0–XW0

X New Technology
W Anatomical Regions
0 Introduction

Definition: Putting in or on a therapeutic, diagnostic, nutritional, physiological, or prophylactic substance except blood or blood products
Explanation: None

XW0 Continued

Body Part Character 4	Approach Character 5	Device/Substance/Technology Character 6	Qualifier Character 7
4 Central Vein	3 Percutaneous	B Cytarabine and Daunorubicin Liposome Antineoplastic	3 New Technology Group 3
4 Central Vein	3 Percutaneous	B Omadacycline Anti-infective	6 New Technology Group 6
4 Central Vein	3 Percutaneous	B Amivantamab Monoclonal Antibody	7 New Technology Group 7
4 Central Vein	3 Percutaneous	B Orca-T Allogeneic T-cell Immunotherapy	A New Technology Group 10
4 Central Vein	3 Percutaneous	C Eculizumab	6 New Technology Group 6
4 Central Vein	3 Percutaneous	C Engineered Chimeric Antigen Receptor T-cell Immunotherapy, Autologous	7 New Technology Group 7
4 Central Vein	3 Percutaneous	C Zanidatamab Antineoplastic	A New Technology Group 10
4 Central Vein	3 Percutaneous	D Atezolizumab Antineoplastic	6 New Technology Group 6
4 Central Vein	3 Percutaneous	E Remdesivir Anti-infective	5 New Technology Group 5
4 Central Vein	3 Percutaneous	E Etesevimab Monoclonal Antibody	6 New Technology Group 6
4 Central Vein	3 Percutaneous	F Other New Technology Therapeutic Substance	3 New Technology Group 3
4 Central Vein	3 Percutaneous	F Other New Technology Therapeutic Substance	5 New Technology Group 5
4 Central Vein	3 Percutaneous	F Bamlanivimab Monoclonal Antibody	6 New Technology Group 6
4 Central Vein	3 Percutaneous	F Non-Chimeric Antigen Receptor T-cell Immune Effector Cell Therapy	A New Technology Group 10
4 Central Vein	3 Percutaneous	G Sarilumab	5 New Technology Group 5
4 Central Vein	3 Percutaneous	G REGN-COV2 Monoclonal Antibody	6 New Technology Group 6
4 Central Vein	3 Percutaneous	G Engineered Chimeric Antigen Receptor T-cell Immunotherapy, Allogeneic	7 New Technology Group 7
4 Central Vein	3 Percutaneous	H Tocilizumab	5 New Technology Group 5
4 Central Vein	3 Percutaneous	H Other New Technology Monoclonal Antibody	6 New Technology Group 6
4 Central Vein	3 Percutaneous	H Axicabtagene Ciloleucel Immunotherapy J Tisagenlecleucel Immunotherapy K Idecabtagene Vicleucel Immunotherapy	7 New Technology Group 7
4 Central Vein	3 Percutaneous	K Sulbactam-Durlobactam [NT]	9 New Technology Group 9
4 Central Vein	3 Percutaneous	L CD24Fc Immunomodulator	6 New Technology Group 6
4 Central Vein	3 Percutaneous	L Lifileucel Immunotherapy M Brexucabtagene Autoleucel Immunotherapy N Lisocabtagene Maraleucel Immunotherapy	7 New Technology Group 7
4 Central Vein	3 Percutaneous	P Glofitamab Antineoplastic [NT]	9 New Technology Group 9
4 Central Vein	3 Percutaneous	Q Tagraxofusp-erzs Antineoplastic	5 New Technology Group 5
4 Central Vein	3 Percutaneous	Q Posoleucel R Rezafungin [NT]	9 New Technology Group 9
4 Central Vein	3 Percutaneous	S Iobenguane I-131 Antineoplastic W Caplacizumab	5 New Technology Group 5
5 Peripheral Artery	3 Percutaneous	T Melphalan Hydrochloride Antineoplastic	9 New Technology Group 9
D Mouth and Pharynx	X External	3 Maribavir Anti-infective	8 New Technology Group 8
D Mouth and Pharynx	X External	6 Lefamulin Anti-infective	6 New Technology Group 6
D Mouth and Pharynx	X External	8 Uridine Triacetate	2 New Technology Group 2
D Mouth and Pharynx	X External	F Other New Technology Therapeutic Substance	5 New Technology Group 5
D Mouth and Pharynx	X External	J Quizartinib Antineoplastic	9 New Technology Group 9
D Mouth and Pharynx	X External	K Sabizabulin	8 New Technology Group 8
D Mouth and Pharynx	X External	M Baricitinib	6 New Technology Group 6
D Mouth and Pharynx	X External	N SER-109 [NT]	9 New Technology Group 9
D Mouth and Pharynx	X External	R Fostamatinib	7 New Technology Group 7
G Upper GI	7 Via Natural or Artificial Opening	3 Maribavir Anti-infective K Sabizabulin	8 New Technology Group 8
G Upper GI	7 Via Natural or Artificial Opening	M Baricitinib	6 New Technology Group 6
G Upper GI	7 Via Natural or Artificial Opening	R Fostamatinib	7 New Technology Group 7
G Upper GI	8 Via Natural or Artificial Opening Endoscopic	8 Mineral-based Topical Hemostatic Agent	6 New Technology Group 6
H Lower GI	7 Via Natural or Artificial Opening	3 Maribavir Anti-infective K Sabizabulin	8 New Technology Group 8

DRG Non-OR XW043C7
DRG Non-OR XW043G7
DRG Non-OR XW043[H,J,K]7
DRG Non-OR XW043[L,M,N]7

[NT] XW043K9 for XACDURO® in combination with one of the following code combinations: J15.61 and Y95 or J95.851 and B96.83
[NT] XW043P9 for EPKINLY™
[NT] XW043R9 for REZZAYO™
[NT] XW0DXN9 for VOWST™

XW0 Continued on next page

XW0–XWH New Technology ICD-10-PCS 2025

XW0 Continued

X New Technology
W Anatomical Regions
0 Introduction Definition: Putting in or on a therapeutic, diagnostic, nutritional, physiological, or prophylactic substance except blood or blood products
  Explanation: None

Body Part Character 4	Approach Character 5	Device/Substance/Technology Character 6	Qualifier Character 7
H Lower GI	7 Via Natural or Artificial Opening	M Baricitinib	6 New Technology Group 6
H Lower GI	7 Via Natural or Artificial Opening	R Fostamatinib	7 New Technology Group 7
H Lower GI	7 Via Natural or Artificial Opening	X Broad Consortium Microbiota-based Live Biotherapeutic Suspension [NT]	8 New Technology Group 8
H Lower GI	8 Via Natural or Artificial Opening Endoscopic	8 Mineral-based Topical Hemostatic Agent	6 New Technology Group 6
J Coronary Artery, One Artery K Coronary Artery, Two Arteries L Coronary Artery, Three Arteries M Coronary Artery, Four or More Arteries	3 Percutaneous	H Paclitaxel-Coated Balloon Technology, One Balloon J Paclitaxel-Coated Balloon Technology, Two Balloons K Paclitaxel-Coated Balloon Technology, Three Balloons L Paclitaxel-Coated Balloon Technology, Four or More Balloons	A New Technology Group 10
Q Cranial Cavity and Brain	3 Percutaneous	1 Eladocagene exuparvovec	6 New Technology Group 6
U Joints	0 Open	G Vancomycin Hydrochloride and Tobramycin Sulfate Anti-Infective, Temporary Irrigation Spacer System	A New Technology Group 10
V Bones	0 Open	P Antibiotic-eluting Bone Void Filler [NT]	7 New Technology Group 7
V Bones	3 Percutaneous	W AGN1 Bone Void Filler	A New Technology Group 10

Valid OR XW0Q316
[NT] XW0H7X8 for REBYOTA™
[NT] XW0V0P7 for Cerament® G

X New Technology
W Anatomical Regions
1 Transfusion Definition: Putting in blood or blood products
  Explanation: None

Body Part Character 4	Approach Character 5	Device/Substance/Technology Character 6	Qualifier Character 7
3 Peripheral Vein	3 Percutaneous	2 Plasma, Convalescent (Nonautologous)	5 New Technology Group 5
3 Peripheral Vein	3 Percutaneous	7 Marnetegragene Autotemcel	A New Technology Group 10
3 Peripheral Vein	3 Percutaneous	B Betibeglogene Autotemcel C Omidubicel	8 New Technology Group 8
3 Peripheral Vein	3 Percutaneous	D High-Dose Intravenous Immune Globulin E Hyperimmune Globulin	7 New Technology Group 7
3 Peripheral Vein	3 Percutaneous	F OTL-103 G OTL-200	8 New Technology Group 8
3 Peripheral Vein	3 Percutaneous	H Lovotibeglogene Autotemcel	9 New Technology Group 9
3 Peripheral Vein	3 Percutaneous	J Exagamglogene Autotemcel	8 New Technology Group 8
4 Central Vein	3 Percutaneous	2 Plasma, Convalescent (Nonautologous)	5 New Technology Group 5
4 Central Vein	3 Percutaneous	7 Marnetegragene Autotemcel	A New Technology Group 10
4 Central Vein	3 Percutaneous	B Betibeglogene Autotemcel C Omidubicel	8 New Technology Group 8
4 Central Vein	3 Percutaneous	D High-Dose Intravenous Immune Globulin E Hyperimmune Globulin	7 New Technology Group 7
4 Central Vein	3 Percutaneous	F OTL-103 G OTL-200	8 New Technology Group 8
4 Central Vein	3 Percutaneous	H Lovotibeglogene Autotemcel	9 New Technology Group 9
4 Central Vein	3 Percutaneous	J Exagamglogene Autotemcel	8 New Technology Group 8

DRG Non-OR XW133[B,C]8
DRG Non-OR XW133[F,G]8
DRG Non-OR XW133H9
DRG Non-OR XW133J8
DRG Non-OR XW143[B,C]8
DRG Non-OR XW143[F,G]8
DRG Non-OR XW143H9
DRG Non-OR XW143J8

X New Technology
W Anatomical Regions
H Insertion Definition: Putting in a nonbiological appliance that monitors, assists, performs, or prevents a physiological function but does not physically take the place of a body part
  Explanation: None

Body Part Character 4	Approach Character 5	Device/Substance/Technology Character 6	Qualifier Character 7
D Mouth and Pharynx	7 Via Natural or Artificial Opening	Q Neurostimulator Lead [NT]	7 New Technology Group 7

[NT] XWHD7Q7 for Phagenyx® System

Non-OR Procedure DRG Non-OR Procedure Valid OR Procedure HAC Associated Procedure Combination Only New/Revised April New/Revised October

New Technology

X New Technology
X Physiological Systems
2 Monitoring   Definition: Determining the level of a physiological or physical function repetitively over a period of time
Explanation: None

Body Part Character 4	Approach Character 5	Device/Substance/Technology Character 6	Qualifier Character 7
0 Central Nervous	X External	8 Brain Electrical Activity, Computer-aided Detection and Notification [NT]	9 New Technology Group 9
5 Ciculatory	X External	0 Blood Flow, Adhesive Ultrasound Patch Technology	A New Technology Group 10
F Musculoskeletal	3 Percutaneous	W Muscle Compartment Pressure, Micro-Electro-Mechanical System	9 New Technology Group 9
K Subcutaneous Tissue	X External	P Interstitial Fluid Volume, Sub-Epidermal Moisture using Electrical Biocapacitance	9 New Technology Group 9

[NT] XX20X89 for Ceribell Status Epilepticus Monitor

X New Technology
X Physiological Systems
A Assistance   Definition: Taking over a portion of a physiological function by extracorporeal means
Explanation: None

Body Part Character 4	Approach Character 5	Device/Substance/Technology Character 6	Qualifier Character 7
5 Ciculatory	3 Percutaneous	6 Filtration, Blood Pathogens	A New Technology Group 10

[NC] Noncovered Procedure [LC] Limited Coverage [QA] Questionable OB Admit [NT] New Tech Add-on ✚ Combination Member ♂ Male ♀ Female

New Technology

- **X** New Technology
- **X** Physiological Systems
- **E** Measurement **Definition:** Determining the level of a physiological or physical function at a point in time
  Explanation: None

Body Part Character 4	Approach Character 5	Device/Substance/Technology Character 6	Qualifier Character 7
0 Central Nervous	X External	0 Intracranial Vascular Activity, Computer-aided Assessment	7 New Technology Group 7
0 Central Nervous	X External	1 Intracranial Cerebrospinal Fluid Flow, Computer-aided Triage and Notification	A New Technology Group 10
0 Central Nervous	X External	4 Brain Electrical Activity, Computer-aided Semiologic Analysis	8 New Technology Group 8
2 Cardiac	X External	1 Output, Computer-aided Assessment [NT]	9 New Technology Group 9
3 Arterial	X External	2 Pulmonary Artery Flow, Computer-aided Triage and Notification	7 New Technology Group 7
3 Arterial	X External	5 Coronary Artery Flow, Quantitative Flow Ratio Analysis 6 Coronary Artery Flow, Computer-aided Valve Modeling and Notification	8 New Technology Group 8
5 Circulatory	X External	2 Infection, Phenotypic Fully Automated Rapid Susceptibility Technology with Controlled Inoculum	A New Technology Group 10
5 Circulatory	X External	3 Infection, Whole Blood Reverse Transcription and Quantitative Real-time Polymerase Chain Reaction	8 New Technology Group 8
5 Circulatory	X External	4 Infection, Positive Blood Culture Small Molecule Sensor Array Technology	A New Technology Group 10
5 Circulatory	X External	N Infection, Positive Blood Culture Fluorescence Hybridization for Organism Identification, Concentration and Susceptibility	6 New Technology Group 6
5 Circulatory	X External	R Infection, Mechanical Initial Specimen Diversion Technique Using Active Negative Pressure T Intracranial Arterial Flow, Whole Blood mRNA V Infection, Serum/Plasma Nanoparticle Fluorescence SARS-CoV-2 Antibody Detection	7 New Technology Group 7
5 Circulatory	X External	Y Infection, Other Positive Blood/Isolated Colonies Bimodal Phenotypic Susceptibility Technology	9 New Technology Group 9
9 Nose	7 Via Natural or Artificial Opening	U Infection, Nasopharyngeal Fluid SARS-CoV-2 Polymerase Chain Reaction	7 New Technology Group 7
B Respiratory	X External	Q Infection, Lower Respiratory Fluid Nucleic Acid-base Microbial Detection	6 New Technology Group 6

[NT] XXE2X19 for EchoGo Heart Failure 1.0

- **X** New Technology
- **Y** Extracorporeal
- **0** Introduction **Definition:** Putting in or on a therapeutic, diagnostic, nutritional, physiological, or prophylactic substance except blood or blood products
  Explanation: None

Body Part Character 4	Approach Character 5	Device/Substance/Technology Character 6	Qualifier Character 7
V Vein Graft	X External	8 Endothelial Damage Inhibitor	3 New Technology Group 3
Y Extracorporeal	X External	2 Taurolidine Anti-infective and Heparin Anticoagulant [NT]	8 New Technology Group 8
Y Extracorporeal	X External	3 Nafamostat Anticoagulant	7 New Technology Group 7

[NT] XY0YX28 for DefenCath™

Appendixes

Appendix A: Components of the Medical and Surgical Approach Definitions

ICD-10-PCS Value	Definition	Access Location	Method	Type of Instrumentation	Example
Open (0)	Cutting through the skin or mucous membrane and any other body layers necessary to expose the site of the procedure	Skin or mucous membrane, any other body layers	Cutting	None	Abdominal hysterectomy
Percutaneous (3)	Entry, by puncture or minor incision, of instrumentation through the skin or mucous membrane and any other body layers necessary to reach the site of the procedure	Skin or mucous membrane, any other body layers	Puncture or minor incision	Without visualization	Needle biopsy of liver, Liposuction
Percutaneous endoscopic (4)	Entry, by puncture or minor incision, of instrumentation through the skin or mucous membrane and any other body layers necessary to reach and visualize the site of the procedure	Skin or mucous membrane, any other body layers	Puncture or minor incision	With visualization	Arthroscopy, Laparoscopic cholecystectomy
Via natural or artificial opening (7)	Entry of instrumentation through a natural or artificial external opening to reach the site of the procedure	Natural or artificial external opening	Direct entry	Without visualization	Endotracheal tube insertion, Foley catheter placement
Via natural or artificial opening endoscopic (8)	Entry of instrumentation through a natural or artificial external opening to reach and visualize the site of the procedure	Natural or artificial external opening	Direct entry	With visualization	Sigmoidoscopy, EGD, ERCP
Via natural or artificial opening with percutaneous endoscopic assistance (F)	Entry of instrumentation through a natural or artificial external opening and entry, by puncture or minor incision, of instrumentation through the skin or mucous membrane and any other body layers necessary to aid in the performance of the procedure	Skin or mucous membrane, any other body layers	Direct entry with puncture or minor incision for instrumentation only	With visualization	Laparoscopic-assisted vaginal hysterectomy
External (X)	Procedures performed directly on the skin or mucous membrane and procedures performed indirectly by the application of external force through the skin or mucous membrane	Skin or mucous membrane	Direct or indirect application	None	Closed fracture reduction, Resection of tonsils

The approach comprises three components: the access location, method, and type of instrumentation.

Access location: For procedures performed on an internal body part, the access location specifies the external site through which the site of the procedure is reached. There are two general types of access locations: skin or mucous membranes, and external orifices. Every approach value except external includes one of these two access locations. The skin or mucous membrane can be cut or punctured to reach the procedure site. All open and percutaneous approach values use this access location. The site of a procedure can also be reached through an external opening. External openings can be natural (e.g., mouth) or artificial (e.g., colostomy stoma).

Method: For procedures performed on an internal body part, the method specifies how the external access location is entered. An open method specifies cutting through the skin or mucous membrane and any other intervening body layers necessary to expose the site of the procedure. An instrumentation method specifies the entry of instrumentation through the access location to the internal procedure site. Instrumentation can be introduced by puncture or minor incision, or through an external opening. The puncture or minor incision does not constitute an open approach because it does not expose the site of the procedure. An approach can define multiple methods. For example, Via Natural or Artificial Opening with Percutaneous Endoscopic Assistance includes both the initial entry of instrumentation to reach the site of the procedure, and the placement of additional percutaneous instrumentation into the body part to visualize and assist in the performance of the procedure.

Type of instrumentation: For procedures performed on an internal body part, instrumentation means that specialized equipment is used to perform the procedure. Instrumentation is used in all internal approaches other than the basic open approach. Instrumentation may or may not include the capacity to visualize the procedure site. For example, the instrumentation used to perform a sigmoidoscopy permits the internal site of the procedure to be visualized, while the instrumentation used to perform a needle biopsy of the liver does not. The term "endoscopic" as used in approach values refers to instrumentation that permits a site to be visualized.

Procedures performed directly on the skin or mucous membrane are identified by the external approach (e.g., skin excision). Procedures performed indirectly by the application of external force are also identified by the external approach (e.g., closed reduction of fracture).

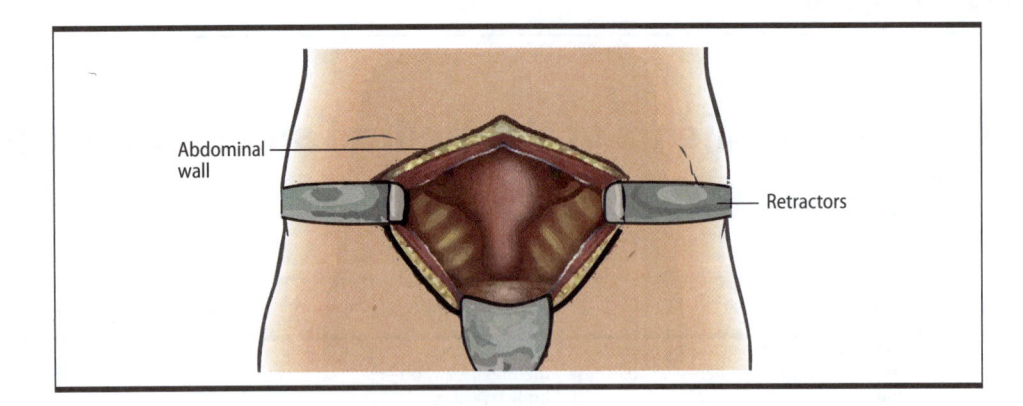

Appendix A: Components of the Medical and Surgical Approach Definitions

Open (0)

Percutaneous (3)

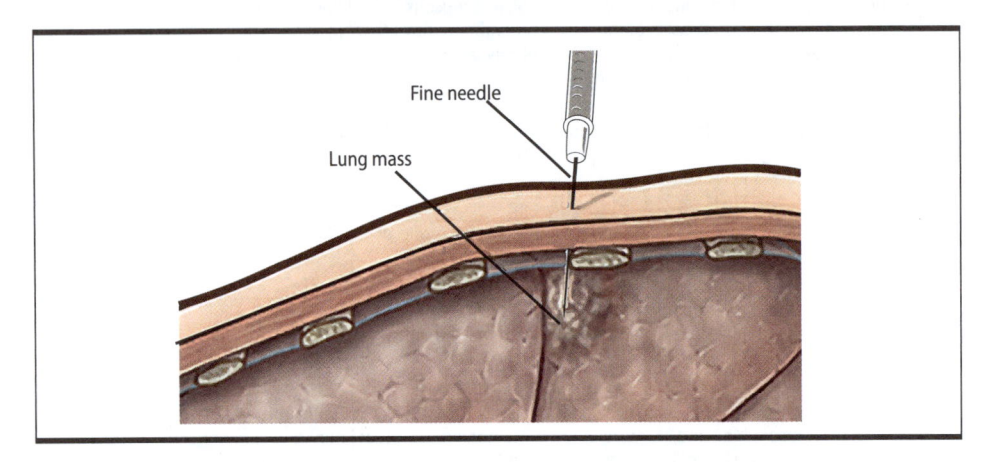

Percutaneous Endoscopic (4)

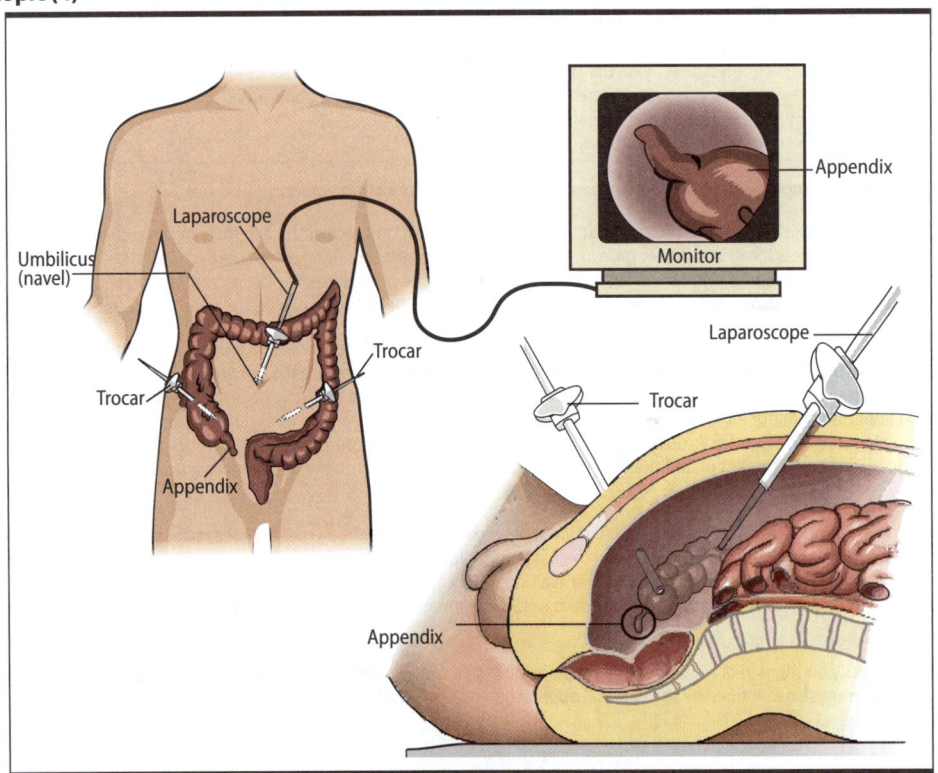

Appendix A: Components of the Medical and Surgical Approach Definitions

Via Natural or Artificial Opening (7)

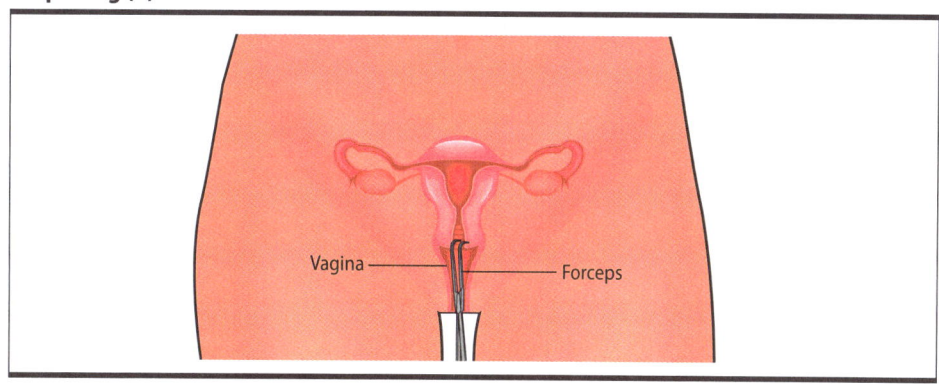

Via Natural or Artificial Opening, Endoscopic (8)

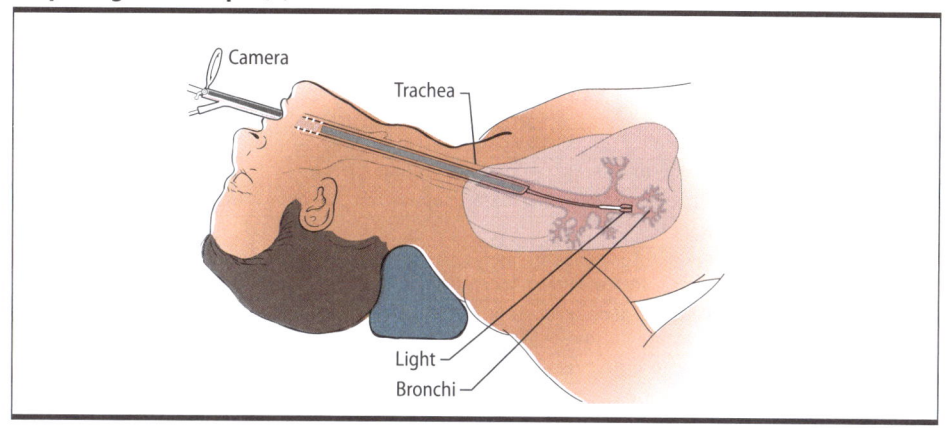

Via Natural or Artificial Opening with Percutaneous Endoscopic Assistance (F)

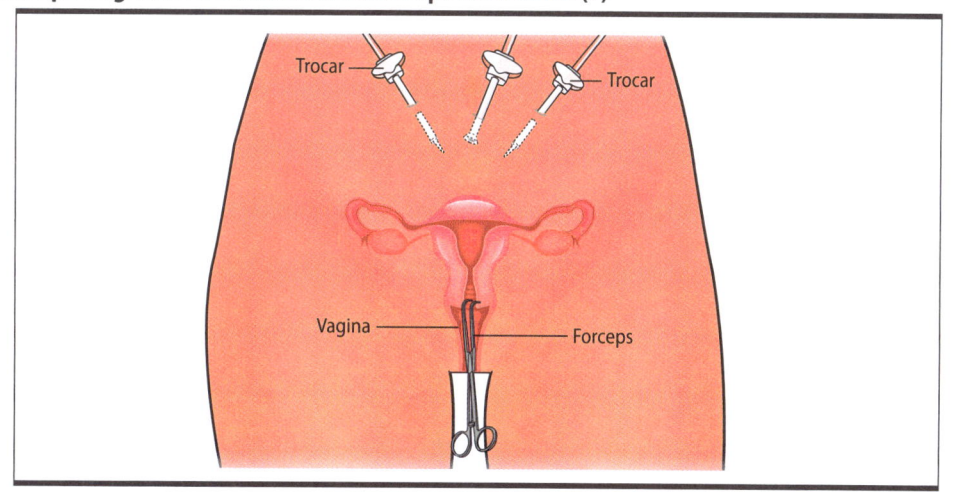

External (X)

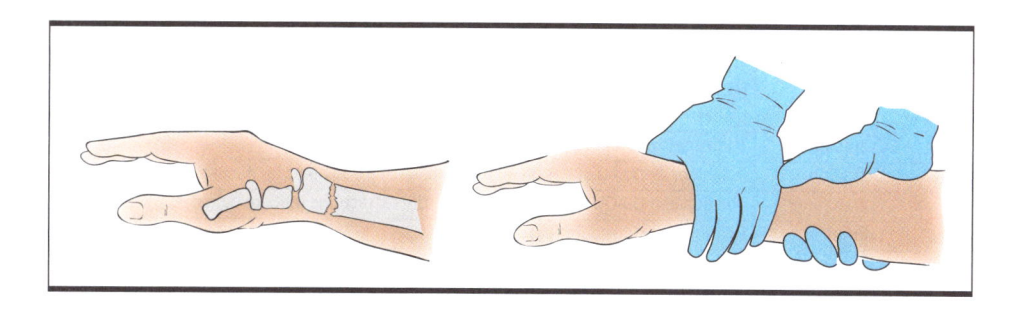

Appendix B: Root Operation Definitions

The character 3 value in the Medical and Surgical section (0) and the Medical and Surgical-related sections (1-9) represents the root operation. This resource provides each root operation (character 3) value, found in sections 0-9, as well as their associated definition, explanation, and examples, where applicable. The Ancillary sections (B-H) do not include root operations; instead, the character 3 value represents the type of procedure performed with additional detail provided by the character 4 or 5 value, when applicable. For the character 3, character 4, and character 5 values used in the Ancillary sections of B-H, along with their definitions, see appendix J.

Ø Medical and Surgical

ICD-10-PCS Value			Definition
Ø	Alteration	Definition:	Modifying the anatomic structure of a body part without affecting the function of the body part
		Explanation:	Principal purpose is to improve appearance
		Examples:	Face lift, breast augmentation
1	Bypass	Definition:	Altering the route of passage of the contents of a tubular body part
		Explanation:	Rerouting contents of a body part to a downstream area of the normal route, to a similar route and body part, or to an abnormal route and dissimilar body part. Includes one or more anastomoses, with or without the use of a device.
		Examples:	Coronary artery bypass, colostomy formation
2	Change	Definition:	Taking out or off a device from a body part and putting back an identical or similar device in or on the same body part without cutting or puncturing the skin or a mucous membrane
		Explanation:	All CHANGE procedures are coded using the approach EXTERNAL
		Examples:	Urinary catheter change, gastrostomy tube change
3	Control	Definition:	Stopping, or attempting to stop, postprocedural or other acute bleeding
		Explanation:	None
		Examples:	Control of post-prostatectomy hemorrhage, control of intracranial subdural hemorrhage, control of bleeding duodenal ulcer, control of retroperitoneal hemorrhage
4	Creation	Definition:	Putting in or on biological or synthetic material to form a new body part that to the extent possible replicates the anatomic structure or function of an absent body part
		Explanation:	Used for gender reassignment surgery and corrective procedures in individuals with congenital anomalies
		Examples:	Creation of vagina in a male, creation of right and left atrioventricular valve from common atrioventricular valve
5	Destruction	Definition:	Physical eradication of all or a portion of a body part by the direct use of energy, force, or a destructive agent
		Explanation:	None of the body part is physically taken out
		Examples:	Fulguration of rectal polyp, cautery of skin lesion
6	Detachment	Definition:	Cutting off all or a portion of the upper or lower extremities
		Explanation:	The body part value is the site of the detachment, with a qualifier if applicable to further specify the level where the extremity was detached
		Examples:	Below knee amputation, disarticulation of shoulder
7	Dilation	Definition:	Expanding an orifice or the lumen of a tubular body part
		Explanation:	The orifice can be a natural orifice or an artificially created orifice. Accomplished by stretching a tubular body part using intraluminal pressure or by cutting part of the orifice or wall of the tubular body part.
		Examples:	Percutaneous transluminal angioplasty, internal urethrotomy
8	Division	Definition:	Cutting into a body part, without draining fluids and/or gases from the body part, in order to separate or transect a body part
		Explanation:	All or a portion of the body part is separated into two or more portions
		Examples:	Spinal cordotomy, osteotomy
9	Drainage	Definition:	Taking or letting out fluids and/or gases from a body part
		Explanation:	The qualifier DIAGNOSTIC is used to identify drainage procedures that are biopsies
		Examples:	Thoracentesis, incision and drainage
B	Excision	Definition:	Cutting out or off, without replacement, a portion of a body part
		Explanation:	The qualifier DIAGNOSTIC is used to identify excision procedures that are biopsies
		Examples:	Partial nephrectomy, liver biopsy
C	Extirpation	Definition:	Taking or cutting out solid matter from a body part
		Explanation:	The solid matter may be an abnormal byproduct of a biological function or a foreign body; it may be imbedded in a body part or in the lumen of a tubular body part. The solid matter may or may not have been previously broken into pieces.
		Examples:	Thrombectomy, choledocholithotomy
D	Extraction	Definition:	Pulling or stripping out or off all or a portion of a body part by the use of force
		Explanation:	The qualifier DIAGNOSTIC is used to identify extractions that are biopsies
		Examples:	Dilation and curettage, vein stripping

Continued on next page

Appendix B: Root Operation Definitions

0 — Medical and Surgical (Continued from previous page)

ICD-10-PCS Value			Definition
F	Fragmentation	Definition:	Breaking solid matter in a body part into pieces
		Explanation:	Physical force (e.g., manual, ultrasonic) applied directly or indirectly is used to break the solid matter into pieces. The solid matter may be an abnormal byproduct of a biological function or a foreign body. The pieces of solid matter are not taken out.
		Examples:	Extracorporeal shockwave lithotripsy, transurethral lithotripsy
G	Fusion	Definition:	Joining together portions of an articular body part rendering the articular body part immobile
		Explanation:	The body part is joined together by fixation device, bone graft, or other means
		Examples:	Spinal fusion, ankle arthrodesis
H	Insertion	Definition:	Putting in a nonbiological appliance that monitors, assists, performs, or prevents a physiological function but does not physically take the place of a body part
		Explanation:	None
		Examples:	Insertion of radioactive implant, insertion of central venous catheter
J	Inspection	Definition:	Visually and/or manually exploring a body part
		Explanation:	Visual exploration may be performed with or without optical instrumentation. Manual exploration may be performed directly or through intervening body layers.
		Examples:	Diagnostic arthroscopy, exploratory laparotomy
K	Map	Definition:	Locating the route of passage of electrical impulses and/or locating functional areas in a body part
		Explanation:	Applicable only to the cardiac conduction mechanism and the central nervous system
		Examples:	Cardiac mapping, cortical mapping
L	Occlusion	Definition:	Completely closing an orifice or lumen of a tubular body part
		Explanation:	The orifice can be a natural orifice or an artificially created orifice
		Examples:	Fallopian tube ligation, ligation of inferior vena cava
M	Reattachment	Definition:	Putting back in or on all or a portion of a separated body part to its normal location or other suitable location
		Explanation:	Vascular circulation and nervous pathways may or may not be reestablished
		Examples:	Reattachment of hand, reattachment of avulsed kidney
N	Release	Definition:	Freeing a body part from an abnormal physical constraint by cutting or by use of force
		Explanation:	Some of the restraining tissue may be taken out but none of the body part is taken out
		Examples:	Adhesiolysis, carpal tunnel release
P	Removal	Definition:	Taking out or off a device from a body part
		Explanation:	If a device is taken out and a similar device put in without cutting or puncturing the skin or mucous membrane, the procedure is coded to the root operation CHANGE. Otherwise, the procedure for taking out a device is coded to the root operation REMOVAL.
		Examples:	Drainage tube removal, cardiac pacemaker removal
Q	Repair	Definition:	Restoring, to the extent possible, a body part to its normal anatomic structure and function
		Explanation:	Used only when the method to accomplish the repair is not one of the other root operations
		Examples:	Colostomy takedown, suture of laceration
R	Replacement	Definition:	Putting in or on biological or synthetic material that physically takes the place and/or function of all or a portion of a body part
		Explanation:	The body part may have been taken out or replaced, or may be taken out, physically eradicated, or rendered nonfunctional during the REPLACEMENT procedure. A REMOVAL procedure is coded for taking out the device used in a previous replacement procedure.
		Examples:	Total hip replacement, bone graft, free skin graft
S	Reposition	Definition:	Moving to its normal location, or other suitable location, all or a portion of a body part
		Explanation:	The body part is moved to a new location from an abnormal location, or from a normal location where it is not functioning correctly. The body part may or may not be cut out or off to be moved to the new location.
		Examples:	Reposition of undescended testicle, fracture reduction
T	Resection	Definition:	Cutting out or off, without replacement, all of a body part
		Explanation:	None
		Examples:	Total nephrectomy, total lobectomy of lung
V	Restriction	Definition:	Partially closing an orifice or the lumen of a tubular body part
		Explanation:	The orifice can be a natural orifice or an artificially created orifice
		Examples:	Esophagogastric fundoplication, cervical cerclage
W	Revision	Definition:	Correcting, to the extent possible, a portion of a malfunctioning device or the position of a displaced device
		Explanation:	Revision can include correcting a malfunctioning or displaced device by taking out or putting in components of the device such as a screw or pin
		Examples:	Adjustment of position of pacemaker lead, recementing of hip prosthesis

Continued on next page

Appendix B: Root Operation Definitions

0 — Medical and Surgical

Continued from previous page

ICD-10-PCS Value			Definition
U	Supplement	Definition:	Putting in or on biological or synthetic material that physically reinforces and/or augments the function of a portion of a body part
		Explanation:	The biological material is non-living, or is living and from the same individual. The body part may have been previously replaced, and the SUPPLEMENT procedure is performed to physically reinforce and/or augment the function of the replaced body part.
		Examples:	Herniorrhaphy using mesh, mitral valve ring annuloplasty, put a new acetabular liner in a previous hip replacement
X	Transfer	Definition:	Moving, without taking out, all or a portion of a body part to another location to take over the function of all or a portion of a body part
		Explanation:	The body part transferred remains connected to its vascular and nervous supply
		Examples:	Tendon transfer, skin pedicle flap transfer
Y	Transplantation	Definition:	Putting in or on all or a portion of a living body part taken from another individual or animal to physically take the place and/or function of all or a portion of a similar body part
		Explanation:	The native body part may or may not be taken out, and the transplanted body part may take over all or a portion of its function
		Examples:	Kidney transplant, heart transplant

Root Operation Definitions for Other Sections

1 — Obstetrics

ICD-10-PCS Value			Definition
2	Change	Definition:	Taking out or off a device from a body part and putting back an identical or similar device in or on the same body part without cutting or puncturing the skin or a mucous membrane
		Explanation:	None
		Example:	Replacement of fetal scalp electrode
9	Drainage	Definition:	Taking or letting out fluids and/or gases from a body part
		Explanation:	None
		Example:	Biopsy of amniotic fluid
A	Abortion	Definition:	Artificially terminating a pregnancy
		Explanation:	None
		Example:	Transvaginal abortion using vacuum aspiration technique
D	Extraction	Definition:	Pulling or stripping out or off all or a portion of a body part by the use of force
		Explanation:	None
		Example:	Low-transverse C-section
E	Delivery	Definition:	Assisting the passage of the products of conception from the genital canal
		Explanation:	None
		Example:	Manually-assisted delivery
H	Insertion	Definition:	Putting in a nonbiological appliance that monitors, assists, performs, or prevents a physiological function but does not physically take the place of a body part
		Explanation:	None
		Example:	Placement of fetal scalp electrode
J	Inspection	Definition:	Visually and/or manually exploring a body part
		Explanation:	Visual exploration may be performed with or without optical instrumentation. Manual exploration may be performed directly or through intervening body layers.
		Example:	Bimanual pregnancy exam
P	Removal	Definition:	Taking out or off a device from a body part, region or orifice
		Explanation:	If a device is taken out and a similar device put in without cutting or puncturing the skin or mucous membrane, the procedure is coded to the root operation CHANGE. Otherwise, the procedure for taking out a device is coded to the root operation REMOVAL.
		Example:	Removal of fetal monitoring electrode
Q	Repair	Definition:	Restoring, to the extent possible, a body part to its normal anatomic structure and function
		Explanation:	Used only when the method to accomplish the repair is not one of the other root operations
		Example:	In utero repair of congenital diaphragmatic hernia
S	Reposition	Definition:	Moving to its normal location, or other suitable location, all or a portion of a body part
		Explanation:	The body part is moved to a new location from an abnormal location, or from a normal location where it is not functioning correctly. The body part may or may not be cut out or off to be moved to the new location.
		Example:	External version of fetus
T	Resection	Definition:	Cutting out or off, without replacement, all of a body part
		Explanation:	None
		Example:	Total excision of tubal pregnancy

Continued on next page

1 Obstetrics

Continued from previous page

ICD-10-PCS Value		Definition
Y Transplantation	Definition:	Putting in or on all or a portion of a living body part taken from another individual or animal to physically take the place and/or function of all or a portion of a similar body part
	Explanation:	The native body part may or may not be taken out, and the transplanted body part may take over all or a portion of its function
	Example:	In utero fetal kidney transplant

2 Placement

ICD-10-PCS Value		Definition
0 Change	Definition:	Taking out or off a device from a body part and putting back an identical or similar device in or on the same body part without cutting or puncturing the skin or a mucous membrane
	Example:	Change of vaginal packing
1 Compression	Definition:	Putting pressure on a body region
	Example:	Placement of pressure dressing on abdominal wall
2 Dressing	Definition:	Putting material on a body region for protection
	Example:	Application of sterile dressing to head wound
3 Immobilization	Definition:	Limiting or preventing motion of a body region
	Example:	Placement of splint on left finger
4 Packing	Definition:	Putting material in a body region or orifice
	Example:	Placement of nasal packing
5 Removal	Definition:	Taking out or off a device from a body part
	Example:	Removal of stereotactic head frame
6 Traction	Definition:	Exerting a pulling force on a body region in a distal direction
	Example:	Lumbar traction using motorized split-traction table

3 Administration

ICD-10-PCS Value		Definition
0 Introduction	Definition:	Putting in or on a therapeutic, diagnostic, nutritional, physiological, or prophylactic substance except blood or blood products
	Example:	Nerve block injection to median nerve
1 Irrigation	Definition:	Putting in or on a cleansing substance
	Example:	Flushing of eye
2 Transfusion	Definition:	Putting in blood or blood products
	Example:	Transfusion of cell saver red cells into central venous line

4 Measurement and Monitoring

ICD-10-PCS Value		Definition
0 Measurement	Definition:	Determining the level of a physiological or physical function at a point in time
	Example:	External electrocardiogram(EKG), single reading
1 Monitoring	Definition:	Determining the level of a physiological or physical function repetitively over a period of time
	Example:	Urinary pressure monitoring

5 Extracorporeal or Systemic Assistance and Performance

ICD-10-PCS Value		Definition
0 Assistance	Definition:	Taking over a portion of a physiological function by extracorporeal means
	Example:	Hyperbaric oxygenation of wound
1 Performance	Definition:	Completely taking over a physiological function by extracorporeal means
	Example:	Cardiopulmonary bypass in conjunction with CABG
2 Restoration	Definition:	Returning, or attempting to return, a physiological function to its original state by extracorporeal means
	Example:	Attempted cardiac defibrillation, unsuccessful

6 Extracorporeal or Systemic Therapies

ICD-10-PCS Value		Definition
0	Atmospheric Control	Definition: Extracorporeal control of atmospheric pressure and composition
		Example: Antigen-free air conditioning, series treatment
1	Decompression	Definition: Extracorporeal elimination of undissolved gas from body fluids
		Example: Hyperbaric decompression treatment, single
2	Electromagnetic Therapy	Definition: Extracorporeal treatment by electromagnetic rays
		Example: TMS (transcranial magnetic stimulation), series treatment
3	Hyperthermia	Definition: Extracorporeal raising of body temperature
		Example: None
4	Hypothermia	Definition: Extracorporeal lowering of body temperature
		Example: Whole body hypothermia treatment for temperature imbalances, series
5	Pheresis	Definition: Extracorporeal separation of blood products
		Example: Therapeutic leukopheresis, single treatment
6	Phototherapy	Definition: Extracorporeal treatment by light rays
		Example: Phototherapy of circulatory system, series treatment
7	Ultrasound Therapy	Definition: Extracorporeal treatment by ultrasound
		Example: Therapeutic ultrasound of peripheral vessels, single treatment
8	Ultraviolet Light Therapy	Definition: Extracorporeal treatment by ultraviolet light
		Example: Ultraviolet light phototherapy, series treatment
9	Shock Wave Therapy	Definition: Extracorporeal treatment by shock waves
		Example: Shockwave therapy of plantar fascia, single treatment
B	Perfusion	Definition: Extracorporeal treatment by diffusion of therapeutic fluid
		Example: Perfusion of donor liver while preparing transplant patient

7 Osteopathic

ICD-10-PCS Value		Definition
0	Treatment	Definition: Manual treatment to eliminate or alleviate somatic dysfunction and related disorders
		Examples: Fascial release of abdomen, osteopathic treatment

8 Other Procedures

ICD-10-PCS Value		Definition
0	Other Procedures	Definition: Methodologies which attempt to remediate or cure a disorder or disease
		Examples: Acupuncture, yoga therapy

9 Chiropractic

ICD-10-PCS Value		Definition
B	Manipulation	Definition: Manual procedure that involves a directed thrust to move a joint past the physiological range of motion, without exceeding the anatomical limit
		Example: Chiropractic treatment of cervical spine, short lever specific contact

Appendix C: Comparison of Medical and Surgical Root Operations

Note: The character associated with each operation appears in parentheses after its title.

Procedures That Take Out Some or All of a Body Part

Root Operation	Objective of Procedure	Site of Procedure	Example
Destruction (5)	Eradicating without taking out or replacement	Some/all of a body part	Fulguration of endometrium
Detachment (6)	Cutting out/off without replacement	Extremity only, any level	Amputation above elbow
Excision (B)	Cutting out/off without replacement	Some of a body part	Breast lumpectomy
Extraction (D)	Pulling out/off without replacement	Some/all of a body part	Suction D&C
Resection (T)	Cutting out/off without replacement	All of a body part	Total mastectomy

Procedures That Put In/Put Back or Move Some/All of a Body Part

Root Operation	Objective of Procedure	Site of Procedure	Example
Reattachment (M)	Putting back a detached body part	Some/all of a body part	Reattach finger
Reposition (S)	Moving a body part to normal or other suitable location	Some/all of a body part	Move undescended testicle
Transfer (X)	Moving a body part to function for a similar body part	Some/all of a body part	Skin pedicle transfer flap
Transplantation (Y)	Putting in a living body part from a person/animal	Some/all of a body part	Kidney transplant

Procedures That Take Out or Eliminate Solid Matter, Fluids, or Gases From a Body Part

Root Operation	Objective of Procedure	Site of Procedure	Example
Drainage (9)	Taking or letting out	Fluids and/or gases from a body part	Incision and drainage
Extirpation (C)	Taking or cutting out	Solid matter in a body part	Thrombectomy
Fragmentation (F)	Breaking into pieces	Solid matter within a body part	Lithotripsy

Procedures That Involve Only Examination of Body Parts and Regions

Root Operation	Objective of Procedure	Site of Procedure	Example
Inspection (J)	Visual/manual exploration	Some/all of a body part	Diagnostic cystoscopy Exploratory laparoscopy
Map (K)	Locating electrical impulse route/functional areas	Brain/cardiac conduction mechanism	Cardiac mapping

Procedures That Alter the Diameter/Route of a Tubular Body Part

Root Operation	Objective of Procedure	Site of Procedure	Example
Bypass (1)	Altering route of passage of contents	Tubular body part	Coronary artery bypass graft (CABG)
Dilation (7)	Expanding natural or artificially created orifice/lumen	Tubular body part	Percutaneous transluminal coronary angioplasty (PTCA)
Occlusion (L)	Completely closing natural or artificially created orifice/lumen	Tubular body part	Fallopian tube ligation
Restriction (V)	Partially closing natural or artificially created orifice/lumen	Tubular body part	Gastroesophageal fundoplication

Appendix C: Comparison of Medical and Surgical Root Operations

Procedures That Always Involve Devices

Root Operation		Objective of Procedure	Site of Procedure	Example
Change (2)	DVC	Exchanging device w/out cutting/puncturing	In/on a body part	Gastrostomy tube change
Insertion (H)	DVC	Putting in nonbiological device	In/on a body part	Central line insertion
Removal (P)	DVC	Taking out device	In/on a body part	Central line removal
Replacement (R)	DVC	Putting in device that replaces a body part	Some/all of a body part	Total hip replacement
Revision (W)	DVC	Correcting a malfunctioning/displaced device	In/on a body part	Revision of pacemaker
Supplement (U)	DVC	Putting in device that reinforces or augments a body part	In/on a body part	Abdominal wall herniorrhaphy using mesh

DVC = Device involved in root operation

Procedures Involving Cutting or Separation Only

Root Operation	Objective of Procedure	Site of Procedure	Example
Division (8)	Cutting into/separating	A body part	Neurotomy
Release (N)	Freeing a body part from constraint	Around a body part	Adhesiolysis

Procedures That Define Other Repairs

Root Operation	Objective of Procedure	Site of Procedure	Example
Control (3)	Stopping/attempting to stop postprocedural or other acute bleeding	Anatomical region or nasal mucosa/soft tissue	Post-prostatectomy bleeding control, control subdural hemorrhage, bleeding ulcer, retroperitoneal hemorrhage
Repair (Q)	Restoring body part to its normal structure/function	Some/all of a body part	Suture laceration

Procedures That Define Other Objectives

Root Operation	Objective of Procedure	Site of Procedure	Example
Alteration (Ø)	Modifying body part for cosmetic purposes without affecting function	Some/all of a body part	Face lift
Creation (4)	Using biological or synthetic material to form a new body part that replicates the anatomic structure or function of a missing body part	Perineum, valve	Sex change/artificial vagina/penis, atrioventricular valve creation
Fusion (G)	Unification or immobilization	Joint or articular body part	Spinal fusion

Appendix D: Body Part Key

Term	ICD-10-PCS Value
Abdominal aortic plexus	Abdominal Sympathetic Nerve
Abdominal cavity	Peritoneal Cavity
Abdominal esophagus	Esophagus, Lower
Abductor hallucis muscle	Foot Muscle, Right
	Foot Muscle, Left
Accessory cephalic vein	Cephalic Vein, Right
	Cephalic Vein, Left
Accessory obturator nerve	Lumbar Plexus
Accessory phrenic nerve	Phrenic nerve
Accessory spleen	Spleen
Acetabulofemoral joint	Hip Joint, Right
	Hip Joint, Left
Achilles tendon	Lower Leg Tendon, Right
	Lower Leg Tendon, Left
Acromioclavicular ligament	Shoulder Bursa and Ligament, Right
	Shoulder Bursa and Ligament, Left
Acromion (process)	Scapula, Right
	Scapula, Left
Adductor brevis muscle	Upper Leg Muscle, Right
	Upper Leg Muscle, Left
Adductor hallucis muscle	Foot Muscle, Right
	Foot Muscle, Left
Adductor longus muscle	Upper Leg Muscle, Right
	Upper Leg Muscle, Left
Adductor magnus muscle	Upper Leg Muscle, Right
	Upper Leg Muscle, Left
Adductor pollicis muscle	Hand Muscle, Right
	Hand Muscle, Left
Adenohypophysis	Pituitary Gland
Alar ligament of axis	Head and Neck Bursa and Ligament
Alveolar process of mandible	Mandible, Right
	Mandible, Left
Alveolar process of maxilla	Maxilla
Anal orifice	Anus
Anatomical snuffbox	Lower Arm and Wrist Muscle, Right
	Lower Arm and Wrist Muscle, Left
Anconeus muscle	Lower Arm and Wrist Muscle, Right
	Lower Arm and Wrist Muscle, Left
Angular artery	Face Artery
Angular vein	Face Vein, Right
	Face Vein, Left
Annular ligament	Elbow Bursa and Ligament, Right
	Elbow Bursa and Ligament, Left
Anorectal junction	Rectum
Ansa cervicalis	Cervical Plexus
Antebrachial fascia	Subcutaneous Tissue and Fascia, Right Lower Arm
	Subcutaneous Tissue and Fascia, Left Lower Arm
Anterior (pectoral) lymph node	Lymphatic, Right Axillary
	Lymphatic, Left Axillary
Anterior cerebral artery	Intracranial Artery
Anterior cerebral vein	Intracranial Vein
Anterior choroidal artery	Intracranial Artery
Anterior circumflex humeral artery	Axillary Artery, Right
	Axillary Artery, Left

Term	ICD-10-PCS Value
Anterior communicating artery	Intracranial Artery
Anterior cruciate ligament (ACL)	Knee Bursa and Ligament, Right
	Knee Bursa and Ligament, Left
Anterior crural nerve	Femoral Nerve
Anterior facial vein	Face Vein, Right
	Face Vein, Left
Anterior intercostal artery	Internal Mammary Artery, Right
	Internal Mammary Artery, Left
Anterior interosseous nerve	Median Nerve
Anterior lateral malleolar artery	Anterior Tibial Artery, Right
	Anterior Tibial Artery, Left
Anterior lingual gland	Minor Salivary Gland
Anterior medial malleolar artery	Anterior Tibial Artery, Right
	Anterior Tibial Artery, Left
Anterior spinal artery	Vertebral Artery, Right
	Vertebral Artery, Left
Anterior tibial recurrent artery	Anterior Tibial Artery, Right
	Anterior Tibial Artery, Left
Anterior ulnar recurrent artery	Ulnar Artery, Right
	Ulnar Artery, Left
Anterior vagal trunk	Vagus Nerve
Anterior vertebral muscle	Neck Muscle, Right
	Neck Muscle, Left
Antihelix	External Ear, Right
	External Ear, Left
	External Ear, Bilateral
Antitragus	External Ear, Right
	External Ear, Left
	External Ear, Bilateral
Antrum of Highmore	Maxillary Sinus, Right
	Maxillary Sinus, Left
Aortic annulus	Aortic Valve
Aortic arch	Thoracic Aorta, Ascending/Arch
Aortic intercostal artery	Upper Artery
Aortic isthmus	Thoracic Aorta, Ascending/Arch
Apical (subclavicular) lymph node	Lymphatic, Right Axillary
	Lymphatic, Left Axillary
Apneustic center	Pons
Appendiceal orifice	Appendix
Aqueduct of Sylvius	Cerebral Ventricle
Aqueous humour	Anterior Chamber, Right
	Anterior Chamber, Left
Arachnoid mater, intracranial	Cerebral Meninges
Arachnoid mater, spinal	Spinal Meninges
Arcuate artery	Foot Artery, Right
	Foot Artery, Left
Areola	Nipple, Right
	Nipple, Left
Arterial canal (duct)	Pulmonary Artery, Left
Aryepiglottic fold	Larynx
Arytenoid cartilage	Larynx
Arytenoid muscle	Neck Muscle, Right
	Neck Muscle, Left
Ascending aorta	Thoracic Aorta, Ascending/Arch
Ascending palatine artery	Face Artery

Appendix D: Body Part Key

Term	ICD-10-PCS Value
Ascending pharyngeal artery	External Carotid Artery, Right
	External Carotid Artery, Left
Atlantoaxial joint	Cervical Vertebral Joint
Atrioventricular node	Conduction Mechanism
Atrium dextrum cordis	Atrium, Right
Atrium pulmonale	Atrium, Left
Auditory tube	Eustachian Tube, Right
	Eustachian Tube, Left
Auerbach's (myenteric) plexus	Abdominal Sympathetic Nerve
Auricle	External Ear, Right
	External Ear, Left
	External Ear, Bilateral
Auricularis muscle	Head Muscle
Axillary fascia	Subcutaneous Tissue and Fascia, Right Upper Arm
	Subcutaneous Tissue and Fascia, Left Upper Arm
Axillary nerve	Brachial Plexus
Bartholin's (greater vestibular) gland	Vestibular Gland
Basal (internal) cerebral vein	Intracranial Vein
Basal nuclei	Basal Ganglia
Base of tongue	Pharynx
Basilar artery	Intracranial Artery
Basis pontis	Pons
Biceps brachii muscle	Upper Arm Muscle, Right
	Upper Arm Muscle, Left
Biceps femoris muscle	Upper Leg Muscle, Right
	Upper Leg Muscle, Left
Bicipital aponeurosis	Subcutaneous Tissue and Fascia, Right Lower Arm
	Subcutaneous Tissue and Fascia, Left Lower Arm
Bicuspid valve	Mitral Valve
Body of femur	Femoral Shaft, Right
	Femoral Shaft, Left
Body of fibula	Fibula, Right
	Fibula, Left
Bony labyrinth	Inner Ear, Right
	Inner Ear, Left
Bony orbit	Orbit, Right
	Orbit, Left
Bony vestibule	Inner Ear, Right
	Inner Ear, Left
Botallo's duct	Pulmonary Artery, Left
Brachial (lateral) lymph node	Lymphatic, Right Axillary
	Lymphatic, Left Axillary
Brachialis muscle	Upper Arm Muscle, Right
	Upper Arm Muscle, Left
Brachiocephalic artery	Innominate Artery
Brachiocephalic trunk	Innominate Artery
Brachiocephalic vein	Innominate Vein, Right
	Innominate Vein, Left
Brachioradialis muscle	Lower Arm and Wrist Muscle, Right
	Lower Arm and Wrist Muscle, Left
Breast procedures, skin only	Skin, Chest
Broad ligament	Uterine Supporting Structure
Bronchial artery	Upper Artery
Bronchus intermedius	Main Bronchus, Right
Buccal gland	Buccal Mucosa

Term	ICD-10-PCS Value
Buccinator lymph node	Lymphatic, Head
Buccinator muscle	Facial Muscle
Bulbospongiosus muscle	Perineum Muscle
Bulbourethral (Cowper's) gland	Urethra
Bundle of His	Conduction Mechanism
Bundle of Kent	Conduction Mechanism
Calcaneocuboid joint	Tarsal Joint, Right
	Tarsal Joint, Left
Calcaneocuboid ligament	Foot Bursa and Ligament, Right
	Foot Bursa and Ligament, Left
Calcaneofibular ligament	Ankle Bursa and Ligament, Right
	Ankle Bursa and Ligament, Left
Calcaneus	Tarsal, Right
	Tarsal, Left
Capitate bone	Carpal, Right
	Carpal, Left
Cardia	Esophagogastric Junction
Cardiac plexus	Thoracic Sympathetic Nerve
Cardioesophageal junction	Esophagogastric Junction
Caroticotympanic artery	Internal Carotid Artery, Right
	Internal Carotid Artery, Left
Carotid glomus	Carotid Body, Right
	Carotid Body, Left
	Carotid Bodies, Bilateral
Carotid sinus	Internal Carotid Artery, Right
	Internal Carotid Artery, Left
Carotid sinus nerve	Glossopharyngeal Nerve
Carpometacarpal ligament	Hand Bursa and Ligament, Right
	Hand Bursa and Ligament, Left
Cauda equina	Lumbar Spinal Cord
Cavernous plexus	Head and Neck Sympathetic Nerve
Cavoatrial junction	Superior Vena Cava
Celiac ganglion	Abdominal Sympathetic Nerve
Celiac (solar) plexus	Abdominal Sympathetic Nerve
Celiac lymph node	Lymphatic, Aortic
Celiac trunk	Celiac Artery
Central axillary lymph node	Lymphatic, Right Axillary
	Lymphatic, Left Axillary
Cerebral aqueduct (Sylvius)	Cerebral Ventricle
Cerebrum	Brain
Cervical esophagus	Esophagus, Upper
Cervical facet joint	Cervical Vertebral Joint
	Cervical Vertebral Joints, 2 or more
Cervical ganglion	Head and Neck Sympathetic Nerve
Cervical interspinous ligament	Head and Neck Bursa and Ligament
Cervical intertransverse ligament	Head and Neck Bursa and Ligament
Cervical ligamentum flavum	Head and Neck Bursa and Ligament
Cervical lymph node	Lymphatic, Right Neck
	Lymphatic, Left Neck
Cervicothoracic facet joint	Cervicothoracic Vertebral Joint
Chin	Subcutaneous Tissue and Fascia, Face
Choana	Nasopharynx
Chondroglossus muscle	Tongue, Palate, Pharynx Muscle
Chorda tympani	Facial Nerve
Choroid plexus	Cerebral Ventricle
Ciliary body	Eye, Right
	Eye, Left
Ciliary ganglion	Head and Neck Sympathetic Nerve

Term	ICD-10-PCS Value
Circle of Willis	Intracranial Artery
Circumflex iliac artery	Femoral Artery, Right
	Femoral Artery, Left
Claustrum	Basal Ganglia
Coccygeal body	Coccygeal Glomus
Coccygeus muscle	Trunk Muscle, Right
	Trunk Muscle, Left
Cochlea	Inner Ear, Right
	Inner Ear, Left
Cochlear nerve	Acoustic Nerve
Columella	Nasal Mucosa and Soft Tissue
Common digital vein	Foot Vein, Right
	Foot Vein, Left
Common facial vein	Face Vein, Right
	Face Vein, Left
Common fibular nerve	Peroneal Nerve
Common hepatic artery	Hepatic Artery
Common iliac (subaortic) lymph node	Lymphatic, Pelvis
Common interosseous artery	Ulnar Artery, Right
	Ulnar Artery, Left
Common peroneal nerve	Peroneal Nerve
Condyloid process	Mandible, Right
	Mandible, Left
Conus arteriosus	Ventricle, Right
Conus medullaris	Lumbar Spinal Cord
Coracoacromial ligament	Shoulder Bursa and Ligament, Right
	Shoulder Bursa and Ligament, Left
Coracobrachialis muscle	Upper Arm Muscle, Right
	Upper Arm Muscle, Left
Coracoclavicular ligament	Shoulder Bursa and Ligament, Right
	Shoulder Bursa and Ligament, Left
Coracohumeral ligament	Shoulder Bursa and Ligament, Right
	Shoulder Bursa and Ligament, Left
Coracoid process	Scapula, Right
	Scapula, Left
Corniculate cartilage	Larynx
Corpus callosum	Brain
Corpus cavernosum	Penis
Corpus spongiosum	Penis
Corpus striatum	Basal Ganglia
Corrugator supercilii muscle	Facial Muscle
Costocervical trunk	Subclavian Artery, Right
	Subclavian Artery, Left
Costoclavicular ligament	Shoulder Bursa and Ligament, Right
	Shoulder Bursa and Ligament, Left
Costotransverse joint	Thoracic Vertebral Joint
Costotransverse ligament	Rib(s) Bursa and Ligament
Costovertebral joint	Thoracic Vertebral Joint
Costoxiphoid ligament	Sternum Bursa and Ligament
Cowper's (bulbourethral) gland	Urethra
Cremaster muscle	Perineum Muscle
Cribriform plate	Ethmoid Bone, Right
	Ethmoid Bone, Left
Cricoid cartilage	Trachea
Cricothyroid artery	Thyroid Artery, Right
	Thyroid Artery, Left
Cricothyroid muscle	Neck Muscle, Right
	Neck Muscle, Left

Term	ICD-10-PCS Value
Crural fascia	Subcutaneous Tissue and Fascia, Right Upper Leg
	Subcutaneous Tissue and Fascia, Left Upper Leg
Cubital lymph node	Lymphatic, Right Upper Extremity
	Lymphatic, Left Upper Extremity
Cubital nerve	Ulnar Nerve
Cuboid bone	Tarsal, Right
	Tarsal, Left
Cuboideonavicular joint	Tarsal Joint, Right
	Tarsal Joint, Left
Culmen	Cerebellum
Cuneiform cartilage	Larynx
Cuneonavicular joint	Tarsal Joint, Right
	Tarsal Joint, Left
Cuneonavicular ligament	Foot Bursa and Ligament, Right
	Foot Bursa and Ligament, Left
Cutaneous (transverse) cervical nerve	Cervical Plexus
Deep cervical fascia	Subcutaneous Tissue and Fascia, Right Neck
	Subcutaneous Tissue and Fascia, Left Neck
Deep cervical vein	Vertebral Vein, Right
	Vertebral Vein, Left
Deep circumflex iliac artery	External Iliac Artery, Right
	External Iliac Artery, Left
Deep facial vein	Face Vein, Right
	Face Vein, Left
Deep femoral artery	Femoral Artery, Right
	Femoral Artery, Left
Deep femoral (profunda femoris) vein	Femoral Vein, Right
	Femoral Vein, Left
Deep palmar arch	Hand Artery, Right
	Hand Artery, Left
Deep transverse perineal muscle	Perineum Muscle
Deferential artery	Internal Iliac Artery, Right
	Internal Iliac Artery, Left
Deltoid fascia	Subcutaneous Tissue and Fascia, Right Upper Arm
	Subcutaneous Tissue and Fascia, Left Upper Arm
Deltoid ligament	Ankle Bursa and Ligament, Right
	Ankle Bursa and Ligament, Left
Deltoid muscle	Shoulder Muscle, Right
	Shoulder Muscle, Left
Deltopectoral (infraclavicular) lymph node	Lymphatic, Right Upper Extremity
	Lymphatic, Left Upper Extremity
Dens	Cervical Vertebra
Denticulate (dentate) ligament	Spinal Meninges
Depressor anguli oris muscle	Facial Muscle
Depressor labii inferioris muscle	Facial Muscle
Depressor septi nasi muscle	Facial Muscle
Depressor supercilii muscle	Facial Muscle
Dermis	Skin
Descending genicular artery	Femoral Artery, Right
	Femoral Artery, Left
Diaphragma sellae	Dura Mater
Distal humerus	Humeral Shaft, Right
	Humeral Shaft, Left

Term	ICD-10-PCS Value
Distal humerus, involving joint	Elbow Joint, Right
	Elbow Joint, Left
Distal radioulnar joint	Wrist Joint, Right
	Wrist Joint, Left
Dorsal digital nerve	Radial Nerve
Dorsal metacarpal vein	Hand Vein, Right
	Hand Vein, Left
Dorsal metatarsal artery	Foot Artery, Right
	Foot Artery, Left
Dorsal metatarsal vein	Foot Vein, Right
	Foot Vein, Left
Dorsal root ganglion	Cervical Spinal Cord
	Lumbar Spinal Cord
	Spinal Cord
	Thoracic Spinal Cord
Dorsal scapular artery	Subclavian Artery, Right
	Subclavian Artery, Left
Dorsal scapular nerve	Brachial Plexus
Dorsal venous arch	Foot Vein, Right
	Foot Vein, Left
Dorsalis pedis artery	Anterior Tibial Artery, Right
	Anterior Tibial Artery, Left
Duct of Santorini	Pancreatic Duct, Accessory
Duct of Wirsung	Pancreatic Duct
Ductus deferens	Vas Deferens, Right
	Vas Deferens, Left
	Vas Deferens, Bilateral
	Vas Deferens
Duodenal ampulla	Ampulla of Vater
Duodenojejunal flexure	Jejunum
Dura mater, intracranial	Dura Mater
Dura mater, spinal	Spinal Meninges
Dural venous sinus	Intracranial Vein
Earlobe	External Ear, Right
	External Ear, Left
	External Ear, Bilateral
Eighth cranial nerve	Acoustic Nerve
Ejaculatory duct	Vas Deferens, Right
	Vas Deferens, Left
	Vas Deferens, Bilateral
	Vas Deferens
Eleventh cranial nerve	Accessory Nerve
Encephalon	Brain
Ependyma	Cerebral Ventricle
Epidermis	Skin
Epidural space, spinal	Spinal Canal
Epiploic foramen	Peritoneum
Epithalamus	Thalamus
Epitrochlear lymph node	Lymphatic, Right Upper Extremity
	Lymphatic, Left Upper Extremity
Erector spinae muscle	Trunk Muscle, Right
	Trunk Muscle, Left
Esophageal artery	Upper Artery
Esophageal plexus	Thoracic Sympathetic Nerve
Ethmoidal air cell	Ethmoid Sinus, Right
	Ethmoid Sinus, Left
Extensor carpi radialis muscle	Lower Arm and Wrist Muscle, Right
	Lower Arm and Wrist Muscle, Left
Extensor carpi ulnaris muscle	Lower Arm and Wrist Muscle, Right
	Lower Arm and Wrist Muscle, Left

Term	ICD-10-PCS Value
Extensor digitorum brevis muscle	Foot Muscle, Right
	Foot Muscle, Left
Extensor digitorum longus muscle	Lower Leg Muscle, Right
	Lower Leg Muscle, Left
Extensor hallucis brevis muscle	Foot Muscle, Right
	Foot Muscle, Left
Extensor hallucis longus muscle	Lower Leg Muscle, Right
	Lower Leg Muscle, Left
External anal sphincter	Anal Sphincter
External auditory meatus	External Auditory Canal, Right
	External Auditory Canal, Left
External maxillary artery	Face Artery
External naris	Nasal Mucosa and Soft Tissue
External oblique aponeurosis	Subcutaneous Tissue and Fascia, Trunk
External oblique muscle	Abdomen Muscle, Right
	Abdomen Muscle, Left
External popliteal nerve	Peroneal Nerve
External pudendal artery	Femoral Artery, Right
	Femoral Artery, Left
External pudendal vein	Saphenous Vein, Right
	Saphenous Vein, Left
External urethral sphincter	Urethra
Extradural space, intracranial	Epidural Space, Intracranial
Extradural space, spinal	Spinal Canal
Facial artery	Face Artery
False vocal cord	Larynx
Falx cerebri	Dura Mater
Fascia lata	Subcutaneous Tissue and Fascia, Right Upper Leg
	Subcutaneous Tissue and Fascia, Left Upper Leg
Femoral head	Upper Femur, Right
	Upper Femur, Left
Femoral lymph node	Lymphatic, Right Lower Extremity
	Lymphatic, Left Lower Extremity
Femoropatellar joint	Knee Joint, Right
	Knee Joint, Left
	Knee Joint, Femoral Surface, Right
	Knee Joint, Femoral Surface, Left
Femorotibial joint	Knee Joint, Right
	Knee Joint, Left
	Knee Joint, Tibial Surface, Right
	Knee Joint, Tibial Surface, Left
Fibular artery	Peroneal Artery, Right
	Peroneal Artery, Left
Fibular sesamoid	Metatarsal, Right
	Metatarsal, Left
Fibularis brevis muscle	Lower Leg Muscle, Right
	Lower Leg Muscle, Left
Fibularis longus muscle	Lower Leg Muscle, Right
	Lower Leg Muscle, Left
Fifth cranial nerve	Trigeminal Nerve
Filum terminale	Spinal Meninges
First cranial nerve	Olfactory Nerve
First intercostal nerve	Brachial Plexus
Flexor carpi radialis muscle	Lower Arm and Wrist Muscle, Right
	Lower Arm and Wrist Muscle, Left
Flexor carpi ulnaris muscle	Lower Arm and Wrist Muscle, Right
	Lower Arm and Wrist Muscle, Left
Flexor digitorum brevis muscle	Foot Muscle, Right
	Foot Muscle, Left

Term	ICD-10-PCS Value
Flexor digitorum longus muscle	Lower Leg Muscle, Right
	Lower Leg Muscle, Left
Flexor hallucis brevis muscle	Foot Muscle, Right
	Foot Muscle, Left
Flexor hallucis longus muscle	Lower Leg Muscle, Right
	Lower Leg Muscle, Left
Flexor pollicis longus muscle	Lower Arm and Wrist Muscle, Right
	Lower Arm and Wrist Muscle, Left
Foramen magnum	Occipital Bone
Foramen of Monro (intraventricular)	Cerebral Ventricle
Foreskin	Prepuce
Fossa of Rosenmuller	Nasopharynx
Fourth cranial nerve	Trochlear Nerve
Fourth ventricle	Cerebral Ventricle
Fovea	Retina, Right
	Retina, Left
Frenulum labii inferioris	Lower Lip
Frenulum labii superioris	Upper Lip
Frenulum linguae	Tongue
Frontal lobe	Cerebral Hemisphere
Frontal vein	Face Vein, Right
	Face Vein, Left
Fundus uteri	Uterus
Galea aponeurotica	Subcutaneous Tissue and Fascia, Scalp
Ganglion impar (ganglion of Walther)	Sacral Sympathetic Nerve
Gasserian ganglion	Trigeminal Nerve
Gastric lymph node	Lymphatic, Aortic
Gastric plexus	Abdominal Sympathetic Nerve
Gastrocnemius muscle	Lower Leg Muscle, Right
	Lower Leg Muscle, Left
Gastrocolic ligament	Omentum
Gastrocolic omentum	Omentum
Gastroduodenal artery	Hepatic Artery
Gastroesophageal (GE) junction	Esophagogastric Junction
Gastrohepatic omentum	Omentum
Gastrophrenic ligament	Omentum
Gastrosplenic ligament	Omentum
Gemellus muscle	Hip Muscle, Right
	Hip Muscle, Left
Geniculate ganglion	Facial Nerve
Geniculate nucleus	Thalamus
Genioglossus muscle	Tongue, Palate, Pharynx Muscle
Genitofemoral nerve	Lumbar Plexus
Glans penis	Prepuce
Glenohumeral joint	Shoulder Joint, Right
	Shoulder Joint, Left
Glenohumeral ligament	Shoulder Bursa and Ligament, Right
	Shoulder Bursa and Ligament, Left
Glenoid fossa (of scapula)	Glenoid Cavity, Right
	Glenoid Cavity, Left
Glenoid ligament (labrum)	Shoulder Joint, Right
	Shoulder Joint, Left
Globus pallidus	Basal Ganglia
Glossoepiglottic fold	Epiglottis
Glottis	Larynx
Gluteal lymph node	Lymphatic, Pelvis
Gluteal vein	Hypogastric Vein, Right
	Hypogastric Vein, Left

Term	ICD-10-PCS Value
Gluteus maximus muscle	Hip Muscle, Right
	Hip Muscle, Left
Gluteus medius muscle	Hip Muscle, Right
	Hip Muscle, Left
Gluteus minimus muscle	Hip Muscle, Right
	Hip Muscle, Left
Gracilis muscle	Upper Leg Muscle, Right
	Upper Leg Muscle, Left
Great auricular nerve	Cervical Plexus
Great cerebral vein	Intracranial Vein
Great(er) saphenous vein	Saphenous Vein, Right
	Saphenous Vein, Left
Greater alar cartilage	Nasal Mucosa and Soft Tissue
Greater occipital nerve	Cervical Nerve
Greater omentum	Omentum
Greater splanchnic nerve	Thoracic Sympathetic Nerve
Greater superficial petrosal nerve	Facial Nerve
Greater trochanter	Upper Femur, Right
	Upper Femur, Left
Greater tuberosity	Humeral Head, Right
	Humeral Head, Left
Greater vestibular (Bartholin's) gland	Vestibular Gland
Greater wing	Sphenoid Bone
Hallux	1st Toe, Right
	1st Toe, Left
Hamate bone	Carpal, Right
	Carpal, Left
Hamstring muscle	Upper Leg Muscle, Right
	Upper Leg Muscle, Left
Head of fibula	Fibula, Right
	Fibula, Left
Helix	External Ear, Right
	External Ear, Left
	External Ear, Bilateral
Hepatic artery proper	Hepatic Artery
Hepatic flexure	Transverse Colon
Hepatic lymph node	Lymphatic, Aortic
Hepatic plexus	Abdominal Sympathetic Nerve
Hepatic portal vein	Portal Vein
Hepatogastric ligament	Omentum
Hepatopancreatic ampulla	Ampulla of Vater
Humeroradial joint	Elbow Joint, Right
	Elbow Joint, Left
Humeroulnar joint	Elbow Joint, Right
	Elbow Joint, Left
Humerus, distal	Humeral Shaft, Right
	Humeral Shaft, Left
Hyoglossus muscle	Tongue, Palate, Pharynx Muscle
Hyoid artery	Thyroid Artery, Right
	Thyroid Artery, Left
Hypogastric artery	Internal Iliac Artery, Right
	Internal Iliac Artery, Left
Hypopharynx	Pharynx
Hypophysis	Pituitary Gland
Hypothenar muscle	Hand Muscle, Right
	Hand Muscle, Left
Ileal artery	Superior Mesenteric Artery
Ileocolic artery	Superior Mesenteric Artery
Ileocolic vein	Colic Vein

Appendix D: Body Part Key

Term	ICD-10-PCS Value
Iliac crest	Pelvic Bone, Right
	Pelvic Bone, Left
Iliac fascia	Subcutaneous Tissue and Fascia, Right Upper Leg
	Subcutaneous Tissue and Fascia, Left Upper Leg
Iliac lymph node	Lymphatic, Pelvis
Iliacus muscle	Hip Muscle, Right
	Hip Muscle, Left
Iliofemoral ligament	Hip Bursa and Ligament, Right
	Hip Bursa and Ligament, Left
Iliohypogastric nerve	Lumbar Plexus
Ilioinguinal nerve	Lumbar Plexus
Iliolumbar artery	Internal Iliac Artery, Right
	Internal Iliac Artery, Left
Iliolumbar ligament	Lower Spine Bursa and Ligament
Iliotibial tract (band)	Subcutaneous Tissue and Fascia, Right Upper Leg
	Subcutaneous Tissue and Fascia, Left Upper Leg
Iliopsoas muscle	Hip Muscle, Right
	Hip Muscle, Left
Ilium	Pelvic Bone, Right
	Pelvic Bone, Left
Incus	Auditory Ossicle, Right
	Auditory Ossicle, Left
Inferior cardiac nerve	Thoracic Sympathetic Nerve
Inferior cerebellar vein	Intracranial Vein
Inferior cerebral vein	Intracranial Vein
Inferior epigastric artery	External Iliac Artery, Right
	External Iliac Artery, Left
Inferior epigastric lymph node	Lymphatic, Pelvis
Inferior genicular artery	Popliteal Artery, Right
	Popliteal Artery, Left
Inferior gluteal artery	Internal Iliac Artery, Right
	Internal Iliac Artery, Left
Inferior gluteal nerve	Sacral Plexus
Inferior hypogastric plexus	Abdominal Sympathetic Nerve
Inferior labial artery	Face Artery
Inferior longitudinal muscle	Tongue, Palate, Pharynx Muscle
Inferior mesenteric ganglion	Abdominal Sympathetic Nerve
Inferior mesenteric lymph node	Lymphatic, Mesenteric
Inferior mesenteric plexus	Abdominal Sympathetic Nerve
Inferior oblique muscle	Extraocular Muscle, Right
	Extraocular Muscle, Left
Inferior pancreaticoduodenal artery	Superior Mesenteric Artery
Inferior phrenic artery	Abdominal Aorta
Inferior rectus muscle	Extraocular Muscle, Right
	Extraocular Muscle, Left
Inferior suprarenal artery	Renal Artery, Right
	Renal Artery, Left
Inferior tarsal plate	Lower Eyelid, Right
	Lower Eyelid, Left
Inferior thyroid vein	Innominate Vein, Right
	Innominate Vein, Left
Inferior tibiofibular joint	Ankle Joint, Right
	Ankle Joint, Left
Inferior turbinate	Nasal Turbinate

Term	ICD-10-PCS Value
Inferior ulnar collateral artery	Brachial Artery, Right
	Brachial Artery, Left
Inferior vesical artery	Internal Iliac Artery, Right
	Internal Iliac Artery, Left
Infraauricular lymph node	Lymphatic, Head
Infraclavicular (deltopectoral) lymph node	Lymphatic, Right Upper Extremity
	Lymphatic, Left Upper Extremity
Infrahyoid muscle	Neck Muscle, Right
	Neck Muscle, Left
Infraparotid lymph node	Lymphatic, Head
Infraspinatus fascia	Subcutaneous Tissue and Fascia, Right Upper Arm
	Subcutaneous Tissue and Fascia, Left Upper Arm
Infraspinatus muscle	Shoulder Muscle, Right
	Shoulder Muscle, Left
Infundibulopelvic ligament	Uterine Supporting Structure
Inguinal canal	Inguinal Region, Right
	Inguinal Region, Left
	Inguinal Region, Bilateral
Inguinal triangle	Inguinal Region, Right
	Inguinal Region, Left
	Inguinal Region, Bilateral
Interatrial septum	Atrial Septum
Intercarpal joint	Carpal Joint, Right
	Carpal Joint, Left
Intercarpal ligament	Hand Bursa and Ligament, Right
	Hand Bursa and Ligament, Left
Interclavicular ligament	Shoulder Bursa and Ligament, Right
	Shoulder Bursa and Ligament, Left
Intercostal lymph node	Lymphatic, Thorax
Intercostal muscle	Thorax Muscle, Right
	Thorax Muscle, Left
Intercostal nerve	Thoracic Nerve
Intercostobrachial nerve	Thoracic Nerve
Intercuneiform joint	Tarsal Joint, Right
	Tarsal Joint, Left
Intercuneiform ligament	Foot Bursa and Ligament, Right
	Foot Bursa and Ligament, Left
Intermediate bronchus	Main Bronchus, Right
Intermediate cuneiform bone	Tarsal, Right
	Tarsal, Left
Internal anal sphincter	Anal Sphincter
Internal (basal) cerebral vein	Intracranial Vein
Internal carotid artery, intracranial portion	Intracranial Artery
Internal carotid plexus	Head and Neck Sympathetic Nerve
Internal iliac vein	Hypogastric Vein, Right
	Hypogastric Vein, Left
Internal maxillary artery	External Carotid Artery, Right
	External Carotid Artery, Left
Internal naris	Nasal Mucosa and Soft Tissue
Internal oblique muscle	Abdomen Muscle, Right
	Abdomen Muscle, Left
Internal pudendal artery	Internal Iliac Artery, Right
	Internal Iliac Artery, Left
Internal pudendal vein	Hypogastric Vein, Right
	Hypogastric Vein, Left

Term	ICD-10-PCS Value
Internal thoracic artery	Internal Mammary Artery, Right
	Internal Mammary Artery, Left
	Subclavian Artery, Right
	Subclavian Artery, Left
Internal urethral sphincter	Urethra
Interphalangeal (IP) joint	Finger Phalangeal Joint, Right
	Finger Phalangeal Joint, Left
	Toe Phalangeal Joint, Right
	Toe Phalangeal Joint, Left
Interphalangeal ligament	Foot Bursa and Ligament, Right
	Foot Bursa and Ligament, Left
	Hand Bursa and Ligament, Right
	Hand Bursa and Ligament, Left
Interspinalis muscle	Trunk Muscle, Right
	Trunk Muscle, Left
Interspinous ligament, cervical	Head and Neck Bursa and Ligament
Interspinous ligament, lumbar	Lower Spine Bursa and Ligament
Interspinous ligament, thoracic	Upper Spine Bursa and Ligament
Intertransversarius muscle	Trunk Muscle, Right
	Trunk Muscle, Left
Intertransverse ligament, cervical	Head and Neck Bursa and Ligament
Intertransverse ligament, lumbar	Lower Spine Bursa and Ligament
Intertransverse ligament, thoracic	Upper Spine Bursa and Ligament
Interventricular foramen (Monro)	Cerebral Ventricle
Interventricular septum	Ventricular Septum
Intestinal lymphatic trunk	Cisterna Chyli
Ischiatic nerve	Sciatic Nerve
Ischiocavernosus muscle	Perineum Muscle
Ischiofemoral ligament	Hip Bursa and Ligament, Right
	Hip Bursa and Ligament, Left
Ischium	Pelvic Bone, Right
	Pelvic Bone, Left
Jejunal artery	Superior Mesenteric Artery
Jugular body	Glomus Jugulare
Jugular lymph node	Lymphatic, Right Neck
	Lymphatic, Left Neck
Juxtaductal aorta	Thoracic Aorta, Ascending/Arch
Labia majora	Vulva
Labia minora	Vulva
Labial gland	Upper Lip
	Lower Lip
Lacrimal canaliculus	Lacrimal Duct, Right
	Lacrimal Duct, Left
Lacrimal punctum	Lacrimal Duct, Right
	Lacrimal Duct, Left
Lacrimal sac	Lacrimal Duct, Right
	Lacrimal Duct, Left
Laryngopharynx	Pharynx
Lateral (brachial) lymph node	Lymphatic, Right Axillary
	Lymphatic, Left Axillary
Lateral canthus	Upper Eyelid, Right
	Upper Eyelid, Left
Lateral collateral ligament (LCL)	Knee Bursa and Ligament, Right
	Knee Bursa and Ligament, Left

Term	ICD-10-PCS Value
Lateral condyle of femur	Lower Femur, Right
	Lower Femur, Left
Lateral condyle of tibia	Tibia, Right
	Tibia, Left
Lateral cuneiform bone	Tarsal, Right
	Tarsal, Left
Lateral epicondyle of femur	Lower Femur, Right
	Lower Femur, Left
Lateral epicondyle of humerus	Humeral Shaft, Right
	Humeral Shaft, Left
Lateral femoral cutaneous nerve	Lumbar Plexus
Lateral malleolus	Fibula, Right
	Fibula, Left
Lateral meniscus	Knee Joint, Right
	Knee Joint, Left
Lateral nasal cartilage	Nasal Mucosa and Soft Tissue
Lateral plantar artery	Foot Artery, Right
	Foot Artery, Left
Lateral plantar nerve	Tibial Nerve
Lateral rectus muscle	Extraocular Muscle, Right
	Extraocular Muscle, Left
Lateral sacral artery	Internal Iliac Artery, Right
	Internal Iliac Artery, Left
Lateral sacral vein	Hypogastric Vein, Right
	Hypogastric Vein, Left
Lateral sural cutaneous nerve	Peroneal Nerve
Lateral tarsal artery	Foot Artery, Right
	Foot Artery, Left
Lateral temporo- mandibular ligament	Head and Neck Bursa and Ligament
Lateral thoracic artery	Axillary Artery, Right
	Axillary Artery, Left
Latissimus dorsi muscle	Trunk Muscle, Right
	Trunk Muscle, Left
Least splanchnic nerve	Thoracic Sympathetic Nerve
Left ascending lumbar vein	Hemiazygos Vein
Left atrioventricular valve	Mitral Valve
Left auricular appendix	Atrium, Left
Left colic vein	Colic Vein
Left coronary sulcus	Heart, Left
Left gastric artery	Gastric Artery
Left gastroepiploic artery	Splenic Artery
Left gastroepiploic vein	Splenic Vein
Left inferior phrenic vein	Renal Vein, Left
Left inferior pulmonary vein	Pulmonary Vein, Left
Left jugular trunk	Thoracic Duct
Left lateral ventricle	Cerebral Ventricle
Left ovarian vein	Renal Vein, Left
Left second lumbar vein	Renal Vein, Left
Left subclavian trunk	Thoracic Duct
Left subcostal vein	Hemiazygos Vein
Left superior pulmonary vein	Pulmonary Vein, Left
Left suprarenal vein	Renal Vein, Left
Left testicular vein	Renal Vein, Left
Leptomeninges, intracranial	Cerebral Meninges
Leptomeninges, spinal	Spinal Meninges
Lesser alar cartilage	Nasal Mucosa and Soft Tissue
Lesser occipital nerve	Cervical Plexus
Lesser omentum	Omentum

Appendix D: Body Part Key

Term	ICD-10-PCS Value
Lesser saphenous vein	Saphenous Vein, Right
	Saphenous Vein, Left
Lesser splanchnic nerve	Thoracic Sympathetic Nerve
Lesser trochanter	Upper Femur, Right
	Upper Femur, Left
Lesser tuberosity	Humeral Head, Right
	Humeral Head, Left
Lesser wing	Sphenoid Bone
Levator anguli oris muscle	Facial Muscle
Levator ani muscle	Perineum Muscle
Levator labii superioris alaeque nasi muscle	Facial Muscle
Levator labii superioris muscle	Facial Muscle
Levator palpebrae superioris muscle	Upper Eyelid, Right
	Upper Eyelid, Left
Levator scapulae muscle	Neck Muscle, Right
	Neck Muscle, Left
Levator veli palatini muscle	Tongue, Palate, Pharynx Muscle
Levatores costarum muscle	Thorax Muscle, Right
	Thorax Muscle, Left
Ligament of head of fibula	Knee Bursa and Ligament, Right
	Knee Bursa and Ligament, Left
Ligament of the lateral malleolus	Ankle Bursa and Ligament, Right
	Ankle Bursa and Ligament, Left
Ligamentum flavum, cervical	Head and Neck Bursa and Ligament
Ligamentum flavum, lumbar	Lower Spine Bursa and Ligament
Ligamentum flavum, thoracic	Upper Spine Bursa and Ligament
Lingual artery	External Carotid Artery, Right
	External Carotid Artery, Left
Lingual tonsil	Pharynx
Locus ceruleus	Pons
Long thoracic nerve	Brachial Plexus
Lumbar artery	Abdominal Aorta
Lumbar facet joint	Lumbar Vertebral Joint
Lumbar ganglion	Lumbar Sympathetic Nerve
Lumbar lymph node	Lymphatic, Aortic
Lumbar lymphatic trunk	Cisterna Chyli
Lumbar splanchnic nerve	Lumbar Sympathetic Nerve
Lumbosacral facet joint	Lumbosacral Joint
Lumbosacral trunk	Lumbar Nerve
Lunate bone	Carpal, Right
	Carpal, Left
Lunotriquetral ligament	Hand Bursa and Ligament, Right
	Hand Bursa and Ligament, Left
Macula	Retina, Right
	Retina, Left
Malleus	Auditory Ossicle, Right
	Auditory Ossicle, Left
Mammary duct	Breast, Right
	Breast, Left
	Breast, Bilateral
Mammary gland	Breast, Right
	Breast, Left
	Breast, Bilateral
Mammillary body	Hypothalamus
Mandibular nerve	Trigeminal Nerve
Mandibular notch	Mandible, Right
	Mandible, Left
Manubrium	Sternum
Masseter muscle	Head Muscle

Term	ICD-10-PCS Value
Masseteric fascia	Subcutaneous Tissue and Fascia, Face
Mastoid (postauricular) lymph node	Lymphatic, Right Neck
	Lymphatic, Left Neck
Mastoid air cells	Mastoid Sinus, Right
	Mastoid Sinus, Left
Mastoid process	Temporal Bone, Right
	Temporal Bone, Left
Maxillary artery	External Carotid Artery, Right
	External Carotid Artery, Left
Maxillary nerve	Trigeminal Nerve
Medial canthus	Lower Eyelid, Right
	Lower Eyelid, Left
Medial collateral ligament (MCL)	Knee Bursa and Ligament, Right
	Knee Bursa and Ligament, Left
Medial condyle of femur	Lower Femur, Right
	Lower Femur, Left
Medial condyle of tibia	Tibia, Right
	Tibia, Left
Medial cuneiform bone	Tarsal, Right
	Tarsal, Left
Medial epicondyle of femur	Lower Femur, Right
	Lower Femur, Left
Medial epicondyle of humerus	Humeral Shaft, Right
	Humeral Shaft, Left
Medial malleolus	Tibia, Right
	Tibia, Left
Medial meniscus	Knee Joint, Right
	Knee Joint, Left
Medial plantar artery	Foot Artery, Right
	Foot Artery, Left
Medial plantar nerve	Tibial Nerve
Medial popliteal nerve	Tibial Nerve
Medial rectus muscle	Extraocular Muscle, Right
	Extraocular Muscle, Left
Medial sural cutaneous nerve	Tibial Nerve
Median antebrachial vein	Basilic Vein, Right
	Basilic Vein, Left
Median cubital vein	Basilic Vein, Right
	Basilic Vein, Left
Median sacral artery	Abdominal Aorta
Mediastinal cavity	Mediastinum
Mediastinal lymph node	Lymphatic, Thorax
Mediastinal space	Mediastinum
Meissner's (submucous) plexus	Abdominal Sympathetic Nerve
Membranous urethra	Urethra
Mental foramen	Mandible, Right
	Mandible, Left
Mentalis muscle	Facial Muscle
Mesoappendix	Mesentery
Mesocolon	Mesentery
Metacarpal ligament	Hand Bursa and Ligament, Right
	Hand Bursa and Ligament, Left
Metacarpophalangeal ligament	Hand Bursa and Ligament, Right
	Hand Bursa and Ligament, Left
Metatarsal ligament	Foot Bursa and Ligament, Right
	Foot Bursa and Ligament, Left
Metatarsophalangeal ligament	Foot Bursa and Ligament, Right
	Foot Bursa and Ligament, Left

Appendix D: Body Part Key

Term	ICD-10-PCS Value
Metatarsophalangeal (MTP) joint	Metatarsal-Phalangeal Joint, Right
	Metatarsal-Phalangeal Joint, Left
Metathalamus	Thalamus
Midcarpal joint	Carpal Joint, Right
	Carpal Joint, Left
Middle cardiac nerve	Thoracic Sympathetic Nerve
Middle cerebral artery	Intracranial Artery
Middle cerebral vein	Intracranial Vein
Middle colic vein	Colic Vein
Middle genicular artery	Popliteal Artery, Right
	Popliteal Artery, Left
Middle hemorrhoidal vein	Hypogastric Vein, Right
	Hypogastric Vein, Left
Middle meningeal artery, intracranial portion	Intracranial Artery
Middle rectal artery	Internal Iliac Artery, Right
	Internal Iliac Artery, Left
Middle suprarenal artery	Abdominal Aorta
Middle temporal artery	Temporal Artery, Right
	Temporal Artery, Left
Middle turbinate	Nasal Turbinate
Mitral annulus	Mitral Valve
Molar gland	Buccal Mucosa
Musculocutaneous nerve	Brachial Plexus
Musculophrenic artery	Internal Mammary Artery, Right
	Internal Mammary Artery, Left
Musculospiral nerve	Radial Nerve
Myelencephalon	Medulla Oblongata
Myenteric (Auerbach's) plexus	Abdominal Sympathetic Nerve
Myometrium	Uterus
Nail bed	Finger Nail
	Toe Nail
Nail plate	Finger Nail
	Toe Nail
Nasal cavity	Nasal Mucosa and Soft Tissue
Nasal concha	Nasal Turbinate
Nasalis muscle	Facial Muscle
Nasolacrimal duct	Lacrimal Duct, Right
	Lacrimal Duct, Left
Navicular bone	Tarsal, Right
	Tarsal, Left
Neck of femur	Upper Femur, Right
	Upper Femur, Left
Neck of humerus (anatomical) (surgical)	Humeral Head, Right
	Humeral Head, Left
Nerve to the stapedius	Facial Nerve
Neurohypophysis	Pituitary Gland
Ninth cranial nerve	Glossopharyngeal Nerve
Nostril	Nasal Mucosa and Soft Tissue
Obturator artery	Internal Iliac Artery, Right
	Internal Iliac Artery, Left
Obturator lymph node	Lymphatic, Pelvis
Obturator muscle	Hip Muscle, Right
	Hip Muscle, Left
Obturator nerve	Lumbar Plexus
Obturator vein	Hypogastric Vein, Right
	Hypogastric Vein, Left
Obtuse margin	Heart, Left

Term	ICD-10-PCS Value
Occipital artery	External Carotid Artery, Right
	External Carotid Artery, Left
Occipital lobe	Cerebral Hemisphere
Occipital lymph node	Lymphatic, Right Neck
	Lymphatic, Left Neck
Occipitofrontalis muscle	Facial Muscle
Odontoid process	Cervical Vertebra
Olecranon bursa	Elbow Bursa and Ligament, Right
	Elbow Bursa and Ligament, Left
Olecranon process	Ulna, Right
	Ulna, Left
Olfactory bulb	Olfactory Nerve
Ophthalmic artery	Intracranial Artery
Ophthalmic nerve	Trigeminal Nerve
Ophthalmic vein	Intracranial Vein
Optic chiasma	Optic Nerve
Optic disc	Retina, Right
	Retina, Left
Optic foramen	Sphenoid Bone
Orbicularis oculi muscle	Upper Eyelid, Right
	Upper Eyelid, Left
Orbicularis oris muscle	Facial Muscle
Orbital fascia	Subcutaneous Tissue and Fascia, Face
Orbital portion of ethmoid bone	Orbit, Right
	Orbit, Left
Orbital portion of frontal bone	Orbit, Right
	Orbit, Left
Orbital portion of lacrimal bone	Orbit, Right
	Orbit, Left
Orbital portion of maxilla	Orbit, Right
	Orbit, Left
Orbital portion of palatine bone	Orbit, Right
	Orbit, Left
Orbital portion of sphenoid bone	Orbit, Right
	Orbit, Left
Orbital portion of zygomatic bone	Orbit, Right
	Orbit, Left
Oropharynx	Pharynx
Otic ganglion	Head and Neck Sympathetic Nerve
Oval window	Middle Ear, Right
	Middle Ear, Left
Ovarian artery	Abdominal Aorta
Ovarian ligament	Uterine Supporting Structure
Oviduct	Fallopian Tube, Right
	Fallopian Tube, Left
Palatine gland	Buccal Mucosa
Palatine tonsil	Tonsils
Palatine uvula	Uvula
Palatoglossal muscle	Tongue, Palate, Pharynx Muscle
Palatopharyngeal muscle	Tongue, Palate, Pharynx Muscle
Palmar (volar) digital vein	Hand Vein, Right
	Hand Vein, Left
Palmar (volar) metacarpal vein	Hand Vein, Right
	Hand Vein, Left
Palmar cutaneous nerve	Median Nerve
	Radial Nerve
Palmar fascia (aponeurosis)	Subcutaneous Tissue and Fascia, Right Hand
	Subcutaneous Tissue and Fascia, Left Hand
Palmar interosseous muscle	Hand Muscle, Right
	Hand Muscle, Left

Appendix D: Body Part Key

Term	ICD-10-PCS Value
Palmar ulnocarpal ligament	Wrist Bursa and Ligament, Right
	Wrist Bursa and Ligament, Left
Palmaris longus muscle	Lower Arm and Wrist Muscle, Right
	Lower Arm and Wrist Muscle, Left
Pancreatic artery	Splenic Artery
Pancreatic plexus	Abdominal Sympathetic Nerve
Pancreatic vein	Splenic Vein
Pancreaticosplenic lymph node	Lymphatic, Aortic
Paraaortic lymph node	Lymphatic, Aortic
Parapharyngeal space	Neck
Pararectal lymph node	Lymphatic, Mesenteric
Parasternal lymph node	Lymphatic, Thorax
Paratracheal lymph node	Lymphatic, Thorax
Paraurethral (Skene's) gland	Vestibular Gland
Parietal lobe	Cerebral Hemisphere
Parotid lymph node	Lymphatic, Head
Parotid plexus	Facial Nerve
Pars flaccida	Tympanic Membrane, Right
	Tympanic Membrane, Left
Patellar ligament	Knee Bursa and Ligament, Right
	Knee Bursa and Ligament, Left
Patellar tendon	Knee Tendon, Right
	Knee Tendon, Left
Patellofemoral joint	Knee Joint, Right
	Knee Joint, Left
	Knee Joint, Femoral Surface, Right
	Knee Joint, Femoral Surface, Left
Pectineus muscle	Upper Leg Muscle, Right
	Upper Leg Muscle, Left
Pectoral (anterior) lymph node	Lymphatic, Right Axillary
	Lymphatic, Left Axillary
Pectoral fascia	Subcutaneous Tissue and Fascia, Chest
Pectoralis major muscle	Thorax Muscle, Right
	Thorax Muscle, Left
Pectoralis minor muscle	Thorax Muscle, Right
	Thorax Muscle, Left
Pelvic splanchnic nerve	Abdominal Sympathetic Nerve
	Sacral Sympathetic Nerve
Penile urethra	Urethra
Perianal skin	Skin, Perineum
Pericardiophrenic artery	Internal Mammary Artery, Right
	Internal Mammary Artery, Left
Perimetrium	Uterus
Peroneus brevis muscle	Lower Leg Muscle, Right
	Lower Leg Muscle, Left
Peroneus longus muscle	Lower Leg Muscle, Right
	Lower Leg Muscle, Left
Petrous part of temporal bone	Temporal Bone, Right
	Temporal Bone, Left
Pharyngeal constrictor muscle	Tongue, Palate, Pharynx Muscle
Pharyngeal plexus	Vagus Nerve
Pharyngeal recess	Nasopharynx
Pharyngeal tonsil	Adenoids
Pharyngotympanic tube	Eustachian Tube, Right
	Eustachian Tube, Left
Pia mater, intracranial	Cerebral Meninges
Pia mater, spinal	Spinal Meninges

Term	ICD-10-PCS Value
Pinna	External Ear, Right
	External Ear, Left
	External Ear, Bilateral
Piriform recess (sinus)	Pharynx
Piriformis muscle	Hip Muscle, Right
	Hip Muscle, Left
Pisiform bone	Carpal, Right
	Carpal, Left
Pisohamate ligament	Hand Bursa and Ligament, Right
	Hand Bursa and Ligament, Left
Pisometacarpal ligament	Hand Bursa and Ligament, Right
	Hand Bursa and Ligament, Left
Plantar digital vein	Foot Vein, Right
	Foot Vein, Left
Plantar fascia (aponeurosis)	Subcutaneous Tissue and Fascia, Right Foot
	Subcutaneous Tissue and Fascia, Left Foot
Plantar metatarsal vein	Foot Vein, Right
	Foot Vein, Left
Plantar venous arch	Foot Vein, Right
	Foot Vein, Left
Plantaris muscle	Lower Leg Muscle, Right
	Lower Leg Muscle, Left
Platysma muscle	Neck Muscle, Right
	Neck Muscle, Left
Plica semilunaris	Conjunctiva, Right
	Conjunctiva, Left
Pneumogastric nerve	Vagus Nerve
Pneumotaxic center	Pons
Pontine tegmentum	Pons
Popliteal fossa	Knee Region, Right
	Knee Region, Left
Popliteal ligament	Knee Bursa and Ligament, Right
	Knee Bursa and Ligament, Left
Popliteal lymph node	Lymphatic, Left Lower Extremity
	Lymphatic, Right Lower Extremity
Popliteal vein	Femoral Vein, Right
	Femoral Vein, Left
Popliteus muscle	Lower Leg Muscle, Right
	Lower Leg Muscle, Left
Postauricular (mastoid) lymph node	Lymphatic, Right Neck
	Lymphatic, Left Neck
Postcava	Inferior Vena Cava
Posterior (subscapular) lymph node	Lymphatic, Right Axillary
	Lymphatic, Left Axillary
Posterior auricular artery	External Carotid Artery, Right
	External Carotid Artery, Left
Posterior auricular nerve	Facial Nerve
Posterior auricular vein	External Jugular Vein, Right
	External Jugular Vein, Left
Posterior cerebral artery	Intracranial Artery
Posterior chamber	Eye, Right
	Eye, Left
Posterior circumflex humeral artery	Axillary Artery, Right
	Axillary Artery, Left
Posterior communicating artery	Intracranial Artery
Posterior cruciate ligament (PCL)	Knee Bursa and Ligament, Right
	Knee Bursa and Ligament, Left
Posterior facial (retromandibular) vein	Face Vein, Right
	Face Vein, Left

Term	ICD-10-PCS Value
Posterior femoral cutaneous nerve	Sacral Plexus
Posterior inferior cerebellar artery (PICA)	Intracranial Artery
Posterior interosseous nerve	Radial Nerve
Posterior labial nerve	Pudendal Nerve
Posterior scrotal nerve	Pudendal Nerve
Posterior spinal artery	Vertebral Artery, Right
	Vertebral Artery, Left
Posterior tibial recurrent artery	Anterior Tibial Artery, Right
	Anterior Tibial Artery, Left
Posterior ulnar recurrent artery	Ulnar Artery, Right
	Ulnar Artery, Left
Posterior vagal trunk	Vagus Nerve
Preauricular lymph node	Lymphatic, Head
Precava	Superior Vena Cava
Prepatellar bursa	Knee Bursa and Ligament, Right
	Knee Bursa and Ligament, Left
Pretracheal fascia	Subcutaneous Tissue and Fascia, Right Neck
	Subcutaneous Tissue and Fascia, Left Neck
Prevertebral fascia	Subcutaneous Tissue and Fascia, Right Neck
	Subcutaneous Tissue and Fascia, Left Neck
Prevesical space	Pelvic Cavity
Princeps pollicis artery	Hand Artery, Right
	Hand Artery, Left
Procerus muscle	Facial Muscle
Profunda brachii	Brachial Artery, Right
	Brachial Artery, Left
Profunda femoris (deep femoral) vein	Femoral Vein, Right
	Femoral Vein, Left
Pronator quadratus muscle	Lower Arm and Wrist Muscle, Right
	Lower Arm and Wrist Muscle, Left
Pronator teres muscle	Lower Arm and Wrist Muscle, Right
	Lower Arm and Wrist Muscle, Left
Prostatic artery	Internal Iliac Artery, Right
	Internal Iliac Artery, Left
Prostatic urethra	Urethra
Proximal radioulnar joint	Elbow Joint, Right
	Elbow Joint, Left
Psoas muscle	Hip Muscle, Right
	Hip Muscle, Left
Pterygoid muscle	Head Muscle
Pterygoid process	Sphenoid Bone
Pterygopalatine (sphenopalatine) ganglion	Head and Neck Sympathetic Nerve
Pubis	Pelvic Bone, Right
	Pelvic Bone, Left
Pubofemoral ligament	Hip Bursa and Ligament, Right
	Hip Bursa and Ligament, Left
Pudendal nerve	Sacral Plexus
Pulmoaortic canal	Pulmonary Artery, Left
Pulmonary annulus	Pulmonary Valve
Pulmonary plexus	Thoracic Sympathetic Nerve
	Vagus Nerve
Pulmonic valve	Pulmonary Valve
Pulvinar	Thalamus
Pyloric antrum	Stomach, Pylorus
Pyloric canal	Stomach, Pylorus
Pyloric sphincter	Stomach, Pylorus
Pyramidalis muscle	Abdomen Muscle, Right
	Abdomen Muscle, Left

Term	ICD-10-PCS Value
Quadrangular cartilage	Nasal Septum
Quadrate lobe	Liver
Quadratus femoris muscle	Hip Muscle, Right
	Hip Muscle, Left
Quadratus lumborum muscle	Trunk Muscle, Right
	Trunk Muscle, Left
Quadratus plantae muscle	Foot Muscle, Right
	Foot Muscle, Left
Quadriceps (femoris)	Upper Leg Muscle, Right
	Upper Leg Muscle, Left
Radial collateral carpal ligament	Wrist Bursa and Ligament, Right
	Wrist Bursa and Ligament, Left
Radial collateral ligament	Elbow Bursa and Ligament, Right
	Elbow Bursa and Ligament, Left
Radial notch	Ulna, Right
	Ulna, Left
Radial recurrent artery	Radial Artery, Right
	Radial Artery, Left
Radial vein	Brachial Vein, Right
	Brachial Vein, Left
Radialis indicis	Hand Artery, Right
	Hand Artery, Left
Radiocarpal joint	Wrist Joint, Right
	Wrist Joint, Left
Radiocarpal ligament	Wrist Bursa and Ligament, Right
	Wrist Bursa and Ligament, Left
Radioulnar ligament	Wrist Bursa and Ligament, Right
	Wrist Bursa and Ligament, Left
Rectosigmoid junction	Sigmoid Colon
Rectus abdominis muscle	Abdomen Muscle, Right
	Abdomen Muscle, Left
Rectus femoris muscle	Upper Leg Muscle, Right
	Upper Leg Muscle, Left
Recurrent laryngeal nerve	Vagus Nerve
Renal calyx	Kidney, Right
	Kidney, Left
	Kidneys, Bilateral
	Kidney
Renal capsule	Kidney, Right
	Kidney, Left
	Kidneys, Bilateral
	Kidney
Renal cortex	Kidney, Right
	Kidney, Left
	Kidneys, Bilateral
	Kidney
Renal nerve	Abdominal sympathetic Nerve
Renal plexus	Abdominal Sympathetic Nerve
Renal segment	Kidney, Right
	Kidney, Left
	Kidneys, Bilateral
	Kidney
Renal segmental artery	Renal Artery, Right
	Renal Artery, Left
Retroperitoneal cavity	Retroperitoneum
Retroperitoneal lymph node	Lymphatic, Aortic
Retroperitoneal space	Retroperitoneum
Retropharyngeal lymph node	Lymphatic, Right Neck
	Lymphatic, Left Neck
Retropharyngeal space	Neck

Appendix D: Body Part Key

Term	ICD-10-PCS Value
Retropubic space	Pelvic Cavity
Rhinopharynx	Nasopharynx
Rhomboid major muscle	Trunk Muscle, Right
	Trunk Muscle, Left
Rhomboid minor muscle	Trunk Muscle, Right
	Trunk Muscle, Left
Right ascending lumbar vein	Azygos Vein
Right atrioventricular valve	Tricuspid Valve
Right auricular appendix	Atrium, Right
Right colic vein	Colic Vein
Right coronary sulcus	Heart, Right
Right gastric artery	Gastric Artery
Right gastroepiploic vein	Superior Mesenteric Vein
Right inferior phrenic vein	Inferior Vena Cava
Right inferior pulmonary vein	Pulmonary Vein, Right
Right jugular trunk	Lymphatic, Right Neck
Right lateral ventricle	Cerebral Ventricle
Right lymphatic duct	Lymphatic, Right Neck
Right ovarian vein	Inferior Vena Cava
Right second lumbar vein	Inferior Vena Cava
Right subclavian trunk	Lymphatic, Right Neck
Right subcostal vein	Azygos Vein
Right superior pulmonary vein	Pulmonary Vein, Right
Right suprarenal vein	Inferior Vena Cava
Right testicular vein	Inferior Vena Cava
Rima glottidis	Larynx
Risorius muscle	Facial Muscle
Round ligament of uterus	Uterine Supporting Structure
Round window	Inner Ear, Right
	Inner Ear, Left
Sacral ganglion	Sacral Sympathetic Nerve
Sacral lymph node	Lymphatic, Pelvis
Sacral splanchnic nerve	Sacral Sympathetic Nerve
Sacrococcygeal ligament	Lower Spine Bursa and Ligament
Sacrococcygeal symphysis	Sacrococcygeal Joint
Sacroiliac ligament	Lower Spine Bursa and Ligament
Sacrospinous ligament	Lower Spine Bursa and Ligament
Sacrotuberous ligament	Lower Spine Bursa and Ligament
Salpingopharyngeus muscle	Tongue, Palate, Pharynx Muscle
Salpinx	Fallopian Tube, Right
	Fallopian Tube, Left
Saphenous nerve	Femoral Nerve
Sartorius muscle	Upper Leg Muscle, Right
	Upper Leg Muscle, Left
Scalene muscle	Neck Muscle, Right
	Neck Muscle, Left
Scaphoid bone	Carpal, Right
	Carpal, Left
Scapholunate ligament	Wrist Bursa and Ligament, Right
	Wrist Bursa and Ligament, Left
Scaphotrapezium ligament	Hand Bursa and Ligament, Right
	Hand Bursa and Ligament, Left
Scarpa's (vestibular) ganglion	Acoustic Nerve
Sebaceous gland	Skin
Second cranial nerve	Optic Nerve
Sella turcica	Sphenoid Bone
Semicircular canal	Inner Ear, Right
	Inner Ear, Left

Term	ICD-10-PCS Value
Semimembranosus muscle	Upper Leg Muscle, Right
	Upper Leg Muscle, Left
Semitendinosus muscle	Upper Leg Muscle, Right
	Upper Leg Muscle, Left
Septal cartilage	Nasal Septum
Serratus anterior muscle	Thorax Muscle, Right
	Thorax Muscle, Left
Serratus posterior muscle	Trunk Muscle, Right
	Trunk Muscle, Left
Seventh cranial nerve	Facial Nerve
Short gastric artery	Splenic Artery
Sigmoid artery	Inferior Mesenteric Artery
Sigmoid flexure	Sigmoid Colon
Sigmoid vein	Inferior Mesenteric Vein
Sinoatrial node	Conduction Mechanism
Sinus venosus	Atrium, Right
Sixth cranial nerve	Abducens Nerve
Skene's (paraurethral) gland	Vestibular Gland
Small saphenous vein	Saphenous Vein, Right
	Saphenous Vein, Left
Solar (celiac) plexus	Abdominal Sympathetic Nerve
Soleus muscle	Lower Leg Muscle, Right
	Lower Leg Muscle, Left
Space of Retzius	Pelvic Cavity
Sphenomandibular ligament	Head and Neck Bursa and Ligament
Sphenopalatine (pterygopalatine) ganglion	Head and Neck Sympathetic Nerve
Spinal nerve, cervical	Cervical Nerve
Spinal nerve, lumbar	Lumbar Nerve
Spinal nerve, sacral	Sacral Nerve
Spinal nerve, thoracic	Thoracic Nerve
Spinous process	Cervical Vertebra
	Lumbar Vertebra
	Thoracic Vertebra
Spiral ganglion	Acoustic Nerve
Splenic flexure	Transverse Colon
Splenic plexus	Abdominal Sympathetic Nerve
Splenius capitis muscle	Head Muscle
Splenius cervicis muscle	Neck Muscle, Right
	Neck Muscle, Left
Stapes	Auditory Ossicle, Right
	Auditory Ossicle, Left
Stellate ganglion	Head and Neck Sympathetic Nerve
Stensen's duct	Parotid Duct, Right
	Parotid Duct, Left
Sternoclavicular ligament	Shoulder Bursa and Ligament, Right
	Shoulder Bursa and Ligament, Left
Sternocleidomastoid artery	Thyroid Artery, Right
	Thyroid Artery, Left
Sternocleidomastoid muscle	Neck Muscle, Right
	Neck Muscle, Left
Sternocostal ligament	Sternum Bursa and Ligament
Styloglossus muscle	Tongue, Palate, Pharynx Muscle
Stylomandibular ligament	Head and Neck Bursa and Ligament
Stylopharyngeus muscle	Tongue, Palate, Pharynx Muscle
Subacromial bursa	Shoulder Bursa and Ligament, Right
	Shoulder Bursa and Ligament, Left
Subaortic (common iliac) lymph node	Lymphatic, Pelvis
Subarachnoid space, spinal	Spinal Canal

Term	ICD-10-PCS Value
Subclavicular (apical) lymph node	Lymphatic, Right Axillary
	Lymphatic, Left Axillary
Subclavius muscle	Thorax Muscle, Right
	Thorax Muscle, Left
Subclavius nerve	Brachial Plexus
Subcostal artery	Upper Artery
Subcostal muscle	Thorax Muscle, Right
	Thorax Muscle, Left
Subcostal nerve	Thoracic Nerve
Subdural space, spinal	Spinal Canal
Submandibular ganglion	Facial Nerve
	Head and Neck Sympathetic Nerve
Submandibular gland	Submaxillary Gland, Right
	Submaxillary Gland, Left
Submandibular lymph node	Lymphatic, Head
Submandibular space	Subcutaneous Tissue and Fascia, Face
Submaxillary ganglion	Head and Neck Sympathetic Nerve
Submaxillary lymph node	Lymphatic, Head
Submental artery	Face Artery
Submental lymph node	Lymphatic, Head
Submucous (Meissner's) plexus	Abdominal Sympathetic Nerve
Suboccipital nerve	Cervical Nerve
Suboccipital venous plexus	Vertebral Vein, Right
	Vertebral Vein, Left
Subparotid lymph node	Lymphatic, Head
Subscapular aponeurosis	Subcutaneous Tissue and Fascia, Right Upper Arm
	Subcutaneous Tissue and Fascia, Left Upper Arm
Subscapular artery	Axillary Artery, Right
	Axillary Artery, Left
Subscapular (posterior) lymph node	Lymphatic, Right Axillary
	Lymphatic, Left Axillary
Subscapularis muscle	Shoulder Muscle, Right
	Shoulder Muscle, Left
Substantia nigra	Basal Ganglia
Subtalar (talocalcaneal) joint	Tarsal Joint, Right
	Tarsal Joint, Left
Subtalar ligament	Foot Bursa and Ligament, Right
	Foot Bursa and Ligament, Left
Subthalamic nucleus	Basal Ganglia
Superficial circumflex iliac vein	Saphenous Vein, Right
	Saphenous Vein, Left
Superficial epigastric artery	Femoral Artery, Right
	Femoral Artery, Left
Superficial epigastric vein	Saphenous Vein, Right
	Saphenous Vein, Left
Superficial palmar arch	Hand Artery, Right
	Hand Artery, Left
Superficial palmar venous arch	Hand Vein, Right
	Hand Vein, Left
Superficial temporal artery	Temporal Artery, Right
	Temporal Artery, Left
Superficial transverse perineal muscle	Perineum Muscle
Superior cardiac nerve	Thoracic Sympathetic Nerve
Superior cerebellar vein	Intracranial Vein
Superior cerebral vein	Intracranial Vein
Superior clunic (cluneal) nerve	Lumbar Nerve

Term	ICD-10-PCS Value
Superior epigastric artery	Internal Mammary Artery, Right
	Internal Mammary Artery, Left
Superior genicular artery	Popliteal Artery, Right
	Popliteal Artery, Left
Superior gluteal artery	Internal Iliac Artery, Right
	Internal Iliac Artery, Left
Superior gluteal nerve	Lumbar Plexus
Superior hypogastric plexus	Abdominal Sympathetic Nerve
Superior labial artery	Face Artery
Superior laryngeal artery	Thyroid Artery, Right
	Thyroid Artery, Left
Superior laryngeal nerve	Vagus Nerve
Superior longitudinal muscle	Tongue, Palate, Pharynx Muscle
Superior mesenteric ganglion	Abdominal Sympathetic Nerve
Superior mesenteric lymph node	Lymphatic, Mesenteric
Superior mesenteric plexus	Abdominal Sympathetic Nerve
Superior oblique muscle	Extraocular Muscle, Right
	Extraocular Muscle, Left
Superior olivary nucleus	Pons
Superior rectal artery	Inferior Mesenteric Artery
Superior rectal vein	Inferior Mesenteric Vein
Superior rectus muscle	Extraocular Muscle, Right
	Extraocular Muscle, Left
Superior tarsal plate	Upper Eyelid, Right
	Upper Eyelid, Left
Superior thoracic artery	Axillary Artery, Right
	Axillary Artery, Left
Superior thyroid artery	External Carotid Artery, Right
	External Carotid Artery, Left
	Thyroid Artery, Right
	Thyroid Artery, Left
Superior turbinate	Nasal Turbinate
Superior ulnar collateral artery	Brachial Artery, Right
	Brachial Artery, Left
Superior vesical artery	Internal Iliac Artery, Right
	Internal Iliac Artery, Left
Supraclavicular nerve	Cervical Plexus
Supraclavicular (Virchow's) lymph node	Lymphatic, Right Neck
	Lymphatic, Left Neck
Suprahyoid lymph node	Lymphatic, Head
Suprahyoid muscle	Neck Muscle, Right
	Neck Muscle, Left
Suprainguinal lymph node	Lymphatic, Pelvis
Supraorbital vein	Face Vein, Right
	Face Vein, Left
Suprarenal gland	Adrenal Gland, Right
	Adrenal Gland, Left
	Adrenal Glands, Bilateral
	Adrenal Gland
Suprarenal plexus	Abdominal Sympathetic Nerve
Suprascapular nerve	Brachial Plexus
Supraspinatus fascia	Subcutaneous Tissue and Fascia, Right Upper Arm
	Subcutaneous Tissue and Fascia, Left Upper Arm
Supraspinatus muscle	Shoulder Muscle, Right
	Shoulder Muscle, Left
Supraspinous ligament	Upper Spine Bursa and Ligament
	Lower Spine Bursa and Ligament

Appendix D: Body Part Key

Term	ICD-10-PCS Value
Suprasternal notch	Sternum
Supratrochlear lymph node	Lymphatic, Right Upper Extremity
	Lymphatic, Left Upper Extremity
Sural artery	Popliteal Artery, Right
	Popliteal Artery, Left
Sweat gland	Skin
Talocalcaneal ligament	Foot Bursa and Ligament, Right
	Foot Bursa and Ligament, Left
Talocalcaneal (subtalar) joint	Tarsal Joint, Right
	Tarsal Joint, Left
Talocalcaneonavicular joint	Tarsal Joint, Right
	Tarsal Joint, Left
Talocalcaneonavicular ligament	Foot Bursa and Ligament, Right
	Foot Bursa and Ligament, Left
Talocrural joint	Ankle Joint, Right
	Ankle Joint, Left
Talofibular ligament	Ankle Bursa and Ligament, Right
	Ankle Bursa and Ligament, Left
Talus bone	Tarsal, Right
	Tarsal, Left
Tarsometatarsal ligament	Foot Bursa and Ligament, Right
	Foot Bursa and Ligament, Left
Temporal lobe	Cerebral Hemisphere
Temporalis muscle	Head Muscle
Temporoparietalis muscle	Head Muscle
Tensor fasciae latae muscle	Hip Muscle, Right
	Hip Muscle, Left
Tensor veli palatini muscle	Tongue, Palate, Pharynx Muscle
Tenth cranial nerve	Vagus Nerve
Tentorium cerebelli	Dura Mater
Teres major muscle	Shoulder Muscle, Right
	Shoulder Muscle, Left
Teres minor muscle	Shoulder Muscle, Right
	Shoulder Muscle, Left
Testicular artery	Abdominal Aorta
Thenar muscle	Hand Muscle, Right
	Hand Muscle, Left
Third cranial nerve	Oculomotor Nerve
Third occipital nerve	Cervical Nerve
Third ventricle	Cerebral Ventricle
Thoracic aortic plexus	Thoracic Sympathetic Nerve
Thoracic esophagus	Esophagus, Middle
Thoracic facet joint	Thoracic Vertebral Joint
Thoracic ganglion	Thoracic Sympathetic Nerve
Thoracoacromial artery	Axillary Artery, Right
	Axillary Artery, Left
Thoracolumbar facet joint	Thoracolumbar Vertebral Joint
Thymus gland	Thymus
Thyroarytenoid muscle	Neck Muscle, Right
	Neck Muscle, Left
Thyrocervical trunk	Thyroid Artery, Right
	Thyroid Artery, Left
Thyroid cartilage	Larynx
Tibial sesamoid	Metatarsal, Right
	Metatarsal, Left
Tibialis anterior muscle	Lower Leg Muscle, Right
	Lower Leg Muscle, Left
Tibialis posterior muscle	Lower Leg Muscle, Right
	Lower Leg Muscle, Left

Term	ICD-10-PCS Value
Tibiofemoral joint	Knee Joint, Right
	Knee Joint, Left
	Knee Joint, Tibial Surface, Right
	Knee Joint, Tibial Surface, Left
Tibioperoneal trunk	Popliteal Artery, Right
	Popliteal Artery, Left
Tongue, base of	Pharynx
Tracheobronchial lymph node	Lymphatic, Thorax
Tragus	External Ear, Right
	External Ear, Left
	External Ear, Bilateral
Transversalis fascia	Subcutaneous Tissue and Fascia, Trunk
Transverse acetabular ligament	Hip Bursa and Ligament, Right
	Hip Bursa and Ligament, Left
Transverse (cutaneous) cervical nerve	Cervical Plexus
Transverse facial artery	Temporal Artery, Right
	Temporal Artery, Left
Transverse foramen	Cervical Vertebra
Transverse humeral ligament	Shoulder Bursa and Ligament, Right
	Shoulder Bursa and Ligament, Left
Transverse ligament of atlas	Head and Neck Bursa and Ligament
Transverse process	Cervical Vertebra
	Thoracic Vertebra
	Lumbar Vertebra
Transverse scapular ligament	Shoulder Bursa and Ligament, Right
	Shoulder Bursa and Ligament, Left
Transverse thoracis muscle	Thorax Muscle, Right
	Thorax Muscle, Left
Transversospinalis muscle	Trunk Muscle, Right
	Trunk Muscle, Left
Transversus abdominis muscle	Abdomen Muscle, Right
	Abdomen Muscle, Left
Trapezium bone	Carpal, Right
	Carpal, Left
Trapezius muscle	Trunk Muscle, Right
	Trunk Muscle, Left
Trapezoid bone	Carpal, Right
	Carpal, Left
Triceps brachii muscle	Upper Arm Muscle, Right
	Upper Arm Muscle, Left
Tricuspid annulus	Tricuspid Valve
Trifacial nerve	Trigeminal Nerve
Trigone of bladder	Bladder
Triquetral bone	Carpal, Right
	Carpal, Left
Trochanteric bursa	Hip Bursa and Ligament, Right
	Hip Bursa and Ligament, Left
Twelfth cranial nerve	Hypoglossal Nerve
Tympanic cavity	Middle Ear, Right
	Middle Ear, Left
Tympanic nerve	Glossopharyngeal Nerve
Tympanic part of temporal bone	Temporal Bone, Right
	Temporal Bone, Left
Ulnar collateral carpal ligament	Wrist Bursa and Ligament, Right
	Wrist Bursa and Ligament, Left
Ulnar collateral ligament	Elbow Bursa and Ligament, Right
	Elbow Bursa and Ligament, Left
Ulnar notch	Radius, Right
	Radius, Left

Term	ICD-10-PCS Value
Ulnar vein	Brachial Vein, Right
	Brachial Vein, Left
Umbilical artery	Internal Iliac Artery, Right
	Internal Iliac Artery, Left
	Lower Artery
Ureteral orifice	Ureter, Right
	Ureter, Left
	Ureters, Bilateral
	Ureter
Ureteropelvic junction (UPJ)	Kidney Pelvis, Right
	Kidney Pelvis, Left
Ureterovesical orifice	Ureter, Right
	Ureter, Left
	Ureters, Bilateral
	Ureter
Uterine artery	Internal Iliac Artery, Right
	Internal Iliac Artery, Left
Uterine cornu	Uterus
Uterine tube	Fallopian Tube, Right
	Fallopian Tube, Left
Uterine vein	Hypogastric Vein, Right
	Hypogastric Vein, Left
Vaginal artery	Internal Iliac Artery, Right
	Internal Iliac Artery, Left
Vaginal vein	Hypogastric Vein, Right
	Hypogastric Vein, Left
Vastus intermedius muscle	Upper Leg Muscle, Right
	Upper Leg Muscle, Left
Vastus lateralis muscle	Upper Leg Muscle, Right
	Upper Leg Muscle, Left
Vastus medialis muscle	Upper Leg Muscle, Right
	Upper Leg Muscle, Left
Ventricular fold	Larynx
Vermiform appendix	Appendix
Vermilion border	Upper Lip
	Lower Lip
Vertebral arch	Cervical Vertebra
	Lumbar Vertebra
	Thoracic Vertebra
Vertebral artery, intracranial portion	Intracranial Artery
Vertebral body	Cervical Vertebra
	Lumbar Vertebra
	Thoracic Vertebra
Vertebral canal	Spinal Canal
Vertebral foramen	Cervical Vertebra
	Lumbar Vertebra
	Thoracic Vertebra
Vertebral lamina	Cervical Vertebra
	Lumbar Vertebra
	Thoracic Vertebra
Vertebral pedicle	Cervical Vertebra
	Lumbar Vertebra
	Thoracic Vertebra
Vesical vein	Hypogastric Vein, Right
	Hypogastric Vein, Left
Vestibular (Scarpa's) ganglion	Acoustic Nerve
Vestibular nerve	Acoustic Nerve
Vestibulocochlear nerve	Acoustic Nerve

Term	ICD-10-PCS Value
Virchow's (supraclavicular) lymph node	Lymphatic, Right Neck
	Lymphatic, Left Neck
Vitreous body	Vitreous, Right
	Vitreous, Left
Vocal fold	Vocal Cord, Right
	Vocal Cord, Left
Volar (palmar) digital vein	Hand Vein, Right
	Hand Vein, Left
Volar (palmar) metacarpal vein	Hand Vein, Right
	Hand Vein, Left
Vomer bone	Nasal Septum
Vomer of nasal septum	Nasal Bone
Xiphoid process	Sternum
Zonule of Zinn	Lens, Right
	Lens, Left
Zygomatic process of frontal bone	Frontal Bone
Zygomatic process of temporal bone	Temporal Bone, Right
	Temporal Bone, Left
Zygomaticus muscle	Facial Muscle

Appendix E: Body Part Definitions

ICD-10-PCS Value	Definition
1st Toe, Left 1st Toe, Right	Hallux
Abdomen Muscle, Left Abdomen Muscle, Right	External oblique muscle Internal oblique muscle Pyramidalis muscle Rectus abdominis muscle Transversus abdominis muscle
Abdominal Aorta	Inferior phrenic artery Lumbar artery Median sacral artery Middle suprarenal artery Ovarian artery Testicular artery
Abdominal Sympathetic Nerve	Abdominal aortic plexus Auerbach's (myenteric) plexus Celiac (solar) plexus Celiac ganglion Gastric plexus Hepatic plexus Inferior hypogastric plexus Inferior mesenteric ganglion Inferior mesenteric plexus Meissner's (submucous) plexus Myenteric (Auerbach's) plexus Pancreatic plexus Pelvic splanchnic nerve Renal nerve Renal plexus Solar (celiac) plexus Splenic plexus Submucous (Meissner's) plexus Superior hypogastric plexus Superior mesenteric ganglion Superior mesenteric plexus Suprarenal plexus
Abducens Nerve	Sixth cranial nerve
Accessory Nerve	Eleventh cranial nerve
Acoustic Nerve	Cochlear nerve Eighth cranial nerve Scarpa's (vestibular) ganglion Spiral ganglion Vestibular (Scarpa's) ganglion Vestibular nerve Vestibulocochlear nerve
Adenoids	Pharyngeal tonsil
Adrenal Gland Adrenal Gland, Left Adrenal Gland, Right Adrenal Glands, Bilateral	Suprarenal gland
Ampulla of Vater	Duodenal ampulla Hepatopancreatic ampulla
Anal Sphincter	External anal sphincter Internal anal sphincter
Ankle Bursa and Ligament, Left Ankle Bursa and Ligament, Right	Calcaneofibular ligament Deltoid ligament Ligament of the lateral malleolus Talofibular ligament
Ankle Joint, Left Ankle Joint, Right	Inferior tibiofibular joint Talocrural joint
Anterior Chamber, Left Anterior Chamber, Right	Aqueous humour
Anterior Tibial Artery, Left Anterior Tibial Artery, Right	Anterior lateral malleolar artery Anterior medial malleolar artery Anterior tibial recurrent artery Dorsalis pedis artery Posterior tibial recurrent artery

ICD-10-PCS Value	Definition
Anus	Anal orifice
Aortic Valve	Aortic annulus
Appendix	Appendiceal orifice Vermiform appendix
Atrial Septum	Interatrial septum
Atrium, Left	Atrium pulmonale Left auricular appendix
Atrium, Right	Atrium dextrum cordis Right auricular appendix Sinus venosus
Auditory Ossicle, Left Auditory Ossicle, Right	Incus Malleus Stapes
Axillary Artery, Left Axillary Artery, Right	Anterior circumflex humeral artery Lateral thoracic artery Posterior circumflex humeral artery Subscapular artery Superior thoracic artery Thoracoacromial artery
Azygos Vein	Right ascending lumbar vein Right subcostal vein
Basal Ganglia	Basal nuclei Claustrum Corpus striatum Globus pallidus Substantia nigra Subthalamic nucleus
Basilic Vein, Left Basilic Vein, Right	Median antebrachial vein Median cubital vein
Bladder	Trigone of bladder
Brachial Artery, Left Brachial Artery, Right	Inferior ulnar collateral artery Profunda brachii Superior ulnar collateral artery
Brachial Plexus	Axillary nerve Dorsal scapular nerve First intercostal nerve Long thoracic nerve Musculocutaneous nerve Subclavius nerve Suprascapular nerve
Brachial Vein, Left Brachial Vein, Right	Radial vein Ulnar vein
Brain	Cerebrum Corpus callosum Encephalon
Breast, Bilateral Breast, Left Breast, Right	Mammary duct Mammary gland
Buccal Mucosa	Buccal gland Molar gland Palatine gland
Carotid Bodies, Bilateral Carotid Body, Left Carotid Body, Right	Carotid glomus
Carpal Joint, Left Carpal Joint, Right	Intercarpal joint Midcarpal joint
Carpal, Left Carpal, Right	Capitate bone Hamate bone Lunate bone Pisiform bone Scaphoid bone Trapezium bone Trapezoid bone Triquetral bone
Celiac Artery	Celiac trunk

ICD-10-PCS Value	Definition
Cephalic Vein, Left Cephalic Vein, Right	Accessory cephalic vein
Cerebellum	Culmen
Cerebral Hemisphere	Frontal lobe Occipital lobe Parietal lobe Temporal lobe
Cerebral Meninges	Arachnoid mater, intracranial Leptomeninges, intracranial Pia mater, intracranial
Cerebral Ventricle	Aqueduct of Sylvius Cerebral aqueduct (Sylvius) Choroid plexus Ependyma Foramen of Monro (intraventricular) Fourth ventricle Interventricular foramen (Monro) Left lateral ventricle Right lateral ventricle Third ventricle
Cervical Nerve	Greater occipital nerve Spinal nerve, cervical Suboccipital nerve Third occipital nerve
Cervical Plexus	Ansa cervicalis Cutaneous (transverse) cervical nerve Great auricular nerve Lesser occipital nerve Supraclavicular nerve Transverse (cutaneous) cervical nerve
Cervical Spinal Cord	Dorsal root ganglion
Cervical Vertebra	Dens Odontoid process Spinous process Transverse foramen Transverse process Vertebral arch Vertebral body Vertebral foramen Vertebral lamina Vertebral pedicle
Cervical Vertebral Joint	Atlantoaxial joint Cervical facet joint
Cervical Vertebral Joints, 2 or more	Cervical facet joint
Cervicothoracic Vertebral Joint	Cervicothoracic facet joint
Cisterna Chyli	Intestinal lymphatic trunk Lumbar lymphatic trunk
Coccygeal Glomus	Coccygeal body
Colic Vein	Ileocolic vein Left colic vein Middle colic vein Right colic vein
Conduction Mechanism	Atrioventricular node Bundle of His Bundle of Kent Sinoatrial node
Conjunctiva, Left Conjunctiva, Right	Plica semilunaris
Dura Mater	Diaphragma sellae Dura mater, intracranial Falx cerebri Tentorium cerebelli
Elbow Bursa and Ligament, Left Elbow Bursa and Ligament, Right	Annular ligament Olecranon bursa Radial collateral ligament Ulnar collateral ligament

ICD-10-PCS Value	Definition
Elbow Joint, Left Elbow Joint, Right	Distal humerus, involving joint Humeroradial joint Humeroulnar joint Proximal radioulnar joint
Epidural Space, Intracranial	Extradural space, intracranial
Epiglottis	Glossoepiglottic fold
Esophagogastric Junction	Cardia Cardioesophageal junction Gastroesophageal (GE) junction
Esophagus, Lower	Abdominal esophagus
Esophagus, Middle	Thoracic esophagus
Esophagus, Upper	Cervical esophagus
Ethmoid Bone, Left Ethmoid Bone, Right	Cribriform plate
Ethmoid Sinus, Left Ethmoid Sinus, Right	Ethmoidal air cell
Eustachian Tube, Left Eustachian Tube, Right	Auditory tube Pharyngotympanic tube
External Auditory Canal, Left External Auditory Canal, Right	External auditory meatus
External Carotid Artery, Left External Carotid Artery, Right	Ascending pharyngeal artery Internal maxillary artery Lingual artery Maxillary artery Occipital artery Posterior auricular artery Superior thyroid artery
External Ear, Bilateral External Ear, Left External Ear, Right	Antihelix Antitragus Auricle Earlobe Helix Pinna Tragus
External Iliac Artery, Left External Iliac Artery, Right	Deep circumflex iliac artery Inferior epigastric artery
External Jugular Vein, Left External Jugular Vein, Right	Posterior auricular vein
Extraocular Muscle, Left Extraocular Muscle, Right	Inferior oblique muscle Inferior rectus muscle Lateral rectus muscle Medial rectus muscle Superior oblique muscle Superior rectus muscle
Eye, Left Eye, Right	Ciliary body Posterior chamber
Face Artery	Angular artery Ascending palatine artery External maxillary artery Facial artery Inferior labial artery Submental artery Superior labial artery
Face Vein, Left Face Vein, Right	Angular vein Anterior facial vein Common facial vein Deep facial vein Frontal vein Posterior facial (retromandibular) vein Supraorbital vein

Appendix E: Body Part Definitions

ICD-10-PCS Value	Definition
Facial Muscle	Buccinator muscle Corrugator supercilii muscle Depressor anguli oris muscle Depressor labii inferioris muscle Depressor septi nasi muscle Depressor supercilii muscle Levator anguli oris muscle Levator labii superioris alaeque nasi muscle Levator labii superioris muscle Mentalis muscle Nasalis muscle Occipitofrontalis muscle Orbicularis oris muscle Procerus muscle Risorius muscle Zygomaticus muscle
Facial Nerve	Chorda tympani Geniculate ganglion Greater superficial petrosal nerve Nerve to the stapedius Parotid plexus Posterior auricular nerve Seventh cranial nerve Submandibular ganglion
Fallopian Tube, Left Fallopian Tube, Right	Oviduct Salpinx Uterine tube
Femoral Artery, Left Femoral Artery, Right	Circumflex iliac artery Deep femoral artery Descending genicular artery External pudendal artery Superficial epigastric artery
Femoral Nerve	Anterior crural nerve Saphenous nerve
Femoral Shaft, Left Femoral Shaft, Right	Body of femur
Femoral Vein, Left Femoral Vein, Right	Deep femoral (profunda femoris) vein Popliteal vein Profunda femoris (deep femoral) vein
Fibula, Left Fibula, Right	Body of fibula Head of fibula Lateral malleolus
Finger Nail	Nail bed Nail plate
Finger Phalangeal Joint, Left Finger Phalangeal Joint, Right	Interphalangeal (IP) joint
Foot Artery, Left Foot Artery, Right	Arcuate artery Dorsal metatarsal artery Lateral plantar artery Lateral tarsal artery Medial plantar artery
Foot Bursa and Ligament, Left Foot Bursa and Ligament, Right	Calcaneocuboid ligament Cuneonavicular ligament Intercuneiform ligament Interphalangeal ligament Metatarsal ligament Metatarsophalangeal ligament Subtalar ligament Talocalcaneal ligament Talocalcaneonavicular ligament Tarsometatarsal ligament
Foot Muscle, Left Foot Muscle, Right	Abductor hallucis muscle Adductor hallucis muscle Extensor digitorum brevis muscle Extensor hallucis brevis muscle Flexor digitorum brevis muscle Flexor hallucis brevis muscle Quadratus plantae muscle

ICD-10-PCS Value	Definition
Foot Vein, Left Foot Vein, Right	Common digital vein Dorsal metatarsal vein Dorsal venous arch Plantar digital vein Plantar metatarsal vein Plantar venous arch
Frontal Bone	Zygomatic process of frontal bone
Gastric Artery	Left gastric artery Right gastric artery
Glenoid Cavity, Left Glenoid Cavity, Right	Glenoid fossa (of scapula)
Glomus Jugulare	Jugular body
Glossopharyngeal Nerve	Carotid sinus nerve Ninth cranial nerve Tympanic nerve
Hand Artery, Left Hand Artery, Right	Deep palmar arch Princeps pollicis artery Radialis indicis Superficial palmar arch
Hand Bursa and Ligament, Left Hand Bursa and Ligament, Right	Carpometacarpal ligament Intercarpal ligament Interphalangeal ligament Lunotriquetral ligament Metacarpal ligament Metacarpophalangeal ligament Pisohamate ligament Pisometacarpal ligament Scaphotrapezium ligament
Hand Muscle, Left Hand Muscle, Right	Adductor pollicis muscle Hypothenar muscle Palmar interosseous muscle Thenar muscle
Hand Vein, Left Hand Vein, Right	Dorsal metacarpal vein Palmar (volar) digital vein Palmar (volar) metacarpal vein Superficial palmar venous arch Volar (palmar) digital vein Volar (palmar) metacarpal vein
Head and Neck Bursa and Ligament	Alar ligament of axis Cervical interspinous ligament Cervical intertransverse ligament Cervical ligamentum flavum Interspinous ligament, cervical Intertransverse ligament, cervical Lateral temporomandibular ligament Ligamentum flavum, cervical Sphenomandibular ligament Stylomandibular ligament Transverse ligament of atlas
Head and Neck Sympathetic Nerve	Cavernous plexus Cervical ganglion Ciliary ganglion Internal carotid plexus Otic ganglion Pterygopalatine (sphenopalatine) ganglion Sphenopalatine (pterygopalatine) ganglion Stellate ganglion Submandibular ganglion Submaxillary ganglion
Head Muscle	Auricularis muscle Masseter muscle Pterygoid muscle Splenius capitis muscle Temporalis muscle Temporoparietalis muscle
Heart, Left	Left coronary sulcus Obtuse margin
Heart, Right	Right coronary sulcus
Hemiazygos Vein	Left ascending lumbar vein Left subcostal vein

ICD-10-PCS Value	Definition
Hepatic Artery	Common hepatic artery Gastroduodenal artery Hepatic artery proper
Hip Bursa and Ligament, Left Hip Bursa and Ligament, Right	Iliofemoral ligament Ischiofemoral ligament Pubofemoral ligament Transverse acetabular ligament Trochanteric bursa
Hip Joint, Left Hip Joint, Right	Acetabulofemoral joint
Hip Muscle, Left Hip Muscle, Right	Gemellus muscle Gluteus maximus muscle Gluteus medius muscle Gluteus minimus muscle Iliacus muscle Iliopsoas muscle Obturator muscle Piriformis muscle Psoas muscle Quadratus femoris muscle Tensor fasciae latae muscle
Humeral Head, Left Humeral Head, Right	Greater tuberosity Lesser tuberosity Neck of humerus (anatomical)(surgical)
Humeral Shaft, Left Humeral Shaft, Right	Distal humerus Humerus, distal Lateral epicondyle of humerus Medial epicondyle of humerus
Hypogastric Vein, Left Hypogastric Vein, Right	Gluteal vein Internal iliac vein Internal pudendal vein Lateral sacral vein Middle hemorrhoidal vein Obturator vein Uterine vein Vaginal vein Vesical vein
Hypoglossal Nerve	Twelfth cranial nerve
Hypothalamus	Mammillary body
Inferior Mesenteric Artery	Sigmoid artery Superior rectal artery
Inferior Mesenteric Vein	Sigmoid vein Superior rectal vein
Inferior Vena Cava	Postcava Right inferior phrenic vein Right ovarian vein Right second lumbar vein Right suprarenal vein Right testicular vein
Inguinal Region, Bilateral Inguinal Region, Left Inguinal Region, Right	Inguinal canal Inguinal triangle
Inner Ear, Left Inner Ear, Right	Bony labyrinth Bony vestibule Cochlea Round window Semicircular canal
Innominate Artery	Brachiocephalic artery Brachiocephalic trunk
Innominate Vein, Left Innominate Vein, Right	Brachiocephalic vein Inferior thyroid vein
Internal Carotid Artery, Left Internal Carotid Artery, Right	Caroticotympanic artery Carotid sinus

ICD-10-PCS Value	Definition
Internal Iliac Artery, Left Internal Iliac Artery, Right	Deferential artery Hypogastric artery Iliolumbar artery Inferior gluteal artery Inferior vesical artery Internal pudendal artery Lateral sacral artery Middle rectal artery Obturator artery Prostatic artery Superior gluteal artery Superior vesical artery Umbilical artery Uterine artery Vaginal artery
Internal Mammary Artery, Left Internal Mammary Artery, Right	Anterior intercostal artery Internal thoracic artery Musculophrenic artery Pericardiophrenic artery Superior epigastric artery
Intracranial Artery	Anterior cerebral artery Anterior choroidal artery Anterior communicating artery Basilar artery Circle of Willis Internal carotid artery, intracranial portion Middle cerebral artery Middle meningeal artery, intracranial portion Ophthalmic artery Posterior cerebral artery Posterior communicating artery Posterior inferior cerebellar artery (PICA) Vertebral artery, intracranial portion
Intracranial Vein	Anterior cerebral vein Basal (internal) cerebral vein Dural venous sinus Great cerebral vein Inferior cerebellar vein Inferior cerebral vein Internal (basal) cerebral vein Middle cerebral vein Ophthalmic vein Superior cerebellar vein Superior cerebral vein
Jejunum	Duodenojejunal flexure
Kidney	Renal calyx Renal capsule Renal cortex Renal segment
Kidney Pelvis, Left Kidney Pelvis, Right	Ureteropelvic junction (UPJ)
Kidney, Left Kidney, Right Kidneys, Bilateral	Renal calyx Renal capsule Renal cortex Renal segment
Knee Bursa and Ligament, Left Knee Bursa and Ligament, Right	Anterior cruciate ligament (ACL) Lateral collateral ligament (LCL) Ligament of head of fibula Medial collateral ligament (MCL) Patellar ligament Popliteal ligament Posterior cruciate ligament (PCL) Prepatellar bursa
Knee Joint, Femoral Surface, Left Knee Joint, Femoral Surface, Right	Femoropatellar joint Patellofemoral joint

Appendix E: Body Part Definitions

ICD-10-PCS Value	Definition
Knee Joint, Left Knee Joint, Right	Femoropatellar joint Femorotibial joint Lateral meniscus Medial meniscus Patellofemoral joint Tibiofemoral joint
Knee Joint, Tibial Surface, Left Knee Joint, Tibial Surface, Right	Femorotibial joint Tibiofemoral joint
Knee Region, Left Knee Region, Right	Popliteal fossa
Knee Tendon, Left Knee Tendon, Right	Patellar tendon
Lacrimal Duct, Left Lacrimal Duct, Right	Lacrimal canaliculus Lacrimal punctum Lacrimal sac Nasolacrimal duct
Larynx	Aryepiglottic fold Arytenoid cartilage Corniculate cartilage Cuneiform cartilage False vocal cord Glottis Rima glottidis Thyroid cartilage Ventricular fold
Lens, Left Lens, Right	Zonule of Zinn
Liver	Quadrate lobe
Lower Arm and Wrist Muscle, Left Lower Arm and Wrist Muscle, Right	Anatomical snuffbox Anconeus muscle Brachioradialis muscle Extensor carpi radialis muscle Extensor carpi ulnaris muscle Flexor carpi radialis muscle Flexor carpi ulnaris muscle Flexor pollicis longus muscle Palmaris longus muscle Pronator quadratus muscle Pronator teres muscle
Lower Artery	Umbilical artery
Lower Eyelid, Left Lower Eyelid, Right	Inferior tarsal plate Medial canthus
Lower Femur, Left Lower Femur, Right	Lateral condyle of femur Lateral epicondyle of femur Medial condyle of femur Medial epicondyle of femur
Lower Leg Muscle, Left Lower Leg Muscle, Right	Extensor digitorum longus muscle Extensor hallucis longus muscle Fibularis brevis muscle Fibularis longus muscle Flexor digitorum longus muscle Flexor hallucis longus muscle Gastrocnemius muscle Peroneus brevis muscle Peroneus longus muscle Plantaris muscle Popliteus muscle Soleus muscle Tibialis anterior muscle Tibialis posterior muscle
Lower Leg Tendon, Left Lower Leg Tendon, Right	Achilles tendon
Lower Lip	Frenulum labii inferioris Labial gland Vermilion border

ICD-10-PCS Value	Definition
Lower Spine Bursa and Ligament	Iliolumbar ligament Interspinous ligament, lumbar Intertransverse ligament, lumbar Ligamentum flavum, lumbar Sacrococcygeal ligament Sacroiliac ligament Sacrospinous ligament Sacrotuberous ligament Supraspinous ligament
Lumbar Nerve	Lumbosacral trunk Spinal nerve, lumbar Superior clunic (cluneal) nerve
Lumbar Plexus	Accessory obturator nerve Genitofemoral nerve Iliohypogastric nerve Ilioinguinal nerve Lateral femoral cutaneous nerve Obturator nerve Superior gluteal nerve
Lumbar Spinal Cord	Cauda equina Conus medullaris Dorsal root ganglion
Lumbar Sympathetic Nerve	Lumbar ganglion Lumbar splanchnic nerve
Lumbar Vertebra	Spinous process Transverse process Vertebral arch Vertebral body Vertebral foramen Vertebral lamina Vertebral pedicle
Lumbar Vertebral Joint	Lumbar facet joint
Lumbosacral Joint	Lumbosacral facet joint
Lymphatic, Aortic	Celiac lymph node Gastric lymph node Hepatic lymph node Lumbar lymph node Pancreaticosplenic lymph node Paraaortic lymph node Retroperitoneal lymph node
Lymphatic, Head	Buccinator lymph node Infraauricular lymph node Infraparotid lymph node Parotid lymph node Preauricular lymph node Submandibular lymph node Submaxillary lymph node Submental lymph node Subparotid lymph node Suprahyoid lymph node
Lymphatic, Left Axillary	Anterior (pectoral) lymph node Apical (subclavicular) lymph node Brachial (lateral) lymph node Central axillary lymph node Lateral (brachial) lymph node Pectoral (anterior) lymph node Posterior (subscapular) lymph node Subclavicular (apical) lymph node Subscapular (posterior) lymph node
Lymphatic, Left Lower Extremity	Femoral lymph node Popliteal lymph node
Lymphatic, Left Neck	Cervical lymph node Jugular lymph node Mastoid (postauricular) lymph node Occipital lymph node Postauricular (mastoid) lymph node Retropharyngeal lymph node Supraclavicular (Virchow's) lymph node Virchow's (supraclavicular) lymph node

ICD-10-PCS Value	Definition
Lymphatic, Left Upper Extremity	Cubital lymph node Deltopectoral (infraclavicular) lymph node Epitrochlear lymph node Infraclavicular (deltopectoral) lymph node Supratrochlear lymph node
Lymphatic, Mesenteric	Inferior mesenteric lymph node Pararectal lymph node Superior mesenteric lymph node
Lymphatic, Pelvis	Common iliac (subaortic) lymph node Gluteal lymph node Iliac lymph node Inferior epigastric lymph node Obturator lymph node Sacral lymph node Subaortic (common iliac) lymph node Suprainguinal lymph node
Lymphatic, Right Axillary	Anterior (pectoral) lymph node Apical (subclavicular) lymph node Brachial (lateral) lymph node Central axillary lymph node Lateral (brachial) lymph node Pectoral (anterior) lymph node Posterior (subscapular) lymph node Subclavicular (apical) lymph node Subscapular (posterior) lymph node
Lymphatic, Right Lower Extremity	Femoral lymph node Popliteal lymph node
Lymphatic, Right Neck	Cervical lymph node Jugular lymph node Mastoid (postauricular) lymph node Occipital lymph node Postauricular (mastoid) lymph node Retropharyngeal lymph node Right jugular trunk Right lymphatic duct Right subclavian trunk Supraclavicular (Virchow's) lymph node Virchow's (supraclavicular) lymph node
Lymphatic, Right Upper Extremity	Cubital lymph node Deltopectoral (infraclavicular) lymph node Epitrochlear lymph node Infraclavicular (deltopectoral) lymph node Supratrochlear lymph node
Lymphatic, Thorax	Intercostal lymph node Mediastinal lymph node Parasternal lymph node Paratracheal lymph node Tracheobronchial lymph node
Main Bronchus, Right	Bronchus intermedius Intermediate bronchus
Mandible, Left Mandible, Right	Alveolar process of mandible Condyloid process Mandibular notch Mental foramen
Mastoid Sinus, Left Mastoid Sinus, Right	Mastoid air cells
Metatarsal, Left Metatarsal, Right	Fibular sesamoid Tibial sesamoid
Maxilla	Alveolar process of maxilla
Maxillary Sinus, Left Maxillary Sinus, Right	Antrum of Highmore
Median Nerve	Anterior interosseous nerve Palmar cutaneous nerve
Mediastinum	Mediastinal cavity Mediastinal space
Medulla Oblongata	Myelencephalon
Mesentery	Mesoappendix Mesocolon
Metatarsal, Right Metatarsal, Left	Fibular sesamoid Tibial sesamoid

ICD-10-PCS Value	Definition
Metatarsal-Phalangeal Joint, Left Metatarsal-Phalangeal Joint, Right	Metatarsophalangeal (MTP) joint
Middle Ear, Left Middle Ear, Right	Oval window Tympanic cavity
Minor Salivary Gland	Anterior lingual gland
Mitral Valve	Bicuspid valve Left atrioventricular valve Mitral annulus
Nasal Bone	Vomer of nasal septum
Nasal Mucosa and Soft Tissue	Columella External naris Greater alar cartilage Internal naris Lateral nasal cartilage Lesser alar cartilage Nasal cavity Nostril
Nasal Septum	Quadrangular cartilage Septal cartilage Vomer bone
Nasal Turbinate	Inferior turbinate Middle turbinate Nasal concha Superior turbinate
Nasopharynx	Choana Fossa of Rosenmuller Pharyngeal recess Rhinopharynx
Neck	Parapharyngeal space Retropharyngeal space
Neck Muscle, Left Neck Muscle, Right	Anterior vertebral muscle Arytenoid muscle Cricothyroid muscle Infrahyoid muscle Levator scapulae muscle Platysma muscle Scalene muscle Splenius cervicis muscle Sternocleidomastoid muscle Suprahyoid muscle Thyroarytenoid muscle
Nipple, Left Nipple, Right	Areola
Occipital Bone	Foramen magnum
Oculomotor Nerve	Third cranial nerve
Olfactory Nerve	First cranial nerve Olfactory bulb
Omentum	Gastrocolic ligament Gastrocolic omentum Gastrohepatic omentum Gastrophrenic ligament Gastrosplenic ligament Greater Omentum Hepatogastric ligament Lesser Omentum
Optic Nerve	Optic chiasma Second cranial nerve
Orbit, Left Orbit, Right	Bony orbit Orbital portion of ethmoid bone Orbital portion of frontal bone Orbital portion of lacrimal bone Orbital portion of maxilla Orbital portion of palatine bone Orbital portion of sphenoid bone Orbital portion of zygomatic bone
Pancreatic Duct	Duct of Wirsung
Pancreatic Duct, Accessory	Duct of Santorini

Appendix E: Body Part Definitions

ICD-10-PCS Value	Definition
Parotid Duct, Left Parotid Duct, Right	Stensen's duct
Pelvic Bone, Left Pelvic Bone, Right	Iliac crest Ilium Ischium Pubis
Pelvic Cavity	Prevesical space Retropubic space Space of Retzius
Penis	Corpus cavernosum Corpus spongiosum
Perineum Muscle	Bulbospongiosus muscle Cremaster muscle Deep transverse perineal muscle Ischiocavernosus muscle Levator ani muscle Superficial transverse perineal muscle
Peritoneal Cavity	Abdominal cavity
Peritoneum	Epiploic foramen
Peroneal Artery, Left Peroneal Artery, Right	Fibular artery
Peroneal Nerve	Common fibular nerve Common peroneal nerve External popliteal nerve Lateral sural cutaneous nerve
Pharynx	Base of Tongue Hypopharynx Laryngopharynx Lingual tonsil Oropharynx Piriform recess (sinus) Tongue, base of
Phrenic Nerve	Accessory phrenic nerve
Pituitary Gland	Adenohypophysis Hypophysis Neurohypophysis
Pons	Apneustic center Basis pontis Locus ceruleus Pneumotaxic center Pontine tegmentum Superior olivary nucleus
Popliteal Artery, Left Popliteal Artery, Right	Inferior genicular artery Middle genicular artery Superior genicular artery Sural artery Tibioperoneal trunk
Portal Vein	Hepatic portal vein
Prepuce	Foreskin Glans penis
Pudendal Nerve	Posterior labial nerve Posterior scrotal nerve
Pulmonary Artery, Left	Arterial canal (duct) Botallo's duct Pulmoaortic canal
Pulmonary Valve	Pulmonary annulus Pulmonic valve
Pulmonary Vein, Left	Left inferior pulmonary vein Left superior pulmonary vein
Pulmonary Vein, Right	Right inferior pulmonary vein Right superior pulmonary vein
Radial Artery, Left Radial Artery, Right	Radial recurrent artery
Radial Nerve	Dorsal digital nerve Musculospiral nerve Palmar cutaneous nerve Posterior interosseous nerve
Radius, Left Radius, Right	Ulnar notch

ICD-10-PCS Value	Definition
Rectum	Anorectal junction
Renal Artery, Left Renal Artery, Right	Inferior suprarenal artery Renal segmental artery
Renal Vein, Left	Left inferior phrenic vein Left ovarian vein Left second lumbar vein Left suprarenal vein Left testicular vein
Retina, Left Retina, Right	Fovea Macula Optic disc
Retroperitoneum	Retroperitoneal cavity Retroperitoneal space
Rib(s) Bursa and Ligament	Costotransverse ligament
Sacral Nerve	Spinal nerve, sacral
Sacral Plexus	Inferior gluteal nerve Posterior femoral cutaneous nerve Pudendal nerve
Sacral Sympathetic Nerve	Ganglion impar (ganglion of Walther) Pelvic splanchnic nerve Sacral ganglion Sacral splanchnic nerve
Sacrococcygeal Joint	Sacrococcygeal symphysis
Saphenous Vein, Left Saphenous Vein, Right	External pudendal vein Great(er) saphenous vein Lesser saphenous vein Small saphenous vein Superficial circumflex iliac vein Superficial epigastric vein
Scapula, Left Scapula, Right	Acromion (process) Coracoid process
Sciatic Nerve	Ischiatic nerve
Shoulder Bursa and Ligament, Left Shoulder Bursa and Ligament, Right	Acromioclavicular ligament Coracoacromial ligament Coracoclavicular ligament Coracohumeral ligament Costoclavicular ligament Glenohumeral ligament Interclavicular ligament Sternoclavicular ligament Subacromial bursa Transverse humeral ligament Transverse scapular ligament
Shoulder Joint, Left Shoulder Joint, Right	Glenohumeral joint Glenoid ligament (labrum)
Shoulder Muscle, Left Shoulder Muscle, Right	Deltoid muscle Infraspinatus muscle Subscapularis muscle Supraspinatus muscle Teres major muscle Teres minor muscle
Sigmoid Colon	Rectosigmoid junction Sigmoid flexure
Skin	Dermis Epidermis Sebaceous gland Sweat gland
Skin, Chest	Breast procedures, skin only
Skin, Perineum	Perianal skin
Sphenoid Bone	Greater wing Lesser wing Optic foramen Pterygoid process Sella turcica

ICD-10-PCS Value	Definition
Spinal Canal	Epidural space, spinal Extradural space, spinal Subarachnoid space, spinal Subdural space, spinal Vertebral canal
Spinal Cord	Dorsal root ganglion
Spinal Meninges	Arachnoid mater, spinal Denticulate (dentate) ligament Dura mater, spinal Filum terminale Leptomeninges, spinal Pia mater, spinal
Spleen	Accessory spleen
Splenic Artery	Left gastroepiploic artery Pancreatic artery Short gastric artery
Splenic Vein	Left gastroepiploic vein Pancreatic vein
Sternum	Manubrium Suprasternal notch Xiphoid process
Sternum Bursa and Ligament	Costoxiphoid ligament Sternocostal ligament
Stomach, Pylorus	Pyloric antrum Pyloric canal Pyloric sphincter
Subclavian Artery, Left Subclavian Artery, Right	Costocervical trunk Dorsal scapular artery Internal thoracic artery
Subcutaneous Tissue and Fascia, Chest	Pectoral fascia
Subcutaneous Tissue and Fascia, Face	Chin Masseteric fascia Orbital fascia Submandibular space
Subcutaneous Tissue and Fascia, Left Foot	Plantar fascia (aponeurosis)
Subcutaneous Tissue and Fascia, Left Hand	Palmar fascia (aponeurosis)
Subcutaneous Tissue and Fascia, Left Lower Arm	Antebrachial fascia Bicipital aponeurosis
Subcutaneous Tissue and Fascia, Left Neck	Deep cervical fascia Pretracheal fascia Prevertebral fascia
Subcutaneous Tissue and Fascia, Left Upper Arm	Axillary fascia Deltoid fascia Infraspinatus fascia Subscapular aponeurosis Supraspinatus fascia
Subcutaneous Tissue and Fascia, Left Upper Leg	Crural fascia Fascia lata Iliac fascia Iliotibial tract (band)
Subcutaneous Tissue and Fascia, Right Foot	Plantar fascia (aponeurosis)
Subcutaneous Tissue and Fascia, Right Hand	Palmar fascia (aponeurosis)
Subcutaneous Tissue and Fascia, Right Lower Arm	Antebrachial fascia Bicipital aponeurosis
Subcutaneous Tissue and Fascia, Right Neck	Deep cervical fascia Pretracheal fascia Prevertebral fascia
Subcutaneous Tissue and Fascia, Right Upper Arm	Axillary fascia Deltoid fascia Infraspinatus fascia Subscapular aponeurosis Supraspinatus fascia

ICD-10-PCS Value	Definition
Subcutaneous Tissue and Fascia, Right Upper Leg	Crural fascia Fascia lata Iliac fascia Iliotibial tract (band)
Subcutaneous Tissue and Fascia, Scalp	Galea aponeurotica
Subcutaneous Tissue and Fascia, Trunk	External oblique aponeurosis Transversalis fascia
Submaxillary Gland, Left Submaxillary Gland, Right	Submandibular gland
Superior Mesenteric Artery	Ileal artery Ileocolic artery Inferior pancreaticoduodenal artery Jejunal artery
Superior Mesenteric Vein	Right gastroepiploic vein
Superior Vena Cava	Cavoatrial junction Precava
Tarsal Joint, Left Tarsal Joint, Right	Calcaneocuboid joint Cuboideonavicular joint Cuneonavicular joint Intercuneiform joint Subtalar (talocalcaneal) joint Talocalcaneal (subtalar) joint Talocalcaneonavicular joint
Tarsal, Left Tarsal, Right	Calcaneus Cuboid bone Intermediate cuneiform bone Lateral cuneiform bone Medial cuneiform bone Navicular bone Talus bone
Temporal Artery, Left Temporal Artery, Right	Middle temporal artery Superficial temporal artery Transverse facial artery
Temporal Bone, Left Temporal Bone, Right	Mastoid process Petrous part of temporal bone Tympanic part of temporal bone Zygomatic process of temporal bone
Thalamus	Epithalamus Geniculate nucleus Metathalamus Pulvinar
Thoracic Aorta, Ascending/Arch	Aortic arch Aortic isthmus Ascending aorta Juxtaductal aorta
Thoracic Duct	Left jugular trunk Left subclavian trunk
Thoracic Nerve	Intercostal nerve Intercostobrachial nerve Spinal nerve, thoracic Subcostal nerve
Thoracic Spinal Cord	Dorsal root ganglion
Thoracic Sympathetic Nerve	Cardiac plexus Esophageal plexus Greater splanchnic nerve Inferior cardiac nerve Least splanchnic nerve Lesser splanchnic nerve Middle cardiac nerve Pulmonary plexus Superior cardiac nerve Thoracic aortic plexus Thoracic ganglion

ICD-10-PCS Value	Definition
Thoracic Vertebra	Spinous process Transverse process Vertebral arch Vertebral body Vertebral foramen Vertebral lamina Vertebral pedicle
Thoracic Vertebral Joint	Costotransverse joint Costovertebral joint Thoracic facet joint
Thoracolumbar Vertebral Joint	Thoracolumbar facet joint
Thorax Muscle, Left Thorax Muscle, Right	Intercostal muscle Levatores costarum muscle Pectoralis major muscle Pectoralis minor muscle Serratus anterior muscle Subclavius muscle Subcostal muscle Transverse thoracis muscle
Thymus	Thymus gland
Thyroid Artery, Left Thyroid Artery, Right	Cricothyroid artery Hyoid artery Sternocleidomastoid artery Superior laryngeal artery Superior thyroid artery Thyrocervical trunk
Tibia, Left Tibia, Right	Lateral condyle of tibia Medial condyle of tibia Medial malleolus
Tibial Nerve	Lateral plantar nerve Medial plantar nerve Medial popliteal nerve Medial sural cutaneous nerve
Toe Nail	Nail bed Nail plate
Toe Phalangeal Joint, Left Toe Phalangeal Joint, Right	Interphalangeal (IP) joint
Tongue	Frenulum linguae
Tongue, Palate, Pharynx Muscle	Chondroglossus muscle Genioglossus muscle Hyoglossus muscle Inferior longitudinal muscle Levator veli palatini muscle Palatoglossal muscle Palatopharyngeal muscle Pharyngeal constrictor muscle Salpingopharyngeus muscle Styloglossus muscle Stylopharyngeus muscle Superior longitudinal muscle Tensor veli palatini muscle
Tonsils	Palatine tonsil
Trachea	Cricoid cartilage
Transverse Colon	Hepatic flexure Splenic flexure
Tricuspid Valve	Right atrioventricular valve Tricuspid annulus
Trigeminal Nerve	Fifth cranial nerve Gasserian ganglion Mandibular nerve Maxillary nerve Ophthalmic nerve Trifacial nerve
Trochlear Nerve	Fourth cranial nerve

ICD-10-PCS Value	Definition
Trunk Muscle, Left Trunk Muscle, Right	Coccygeus muscle Erector spinae muscle Interspinalis muscle Intertransversarius muscle Latissimus dorsi muscle Quadratus lumborum muscle Rhomboid major muscle Rhomboid minor muscle Serratus posterior muscle Transversospinalis muscle Trapezius muscle
Tympanic Membrane, Left Tympanic Membrane, Right	Pars flaccida
Ulna, Left Ulna, Right	Olecranon process Radial notch
Ulnar Artery, Left Ulnar Artery, Right	Anterior ulnar recurrent artery Common interosseous artery Posterior ulnar recurrent artery
Ulnar Nerve	Cubital nerve
Upper Arm Muscle, Left Upper Arm Muscle, Right	Biceps brachii muscle Brachialis muscle Coracobrachialis muscle Triceps brachii muscle
Upper Artery	Aortic intercostal artery Bronchial artery Esophageal artery Subcostal artery
Upper Eyelid, Left Upper Eyelid, Right	Lateral canthus Levator palpebrae superioris muscle Orbicularis oculi muscle Superior tarsal plate
Upper Femur, Left Upper Femur, Right	Femoral head Greater trochanter Lesser trochanter Neck of femur
Upper Leg Muscle, Left Upper Leg Muscle, Right	Adductor brevis muscle Adductor longus muscle Adductor magnus muscle Biceps femoris muscle Gracilis muscle Hamstring muscle Pectineus muscle Quadriceps (femoris) Rectus femoris muscle Sartorius muscle Semimembranosus muscle Semitendinosus muscle Vastus intermedius muscle Vastus lateralis muscle Vastus medialis muscle
Upper Lip	Frenulum labii superioris Labial gland Vermilion border
Upper Spine Bursa and Ligament	Interspinous ligament, thoracic Intertransverse ligament, thoracic Ligamentum flavum, thoracic Supraspinous ligament
Ureter Ureter, Left Ureter, Right Ureters, Bilateral	Ureteral orifice Ureterovesical orifice
Urethra	Bulbourethral (Cowper's) gland Cowper's (bulbourethral) gland External urethral sphincter Internal urethral sphincter Membranous urethra Penile urethra Prostatic urethra

ICD-10-PCS Value	Definition
Uterine Supporting Structure	Broad ligament Infundibulopelvic ligament Ovarian ligament Round ligament of uterus
Uterus	Fundus uteri Myometrium Perimetrium Uterine cornu
Uvula	Palatine uvula
Vagus Nerve	Anterior vagal trunk Pharyngeal plexus Pneumogastric nerve Posterior vagal trunk Pulmonary plexus Recurrent laryngeal nerve Superior laryngeal nerve Tenth cranial nerve
Vas Deferens Vas Deferens, Bilateral Vas Deferens, Left Vas Deferens, Right	Ductus deferens Ejaculatory duct
Ventricle, Right	Conus arteriosus
Ventricular Septum	Interventricular septum
Vertebral Artery, Left Vertebral Artery, Right	Anterior spinal artery Posterior spinal artery
Vertebral Vein, Left Vertebral Vein, Right	Deep cervical vein Suboccipital venous plexus
Vestibular Gland	Bartholin's (greater vestibular) gland Greater vestibular (Bartholin's) gland Paraurethral (Skene's) gland Skene's (paraurethral) gland
Vitreous, Left Vitreous, Right	Vitreous body
Vocal Cord, Left Vocal Cord, Right	Vocal fold
Vulva	Labia majora Labia minora
Wrist Bursa and Ligament, Left Wrist Bursa and Ligament, Right	Palmar ulnocarpal ligament Radial collateral carpal ligament Radiocarpal ligament Radioulnar ligament Scapholunate ligament Ulnar collateral carpal ligament
Wrist Joint, Left Wrist Joint, Right	Distal radioulnar joint Radiocarpal joint

Appendix F: Device Classification

In most PCS codes, the sixth character of the code classifies the device. The sixth character device value "defines the material or appliance used to accomplish the objective of the procedure that remains in or on the procedure site at the end of the procedure." If the device is the means by which the procedural objective is accomplished, then a specific device value is coded in the sixth character. If no device is used to accomplish the objective of the procedure, the device value *No Device* is coded in the sixth character. In limited root operations, the classification provides the qualifier values *Temporary* and *Intraoperative*, for specific procedures involving clinically significant devices whose purpose is brief use during the procedure or current inpatient stay.

Material that is classified as a PCS device is distinguished from material classified as a PCS substance by its having a specific location. A device is intended to maintain a fixed location at the procedure site where it was put, whereas a substance is intended to disperse or be absorbed in the body. There are circumstances in which a device does not stay where it was put and may need to be "revised" in a subsequent procedure to move the device back to its intended location.

Material classified as a PCS device is also distinguishable by the fact that it is removable. Although it may not be practical to remove some types of devices, once they become established at the site, it is physically possible to remove a device for some time after the procedure. A skin graft, for example, once it "takes," may be nearly indistinguishable from the surrounding skin and so is no longer clearly identifiable as a device. Nevertheless, procedures that involve material coded as a device can for the most part be "reversed" by removing the device from the procedure site.

General Device Types

Device Type	Definition	Examples
Grafts	Biological or synthetic material that **takes the place of all or a portion of a body part.**	Full- or partial-thickness skin grafts: • Autologous • Nonautologous • Synthetic • Zooplastic Other tissue grafts: • Bone • Tendon • Vascular
Prosthesis	Biological or synthetic material that **takes the place of all or a portion of a body part.**	Joint prosthesis: • Autologous • Nonautologous • Synthetic
Implants	**Therapeutic** material that is not absorbed by, eliminated by, or incorporated into a body part.	External fixation device Internal fixation device: • Orthopaedic pins • Intramedullary rods Radioactive element implant Mesh
Simple or mechanical appliances	Biological or synthetic material that **assists or prevents a physiological function.**	Drainage device Extraluminal device Endobrachial device Fusion device Intraluminal device (can be temporary) Tracheostomy device IUD
Electronic appliances	Electronic appliances used to **assist, monitor, take the pace of, or prevent a physiological function.**	Cardiac leads Diaphragmatic pacemaker External heart assist system Short-term external heart assist system (Intraoperative) Fetal monitoring Hearing device Monitoring device Neurostimulator
External appliances	Performed without making an incision or a puncture, external appliances are used for the purpose of **protection, immobilization, stretching, compression, or packing.**	Bandage Cast Packing material Pressure dressing Traction apparatus

Transplant/Grafting Tissue Type Terminology

Tissue Type	Terminology
Tissue or organ transferred into a new position in **the body of the same individual**	Autograft Autologous Autoplastic
Having to do with individuals or tissues that have **identical genes**, such as identical twins	Isograft Isologous Syngeneic Syngraft
Tissue or organ taken from **different individuals** of the same species	Allogeneic Allograft Homologous Homograft
Tissue or organ from a **cadaver**	Nonautologous
Tissue or organ from individuals of **different species**	Heterogeneic Heterologous Xenogeneic Xenograft Zooplastic

Appendix G: Device Key and Aggregation Table

This [NT] symbol next to a device in the Term column identifies that the device has been approved for NTAP (new technology add-on payment). CMS provides incremental payment, in addition to the DRG payment, for technologies that have received an NTAP designation.

Device Key

Terms	ICD-10-PCS Value
3f (Aortic) Bioprosthesis valve	Zooplastic Tissue in Heart and Great Vessels
AbioCor® Total Replacement Heart	Synthetic Substitute
Absolute Pro Vascular (OTW) Self-Expanding Stent System	Intraluminal Device
Acculink (RX) Carotid Stent System	Intraluminal Device
Acellular Hydrated Dermis	Nonautologous Tissue Substitute
Acetabular cup	Liner in Lower Joints
Activa PC neurostimulator	Stimulator Generator, Multiple Array for Insertion in Subcutaneous Tissue and Fascia
Activa RC neurostimulator	Stimulator Generator, Multiple Array Rechargeable for Insertion in Subcutaneous Tissue and Fascia
Activa SC neurostimulator	Stimulator Generator, Single Array for Insertion in Subcutaneous Tissue and Fascia
ACUITY™ Steerable Lead	Cardiac Lead, Pacemaker for Insertion in Heart and Great Vessels Cardiac Lead, Defibrillator for Insertion in Heart and Great Vessels
Advisa (MRI)	Pacemaker, Dual Chamber for Insertion in Subcutaneous Tissue and Fascia
AFX® Endovascular AAA System	Intraluminal Device
Alfapump® system	Other Device
AMPLATZER® Muscular VSD Occluder	Synthetic Substitute
AMS 800® Urinary Control System	Artificial Sphincter in Urinary System
AneuRx® AAA Advantage®	Intraluminal Device
Ankle Truss System™ (ATS)	Internal Fixation Device, Open-truss Design in New Technology
Annuloplasty ring	Synthetic Substitute
Aortix™ System	Short-term External Heart Assist System in Heart and Great Vessels
ApiFix® Minimally Invasive Deformity Correction (MID-C) System (C)	Posterior (Dynamic) Distraction Device in New Technology
aprevo™	Interbody Fusion Device, Custom-made Anatomically Designed in New Technology
Articulating Spacer (Antibiotic)	Articulating Spacer in Lower Joints
Artificial anal sphincter (AAS)	Artificial Sphincter in Gastrointestinal System
Artificial bowel sphincter (neosphincter)	Artificial Sphincter in Gastrointestinal System
Artificial urinary sphincter (AUS)	Artificial Sphincter in Urinary System
Ascenda Intrathecal Catheter	Infusion Device
Assurant (Cobalt) stent	Intraluminal Device
AtriClip LAA Exclusion System	Extraluminal Device
Attain Ability® Lead	Cardiac Lead, Pacemaker for Insertion in Heart and Great Vessels Cardiac Lead, Defibrillator for Insertion in Heart and Great Vessels
Attain StarFix® (OTW) Lead	Cardiac Lead, Pacemaker for Insertion in Heart and Great Vessels Cardiac Lead, Defibrillator for Insertion in Heart and Great Vessels

Terms	ICD-10-PCS Value
Autograft	Autologous Tissue Substitute
Autologous artery graft	Autologous Arterial Tissue in Heart and Great Vessels Autologous Arterial Tissue in Upper Arteries Autologous Arterial Tissue in Lower Arteries Autologous Arterial Tissue in Upper Veins Autologous Arterial Tissue in Lower Veins
Autologous vein graft	Autologous Venous Tissue in Heart and Great Vessels Autologous Venous Tissue in Upper Arteries Autologous Venous Tissue in Lower Arteries Autologous Venous Tissue in Upper Veins Autologous Venous Tissue in Lower Veins
Aveir™ AR, as dual chamber [NT]	Intracardiac Pacemaker, Dual-Chamber in New Technology
Aveir™ DR, dual chamber [NT]	Intracardiac Pacemaker, Dual-Chamber in New Technology
Aveir™ VR, as single chamber	Intracardiac Pacemaker in the Heart and Great Vessels
Axial Lumbar Interbody Fusion System	Interbody Fusion Device in Lower Joints
AxiaLIF® System	Interbody Fusion Device in Lower Joints
BAK/C® Interbody Cervical Fusion System	Interbody Fusion Device in Upper Joints
Bard® Composix® (E/X)(LP) mesh	Synthetic Substitute
Bard® Composix® Kugel® patch	Synthetic Substitute
Bard® Dulex™ mesh	Synthetic Substitute
Bard® Ventralex™ hernia patch	Synthetic Substitute
Baroreflex Activation Therapy® (BAT®)	Stimulator Lead in Upper Arteries Stimulator Generator in Subcutaneous Tissue and Fascia
Barricaid® Annular Closure Device (ACD)	Synthetic Substitute
Berlin Heart Ventricular Assist Device	Implantable Heart Assist System in Heart and Great Vessels
Bioactive embolization coil(s)	Intraluminal Device, Bioactive in Upper Arteries
Biventricular external heart assist system	Short-term External Heart Assist System in Heart and Great Vessels
BlackArmor® Carbon/PEEK fixation system	Carbon/PEEK Spinal Stabilization Device, Pedicle Based in New Technology
Blood glucose monitoring system	Monitoring Device
Bone anchored hearing device	Hearing Device, Bone Conduction for Insertion in Ear, Nose, Sinus Hearing Device, in Head and Facial Bones
Bone bank bone graft	Nonautologous Tissue Substitute
Bone screw (interlocking)(lag)(pedicle)(recessed)	Internal Fixation Device in Head and Facial Bones Internal Fixation Device in Upper Bones Internal Fixation Device in Lower Bones
Bovine pericardial valve	Zooplastic Tissue in Heart and Great Vessels
Bovine pericardium graft	Zooplastic Tissue in Heart and Great Vessels
Brachytherapy seeds	Radioactive Element
BRYAN® Cervical Disc System	Synthetic Substitute
BVS 5000 Ventricular Assist Device	Short-term External Heart Assist System in Heart and Great Vessels
Canturio™ te (Tibial Extension)	Tibial Extension with Motion Sensors in New Technology

Terms	ICD-10-PCS Value
Cardiac contractility modulation lead	Cardiac Lead in Heart and Great Vessels
Cardiac event recorder	Monitoring Device
Cardiac resynchronization therapy (CRT) lead	Cardiac Lead, Pacemaker for Insertion in Heart and Great Vessels Cardiac Lead, Defibrillator for Insertion in Heart and Great Vessels
CardioMEMS® pressure sensor	Monitoring Device, Pressure Sensor for Insertion in Heart and Great Vessels
Carmat total artificial heart (TAH)	Biologic with Synthetic Substitute, Autoregulated Electrohydraulic for Replacement in Heart and Great Vessels
Carotid (artery) sinus (baroreceptor) lead	Stimulator Lead in Upper Arteries
Carotid WALLSTENT® Monorail® Endoprosthesis	Intraluminal Device
Centrimag® Blood Pump	Short-term External Heart Assist System in Heart and Great Vessels
Ceramic on ceramic bearing surface	Synthetic Substitute, Ceramic for Replacement in Lower Joints
Cesium-131 Collagen Implant	Radioactive Element, Cesium-131 Collagen Implant for Insertion in Central Nervous System and Cranial Nerves
CivaSheet®	Radioactive Element
Clamp and rod internal fixation system (CRIF)	Internal Fixation Device in Upper Bones Internal Fixation Device in Lower Bones
COALESCE® radiolucent interbody fusion device	Interbody Fusion Device in Upper Joints Interbody Fusion Device in Lower Joints
CoAxia NeuroFlo catheter	Intraluminal Device
Cobalt/chromium head and polyethylene socket	Synthetic Substitute, Metal on Polyethylene for Replacement in Lower Joints
Cobalt/chromium head and socket	Synthetic Substitute, Metal for Replacement in Lower Joints
Cochlear implant (CI), multiple channel (electrode)	Hearing Device, Multiple Channel Cochlear Prosthesis for Insertion in Ear, Nose, Sinus
Cochlear implant (CI), single channel (electrode)	Hearing Device, Single Channel Cochlear Prosthesis for Insertion in Ear, Nose, Sinus
COGNIS® CRT-D	Cardiac Resynchronization Defibrillator Pulse Generator for Insertion in Subcutaneous Tissue and Fascia
COHERE® radiolucent interbody fusion device	Interbody Fusion Device in Upper Joints Interbody Fusion Device in Lower Joints
Colonic Z-Stent®	Intraluminal Device
Complete (SE) stent	Intraluminal Device
Concerto II CRT-D	Cardiac Resynchronization Defibrillator Pulse Generator for Insertion in Subcutaneous Tissue and Fascia
CONSERVE® PLUS Total Resurfacing Hip System	Resurfacing Device in Lower Joints
Consulta CRT-D	Cardiac Resynchronization Defibrillator Pulse Generator for Insertion in Subcutaneous Tissue and Fascia
Consulta CRT-P	Cardiac Resynchronization Pacemaker Pulse Generator for Insertion in Subcutaneous Tissue and Fascia
CONTAK RENEWAL® 3 RF (HE) CRT-D	Cardiac Resynchronization Defibrillator Pulse Generator for Insertion in Subcutaneous Tissue and Fascia
Contegra Pulmonary Valved Conduit	Zooplastic Tissue in Heart and Great Vessels
Continuous Glucose Monitoring (CGM) device	Monitoring Device
Cook Biodesign® Fistula Plug(s)	Nonautologous Tissue Substitute
Cook Biodesign® Hernia Graft(s)	Nonautologous Tissue Substitute
Cook Biodesign® Layered Graft(s)	Nonautologous Tissue Substitute

Terms	ICD-10-PCS Value
Cook Zenapro™ Layered Graft(s)	Nonautologous Tissue Substitute
Cook Zenith AAA Endovascular Graft	Intraluminal Device
Cook Zenith® Fenestrated AAA Endovascular Graft	Intraluminal Device, Branched or Fenestrated, One or Two Arteries for Restriction in Lower Arteries Intraluminal Device, Branched or Fenestrated, Three or More Arteries for Restriction in Lower Arteries
CoreValve transcatheter aortic valve	Zooplastic Tissue in Heart and Great Vessels
Cormet Hip Resurfacing System	Resurfacing Device in Lower Joints
CoRoent® XL	Interbody Fusion Device in Lower Joints
Corox (OTW) Bipolar Lead	Cardiac Lead, Pacemaker for Insertion in Heart and Great Vessels Cardiac Lead, Defibrillator for Insertion in Heart and Great Vessels
Cortical strip neurostimulator lead	Neurostimulator Lead in Central Nervous System and Cranial Nerves
Corvia IASD®	Synthetic Substitute
Cultured epidermal cell autograft	Autologous Tissue Substitute
CYPHER® Stent	Intraluminal Device, Drug-eluting in Heart and Great Vessels
Cystostomy tube	Drainage Device
DBS lead	Neurostimulator Lead in Central Nervous System and Cranial Nerves
DeBakey Left Ventricular Assist Device	Implantable Heart Assist System in Heart and Great Vessels
Deep brain neurostimulator lead	Neurostimulator Lead in Central Nervous System and Cranial Nerves
Delta frame external fixator	External Fixation Device, Hybrid for Insertion in Upper Bones External Fixation Device, Hybrid for Reposition in Upper Bones External Fixation Device, Hybrid for Insertion in Lower Bones External Fixation Device, Hybrid for Reposition in Lower Bones
Delta III Reverse shoulder prosthesis	Synthetic Substitute, Reverse Ball and Socket for Replacement in Upper Joints
DETOUR® System [NT]	Conduit through Femoral Vein to Popliteal Artery in New Technology Conduit through Femoral Vein to Superficial Femoral Artery in New Technology
Diaphragmatic pacemaker generator	Stimulator Generator in Subcutaneous Tissue and Fascia
Direct Lateral Interbody Fusion (DLIF) device	Interbody Fusion Device in Lower Joints
Driver stent (RX) (OTW)	Intraluminal Device
Drug-eluting resorbable scaffold intraluminal device	Intraluminal Device, Everolimus-eluting Resorbable Scaffold(s) in New Technology
DuraHeart Left Ventricular Assist System	Implantable Heart Assist System in Heart and Great Vessels
Durata® Defibrillation Lead	Cardiac Lead, Defibrillator for Insertion in Heart and Great Vessels
DynaClip® (Delta) (Forte) (Quattro)	Internal Fixation Device, Sustained Compression for Fusion in Upper Joints Internal Fixation Device, Sustained Compression for Fusion in Lower Joints
DynaNail® (Helix) (Hybrid) (Mini)	Internal Fixation Device, Sustained Compression for Fusion in Upper Joints Internal Fixation Device, Sustained Compression for Fusion in Lower Joints

Appendix G: Device Key and Aggregation Table

Terms	ICD-10-PCS Value
Dynesys® Dynamic Stabilization System	Spinal Stabilization Device, Pedicle-Based for Insertion in Upper Joints Spinal Stabilization Device, Pedicle-Based for Insertion in Lower Joints
EB-101 gene-corrected autologous cell therapy	Prademagene Zamikeracel, Genetically Engineered Autologous Cell Therapy in New Technology
EB-101 gene-corrected keratinocyte sheets	Prademagene Zamikeracel, Genetically Engineered Autologous Cell Therapy in New Technology
Edwards EVOQUE tricuspid valve replacement system	Multi-plane Flex Technology Bioprosthetic Valve in New Technology
E-Luminexx™ (Biliary) (Vascular) Stent	Intraluminal Device
Electrical bone growth stimulator (EBGS)	Bone Growth Stimulator in Head and Facial Bones Bone Growth Stimulator in Upper Bones Bone Growth Stimulator in Lower Bones
Electrical muscle stimulation (EMS) lead	Stimulator Lead in Muscles
Electronic muscle stimulator lead	Stimulator Lead in Muscles
Eluvia™ Drug-eluting Vascular Stent System	Intraluminal Device, Drug-eluting, Four or More in Lower Arteries Intraluminal Device, Drug-eluting in Lower Arteries Intraluminal Device, Drug-eluting, Three in Lower Arteries Intraluminal Device, Drug-eluting, Two in Lower Arteries
Embolization coil(s)	Intraluminal Device
Endeavor® (III) (IV) (Sprint) Zotarolimus-eluting Coronary Stent System	Intraluminal Device, Drug-eluting in Heart and Great Vessels
Endologix AFX® Endovascular AAA System	Intraluminal Device
EndoSure® sensor	Monitoring Device, Pressure Sensor for Insertion in Heart and Great Vessels
ENDOTAK RELIANCE® (G) Defibrillation Lead	Cardiac Lead, Defibrillator for Insertion in Heart and Great Vessels
Endotracheal tube (cuffed) (double-lumen)	Intraluminal Device, Endotracheal Airway in Respiratory System
Endurant® Endovascular Stent Graft	Intraluminal Device
Endurant® II AAA stent graft system	Intraluminal Device
EnRhythm	Pacemaker, Dual Chamber for Insertion in Subcutaneous Tissue and Fascia
Enterra gastric neurostimulator	Stimulator Generator, Multiple Array for Insertion in Subcutaneous Tissue and Fascia
Epic™ Stented Tissue Valve (aortic)	Zooplastic Tissue in Heart and Great Vessels
Epicel® cultured epidermal autograft	Autologous Tissue Substitute
Esophageal obturator airway (EOA)	Intraluminal Device, Airway in Gastrointestinal System
Esprit™ BTK (scaffold) (stent)	Intraluminal Device, Everolimus-eluting Resorbable Scaffold(s) in New Technology
Esteem® implantable hearing system	Hearing Device in Ear, Nose, Sinus
EV ICD System (Extravascular implantable defibrillator lead)	Defibrillator Lead in Anatomical Regions, General
Evera (XT)(S)(DR/VR)	Defibrillator Generator for Insertion in Subcutaneous Tissue and Fascia
Everolimus-eluting coronary stent	Intraluminal Device, Drug-eluting in Heart and Great Vessels

Terms	ICD-10-PCS Value
Everolimus Eluting Resorbable Scaffold System	Intraluminal Device, Everolimus-eluting Resorbable Scaffold(s) in New Technology
Ex-PRESS™ mini glaucoma shunt	Synthetic Substitute
EXCLUDER® AAA Endoprosthesis	Intraluminal Device Intraluminal Device, Branched or Fenestrated, One or Two Arteries for Restriction in Lower Arteries Intraluminal Device, Branched or Fenestrated, Three or More Arteries for Restriction in Lower Arteries
EXCLUDER® IBE Endoprosthesis	Intraluminal Device, Branched or Fenestrated, One or Two Arteries for Restriction in Lower Arteries
Express® (LD) Premounted Stent System	Intraluminal Device
Express® Biliary SD Monorail® Premounted Stent System	Intraluminal Device
Express® SD Renal Monorail® Premounted Stent System	Intraluminal Device
External fixator	External Fixation Device in Head and Facial Bones External Fixation Device in Upper Bones External Fixation Device in Lower Bones External Fixation Device in Upper Joints External Fixation Device in Lower Joints
EXtreme Lateral Interbody Fusion (XLIF) device	Interbody Fusion Device in Lower Joints
Facet FiXation implant	Facet Joint Fusion Device Paired Titanium Cages in New Technology
Facet replacement spinal stabilization device	Spinal Stabilization Device, Facet Replacement for Insertion in Upper Joints Spinal Stabilization Device, Facet Replacement for Insertion in Lower Joints
Fish skin	Nonautologous Tissue Substitute
FLAIR® Endovascular Stent Graft	Intraluminal Device
Flexible Composite Mesh	Synthetic Substitute
Flourish® Pediatric Esophageal Atresia Device	Magnetic Lengthening Device in Gastrointestinal System
Flow Diverter embolization device	Intraluminal Device, Flow Diverter for Restriction in Upper Arteries
Foley catheter	Drainage Device
Formula™ Balloon-Expandable Renal Stent System	Intraluminal Device
Freestyle (Stentless) Aortic Root Bioprosthesis	Zooplastic Tissue in Heart and Great Vessels
Fusion screw (compression)(lag)(locking)	Internal Fixation Device in Upper Joints Internal Fixation Device in Lower Joints
FFX® (Facet FiXation) implant	Facet Joint Fusion Device Paired Titanium Cages in New Technology
GammaTile™	Radioactive Element, Cesium-131 Collagen Implant for Insertion in Central Nervous System and Cranial Nerves Radioactive Element, Palladium-103 Collagen Implant for Insertion in the Central Nervous System and Cranial Nerves
Gastric electrical stimulation (GES) lead	Stimulator Lead in Gastrointestinal System
Gastric pacemaker lead	Stimulator Lead in Gastrointestinal System
GORE EXCLUDER® AAA Endoprosthesis	Intraluminal Device Intraluminal Device, Branched or Fenestrated, One or Two Arteries for Restriction in Lower Arteries Intraluminal Device, Branched or Fenestrated, Three or More Arteries for Restriction in Lower Arteries

Terms	ICD-10-PCS Value
GORE EXCLUDER® IBE Endoprosthesis	Intraluminal Device, Branched or Fenestrated, One or Two Arteries for Restriction in Lower Arteries
GORE® EXCLUDER® TAMBE Device (Thoracoabdominal Branch Endoprosthesis)	Branched Intraluminal Device, Manufactured Integrated System, Four or More Arteries in New Technology
GORE TAG® Thoracic Endoprosthesis NT	Intraluminal Device
GORE® DUALMESH®	Synthetic Substitute
Guedel airway	Intraluminal Device, Airway in Mouth and Throat
Hancock Bioprosthesis (aortic)(mitral) valve	Zooplastic Tissue in Heart and Great Vessels
Hancock Bioprosthetic Valved Conduit	Zooplastic Tissue in Heart and Great Vessels
HAV™ (Human Acellular Vessel)	Bioengineered Human Acellular Vessel in New Technology
HeartMate 3™ LVAS	Implantable Heart Assist System in Heart and Great Vessels
HeartMate II® Left Ventricular Assist Device (LVAD)	Implantable Heart Assist System in Heart and Great Vessels
HeartMate XVE® Left Ventricular Assist Device (LVAD)	Implantable Heart Assist System in Heart and Great Vessels
Herculink (RX) Elite Renal Stent System	Intraluminal Device
Hip (joint) liner	Liner in Lower Joints
Holter valve ventricular shunt	Synthetic Substitute
Human Acellular Vessel™ (HAV)	Bioengineered Human Acellular Vessel in New Technology
IASD® (InterAtrial Shunt Device), Corvia	Synthetic Substitute
iFuse Bedrock™ Granite Implant System NT	Internal Fixation Device with Tulip Connector in New Technology
Ilizarov external fixator	External Fixation Device, Ring for Insertion in Upper Bones External Fixation Device, Ring for Reposition in Upper Bones External Fixation Device, Ring for Insertion in Lower Bones External Fixation Device, Ring for Reposition in Lower Bones
Ilizarov-Vecklich device	External Fixation Device, Limb Lengthening for Insertion in Upper Bones External Fixation Device, Limb Lengthening for Insertion in Lower Bones
Impella® 5.5 with SmartAssist® System	Conduit To Short-term External Heart Assist System in New Technology
Impella® heart pump	Short-term External Heart Assist System in Heart and Great Vessels
Implantable cardioverter-defibrillator (ICD)	Defibrillator Generator for Insertion in Subcutaneous Tissue and Fascia
Implantable drug infusion pump (anti-spasmodic) (chemotherapy)(pain)	Infusion Device, Pump in Subcutaneous Tissue and Fascia
Implantable glucose monitoring device	Monitoring Device
Implantable hemodynamic monitor (IHM)	Monitoring Device, Hemodynamic for Insertion in Subcutaneous Tissue and Fascia
Implantable hemodynamic monitoring system (IHMS)	Monitoring Device, Hemodynamic for Insertion in Subcutaneous Tissue and Fascia
Implantable Miniature Telescope™ (IMT)	Synthetic Substitute, Intraocular Telescope for Replacement in Eye
Implanted (venous)(access) port	Vascular Access Device, Totally Implantable in Subcutaneous Tissue and Fascia
InDura, intrathecal catheter (1P) (spinal)	Infusion Device

Terms	ICD-10-PCS Value
Injection reservoir, port	Vascular Access Device, Totally Implantable in Subcutaneous Tissue and Fascia
Injection reservoir, pump	Infusion Device, Pump in Subcutaneous Tissue and Fascia
Innova™ stent	Intraluminal Device
Inspiris Resilia valve	Zooplastic Tissue in Heart and Great Vessels
Intellis™ neurostimulator	Stimulator Generator, Multiple Array Rechargeable for Insertion in Subcutaneous Tissue and Fascia
InterAtrial Shunt Device IASD®, Corvia	Synthetic Substitute
Interbody fusion (spine) cage	Interbody Fusion Device in Upper Joints Interbody Fusion Device in Lower Joints
Interspinous process spinal stabilization device	Spinal Stabilization Device, Interspinous Process for Insertion in Upper Joints Spinal Stabilization Device, Interspinous Process for Insertion in Lower Joints
InterStim™ Micro Therapy neurostimulator	Stimulator Generator, Single Array Rechargeable for Insertion in Subcutaneous Tissue and Fascia
InterStim® Therapy lead	Neurostimulator Lead in Peripheral Nervous System
InterStim™ II Therapy neurostimulator	Stimulator Generator, Single Array for Insertion in Subcutaneous Tissue and Fascia
Intramedullary (IM) rod (nail)	Internal Fixation Device, Intramedullary in Upper Bones Internal Fixation Device, Intramedullary in Lower Bones
Intramedullary skeletal kinetic distractor (ISKD)	Internal Fixation Device, Intramedullary in Upper Bones Internal Fixation Device, Intramedullary in Lower Bones
Intrauterine Device (IUD)	Contraceptive Device in Female Reproductive System
Ischemic Stroke System (ISS500)	Neurostimulator Lead in New Technology
ISS500 (Ischemic Stroke System)	Neurostimulator Lead in New Technology
Itrel (3)(4) neurostimulator	Stimulator Generator, Single Array for Insertion in Subcutaneous Tissue and Fascia
Joint fixation plate	Internal Fixation Device in Upper Joints Internal Fixation Device in Lower Joints
Joint liner (insert)	Liner in Lower Joints
Joint spacer (antibiotic)	Spacer in Upper Joints Spacer in Lower Joints
Kappa	Pacemaker, Dual Chamber for Insertion in Subcutaneous Tissue and Fascia
Kerecis® (GraftGuide) (MariGen) (SurgiBind) (SurgiClose)	Nonautologous Tissue Substitute
Kirschner wire (K-wire)	Internal Fixation Device in Head and Facial Bones Internal Fixation Device in Upper Bones Internal Fixation Device in Lower Bones Internal Fixation Device in Upper Joints Internal Fixation Device in Lower Joints
Knee (implant) insert	Liner in Lower Joints
Kuntscher nail	Internal Fixation Device, Intramedullary in Upper Bones Internal Fixation Device, Intramedullary in Lower Bones
LAP-BAND® adjustable gastric banding system	Extraluminal Device
LifeStent® (Flexstar)(XL) Vascular Stent System	Intraluminal Device
LigaPASS 2.0™ PJK Prevention System	Posterior Vertebral Tether in New Technology

Appendix G: Device Key and Aggregation Table

Terms	ICD-10-PCS Value
LimFlow™ Transcatheter Arterialization of the Deep Veins (TADV) System	Synthetic Substitute
LIVIAN™ CRT-D	Cardiac Resynchronization Defibrillator Pulse Generator for Insertion in Subcutaneous Tissue and Fascia
Longeviti ClearFit® Cranial Implant	Synthetic Substitute, Ultrasound Penetrable in New Technology
Longeviti ClearFit® OTS Cranial Implant	Synthetic Substitute, Ultrasound Penetrable in New Technology
Loop recorder, implantable	Monitoring Device
LZRSE-COL7A1 engineered autologous epidermal sheets	Prademagene Zamikeracel, Genetically Engineered Autologous Cell Therapy in New Technology
MAGEC® Spinal Bracing and Distraction System	Magnetically Controlled Growth Rod(s) in New Technology
Mark IV Breathing Pacemaker System	Stimulator Generator in Subcutaneous Tissue and Fascia
Maximo II DR (VR)	Defibrillator Generator for Insertion in Subcutaneous Tissue and Fascia
Maximo II DR CRT-D	Cardiac Resynchronization Defibrillator Pulse Generator for Insertion in Subcutaneous Tissue and Fascia
Medtronic Endurant® II AAA stent graft system	Intraluminal Device
Melody® transcatheter pulmonary valve	Zooplastic Tissue in Heart and Great Vessels
Metal on metal bearing surface	Synthetic Substitute, Metal for Replacement in Lower Joints
Micro-Driver stent (RX) (OTW)	Intraluminal Device
MicroMed HeartAssist	Implantable Heart Assist System in Heart and Great Vessels
Micrus CERECYTE microcoil	Intraluminal Device, Bioactive in Upper Arteries
MIRODERM™ Biologic Wound Matrix	Nonautologous Tissue Substitute
MitraClip valve repair system	Synthetic Substitute
Mitroflow® Aortic Pericardial Heart Valve	Zooplastic Tissue in Heart and Great Vessels
Mosaic Bioprosthesis (aortic) (mitral) valve	Zooplastic Tissue in Heart and Great Vessels
MULTI-LINK (VISION)(MINI-VISION)(ULTRA) Coronary Stent System	Intraluminal Device
nanoLOCK™ interbody fusion device	Interbody Fusion Device in Upper Joints Interbody Fusion Device in Lower Joints
Nasopharyngeal airway (NPA)	Intraluminal Device, Airway in Ear, Nose, Sinus
Neovasc Reducer™	Reduction Device in New Technology
Neuromuscular electrical stimulation (NEMS) lead	Stimulator Lead in Muscles
Neurostimulator generator, multiple channel	Stimulator Generator, Multiple Array for Insertion in Subcutaneous Tissue and Fascia
Neurostimulator generator, multiple channel rechargeable	Stimulator Generator, Multiple Array Rechargeable for Insertion in Subcutaneous Tissue and Fascia
Neurostimulator generator, single channel	Stimulator Generator, Single Array for Insertion in Subcutaneous Tissue and Fascia
Neurostimulator generator, single channel rechargeable	Stimulator Generator, Single Array Rechargeable for Insertion in Subcutaneous Tissue and Fascia
Neutralization plate	Internal Fixation Device in Head and Facial Bones Internal Fixation Device in Upper Bones Internal Fixation Device in Lower Bones
Nitinol framed polymer mesh	Synthetic Substitute
Non-tunneled central venous catheter	Infusion Device

Terms	ICD-10-PCS Value
Novacor Left Ventricular Assist Device	Implantable Heart Assist System in Heart and Great Vessels
Novation® Ceramic AHS® (Articulation Hip System)	Synthetic Substitute, Ceramic for Replacement in Lower Joints
NUsurface® Meniscus Implant	Synthetic Substitute, Lateral Meniscus in New Technology Synthetic Substitute, Medial Meniscus in New Technology
Omnilink Elite Vascular Balloon Expandable Stent System	Intraluminal Device
Open Pivot Aortic Valve Graft (AVG)	Synthetic Substitute
Open Pivot (mechanical) Valve	Synthetic Substitute
Optimizer™ III implantable pulse generator	Contractility Modulation Device for Insertion in Subcutaneous Tissue and Fascia
Oropharyngeal airway (OPA)	Intraluminal Device, Airway in Mouth and Throat
Ovatio™ CRT-D	Cardiac Resynchronization Defibrillator Pulse Generator for Insertion in Subcutaneous Tissue and Fascia
OXINIUM	Synthetic Substitute, Oxidized Zirconium on Polyethylene for Replacement in Lower Joints
Paclitaxel-eluting coronary stent	Intraluminal Device, Drug-eluting in Heart and Great Vessels
Paclitaxel-eluting peripheral stent	Intraluminal Device, Drug-eluting in Upper Arteries Intraluminal Device, Drug-eluting in Lower Arteries
Palladium-103 Collagen Implant	Radioactive Element, Palladium-103 Collagen Implant for Insertion in Central Nervous System and Cranial Nerves
Partially absorbable mesh	Synthetic Substitute
Pedicle-based dynamic stabilization device	Spinal Stabilization Device, Pedicle-Based for Insertion in Upper Joints Spinal Stabilization Device, Pedicle-Based for Insertion in Lower Joints
PERCEPT™ PC neurostimulator	Stimulator Generator, Multiple Array for Insertion in Subcutaneous Tissue and Fascia
Percutaneous endoscopic gastrojejunostomy (PEG/J) tube	Feeding Device in Gastrointestinal System
Percutaneous endoscopic gastrostomy (PEG) tube	Feeding Device in Gastrointestinal System
Percutaneous nephrostomy catheter	Drainage Device
Peripherally inserted central catheter (PICC)	Infusion Device
Pessary ring	Intraluminal Device, Pessary in Female Reproductive System
Phrenic nerve stimulator generator	Stimulator Generator in Subcutaneous Tissue and Fascia
Phrenic nerve stimulator lead	Diaphragmatic Pacemaker Lead in Respiratory System
PHYSIOMESH™ Flexible Composite Mesh	Synthetic Substitute
Pipeline™ (Flex) embolization device	Intraluminal Device, Flow Diverter for Restriction in Upper Arteries
Piscine skin	Nonautologous Tissue Substitute
Polyethylene socket	Synthetic Substitute, Polyethylene for Replacement in Lower Joints
Polymethylmethacrylate (PMMA)	Synthetic Substitute
Polypropylene mesh	Synthetic Substitute
Porcine (bioprosthetic) valve	Zooplastic Tissue in Heart and Great Vessels

Terms	ICD-10-PCS Value
PRECICE intramedullary limb lengthening system	Internal Fixation Device, Intramedullary Limb Lengthening for Insertion in Upper Bones Internal Fixation Device, Intramedullary Limb Lengthening for Insertion in Lower Bones
PRESTIGE® Cervical Disc	Synthetic Substitute
PrimeAdvanced neurostimulator (SureScan)(MRI Safe)	Stimulator Generator, Multiple Array for Insertion in Subcutaneous Tissue and Fascia
PROCEED™ Ventral Patch	Synthetic Substitute
Prodisc-C	Synthetic Substitute
Prodisc-L	Synthetic Substitute
PROLENE Polypropylene Hernia System (PHS)	Synthetic Substitute
Protecta XT CRT-D	Cardiac Resynchronization Defibrillator Pulse Generator for Insertion in Subcutaneous Tissue and Fascia
Protecta XT DR (XT VR)	Defibrillator Generator for Insertion in Subcutaneous Tissue and Fascia
Protégé® RX Carotid Stent System	Intraluminal Device
Pump reservoir	Infusion Device, Pump in Subcutaneous Tissue and Fascia
Pz-cel	Prademagene Zamikeracel, Genetically Engineered Autologous Cell Therapy in New Technology
REALIZE® Adjustable Gastric Band	Extraluminal Device
Rebound HRD® (Hernia Repair Device)	Synthetic Substitute
Reducer™ System	Reduction Device in New Technology
RestoreAdvanced neurostimulator (SureScan)(MRI Safe)	Stimulator Generator, Multiple Array Rechargeable for Insertion in Subcutaneous Tissue and Fascia
Restor3d TIDAL™ Fusion Cage	Internal Fixation Device, Gyroid-Sheet Lattice Design in New Technology
RestoreSensor neurostimulator (SureScan)(MRI Safe)	Stimulator Generator, Multiple Array Rechargeable for Insertion in Subcutaneous Tissue and Fascia
RestoreUltra neurostimulator (SureScan)(MRI Safe)	Stimulator Generator, Multiple Array Rechargeable for Insertion in Subcutaneous Tissue and Fascia
Reveal (LINQ)(DX)(XT)	Monitoring Device
Reverse® Shoulder Prosthesis	Synthetic Substitute, Reverse Ball and Socket for Replacement in Upper Joints
Revo MRI™ SureScan® pacemaker	Pacemaker, Dual Chamber for Insertion in Subcutaneous Tissue and Fascia
Rheos® System device	Stimulator Generator in Subcutaneous Tissue and Fascia
Rheos® System lead	Stimulator Lead in Upper Arteries
RNS System lead	Neurostimulator Lead in Central Nervous System and Cranial Nerves
RNS system neurostimulator generator	Neurostimulator Generator in Head and Facial Bones
S-ICD™ lead	Subcutaneous Defibrillator Lead in Subcutaneous Tissue and Fascia
Sacral nerve modulation (SNM) lead	Stimulator Lead in Urinary System
Sacral neuromodulation lead	Stimulator Lead in Urinary System
SAPIEN transcatheter aortic valve	Zooplastic Tissue in Heart and Great Vessels

Terms	ICD-10-PCS Value
SAVAL below-the-knee (BTK) drug-eluting stent system	Intraluminal Device, Drug-eluting, Four or More in Lower Arteries Intraluminal Device, Drug-eluting in Lower Arteries Intraluminal Device, Drug-eluting, Three in Lower Arteries Intraluminal Device, Drug-eluting, Two in Lower Arteries
Secura (DR) (VR)	Defibrillator Generator for Insertion in Subcutaneous Tissue and Fascia
Sheffield hybrid external fixator	External Fixation Device, Hybrid for Insertion in Upper Bones External Fixation Device, Hybrid for Reposition in Upper Bones External Fixation Device, Hybrid for Insertion in Lower Bones External Fixation Device, Hybrid for Reposition in Lower Bones
Sheffield ring external fixator	External Fixation Device, Ring for Insertion in Upper Bones External Fixation Device, Ring for Reposition in Upper Bones External Fixation Device, Ring for Insertion in Lower Bones External Fixation Device, Ring for Reposition in Lower Bones
Single lead pacemaker (atrium)(ventricle)	Pacemaker, Single Chamber for Insertion in Subcutaneous Tissue and Fascia
Single lead rate responsive pacemaker (atrium)(ventricle)	Pacemaker, Single Chamber Rate Responsive for Insertion in Subcutaneous Tissue and Fascia
Sirolimus-eluting coronary stent	Intraluminal Device, Drug-eluting in Heart and Great Vessels
SJM Biocor® Stented Valve System	Zooplastic Tissue in Heart and Great Vessels
Spacer, Articulating (Antibiotic)	Articulating Spacer in Lower Joints
Spacer, Static (Antibiotic)	Spacer in Lower Joints
Spinal cord neurostimulator lead	Neurostimulator Lead in Central Nervous System and Cranial Nerves
Spinal growth rods, magnetically controlled	Magnetically Controlled Growth Rod(s) in New Technology
SpineJack® system	Synthetic Substitute, Mechanically Expandable (Paired) in New Technology
Spiration IBV™ Valve System	Intraluminal Device, Endobronchial Valve in Respiratory System
Static Spacer (Antibiotic)	Spacer in Lower Joints
Stent, intraluminal (cardiovascular) (gastrointestinal) (hepatobiliary)(urinary)	Intraluminal Device
Stented tissue valve	Zooplastic Tissue in Heart and Great Vessels
Stratos LV	Cardiac Resynchronization Pacemaker Pulse Generator for Insertion in Subcutaneous Tissue and Fascia
Subcutaneous injection reservoir, port	Vascular Access Device, Totally Implantable in Subcutaneous Tissue and Fascia
Subcutaneous injection reservoir, pump	Infusion Device, Pump in Subcutaneous Tissue and Fascia
Subdermal progesterone implant	Contraceptive Device in Subcutaneous Tissue and Fascia
Surpass Streamline™ Flow Diverter	Intraluminal Device, Flow Diverter for Restriction in Upper Arteries
SynCardia (temporary) Total Artificial Heart (TAH)	Synthetic Substitute, Pneumatic for Replacement in Heart and Great Vessels
SynCardia Total Artificial Heart	Synthetic Substitute
Syncra CRT-P	Cardiac Resynchronization Pacemaker Pulse Generator for Insertion in Subcutaneous Tissue and Fascia

Appendix G: Device Key and Aggregation Table

Terms	ICD-10-PCS Value
SynchroMed Pump	Infusion Device, Pump in Subcutaneous Tissue and Fascia
Talent® Converter	Intraluminal Device
Talent® Occluder	Intraluminal Device
Talent® Stent Graft (abdominal)(thoracic)	Intraluminal Device
TAMBE Device (Thoracoabdominal Branch Endoprosthesis), GORE® EXCLUDER®	Branched Intraluminal Device, Manufactured Integrated System, Four or More Arteries in New Technology
TandemHeart® System	Short-term External Heart Assist System in Heart and Great Vessels
TAXUS® Liberté® Paclitaxel-eluting Coronary Stent System	Intraluminal Device, Drug-eluting in Heart and Great Vessels
Therapeutic occlusion coil(s)	Intraluminal Device
Thoracostomy tube	Drainage Device
Thoraflex™ Hybrid device [NT]	Branched Synthetic Substitute with Intraluminal Device in New Technology
Thoratec IVAD (Implantable Ventricular Assist Device)	Implantable Heart Assist System in Heart and Great Vessels
Thoratec Paracorporeal Ventricular Assist Device	Short-term External Heart Assist System in Heart and Great Vessels
Tibial insert	Liner in Lower Joints
Tissue bank graft	Nonautologous Tissue Substitute
Tissue expander (inflatable)(injectable)	Tissue Expander in Skin and Breast Tissue Expander in Subcutaneous Tissue and Fascia
Titan Endoskeleton™	Interbody Fusion Device in Upper Joints Interbody Fusion Device in Lower Joints
Titanium Sternal Fixation System (TSFS)	Internal Fixation Device, Rigid Plate for Insertion in Upper Bones Internal Fixation Device, Rigid Plate for Reposition in Upper Bones
TOPS™ System [NT]	Posterior Spinal Motion Preservation Device in New Technology
Total Ankle Talar Replacement™ (TATR)	Synthetic Substitute, Talar Prosthesis in New Technology
Total artificial (replacement) heart	Synthetic Substitute
Tracheostomy tube	Tracheostomy Device in Respiratory System
TricValve® Transcatheter Bicaval Valve System	Intraluminal Device, Bioprosthetic Valve in New Technology
Trifecta™ Valve (aortic)	Zooplastic Tissue in Heart and Great Vessels
Tunneled central venous catheter	Vascular Access Device, Tunneled in Subcutaneous Tissue and Fascia
Tunneled spinal (intrathecal) catheter	Infusion Device
Two lead pacemaker	Pacemaker, Dual Chamber for Insertion in Subcutaneous Tissue and Fascia
Ultraflex™ Precision Colonic Stent System	Intraluminal Device
ULTRAPRO Hernia System (UHS)	Synthetic Substitute
ULTRAPRO Partially Absorbable Lightweight Mesh	Synthetic Substitute
ULTRAPRO Plug	Synthetic Substitute
Ultrasonic osteogenic stimulator	Bone Growth Stimulator in Head and Facial Bones Bone Growth Stimulator in Upper Bones Bone Growth Stimulator in Lower Bones
Ultrasound bone healing system	Bone Growth Stimulator in Head and Facial Bones Bone Growth Stimulator in Upper Bones Bone Growth Stimulator in Lower Bones

Terms	ICD-10-PCS Value
Uniplanar external fixator	External Fixation Device, Monoplanar for Insertion in Upper Bones External Fixation Device, Monoplanar for Reposition in Upper Bones External Fixation Device, Monoplanar for Insertion in Lower Bones External Fixation Device, Monoplanar for Reposition in Lower Bones
Urinary incontinence stimulator lead	Stimulator Lead in Urinary System
V-Wave Interatrial Shunt System	Synthetic Substitute
VADER® Pedicle System	Carbon/PEEK Spinal Stabilization Device, Pedicle Based in New Technology
Vaginal pessary	Intraluminal Device, Pessary in Female Reproductive System
Valiant Thoracic Stent Graft	Intraluminal Device
Vanta™ PC neurostimulator	Stimulator Generator, Multiple Array for Insertion in Subcutaneous Tissue and Fascia
VasQ™ External Support device	Synthetic Substitute, Extraluminal Support Device in New Technology
Vectra® Vascular Access Graft	Vascular Access Device, Tunneled in Subcutaneous Tissue and Fascia
VenoValve®	Intraluminal Device, Bioprosthetic Valve in New Technology
Ventrio™ Hernia Patch	Synthetic Substitute
Versa	Pacemaker, Dual Chamber for Insertion in Subcutaneous Tissue and Fascia
VEST™ Venous External Support device	Vein Graft Extraluminal Support Device(s) in New Technology
Virtuoso (II) (DR) (VR)	Defibrillator Generator for Insertion in Subcutaneous Tissue and Fascia
Viva(XT)(S)	Cardiac Resynchronization Defibrillator Pulse Generator for Insertion in Subcutaneous Tissue and Fascia
Vivistim® Paired VNS System Lead [NT]	Neurostimulator Lead with Paired Stimulation System in New Technology
WALLSTENT® Endoprosthesis	Intraluminal Device
X-Spine Axle Cage	Spinal Stabilization Device, Interspinous Process for Insertion in Upper Joints Spinal Stabilization Device, Interspinous Process for Insertion in Lower Joints
X-STOP® Spacer	Spinal Stabilization Device, Interspinous Process for Insertion in Upper Joints Spinal Stabilization Device, Interspinous Process for Insertion in Lower Joints
Xact Carotid Stent System	Intraluminal Device
Xenograft	Zooplastic Tissue in Heart and Great Vessels
XIENCE Everolimus Eluting Coronary Stent System	Intraluminal Device, Drug-eluting in Heart and Great Vessels
XLIF® System	Interbody Fusion Device in Lower Joints
Zenith AAA Endovascular Graft	Intraluminal Device
Zenith® Fenestrated AAA Endovascular Graft	Intraluminal Device, Branched or Fenestrated, One or Two Arteries for Restriction in Lower Arteries Intraluminal Device, Branched or Fenestrated, Three or More Arteries for Restriction in Lower Arteries
Zenith Flex® AAA Endovascular Graft	Intraluminal Device
Zenith® Renu™ AAA Ancillary Graft	Intraluminal Device
Zenith TX2® TAA Endovascular Graft	Intraluminal Device

Terms	ICD-10-PCS Value
Zilver® PTX® (paclitaxel) Drug-Eluting Peripheral Stent	Intraluminal Device, Drug-eluting in Upper Arteries Intraluminal Device, Drug-eluting in Lower Arteries
Zimmer® NexGen® LPS Mobile Bearing Knee	Synthetic Substitute
Zimmer® NexGen® LPS-Flex Mobile Knee	Synthetic Substitute
Zotarolimus-eluting coronary stent	Intraluminal Device, Drug-eluting in Heart and Great Vessels

Device Aggregation Table

This table crosswalks specific device character value definitions for specific root operations in a specific body system to the more general device character value to be used when the root operation covers a wide range of body parts and the device character represents an entire family of devices.

Specific Device	for Operation	in Body System	General Device	
Autologous Arterial Tissue (A)	All applicable	Heart and Great Vessels Lower Arteries Lower Veins Upper Arteries Upper Veins	7	Autologous Tissue Substitute
Autologous Venous Tissue (9)	All applicable	Heart and Great Vessels Lower Arteries Lower Veins Upper Arteries Upper Veins	7	Autologous Tissue Substitute
Cardiac Lead, Defibrillator (K)	Insertion	Heart and Great Vessels	M	Cardiac Lead
Cardiac Lead, Pacemaker (J)	Insertion	Heart and Great Vessels	M	Cardiac Lead
Cardiac Resynchronization Defibrillator Pulse Generator (9)	Insertion	Subcutaneous Tissue and Fascia	P	Cardiac Rhythm Related Device
Cardiac Resynchronization Pacemaker Pulse Generator (7)	Insertion	Subcutaneous Tissue and Fascia	P	Cardiac Rhythm Related Device
Contractility Modulation Device (A)	Insertion	Subcutaneous Tissue and Fascia	P	Cardiac Rhythm Related Device
Defibrillator Generator (8)	Insertion	Subcutaneous Tissue and Fascia	P	Cardiac Rhythm Related Device
Epiretinal Visual Prosthesis (5)	All applicable	Eye	J	Synthetic Substitute
External Fixation Device, Hybrid (D)	Insertion	Lower Bones Upper Bones	5	External Fixation Device
External Fixation Device, Hybrid (D)	Reposition	Lower Bones Upper Bones	5	External Fixation Device
External Fixation Device, Limb Lengthening (8)	Insertion	Lower Bones Upper Bones	5	External Fixation Device
External Fixation Device, Monoplanar (B)	Insertion	Lower Bones Upper Bones	5	External Fixation Device
External Fixation Device, Monoplanar (B)	Reposition	Lower Bones Upper Bones	5	External Fixation Device
External Fixation Device, Ring (C)	Insertion	Lower Bones Upper Bones	5	External Fixation Device
External Fixation Device, Ring (C)	Reposition	Lower Bones Upper Bones	5	External Fixation Device
Hearing Device, Bone Conduction (4)	Insertion	Ear, Nose, Sinus	S	Hearing Device
Hearing Device, Multiple Channel Cochlear Prosthesis (6)	Insertion	Ear, Nose, Sinus	S	Hearing Device
Hearing Device, Single Channel Cochlear Prosthesis (5)	Insertion	Ear, Nose, Sinus	S	Hearing Device
Internal Fixation Device, Intramedullary (6)	All applicable	Lower Bones Upper Bones	4	Internal Fixation Device
Internal Fixation Device, Intramedullary Limb Lengthening (7)	Insertion	Lower Bones Upper Bones	6	Internal Fixation Device, Intramedullary
Internal Fixation Device, Rigid Plate (0)	Insertion	Upper Bones	4	Internal Fixation Device
Internal Fixation Device, Rigid Plate (0)	Reposition	Upper Bones	4	Internal Fixation Device
Intraluminal Device, Airway (B)	All applicable	Ear, Nose, Sinus Gastrointestinal System Mouth and Throat	D	Intraluminal Device
Intraluminal Device, Bioactive (B)	All applicable	Upper Arteries	D	Intraluminal Device
Intraluminal Device, Branched or Fenestrated, One or Two Arteries (E)	Restriction	Heart and Great Vessels Lower Arteries	D	Intraluminal Device
Intraluminal Device, Branched or Fenestrated, Three or More Arteries (F)	Restriction	Heart and Great Vessels Lower Arteries	D	Intraluminal Device

Appendix G: Device Key and Aggregation Table

Specific Device	for Operation	in Body System	General Device	
Intraluminal Device, Drug-eluting (4)	All applicable	Heart and Great Vessels Lower Arteries Upper Arteries	D	Intraluminal Device
Intraluminal Device, Drug-eluting, Four or More (7)	All applicable	Heart and Great Vessels Lower Arteries Upper Arteries	D	Intraluminal Device
Intraluminal Device, Drug-eluting, Three (6)	All applicable	Heart and Great Vessels Lower Arteries Upper Arteries	D	Intraluminal Device
Intraluminal Device, Drug-eluting, Two (5)	All applicable	Heart and Great Vessels Lower Arteries Upper Arteries	D	Intraluminal Device
Intraluminal Device, Endobronchial Valve (G)	All applicable	Respiratory System	D	Intraluminal Device
Intraluminal Device, Endotracheal Airway (E)	All applicable	Respiratory System	D	Intraluminal Device
Intraluminal Device, Flow Diverter (H)	Restriction	Upper Arteries	D	Intraluminal Device
Intraluminal Device, Four or More (G)	All applicable	Heart and Great Vessels Lower Arteries Upper Arteries	D	Intraluminal Device
Intraluminal Device, Pessary (G)	All applicable	Female Reproductive System	D	Intraluminal Device
Intraluminal Device, Radioactive (T)	All applicable	Heart and Great Vessels	D	Intraluminal Device
Intraluminal Device, Three (F)	All applicable	Heart and Great Vessels Lower Arteries Upper Arteries	D	Intraluminal Device
Intraluminal Device, Two (E)	All applicable	Heart and Great Vessels Lower Arteries Upper Arteries	D	Intraluminal Device
Monitoring Device, Hemodynamic (Ø)	Insertion	Subcutaneous Tissue and Fascia	2	Monitoring Device
Monitoring Device, Pressure Sensor (Ø)	Insertion	Heart and Great Vessels	2	Monitoring Device
Pacemaker, Dual Chamber (6)	Insertion	Subcutaneous Tissue and Fascia	P	Cardiac Rhythm Related Device
Pacemaker, Single Chamber (4)	Insertion	Subcutaneous Tissue and Fascia	P	Cardiac Rhythm Related Device
Pacemaker, Single Chamber Rate Responsive (5)	Insertion	Subcutaneous Tissue and Fascia	P	Cardiac Rhythm Related Device
Spinal Stabilization Device, Facet Replacement (D)	Insertion	Lower Joints Upper Joints	4	Internal Fixation Device
Spinal Stabilization Device, Interspinous Process (B)	Insertion	Lower Joints Upper Joints	4	Internal Fixation Device
Spinal Stabilization Device, Pedicle-Based (C)	Insertion	Lower Joints Upper Joints	4	Internal Fixation Device
Spinal Stabilization Device, Vertebral Body Tether (3)	Reposition	Lower Bones Upper Bones	4	Internal Fixation Device
Stimulator Generator, Multiple Array (D)	Insertion	Subcutaneous Tissue and Fascia	M	Stimulator Generator
Stimulator Generator, Multiple Array Rechargeable (E)	Insertion	Subcutaneous Tissue and Fascia	M	Stimulator Generator
Stimulator Generator, Single Array (B)	Insertion	Subcutaneous Tissue and Fascia	M	Stimulator Generator
Stimulator Generator, Single Array Rechargeable (C)	Insertion	Subcutaneous Tissue and Fascia	M	Stimulator Generator
Synthetic Substitute, Ceramic (3)	Replacement	Lower Joints	J	Synthetic Substitute
Synthetic Substitute, Ceramic on Polyethylene (4)	Replacement	Lower Joints	J	Synthetic Substitute
Synthetic Substitute, Intraocular Telescope (Ø)	Replacement	Eye	J	Synthetic Substitute
Synthetic Substitute, Metal (1)	Replacement	Lower Joints	J	Synthetic Substitute
Synthetic Substitute, Metal on Polyethylene (2)	Replacement	Lower Joints	J	Synthetic Substitute
Synthetic Substitute, Oxidized Zirconium on Polyethylene (6)	Replacement	Lower Joints	J	Synthetic Substitute
Synthetic Substitute, Polyethylene (Ø)	Replacement	Lower Joints	J	Synthetic Substitute
Synthetic Substitute, Reverse Ball and Socket (Ø)	Replacement	Upper Joints	J	Synthetic Substitute

Appendix H: Device Definitions

This **NT** symbol next to a device in the Definition column identifies that the device has been approved for NTAP (new technology add-on payment). CMS provides incremental payment, in addition to the DRG payment, for technologies that have received an NTAP designation.

ICD-10-PCS Value	Definition
Articulating Spacer in Lower Joints	Articulating Spacer (Antibiotic) Spacer, Articulating (Antibiotic)
Artificial Sphincter in Gastrointestinal System	Artificial anal sphincter (AAS) Artificial bowel sphincter (neosphincter)
Artificial Sphincter in Urinary System	AMS 800® Urinary Control System Artificial urinary sphincter (AUS)
Autologous Arterial Tissue in Heart and Great Vessels	Autologous artery graft
Autologous Arterial Tissue in Lower Arteries	Autologous artery graft
Autologous Arterial Tissue in Lower Veins	Autologous artery graft
Autologous Arterial Tissue in Upper Arteries	Autologous artery graft
Autologous Arterial Tissue in Upper Veins	Autologous artery graft
Autologous Tissue Substitute	Autograft Cultured epidermal cell autograft Epicel® cultured epidermal autograft
Autologous Venous Tissue in Heart and Great Vessels	Autologous vein graft
Autologous Venous Tissue in Lower Arteries	Autologous vein graft
Autologous Venous Tissue in Lower Veins	Autologous vein graft
Autologous Venous Tissue in Upper Arteries	Autologous vein graft
Autologous Venous Tissue in Upper Veins	Autologous vein graft
Bioengineered Human Acellular Vessel in New Technology	HAV™ (Human Acellular Vessel) Human Acellular Vessel™ (HAV)
Biologic with Synthetic Substitute, Autoregulated Electrohydraulic for Replacement in Heart and Great Vessels	Carmat total artificial heart (TAH)
Bone Growth Stimulator in Head and Facial Bones	Electrical bone growth stimulator (EBGS) Ultrasonic osteogenic stimulator Ultrasound bone healing system
Bone Growth Stimulator in Lower Bones	Electrical bone growth stimulator (EBGS) Ultrasonic osteogenic stimulator Ultrasound bone healing system
Bone Growth Stimulator in Upper Bones	Electrical bone growth stimulator (EBGS) Ultrasonic osteogenic stimulator Ultrasound bone healing system
Branched Intraluminal Device, Manufactured Integrated System, Four or More Arteries in New Technology	GORE® EXCLUDER® TAMBE Device (Thoracoabdominal Branch Endoprosthesis) TAMBE Device (Thoracoabdominal Branch Endoprosthesis), GORE® EXCLUDER®
Branched Synthetic Substitute with Intraluminal Device in New Technology	Thoraflex™ Hybrid device **NT**
Carbon/PEEK Spinal Stabilization Device, Pedicle Based in New Technology	BlackArmor® Carbon/PEEK fixation system VADER® Pedicle System
Cardiac Lead in Heart and Great Vessels	Cardiac contractility modulation lead

ICD-10-PCS Value	Definition
Cardiac Lead, Defibrillator for Insertion in Heart and Great Vessels	ACUITY™ Steerable Lead Attain Ability® lead Attain StarFix® (OTW) lead Cardiac resynchronization therapy (CRT) lead Corox (OTW) Bipolar Lead Durata® Defibrillation Lead ENDOTAK RELIANCE® (G) Defibrillation Lead
Cardiac Lead, Pacemaker for Insertion in Heart and Great Vessels	ACUITY™ Steerable Lead Attain Ability® lead Attain StarFix® (OTW) lead Cardiac resynchronization therapy (CRT) lead Corox (OTW) Bipolar Lead
Cardiac Resynchronization Defibrillator Pulse Generator for Insertion in Subcutaneous Tissue and Fascia	COGNIS® CRT-D Concerto II CRT-D Consulta CRT-D CONTAK RENEWA® 3 RF (HE) CRT-D LIVIAN™ CRT-D Maximo II DR CRT-D Ovatio™ CRT-D Protecta XT CRT-D Viva (XT)(S)
Cardiac Resynchronization Pacemaker Pulse Generator for Insertion in Subcutaneous Tissue and Fascia	Consulta CRT-P Stratos LV Syncra CRT-P
Conduit through Femoral Vein to Popliteal Artery in New Technology	DETOUR® System **NT**
Conduit through Femoral Vein to Superficial Femoral Artery in New Technology	DETOUR® System **NT**
Conduit to Short-term External Heart Assist System in New Technology	Impella® 5.5 with SmartAssist® System
Contraceptive Device in Female Reproductive System	Intrauterine device (IUD)
Contraceptive Device in Subcutaneous Tissue and Fascia	Subdermal progesterone implant
Contractility Modulation Device for Insertion in Subcutaneous Tissue and Fascia	Optimizer™ III implantable pulse generator
Defibrillator Generator for Insertion in Subcutaneous Tissue and Fascia	Evera (XT)(S)(DR/VR) Implantable cardioverter-defibrillator (ICD) Maximo II DR (VR) Protecta XT DR (XT VR) Secura (DR) (VR) Virtuoso (II) (DR) (VR)
Defibrillator Lead in Anatomical Regions, General	EV ICD System (Extravascular implantable defibrillator lead)
Diaphragmatic Pacemaker Lead in Respiratory System	Phrenic nerve stimulator lead
Drainage Device	Cystostomy tube Foley catheter Percutaneous nephrostomy catheter Thoracostomy tube
External Fixation Device in Head and Facial Bones	External fixator
External Fixation Device in Lower Bones	External fixator

Appendix H: Device Definitions

ICD-10-PCS Value	Definition
External Fixation Device in Lower Joints	External fixator
External Fixation Device in Upper Bones	External fixator
External Fixation Device in Upper Joints	External fixator
External Fixation Device, Hybrid for Insertion in Lower Bones	Delta frame external fixator Sheffield hybrid external fixator
External Fixation Device, Hybrid for Insertion in Upper Bones	Delta frame external fixator Sheffield hybrid external fixator
External Fixation Device, Hybrid for Reposition in Lower Bones	Delta frame external fixator Sheffield hybrid external fixator
External Fixation Device, Hybrid for Reposition in Upper Bones	Delta frame external fixator Sheffield hybrid external fixator
External Fixation Device, Limb Lengthening for Insertion in Lower Bones	Ilizarov-Vecklich device
External Fixation Device, Limb Lengthening for Insertion in Upper Bones	Ilizarov-Vecklich device
External Fixation Device, Monoplanar for Insertion in Lower Bones	Uniplanar external fixator
External Fixation Device, Monoplanar for Insertion in Upper Bones	Uniplanar external fixator
External Fixation Device, Monoplanar for Reposition in Lower Bones	Uniplanar external fixator
External Fixation Device, Monoplanar for Reposition in Upper Bones	Uniplanar external fixator
External Fixation Device, Ring for Insertion in Lower Bones	Ilizarov external fixator Sheffield ring external fixator
External Fixation Device, Ring for Insertion in Upper Bones	Ilizarov external fixator Sheffield ring external fixator
External Fixation Device, Ring for Reposition in Lower Bones	Ilizarov external fixator Sheffield ring external fixator
External Fixation Device, Ring for Reposition in Upper Bones	Ilizarov external fixator Sheffield ring external fixator
Extraluminal Device	AtriClip LAA Exclusion System LAP-BAND® adjustable gastric banding system REALIZE® Adjustable Gastric Band
Facet Joint Fusion Device, Paired Titanium Cages in New Technology	Facet FiXation implant FFX® (Facet FiXation) implant
Feeding Device in Gastrointestinal System	Percutaneous endoscopic gastrojejunostomy (PEG/J) tube Percutaneous endoscopic gastrostomy (PEG) tube
Hearing Device in Ear, Nose, Sinus	Esteem® implantable hearing system
Hearing Device in Head and Facial Bones	Bone anchored hearing device
Hearing Device, Bone Conduction for Insertion in Ear, Nose, Sinus	Bone anchored hearing device

ICD-10-PCS Value	Definition
Hearing Device, Multiple Channel Cochlear Prosthesis for Insertion in Ear, Nose, Sinus	Cochlear implant (CI), multiple channel (electrode)
Hearing Device, Single Channel Cochlear Prosthesis for Insertion in Ear, Nose, Sinus	Cochlear implant (CI), single channel (electrode)
Implantable Heart Assist System in Heart and Great Vessels	Berlin Heart Ventricular Assist Device DeBakey Left Ventricular Assist Device DuraHeart Left Ventricular Assist System HeartMate 3™ LVAS HeartMate II® Left Ventricular Assist Device (LVAD) HeartMate XVE® Left Ventricular Assist Device (LVAD) MicroMed Heart Assist Novacor Left Ventricular Assist Device Thoratec IVAD (Implantable Ventricular Assist Device)
Infusion Device	Ascenda Intrathecal Catheter InDura, intrathecal catheter (1P) (spinal) Non-tunneled central venous catheter Peripherally inserted central catheter (PICC) Tunneled spinal (intrathecal) catheter
Infusion Device, Pump in Subcutaneous Tissue and Fascia	Implantable drug infusion pump (anti-spasmodic)(chemotherapy)(pain) Injection reservoir, pump Pump reservoir Subcutaneous injection reservoir, pump SynchroMed pump
Interbody Fusion Device, Custom-made Anatomically Designed in New Technology	aprevo™
Interbody Fusion Device in Lower Joints	Axial Lumbar Interbody Fusion System AxiaLIF® System COALESCE® radiolucent interbody fusion device COHERE® radiolucent interbody fusion device CoRoent® XL Direct Lateral Interbody Fusion (DLIF) device EXtreme Lateral Interbody Fusion (XLIF) device Interbody fusion (spine) cage nanoLOCK™ interbody fusion device Titan Endoskeleton™ XLIF® System
Interbody Fusion Device in Upper Joints	BAK/C® Interbody Cervical Fusion System COALESCE® radiolucent interbody fusion device COHERE® radiolucent interbody fusion device Interbody fusion (spine) cage nanoLOCK™ interbody fusion device Titan Endoskeleton™
Internal Fixation Device, Gyroid-Sheet Lattice Design in New Technology	restor3d TIDAL™ Fusion Cage
Internal Fixation Device in Head and Facial Bones	Bone screw (interlocking)(lag)(pedicle)(recessed) Kirschner wire (K-wire) Neutralization plate
Internal Fixation Device in Lower Bones	Bone screw (interlocking)(lag)(pedicle)(recessed) Clamp and rod internal fixation system (CRIF) Kirschner wire (K-wire) Neutralization plate
Internal Fixation Device in Lower Joints	Fusion screw (compression)(lag)(locking) Joint fixation plate Kirschner wire (K-wire)

ICD-10-PCS Value	Definition
Internal Fixation Device in Upper Bones	Bone screw (interlocking)(lag)(pedicle) (recessed) Clamp and rod internal fixation system (CRIF) Kirschner wire (K-wire) Neutralization plate
Internal Fixation Device in Upper Joints	Fusion screw (compression)(lag)(locking) Joint fixation plate Kirschner wire (K-wire)
Internal Fixation Device, Intramedullary in Lower Bones	Intramedullary (IM) rod (nail) Intramedullary skeletal kinetic distractor (ISKD) Kuntscher nail
Internal Fixation Device, Intramedullary in Upper Bones	Intramedullary (IM) rod (nail) Intramedullary skeletal kinetic distractor (ISKD) Kuntscher nail
Internal Fixation Device Intramedullary Limb Lengthening for Insertion in Lower Bones	PRECICE intramedullary limb lengthening system
Internal Fixation Device Intramedullary Limb Lengthening for Insertion in Upper Bones	PRECICE intramedullary limb lengthening system
Internal Fixation Device, Open-truss Design in New Technology	Ankle Truss System™ (ATS)
Internal Fixation Device, Rigid Plate for Insertion in Upper Bones	Titanium Sternal Fixation System (TSFS)
Internal Fixation Device, Rigid Plate for Reposition in Upper Bones	Titanium Sternal Fixation System (TSFS)
Internal Fixation Device, Sustained Compression for Fusion in Lower Joints	DynaClip® (Delta) (Forte) (Quattro) DynaNail® (Helix) (Hybrid) (Mini)
Internal Fixation Device, Sustained Compression for Fusion in Upper Joints	DynaClip® (Delta) (Forte) (Quattro) DynaNail® (Helix) (Hybrid) (Mini)
Internal Fixation Device with Tulip Connector in New Technology	iFuse Bedrock™ Granite Implant System [NT]
Intracardiac Pacemaker, Dual-Chamber in New Technology	Aveir™ AR, as dual chamber [NT] Aveir™ DR, dual chamber [NT]
Intracardiac Pacemaker in Heart and Great Vessels	Aveir™ VR, as single chamber
Intraluminal Device	Absolute Pro Vascular (OTW) Self-Expanding Stent System Acculink (RX) Carotid Stent System AFX® Endovascular AAA System AneuRx® AAA Advantage® Assurant (Cobalt) stent Carotid WALLSTENT® Monorail® Endoprosthesis CoAxia NeuroFlo catheter Colonic Z-Stent® Complete (SE) stent Cook Zenith AAA Endovascular Graft Driver stent (RX) (OTW) E-Luminexx™ (Biliary)(Vascular) Stent Embolization coil(s) Endologix AFX® Endovascular AAA System Endurant® Endovascular Stent Graft Endurant® II AAA stent graft system EXCLUDER® AAA Endoprosthesis Express® (LD) Premounted Stent System Express® Biliary SD Monorail® Premounted Stent System Express® SD Renal Monorail® Premounted Stent System FLAIR® Endovascular Stent Graft Formula™ Balloon-Expandable Renal Stent System GORE EXCLUDER® AAA Endoprosthesis GORE TAG® Thoracic Endoprosthesis [NT] Herculink (RX) Elite Renal Stent System Innova™ stent LifeStent® (Flexstar)(XL) Vascular Stent System Medtronic Endurant® II AAA stent graft system Micro-Driver stent (RX) (OTW) MULTI-LINK (VISION)(MINI-VISION)(ULTRA) Coronary Stent System Omnilink Elite Vascular Balloon Expandable Stent System Protege® RX Carotid Stent System Stent, intraluminal (cardiovascular) (gastrointestinal)(hepatobiliary) (urinary) Talent® Converter Talent® Occluder Talent® Stent Graft (abdominal)(thoracic) Therapeutic occlusion coil(s) Ultraflex™ Precision Colonic Stent System Valiant Thoracic Stent Graft WALLSTENT® Endoprosthesis Xact Carotid Stent System Zenith AAA Endovascular Graft Zenith Flex® AAA Endovascular Graft Zenith TX2® TAA Endovascular Graft Zenith® Renu™ AAA Ancillary Graft
Intraluminal Device, Airway in Ear, Nose, Sinus	Nasopharyngeal airway (NPA)
Intraluminal Device, Airway in Gastrointestinal System	Esophageal obturator airway (EOA)
Intraluminal Device, Airway in Mouth and Throat	Guedel airway Oropharyngeal airway (OPA)
Intraluminal Device, Bioactive in Upper Arteries	Bioactive embolization coil(s) Micrus CERECYTE microcoil
Intraluminal Device, Bioprosthetic Valve in New Technology	TricValve® Transcatheter Bicaval Valve System VenoValve®

Appendix H: Device Definitions

ICD-10-PCS Value	Definition
Intraluminal Device, Branched or Fenestrated, One or Two Arteries for Restriction in Lower Arteries	Cook Zenith® Fenestrated AAA Endovascular Graft EXCLUDER® AAA Endoprosthesis EXCLUDER® IBE Endoprosthesis GORE EXCLUDER® AAA Endoprosthesis GORE EXCLUDER®IBE Endoprosthesis Zenith® Fenestrated AAA Endovascular Graft
Intraluminal Device, Branched or Fenestrated, Three or More Arteries for Restriction in Lower Arteries	Cook Zenith® Fenestrated AAA Endovascular Graft EXCLUDER® AAA Endoprosthesis GORE EXCLUDER® AAA Endoprosthesis Zenith® Fenestrated AAA Endovascular Graft
Intraluminal Device, Drug-eluting in Heart and Great Vessels	CYPHER® Stent Endeavor® (III)(IV) (Sprint) Zotarolimus-eluting Coronary Stent System Everolimus-eluting coronary stent Paclitaxel-eluting coronary stent Sirolimus-eluting coronary stent TAXUS® Liberte® Paclitaxel-eluting Coronary Stent System XIENCE Everolimus Eluting Coronary Stent System Zotarolimus-eluting coronary stent
Intraluminal Device, Drug-eluting in Lower Arteries	Eluvia™ Drug-eluting Vascular Stent System Paclitaxel-eluting peripheral stent SAVAL below-the-knee (BTK) drug-eluting stent system Zilver® PTX® (paclitaxel) Drug-Eluting Peripheral Stent
Intraluminal Device, Drug-eluting, Four or More in Lower Arteries	Eluvia™ Drug-eluting Vascular Stent System SAVAL below-the-knee (BTK) drug-eluting stent system
Intraluminal Device, Drug-eluting, Three in Lower Arteries	Eluvia™ Drug-eluting Vascular Stent System SAVAL below-the-knee (BTK) drug-eluting stent system
Intraluminal Device, Drug-eluting, Two in Lower Arteries	Eluvia™ Drug-eluting Vascular Stent System SAVAL below-the-knee (BTK) drug-eluting stent system
Intraluminal Device, Drug-eluting in Upper Arteries	Paclitaxel-eluting peripheral stent Zilver® PTX® (paclitaxel) Drug-Eluting Peripheral Stent
Intraluminal Device, Endobronchial Valve in Respiratory System	Spiration IBV™ Valve System
Intraluminal Device, Endotracheal Airway in Respiratory System	Endotracheal tube (cuffed)(double-lumen)
Intraluminal Device, Everolimus-eluting Resorbable Scaffold(s) in New Technology	Drug-eluting resorbable scaffold intraluminal device Esprit™ BTK (scaffold) (stent) Everolimus Eluting Resorbable Scaffold System
Intraluminal Device, Flow Diverter for Restriction in Upper Arteries	Flow Diverter embolization device Pipeline™ (Flex) embolization device Surpass Streamline™ Flow Diverter
Intraluminal Device, Pessary in Female Reproductive System	Pessary ring Vaginal pessary
Liner in Lower Joints	Acetabular cup Hip (joint) liner Joint liner (insert) Knee (implant) insert Tibial insert
Magnetically Controlled Growth Rod(s) in New Technology	MAGEC® Spinal Bracing and Distraction System Spinal growth rods, magnetically controlled
Magnetic Lengthening Device in Gastrointestinal System	Flourish® Pediatric Esophageal Atresia Device

ICD-10-PCS Value	Definition
Monitoring Device	Blood glucose monitoring system Cardiac event recorder Continuous Glucose Monitoring (CGM) device Implantable glucose monitoring device Loop recorder, implantable Reveal (LINQ)(DX)(XT)
Monitoring Device, Hemodynamic for Insertion in Subcutaneous Tissue and Fascia	Implantable hemodynamic monitor (IHM) Implantable hemodynamic monitoring system (IHMS)
Monitoring Device, Pressure Sensor for Insertion in Heart and Great Vessels	CardioMEMS® pressure sensor EndoSure® sensor
Multi-plane Flex Technology Bioprosthetic Valve in New Technology	Edwards EVOQUE tricuspid valve replacement system
Neurostimulator Generator in Head and Facial Bones	RNS system neurostimulator generator
Neurostimulator Lead in Central Nervous System and Cranial Nerves	Cortical strip neurostimulator lead DBS lead Deep brain neurostimulator lead RNS System lead Spinal cord neurostimulator lead
Neurostimulator Lead in Peripheral Nervous System	InterStim® Therapy lead
Neurostimulator Lead in New Technology	Ischemic Stroke System (ISS500) ISS500 (Ischemic Stroke System)
Neurostimulator Lead with Paired Stimulation System in New Technology	Vivistim® Paired VNS System Lead
Nonautologous Tissue Substitute	Acellular Hydrated Dermis Bone bank bone graft Cook Biodesign® Fistula Plug(s) Cook Biodesign® Hernia Graft(s) Cook Biodesign® Layered Graft(s) Cook Zenapro™ Layered Graft(s) Fish skin Kerecis® (GraftGuide) (MariGen) (SurgiBind) (SurgiClose) MIRODERM™ Biologic Wound Matrix Piscine skin Tissue bank graft
Other Device	Alfapump® system
Pacemaker, Dual Chamber for Insertion in Subcutaneous Tissue and Fascia	Advisa (MRI) EnRhythm Kappa Revo MRI™ SureScan® pacemaker Two lead pacemaker Versa
Pacemaker, Single Chamber for Insertion in Subcutaneous Tissue and Fascia	Single lead pacemaker (atrium)(ventricle)
Pacemaker, Single Chamber Rate Responsive for Insertion in Subcutaneous Tissue and Fascia	Single lead rate responsive pacemaker (atrium)(ventricle)
Posterior (Dynamic) Distraction Device in New Technology	ApiFix® Minimally Invasive Deformity Correction (MID-C) System
Posterior Spinal Motion Preservation Device in New Technology	TOPS™ System
Posterior Vertebral Tether in New Technology	LigaPASS 2.0™ PJK Prevention System

ICD-10-PCS Value	Definition
Prademagene Zamikeracel, Genetically Engineered Autologous Cell Therapy in New Technology	EB-101 gene-corrected autologous cell therapy EB-101 gene-corrected keratinocyte sheets LZRSE-COL7A1 engineered autologous epidermal sheets pz-cel
Radioactive Element	Brachytherapy seeds CivaSheet®
Radioactive Element, Cesium-131 Collagen Implant for Insertion in Central Nervous System and Cranial Nerves	Cesium-131 Collagen Implant GammaTile™
Radioactive Element, Palladium-103 Collagen Implant for Insertion in Central Nervous System and Cranial Nerves	GammaTile™ Palladium-103 Collagen Implant
Reduction Device in New Technology	Neovasc Reducer™ Reducer™ System
Resurfacing Device in Lower Joints	CONSERVE® PLUS Total Resurfacing Hip System Cormet Hip Resurfacing System
Short-term External Heart Assist System in Heart and Great Vessels	Aortix™ System Biventricular external heart assist system BVS 5000 Ventricular Assist Device Centrimag® Blood Pump Impella® heart pump TandemHeart® System Thoratec Paracorporeal Ventricular Assist Device
Spacer in Lower Joints	Joint spacer (antibiotic) Spacer, Static (Antibiotic) Static Spacer (Antibiotic)
Spacer in Upper Joints	Joint spacer (antibiotic)
Spinal Stabilization Device, Facet Replacement for Insertion in Lower Joints	Facet replacement spinal stabilization device
Spinal Stabilization Device, Facet Replacement for Insertion in Upper Joints	Facet replacement spinal stabilization device
Spinal Stabilization Device, Interspinous Process for Insertion in Lower Joints	Interspinous process spinal stabilization device X-Spine Axle Cage X-STOP® Spacer
Spinal Stabilization Device, Interspinous Process for Insertion in Upper Joints	Interspinous process spinal stabilization device X-Spine Axle Cage X-STOP® Spacer
Spinal Stabilization Device, Pedicle- Based for Insertion in Lower Joints	Dynesys® Dynamic Stabilization System Pedicle-based dynamic stabilization device
Spinal Stabilization Device, Pedicle-Based for Insertion in Upper Joints	Dynesys® Dynamic Stabilization System Pedicle-based dynamic stabilization device
Stimulator Generator in Subcutaneous Tissue and Fascia	Baroreflex Activation Therapy® (BAT®) Diaphragmatic pacemaker generator Mark IV Breathing Pacemaker System Phrenic nerve stimulator generator Rheos® System device
Stimulator Generator, Multiple Array for Insertion in Subcutaneous Tissue and Fascia	Activa PC neurostimulator Enterra gastric neurostimulator Neurostimulator generator, multiple channel PERCEPT™ PC neurostimulator PrimeAdvanced neurostimulator (SureScan)(MRI Safe) Vanta™ PC neurostimulator

ICD-10-PCS Value	Definition
Stimulator Generator, Multiple Array Rechargeable for Insertion in Subcutaneous Tissue and Fascia	Activa RC neurostimulator Intellis™ neurostimulator Neurostimulator generator, multiple channel rechargeable RestoreAdvanced neurostimulator (SureScan)(MRI Safe) RestoreSensor neurostimulator (SureScan)(MRI Safe) RestoreUltra neurostimulator (SureScan)(MRI Safe)
Stimulator Generator, Single Array for Insertion in Subcutaneous Tissue and Fascia	Activa SC neurostimulator InterStim™ II Therapy neurostimulator Itrel (3)(4) neurostimulator Neurostimulator generator, single channel
Stimulator Generator, Single Array Rechargeable for Insertion in Subcutaneous Tissue and Fascia	InterStim™ Micro Therapy neurostimulator Neurostimulator generator, single channel rechargeable
Stimulator Lead in Gastrointestinal System	Gastric electrical stimulation (GES) lead Gastric pacemaker lead
Stimulator Lead in Muscles	Electrical muscle stimulation (EMS) lead Electronic muscle stimulator lead Neuromuscular electrical stimulation (NEMS) lead
Stimulator Lead in Upper Arteries	Baroreflex Activation Therapy® (BAT®) Carotid (artery) sinus (baroreceptor) lead Rheos® System lead
Stimulator Lead in Urinary System	Sacral nerve modulation (SNM) lead Sacral neuromodulation lead Urinary incontinence stimulator lead
Subcutaneous Defibrillator Lead in Subcutaneous Tissue and Fascia	S-ICD™ lead

Appendix H: Device Definitions

ICD-10-PCS Value	Definition
Synthetic Substitute	AbioCor® Total Replacement Heart AMPLATZER® Muscular VSD Occluder Annuloplasty ring Bard® Composix® (E/X) (LP) mesh Bard® Composix® Kugel® patch Bard® Dulex™ mesh Bard® Ventralex™ hernia patch Barricaid® Annular Closure Device (ACD) BRYAN® Cervical Disc System Corvia IASD® Ex-PRESS™ mini glaucoma shunt Flexible Composite Mesh GORE® DUALMESH® Holter valve ventricular shunt IASD® (InterAtrial Shunt Device), Corvia InterAtrial Shunt Device IASD®, Corvia LimFlow™ Transcatheter Arterialization of the Deep Veins (TADV) System MitraClip valve repair system Nitinol framed polymer mesh Open Pivot (mechanical) valve Open Pivot Aortic Valve Graft (AVG) Partially absorbable mesh PHYSIOMESH™ Flexible Composite Mesh Polymethylmethacrylate (PMMA) Polypropylene mesh PRESTIGE® Cervical Disc PROCEED™ Ventral Patch Prodisc-C Prodisc-L PROLENE Polypropylene Hernia System (PHS) Rebound HRD® (Hernia Repair Device) SynCardia Total Artificial Heart Total artificial (replacement) heart ULTRAPRO Hernia System (UHS) ULTRAPRO Partially Absorbable Lightweight Mesh ULTRAPRO Plug V-Wave Interatrial Shunt System Ventrio™ Hernia Patch Zimmer® NexGen® LPS Mobile Bearing Knee Zimmer® NexGen® LPS-Flex Mobile Knee
Synthetic Substitute, Ceramic for Replacement in Lower Joints	Ceramic on ceramic bearing surface Novation® Ceramic AHS® (Articulation Hip System)
Synthetic Substitute, Extraluminal Support Device in New Technology	VasQ™ External Support device
Synthetic Substitute, Intraocular Telescope for Replacement in Eye	Implantable Miniature Telescope™ (IMT)
Synthetic Substitute, Lateral Meniscus in New Technology	NUsurface® Meniscus Implant
Synthetic Substitute, Mechanically Expandable (Paired) in New Technology	SpineJack® system
Synthetic Substitute, Medial Meniscus in New Technology	NUsurface® Meniscus Implant
Synthetic Substitute, Metal for Replacement in Lower Joints	Cobalt/chromium head and socket Metal on metal bearing surface
Synthetic Substitute, Metal on Polyethylene for Replacement in Lower Joints	Cobalt/chromium head and polyethylene socket
Synthetic Substitute, Oxidized Zirconium on Polyethylene for Replacement in Lower Joints	OXINIUM
Synthetic Substitute, Pneumatic for Replacement in Heart and Great Vessels	SynCardia (temporary) total artificial heart (TAH)

ICD-10-PCS Value	Definition
Synthetic Substitute, Polyethylene for Replacement in Lower Joints	Polyethylene socket
Synthetic Substitute, Reverse Ball and Socket for Replacement in Upper Joints	Delta III Reverse shoulder prosthesis Reverse® Shoulder Prosthesis
Synthetic Substitute, Talar Prosthesis in New Technology	Total Ankle Talar Replacement™ (TATR)
Synthetic Substitute, Ultrasound Penetrable in New Technology	Longeviti ClearFit® Cranial Implant Longeviti ClearFit® OTS Cranial Implant
Tibial Extension with Motion Sensors in New Technology	Canturio™ te (Tibial Extension)
Tissue Expander in Skin and Breast	Tissue expander (inflatable) (injectable)
Tissue Expander in Subcutaneous Tissue and Fascia	Tissue expander (inflatable) (injectable)
Tracheostomy Device in Respiratory System	Tracheostomy tube
Vascular Access Device, Totally Implantable in Subcutaneous Tissue and Fascia	Implanted (venous)(access) port Injection reservoir, port Subcutaneous injection reservoir, port
Vascular Access Device, Tunneled in Subcutaneous Tissue and Fascia	Tunneled central venous catheter Vectra® Vascular Access Graft
Vein Graft Extraluminal Support Device(s) in New Technology	VEST™ Venous External Support device
Zooplastic Tissue in Heart and Great Vessels	3f (Aortic) Bioprosthesis valve Bovine pericardial valve Bovine pericardium graft Contegra Pulmonary Valved Conduit CoreValve transcatheter aortic valve Epic™ Stented Tissue Valve (aortic) Freestyle (Stentless) Aortic Root Bioprosthesis Hancock Bioprosthesis (aortic) (mitral) valve Hancock Bioprosthetic Valved Conduit Inspiris Resilia valve Melody® transcatheter pulmonary valve Mitroflow® Aortic Pericardial Heart Valve Mosaic Bioprosthesis (aortic) (mitral) valve Porcine (bioprosthetic) valve SAPIEN transcatheter aortic valve SJM Biocor® Stented Valve System Stented tissue valve Trifecta™ Valve (aortic) Xenograft

Appendix I: Substance Key/Substance Definitions

Substance Key

This table crosswalks a specific substance, listed by trade name or synonym, to the PCS value that would be used to represent that substance in either the Administration or New Technology section. The ICD-10-PCS value may be located in either the 6th-character Substance column or the 7th-character Qualifier column depending on the section/table to which it is classified. The most specific character is listed in the table.

This **NT** symbol next to a substance/technology in the Trade Name or Synonym column identifies that the substance/technology has been approved for NTAP (new technology add-on payment). CMS provides incremental payment, in addition to the DRG payment, for technologies that have received an NTAP designation.

Substances denoted by an asterisk (*) in the Trade Name or Synonym column, although not included in the official ICD-10-PCS classification, were added based on information provided in the IPPS proposed and final rules.

Trade Name or Synonym	ICD-10-PCS Value	PCS Section
ABECMA®	Idecabtagene Vicleucel Immunotherapy (K)	New Technology (XW0)
ACTEMRA®	Tocilizumab (H)	New Technology (XW0)
afami-cel	Afamitresgene Autoleucel Immunotherapy (6)	New Technology (XW0)
AIGISRx Antibacterial Envelope	Anti-Infective Envelope (A)	Administration (3E0)
AMTAGVI™	Lifileucel Immunotherapy (L)	New Technology (XW0)
Andexanet Alfa, Factor Xa Inhibitor Reversal Agent	Coagulation Factor Xa, Inactivated (7)	New Technology (XW0)
Andexxa	Coagulation Factor Xa, Inactivated (7)	New Technology (XW0)
Angiotensin II	Vasopressor (X)	Administration (3E0)
Antibacterial Envelope (TYRX) (AIGISRx)	Anti-Infective Envelope (A)	Administration (3E0)
Antimicrobial envelope	Anti-Infective Envelope (A)	Administration (3E0)
Anti-SARS-CoV-2 hyperimmune globulin	Hyperimmune Globulin (E)	New Technology (XW0)
Apalutamide Antineoplastic	Other Antineoplastic (5)	Administration (3E0)
AVYCAZ® (ceftazidime-avibactam)	Other Anti-infective (9)	Administration (3E0)
Axicabtagene Ciloleucel	Axicabtagene Ciloleucel Immunotherapy (H)	New Technology (XW0)
AZEDRA®	Iobenguane I-131 Antineoplastic (S)	New Technology (XW0)
Balversa™ (Erdafitinib Antineoplastic)	Other Antineoplastic (5)	Administration (3E0)
beti-cel	Betibeglogene Autotemcel (B)	New Technology (XW1)
Blinatumomab	Other Antineoplastic (5)	Administration (3E0)
BLINCYTO® (blinatumomab)	Other Antineoplastic (5)	Administration (3E0)
Bone morphogenetic protein 2 (BMP 2)	Recombinant Bone Morphogenetic Protein (B)	Administration (3E0)
Brexucabtagene Autoleucel	Brexucabtagene Autoleucel Immunotherapy (4)	New Technology (XW0)
Breyanzi®	Lisocabtagene Maraleucel Immunotherapy (N)	New Technology (XW0)
Bromelain-enriched Proteolytic Enzyme	Anacaulase-bcdb (2)	New Technology (XW0)
*CABLIVI®	Caplacizumab (W)	New Technology (XW0)
CARVYKTI™	Ciltacabtagene Autoleucel (A)	New Technology (XW0)
CASGEVY™	Exagamglogene Autotemcel (J)	New Technology (XW1)
Casirivimab (REGN10933) and Imdevimab (REGN10987)	REGN-COV2 Monoclonal Antibody (G)	New Technology (XW0)
CBMA (Concentrated Bone Marrow Aspirate)	Other Substance (C)	Administration (3E0)
Ceftazidime-avibactam	Other Anti-infective (9)	Administration (3E0)
CERAMENT® G **NT**	Antibiotic-eluting Bone Void Filler (P)	New Technology (XW0)
cilta-cel	Ciltacabtagene Autoleucel (A)	New Technology (XW0)
Clolar	Clofarabine (P)	Administration (3E0)
Columvi™ **NT**	Glofitamab Antineoplastic (P)	New Technology (XW0)
Coagulation Factor Xa, (Recombinant) Inactivated	Coagulation Factor Xa, Inactivated (7)	New Technology (XW0)
COMIRNATY®	COVID-19 Vaccine (U) COVID-19 Vaccine Dose 2 (T) COVID-19 Booster (W) COVID-19 Vaccine Dose 3 (V) COVID-19 Vaccine Dose 1 (S)	New Technology (XW0)
CONTEPO™ (Fosfomycin Anti-infective)	Other Anti-infective (9)	Administration (3E0)
COSELA™	Trilaciclib (7)	New Technology (XW0)
CRESEMBA® (isavuconazonium sulfate)	Other Anti-infective (9)	Administration (3E0)
CTX001™	Exagamglogene Autotemcel (J)	New Technology (XW1)
Darzalex Faspro®	Daratumumab and Hyaluronidase-fihj (1)	New Technology (XW0)
DefenCath™ **NT**	Taurolidine Anti-infective and Heparin Anticoagulant (2)	New Technology (XY0)
Defitelio	Other Substance (C)	Administration (3E0)
Dnase (Deoxyribonuclease)	Other Substance (C)	Administration (3E0)
DuraGraft® Endothelial Damage Inhibitor	Endothelial Damage Inhibitor (8)	New Technology (XY0)
EBVALLO™	Tabelecleucel Immunotherapy (7)	New Technology (XW0)
ELREXFIO™	Elranatamab Antineoplastic (L)	New Technology (XW0)
ELZONRIS™	Tagraxofusp-erzs Antineoplastic (Q)	New Technology (XW0)
ENSPRYNG™	Satralizumab-mwge (9)	New Technology (XW0)

Appendix I: Substance Key/Substance Definitions

Trade Name or Synonym	ICD-10-PCS Value	PCS Section
EPKINLY™ [NT]	Epcoritamab Monoclonal Antibody (S)	New Technology (XW0)
Erdafitinib Antineoplastic	Other Antineoplastic (5)	Administration (3E0)
ERLEADA™ (Apalutamide Antineoplastic)	Other Antineoplastic (5)	Administration (3E0)
Esketamine Hydrochloride	Other Substance (C)	Administration (3E0)
EVUSHELD™ (Apalutamide Antineoplastic)	Other Antineoplastic (5)	Administration (3E0)
Factor Xa Inhibitor Reversal Agent, Andexanet Alfa	Coagulation Factor Xa, Inactivated (7)	New Technology (XW0)
FETROJA®	Cefiderocol Anti-infective (A)	New Technology (XW0)
Fosfomycin Anti-infective	Other Anti-infective (9)	Administration (3E0)
Gammaglobulin	Globulin (S)	Administration (3E0)
GAMUNEX-C, for COVID-19 treatment	High-Dose Intravenous Immune Globulin (D)	New Technology (XW1)
GIAPREZA™	Vasopressor (X)	Administration (3E0)
Gilteritinib	Other Antineoplastic (5)	Administration (3E0)
GS-5734	Remdesivir Anti-infective (E)	New Technology (XW0)
hdIVIG (high-dose intravenous immunoglobulin), for COVID-19 treatment	High-Dose Intravenous Immune Globulin (D)	New Technology (XW1)
Hemospray® Endoscopic Hemostat	Mineral-based Topical Hemostatic Agent (8)	New Technology (XW0)
HEPZATO™ KIT (melphalan hydrochloride Hepatic Delivery System)	Melphalan Hydrochloride Antineoplastic (T)	New Technology (XW0)
HIG (hyperimmune globulin), for COVID-19 treatment	Hyperimmune Globulin (E)	New Technology (XW1)
High-dose intravenous immunoglobulin (hdIVIG), for COVID-19 treatment	High-Dose Intravenous Immune Globulin (D)	New Technology (XW1)
hIVIG (hyperimmune intravenous immunoglobulin), for COVID-19 treatment	Hyperimmune Globulin (E)	New Technology (XW1)
Human angiotensin II, synthetic	Vasopressor (X)	Administration (3E0)
Hyperimmune globulin	Globulin (S)	Administration (3E0)
Hyperimmune intravenous immunoglobulin (hIVIG), for COVID-19 treatment	Hyperimmune Globulin (E)	New Technology (XW1)
Idarucizumab, Pradaxa® (dabigatran) reversal agent	Other Therapeutic Substance (G)	Administration (3E0)
Idecabtagene Vicleucel	Idecabtagene Vicleucel Immunotherapy (K)	New Technology (XW0)
Ide-cel	Idecabtagene Vicleucel Immunotherapy (K)	New Technology (XW0)
IGIV-C, for COVID-19 treatment	Hyperimmune Globulin (E)	New Technology (XW1)
Imdevimab (REGN10987) and Casirivimab (REGN10933)	REGN-COV2 Monoclonal Antibody (G)	New Technology (XW0)
IMFINZI®	Durvalumab Antineoplastic (3)	New Technology (XW0)
IMI/REL	Other Anti-infective (9)	Administration (3E0)
Imipenem-cilastatin-relebactam Anti-infective	Other Anti-infective (9)	Administration (3E0)
Immunoglobulin	Globulin (S)	Administration (3E0)
INTERCEPT Blood System for Plasma Pathogen Reduced Cryoprecipitated Fibrinogen Complex	Pathogen Reduced Cryoprecipitated Fibrinogen Complex (D)	Administration (302)
INTERCEPT Fibrinogen Complex	Pathogen Reduced Cryoprecipitated Fibrinogen Complex (D)	Administration (302)
Iobenguane I-131, High Specific Activity (HSA)	Iobenguane I-131 Antineoplastic (S)	New Technology (XW0)
Isavuconazole (isavuconazonium sulfate)	Other Anti-infective (9)	Administration (3E0)
Jakafi® (Ruxolitinib)	Other Substance (C)	Administration (3E0)
Kcentra	4-Factor Prothrombin Complex Concentrate (B)	Administration (3E0)
KEVZARA®	Sarilumab (G)	New Technology (XW0)
KYMRIAH®	Tisagenlecleucel Immunotherapy (J)	New Technology (XW0)
Lantidra™	Donislecel-jujn Allogeneic Pancreatic Islet Cellular Suspension (D)	New Technology (XW0)
Lifileucel	Lifileucel Immunotherapy (L)	New Technology (XW0)
Lisocabtagene Maraleucel	Lisocabtagene Maraleucel Immunotherapy (7)	New Technology (XW0)
LIVTENCITY™	Maribavir Anti-infective (3)	New Technology (XW0)
LTX Regional Anticoagulant	Nafamostat Anticoagulant (3)	New Technology (XW0)
LUNSUMIO™ [NT]	Mosunetuzumab Antineoplastic (5)	New Technology (XW0)
LYFGENIA™	Lovotibeglogene autotemcel (H)	New Technology (XW1)
MarrowStim™ PAD Kit for CBMA (Concentrated Bone Marrow Aspirate)	Other Substance (C)	Administration (3E0)
Meropenem-vaborbactam Anti-infective	Other Anti-infective (9)	Administration (3E0)
NA-1 (Nerinitide)	Nerinitide (2)	New Technology (XW0)
Nesiritide	Human B-type Natriuretic Peptide (H)	Administration (3E0)
NexoBrid™	Anacaulase-bcdb (2)	New Technology (XW0)
Niyad™	Nafamostat Anticoagulant (3)	New Technology (XW0)
NUZYRA™	Omadacycline Anti-infective (B)	New Technology (XW0)
Obe-cel	Obecabtagene Autoleucel (8)	New Technology (XW0)
Octagam 10%, for COVID-19 treatment	High-Dose Intravenous Immune Globulin (D)	New Technology (XW1)
Olumiant®	Baricitinib (M)	New Technology (XW0)

Appendix I: Substance Key/Substance Definitions

Trade Name or Synonym	ICD-10-PCS Value	PCS Section
Omisirge®	Omidubicel (C)	New Technology (XW1)
OSSURE™ implant material	AGN1 Bone Void Filler (W)	New Technology (XW0)
OTL-101	Hematopoietic Stem/Progenitor Cells, Genetically Modified (C)	Administration (3E0)
Plazomicin	Other Anti-infective (9)	Administration (3E0)
Polyclonal hyperimmune globulin	Globulin (S)	Administration (3E0)
Praxbind® (idarucizumab), Pradaxa® (dabigatran) reversal agent	Other Therapeutic Substance (G)	Administration (3E0)
REBYOTA® **NT**	Broad Consortium Microbiota-based Live Biotherapeutic Suspension (X)	New Technology (XW0)
RECARBRIO™ (Imipenem-cilastatin-relebactam Anti-infective)	Other Anti-infective (9)	Administration (3E0)
RETHYMIC®	Engineered Allogeneic Thymus Tissue (D)	New Technology (XW0)
*REZZAYO™ **NT**	Rezafungin (R)	New Technology (XW0)
rhBMP-2	Recombinant Bone Morphogenetic Protein (B)	Administration (3E0)
RP-L201	Marnetegragene Autotemcel (7)	New Technology (XW1)
Ruxolitinib	Other Substance (C)	Administration (3E0)
RYBREVANT™	Amivantamab Monoclonal Antibody (B)	New Technology (XW0)
Seprafilm	Adhesion Barrier (5)	Administration (3E0)
Soliris®	Eculizumab (C)	New Technology (XW0)
SPEVIGO® **NT**	Spesolimab Monoclonal Antibody (0)	New Technology (XW0)
SPIKEVAX™	COVID-19 Vaccine (U) COVID-19 Vaccine Dose 2 (T) COVID-19 Booster (W) COVID-19 Vaccine Dose 3 (V) COVID-19 Vaccine Dose 1 (S)	New Technology (XW0)
SPRAVATO™ (Esketamine Hydrochloride)	Other Substance (C)	Administration (3E0)
STELARA®	Other New Technology Therapeutic Substance (F)	New Technology (XW0)
SUL-DUR	Sulbactam-Durlobactam (K)	New Technology (XW0)
tab-cel®	Tabelecleucel Immunotherapy (7)	New Technology (XW0)
TALVEY™	Talquetamab Antineoplastic (2)	New Technology (XW0)
T-cell Antigen Coupler T-cell (TAC-T) Therapy	Non-Chimeric Antigen Receptor T-cell Immune Effector Cell Therapy (F)	New Technology (XW0)
T-cell Receptor-Engineered T-cell (TCR-T) Therapy	Non-Chimeric Antigen Receptor T-cell Immune Effector Cell Therapy (F)	New Technology (XW0)
TECARTUS™	Brexucabtagene Autoleucel Immunotherapy (M)	New Technology (XW0)
TECENTRIQ®	Atezolizumab Antineoplastic (D)	New Technology (XW0)
TECVAYLI™ **NT**	Teclistamab Antineoplastic (4)	New Technology (XW0)
TERLIVAZ® **NT**	Terlipressin (6)	New Technology (XW0)
Tisagenlecleucel	Tisagenlecleucel Immunotherapy (J)	New Technology (XW0)
Tissue Plasminogen Activator (tPA)(r-tPA)	Other Thrombolytic (7)	Administration (3E0)
Tumor-Infiltrating Lymphocyte (TIL) Therapy	Non-Chimeric Antigen Receptor T-cell Immune Effector Cell Therapy (F)	New Technology (XW0)
TYRX Antibacterial Envelope	Anti-Infective Envelope (A)	Administration (3E0)
UPLIZNA®	Inebilizumab-cdon (9)	New Technology (XW0)
Ustekinumab	Other New Technology Therapeutic Substance (F)	New Technology (XW0)
VABOMERE™ (Meropenem-vaborbactam Anti-infective)	Other Anti-infective (9)	Administration (3E0)
Veklury	Remdesivir Anti-infective (E)	New Technology (XW0)
Venclexta® (Venetoclax Antineoplastic tablets)	Other Antineoplastic (5)	Administration (3E0)
Venetoclax Antineoplastic (tablets)	Other Antineoplastic (5)	Administration (3E0)
Vistogard®	Uridine Triacetate (8)	New Technology (XW0)
Voraxaze	Glucarpidase (Q)	Administration (3E0)
VOWST™ **NT**	SER-109 (N)	New Technology (XW0)
VT-X7 (Irrigation System) (Spacer)	Vancomycin Hydrochloride and Tobramycin Sulfate Anti-Infective, Temporary Irrigation Spacer System (G)	New Technology (XW0)
VYXEOS™	Cytarabine and Daunorubicin Liposome Antineoplastic (B)	New Technology (XW0)
XACDURO® **NT**	Sulbactam-Durlobactam (K)	New Technology (XW0)
XENLETA™	Lefamulin Anti-infective (6)	New Technology (XW0)
XOSPATA® (Gilteritinib)	Other Antineoplastic (5)	Administration (3E0)
Yescarta®	Axicabtagene Ciloleucel Immunotherapy (H)	New Technology (XW0)
*ZEMDRI®	Plazomicin Anti-infective (6)	New Technology (XW0)
ZEPZELCA™	Lurbinectedin (8)	New Technology (XW0)
ZERBAXA®	Ceftolozane/Tazobactam Anti-infective (9)	New Technology (XW0)
ZULRESSO™	Brexanolone (0)	New Technology (XW0)
ZYNTEGLO®	Betibeglogene Autotemcel (B)	New Technology (XW1)
Zyvox	Oxazolidinones (8)	Administration (3E0)

Appendix I: Substance Key/Substance Definitions

Substance Definitions

This table crosswalks a PCS value, used in the Administration or New Technology section, to a specific substance. The specific substances are listed by trade name or synonym. The ICD-10-PCS value may be located in either the 6th-character Substance column or the 7th-character Qualifier column depending on the section/table to which it is classified.

Substances denoted by an asterisk (*) in the Trade Name or Synonym column, although not included in the official ICD-10-PCS classification, were added based on information provided in the IPPS proposed and final rules.

ICD-10-PCS Value	Trade Name or Synonym	PCS Section
4-Factor Prothrombin Complex Concentrate (B)	Kcentra	Administration (3E0)
Afamitresgene Autoleucel Immunotherapy (6)	afami-cel	New Technology (XW0)
Adhesion Barrier (5)	Seprafilm	Administration (3E0)
AGN1 Bone Void Filler (W)	OSSURE™ implant material	New Technnology (XW0)
Amivantamab Monoclonal Antibody (B)	RYBREVANT™	New Technology (XW0)
Anacaulase-bcdb (2)	Bromelain-enriched Proteolytic Enzyme NexoBrid™	New Technology (XW0)
Antibiotic-eluting Bone Void Filler (P)	CERAMENT® G	New Technology (XW0)
Anti-Infective Envelope (A)	AIGISRx Antibacterial Envelope Antibacterial Envelope (TYRX) (AIGISRx) Antimicrobial envelope TYRX Antibacterial Envelope	Administration (3E0)
Atezolizumab Antineoplastic (D)	TECENTRIQ®	New Technology (XW0)
Axicabtagene Ciloleucel Immunotherapy (H)	Axicabtagene Ciloleucel Yescarta®	New Technology (XW0)
Baricitinib (M)	Olumiant®	New Technology (XW0)
Betibeglogene Autotemcel (B)	beti-cel ZYNTEGLO®	New Technology (XW1)
Brexanolone (0)	ZULRESSO™	New Technology (XW0)
Brexucabtagene Autoleucel Immunotherapy (M)	TECARTUS™	New Technology (XW0)
Broad Consortium Microbiota-based Live Biotherapeutic Suspension (X)	REBYOTA®	New Technology (XW0)
Caplacizumab (W)	*CABLIVI®	New Technology (XW0)
Cefiderocol Anti-infective (A)	FETROJA®	New Technology (XW0)
Ceftolozane/Tazobactam Anti- infective (9)	ZERBAXA®	New Technology (XW0)
Ciltacabtagene Autoleucel (A)	CARVYKTI™ cilta-cel	New Technology (XW0)
Clofarabine (P)	Clolar	Administration (3E0)
Coagulation Factor Xa, Inactivated (7)	Andexanet Alfa, Factor Xa Inhibitor Reversal Agent Andexxa Coagulation Factor Xa, (Recombinant) Inactivated Factor Xa Inhibitor Reversal Agent, Andexanet Alfa	New Technology (XW0)
COVID-19 Vaccine (U)	COMIRNATY® SPIKEVAX™	New Technology (XW0)
COVID-19 Booster (W)	COMIRNATY® SPIKEVAX™	New Technology (XW0)
COVID-19 Vaccine Dose 1 (S)	COMIRNATY® SPIKEVAX™	New Technology (XW0)
COVID-19 Vaccine Dose 2 (T)	COMIRNATY® SPIKEVAX™	New Technology (XW0)
COVID-19 Vaccine Dose 3 (V)	COMIRNATY® SPIKEVAX™	New Technology (XW0)
Cytarabine and Daunorubicin Liposome Antineoplastic (B)	VYXEOS™	New Technology (XW0)
Daratumumab and Hyaluronidase-fihj (1)	Darzalex Faspro®	New Technology (XW0)
Donislecel-jujn Allogeneic Pancreatic Islet Cellular Suspension (D)	Lantidra™	New Technology (XW0)
Durvalumab Antineoplastic (3)	IMFINZI®	New Technology (XW0)
Eculizumab (C)	Soliris®	New Technology (XW0)
Elranatamab Antineoplastic (L)	ELREXFIO™	New Technology (XW0)
Endothelial Damage Inhibitor (8)	DuraGraft® Endothelial Damage Inhibitor	New Technology (XY0)
Engineered Allogeneic Thymus Tissue (D)	RETHYMIC®	New Technology (XW0)
Epcoritamab Monoclonal Antibody (S)	EPKINLY™	New Technology (XW0)
Exagamglogene Autotemcel (J)	CASGEVY™ CTX001™	New Technology (XW1)
Globulin (S)	Gammaglobulin Hyperimmune globulin Immunoglobulin Polyclonal hyperimmune globulin	Administration (3E0)

ICD-10-PCS Value	Trade Name or Synonym	PCS Section
Glofitamab Antineoplastic (P)	Columvi™	New Technology (XW0)
Glucarpidase (Q)	Voraxaze	Administration (3E0)
Hematopoietic Stem/Progenitor Cells, Genetically Modified (C)	OTL-101	Administration (3E0)
High-Dose Intravenous Immune Globulin (D)	GAMUNEX-C, for COVID-19 treatment hdIVIG (high-dose intravenous immunoglobulin), for COVID-19 treatment High-dose intravenous immunoglobulin (hdIVIG), for COVID-19 treatment Octagam 10%, for COVID-19 treatment	New Technology (XW1)
Human B-type Natriuretic Peptide (H)	Nesiritide	Administration (3E0)
Hyperimmune Globulin (E)	Anti-SARS-CoV-2 hyperimmune globulin HIG (hyperimmune globulin), for COVID-19 treatment hIVIG (hyperimmune intravenous immunoglobulin), for COVID-19 treatment Hyperimmune intravenous immunoglobulin (hIVIG), for COVID-19 treatment IGIV-C, for COVID-19 treatment	New Technology (XW1)
Idecabtagene Vicleucel Immunotherapy (K)	ABECMA® Idecabtagene Vicleucel Ide-cel	New Technology (XW0)
Inebilizumab-cdon (9)	UPLIZNA®	New Technology (XW0)
Iobenguane I-131 Antineoplastic (S)	AZEDRA® Iobenguane I-131, High Specific Activity (HSA)	New Technology (XW0)
Lefamulin Anti-infective (6)	XENLETA™	New Technology (XW0)
Lifileucel Immunotherapy (L)	AMTAGVI™ Lifileucel	New Technology (XW0)
Lisocabtagene Maraleucel Immunotherapy (7)	Breyanzi® Lisocabtagene Maraleucel	New Technology (XW0)
Lovotibeglogene Autotemcel (H)	LYFGENIA™	New Technology (XW1)
Lurbinectedin (8)	ZEPZELCA™	New Technology (XW0)
Maribavir Anti-infective (3)	LIVTENCITY™	New Technology (XW0)
Marnetegragene Autotemcel (7)	RP-L201	New Technology (XW1)
Melphalan Hydrochloride Antineoplastic (T)	HEPZATO™ KIT (melphalan hydrochloride Hepatic Delivery System)	New Technology (XW0)
Mineral-based Topical Hemostatic Agent (8)	Hemospray® Endoscopic Hemostat	New Technology (XW0)
Mosunetuzumab Antineoplastic (5)	LUNSUMIO™	New Technology (XW0)
Nafamostat Anticoagulant (3)	LTX Regional Anticoagulant Niyad™	New Technology (XY0)
Nerinitide (2)	NA-1 (Nerinitide)	New Technology (XW0)
Non-Chimeric Antigen Receptor T-cell Immune Effector Cell Therapy (F)	T-cell Antigen Coupler T-cell (TAC-T) Therapy T-cell Receptor-Engineered T-cell (TCR-T) Therapy Tumor-Infiltrating Lymphocyte (TIL) Therapy	New Technology (XW0)
Obecabtagene Autoleucel (8)	obe-cel	New Technology (XW0)
Omadacycline Anti-infective (B)	NUZYRA™	New Technology (XW0)
Omidubicel (C)	Omisirge®	New Technology (XW1)
Other Anti-infective (9)	AVYCAZ® (ceftazidime-avibactam) Ceftazidime-avibactam CONTEPO™ (Fosfomycin Anti-infective) Fosfomycin Anti-infective CRESEMBA® (isavuconazonium sulfate) IMI/REL Imipenem-cilastatin-relebactam Anti-infective Meropenem-vaborbactam Anti-infective Isavuconazole (isavuconazonium sulfate) Plazomicin RECARBRIO™ (Imipenem-cilastatin-relebactam Anti-infective) VABOMERE™ (Meropenem-vaborbactam Anti-infective) *ZEMDRI	Administration (3E0)
Other Antineoplastic (5)	Apalutamide Antineoplastic Balversa™ (Erdafitinib Antineoplastic) Blinatumomab BLINCYTO® (blinatumomab) Erdafitinib Antineoplastic ERLEADA™ (Apalutamide Antineoplastic) Gilteritinib Venclexta® (Venetoclax Antineoplastic tablets) Venetoclax Antineoplastic (tablets) XOSPATA® (Gilteritinib)	Administration (3E0)

Appendix I: Substance Key/Substance Definitions

ICD-10-PCS Value	Trade Name or Synonym	PCS Section
Other New Technology Therapeutic Substance (F)	STELARA® Ustekinumab	New Technology (XW0)
Other Substance (C)	CBMA (Concentrated Bone Marrow Aspirate) Defitelio Dnase (Deoxyribonuclease) Esketamine Hydrochloride JAKAFI® (Ruxolitinib) MarrowStim™ PAD Kit for CBMA (Concentrated Bone Marrow Aspirate) Ruxolitinib SPRAVATO™ (Esketamine Hydrochloride)	Administration (3E0)
Other Therapeutic Substance (G)	Idarucizumab, Pradaxa® (dabigatran) reversal agent Praxbind® (idarucizumab), Pradaxa® (dabigatran) reversal agent	Administration (3E0)
Other Thrombolytic (7)	Tissue Plasminogen Activator (tPA)(r-tPA)	Administration (3E0)
Oxazolidinones (8)	Zyvox	Administration (3E0)
Pathogen Reduced Cryoprecipitated Fibrinogen Complex (D)	INTERCEPT Blood System for Plasma Pathogen Reduced Cryoprecipitated Fibrinogen Complex INTERCEPT Fibrinogen Complex	Administration (302)
Recombinant Bone Morphogenetic Protein (B)	Bone morphogenetic protein 2 (BMP 2) rhBMP-2	Administration (3E0)
REGN-COV2 Monoclonal Antibody (G)	Casirivimab (REGN10933) and Imdevimab (REGN10987) Imdevimab (REGN10987) and Casirivimab (REGN10933)	New Technology (XW0)
Remdesivir Anti-infective (E)	GS-5734 Veklury	New Technology (XW0)
Rezafungin (R)	*REZZAYO™	New Technology (XW0)
Sarilumab (G)	KEVZARA®	New Technology (XW0)
Satralizumab-mwge (9)	ENSPRYNG™	New Technology (XW0)
SER-109 (N)	VOWST™	New Technology (XW0)
Spesolimab Monoclonal Antibody (0)	SPEVIGO®	New Technology (XW0)
Sulbactam-Durlobactam (K)	SUL-DUR Xacduro®	New Technology (XW0)
Tabelecleucel Immunotherapy (7)	EBVALLO™ tab-cel®	New Technology (XW0)
Tagraxofusp-erzs Antineoplastic (Q)	ELZONRIS™	New Technology (XW0)
Talquetamab Antineoplastic (2)	TALVEY™	New Technology (XW0)
Taurolidine Anti-infective and Heparin Anticoagulant (2)	DefenCath™	New Technology (XY0)
Teclistamab Antineoplastic (4)	TECVAYLI™	New Technology (XW0)
Terlipressin (6)	TERLIVAZ®	New Technology (XW0)
Tisagenlecleucel Immunotherapy (J)	KYMRIAH® Tisagenlecleucel	New Technology (XW0)
Tixagevimab and Cilgavimab Monoclonal Antibody (X)	EVUSHELD™	New Technology (XW0)
Tocilizumab (H)	ACTEMRA®	New Technology (XW0)
Trilaciclib (7)	COSELA™	New Technology (XW0)
Uridine Triacetate (8)	Vistogard®	New Technology (XW0)
Vancomycin Hydrochloride and Tobramycin Sulfate Anti-Infective, Temporary Irrigation Spacer System (G)	VT-X7 (Irrigation System) (Spacer)	New Technology (XW0)
Vasopressor (X)	Angiotensin II GIAPREZA™ Human angiotensin II, synthetic	Administration (3E0)

Appendix J: Sections B–H Character Definitions

Sections B-H (Imaging through Substance Abuse Treatment) do not include root operations. Instead, the character 3 value represents the type of procedure performed with additional details about that procedure provided by the character 4 or 5 value, when appropriate. This resource provides the specific ICD-10-PCS value and its associated definition for the character 3, character 4, and character 5 values in the ancillary sections of B-H.

Section B–Imaging

ICD-10-PCS Value (Character 3)	Definition
Computerized Tomography (CT Scan) (2)	Computer reformatted digital display of multiplanar images developed from the capture of multiple exposures of external ionizing radiation
Fluoroscopy (1)	Single plane or bi-plane real time display of an image developed from the capture of external ionizing radiation on a fluorescent screen. The image may also be stored by either digital or analog means.
Magnetic Resonance Imaging (MRI) (3)	Computer reformatted digital display of multiplanar images developed from the capture of radiofrequency signals emitted by nuclei in a body site excited within a magnetic field
Other Imaging (5)	Other specified modality for visualizing a body part
Plain Radiography (0)	Planar display of an image developed from the capture of external ionizing radiation on photographic or photoconductive plate
Ultrasonography (4)	Real time display of images of anatomy or flow information developed from the capture of reflected and attenuated high frequency sound waves

Section C–Nuclear Medicine

ICD-10-PCS Value (Character 3)	Definition
Nonimaging Nuclear Medicine Assay (6)	Introduction of radioactive materials into the body for the study of body fluids and blood elements, by the detection of radioactive emissions
Nonimaging Nuclear Medicine Probe (5)	Introduction of radioactive materials into the body for the study of distribution and fate of certain substances by the detection of radioactive emissions; or, alternatively, measurement of absorption of radioactive emissions from an external source
Nonimaging Nuclear Medicine Uptake (4)	Introduction of radioactive materials into the body for measurements of organ function, from the detection of radioactive emissions
Planar Nuclear Medicine Imaging (1)	Introduction of radioactive materials into the body for single plane display of images developed from the capture of radioactive emissions
Positron Emission Tomographic (PET) Imaging (3)	Introduction of radioactive materials into the body for three dimensional display of images developed from the simultaneous capture, 180 degrees apart, of radioactive emissions
Systemic Nuclear Medicine Therapy (7)	Introduction of unsealed radioactive materials into the body for treatment
Tomographic (Tomo) Nuclear Medicine Imaging (2)	Introduction of radioactive materials into the body for three dimensional display of images developed from the capture of radioactive emissions

Section F–Physical Rehabilitation and Diagnostic Audiology

ICD-10-PCS Value (Character 3)	Definition
Activities of Daily Living Assessment (2)	Measurement of functional level for activities of daily living
Activities of Daily Living Treatment (8)	Exercise or activities to facilitate functional competence for activities of daily living
Caregiver Training (F)	Training in activities to support patient's optimal level of function
Cochlear Implant Treatment (B)	Application of techniques to improve the communication abilities of individuals with cochlear implant
Device Fitting (D)	Fitting of a device designed to facilitate or support achievement of a higher level of function
Hearing Aid Assessment (4)	Measurement of the appropriateness and/or effectiveness of a hearing device
Hearing Assessment (3)	Measurement of hearing and related functions
Hearing Treatment (9)	Application of techniques to improve, augment, or compensate for hearing and related functional impairment
Motor and/or Nerve Function Assessment (1)	Measurement of motor, nerve, and related functions
Motor Treatment (7)	Exercise or activities to increase or facilitate motor function
Speech Assessment (0)	Measurement of speech and related functions

Continued on next page

Appendix J: Sections B–H Character Definitions

Section F–Physical Rehabilitation and Diagnostic Audiology

Continued from previous page

ICD-10-PCS Value (Character 3)	Definition
Speech Treatment (6)	Application of techniques to improve, augment, or compensate for speech and related functional impairment
Vestibular Assessment (5)	Measurement of the vestibular system and related functions
Vestibular Treatment (C)	Application of techniques to improve, augment, or compensate for vestibular and related functional impairment

Section F–Physical Rehabilitation and Diagnostic Audiology

ICD-10-PCS Value Qualifier (Character 5)	Definition
Acoustic Reflex Decay (J)	Measures reduction in size/strength of acoustic reflex over time Includes/Examples: Includes site of lesion test
Acoustic Reflex Patterns (G)	Defines site of lesion based upon presence/absence of acoustic reflexes with ipsilateral vs. contralateral stimulation
Acoustic Reflex Threshold (H)	Determines minimal intensity that acoustic reflex occurs with ipsilateral and/or contralateral stimulation
Aerobic Capacity and Endurance (7)	Measures autonomic responses to positional changes; perceived exertion, dyspnea or angina during activity; performance during exercise protocols; standard vital signs; and blood gas analysis or oxygen consumption
Alternate Binaural or Monaural Loudness Balance (7)	Determines auditory stimulus parameter that yields the same objective sensation Includes/Examples: Sound intensities that yield same loudness perception
Anthropometric Characteristics (B)	Measures edema, body fat composition, height, weight, length and girth
Aphasia (Assessment) (C)	Measures expressive and receptive speech and language function including reading and writing
Aphasia (Treatment) (3)	Applying techniques to improve, augment, or compensate for receptive/ expressive language impairments
Articulation/Phonology (Assessment) (9)	Measures speech production
Articulation/Phonology (Treatment) (4)	Applying techniques to correct, improve, or compensate for speech productive impairment
Assistive Listening Device (5)	Assists in use of effective and appropriate assistive listening device/system
Assistive Listening System/Device Selection (4)	Measures the effectiveness and appropriateness of assistive listening systems/devices
Assistive, Adaptive, Supportive or Protective Devices (9)	Explanation: Devices to facilitate or support achievement of a higher level of function in wheelchair mobility; bed mobility; transfer or ambulation ability; bath and showering ability; dressing; grooming; personal hygiene; play or leisure
Auditory Evoked Potentials (L)	Measures electric responses produced by the VIIIth cranial nerve and brainstem following auditory stimulation
Auditory Processing (Assessment) (Q)	Evaluates ability to receive and process auditory information and comprehension of spoken language
Auditory Processing (Treatment) (2)	Applying techniques to improve the receiving and processing of auditory information and comprehension of spoken language
Augmentative/Alternative Communication System (Assessment) (L)	Determines the appropriateness of aids, techniques, symbols, and/or strategies to augment or replace speech and enhance communication Includes/Examples: Includes the use of telephones, writing equipment, emergency equipment, and TDD
Augmentative/Alternative Communication System (Treatment) (3)	Includes/Examples: Includes augmentative communication devices and aids
Aural Rehabilitation (5)	Applying techniques to improve the communication abilities associated with hearing loss
Aural Rehabilitation Status (P)	Measures impact of a hearing loss including evaluation of receptive and expressive communication skills
Bathing/Showering (0)	Includes/Examples: Includes obtaining and using supplies; soaping, rinsing, and drying body parts; maintaining bathing position; and transferring to and from bathing positions
Bathing/Showering Techniques (0)	Activities to facilitate obtaining and using supplies, soaping, rinsing and drying body parts, maintaining bathing position, and transferring to and from bathing positions
Bed Mobility (Assessment) (B)	Transitional movement within bed
Bed Mobility (Treatment) (5)	Exercise or activities to facilitate transitional movements within bed
Bedside Swallowing and Oral Function (H)	Includes/Examples: Bedside swallowing includes assessment of sucking, masticating, coughing, and swallowing. Oral function includes assessment of musculature for controlled movements, structures, and functions to determine coordination and phonation.

Continued on next page

Section F–Physical Rehabilitation and Diagnostic Audiology

Continued from previous page

ICD-10-PCS Value Qualifier (Character 5)	Definition
Bekesy Audiometry (3)	Uses an instrument that provides a choice of discrete or continuously varying pure tones; choice of pulsed or continuous signal
Binaural Electroacoustic Hearing Aid Check (6)	Determines mechanical and electroacoustic function of bilateral hearing aids using hearing aid test box
Binaural Hearing Aid (Assessment) (3)	Measures the candidacy, effectiveness, and appropriateness of a hearing aid Explanation: Measures bilateral fit
Binaural Hearing Aid (Treatment) (2)	Explanation: Assists in achieving maximum understanding and performance
Bithermal, Binaural Caloric Irrigation (Ø)	Measures the rhythmic eye movements stimulated by changing the temperature of the vestibular system
Bithermal, Monaural Caloric Irrigation (1)	Measures the rhythmic eye movements stimulated by changing the temperature of the vestibular system in one ear
Brief Tone Stimuli (R)	Measures specific central auditory process
Cerumen Management (3)	Includes examination of external auditory canal and tympanic membrane and removal of cerumen from external ear canal
Cochlear Implant (Ø)	Measures candidacy for cochlear implant
Cochlear Implant Rehabilitation (Ø)	Applying techniques to improve the communication abilities of individuals with cochlear implant; includes programming the device, providing patients/families with information
Communicative/Cognitive Integration Skills (Assessment) (G)	Measures ability to use higher cortical functions Includes/Examples: Includes orientation, recognition, attention span, initiation and termination of activity, memory, sequencing, categorizing, concept formation, spatial operations, judgment, problem solving, generalization and pragmatic communication
Communicative/Cognitive Integration Skills (Treatment) (6)	Activities to facilitate the use of higher cortical functions Includes/Examples: Includes level of arousal, orientation, recognition, attention span, initiation and termination of activity, memory sequencing, judgment and problem solving, learning and generalization, and pragmatic communication
Computerized Dynamic Posturography (6)	Measures the status of the peripheral and central vestibular system and the sensory/motor component of balance; evaluates the efficacy of vestibular rehabilitation
Conditioned Play Audiometry (4)	Behavioral measures using nonspeech and speech stimuli to obtain frequency-specific and ear-specific information on auditory status from the patient Explanation: Obtains speech reception threshold by having patient point to pictures of spondaic words
Coordination/Dexterity (Assessment) (3)	Measures large and small muscle groups for controlled goal-directed movements Explanation: Dexterity includes object manipulation
Coordination/Dexterity (Treatment) (2)	Exercise or activities to facilitate gross coordination and fine coordination
Cranial Nerve Integrity (9)	Measures cranial nerve sensory and motor functions, including tastes, smell and facial expression
Dichotic Stimuli (T)	Measures specific central auditory process
Distorted Speech (S)	Measures specific central auditory process
Dix-Hallpike Dynamic (5)	Measures nystagmus following Dix-Hallpike maneuver
Dressing (1)	Includes/Examples: Includes selecting clothing and accessories, obtaining clothing from storage, dressing, fastening and adjusting clothing and shoes, and applying and removing personal devices, prosthesis or orthosis
Dressing Techniques (1)	Activities to facilitate selecting clothing and accessories, dressing and undressing, adjusting clothing and shoes, applying and removing devices, prostheses or orthoses
Dynamic Orthosis (6)	Includes/Examples: Includes customized and prefabricated splints, inhibitory casts, spinal and other braces, and protective devices; allows motion through transfer of movement from other body parts or by use of outside forces
Ear Canal Probe Microphone (1)	Real ear measures
Ear Protector Attentuation (7)	Measures ear protector fit and effectiveness
Electrocochleography (K)	Measures the VIIIth cranial nerve action potential
Environmental, Home, Work Barriers (B)	Measures current and potential barriers to optimal function, including safety hazards, access problems and home or office design
Ergonomics and Body Mechanics (C)	Ergonomic measurement of job tasks, work hardening or work conditioning needs; functional capacity; and body mechanics
Eustachian Tube Function (F)	Measures eustachian tube function and patency of eustachian tube

Continued on next page

Section F–Physical Rehabilitation and Diagnostic Audiology

ICD-10-PCS Value Qualifier (Character 5)	Definition
Evoked Otoacoustic Emissions, Diagnostic (N)	Measures auditory evoked potentials in a diagnostic format
Evoked Otoacoustic Emissions, Screening (M)	Measures auditory evoked potentials in a screening format
Facial Nerve Function (7)	Measures electrical activity of the VIIth cranial nerve (facial nerve)
Feeding/Eating (Assessment) (2)	Includes/Examples: Includes setting up food, selecting and using utensils and tableware, bringing food or drink to mouth, cleaning face, hands, and clothing, and management of alternative methods of nourishment
Feeding/Eating (Treatment) (3)	Exercise or activities to facilitate setting up food, selecting and using utensils and tableware, bringing food or drink to mouth, cleaning face, hands, and clothing, and management of alternative methods of nourishment
Filtered Speech (0)	Uses high or low pass filtered speech stimuli to assess central auditory processing disorders, site of lesion testing
Fluency (Assessment) (D)	Measures speech fluency or stuttering
Fluency (Treatment) (7)	Applying techniques to improve and augment fluent speech
Gait and/or Balance (D)	Measures biomechanical, arthrokinematic and other spatial and temporal characteristics of gait and balance
Gait Training/Functional Ambulation (9)	Exercise or activities to facilitate ambulation on a variety of surfaces and in a variety of environments
Grooming/Personal Hygiene (Assessment) (3)	Includes/Examples: Includes ability to obtain and use supplies in a sequential fashion, general grooming, oral hygiene, toilet hygiene, personal care devices, including care for artificial airways
Grooming/Personal Hygiene (Treatment) (2)	Activities to facilitate obtaining and using supplies in a sequential fashion: general grooming, oral hygiene, toilet hygiene, cleaning body, and personal care devices, including artificial airways
Hearing and Related Disorders Counseling (0)	Provides patients/families/caregivers with information, support, referrals to facilitate recovery from a communication disorder Includes/Examples: Includes strategies for psychosocial adjustment to hearing loss for clients and families/caregivers
Hearing and Related Disorders Prevention (1)	Provides patients/families/caregivers with information and support to prevent communication disorders
Hearing Screening (0)	Pass/refer measures designed to identify need for further audiologic assessment
Home Management (Assessment) (4)	Obtaining and maintaining personal and household possessions and environment Includes/Examples: Includes clothing care, cleaning, meal preparation and cleanup, shopping, money management, household maintenance, safety procedures, and childcare/parenting
Home Management (Treatment) (4)	Activities to facilitate obtaining and maintaining personal household possessions and environment Includes/Examples: Includes clothing care, cleaning, meal preparation and clean-up, shopping, money management, household maintenance, safety procedures, childcare/parenting
Instrumental Swallowing and Oral Function (J)	Measures swallowing function using instrumental diagnostic procedures Explanation: Methods include videofluoroscopy, ultrasound, manometry, endoscopy
Integumentary Integrity (1)	Includes/Examples: Includes burns, skin conditions, ecchymosis, bleeding, blisters, scar tissue, wounds and other traumas, tissue mobility, turgor and texture
Manual Therapy Techniques (7)	Techniques in which the therapist uses his/her hands to administer skilled movements Includes/Examples: Includes connective tissue massage, joint mobilization and manipulation, manual lymph drainage, manual traction, soft tissue mobilization and manipulation
Masking Patterns (W)	Measures central auditory processing status
Monaural Electroacoustic Hearing Aid Check (8)	Determines mechanical and electroacoustic function of one hearing aid using hearing aid test box
Monaural Hearing Aid (Assessment) (2)	Measures the candidacy, effectiveness, and appropriateness of a hearing aid Explanation: Measures unilateral fit
Monaural Hearing Aid (Treatment) (1)	Explanation: Assists in achieving maximum understanding and performance
Motor Function (Assessment) (4)	Measures the body's functional and versatile movement patterns Includes/Examples: Includes motor assessment scales, analysis of head, trunk and limb movement, and assessment of motor learning
Motor Function (Treatment) (3)	Exercise or activities to facilitate crossing midline, laterality, bilateral integration, praxis, neuromuscular relaxation, inhibition, facilitation, motor function and motor learning
Motor Speech (Assessment) (B)	Measures neurological motor aspects of speech production
Motor Speech (Treatment) (8)	Applying techniques to improve and augment the impaired neurological motor aspects of speech production

Section F–Physical Rehabilitation and Diagnostic Audiology

ICD-10-PCS Value Qualifier (Character 5)	Definition
Muscle Performance (Assessment) (0)	Measures muscle strength, power and endurance using manual testing, dynamometry or computer-assisted electromechanical muscle test; functional muscle strength, power and endurance; muscle pain, tone, or soreness; or pelvic-floor musculature Explanation: Muscle endurance refers to the ability to contract a muscle repeatedly over time
Muscle Performance (Treatment) (1)	Exercise or activities to increase the capacity of a muscle to do work in terms of strength, power, and/or endurance Explanation: Muscle strength is the force exerted to overcome resistance in one maximal effort. Muscle power is work produced per unit of time, or the product of strength and speed. Muscle endurance is the ability to contract a muscle repeatedly over time.
Neuromotor Development (D)	Measures motor development, righting and equilibrium reactions, and reflex and equilibrium reactions
Non-invasive Instrumental Status (N)	Instrumental measures of oral, nasal, vocal, and velopharyngeal functions as they pertain to speech production
Nonspoken Language (Assessment) (7)	Measures nonspoken language (print, sign, symbols) for communication
Nonspoken Language (Treatment) (0)	Applying techniques that improve, augment, or compensate spoken communication
Oral Peripheral Mechanism (P)	Structural measures of face, jaw, lips, tongue, teeth, hard and soft palate, pharynx as related to speech production
Orofacial Myofunctional (Assessment) (K)	Measures orofacial myofunctional patterns for speech and related functions
Orofacial Myofunctional (Treatment) (9)	Applying techniques to improve, alter, or augment impaired orofacial myofunctional patterns and related speech production errors
Oscillating Tracking (3)	Measures ability to visually track
Pain (F)	Measures muscle soreness, pain and soreness with joint movement, and pain perception Includes/Examples: Includes questionnaires, graphs, symptom magnification scales or visual analog scales
Perceptual Processing (Assessment) (5)	Measures stereognosis, kinesthesia, body schema, right-left discrimination, form constancy, position in space, visual closure, figure-ground, depth perception, spatial relations and topographical orientation
Perceptual Processing (Treatment) (1)	Exercise and activities to facilitate perceptual processing Explanation: Includes stereognosis, kinesthesia, body schema, right-left discrimination, form constancy, position in space, visual closure, figure-ground, depth perception, spatial relations, and topographical orientation Includes/Examples: Includes stereognosis, kinesthesia, body schema, right-left discrimination, form constancy, position in space, visual closure, figure-ground, depth perception, spatial relations, and topographical orientation
Performance Intensity Phonetically Balanced Speech Discrimination (Q)	Measures word recognition over varying intensity levels
Postural Control (3)	Exercise or activities to increase postural alignment and control
Prosthesis (8)	Explanation: Artificial substitutes for missing body parts that augment performance or function Includes/Examples: Limb prosthesis, ocular prosthesis
Psychosocial Skills (Assessment) (6)	The ability to interact in society and to process emotions Includes/Examples: Includes psychological (values, interests, self-concept); social (role performance, social conduct, interpersonal skills, self expression); self-management (coping skills, time management, self-control)
Psychosocial Skills (Treatment) (6)	The ability to interact in society and to process emotions Includes/Examples: Includes psychological (values, interests, self-concept); social (role performance, social conduct, interpersonal skills, self expression); self-management (coping skills, time management, self-control)
Pure Tone Audiometry, Air (1)	Air-conduction pure tone threshold measures with appropriate masking
Pure Tone Audiometry, Air and Bone (2)	Air-conduction and bone-conduction pure tone threshold measures with appropriate masking
Pure Tone Stenger (C)	Measures unilateral nonorganic hearing loss based on simultaneous presentation of pure tones of differing volume
Range of Motion and Joint Integrity (5)	Measures quantity, quality, grade, and classification of joint movement and/or mobility Explanation: Range of Motion is the space, distance or angle through which movement occurs at a joint or series of joints. Joint integrity is the conformance of joints to expected anatomic, biomechanical and kinematic norms.
Range of Motion and Joint Mobility (0)	Exercise or activities to increase muscle length and joint mobility
Receptive/Expressive Language (Assessment) (8)	Measures receptive and expressive language
Receptive/Expressive Language (Treatment) (B)	Applying techniques to improve and augment receptive/expressive language
Reflex Integrity (G)	Measures the presence, absence, or exaggeration of developmentally appropriate, pathologic or normal reflexes

Continued on next page

Section F–Physical Rehabilitation and Diagnostic Audiology

Continued from previous page

ICD-10-PCS Value Qualifier (Character 5)	Definition
Select Picture Audiometry (5)	Establishes hearing threshold levels for speech using pictures
Sensorineural Acuity Level (4)	Measures sensorineural acuity masking presented via bone conduction
Sensory Aids (5)	Determines the appropriateness of a sensory prosthetic device, other than a hearing aid or assistive listening system/device
Sensory Awareness/ Processing/ Integrity (6)	Includes/Examples: Includes light touch, pressure, temperature, pain, sharp/dull, proprioception, vestibular, visual, auditory, gustatory, and olfactory
Short Increment Sensitivity Index (9)	Measures the ear's ability to detect small intensity changes; site of lesion test requiring a behavioral response
Sinusoidal Vertical Axis Rotational (4)	Measures nystagmus following rotation
Somatosensory Evoked Potentials (9)	Measures neural activity from sites throughout the body
Speech/Language Screening (6)	Identifies need for further speech and/or language evaluation
Speech Threshold (1)	Measures minimal intensity needed to repeat spondaic words
Speech-Language Pathology and Related Disorders Counseling (1)	Provides patients/families with information, support, referrals to facilitate recovery from a communication disorder
Speech-Language Pathology and Related Disorders Prevention (2)	Applying techniques to avoid or minimize onset and/or development of a communication disorder
Speech/Word Recognition (2)	Measures ability to repeat/identify single syllable words; scores given as a percentage; includes word recognition/speech discrimination
Staggered Spondaic Word (3)	Measures central auditory processing site of lesion based upon dichotic presentation of spondaic words
Static Orthosis (7)	Includes/Examples: Includes customized and prefabricated splints, inhibitory casts, spinal and other braces, and protective devices; has no moving parts, maintains joint(s) in desired position
Stenger (B)	Measures unilateral nonorganic hearing loss based on simultaneous presentation of signals of differing volume
Swallowing Dysfunction (D)	Activities to improve swallowing function in coordination with respiratory function Includes/Examples: Includes function and coordination of sucking, mastication, coughing, swallowing
Synthetic Sentence Identification (5)	Measures central auditory dysfunction using identification of third order approximations of sentences and competing messages
Temporal Ordering of Stimuli (V)	Measures specific central auditory process
Therapeutic Exercise (6)	Exercise or activities to facilitate sensory awareness, sensory processing, sensory integration, balance training, conditioning, reconditioning Includes/Examples: Includes developmental activities, breathing exercises, aerobic endurance activities, aquatic exercises, stretching and ventilatory muscle training
Tinnitus Masker (Assessment) (7)	Determines candidacy for tinnitus masker
Tinnitus Masker (Treatment) (Ø)	Explanation: Used to verify physical fit, acoustic appropriateness, and benefit; assists in achieving maximum benefit
Tone Decay (8)	Measures decrease in hearing sensitivity to a tone; site of lesion test requiring a behavioral response
Transfer (C)	Transitional movement from one surface to another
Transfer Training (8)	Exercise or activities to facilitate movement from one surface to another
Tympanometry (D)	Measures the integrity of the middle ear; measures ease at which sound flows through the tympanic membrane while air pressure against the membrane is varied
Unithermal Binaural Screen (2)	Measures the rhythmic eye movements stimulated by changing the temperature of the vestibular system in both ears using warm water, screening format
Ventilation/Respiration/Circulation (G)	Measures ventilatory muscle strength, power and endurance, pulmonary function and ventilatory mechanics Includes/Examples: Includes ability to clear airway, activities that aggravate or relieve edema, pain, dyspnea or other symptoms, chest wall mobility, cardiopulmonary response to performance of ADL and IAD, cough and sputum, standard vital signs
Vestibular (Ø)	Applying techniques to compensate for balance disorders; includes habituation, exercise therapy, and balance retraining
Visual Motor Integration (Assessment) (2)	Coordinating the interaction of information from the eyes with body movement during activity

Continued on next page

Section F–Physical Rehabilitation and Diagnostic Audiology

Continued from previous page

ICD-10-PCS Value Qualifier (Character 5)	Definition
Visual Motor Integration (Treatment) (2)	Exercise or activities to facilitate coordinating the interaction of information from eyes with body movement during activity
Visual Reinforcement Audiometry (6)	Behavioral measures using nonspeech and speech stimuli to obtain frequency/ear-specific information on auditory status Includes/Examples: Includes a conditioned response of looking toward a visual reinforcer (e.g., lights, animated toy) every time auditory stimuli are heard
Vocational Activities and Functional Community or Work Reintegration Skills (Assessment) (H)	Measures environmental, home, work (job/school/play) barriers that keep patients from functioning optimally in their environment Includes/Examples: Includes assessment of vocational skills and interests, environment of work (job/school/play), injury potential and injury prevention or reduction, ergonomic stressors, transportation skills, and ability to access and use community resources
Vocational Activities and Functional Community or Work Reintegration Skills (Treatment) (7)	Activities to facilitate vocational exploration, body mechanics training, job acquisition, and environmental or work (job/school/play) task adaptation Includes/Examples: Includes injury prevention and reduction, ergonomic stressor reduction, job coaching and simulation, work hardening and conditioning, driving training, transportation skills, and use of community resources
Voice (Assessment) (F)	Measures vocal structure, function and production
Voice (Treatment) (C)	Applying techniques to improve voice and vocal function
Voice Prosthetic (Assessment) (M)	Determines the appropriateness of voice prosthetic/adaptive device to enhance or facilitate communication
Voice Prosthetic (Treatment) (4)	Includes/Examples: Includes electrolarynx, and other assistive, adaptive, supportive devices
Wheelchair Mobility (Assessment) (F)	Measures fit and functional abilities within wheelchair in a variety of environments
Wheelchair Mobility (Treatment) (4)	Management, maintenance and controlled operation of a wheelchair, scooter or other device, in and on a variety of surfaces and environments
Wound Management (5)	Includes/Examples: Includes non-selective and selective debridement (enzymes, autolysis, sharp debridement), dressings (wound coverings, hydrogel, vacuum-assisted closure), topical agents, etc.

Section G–Mental Health

ICD-10-PCS Value (Character 4)	Definition
Biofeedback (C)	Provision of information from the monitoring and regulating of physiological processes in conjunction with cognitive-behavioral techniques to improve patient functioning or well-being Includes/Examples: Includes EEG, blood pressure, skin temperature or peripheral blood flow, ECG, electrooculogram, EMG, respirometry or capnometry, GSR/EDR, perineometry to monitor/regulate bowel/bladder activity, electrogastrogram to monitor/regulate gastric motility
Counseling (6)	The application of psychological methods to treat an individual with normal developmental issues and psychological problems in order to increase function, improve well-being, alleviate distress, maladjustment or resolve crises
Crisis Intervention (2)	Treatment of a traumatized, acutely disturbed or distressed individual for the purpose of short-term stabilization Includes/Examples: Includes defusing, debriefing, counseling, psychotherapy and/or coordination of care with other providers or agencies
Electroconvulsive Therapy (B)	The application of controlled electrical voltages to treat a mental health disorder Includes/Examples: Includes appropriate sedation and other preparation of the individual
Family Psychotherapy (7)	Treatment that includes one or more family members of an individual with a mental health disorder by behavioral, cognitive, psychoanalytic, psychodynamic or psychophysiological means to improve functioning or well-being Explanation: Remediation of emotional or behavioral problems presented by one or more family members in cases where psychotherapy with more than one family member is indicated
Group Psychotherapy (H)	Treatment of two or more individuals with a mental health disorder by behavioral, cognitive, psychoanalytic, psychodynamic or psychophysiological means to improve functioning or well-being
Hypnosis (F)	Induction of a state of heightened suggestibility by auditory, visual and tactile techniques to elicit an emotional or behavioral response
Individual Psychotherapy (5)	Treatment of an individual with a mental health disorder by behavioral, cognitive, psychoanalytic, psychodynamic or psychophysiological means to improve functioning or well-being
Light Therapy (J)	Application of specialized light treatments to improve functioning or well-being
Medication Management (3)	Monitoring and adjusting the use of medications for the treatment of a mental health disorder
Narcosynthesis (G)	Administration of intravenous barbiturates in order to release suppressed or repressed thoughts
Psychological Tests (1)	The administration and interpretation of standardized psychological tests and measurement instruments for the assessment of psychological function

Continued on next page

Section G–Mental Health

Continued from previous page

ICD-10-PCS Value (Character 4)	Definition
Behavioral (1)	Primarily to modify behavior Includes/Examples: Includes modeling and role playing, positive reinforcement of target behaviors, response cost, and training of self-management skills
Cognitive (2)	Primarily to correct cognitive distortions and errors
Cognitive-Behavioral (8)	Combining cognitive and behavioral treatment strategies to improve functioning Explanation: Maladaptive responses are examined to determine how cognitions relate to behavior patterns in response to an event. Uses learning principles and information-processing models.
Developmental (0)	Age-normed developmental status of cognitive, social and adaptive behavior skills
Intellectual and Psychoeducational (2)	Intellectual abilities, academic achievement and learning capabilities (including behaviors and emotional factors affecting learning)
Interactive (0)	Uses primarily physical aids and other forms of non-oral interaction with a patient who is physically, psychologically or developmentally unable to use ordinary language for communication Includes/Examples: Includes the use of toys in symbolic play
Interpersonal (3)	Helps an individual make changes in interpersonal behaviors to reduce psychological dysfunction Includes/Examples: Includes exploratory techniques, encouragement of affective expression, clarification of patient statements, analysis of communication patterns, use of therapy relationship and behavior change techniques
Neurobehavioral and Cognitive Status (4)	Includes neurobehavioral status exam, interview(s), and observation for the clinical assessment of thinking, reasoning and judgment, acquired knowledge, attention, memory, visual spatial abilities, language functions, and planning
Neuropsychological (3)	Thinking, reasoning and judgment, acquired knowledge, attention, memory, visual spatial abilities, language functions, planning
Personality and Behavioral (1)	Mood, emotion, behavior, social functioning, psychopathological conditions, personality traits and characteristics
Psychoanalysis (4)	Methods of obtaining a detailed account of past and present mental and emotional experiences to determine the source and eliminate or diminish the undesirable effects of unconscious conflicts Explanation: Accomplished by making the individual aware of their existence, origin, and inappropriate expression in emotions and behavior
Psychodynamic (5)	Exploration of past and present emotional experiences to understand motives and drives using insight-oriented techniques to reduce the undesirable effects of internal conflicts on emotions and behavior Explanation: Techniques include empathetic listening, clarifying self-defeating behavior patterns, and exploring adaptive alternatives
Psychophysiological (9)	Monitoring and alteration of physiological processes to help the individual associate physiological reactions combined with cognitive and behavioral strategies to gain improved control of these processes to help the individual cope more effectively
Supportive (6)	Formation of therapeutic relationship primarily for providing emotional support to prevent further deterioration in functioning during periods of particular stress Explanation: Often used in conjunction with other therapeutic approaches
Vocational (1)	Exploration of vocational interests, aptitudes and required adaptive behavior skills to develop and carry out a plan for achieving a successful vocational placement Includes/Examples: Includes enhancing work related adjustment and/or pursuing viable options in training education or preparation

Section H–Substance Abuse Treatment

ICD-10-PCS Value (Character 3)	Definition
Detoxification Services (2)	Detoxification from alcohol and/or drugs Explanation: Not a treatment modality, but helps the patient stabilize physically and psychologically until the body becomes free of drugs and the effects of alcohol
Family Counseling (6)	The application of psychological methods that includes one or more family members to treat an individual with addictive behavior Explanation: Provides support and education for family members of addicted individuals. Family member participation is seen as a critical area of substance abuse treatment.
Group Counseling (4)	The application of psychological methods to treat two or more individuals with addictive behavior Explanation: Provides structured group counseling sessions and healing power through the connection with others
Individual Counseling (3)	The application of psychological methods to treat an individual with addictive behavior Explanation: Comprised of several different techniques, which apply various strategies to address drug addiction
Individual Psychotherapy (5)	Treatment of an individual with addictive behavior by behavioral, cognitive, psychoanalytic, psychodynamic or psychophysiological means
Medication Management (8)	Monitoring and adjusting the use of replacement medications for the treatment of addiction
Pharmacotherapy (9)	The use of replacement medications for the treatment of addiction

Appendix K: Hospital Acquired Conditions

Hospital acquired conditions (HACs) are conditions considered reasonably preventable through the application of evidence-based guidelines. Although it is the ICD-10-CM diagnosis code that drives a HAC designation, in some cases a specific ICD-10-PCS procedure code must also be present before that diagnosis code can be considered a HAC. This resource provides only those HAC categories that require both an ICD-10-PCS code and an ICD-10-CM diagnosis code. The official descriptions for each code are also provided. To see all 14 HAC categories and their corresponding codes, refer to Optum's *ICD-10-CM Expert for Hospitals*.

Note: The resource used to compile this list is the proposed, version 42, MS-DRG Grouper software and Definitions Manual files published with the fiscal 2025 IPPS proposed rule. For the most current files, refer to the following:
https://www.cms.gov/Medicare/Medicare-Fee-for-Service-Payment/AcuteInpatientPPS/MS-DRG-Classifications-and-Software.

HAC 08: Surgical Site Infection of Mediastinitis After Coronary Bypass Graft (CABG) Procedures
Secondary diagnosis not POA:
- J98.51   Mediastinitis
- J98.59   Other diseases of mediastinum, not elsewhere classified

AND

Any of the following procedures:
- 0210083 Bypass Coronary Artery, One Artery from Coronary Artery with Zooplastic Tissue, Open Approach
- 0210088 Bypass Coronary Artery, One Artery from Right Internal Mammary with Zooplastic Tissue, Open Approach
- 0210089 Bypass Coronary Artery, One Artery from Left Internal Mammary with Zooplastic Tissue, Open Approach
- 021008C Bypass Coronary Artery, One Artery from Thoracic Artery with Zooplastic Tissue, Open Approach
- 021008F Bypass Coronary Artery, One Artery from Abdominal Artery with Zooplastic Tissue, Open Approach
- 021008W Bypass Coronary Artery, One Artery from Aorta with Zooplastic Tissue, Open Approach
- 0210093 Bypass Coronary Artery, One Artery from Coronary Artery with Autologous Venous Tissue, Open Approach
- 0210098 Bypass Coronary Artery, One Artery from Right Internal Mammary with Autologous Venous Tissue, Open Approach
- 0210099 Bypass Coronary Artery, One Artery from Left Internal Mammary with Autologous Venous Tissue, Open Approach
- 021009C Bypass Coronary Artery, One Artery from Thoracic Artery with Autologous Venous Tissue, Open Approach
- 021009F Bypass Coronary Artery, One Artery from Abdominal Artery with Autologous Venous Tissue, Open Approach
- 021009W Bypass Coronary Artery, One Artery from Aorta with Autologous Venous Tissue, Open Approach
- 02100A3 Bypass Coronary Artery, One Artery from Coronary Artery with Autologous Arterial Tissue, Open Approach
- 02100A8 Bypass Coronary Artery, One Artery from Right Internal Mammary with Autologous Arterial Tissue, Open Approach
- 02100A9 Bypass Coronary Artery, One Artery from Left Internal Mammary with Autologous Arterial Tissue, Open Approach
- 02100AC Bypass Coronary Artery, One Artery from Thoracic Artery with Autologous Arterial Tissue, Open Approach
- 02100AF Bypass Coronary Artery, One Artery from Abdominal Artery with Autologous Arterial Tissue, Open Approach
- 02100AW Bypass Coronary Artery, One Artery from Aorta with Autologous Arterial Tissue, Open Approach
- 02100J3 Bypass Coronary Artery, One Artery from Coronary Artery with Synthetic Substitute, Open Approach
- 02100J8 Bypass Coronary Artery, One Artery from Right Internal Mammary with Synthetic Substitute, Open Approach
- 02100J9 Bypass Coronary Artery, One Artery from Left Internal Mammary with Synthetic Substitute, Open Approach
- 02100JC Bypass Coronary Artery, One Artery from Thoracic Artery with Synthetic Substitute, Open Approach
- 02100JF Bypass Coronary Artery, One Artery from Abdominal Artery with Synthetic Substitute, Open Approach
- 02100JW Bypass Coronary Artery, One Artery from Aorta with Synthetic Substitute, Open Approach
- 02100K3 Bypass Coronary Artery, One Artery from Coronary Artery with Nonautologous Tissue Substitute, Open Approach
- 02100K8 Bypass Coronary Artery, One Artery from Right Internal Mammary with Nonautologous Tissue Substitute, Open Approach
- 02100K9 Bypass Coronary Artery, One Artery from Left Internal Mammary with Nonautologous Tissue Substitute, Open Approach
- 02100KC Bypass Coronary Artery, One Artery from Thoracic Artery with Nonautologous Tissue Substitute, Open Approach
- 02100KF Bypass Coronary Artery, One Artery from Abdominal Artery with Nonautologous Tissue Substitute, Open Approach
- 02100KW Bypass Coronary Artery, One Artery from Aorta with Nonautologous Tissue Substitute, Open Approach
- 02100Z3 Bypass Coronary Artery, One Artery from Coronary Artery, Open Approach
- 02100Z8 Bypass Coronary Artery, One Artery from Right Internal Mammary, Open Approach
- 02100Z9 Bypass Coronary Artery, One Artery from Left Internal Mammary, Open Approach
- 02100ZC Bypass Coronary Artery, One Artery from Thoracic Artery, Open Approach
- 02100ZF Bypass Coronary Artery, One Artery from Abdominal Artery, Open Approach
- 0210483 Bypass Coronary Artery, One Artery from Coronary Artery with Zooplastic Tissue, Percutaneous Endoscopic Approach
- 0210488 Bypass Coronary Artery, One Artery from Right Internal Mammary with Zooplastic Tissue, Percutaneous Endoscopic Approach
- 0210489 Bypass Coronary Artery, One Artery from Left Internal Mammary with Zooplastic Tissue, Percutaneous Endoscopic Approach
- 021048C Bypass Coronary Artery, One Artery from Thoracic Artery with Zooplastic Tissue, Percutaneous Endoscopic Approach
- 021048F Bypass Coronary Artery, One Artery from Abdominal Artery with Zooplastic Tissue, Percutaneous Endoscopic Approach
- 021048W Bypass Coronary Artery, One Artery from Aorta with Zooplastic Tissue, Percutaneous Endoscopic Approach
- 0210493 Bypass Coronary Artery, One Artery from Coronary Artery with Autologous Venous Tissue, Percutaneous Endoscopic Approach
- 0210498 Bypass Coronary Artery, One Artery from Right Internal Mammary with Autologous Venous Tissue, Percutaneous Endoscopic Approach
- 0210499 Bypass Coronary Artery, One Artery from Left Internal Mammary with Autologous Venous Tissue, Percutaneous Endoscopic Approach
- 021049C Bypass Coronary Artery, One Artery from Thoracic Artery with Autologous Venous Tissue, Percutaneous Endoscopic Approach
- 021049F Bypass Coronary Artery, One Artery from Abdominal Artery with Autologous Venous Tissue, Percutaneous Endoscopic Approach
- 021049W Bypass Coronary Artery, One Artery from Aorta with Autologous Venous Tissue, Percutaneous Endoscopic Approach
- 02104A3 Bypass Coronary Artery, One Artery from Coronary Artery with Autologous Arterial Tissue, Percutaneous Endoscopic Approach
- 02104A8 Bypass Coronary Artery, One Artery from Right Internal Mammary with Autologous Arterial Tissue, Percutaneous Endoscopic Approach
- 02104A9 Bypass Coronary Artery, One Artery from Left Internal Mammary with Autologous Arterial Tissue, Percutaneous Endoscopic Approach
- 02104AC Bypass Coronary Artery, One Artery from Thoracic Artery with Autologous Arterial Tissue, Percutaneous Endoscopic Approach
- 02104AF Bypass Coronary Artery, One Artery from Abdominal Artery with Autologous Arterial Tissue, Percutaneous Endoscopic Approach
- 02104AW Bypass Coronary Artery, One Artery from Aorta with Autologous Arterial Tissue, Percutaneous Endoscopic Approach
- 02104J3 Bypass Coronary Artery, One Artery from Coronary Artery with Synthetic Substitute, Percutaneous Endoscopic Approach
- 02104J8 Bypass Coronary Artery, One Artery from Right Internal Mammary with Synthetic Substitute, Percutaneous Endoscopic Approach
- 02104J9 Bypass Coronary Artery, One Artery from Left Internal Mammary with Synthetic Substitute, Percutaneous Endoscopic Approach

Appendix K: Hospital Acquired Conditions

HAC 08: Surgical Site Infection of Mediastinitis After Coronary Bypass Graft (CABG) Procedures (continued)

Code	Description
02104JC	Bypass Coronary Artery, One Artery from Thoracic Artery with Synthetic Substitute, Percutaneous Endoscopic Approach
02104JF	Bypass Coronary Artery, One Artery from Abdominal Artery with Synthetic Substitute, Percutaneous Endoscopic Approach
02104JW	Bypass Coronary Artery, One Artery from Aorta with Synthetic Substitute, Percutaneous Endoscopic Approach
02104K3	Bypass Coronary Artery, One Artery from Coronary Artery with Nonautologous Tissue Substitute, Percutaneous Endoscopic Approach
02104K8	Bypass Coronary Artery, One Artery from Right Internal Mammary with Nonautologous Tissue Substitute, Percutaneous Endoscopic Approach
02104K9	Bypass Coronary Artery, One Artery from Left Internal Mammary with Nonautologous Tissue Substitute, Percutaneous Endoscopic Approach
02104KC	Bypass Coronary Artery, One Artery from Thoracic Artery with Nonautologous Tissue Substitute, Percutaneous Endoscopic Approach
02104KF	Bypass Coronary Artery, One Artery from Abdominal Artery with Nonautologous Tissue Substitute, Percutaneous Endoscopic Approach
02104KW	Bypass Coronary Artery, One Artery from Aorta with Nonautologous Tissue Substitute, Percutaneous Endoscopic Approach
02104Z3	Bypass Coronary Artery, One Artery from Coronary Artery, Percutaneous Endoscopic Approach
02104Z8	Bypass Coronary Artery, One Artery from Right Internal Mammary, Percutaneous Endoscopic Approach
02104Z9	Bypass Coronary Artery, One Artery from Left Internal Mammary, Percutaneous Endoscopic Approach
02104ZC	Bypass Coronary Artery, One Artery from Thoracic Artery, Percutaneous Endoscopic Approach
02104ZF	Bypass Coronary Artery, One Artery from Abdominal Artery, Percutaneous Endoscopic Approach
0211083	Bypass Coronary Artery, Two Arteries from Coronary Artery with Zooplastic Tissue, Open Approach
0211088	Bypass Coronary Artery, Two Arteries from Right Internal Mammary with Zooplastic Tissue, Open Approach
0211089	Bypass Coronary Artery, Two Arteries from Left Internal Mammary with Zooplastic Tissue, Open Approach
021108C	Bypass Coronary Artery, Two Arteries from Thoracic Artery with Zooplastic Tissue, Open Approach
021108F	Bypass Coronary Artery, Two Arteries from Abdominal Artery with Zooplastic Tissue, Open Approach
021108W	Bypass Coronary Artery, Two Arteries from Aorta with Zooplastic Tissue, Open Approach
0211093	Bypass Coronary Artery, Two Arteries from Coronary Artery with Autologous Venous Tissue, Open Approach
0211098	Bypass Coronary Artery, Two Arteries from Right Internal Mammary with Autologous Venous Tissue, Open Approach
0211099	Bypass Coronary Artery, Two Arteries from Left Internal Mammary with Autologous Venous Tissue, Open Approach
021109C	Bypass Coronary Artery, Two Arteries from Thoracic Artery with Autologous Venous Tissue, Open Approach
021109F	Bypass Coronary Artery, Two Arteries from Abdominal Artery with Autologous Venous Tissue, Open Approach
021109W	Bypass Coronary Artery, Two Arteries from Aorta with Autologous Venous Tissue, Open Approach
02110A3	Bypass Coronary Artery, Two Arteries from Coronary Artery with Autologous Arterial Tissue, Open Approach
02110A8	Bypass Coronary Artery, Two Arteries from Right Internal Mammary with Autologous Arterial Tissue, Open Approach
02110A9	Bypass Coronary Artery, Two Arteries from Left Internal Mammary with Autologous Arterial Tissue, Open Approach
02110AC	Bypass Coronary Artery, Two Arteries from Thoracic Artery with Autologous Arterial Tissue, Open Approach
02110AF	Bypass Coronary Artery, Two Arteries from Abdominal Artery with Autologous Arterial Tissue, Open Approach
02110AW	Bypass Coronary Artery, Two Arteries from Aorta with Autologous Arterial Tissue, Open Approach
02110J3	Bypass Coronary Artery, Two Arteries from Coronary Artery with Synthetic Substitute, Open Approach
02110J8	Bypass Coronary Artery, Two Arteries from Right Internal Mammary with Synthetic Substitute, Open Approach
02110J9	Bypass Coronary Artery, Two Arteries from Left Internal Mammary with Synthetic Substitute, Open Approach
02110JC	Bypass Coronary Artery, Two Arteries from Thoracic Artery with Synthetic Substitute, Open Approach
02110JF	Bypass Coronary Artery, Two Arteries from Abdominal Artery with Synthetic Substitute, Open Approach
02110JW	Bypass Coronary Artery, Two Arteries from Aorta with Synthetic Substitute, Open Approach
02110K3	Bypass Coronary Artery, Two Arteries from Coronary Artery with Nonautologous Tissue Substitute, Open Approach
02110K8	Bypass Coronary Artery, Two Arteries from Right Internal Mammary with Nonautologous Tissue Substitute, Open Approach
02110K9	Bypass Coronary Artery, Two Arteries from Left Internal Mammary with Nonautologous Tissue Substitute, Open Approach
02110KC	Bypass Coronary Artery, Two Arteries from Thoracic Artery with Nonautologous Tissue Substitute, Open Approach
02110KF	Bypass Coronary Artery, Two Arteries from Abdominal Artery with Nonautologous Tissue Substitute, Open Approach
02110KW	Bypass Coronary Artery, Two Arteries from Aorta with Nonautologous Tissue Substitute, Open Approach
02110Z3	Bypass Coronary Artery, Two Arteries from Coronary Artery, Open Approach
02110Z8	Bypass Coronary Artery, Two Arteries from Right Internal Mammary, Open Approach
02110Z9	Bypass Coronary Artery, Two Arteries from Left Internal Mammary, Open Approach
02110ZC	Bypass Coronary Artery, Two Arteries from Thoracic Artery, Open Approach
02110ZF	Bypass Coronary Artery, Two Arteries from Abdominal Artery, Open Approach
0211483	Bypass Coronary Artery, Two Arteries from Coronary Artery with Zooplastic Tissue, Percutaneous Endoscopic Approach
0211488	Bypass Coronary Artery, Two Arteries from Right Internal Mammary with Zooplastic Tissue, Percutaneous Endoscopic Approach
0211489	Bypass Coronary Artery, Two Arteries from Left Internal Mammary with Zooplastic Tissue, Percutaneous Endoscopic Approach
021148C	Bypass Coronary Artery, Two Arteries from Thoracic Artery with Zooplastic Tissue, Percutaneous Endoscopic Approach
021148F	Bypass Coronary Artery, Two Arteries from Abdominal Artery with Zooplastic Tissue, Percutaneous Endoscopic Approach
021148W	Bypass Coronary Artery, Two Arteries from Aorta with Zooplastic Tissue, Percutaneous Endoscopic Approach
0211493	Bypass Coronary Artery, Two Arteries from Coronary Artery with Autologous Venous Tissue, Percutaneous Endoscopic Approach
0211498	Bypass Coronary Artery, Two Arteries from Right Internal Mammary with Autologous Venous Tissue, Percutaneous Endoscopic Approach
0211499	Bypass Coronary Artery, Two Arteries from Left Internal Mammary with Autologous Venous Tissue, Percutaneous Endoscopic Approach
021149C	Bypass Coronary Artery, Two Arteries from Thoracic Artery with Autologous Venous Tissue, Percutaneous Endoscopic Approach
021149F	Bypass Coronary Artery, Two Arteries from Abdominal Artery with Autologous Venous Tissue, Percutaneous Endoscopic Approach
021149W	Bypass Coronary Artery, Two Arteries from Aorta with Autologous Venous Tissue, Percutaneous Endoscopic Approach
02114A3	Bypass Coronary Artery, Two Arteries from Coronary Artery with Autologous Arterial Tissue, Percutaneous Endoscopic Approach
02114A8	Bypass Coronary Artery, Two Arteries from Right Internal Mammary with Autologous Arterial Tissue, Percutaneous Endoscopic Approach
02114A9	Bypass Coronary Artery, Two Arteries from Left Internal Mammary with Autologous Arterial Tissue, Percutaneous Endoscopic Approach
02114AC	Bypass Coronary Artery, Two Arteries from Thoracic Artery with Autologous Arterial Tissue, Percutaneous Endoscopic Approach
02114AF	Bypass Coronary Artery, Two Arteries from Abdominal Artery with Autologous Arterial Tissue, Percutaneous Endoscopic Approach
02114AW	Bypass Coronary Artery, Two Arteries from Aorta with Autologous Arterial Tissue, Percutaneous Endoscopic Approach
02114J3	Bypass Coronary Artery, Two Arteries from Coronary Artery with Synthetic Substitute, Percutaneous Endoscopic Approach
02114J8	Bypass Coronary Artery, Two Arteries from Right Internal Mammary with Synthetic Substitute, Percutaneous Endoscopic Approach

HAC 08: Surgical Site Infection of Mediastinitis After Coronary Bypass Graft (CABG) Procedures (continued)

Code	Description
02114J9	Bypass Coronary Artery, Two Arteries from Left Internal Mammary with Synthetic Substitute, Percutaneous Endoscopic Approach
02114JC	Bypass Coronary Artery, Two Arteries from Thoracic Artery with Synthetic Substitute, Percutaneous Endoscopic Approach
02114JF	Bypass Coronary Artery, Two Arteries from Abdominal Artery with Synthetic Substitute, Percutaneous Endoscopic Approach
02114JW	Bypass Coronary Artery, Two Arteries from Aorta with Synthetic Substitute, Percutaneous Endoscopic Approach
02114K3	Bypass Coronary Artery, Two Arteries from Coronary Artery with Nonautologous Tissue Substitute, Percutaneous Endoscopic Approach
02114K8	Bypass Coronary Artery, Two Arteries from Right Internal Mammary with Nonautologous Tissue Substitute, Percutaneous Endoscopic Approach
02114K9	Bypass Coronary Artery, Two Arteries from Left Internal Mammary with Nonautologous Tissue Substitute, Percutaneous Endoscopic Approach
02114KC	Bypass Coronary Artery, Two Arteries from Thoracic Artery with Nonautologous Tissue Substitute, Percutaneous Endoscopic Approach
02114KF	Bypass Coronary Artery, Two Arteries from Abdominal Artery with Nonautologous Tissue Substitute, Percutaneous Endoscopic Approach
02114KW	Bypass Coronary Artery, Two Arteries from Aorta with Nonautologous Tissue Substitute, Percutaneous Endoscopic Approach
02114Z3	Bypass Coronary Artery, Two Arteries from Coronary Artery, Percutaneous Endoscopic Approach
02114Z8	Bypass Coronary Artery, Two Arteries from Right Internal Mammary, Percutaneous Endoscopic Approach
02114Z9	Bypass Coronary Artery, Two Arteries from Left Internal Mammary, Percutaneous Endoscopic Approach
02114ZC	Bypass Coronary Artery, Two Arteries from Thoracic Artery, Percutaneous Endoscopic Approach
02114ZF	Bypass Coronary Artery, Two Arteries from Abdominal Artery, Percutaneous Endoscopic Approach
0212083	Bypass Coronary Artery, Three Arteries from Coronary Artery with Zooplastic Tissue, Open Approach
0212088	Bypass Coronary Artery, Three Arteries from Right Internal Mammary with Zooplastic Tissue, Open Approach
0212089	Bypass Coronary Artery, Three Arteries from Left Internal Mammary with Zooplastic Tissue, Open Approach
021208C	Bypass Coronary Artery, Three Arteries from Thoracic Artery with Zooplastic Tissue, Open Approach
021208F	Bypass Coronary Artery, Three Arteries from Abdominal Artery with Zooplastic Tissue, Open Approach
021208W	Bypass Coronary Artery, Three Arteries from Aorta with Zooplastic Tissue, Open Approach
0212093	Bypass Coronary Artery, Three Arteries from Coronary Artery with Autologous Venous Tissue, Open Approach
0212098	Bypass Coronary Artery, Three Arteries from Right Internal Mammary with Autologous Venous Tissue, Open Approach
0212099	Bypass Coronary Artery, Three Arteries from Left Internal Mammary with Autologous Venous Tissue, Open Approach
021209C	Bypass Coronary Artery, Three Arteries from Thoracic Artery with Autologous Venous Tissue, Open Approach
021209F	Bypass Coronary Artery, Three Arteries from Abdominal Artery with Autologous Venous Tissue, Open Approach
021209W	Bypass Coronary Artery, Three Arteries from Aorta with Autologous Venous Tissue, Open Approach
02120A3	Bypass Coronary Artery, Three Arteries from Coronary Artery with Autologous Arterial Tissue, Open Approach
02120A8	Bypass Coronary Artery, Three Arteries from Right Internal Mammary with Autologous Arterial Tissue, Open Approach
02120A9	Bypass Coronary Artery, Three Arteries from Left Internal Mammary with Autologous Arterial Tissue, Open Approach
02120AC	Bypass Coronary Artery, Three Arteries from Thoracic Artery with Autologous Arterial Tissue, Open Approach
02120AF	Bypass Coronary Artery, Three Arteries from Abdominal Artery with Autologous Arterial Tissue, Open Approach
02120AW	Bypass Coronary Artery, Three Arteries from Aorta with Autologous Arterial Tissue, Open Approach
02120J3	Bypass Coronary Artery, Three Arteries from Coronary Artery with Synthetic Substitute, Open Approach
02120J8	Bypass Coronary Artery, Three Arteries from Right Internal Mammary with Synthetic Substitute, Open Approach
02120J9	Bypass Coronary Artery, Three Arteries from Left Internal Mammary with Synthetic Substitute, Open Approach
02120JC	Bypass Coronary Artery, Three Arteries from Thoracic Artery with Synthetic Substitute, Open Approach
02120JF	Bypass Coronary Artery, Three Arteries from Abdominal Artery with Synthetic Substitute, Open Approach
02120JW	Bypass Coronary Artery, Three Arteries from Aorta with Synthetic Substitute, Open Approach
02120K3	Bypass Coronary Artery, Three Arteries from Coronary Artery with Nonautologous Tissue Substitute, Open Approach
02120K8	Bypass Coronary Artery, Three Arteries from Right Internal Mammary with Nonautologous Tissue Substitute, Open Approach
02120K9	Bypass Coronary Artery, Three Arteries from Left Internal Mammary with Nonautologous Tissue Substitute, Open Approach
02120KC	Bypass Coronary Artery, Three Arteries from Thoracic Artery with Nonautologous Tissue Substitute, Open Approach
02120KF	Bypass Coronary Artery, Three Arteries from Abdominal Artery with Nonautologous Tissue Substitute, Open Approach
02120KW	Bypass Coronary Artery, Three Arteries from Aorta with Nonautologous Tissue Substitute, Open Approach
02120Z3	Bypass Coronary Artery, Three Arteries from Coronary Artery, Open Approach
02120Z8	Bypass Coronary Artery, Three Arteries from Right Internal Mammary, Open Approach
02120Z9	Bypass Coronary Artery, Three Arteries from Left Internal Mammary, Open Approach
02120ZC	Bypass Coronary Artery, Three Arteries from Thoracic Artery, Open Approach
02120ZF	Bypass Coronary Artery, Three Arteries from Abdominal Artery, Open Approach
0212483	Bypass Coronary Artery, Three Arteries from Coronary Artery with Zooplastic Tissue, Percutaneous Endoscopic Approach
0212488	Bypass Coronary Artery, Three Arteries from Right Internal Mammary with Zooplastic Tissue, Percutaneous Endoscopic Approach
0212489	Bypass Coronary Artery, Three Arteries from Left Internal Mammary with Zooplastic Tissue, Percutaneous Endoscopic Approach
021248C	Bypass Coronary Artery, Three Arteries from Thoracic Artery with Zooplastic Tissue, Percutaneous Endoscopic Approach
021248F	Bypass Coronary Artery, Three Arteries from Abdominal Artery with Zooplastic Tissue, Percutaneous Endoscopic Approach
021248W	Bypass Coronary Artery, Three Arteries from Aorta with Zooplastic Tissue, Percutaneous Endoscopic Approach
0212493	Bypass Coronary Artery, Three Arteries from Coronary Artery with Autologous Venous Tissue, Percutaneous Endoscopic Approach
0212498	Bypass Coronary Artery, Three Arteries from Right Internal Mammary with Autologous Venous Tissue, Percutaneous Endoscopic Approach
0212499	Bypass Coronary Artery, Three Arteries from Left Internal Mammary with Autologous Venous Tissue, Percutaneous Endoscopic Approach
021249C	Bypass Coronary Artery, Three Arteries from Thoracic Artery with Autologous Venous Tissue, Percutaneous Endoscopic Approach
021249F	Bypass Coronary Artery, Three Arteries from Abdominal Artery with Autologous Venous Tissue, Percutaneous Endoscopic Approach
021249W	Bypass Coronary Artery, Three Arteries from Aorta with Autologous Venous Tissue, Percutaneous Endoscopic Approach
02124A3	Bypass Coronary Artery, Three Arteries from Coronary Artery with Autologous Arterial Tissue, Percutaneous Endoscopic Approach
02124A8	Bypass Coronary Artery, Three Arteries from Right Internal Mammary with Autologous Arterial Tissue, Percutaneous Endoscopic Approach
02124A9	Bypass Coronary Artery, Three Arteries from Left Internal Mammary with Autologous Arterial Tissue, Percutaneous Endoscopic Approach

Appendix K: Hospital Acquired Conditions

HAC 08: Surgical Site Infection of Mediastinitis After Coronary Bypass Graft (CABG) Procedures (continued)

Code	Description
02124AC	Bypass Coronary Artery, Three Arteries from Thoracic Artery with Autologous Arterial Tissue, Percutaneous Endoscopic Approach
02124AF	Bypass Coronary Artery, Three Arteries from Abdominal Artery with Autologous Arterial Tissue, Percutaneous Endoscopic Approach
02124AW	Bypass Coronary Artery, Three Arteries from Aorta with Autologous Arterial Tissue, Percutaneous Endoscopic Approach
02124J3	Bypass Coronary Artery, Three Arteries from Coronary Artery with Synthetic Substitute, Percutaneous Endoscopic Approach
02124J8	Bypass Coronary Artery, Three Arteries from Right Internal Mammary with Synthetic Substitute, Percutaneous Endoscopic Approach
02124J9	Bypass Coronary Artery, Three Arteries from Left Internal Mammary with Synthetic Substitute, Percutaneous Endoscopic Approach
02124JC	Bypass Coronary Artery, Three Arteries from Thoracic Artery with Synthetic Substitute, Percutaneous Endoscopic Approach
02124JF	Bypass Coronary Artery, Three Arteries from Abdominal Artery with Synthetic Substitute, Percutaneous Endoscopic Approach
02124JW	Bypass Coronary Artery, Three Arteries from Aorta with Synthetic Substitute, Percutaneous Endoscopic Approach
02124K3	Bypass Coronary Artery, Three Arteries from Coronary Artery with Nonautologous Tissue Substitute, Percutaneous Endoscopic Approach
02124K8	Bypass Coronary Artery, Three Arteries from Right Internal Mammary with Nonautologous Tissue Substitute, Percutaneous Endoscopic Approach
02124K9	Bypass Coronary Artery, Three Arteries from Left Internal Mammary with Nonautologous Tissue Substitute, Percutaneous Endoscopic Approach
02124KC	Bypass Coronary Artery, Three Arteries from Thoracic Artery with Nonautologous Tissue Substitute, Percutaneous Endoscopic Approach
02124KF	Bypass Coronary Artery, Three Arteries from Abdominal Artery with Nonautologous Tissue Substitute, Percutaneous Endoscopic Approach
02124KW	Bypass Coronary Artery, Three Arteries from Aorta with Nonautologous Tissue Substitute, Percutaneous Endoscopic Approach
02124Z3	Bypass Coronary Artery, Three Arteries from Coronary Artery, Percutaneous Endoscopic Approach
02124Z8	Bypass Coronary Artery, Three Arteries from Right Internal Mammary, Percutaneous Endoscopic Approach
02124Z9	Bypass Coronary Artery, Three Arteries from Left Internal Mammary, Percutaneous Endoscopic Approach
02124ZC	Bypass Coronary Artery, Three Arteries from Thoracic Artery, Percutaneous Endoscopic Approach
02124ZF	Bypass Coronary Artery, Three Arteries from Abdominal Artery, Percutaneous Endoscopic Approach
0213083	Bypass Coronary Artery, Four or More Arteries from Coronary Artery with Zooplastic Tissue, Open Approach
0213088	Bypass Coronary Artery, Four or More Arteries from Right Internal Mammary with Zooplastic Tissue, Open Approach
0213089	Bypass Coronary Artery, Four or More Arteries from Left Internal Mammary with Zooplastic Tissue, Open Approach
021308C	Bypass Coronary Artery, Four or More Arteries from Thoracic Artery with Zooplastic Tissue, Open Approach
021308F	Bypass Coronary Artery, Four or More Arteries from Abdominal Artery with Zooplastic Tissue, Open Approach
021308W	Bypass Coronary Artery, Four or More Arteries from Aorta with Zooplastic Tissue, Open Approach
0213093	Bypass Coronary Artery, Four or More Arteries from Coronary Artery with Autologous Venous Tissue, Open Approach
0213098	Bypass Coronary Artery, Four or More Arteries from Right Internal Mammary with Autologous Venous Tissue, Open Approach
0213099	Bypass Coronary Artery, Four or More Arteries from Left Internal Mammary with Autologous Venous Tissue, Open Approach
021309C	Bypass Coronary Artery, Four or More Arteries from Thoracic Artery with Autologous Venous Tissue, Open Approach
021309F	Bypass Coronary Artery, Four or More Arteries from Abdominal Artery with Autologous Venous Tissue, Open Approach
021309W	Bypass Coronary Artery, Four or More Arteries from Aorta with Autologous Venous Tissue, Open Approach
02130A3	Bypass Coronary Artery, Four or More Arteries from Coronary Artery with Autologous Arterial Tissue, Open Approach
02130A8	Bypass Coronary Artery, Four or More Arteries from Right Internal Mammary with Autologous Arterial Tissue, Open Approach
02130A9	Bypass Coronary Artery, Four or More Arteries from Left Internal Mammary with Autologous Arterial Tissue, Open Approach
02130AC	Bypass Coronary Artery, Four or More Arteries from Thoracic Artery with Autologous Arterial Tissue, Open Approach
02130AF	Bypass Coronary Artery, Four or More Arteries from Abdominal Artery with Autologous Arterial Tissue, Open Approach
02130AW	Bypass Coronary Artery, Four or More Arteries from Aorta with Autologous Arterial Tissue, Open Approach
02130J3	Bypass Coronary Artery, Four or More Arteries from Coronary Artery with Synthetic Substitute, Open Approach
02130J8	Bypass Coronary Artery, Four or More Arteries from Right Internal Mammary with Synthetic Substitute, Open Approach
02130J9	Bypass Coronary Artery, Four or More Arteries from Left Internal Mammary with Synthetic Substitute, Open Approach
02130JC	Bypass Coronary Artery, Four or More Arteries from Thoracic Artery with Synthetic Substitute, Open Approach
02130JF	Bypass Coronary Artery, Four or More Arteries from Abdominal Artery with Synthetic Substitute, Open Approach
02130JW	Bypass Coronary Artery, Four or More Arteries from Aorta with Synthetic Substitute, Open Approach
02130K3	Bypass Coronary Artery, Four or More Arteries from Coronary Artery with Nonautologous Tissue Substitute, Open Approach
02130K8	Bypass Coronary Artery, Four or More Arteries from Right Internal Mammary with Nonautologous Tissue Substitute, Open Approach
02130K9	Bypass Coronary Artery, Four or More Arteries from Left Internal Mammary with Nonautologous Tissue Substitute, Open Approach
02130KC	Bypass Coronary Artery, Four or More Arteries from Thoracic Artery with Nonautologous Tissue Substitute, Open Approach
02130KF	Bypass Coronary Artery, Four or More Arteries from Abdominal Artery with Nonautologous Tissue Substitute, Open Approach
02130KW	Bypass Coronary Artery, Four or More Arteries from Aorta with Nonautologous Tissue Substitute, Open Approach
02130Z3	Bypass Coronary Artery, Four or More Arteries from Coronary Artery, Open Approach
02130Z8	Bypass Coronary Artery, Four or More Arteries from Right Internal Mammary, Open Approach
02130Z9	Bypass Coronary Artery, Four or More Arteries from Left Internal Mammary, Open Approach
02130ZC	Bypass Coronary Artery, Four or More Arteries from Thoracic Artery, Open Approach
02130ZF	Bypass Coronary Artery, Four or More Arteries from Abdominal Artery, Open Approach
0213483	Bypass Coronary Artery, Four or More Arteries from Coronary Artery with Zooplastic Tissue, Percutaneous Endoscopic Approach
0213488	Bypass Coronary Artery, Four or More Arteries from Right Internal Mammary with Zooplastic Tissue, Percutaneous Endoscopic Approach
0213489	Bypass Coronary Artery, Four or More Arteries from Left Internal Mammary with Zooplastic Tissue, Percutaneous Endoscopic Approach
021348C	Bypass Coronary Artery, Four or More Arteries from Thoracic Artery with Zooplastic Tissue, Percutaneous Endoscopic Approach
021348F	Bypass Coronary Artery, Four or More Arteries from Abdominal Artery with Zooplastic Tissue, Percutaneous Endoscopic Approach
021348W	Bypass Coronary Artery, Four or More Arteries from Aorta with Zooplastic Tissue, Percutaneous Endoscopic Approach
0213493	Bypass Coronary Artery, Four or More Arteries from Coronary Artery with Autologous Venous Tissue, Percutaneous Endoscopic Approach

HAC 08: Surgical Site Infection of Mediastinitis After Coronary Bypass Graft (CABG) Procedures (continued)

Code	Description
0213498	Bypass Coronary Artery, Four or More Arteries from Right Internal Mammary with Autologous Venous Tissue, Percutaneous Endoscopic Approach
0213499	Bypass Coronary Artery, Four or More Arteries from Left Internal Mammary with Autologous Venous Tissue, Percutaneous Endoscopic Approach
021349C	Bypass Coronary Artery, Four or More Arteries from Thoracic Artery with Autologous Venous Tissue, Percutaneous Endoscopic Approach
021349F	Bypass Coronary Artery, Four or More Arteries from Abdominal Artery with Autologous Venous Tissue, Percutaneous Endoscopic Approach
021349W	Bypass Coronary Artery, Four or More Arteries from Aorta with Autologous Venous Tissue, Percutaneous Endoscopic Approach
02134A3	Bypass Coronary Artery, Four or More Arteries from Coronary Artery with Autologous Arterial Tissue, Percutaneous Endoscopic Approach
02134A8	Bypass Coronary Artery, Four or More Arteries from Right Internal Mammary with Autologous Arterial Tissue, Percutaneous Endoscopic Approach
02134A9	Bypass Coronary Artery, Four or More Arteries from Left Internal Mammary with Autologous Arterial Tissue, Percutaneous Endoscopic Approach
02134AC	Bypass Coronary Artery, Four or More Arteries from Thoracic Artery with Autologous Arterial Tissue, Percutaneous Endoscopic Approach
02134AF	Bypass Coronary Artery, Four or More Arteries from Abdominal Artery with Autologous Arterial Tissue, Percutaneous Endoscopic Approach
02134AW	Bypass Coronary Artery, Four or More Arteries from Aorta with Autologous Arterial Tissue, Percutaneous Endoscopic Approach
02134J3	Bypass Coronary Artery, Four or More Arteries from Coronary Artery with Synthetic Substitute, Percutaneous Endoscopic Approach
02134J8	Bypass Coronary Artery, Four or More Arteries from Right Internal Mammary with Synthetic Substitute, Percutaneous Endoscopic Approach
02134J9	Bypass Coronary Artery, Four or More Arteries from Left Internal Mammary with Synthetic Substitute, Percutaneous Endoscopic Approach
02134JC	Bypass Coronary Artery, Four or More Arteries from Thoracic Artery with Synthetic Substitute, Percutaneous Endoscopic Approach
02134JF	Bypass Coronary Artery, Four or More Arteries from Abdominal Artery with Synthetic Substitute, Percutaneous Endoscopic Approach
02134JW	Bypass Coronary Artery, Four or More Arteries from Aorta with Synthetic Substitute, Percutaneous Endoscopic Approach
02134K3	Bypass Coronary Artery, Four or More Arteries from Coronary Artery with Nonautologous Tissue Substitute, Percutaneous Endoscopic Approach
02134K8	Bypass Coronary Artery, Four or More Arteries from Right Internal Mammary with Nonautologous Tissue Substitute, Percutaneous Endoscopic Approach
02134K9	Bypass Coronary Artery, Four or More Arteries from Left Internal Mammary with Nonautologous Tissue Substitute, Percutaneous Endoscopic Approach
02134KC	Bypass Coronary Artery, Four or More Arteries from Thoracic Artery with Nonautologous Tissue Substitute, Percutaneous Endoscopic Approach
02134KF	Bypass Coronary Artery, Four or More Arteries from Abdominal Artery with Nonautologous Tissue Substitute, Percutaneous Endoscopic Approach
02134KW	Bypass Coronary Artery, Four or More Arteries from Aorta with Nonautologous Tissue Substitute, Percutaneous Endoscopic Approach
02134Z3	Bypass Coronary Artery, Four or More Arteries from Coronary Artery, Percutaneous Endoscopic Approach
02134Z8	Bypass Coronary Artery, Four or More Arteries from Right Internal Mammary, Percutaneous Endoscopic Approach
02134Z9	Bypass Coronary Artery, Four or More Arteries from Left Internal Mammary, Percutaneous Endoscopic Approach
02134ZC	Bypass Coronary Artery, Four or More Arteries from Thoracic Artery, Percutaneous Endoscopic Approach
02134ZF	Bypass Coronary Artery, Four or More Arteries from Abdominal Artery, Percutaneous Endoscopic Approach

HAC 10: Deep Vein Thrombosis (DVT) or Pulmonary Embolism (PE) with Total Knee or Hip Replacement

Secondary diagnosis not POA:

Code	Description
I26.02	Saddle embolus of pulmonary artery with acute cor pulmonale
I26.03	Cement embolism of pulmonary artery with acute cor pulmonale
I26.04	Fat embolism of pulmonary artery with acute core pulmonale
I26.09	Other pulmonary embolism with acute cor pulmonale
I26.92	Saddle embolus of pulmonary artery without acute cor pulmonale
I26.93	Single subsegmental thrombotic pulmonary embolism without acute cor pulmonale
I26.94	Multiple subsegmental thrombotic pulmonary emboli without acute cor pulmonale
I26.95	Cement embolism of pulmonary artery without acute cor pulmonale
I26.96	Fat embolism of pulmonary artery without acute cor pulmonale
I26.99	Other pulmonary embolism without acute cor pulmonale
I82.401	Acute embolism and thrombosis of unspecified deep veins of right lower extremity
I82.402	Acute embolism and thrombosis of unspecified deep veins of left lower extremity
I82.403	Acute embolism and thrombosis of unspecified deep veins of lower extremity, bilateral
I82.409	Acute embolism and thrombosis of unspecified deep veins of unspecified lower extremity
I82.411	Acute embolism and thrombosis of right femoral vein
I82.412	Acute embolism and thrombosis of left femoral vein
I82.413	Acute embolism and thrombosis of femoral vein, bilateral
I82.419	Acute embolism and thrombosis of unspecified femoral vein
I82.421	Acute embolism and thrombosis of right iliac vein
I82.422	Acute embolism and thrombosis of left iliac vein
I82.423	Acute embolism and thrombosis of iliac vein, bilateral
I82.429	Acute embolism and thrombosis of unspecified iliac vein
I82.431	Acute embolism and thrombosis of right popliteal vein
I82.432	Acute embolism and thrombosis of left popliteal vein
I82.433	Acute embolism and thrombosis of popliteal vein, bilateral
I82.439	Acute embolism and thrombosis of unspecified popliteal vein
I82.441	Acute embolism and thrombosis of right tibial vein
I82.442	Acute embolism and thrombosis of left tibial vein
I82.443	Acute embolism and thrombosis of tibial vein, bilateral
I82.449	Acute embolism and thrombosis of unspecified tibial vein
I82.451	Acute embolism and thrombosis of right peroneal vein
I82.452	Acute embolism and thrombosis of left peroneal vein
I82.453	Acute embolism and thrombosis of peroneal vein, bilateral
I82.459	Acute embolism and thrombosis of unspecified peroneal vein
I82.491	Acute embolism and thrombosis of other specified deep vein of right lower extremity
I82.492	Acute embolism and thrombosis of other specified deep vein of left lower extremity
I82.493	Acute embolism and thrombosis of other specified deep vein of lower extremity, bilateral
I82.499	Acute embolism and thrombosis of other specified deep vein of unspecified lower extremity
I82.4Y1	Acute embolism and thrombosis of unspecified deep veins of right proximal lower extremity
I82.4Y2	Acute embolism and thrombosis of unspecified deep veins of left proximal lower extremity
I82.4Y3	Acute embolism and thrombosis of unspecified deep veins of proximal lower extremity, bilateral
I82.4Y9	Acute embolism and thrombosis of unspecified deep veins of unspecified proximal lower extremity
I82.4Z1	Acute embolism and thrombosis of unspecified deep veins of right distal lower extremity
I82.4Z2	Acute embolism and thrombosis of unspecified deep veins of left distal lower extremity
I82.4Z3	Acute embolism and thrombosis of unspecified deep veins of distal lower extremity, bilateral
I82.4Z9	Acute embolism and thrombosis of unspecified deep veins of unspecified distal lower extremity

AND

Any of the following procedures:

Appendix K: Hospital Acquired Conditions

HAC 10: Deep Vein Thrombosis (DVT) or Pulmonary Embolism (PE) with Total Knee or Hip Replacement (continued)

Code	Description
0SR9019	Replacement of Right Hip Joint with Metal Synthetic Substitute, Cemented, Open Approach
0SR901A	Replacement of Right Hip Joint with Metal Synthetic Substitute, Uncemented, Open Approach
0SR901Z	Replacement of Right Hip Joint with Metal Synthetic Substitute, Open Approach
0SR9029	Replacement of Right Hip Joint with Metal on Polyethylene Synthetic Substitute, Cemented, Open Approach
0SR902A	Replacement of Right Hip Joint with Metal on Polyethylene Synthetic Substitute, Uncemented, Open Approach
0SR902Z	Replacement of Right Hip Joint with Metal on Polyethylene Synthetic Substitute, Open Approach
0SR9039	Replacement of Right Hip Joint with Ceramic Synthetic Substitute, Cemented, Open Approach
0SR903A	Replacement of Right Hip Joint with Ceramic Synthetic Substitute, Uncemented, Open Approach
0SR903Z	Replacement of Right Hip Joint with Ceramic Synthetic Substitute, Open Approach
0SR9049	Replacement of Right Hip Joint with Ceramic on Polyethylene Synthetic Substitute, Cemented, Open Approach
0SR904A	Replacement of Right Hip Joint with Ceramic on Polyethylene Synthetic Substitute, Uncemented, Open Approach
0SR904Z	Replacement of Right Hip Joint with Ceramic on Polyethylene Synthetic Substitute, Open Approach
0SR9069	Replacement of Right Hip Joint with Oxidized Zirconium on Polyethylene Synthetic Substitute, Cemented, Open Approach
0SR906A	Replacement of Right Hip Joint with Oxidized Zirconium on Polyethylene Synthetic Substitute, Uncemented, Open Approach
0SR906Z	Replacement of Right Hip Joint with Oxidized Zirconium on Polyethylene Synthetic Substitute, Open Approach
0SR907Z	Replacement of Right Hip Joint with Autologous Tissue Substitute, Open Approach
0SR90EZ	Replacement of Right Hip Joint with Articulating Spacer, Open Approach
0SR90J9	Replacement of Right Hip Joint with Synthetic Substitute, Cemented, Open Approach
0SR90JA	Replacement of Right Hip Joint with Synthetic Substitute, Uncemented, Open Approach
0SR90JZ	Replacement of Right Hip Joint with Synthetic Substitute, Open Approach
0SR90KZ	Replacement of Right Hip Joint with Nonautologous Tissue Substitute, Open Approach
0SRA009	Replacement of Right Hip Joint, Acetabular Surface with Polyethylene Synthetic Substitute, Cemented, Open Approach
0SRA00A	Replacement of Right Hip Joint, Acetabular Surface with Polyethylene Synthetic Substitute, Uncemented, Open Approach
0SRA00Z	Replacement of Right Hip Joint, Acetabular Surface with Polyethylene Synthetic Substitute, Open Approach
0SRA019	Replacement of Right Hip Joint, Acetabular Surface with Metal Synthetic Substitute, Cemented, Open Approach
0SRA01A	Replacement of Right Hip Joint, Acetabular Surface with Metal Synthetic Substitute, Uncemented, Open Approach
0SRA01Z	Replacement of Right Hip Joint, Acetabular Surface with Metal Synthetic Substitute, Open Approach
0SRA039	Replacement of Right Hip Joint, Acetabular Surface with Ceramic Synthetic Substitute, Cemented, Open Approach
0SRA03A	Replacement of Right Hip Joint, Acetabular Surface with Ceramic Synthetic Substitute, Uncemented, Open Approach
0SRA03Z	Replacement of Right Hip Joint, Acetabular Surface with Ceramic Synthetic Substitute, Open Approach
0SRA07Z	Replacement of Right Hip Joint, Acetabular Surface with Autologous Tissue Substitute, Open Approach
0SRA0J9	Replacement of Right Hip Joint, Acetabular Surface with Synthetic Substitute, Cemented, Open Approach
0SRA0JA	Replacement of Right Hip Joint, Acetabular Surface with Synthetic Substitute, Uncemented, Open Approach
0SRA0JZ	Replacement of Right Hip Joint, Acetabular Surface with Synthetic Substitute, Open Approach
0SRA0KZ	Replacement of Right Hip Joint, Acetabular Surface with Nonautologous Tissue Substitute, Open Approach
0SRB019	Replacement of Left Hip Joint with Metal Synthetic Substitute, Cemented, Open Approach
0SRB01A	Replacement of Left Hip Joint with Metal Synthetic Substitute, Uncemented, Open Approach
0SRB01Z	Replacement of Left Hip Joint with Metal Synthetic Substitute, Open Approach
0SRB029	Replacement of Left Hip Joint with Metal on Polyethylene Synthetic Substitute, Cemented, Open Approach
0SRB02A	Replacement of Left Hip Joint with Metal on Polyethylene Synthetic Substitute, Uncemented, Open Approach
0SRB02Z	Replacement of Left Hip Joint with Metal on Polyethylene Synthetic Substitute, Open Approach
0SRB039	Replacement of Left Hip Joint with Ceramic Synthetic Substitute, Cemented, Open Approach
0SRB03A	Replacement of Left Hip Joint with Ceramic Synthetic Substitute, Uncemented, Open Approach
0SRB03Z	Replacement of Left Hip Joint with Ceramic Synthetic Substitute, Open Approach
0SRB049	Replacement of Left Hip Joint with Ceramic on Polyethylene Synthetic Substitute, Cemented, Open Approach
0SRB04A	Replacement of Left Hip Joint with Ceramic on Polyethylene Synthetic Substitute, Uncemented, Open Approach
0SRB04Z	Replacement of Left Hip Joint with Ceramic on Polyethylene Synthetic Substitute, Open Approach
0SRB069	Replacement of Left Hip Joint with Oxidized Zirconium on Polyethylene Synthetic Substitute, Cemented, Open Approach
0SRB06A	Replacement of Left Hip Joint with Oxidized Zirconium on Polyethylene Synthetic Substitute, Uncemented, Open Approach
0SRB06Z	Replacement of Left Hip Joint with Oxidized Zirconium on Polyethylene Synthetic Substitute, Open Approach
0SRB07Z	Replacement of Left Hip Joint with Autologous Tissue Substitute, Open Approach
0SRB0EZ	Replacement of Left Hip Joint with Articulating Spacer, Open Approach
0SRB0J9	Replacement of Left Hip Joint with Synthetic Substitute, Cemented, Open Approach
0SRB0JA	Replacement of Left Hip Joint with Synthetic Substitute, Uncemented, Open Approach
0SRB0JZ	Replacement of Left Hip Joint with Synthetic Substitute, Open Approach
0SRB0KZ	Replacement of Left Hip Joint with Nonautologous Tissue Substitute, Open Approach
0SRC069	Replacement of Right Knee Joint with Oxidized Zirconium on Polyethylene Synthetic Substitute, Cemented, Open Approach
0SRC06A	Replacement of Right Knee Joint with Oxidized Zirconium on Polyethylene Synthetic Substitute, Uncemented, Open Approach
0SRC06Z	Replacement of Right Knee Joint with Oxidized Zirconium on Polyethylene Synthetic Substitute, Open Approach
0SRC07Z	Replacement of Right Knee Joint with Autologous Tissue Substitute, Open Approach
0SRC0EZ	Replacement of Right Knee Joint with Articulating Spacer, Open Approach
0SRC0J9	Replacement of Right Knee Joint with Synthetic Substitute, Cemented, Open Approach
0SRC0JA	Replacement of Right Knee Joint with Synthetic Substitute, Uncemented, Open Approach
0SRC0JZ	Replacement of Right Knee Joint with Synthetic Substitute, Open Approach
0SRC0KZ	Replacement of Right Knee Joint with Nonautologous Tissue Substitute, Open Approach
0SRC0L9	Replacement of Right Knee Joint with Medial Unicondylar Synthetic Substitute, Cemented, Open Approach
0SRC0LA	Replacement of Right Knee Joint with Medial Unicondylar Synthetic Substitute, Uncemented, Open Approach
0SRC0LZ	Replacement of Right Knee Joint with Medial Unicondylar Synthetic Substitute, Open Approach
0SRC0M9	Replacement of Right Knee Joint with Lateral Unicondylar Synthetic Substitute, Cemented, Open Approach
0SRC0MA	Replacement of Right Knee Joint with Lateral Unicondylar Synthetic Substitute, Uncemented, Open Approach
0SRC0MZ	Replacement of Right Knee Joint with Lateral Unicondylar Synthetic Substitute, Open Approach
0SRC0N9	Replacement of Right Knee Joint with Patellofemoral Synthetic Substitute, Cemented, Open Approach
0SRC0NA	Replacement of Right Knee Joint with Patellofemoral Synthetic Substitute, Uncemented, Open Approach
0SRC0NZ	Replacement of Right Knee Joint with Patellofemoral Synthetic Substitute, Open Approach

HAC 10: Deep Vein Thrombosis (DVT) or Pulmonary Embolism (PE) with Total Knee or Hip Replacement (continued)

Code	Description
0SRD069	Replacement of Left Knee Joint with Oxidized Zirconium on Polyethylene Synthetic Substitute, Cemented, Open Approach
0SRD06A	Replacement of Left Knee Joint with Oxidized Zirconium on Polyethylene Synthetic Substitute, Uncemented, Open Approach
0SRD06Z	Replacement of Left Knee Joint with Oxidized Zirconium on Polyethylene Synthetic Substitute, Open Approach
0SRD07Z	Replacement of Left Knee Joint with Autologous Tissue Substitute, Open Approach
0SRD0EZ	Replacement of Left Knee Joint with Articulating Spacer, Open Approach
0SRD0J9	Replacement of Left Knee Joint with Synthetic Substitute, Cemented, Open Approach
0SRD0JA	Replacement of Left Knee Joint with Synthetic Substitute, Uncemented, Open Approach
0SRD0JZ	Replacement of Left Knee Joint with Synthetic Substitute, Open Approach
0SRD0KZ	Replacement of Left Knee Joint with Nonautologous Tissue Substitute, Open Approach
0SRD0L9	Replacement of Left Knee Joint with Medial Unicondylar Synthetic Substitute, Cemented, Open Approach
0SRD0LA	Replacement of Left Knee Joint with Medial Unicondylar Synthetic Substitute, Uncemented, Open Approach
0SRD0LZ	Replacement of Left Knee Joint with Medial Unicondylar Synthetic Substitute, Open Approach
0SRD0M9	Replacement of Left Knee Joint with Lateral Unicondylar Synthetic Substitute, Cemented, Open Approach
0SRD0MA	Replacement of Left Knee Joint with Lateral Unicondylar Synthetic Substitute, Uncemented, Open Approach
0SRD0MZ	Replacement of Left Knee Joint with Lateral Unicondylar Synthetic Substitute, Open Approach
0SRD0N9	Replacement of Left Knee Joint with Patellofemoral Synthetic Substitute, Cemented, Open Approach
0SRD0NA	Replacement of Left Knee Joint with Patellofemoral Synthetic Substitute, Uncemented, Open Approach
0SRD0NZ	Replacement of Left Knee Joint with Patellofemoral Synthetic Substitute, Open Approach
0SRE009	Replacement of Left Hip Joint, Acetabular Surface with Polyethylene Synthetic Substitute, Cemented, Open Approach
0SRE00A	Replacement of Left Hip Joint, Acetabular Surface with Polyethylene Synthetic Substitute, Uncemented, Open Approach
0SRE00Z	Replacement of Left Hip Joint, Acetabular Surface with Polyethylene Synthetic Substitute, Open Approach
0SRE019	Replacement of Left Hip Joint, Acetabular Surface with Metal Synthetic Substitute, Cemented, Open Approach
0SRE01A	Replacement of Left Hip Joint, Acetabular Surface with Metal Synthetic Substitute, Uncemented, Open Approach
0SRE01Z	Replacement of Left Hip Joint, Acetabular Surface with Metal Synthetic Substitute, Open Approach
0SRE039	Replacement of Left Hip Joint, Acetabular Surface with Ceramic Synthetic Substitute, Cemented, Open Approach
0SRE03A	Replacement of Left Hip Joint, Acetabular Surface with Ceramic Synthetic Substitute, Uncemented, Open Approach
0SRE03Z	Replacement of Left Hip Joint, Acetabular Surface with Ceramic Synthetic Substitute, Open Approach
0SRE07Z	Replacement of Left Hip Joint, Acetabular Surface with Autologous Tissue Substitute, Open Approach
0SRE0J9	Replacement of Left Hip Joint, Acetabular Surface with Synthetic Substitute, Cemented, Open Approach
0SRE0JA	Replacement of Left Hip Joint, Acetabular Surface with Synthetic Substitute, Uncemented, Open Approach
0SRE0JZ	Replacement of Left Hip Joint, Acetabular Surface with Synthetic Substitute, Open Approach
0SRE0KZ	Replacement of Left Hip Joint, Acetabular Surface with Nonautologous Tissue Substitute, Open Approach
0SRR019	Replacement of Right Hip Joint, Femoral Surface with Metal Synthetic Substitute, Cemented, Open Approach
0SRR01A	Replacement of Right Hip Joint, Femoral Surface with Metal Synthetic Substitute, Uncemented, Open Approach
0SRR01Z	Replacement of Right Hip Joint, Femoral Surface with Metal Synthetic Substitute, Open Approach
0SRR039	Replacement of Right Hip Joint, Femoral Surface with Ceramic Synthetic Substitute, Cemented, Open Approach
0SRR03A	Replacement of Right Hip Joint, Femoral Surface with Ceramic Synthetic Substitute, Uncemented, Open Approach
0SRR03Z	Replacement of Right Hip Joint, Femoral Surface with Ceramic Synthetic Substitute, Open Approach
0SRR07Z	Replacement of Right Hip Joint, Femoral Surface with Autologous Tissue Substitute, Open Approach
0SRR0J9	Replacement of Right Hip Joint, Femoral Surface with Synthetic Substitute, Cemented, Open Approach
0SRR0JA	Replacement of Right Hip Joint, Femoral Surface with Synthetic Substitute, Uncemented, Open Approach
0SRR0JZ	Replacement of Right Hip Joint, Femoral Surface with Synthetic Substitute, Open Approach
0SRR0KZ	Replacement of Right Hip Joint, Femoral Surface with Nonautologous Tissue Substitute, Open Approach
0SRS019	Replacement of Left Hip Joint, Femoral Surface with Metal Synthetic Substitute, Cemented, Open Approach
0SRS01A	Replacement of Left Hip Joint, Femoral Surface with Metal Synthetic Substitute, Uncemented, Open Approach
0SRS01Z	Replacement of Left Hip Joint, Femoral Surface with Metal Synthetic Substitute, Open Approach
0SRS039	Replacement of Left Hip Joint, Femoral Surface with Ceramic Synthetic Substitute, Cemented, Open Approach
0SRS03A	Replacement of Left Hip Joint, Femoral Surface with Ceramic Synthetic Substitute, Uncemented, Open Approach
0SRS03Z	Replacement of Left Hip Joint, Femoral Surface with Ceramic Synthetic Substitute, Open Approach
0SRS07Z	Replacement of Left Hip Joint, Femoral Surface with Autologous Tissue Substitute, Open Approach
0SRS0J9	Replacement of Left Hip Joint, Femoral Surface with Synthetic Substitute, Cemented, Open Approach
0SRS0JA	Replacement of Left Hip Joint, Femoral Surface with Synthetic Substitute, Uncemented, Open Approach
0SRS0JZ	Replacement of Left Hip Joint, Femoral Surface with Synthetic Substitute, Open Approach
0SRS0KZ	Replacement of Left Hip Joint, Femoral Surface with Nonautologous Tissue Substitute, Open Approach
0SRT07Z	Replacement of Right Knee Joint, Femoral Surface with Autologous Tissue Substitute, Open Approach
0SRT0J9	Replacement of Right Knee Joint, Femoral Surface with Synthetic Substitute, Cemented, Open Approach
0SRT0JA	Replacement of Right Knee Joint, Femoral Surface with Synthetic Substitute, Uncemented, Open Approach
0SRT0JZ	Replacement of Right Knee Joint, Femoral Surface with Synthetic Substitute, Open Approach
0SRT0KZ	Replacement of Right Knee Joint, Femoral Surface with Nonautologous Tissue Substitute, Open Approach
0SRU07Z	Replacement of Left Knee Joint, Femoral Surface with Autologous Tissue Substitute, Open Approach
0SRU0J9	Replacement of Left Knee Joint, Femoral Surface with Synthetic Substitute, Cemented, Open Approach
0SRU0JA	Replacement of Left Knee Joint, Femoral Surface with Synthetic Substitute, Uncemented, Open Approach
0SRU0JZ	Replacement of Left Knee Joint, Femoral Surface with Synthetic Substitute, Open Approach
0SRU0KZ	Replacement of Left Knee Joint, Femoral Surface with Nonautologous Tissue Substitute, Open Approach
0SRV07Z	Replacement of Right Knee Joint, Tibial Surface with Autologous Tissue Substitute, Open Approach
0SRV0J9	Replacement of Right Knee Joint, Tibial Surface with Synthetic Substitute, Cemented, Open Approach
0SRV0JA	Replacement of Right Knee Joint, Tibial Surface with Synthetic Substitute, Uncemented, Open Approach
0SRV0JZ	Replacement of Right Knee Joint, Tibial Surface with Synthetic Substitute, Open Approach
0SRV0KZ	Replacement of Right Knee Joint, Tibial Surface with Nonautologous Tissue Substitute, Open Approach
0SRW07Z	Replacement of Left Knee Joint, Tibial Surface with Autologous Tissue Substitute, Open Approach
0SRW0J9	Replacement of Left Knee Joint, Tibial Surface with Synthetic Substitute, Cemented, Open Approach
0SRW0JA	Replacement of Left Knee Joint, Tibial Surface with Synthetic Substitute, Uncemented, Open Approach
0SRW0JZ	Replacement of Left Knee Joint, Tibial Surface with Synthetic Substitute, Open Approach
0SRW0KZ	Replacement of Left Knee Joint, Tibial Surface with Nonautologous Tissue Substitute, Open Approach

Appendix K: Hospital Acquired Conditions

HAC 10: Deep Vein Thrombosis (DVT) or Pulmonary Embolism (PE) with Total Knee or Hip Replacement (continued)

Code	Description
0SU90BZ	Supplement Right Hip Joint with Resurfacing Device, Open Approach
0SUA0BZ	Supplement Right Hip Joint, Acetabular Surface with Resurfacing Device, Open Approach
0SUB0BZ	Supplement Left Hip Joint with Resurfacing Device, Open Approach
0SUE0BZ	Supplement Left Hip Joint, Acetabular Surface with Resurfacing Device, Open Approach
0SUR0BZ	Supplement Right Hip Joint, Femoral Surface with Resurfacing Device, Open Approach
0SUS0BZ	Supplement Left Hip Joint, Femoral Surface with Resurfacing Device, Open Approach
XRRG0L8	Replacement of Right Knee Joint with Synthetic Substitute, Lateral Meniscus, Open Approach, New Technology Group 8
XRRG0M8	Replacement of Right Knee Joint with Synthetic Substitute, Medial Meniscus, Open Approach, New Technology Group 8
XRRH0L8	Replacement of Left Knee Joint with Synthetic Substitute, Lateral Meniscus, Open Approach, New Technology Group 8
XRRH0M8	Replacement of Left Knee Joint with Synthetic Substitute, Medial Meniscus, Open Approach, New Technology Group 8

HAC 11: Surgical Site Infection-Bariatric Surgery

Principal diagnosis of:

Code	Description
E66.01	Morbid (severe) obesity due to excess calories

AND

Secondary diagnosis not POA:

Code	Description
K68.11	Postprocedural retroperitoneal abscess
K95.01	Infection due to gastric band procedure
K95.81	Infection due to other bariatric procedure
T81.40XA	Infection following a procedure, unspecified, initial encounter
T81.41XA	Infection following a procedure, superficial incisional surgical site, initial encounter
T81.42XA	Infection following a procedure, deep incisional surgical site, initial encounter
T81.43XA	Infection following a procedure, organ and space surgical site, initial encounter
T81.44XA	Sepsis following a procedure, initial encounter
T81.49XA	Infection following a procedure, other surgical site, initial encounter

AND

Any of the following procedures:

Code	Description
0D16079	Bypass Stomach to Duodenum with Autologous Tissue Substitute, Open Approach
0D1607A	Bypass Stomach to Jejunum with Autologous Tissue Substitute, Open Approach
0D1607B	Bypass Stomach to Ileum with Autologous Tissue Substitute, Open Approach
0D1607L	Bypass Stomach to Transverse Colon with Autologous Tissue Substitute, Open Approach
0D160J9	Bypass Stomach to Duodenum with Synthetic Substitute, Open Approach
0D160JA	Bypass Stomach to Jejunum with Synthetic Substitute, Open Approach
0D160JB	Bypass Stomach to Ileum with Synthetic Substitute, Open Approach
0D160JL	Bypass Stomach to Transverse Colon with Synthetic Substitute, Open Approach
0D160K9	Bypass Stomach to Duodenum with Nonautologous Tissue Substitute, Open Approach
0D160KA	Bypass Stomach to Jejunum with Nonautologous Tissue Substitute, Open Approach
0D160KB	Bypass Stomach to Ileum with Nonautologous Tissue Substitute, Open Approach
0D160KL	Bypass Stomach to Transverse Colon with Nonautologous Tissue Substitute, Open Approach
0D160Z9	Bypass Stomach to Duodenum, Open Approach
0D160ZA	Bypass Stomach to Jejunum, Open Approach
0D160ZB	Bypass Stomach to Ileum, Open Approach
0D160ZL	Bypass Stomach to Transverse Colon, Open Approach
0D16479	Bypass Stomach to Duodenum with Autologous Tissue Substitute, Percutaneous Endoscopic Approach
0D1647A	Bypass Stomach to Jejunum with Autologous Tissue Substitute, Percutaneous Endoscopic Approach
0D1647B	Bypass Stomach to Ileum with Autologous Tissue Substitute, Percutaneous Endoscopic Approach
0D1647L	Bypass Stomach to Transverse Colon with Autologous Tissue Substitute, Percutaneous Endoscopic Approach
0D164J9	Bypass Stomach to Duodenum with Synthetic Substitute, Percutaneous Endoscopic Approach
0D164JA	Bypass Stomach to Jejunum with Synthetic Substitute, Percutaneous Endoscopic Approach
0D164JB	Bypass Stomach to Ileum with Synthetic Substitute, Percutaneous Endoscopic Approach
0D164JL	Bypass Stomach to Transverse Colon with Synthetic Substitute, Percutaneous Endoscopic Approach
0D164K9	Bypass Stomach to Duodenum with Nonautologous Tissue Substitute, Percutaneous Endoscopic Approach
0D164KA	Bypass Stomach to Jejunum with Nonautologous Tissue Substitute, Percutaneous Endoscopic Approach
0D164KB	Bypass Stomach to Ileum with Nonautologous Tissue Substitute, Percutaneous Endoscopic Approach
0D164KL	Bypass Stomach to Transverse Colon with Nonautologous Tissue Substitute, Percutaneous Endoscopic Approach
0D164Z9	Bypass Stomach to Duodenum, Percutaneous Endoscopic Approach
0D164ZA	Bypass Stomach to Jejunum, Percutaneous Endoscopic Approach
0D164ZB	Bypass Stomach to Ileum, Percutaneous Endoscopic Approach
0D164ZL	Bypass Stomach to Transverse Colon, Percutaneous Endoscopic Approach
0D16879	Bypass Stomach to Duodenum with Autologous Tissue Substitute, Via Natural or Artificial Opening Endoscopic
0D1687A	Bypass Stomach to Jejunum with Autologous Tissue Substitute, Via Natural or Artificial Opening Endoscopic
0D1687B	Bypass Stomach to Ileum with Autologous Tissue Substitute, Via Natural or Artificial Opening Endoscopic
0D1687L	Bypass Stomach to Transverse Colon with Autologous Tissue Substitute, Via Natural or Artificial Opening Endoscopic
0D168J9	Bypass Stomach to Duodenum with Synthetic Substitute, Via Natural or Artificial Opening Endoscopic
0D168JA	Bypass Stomach to Jejunum with Synthetic Substitute, Via Natural or Artificial Opening Endoscopic
0D168JB	Bypass Stomach to Ileum with Synthetic Substitute, Via Natural or Artificial Opening Endoscopic
0D168JL	Bypass Stomach to Transverse Colon with Synthetic Substitute, Via Natural or Artificial Opening Endoscopic
0D168K9	Bypass Stomach to Duodenum with Nonautologous Tissue Substitute, Via Natural or Artificial Opening Endoscopic
0D168KA	Bypass Stomach to Jejunum with Nonautologous Tissue Substitute, Via Natural or Artificial Opening Endoscopic
0D168KB	Bypass Stomach to Ileum with Nonautologous Tissue Substitute, Via Natural or Artificial Opening Endoscopic
0D168KL	Bypass Stomach to Transverse Colon with Nonautologous Tissue Substitute, Via Natural or Artificial Opening Endoscopic
0D168Z9	Bypass Stomach to Duodenum, Via Natural or Artificial Opening Endoscopic
0D168ZA	Bypass Stomach to Jejunum, Via Natural or Artificial Opening Endoscopic
0D168ZB	Bypass Stomach to Ileum, Via Natural or Artificial Opening Endoscopic
0D168ZL	Bypass Stomach to Transverse Colon, Via Natural or Artificial Opening Endoscopic
0DV64CZ	Restriction of Stomach with Extraluminal Device, Percutaneous Endoscopic Approach

HAC 12: Surgical Site Infection-Certain Orthopedic Procedures of the Spine, Shoulder, and Elbow

Secondary diagnosis not POA:

Code	Description
K68.11	Postprocedural retroperitoneal abscess
T81.40XA	Infection following a procedure, unspecified, initial encounter
T81.41XA	Infection following a procedure, superficial incisional surgical site, initial encounter
T81.42XA	Infection following a procedure, deep incisional surgical site, initial encounter
T81.43XA	Infection following a procedure, organ and space surgical site, initial encounter
T81.44XA	Sepsis following a procedure, initial encounter
T81.49XA	Infection following a procedure, other surgical site, initial encounter
T84.60XA	Infection and inflammatory reaction due to internal fixation device of unspecified site, initial encounter
T84.610A	Infection and inflammatory reaction due to internal fixation device of right humerus, initial encounter
T84.611A	Infection and inflammatory reaction due to internal fixation device of left humerus, initial encounter
T84.612A	Infection and inflammatory reaction due to internal fixation device of right radius, initial encounter
T84.613A	Infection and inflammatory reaction due to internal fixation device of left radius, initial encounter
T84.614A	Infection and inflammatory reaction due to internal fixation device of right ulna, initial encounter
T84.615A	Infection and inflammatory reaction due to internal fixation device of left ulna, initial encounter

HAC 12: Surgical Site Infection-Certain Orthopedic Procedures of the Spine, Shoulder, and Elbow (continued)

Code	Description
T84.619A	Infection and inflammatory reaction due to internal fixation device of unspecified bone of arm, initial encounter
T84.63XA	Infection and inflammatory reaction due to internal fixation device of spine, initial encounter
T84.69XA	Infection and inflammatory reaction due to internal fixation device of other site, initial encounter
T84.7XXA	Infection and inflammatory reaction due to other internal orthopedic prosthetic devices, implants and grafts, initial encounter

AND

Any of the following procedures:

Code	Description
0RG0070	Fusion of Occipital-cervical Joint with Autologous Tissue Substitute, Anterior Approach, Anterior Column, Open Approach
0RG0071	Fusion of Occipital-cervical Joint with Autologous Tissue Substitute, Posterior Approach, Posterior Column, Open Approach
0RG007J	Fusion of Occipital-cervical Joint with Autologous Tissue Substitute, Posterior Approach, Anterior Column, Open Approach
0RG00A0	Fusion of Occipital-cervical Joint with Interbody Fusion Device, Anterior Approach, Anterior Column, Open Approach
0RG00AJ	Fusion of Occipital-cervical Joint with Interbody Fusion Device, Posterior Approach, Anterior Column, Open Approach
0RG00J0	Fusion of Occipital-cervical Joint with Synthetic Substitute, Anterior Approach, Anterior Column, Open Approach
0RG00J1	Fusion of Occipital-cervical Joint with Synthetic Substitute, Posterior Approach, Posterior Column, Open Approach
0RG00JJ	Fusion of Occipital-cervical Joint with Synthetic Substitute, Posterior Approach, Anterior Column, Open Approach
0RG00K0	Fusion of Occipital-cervical Joint with Nonautologous Tissue Substitute, Anterior Approach, Anterior Column, Open Approach
0RG00K1	Fusion of Occipital-cervical Joint with Nonautologous Tissue Substitute, Posterior Approach, Posterior Column, Open Approach
0RG00KJ	Fusion of Occipital-cervical Joint with Nonautologous Tissue Substitute, Posterior Approach, Anterior Column, Open Approach
0RG0370	Fusion of Occipital-cervical Joint with Autologous Tissue Substitute, Anterior Approach, Anterior Column, Percutaneous Approach
0RG0371	Fusion of Occipital-cervical Joint with Autologous Tissue Substitute, Posterior Approach, Posterior Column, Percutaneous Approach
0RG037J	Fusion of Occipital-cervical Joint with Autologous Tissue Substitute, Posterior Approach, Anterior Column, Percutaneous Approach
0RG03A0	Fusion of Occipital-cervical Joint with Interbody Fusion Device, Anterior Approach, Anterior Column, Percutaneous Approach
0RG03AJ	Fusion of Occipital-cervical Joint with Interbody Fusion Device, Posterior Approach, Anterior Column, Percutaneous Approach
0RG03J0	Fusion of Occipital-cervical Joint with Synthetic Substitute, Anterior Approach, Anterior Column, Percutaneous Approach
0RG03J1	Fusion of Occipital-cervical Joint with Synthetic Substitute, Posterior Approach, Posterior Column, Percutaneous Approach
0RG03JJ	Fusion of Occipital-cervical Joint with Synthetic Substitute, Posterior Approach, Anterior Column, Percutaneous Approach
0RG03K0	Fusion of Occipital-cervical Joint with Nonautologous Tissue Substitute, Anterior Approach, Anterior Column, Percutaneous Approach
0RG03K1	Fusion of Occipital-cervical Joint with Nonautologous Tissue Substitute, Posterior Approach, Posterior Column, Percutaneous Approach
0RG03KJ	Fusion of Occipital-cervical Joint with Nonautologous Tissue Substitute, Posterior Approach, Anterior Column, Percutaneous Approach
0RG0470	Fusion of Occipital-cervical Joint with Autologous Tissue Substitute, Anterior Approach, Anterior Column, Percutaneous Endoscopic Approach
0RG0471	Fusion of Occipital-cervical Joint with Autologous Tissue Substitute, Posterior Approach, Posterior Column, Percutaneous Endoscopic Approach
0RG047J	Fusion of Occipital-cervical Joint with Autologous Tissue Substitute, Posterior Approach, Anterior Column, Percutaneous Endoscopic Approach
0RG04A0	Fusion of Occipital-cervical Joint with Interbody Fusion Device, Anterior Approach, Anterior Column, Percutaneous Endoscopic Approach
0RG04AJ	Fusion of Occipital-cervical Joint with Interbody Fusion Device, Posterior Approach, Anterior Column, Percutaneous Endoscopic Approach
0RG04J0	Fusion of Occipital-cervical Joint with Synthetic Substitute, Anterior Approach, Anterior Column, Percutaneous Endoscopic Approach
0RG04J1	Fusion of Occipital-cervical Joint with Synthetic Substitute, Posterior Approach, Posterior Column, Percutaneous Endoscopic Approach
0RG04JJ	Fusion of Occipital-cervical Joint with Synthetic Substitute, Posterior Approach, Anterior Column, Percutaneous Endoscopic Approach
0RG04K0	Fusion of Occipital-cervical Joint with Nonautologous Tissue Substitute, Anterior Approach, Anterior Column, Percutaneous Endoscopic Approach
0RG04K1	Fusion of Occipital-cervical Joint with Nonautologous Tissue Substitute, Posterior Approach, Posterior Column, Percutaneous Endoscopic Approach
0RG04KJ	Fusion of Occipital-cervical Joint with Nonautologous Tissue Substitute, Posterior Approach, Anterior Column, Percutaneous Endoscopic Approach
0RG1070	Fusion of Cervical Vertebral Joint with Autologous Tissue Substitute, Anterior Approach, Anterior Column, Open Approach
0RG1071	Fusion of Cervical Vertebral Joint with Autologous Tissue Substitute, Posterior Approach, Posterior Column, Open Approach
0RG107J	Fusion of Cervical Vertebral Joint with Autologous Tissue Substitute, Posterior Approach, Anterior Column, Open Approach
0RG10A0	Fusion of Cervical Vertebral Joint with Interbody Fusion Device, Anterior Approach, Anterior Column, Open Approach
0RG10AJ	Fusion of Cervical Vertebral Joint with Interbody Fusion Device, Posterior Approach, Anterior Column, Open Approach
0RG10J0	Fusion of Cervical Vertebral Joint with Synthetic Substitute, Anterior Approach, Anterior Column, Open Approach
0RG10J1	Fusion of Cervical Vertebral Joint with Synthetic Substitute, Posterior Approach, Posterior Column, Open Approach
0RG10JJ	Fusion of Cervical Vertebral Joint with Synthetic Substitute, Posterior Approach, Anterior Column, Open Approach
0RG10K0	Fusion of Cervical Vertebral Joint with Nonautologous Tissue Substitute, Anterior Approach, Anterior Column, Open Approach
0RG10K1	Fusion of Cervical Vertebral Joint with Nonautologous Tissue Substitute, Posterior Approach, Posterior Column, Open Approach
0RG10KJ	Fusion of Cervical Vertebral Joint with Nonautologous Tissue Substitute, Posterior Approach, Anterior Column, Open Approach
0RG1370	Fusion of Cervical Vertebral Joint with Autologous Tissue Substitute, Anterior Approach, Anterior Column, Percutaneous Approach
0RG1371	Fusion of Cervical Vertebral Joint with Autologous Tissue Substitute, Posterior Approach, Posterior Column, Percutaneous Approach
0RG137J	Fusion of Cervical Vertebral Joint with Autologous Tissue Substitute, Posterior Approach, Anterior Column, Percutaneous Approach
0RG13A0	Fusion of Cervical Vertebral Joint with Interbody Fusion Device, Anterior Approach, Anterior Column, Percutaneous Approach
0RG13AJ	Fusion of Cervical Vertebral Joint with Interbody Fusion Device, Posterior Approach, Anterior Column, Percutaneous Approach
0RG13J0	Fusion of Cervical Vertebral Joint with Synthetic Substitute, Anterior Approach, Anterior Column, Percutaneous Approach
0RG13J1	Fusion of Cervical Vertebral Joint with Synthetic Substitute, Posterior Approach, Posterior Column, Percutaneous Approach
0RG13JJ	Fusion of Cervical Vertebral Joint with Synthetic Substitute, Posterior Approach, Anterior Column, Percutaneous Approach
0RG13K0	Fusion of Cervical Vertebral Joint with Nonautologous Tissue Substitute, Anterior Approach, Anterior Column, Percutaneous Approach
0RG13K1	Fusion of Cervical Vertebral Joint with Nonautologous Tissue Substitute, Posterior Approach, Posterior Column, Percutaneous Approach

Appendix K: Hospital Acquired Conditions

HAC 12: Surgical Site Infection-Certain Orthopedic Procedures of the Spine, Shoulder, and Elbow (continued)

ØRG13KJ Fusion of Cervical Vertebral Joint with Nonautologous Tissue Substitute, Posterior Approach, Anterior Column, Percutaneous Approach
ØRG147Ø Fusion of Cervical Vertebral Joint with Autologous Tissue Substitute, Anterior Approach, Anterior Column, Percutaneous Endoscopic Approach
ØRG1471 Fusion of Cervical Vertebral Joint with Autologous Tissue Substitute, Posterior Approach, Posterior Column, Percutaneous Endoscopic Approach
ØRG147J Fusion of Cervical Vertebral Joint with Autologous Tissue Substitute, Posterior Approach, Anterior Column, Percutaneous Endoscopic Approach
ØRG14AØ Fusion of Cervical Vertebral Joint with Interbody Fusion Device, Anterior Approach, Anterior Column, Percutaneous Endoscopic Approach
ØRG14AJ Fusion of Cervical Vertebral Joint with Interbody Fusion Device, Posterior Approach, Anterior Column, Percutaneous Endoscopic Approach
ØRG14JØ Fusion of Cervical Vertebral Joint with Synthetic Substitute, Anterior Approach, Anterior Column, Percutaneous Endoscopic Approach
ØRG14J1 Fusion of Cervical Vertebral Joint with Synthetic Substitute, Posterior Approach, Posterior Column, Percutaneous Endoscopic Approach
ØRG14JJ Fusion of Cervical Vertebral Joint with Synthetic Substitute, Posterior Approach, Anterior Column, Percutaneous Endoscopic Approach
ØRG14KØ Fusion of Cervical Vertebral Joint with Nonautologous Tissue Substitute, Anterior Approach, Anterior Column, Percutaneous Endoscopic Approach
ØRG14K1 Fusion of Cervical Vertebral Joint with Nonautologous Tissue Substitute, Posterior Approach, Posterior Column, Percutaneous Endoscopic Approach
ØRG14KJ Fusion of Cervical Vertebral Joint with Nonautologous Tissue Substitute, Posterior Approach, Anterior Column, Percutaneous Endoscopic Approach
ØRG2Ø7Ø Fusion of 2 or more Cervical Vertebral Joints with Autologous Tissue Substitute, Anterior Approach, Anterior Column, Open Approach
ØRG2Ø71 Fusion of 2 or more Cervical Vertebral Joints with Autologous Tissue Substitute, Posterior Approach, Posterior Column, Open Approach
ØRG2Ø7J Fusion of 2 or more Cervical Vertebral Joints with Autologous Tissue Substitute, Posterior Approach, Anterior Column, Open Approach
ØRG2ØAØ Fusion of 2 or more Cervical Vertebral Joints with Interbody Fusion Device, Anterior Approach, Anterior Column, Open Approach
ØRG2ØAJ Fusion of 2 or more Cervical Vertebral Joints with Interbody Fusion Device, Posterior Approach, Anterior Column, Open Approach
ØRG2ØJØ Fusion of 2 or more Cervical Vertebral Joints with Synthetic Substitute, Anterior Approach, Anterior Column, Open Approach
ØRG2ØJ1 Fusion of 2 or more Cervical Vertebral Joints with Synthetic Substitute, Posterior Approach, Posterior Column, Open Approach
ØRG2ØJJ Fusion of 2 or more Cervical Vertebral Joints with Synthetic Substitute, Posterior Approach, Anterior Column, Open Approach
ØRG2ØKØ Fusion of 2 or more Cervical Vertebral Joints with Nonautologous Tissue Substitute, Anterior Approach, Anterior Column, Open Approach
ØRG2ØK1 Fusion of 2 or more Cervical Vertebral Joints with Nonautologous Tissue Substitute, Posterior Approach, Posterior Column, Open Approach
ØRG2ØKJ Fusion of 2 or more Cervical Vertebral Joints with Nonautologous Tissue Substitute, Posterior Approach, Anterior Column, Open Approach
ØRG237Ø Fusion of 2 or more Cervical Vertebral Joints with Autologous Tissue Substitute, Anterior Approach, Anterior Column, Percutaneous Approach
ØRG2371 Fusion of 2 or more Cervical Vertebral Joints with Autologous Tissue Substitute, Posterior Approach, Posterior Column, Percutaneous Approach
ØRG237J Fusion of 2 or more Cervical Vertebral Joints with Autologous Tissue Substitute, Posterior Approach, Anterior Column, Percutaneous Approach
ØRG23AØ Fusion of 2 or more Cervical Vertebral Joints with Interbody Fusion Device, Anterior Approach, Anterior Column, Percutaneous Approach
ØRG23AJ Fusion of 2 or more Cervical Vertebral Joints with Interbody Fusion Device, Posterior Approach, Anterior Column, Percutaneous Approach
ØRG23JØ Fusion of 2 or more Cervical Vertebral Joints with Synthetic Substitute, Anterior Approach, Anterior Column, Percutaneous Approach
ØRG23J1 Fusion of 2 or more Cervical Vertebral Joints with Synthetic Substitute, Posterior Approach, Posterior Column, Percutaneous Approach
ØRG23JJ Fusion of 2 or more Cervical Vertebral Joints with Synthetic Substitute, Posterior Approach, Anterior Column, Percutaneous Approach
ØRG23KØ Fusion of 2 or more Cervical Vertebral Joints with Nonautologous Tissue Substitute, Anterior Approach, Anterior Column, Percutaneous Approach
ØRG23K1 Fusion of 2 or more Cervical Vertebral Joints with Nonautologous Tissue Substitute, Posterior Approach, Posterior Column, Percutaneous Approach
ØRG23KJ Fusion of 2 or more Cervical Vertebral Joints with Nonautologous Tissue Substitute, Posterior Approach, Anterior Column, Percutaneous Approach
ØRG247Ø Fusion of 2 or more Cervical Vertebral Joints with Autologous Tissue Substitute, Anterior Approach, Anterior Column, Percutaneous Endoscopic Approach
ØRG2471 Fusion of 2 or more Cervical Vertebral Joints with Autologous Tissue Substitute, Posterior Approach, Posterior Column, Percutaneous Endoscopic Approach
ØRG247J Fusion of 2 or more Cervical Vertebral Joints with Autologous Tissue Substitute, Posterior Approach, Anterior Column, Percutaneous Endoscopic Approach
ØRG24AØ Fusion of 2 or more Cervical Vertebral Joints with Interbody Fusion Device, Anterior Approach, Anterior Column, Percutaneous Endoscopic Approach
ØRG24AJ Fusion of 2 or more Cervical Vertebral Joints with Interbody Fusion Device, Posterior Approach, Anterior Column, Percutaneous Endoscopic Approach
ØRG24JØ Fusion of 2 or more Cervical Vertebral Joints with Synthetic Substitute, Anterior Approach, Anterior Column, Percutaneous Endoscopic Approach
ØRG24J1 Fusion of 2 or more Cervical Vertebral Joints with Synthetic Substitute, Posterior Approach, Posterior Column, Percutaneous Endoscopic Approach
ØRG24JJ Fusion of 2 or more Cervical Vertebral Joints with Synthetic Substitute, Posterior Approach, Anterior Column, Percutaneous Endoscopic Approach
ØRG24KØ Fusion of 2 or more Cervical Vertebral Joints with Nonautologous Tissue Substitute, Anterior Approach, Anterior Column, Percutaneous Endoscopic Approach
ØRG24K1 Fusion of 2 or more Cervical Vertebral Joints with Nonautologous Tissue Substitute, Posterior Approach, Posterior Column, Percutaneous Endoscopic Approach
ØRG24KJ Fusion of 2 or more Cervical Vertebral Joints with Nonautologous Tissue Substitute, Posterior Approach, Anterior Column, Percutaneous Endoscopic Approach
ØRG4Ø7Ø Fusion of Cervicothoracic Vertebral Joint with Autologous Tissue Substitute, Anterior Approach, Anterior Column, Open Approach
ØRG4Ø71 Fusion of Cervicothoracic Vertebral Joint with Autologous Tissue Substitute, Posterior Approach, Posterior Column, Open Approach
ØRG4Ø7J Fusion of Cervicothoracic Vertebral Joint with Autologous Tissue Substitute, Posterior Approach, Anterior Column, Open Approach
ØRG4ØAØ Fusion of Cervicothoracic Vertebral Joint with Interbody Fusion Device, Anterior Approach, Anterior Column, Open Approach
ØRG4ØAJ Fusion of Cervicothoracic Vertebral Joint with Interbody Fusion Device, Posterior Approach, Anterior Column, Open Approach
ØRG4ØJØ Fusion of Cervicothoracic Vertebral Joint with Synthetic Substitute, Anterior Approach, Anterior Column, Open Approach
ØRG4ØJ1 Fusion of Cervicothoracic Vertebral Joint with Synthetic Substitute, Posterior Approach, Posterior Column, Open Approach
ØRG4ØJJ Fusion of Cervicothoracic Vertebral Joint with Synthetic Substitute, Posterior Approach, Anterior Column, Open Approach
ØRG4ØKØ Fusion of Cervicothoracic Vertebral Joint with Nonautologous Tissue Substitute, Anterior Approach, Anterior Column, Open Approach
ØRG4ØK1 Fusion of Cervicothoracic Vertebral Joint with Nonautologous Tissue Substitute, Posterior Approach, Posterior Column, Open Approach

HAC 12: Surgical Site Infection-Certain Orthopedic Procedures of the Spine, Shoulder, and Elbow (continued)

Code	Description
0RG40KJ	Fusion of Cervicothoracic Vertebral Joint with Nonautologous Tissue Substitute, Posterior Approach, Anterior Column, Open Approach
0RG4370	Fusion of Cervicothoracic Vertebral Joint with Autologous Tissue Substitute, Anterior Approach, Anterior Column, Percutaneous Approach
0RG4371	Fusion of Cervicothoracic Vertebral Joint with Autologous Tissue Substitute, Posterior Approach, Posterior Column, Percutaneous Approach
0RG437J	Fusion of Cervicothoracic Vertebral Joint with Autologous Tissue Substitute, Posterior Approach, Anterior Column, Percutaneous Approach
0RG43A0	Fusion of Cervicothoracic Vertebral Joint with Interbody Fusion Device, Anterior Approach, Anterior Column, Percutaneous Approach
0RG43AJ	Fusion of Cervicothoracic Vertebral Joint with Interbody Fusion Device, Posterior Approach, Anterior Column, Percutaneous Approach
0RG43J0	Fusion of Cervicothoracic Vertebral Joint with Synthetic Substitute, Anterior Approach, Anterior Column, Percutaneous Approach
0RG43J1	Fusion of Cervicothoracic Vertebral Joint with Synthetic Substitute, Posterior Approach, Posterior Column, Percutaneous Approach
0RG43JJ	Fusion of Cervicothoracic Vertebral Joint with Synthetic Substitute, Posterior Approach, Anterior Column, Percutaneous Approach
0RG43K0	Fusion of Cervicothoracic Vertebral Joint with Nonautologous Tissue Substitute, Anterior Approach, Anterior Column, Percutaneous Approach
0RG43K1	Fusion of Cervicothoracic Vertebral Joint with Nonautologous Tissue Substitute, Posterior Approach, Posterior Column, Percutaneous Approach
0RG43KJ	Fusion of Cervicothoracic Vertebral Joint with Nonautologous Tissue Substitute, Posterior Approach, Anterior Column, Percutaneous Approach
0RG4470	Fusion of Cervicothoracic Vertebral Joint with Autologous Tissue Substitute, Anterior Approach, Anterior Column, Percutaneous Endoscopic Approach
0RG4471	Fusion of Cervicothoracic Vertebral Joint with Autologous Tissue Substitute, Posterior Approach, Posterior Column, Percutaneous Endoscopic Approach
0RG447J	Fusion of Cervicothoracic Vertebral Joint with Autologous Tissue Substitute, Posterior Approach, Anterior Column, Percutaneous Endoscopic Approach
0RG44A0	Fusion of Cervicothoracic Vertebral Joint with Interbody Fusion Device, Anterior Approach, Anterior Column, Percutaneous Endoscopic Approach
0RG44AJ	Fusion of Cervicothoracic Vertebral Joint with Interbody Fusion Device, Posterior Approach, Anterior Column, Percutaneous Endoscopic Approach
0RG44J0	Fusion of Cervicothoracic Vertebral Joint with Synthetic Substitute, Anterior Approach, Anterior Column, Percutaneous Endoscopic Approach
0RG44J1	Fusion of Cervicothoracic Vertebral Joint with Synthetic Substitute, Posterior Approach, Posterior Column, Percutaneous Endoscopic Approach
0RG44JJ	Fusion of Cervicothoracic Vertebral Joint with Synthetic Substitute, Posterior Approach, Anterior Column, Percutaneous Endoscopic Approach
0RG44K0	Fusion of Cervicothoracic Vertebral Joint with Nonautologous Tissue Substitute, Anterior Approach, Anterior Column, Percutaneous Endoscopic Approach
0RG44K1	Fusion of Cervicothoracic Vertebral Joint with Nonautologous Tissue Substitute, Posterior Approach, Posterior Column, Percutaneous Endoscopic Approach
0RG44KJ	Fusion of Cervicothoracic Vertebral Joint with Nonautologous Tissue Substitute, Posterior Approach, Anterior Column, Percutaneous Endoscopic Approach
0RG6070	Fusion of Thoracic Vertebral Joint with Autologous Tissue Substitute, Anterior Approach, Anterior Column, Open Approach
0RG6071	Fusion of Thoracic Vertebral Joint with Autologous Tissue Substitute, Posterior Approach, Posterior Column, Open Approach
0RG607J	Fusion of Thoracic Vertebral Joint with Autologous Tissue Substitute, Posterior Approach, Anterior Column, Open Approach
0RG60A0	Fusion of Thoracic Vertebral Joint with Interbody Fusion Device, Anterior Approach, Anterior Column, Open Approach
0RG60AJ	Fusion of Thoracic Vertebral Joint with Interbody Fusion Device, Posterior Approach, Anterior Column, Open Approach
0RG60J0	Fusion of Thoracic Vertebral Joint with Synthetic Substitute, Anterior Approach, Anterior Column, Open Approach
0RG60J1	Fusion of Thoracic Vertebral Joint with Synthetic Substitute, Posterior Approach, Posterior Column, Open Approach
0RG60JJ	Fusion of Thoracic Vertebral Joint with Synthetic Substitute, Posterior Approach, Anterior Column, Open Approach
0RG60K0	Fusion of Thoracic Vertebral Joint with Nonautologous Tissue Substitute, Anterior Approach, Anterior Column, Open Approach
0RG60K1	Fusion of Thoracic Vertebral Joint with Nonautologous Tissue Substitute, Posterior Approach, Posterior Column, Open Approach
0RG60KJ	Fusion of Thoracic Vertebral Joint with Nonautologous Tissue Substitute, Posterior Approach, Anterior Column, Open Approach
0RG6370	Fusion of Thoracic Vertebral Joint with Autologous Tissue Substitute, Anterior Approach, Anterior Column, Percutaneous Approach
0RG6371	Fusion of Thoracic Vertebral Joint with Autologous Tissue Substitute, Posterior Approach, Posterior Column, Percutaneous Approach
0RG637J	Fusion of Thoracic Vertebral Joint with Autologous Tissue Substitute, Posterior Approach, Anterior Column, Percutaneous Approach
0RG63A0	Fusion of Thoracic Vertebral Joint with Interbody Fusion Device, Anterior Approach, Anterior Column, Percutaneous Approach
0RG63AJ	Fusion of Thoracic Vertebral Joint with Interbody Fusion Device, Posterior Approach, Anterior Column, Percutaneous Approach
0RG63J0	Fusion of Thoracic Vertebral Joint with Synthetic Substitute, Anterior Approach, Anterior Column, Percutaneous Approach
0RG63J1	Fusion of Thoracic Vertebral Joint with Synthetic Substitute, Posterior Approach, Posterior Column, Percutaneous Approach
0RG63JJ	Fusion of Thoracic Vertebral Joint with Synthetic Substitute, Posterior Approach, Anterior Column, Percutaneous Approach
0RG63K0	Fusion of Thoracic Vertebral Joint with Nonautologous Tissue Substitute, Anterior Approach, Anterior Column, Percutaneous Approach
0RG63K1	Fusion of Thoracic Vertebral Joint with Nonautologous Tissue Substitute, Posterior Approach, Posterior Column, Percutaneous Approach
0RG63KJ	Fusion of Thoracic Vertebral Joint with Nonautologous Tissue Substitute, Posterior Approach, Anterior Column, Percutaneous Approach
0RG6470	Fusion of Thoracic Vertebral Joint with Autologous Tissue Substitute, Anterior Approach, Anterior Column, Percutaneous Endoscopic Approach
0RG6471	Fusion of Thoracic Vertebral Joint with Autologous Tissue Substitute, Posterior Approach, Posterior Column, Percutaneous Endoscopic Approach
0RG647J	Fusion of Thoracic Vertebral Joint with Autologous Tissue Substitute, Posterior Approach, Anterior Column, Percutaneous Endoscopic Approach
0RG64A0	Fusion of Thoracic Vertebral Joint with Interbody Fusion Device, Anterior Approach, Anterior Column, Percutaneous Endoscopic Approach
0RG64AJ	Fusion of Thoracic Vertebral Joint with Interbody Fusion Device, Posterior Approach, Anterior Column, Percutaneous Endoscopic Approach
0RG64J0	Fusion of Thoracic Vertebral Joint with Synthetic Substitute, Anterior Approach, Anterior Column, Percutaneous Endoscopic Approach
0RG64J1	Fusion of Thoracic Vertebral Joint with Synthetic Substitute, Posterior Approach, Posterior Column, Percutaneous Endoscopic Approach
0RG64JJ	Fusion of Thoracic Vertebral Joint with Synthetic Substitute, Posterior Approach, Anterior Column, Percutaneous Endoscopic Approach
0RG64K0	Fusion of Thoracic Vertebral Joint with Nonautologous Tissue Substitute, Anterior Approach, Anterior Column, Percutaneous Endoscopic Approach
0RG64K1	Fusion of Thoracic Vertebral Joint with Nonautologous Tissue Substitute, Posterior Approach, Posterior Column, Percutaneous Endoscopic Approach
0RG64KJ	Fusion of Thoracic Vertebral Joint with Nonautologous Tissue Substitute, Posterior Approach, Anterior Column, Percutaneous Endoscopic Approach

Appendix K: Hospital Acquired Conditions

HAC 12: Surgical Site Infection-Certain Orthopedic Procedures of the Spine, Shoulder, and Elbow (continued)

Code	Description
0RG7070	Fusion of 2 to 7 Thoracic Vertebral Joints with Autologous Tissue Substitute, Anterior Approach, Anterior Column, Open Approach
0RG7071	Fusion of 2 to 7 Thoracic Vertebral Joints with Autologous Tissue Substitute, Posterior Approach, Posterior Column, Open Approach
0RG707J	Fusion of 2 to 7 Thoracic Vertebral Joints with Autologous Tissue Substitute, Posterior Approach, Anterior Column, Open Approach
0RG70A0	Fusion of 2 to 7 Thoracic Vertebral Joints with Interbody Fusion Device, Anterior Approach, Anterior Column, Open Approach
0RG70AJ	Fusion of 2 to 7 Thoracic Vertebral Joints with Interbody Fusion Device, Posterior Approach, Anterior Column, Open Approach
0RG70J0	Fusion of 2 to 7 Thoracic Vertebral Joints with Synthetic Substitute, Anterior Approach, Anterior Column, Open Approach
0RG70J1	Fusion of 2 to 7 Thoracic Vertebral Joints with Synthetic Substitute, Posterior Approach, Posterior Column, Open Approach
0RG70JJ	Fusion of 2 to 7 Thoracic Vertebral Joints with Synthetic Substitute, Posterior Approach, Anterior Column, Open Approach
0RG70K0	Fusion of 2 to 7 Thoracic Vertebral Joints with Nonautologous Tissue Substitute, Anterior Approach, Anterior Column, Open Approach
0RG70K1	Fusion of 2 to 7 Thoracic Vertebral Joints with Nonautologous Tissue Substitute, Posterior Approach, Posterior Column, Open Approach
0RG70KJ	Fusion of 2 to 7 Thoracic Vertebral Joints with Nonautologous Tissue Substitute, Posterior Approach, Anterior Column, Open Approach
0RG7370	Fusion of 2 to 7 Thoracic Vertebral Joints with Autologous Tissue Substitute, Anterior Approach, Anterior Column, Percutaneous Approach
0RG7371	Fusion of 2 to 7 Thoracic Vertebral Joints with Autologous Tissue Substitute, Posterior Approach, Posterior Column, Percutaneous Approach
0RG737J	Fusion of 2 to 7 Thoracic Vertebral Joints with Autologous Tissue Substitute, Posterior Approach, Anterior Column, Percutaneous Approach
0RG73A0	Fusion of 2 to 7 Thoracic Vertebral Joints with Interbody Fusion Device, Anterior Approach, Anterior Column, Percutaneous Approach
0RG73AJ	Fusion of 2 to 7 Thoracic Vertebral Joints with Interbody Fusion Device, Posterior Approach, Anterior Column, Percutaneous Approach
0RG73J0	Fusion of 2 to 7 Thoracic Vertebral Joints with Synthetic Substitute, Anterior Approach, Anterior Column, Percutaneous Approach
0RG73J1	Fusion of 2 to 7 Thoracic Vertebral Joints with Synthetic Substitute, Posterior Approach, Posterior Column, Percutaneous Approach
0RG73JJ	Fusion of 2 to 7 Thoracic Vertebral Joints with Synthetic Substitute, Posterior Approach, Anterior Column, Percutaneous Approach
0RG73K0	Fusion of 2 to 7 Thoracic Vertebral Joints with Nonautologous Tissue Substitute, Anterior Approach, Anterior Column, Percutaneous Approach
0RG73K1	Fusion of 2 to 7 Thoracic Vertebral Joints with Nonautologous Tissue Substitute, Posterior Approach, Posterior Column, Percutaneous Approach
0RG73KJ	Fusion of 2 to 7 Thoracic Vertebral Joints with Nonautologous Tissue Substitute, Posterior Approach, Anterior Column, Percutaneous Approach
0RG7470	Fusion of 2 to 7 Thoracic Vertebral Joints with Autologous Tissue Substitute, Anterior Approach, Anterior Column, Percutaneous Endoscopic Approach
0RG7471	Fusion of 2 to 7 Thoracic Vertebral Joints with Autologous Tissue Substitute, Posterior Approach, Posterior Column, Percutaneous Endoscopic Approach
0RG747J	Fusion of 2 to 7 Thoracic Vertebral Joints with Autologous Tissue Substitute, Posterior Approach, Anterior Column, Percutaneous Endoscopic Approach
0RG74A0	Fusion of 2 to 7 Thoracic Vertebral Joints with Interbody Fusion Device, Anterior Approach, Anterior Column, Percutaneous Endoscopic Approach
0RG74AJ	Fusion of 2 to 7 Thoracic Vertebral Joints with Interbody Fusion Device, Posterior Approach, Anterior Column, Percutaneous Endoscopic Approach
0RG74J0	Fusion of 2 to 7 Thoracic Vertebral Joints with Synthetic Substitute, Anterior Approach, Anterior Column, Percutaneous Endoscopic Approach
0RG74J1	Fusion of 2 to 7 Thoracic Vertebral Joints with Synthetic Substitute, Posterior Approach, Posterior Column, Percutaneous Endoscopic Approach
0RG74JJ	Fusion of 2 to 7 Thoracic Vertebral Joints with Synthetic Substitute, Posterior Approach, Anterior Column, Percutaneous Endoscopic Approach
0RG74K0	Fusion of 2 to 7 Thoracic Vertebral Joints with Nonautologous Tissue Substitute, Anterior Approach, Anterior Column, Percutaneous Endoscopic Approach
0RG74K1	Fusion of 2 to 7 Thoracic Vertebral Joints with Nonautologous Tissue Substitute, Posterior Approach, Posterior Column, Percutaneous Endoscopic Approach
0RG74KJ	Fusion of 2 to 7 Thoracic Vertebral Joints with Nonautologous Tissue Substitute, Posterior Approach, Anterior Column, Percutaneous Endoscopic Approach
0RG8070	Fusion of 8 or More Thoracic Vertebral Joints with Autologous Tissue Substitute, Anterior Approach, Anterior Column, Open Approach
0RG8071	Fusion of 8 or More Thoracic Vertebral Joints with Autologous Tissue Substitute, Posterior Approach, Posterior Column, Open Approach
0RG807J	Fusion of 8 or More Thoracic Vertebral Joints with Autologous Tissue Substitute, Posterior Approach, Anterior Column, Open Approach
0RG80A0	Fusion of 8 or More Thoracic Vertebral Joints with Interbody Fusion Device, Anterior Approach, Anterior Column, Open Approach
0RG80AJ	Fusion of 8 or More Thoracic Vertebral Joints with Interbody Fusion Device, Posterior Approach, Anterior Column, Open Approach
0RG80J0	Fusion of 8 or More Thoracic Vertebral Joints with Synthetic Substitute, Anterior Approach, Anterior Column, Open Approach
0RG80J1	Fusion of 8 or More Thoracic Vertebral Joints with Synthetic Substitute, Posterior Approach, Posterior Column, Open Approach
0RG80JJ	Fusion of 8 or More Thoracic Vertebral Joints with Synthetic Substitute, Posterior Approach, Anterior Column, Open Approach
0RG80K0	Fusion of 8 or More Thoracic Vertebral Joints with Nonautologous Tissue Substitute, Anterior Approach, Anterior Column, Open Approach
0RG80K1	Fusion of 8 or More Thoracic Vertebral Joints with Nonautologous Tissue Substitute, Posterior Approach, Posterior Column, Open Approach
0RG80KJ	Fusion of 8 or More Thoracic Vertebral Joints with Nonautologous Tissue Substitute, Posterior Approach, Anterior Column, Open Approach
0RG8370	Fusion of 8 or More Thoracic Vertebral Joints with Autologous Tissue Substitute, Anterior Approach, Anterior Column, Percutaneous Approach
0RG8371	Fusion of 8 or More Thoracic Vertebral Joints with Autologous Tissue Substitute, Posterior Approach, Posterior Column, Percutaneous Approach
0RG837J	Fusion of 8 or More Thoracic Vertebral Joints with Autologous Tissue Substitute, Posterior Approach, Anterior Column, Percutaneous Approach
0RG83A0	Fusion of 8 or More Thoracic Vertebral Joints with Interbody Fusion Device, Anterior Approach, Anterior Column, Percutaneous Approach
0RG83AJ	Fusion of 8 or More Thoracic Vertebral Joints with Interbody Fusion Device, Posterior Approach, Anterior Column, Percutaneous Approach
0RG83J0	Fusion of 8 or More Thoracic Vertebral Joints with Synthetic Substitute, Anterior Approach, Anterior Column, Percutaneous Approach
0RG83J1	Fusion of 8 or More Thoracic Vertebral Joints with Synthetic Substitute, Posterior Approach, Posterior Column, Percutaneous Approach
0RG83JJ	Fusion of 8 or More Thoracic Vertebral Joints with Synthetic Substitute, Posterior Approach, Anterior Column, Percutaneous Approach
0RG83K0	Fusion of 8 or More Thoracic Vertebral Joints with Nonautologous Tissue Substitute, Anterior Approach, Anterior Column, Percutaneous Approach
0RG83K1	Fusion of 8 or More Thoracic Vertebral Joints with Nonautologous Tissue Substitute, Posterior Approach, Posterior Column, Percutaneous Approach
0RG83KJ	Fusion of 8 or More Thoracic Vertebral Joints with Nonautologous Tissue Substitute, Posterior Approach, Anterior Column, Percutaneous Approach
0RG8470	Fusion of 8 or More Thoracic Vertebral Joints with Autologous Tissue Substitute, Anterior Approach, Anterior Column, Percutaneous Endoscopic Approach

HAC 12: Surgical Site Infection-Certain Orthopedic Procedures of the Spine, Shoulder, and Elbow (continued)

ØRG8471 Fusion of 8 or More Thoracic Vertebral Joints with Autologous Tissue Substitute, Posterior Approach, Posterior Column, Percutaneous Endoscopic Approach
ØRG847J Fusion of 8 or More Thoracic Vertebral Joints with Autologous Tissue Substitute, Posterior Approach, Anterior Column, Percutaneous Endoscopic Approach
ØRG84AØ Fusion of 8 or More Thoracic Vertebral Joints with Interbody Fusion Device, Anterior Approach, Anterior Column, Percutaneous Endoscopic Approach
ØRG84AJ Fusion of 8 or More Thoracic Vertebral Joints with Interbody Fusion Device, Posterior Approach, Anterior Column, Percutaneous Endoscopic Approach
ØRG84JØ Fusion of 8 or More Thoracic Vertebral Joints with Synthetic Substitute, Anterior Approach, Anterior Column, Percutaneous Endoscopic Approach
ØRG84J1 Fusion of 8 or More Thoracic Vertebral Joints with Synthetic Substitute, Posterior Approach, Posterior Column, Percutaneous Endoscopic Approach
ØRG84JJ Fusion of 8 or More Thoracic Vertebral Joints with Synthetic Substitute, Posterior Approach, Anterior Column, Percutaneous Endoscopic Approach
ØRG84KØ Fusion of 8 or More Thoracic Vertebral Joints with Nonautologous Tissue Substitute, Anterior Approach, Anterior Column, Percutaneous Endoscopic Approach
ØRG84K1 Fusion of 8 or More Thoracic Vertebral Joints with Nonautologous Tissue Substitute, Posterior Approach, Posterior Column, Percutaneous Endoscopic Approach
ØRG84KJ Fusion of 8 or More Thoracic Vertebral Joints with Nonautologous Tissue Substitute, Posterior Approach, Anterior Column, Percutaneous Endoscopic Approach
ØRGAØ7Ø Fusion of Thoracolumbar Vertebral Joint with Autologous Tissue Substitute, Anterior Approach, Anterior Column, Open Approach
ØRGAØ71 Fusion of Thoracolumbar Vertebral Joint with Autologous Tissue Substitute, Posterior Approach, Posterior Column, Open Approach
ØRGAØ7J Fusion of Thoracolumbar Vertebral Joint with Autologous Tissue Substitute, Posterior Approach, Anterior Column, Open Approach
ØRGAØAØ Fusion of Thoracolumbar Vertebral Joint with Interbody Fusion Device, Anterior Approach, Anterior Column, Open Approach
ØRGAØAJ Fusion of Thoracolumbar Vertebral Joint with Interbody Fusion Device, Posterior Approach, Anterior Column, Open Approach
ØRGAØJØ Fusion of Thoracolumbar Vertebral Joint with Synthetic Substitute, Anterior Approach, Anterior Column, Open Approach
ØRGAØJ1 Fusion of Thoracolumbar Vertebral Joint with Synthetic Substitute, Posterior Approach, Posterior Column, Open Approach
ØRGAØJJ Fusion of Thoracolumbar Vertebral Joint with Synthetic Substitute, Posterior Approach, Anterior Column, Open Approach
ØRGAØKØ Fusion of Thoracolumbar Vertebral Joint with Nonautologous Tissue Substitute, Anterior Approach, Anterior Column, Open Approach
ØRGAØK1 Fusion of Thoracolumbar Vertebral Joint with Nonautologous Tissue Substitute, Posterior Approach, Posterior Column, Open Approach
ØRGAØKJ Fusion of Thoracolumbar Vertebral Joint with Nonautologous Tissue Substitute, Posterior Approach, Anterior Column, Open Approach
ØRGA37Ø Fusion of Thoracolumbar Vertebral Joint with Autologous Tissue Substitute, Anterior Approach, Anterior Column, Percutaneous Approach
ØRGA371 Fusion of Thoracolumbar Vertebral Joint with Autologous Tissue Substitute, Posterior Approach, Posterior Column, Percutaneous Approach
ØRGA37J Fusion of Thoracolumbar Vertebral Joint with Autologous Tissue Substitute, Posterior Approach, Anterior Column, Percutaneous Approach
ØRGA3AØ Fusion of Thoracolumbar Vertebral Joint with Interbody Fusion Device, Anterior Approach, Anterior Column, Percutaneous Approach
ØRGA3AJ Fusion of Thoracolumbar Vertebral Joint with Interbody Fusion Device, Posterior Approach, Anterior Column, Percutaneous Approach
ØRGA3JØ Fusion of Thoracolumbar Vertebral Joint with Synthetic Substitute, Anterior Approach, Anterior Column, Percutaneous Approach
ØRGA3J1 Fusion of Thoracolumbar Vertebral Joint with Synthetic Substitute, Posterior Approach, Posterior Column, Percutaneous Approach
ØRGA3JJ Fusion of Thoracolumbar Vertebral Joint with Synthetic Substitute, Posterior Approach, Anterior Column, Percutaneous Approach
ØRGA3KØ Fusion of Thoracolumbar Vertebral Joint with Nonautologous Tissue Substitute, Anterior Approach, Anterior Column, Percutaneous Approach
ØRGA3K1 Fusion of Thoracolumbar Vertebral Joint with Nonautologous Tissue Substitute, Posterior Approach, Posterior Column, Percutaneous Approach
ØRGA3KJ Fusion of Thoracolumbar Vertebral Joint with Nonautologous Tissue Substitute, Posterior Approach, Anterior Column, Percutaneous Approach
ØRGA47Ø Fusion of Thoracolumbar Vertebral Joint with Autologous Tissue Substitute, Anterior Approach, Anterior Column, Percutaneous Endoscopic Approach
ØRGA471 Fusion of Thoracolumbar Vertebral Joint with Autologous Tissue Substitute, Posterior Approach, Posterior Column, Percutaneous Endoscopic Approach
ØRGA47J Fusion of Thoracolumbar Vertebral Joint with Autologous Tissue Substitute, Posterior Approach, Anterior Column, Percutaneous Endoscopic Approach
ØRGA4AØ Fusion of Thoracolumbar Vertebral Joint with Interbody Fusion Device, Anterior Approach, Anterior Column, Percutaneous Endoscopic Approach
ØRGA4AJ Fusion of Thoracolumbar Vertebral Joint with Interbody Fusion Device, Posterior Approach, Anterior Column, Percutaneous Endoscopic Approach
ØRGA4JØ Fusion of Thoracolumbar Vertebral Joint with Synthetic Substitute, Anterior Approach, Anterior Column, Percutaneous Endoscopic Approach
ØRGA4J1 Fusion of Thoracolumbar Vertebral Joint with Synthetic Substitute, Posterior Approach, Posterior Column, Percutaneous Endoscopic Approach
ØRGA4JJ Fusion of Thoracolumbar Vertebral Joint with Synthetic Substitute, Posterior Approach, Anterior Column, Percutaneous Endoscopic Approach
ØRGA4KØ Fusion of Thoracolumbar Vertebral Joint with Nonautologous Tissue Substitute, Anterior Approach, Anterior Column, Percutaneous Endoscopic Approach
ØRGA4K1 Fusion of Thoracolumbar Vertebral Joint with Nonautologous Tissue Substitute, Posterior Approach, Posterior Column, Percutaneous Endoscopic Approach
ØRGA4KJ Fusion of Thoracolumbar Vertebral Joint with Nonautologous Tissue Substitute, Posterior Approach, Anterior Column, Percutaneous Endoscopic Approach
ØRGEØ4Z Fusion of Right Sternoclavicular Joint with Internal Fixation Device, Open Approach
ØRGEØ7Z Fusion of Right Sternoclavicular Joint with Autologous Tissue Substitute, Open Approach
ØRGEØJZ Fusion of Right Sternoclavicular Joint with Synthetic Substitute, Open Approach
ØRGEØKZ Fusion of Right Sternoclavicular Joint with Nonautologous Tissue Substitute, Open Approach
ØRGE34Z Fusion of Right Sternoclavicular Joint with Internal Fixation Device, Percutaneous Approach
ØRGE37Z Fusion of Right Sternoclavicular Joint with Autologous Tissue Substitute, Percutaneous Approach
ØRGE3JZ Fusion of Right Sternoclavicular Joint with Synthetic Substitute, Percutaneous Approach
ØRGE3KZ Fusion of Right Sternoclavicular Joint with Nonautologous Tissue Substitute, Percutaneous Approach
ØRGE44Z Fusion of Right Sternoclavicular Joint with Internal Fixation Device, Percutaneous Endoscopic Approach
ØRGE47Z Fusion of Right Sternoclavicular Joint with Autologous Tissue Substitute, Percutaneous Endoscopic Approach
ØRGE4JZ Fusion of Right Sternoclavicular Joint with Synthetic Substitute, Percutaneous Endoscopic Approach
ØRGE4KZ Fusion of Right Sternoclavicular Joint with Nonautologous Tissue Substitute, Percutaneous Endoscopic Approach
ØRGFØ4Z Fusion of Left Sternoclavicular Joint with Internal Fixation Device, Open Approach
ØRGFØ7Z Fusion of Left Sternoclavicular Joint with Autologous Tissue Substitute, Open Approach
ØRGFØJZ Fusion of Left Sternoclavicular Joint with Synthetic Substitute, Open Approach
ØRGFØKZ Fusion of Left Sternoclavicular Joint with Nonautologous Tissue Substitute, Open Approach
ØRGF34Z Fusion of Left Sternoclavicular Joint with Internal Fixation Device, Percutaneous Approach

Appendix K: Hospital Acquired Conditions

HAC 12: Surgical Site Infection-Certain Orthopedic Procedures of the Spine, Shoulder, and Elbow (continued)

0RGF37Z Fusion of Left Sternoclavicular Joint with Autologous Tissue Substitute, Percutaneous Approach
0RGF3JZ Fusion of Left Sternoclavicular Joint with Synthetic Substitute, Percutaneous Approach
0RGF3KZ Fusion of Left Sternoclavicular Joint with Nonautologous Tissue Substitute, Percutaneous Approach
0RGF44Z Fusion of Left Sternoclavicular Joint with Internal Fixation Device, Percutaneous Endoscopic Approach
0RGF47Z Fusion of Left Sternoclavicular Joint with Autologous Tissue Substitute, Percutaneous Endoscopic Approach
0RGF4JZ Fusion of Left Sternoclavicular Joint with Synthetic Substitute, Percutaneous Endoscopic Approach
0RGF4KZ Fusion of Left Sternoclavicular Joint with Nonautologous Tissue Substitute, Percutaneous Endoscopic Approach
0RGG04Z Fusion of Right Acromioclavicular Joint with Internal Fixation Device, Open Approach
0RGG07Z Fusion of Right Acromioclavicular Joint with Autologous Tissue Substitute, Open Approach
0RGG0JZ Fusion of Right Acromioclavicular Joint with Synthetic Substitute, Open Approach
0RGG0KZ Fusion of Right Acromioclavicular Joint with Nonautologous Tissue Substitute, Open Approach
0RGG34Z Fusion of Right Acromioclavicular Joint with Internal Fixation Device, Percutaneous Approach
0RGG37Z Fusion of Right Acromioclavicular Joint with Autologous Tissue Substitute, Percutaneous Approach
0RGG3JZ Fusion of Right Acromioclavicular Joint with Synthetic Substitute, Percutaneous Approach
0RGG3KZ Fusion of Right Acromioclavicular Joint with Nonautologous Tissue Substitute, Percutaneous Approach
0RGG44Z Fusion of Right Acromioclavicular Joint with Internal Fixation Device, Percutaneous Endoscopic Approach
0RGG47Z Fusion of Right Acromioclavicular Joint with Autologous Tissue Substitute, Percutaneous Endoscopic Approach
0RGG4JZ Fusion of Right Acromioclavicular Joint with Synthetic Substitute, Percutaneous Endoscopic Approach
0RGG4KZ Fusion of Right Acromioclavicular Joint with Nonautologous Tissue Substitute, Percutaneous Endoscopic Approach
0RGH04Z Fusion of Left Acromioclavicular Joint with Internal Fixation Device, Open Approach
0RGH07Z Fusion of Left Acromioclavicular Joint with Autologous Tissue Substitute, Open Approach
0RGH0JZ Fusion of Left Acromioclavicular Joint with Synthetic Substitute, Open Approach
0RGH0KZ Fusion of Left Acromioclavicular Joint with Nonautologous Tissue Substitute, Open Approach
0RGH34Z Fusion of Left Acromioclavicular Joint with Internal Fixation Device, Percutaneous Approach
0RGH37Z Fusion of Left Acromioclavicular Joint with Autologous Tissue Substitute, Percutaneous Approach
0RGH3JZ Fusion of Left Acromioclavicular Joint with Synthetic Substitute, Percutaneous Approach
0RGH3KZ Fusion of Left Acromioclavicular Joint with Nonautologous Tissue Substitute, Percutaneous Approach
0RGH44Z Fusion of Left Acromioclavicular Joint with Internal Fixation Device, Percutaneous Endoscopic Approach
0RGH47Z Fusion of Left Acromioclavicular Joint with Autologous Tissue Substitute, Percutaneous Endoscopic Approach
0RGH4JZ Fusion of Left Acromioclavicular Joint with Synthetic Substitute, Percutaneous Endoscopic Approach
0RGH4KZ Fusion of Left Acromioclavicular Joint with Nonautologous Tissue Substitute, Percutaneous Endoscopic Approach
0RGJ04Z Fusion of Right Shoulder Joint with Internal Fixation Device, Open Approach
0RGJ07Z Fusion of Right Shoulder Joint with Autologous Tissue Substitute, Open Approach
0RGJ0JZ Fusion of Right Shoulder Joint with Synthetic Substitute, Open Approach
0RGJ0KZ Fusion of Right Shoulder Joint with Nonautologous Tissue Substitute, Open Approach
0RGJ34Z Fusion of Right Shoulder Joint with Internal Fixation Device, Percutaneous Approach
0RGJ37Z Fusion of Right Shoulder Joint with Autologous Tissue Substitute, Percutaneous Approach
0RGJ3JZ Fusion of Right Shoulder Joint with Synthetic Substitute, Percutaneous Approach
0RGJ3KZ Fusion of Right Shoulder Joint with Nonautologous Tissue Substitute, Percutaneous Approach
0RGJ44Z Fusion of Right Shoulder Joint with Internal Fixation Device, Percutaneous Endoscopic Approach
0RGJ47Z Fusion of Right Shoulder Joint with Autologous Tissue Substitute, Percutaneous Endoscopic Approach
0RGJ4JZ Fusion of Right Shoulder Joint with Synthetic Substitute, Percutaneous Endoscopic Approach
0RGJ4KZ Fusion of Right Shoulder Joint with Nonautologous Tissue Substitute, Percutaneous Endoscopic Approach
0RGK04Z Fusion of Left Shoulder Joint with Internal Fixation Device, Open Approach
0RGK07Z Fusion of Left Shoulder Joint with Autologous Tissue Substitute, Open Approach
0RGK0JZ Fusion of Left Shoulder Joint with Synthetic Substitute, Open Approach
0RGK0KZ Fusion of Left Shoulder Joint with Nonautologous Tissue Substitute, Open Approach
0RGK34Z Fusion of Left Shoulder Joint with Internal Fixation Device, Percutaneous Approach
0RGK37Z Fusion of Left Shoulder Joint with Autologous Tissue Substitute, Percutaneous Approach
0RGK3JZ Fusion of Left Shoulder Joint with Synthetic Substitute, Percutaneous Approach
0RGK3KZ Fusion of Left Shoulder Joint with Nonautologous Tissue Substitute, Percutaneous Approach
0RGK44Z Fusion of Left Shoulder Joint with Internal Fixation Device, Percutaneous Endoscopic Approach
0RGK47Z Fusion of Left Shoulder Joint with Autologous Tissue Substitute, Percutaneous Endoscopic Approach
0RGK4JZ Fusion of Left Shoulder Joint with Synthetic Substitute, Percutaneous Endoscopic Approach
0RGK4KZ Fusion of Left Shoulder Joint with Nonautologous Tissue Substitute, Percutaneous Endoscopic Approach
0RGL03Z Fusion of Right Elbow Joint with Sustained Compression Internal Fixation Device, Open Approach
0RGL04Z Fusion of Right Elbow Joint with Internal Fixation Device, Open Approach
0RGL05Z Fusion of Right Elbow Joint with External Fixation Device, Open Approach
0RGL07Z Fusion of Right Elbow Joint with Autologous Tissue Substitute, Open Approach
0RGL0JZ Fusion of Right Elbow Joint with Synthetic Substitute, Open Approach
0RGL0KZ Fusion of Right Elbow Joint with Nonautologous Tissue Substitute, Open Approach
0RGL33Z Fusion of Right Elbow Joint with Sustained Compression Internal Fixation Device, Percutaneous Approach
0RGL34Z Fusion of Right Elbow Joint with Internal Fixation Device, Percutaneous Approach
0RGL35Z Fusion of Right Elbow Joint with External Fixation Device, Percutaneous Approach
0RGL37Z Fusion of Right Elbow Joint with Autologous Tissue Substitute, Percutaneous Approach
0RGL3JZ Fusion of Right Elbow Joint with Synthetic Substitute, Percutaneous Approach
0RGL3KZ Fusion of Right Elbow Joint with Nonautologous Tissue Substitute, Percutaneous Approach
0RGL43Z Fusion of Right Elbow Joint with Sustained Compression Internal Fixation Device, Percutaneous Endoscopic Approach
0RGL44Z Fusion of Right Elbow Joint with Internal Fixation Device, Percutaneous Endoscopic Approach
0RGL45Z Fusion of Right Elbow Joint with External Fixation Device, Percutaneous Endoscopic Approach
0RGL47Z Fusion of Right Elbow Joint with Autologous Tissue Substitute, Percutaneous Endoscopic Approach
0RGL4JZ Fusion of Right Elbow Joint with Synthetic Substitute, Percutaneous Endoscopic Approach
0RGL4KZ Fusion of Right Elbow Joint with Nonautologous Tissue Substitute, Percutaneous Endoscopic Approach
0RGM03Z Fusion of Left Elbow Joint with Sustained Compression Internal Fixation Device, Open Approach
0RGM04Z Fusion of Left Elbow Joint with Internal Fixation Device, Open Approach
0RGM05Z Fusion of Left Elbow Joint with External Fixation Device, Open Approach
0RGM07Z Fusion of Left Elbow Joint with Autologous Tissue Substitute, Open Approach
0RGM0JZ Fusion of Left Elbow Joint with Synthetic Substitute, Open Approach
0RGM0KZ Fusion of Left Elbow Joint with Nonautologous Tissue Substitute, Open Approach
0RGM33Z Fusion of Left Elbow Joint with Sustained Compression Internal Fixation Device, Percutaneous Approach
0RGM34Z Fusion of Left Elbow Joint with Internal Fixation Device, Percutaneous Approach

HAC 12: Surgical Site Infection-Certain Orthopedic Procedures of the Spine, Shoulder, and Elbow (continued)

Code	Description
0RGM35Z	Fusion of Left Elbow Joint with External Fixation Device, Percutaneous Approach
0RGM37Z	Fusion of Left Elbow Joint with Autologous Tissue Substitute, Percutaneous Approach
0RGM3JZ	Fusion of Left Elbow Joint with Synthetic Substitute, Percutaneous Approach
0RGM3KZ	Fusion of Left Elbow Joint with Nonautologous Tissue Substitute, Percutaneous Approach
0RGM43Z	Fusion of Left Elbow Joint with Sustained Compression Internal Fixation Device, Percutaneous Endoscopic Approach
0RGM44Z	Fusion of Left Elbow Joint with Internal Fixation Device, Percutaneous Endoscopic Approach
0RGM45Z	Fusion of Left Elbow Joint with External Fixation Device, Percutaneous Endoscopic Approach
0RGM47Z	Fusion of Left Elbow Joint with Autologous Tissue Substitute, Percutaneous Endoscopic Approach
0RGM4JZ	Fusion of Left Elbow Joint with Synthetic Substitute, Percutaneous Endoscopic Approach
0RGM4KZ	Fusion of Left Elbow Joint with Nonautologous Tissue Substitute, Percutaneous Endoscopic Approach
0RQE0ZZ	Repair Right Sternoclavicular Joint, Open Approach
0RQE3ZZ	Repair Right Sternoclavicular Joint, Percutaneous Approach
0RQE4ZZ	Repair Right Sternoclavicular Joint, Percutaneous Endoscopic Approach
0RQEXZZ	Repair Right Sternoclavicular Joint, External Approach
0RQF0ZZ	Repair Left Sternoclavicular Joint, Open Approach
0RQF3ZZ	Repair Left Sternoclavicular Joint, Percutaneous Approach
0RQF4ZZ	Repair Left Sternoclavicular Joint, Percutaneous Endoscopic Approach
0RQFXZZ	Repair Left Sternoclavicular Joint, External Approach
0RQG0ZZ	Repair Right Acromioclavicular Joint, Open Approach
0RQG3ZZ	Repair Right Acromioclavicular Joint, Percutaneous Approach
0RQG4ZZ	Repair Right Acromioclavicular Joint, Percutaneous Endoscopic Approach
0RQGXZZ	Repair Right Acromioclavicular Joint, External Approach
0RQH0ZZ	Repair Left Acromioclavicular Joint, Open Approach
0RQH3ZZ	Repair Left Acromioclavicular Joint, Percutaneous Approach
0RQH4ZZ	Repair Left Acromioclavicular Joint, Percutaneous Endoscopic Approach
0RQHXZZ	Repair Left Acromioclavicular Joint, External Approach
0RQJ0ZZ	Repair Right Shoulder Joint, Open Approach
0RQJ3ZZ	Repair Right Shoulder Joint, Percutaneous Approach
0RQJ4ZZ	Repair Right Shoulder Joint, Percutaneous Endoscopic Approach
0RQJXZZ	Repair Right Shoulder Joint, External Approach
0RQK0ZZ	Repair Left Shoulder Joint, Open Approach
0RQK3ZZ	Repair Left Shoulder Joint, Percutaneous Approach
0RQK4ZZ	Repair Left Shoulder Joint, Percutaneous Endoscopic Approach
0RQKXZZ	Repair Left Shoulder Joint, External Approach
0RQL0ZZ	Repair Right Elbow Joint, Open Approach
0RQL3ZZ	Repair Right Elbow Joint, Percutaneous Approach
0RQL4ZZ	Repair Right Elbow Joint, Percutaneous Endoscopic Approach
0RQLXZZ	Repair Right Elbow Joint, External Approach
0RQM0ZZ	Repair Left Elbow Joint, Open Approach
0RQM3ZZ	Repair Left Elbow Joint, Percutaneous Approach
0RQM4ZZ	Repair Left Elbow Joint, Percutaneous Endoscopic Approach
0RQMXZZ	Repair Left Elbow Joint, External Approach
0RUE07Z	Supplement Right Sternoclavicular Joint with Autologous Tissue Substitute, Open Approach
0RUE0JZ	Supplement Right Sternoclavicular Joint with Synthetic Substitute, Open Approach
0RUE0KZ	Supplement Right Sternoclavicular Joint with Nonautologous Tissue Substitute, Open Approach
0RUE37Z	Supplement Right Sternoclavicular Joint with Autologous Tissue Substitute, Percutaneous Approach
0RUE3JZ	Supplement Right Sternoclavicular Joint with Synthetic Substitute, Percutaneous Approach
0RUE3KZ	Supplement Right Sternoclavicular Joint with Nonautologous Tissue Substitute, Percutaneous Approach
0RUE47Z	Supplement Right Sternoclavicular Joint with Autologous Tissue Substitute, Percutaneous Endoscopic Approach
0RUE4JZ	Supplement Right Sternoclavicular Joint with Synthetic Substitute, Percutaneous Endoscopic Approach
0RUE4KZ	Supplement Right Sternoclavicular Joint with Nonautologous Tissue Substitute, Percutaneous Endoscopic Approach
0RUF07Z	Supplement Left Sternoclavicular Joint with Autologous Tissue Substitute, Open Approach
0RUF0JZ	Supplement Left Sternoclavicular Joint with Synthetic Substitute, Open Approach
0RUF0KZ	Supplement Left Sternoclavicular Joint with Nonautologous Tissue Substitute, Open Approach
0RUF37Z	Supplement Left Sternoclavicular Joint with Autologous Tissue Substitute, Percutaneous Approach
0RUF3JZ	Supplement Left Sternoclavicular Joint with Synthetic Substitute, Percutaneous Approach
0RUF3KZ	Supplement Left Sternoclavicular Joint with Nonautologous Tissue Substitute, Percutaneous Approach
0RUF47Z	Supplement Left Sternoclavicular Joint with Autologous Tissue Substitute, Percutaneous Endoscopic Approach
0RUF4JZ	Supplement Left Sternoclavicular Joint with Synthetic Substitute, Percutaneous Endoscopic Approach
0RUF4KZ	Supplement Left Sternoclavicular Joint with Nonautologous Tissue Substitute, Percutaneous Endoscopic Approach
0RUG07Z	Supplement Right Acromioclavicular Joint with Autologous Tissue Substitute, Open Approach
0RUG0JZ	Supplement Right Acromioclavicular Joint with Synthetic Substitute, Open Approach
0RUG0KZ	Supplement Right Acromioclavicular Joint with Nonautologous Tissue Substitute, Open Approach
0RUG37Z	Supplement Right Acromioclavicular Joint with Autologous Tissue Substitute, Percutaneous Approach
0RUG3JZ	Supplement Right Acromioclavicular Joint with Synthetic Substitute, Percutaneous Approach
0RUG3KZ	Supplement Right Acromioclavicular Joint with Nonautologous Tissue Substitute, Percutaneous Approach
0RUG47Z	Supplement Right Acromioclavicular Joint with Autologous Tissue Substitute, Percutaneous Endoscopic Approach
0RUG4JZ	Supplement Right Acromioclavicular Joint with Synthetic Substitute, Percutaneous Endoscopic Approach
0RUG4KZ	Supplement Right Acromioclavicular Joint with Nonautologous Tissue Substitute, Percutaneous Endoscopic Approach
0RUH07Z	Supplement Left Acromioclavicular Joint with Autologous Tissue Substitute, Open Approach
0RUH0JZ	Supplement Left Acromioclavicular Joint with Synthetic Substitute, Open Approach
0RUH0KZ	Supplement Left Acromioclavicular Joint with Nonautologous Tissue Substitute, Open Approach
0RUH37Z	Supplement Left Acromioclavicular Joint with Autologous Tissue Substitute, Percutaneous Approach
0RUH3JZ	Supplement Left Acromioclavicular Joint with Synthetic Substitute, Percutaneous Approach
0RUH3KZ	Supplement Left Acromioclavicular Joint with Nonautologous Tissue Substitute, Percutaneous Approach
0RUH47Z	Supplement Left Acromioclavicular Joint with Autologous Tissue Substitute, Percutaneous Endoscopic Approach
0RUH4JZ	Supplement Left Acromioclavicular Joint with Synthetic Substitute, Percutaneous Endoscopic Approach
0RUH4KZ	Supplement Left Acromioclavicular Joint with Nonautologous Tissue Substitute, Percutaneous Endoscopic Approach
0RUJ07Z	Supplement Right Shoulder Joint with Autologous Tissue Substitute, Open Approach
0RUJ0JZ	Supplement Right Shoulder Joint with Synthetic Substitute, Open Approach
0RUJ0KZ	Supplement Right Shoulder Joint with Nonautologous Tissue Substitute, Open Approach
0RUJ37Z	Supplement Right Shoulder Joint with Autologous Tissue Substitute, Percutaneous Approach
0RUJ3JZ	Supplement Right Shoulder Joint with Synthetic Substitute, Percutaneous Approach
0RUJ3KZ	Supplement Right Shoulder Joint with Nonautologous Tissue Substitute, Percutaneous Approach
0RUJ47Z	Supplement Right Shoulder Joint with Autologous Tissue Substitute, Percutaneous Endoscopic Approach
0RUJ4JZ	Supplement Right Shoulder Joint with Synthetic Substitute, Percutaneous Endoscopic Approach
0RUJ4KZ	Supplement Right Shoulder Joint with Nonautologous Tissue Substitute, Percutaneous Endoscopic Approach
0RUK07Z	Supplement Left Shoulder Joint with Autologous Tissue Substitute, Open Approach
0RUK0JZ	Supplement Left Shoulder Joint with Synthetic Substitute, Open Approach

Appendix K: Hospital Acquired Conditions

HAC 12: Surgical Site Infection-Certain Orthopedic Procedures of the Spine, Shoulder, and Elbow (continued)

Code	Description
0RUK0KZ	Supplement Left Shoulder Joint with Nonautologous Tissue Substitute, Open Approach
0RUK37Z	Supplement Left Shoulder Joint with Autologous Tissue Substitute, Percutaneous Approach
0RUK3JZ	Supplement Left Shoulder Joint with Synthetic Substitute, Percutaneous Approach
0RUK3KZ	Supplement Left Shoulder Joint with Nonautologous Tissue Substitute, Percutaneous Approach
0RUK47Z	Supplement Left Shoulder Joint with Autologous Tissue Substitute, Percutaneous Endoscopic Approach
0RUK4JZ	Supplement Left Shoulder Joint with Synthetic Substitute, Percutaneous Endoscopic Approach
0RUK4KZ	Supplement Left Shoulder Joint with Nonautologous Tissue Substitute, Percutaneous Endoscopic Approach
0RUL07Z	Supplement Right Elbow Joint with Autologous Tissue Substitute, Open Approach
0RUL0JZ	Supplement Right Elbow Joint with Synthetic Substitute, Open Approach
0RUL0KZ	Supplement Right Elbow Joint with Nonautologous Tissue Substitute, Open Approach
0RUL37Z	Supplement Right Elbow Joint with Autologous Tissue Substitute, Percutaneous Approach
0RUL3JZ	Supplement Right Elbow Joint with Synthetic Substitute, Percutaneous Approach
0RUL3KZ	Supplement Right Elbow Joint with Nonautologous Tissue Substitute, Percutaneous Approach
0RUL47Z	Supplement Right Elbow Joint with Autologous Tissue Substitute, Percutaneous Endoscopic Approach
0RUL4JZ	Supplement Right Elbow Joint with Synthetic Substitute, Percutaneous Endoscopic Approach
0RUL4KZ	Supplement Right Elbow Joint with Nonautologous Tissue Substitute, Percutaneous Endoscopic Approach
0RUM07Z	Supplement Left Elbow Joint with Autologous Tissue Substitute, Open Approach
0RUM0JZ	Supplement Left Elbow Joint with Synthetic Substitute, Open Approach
0RUM0KZ	Supplement Left Elbow Joint with Nonautologous Tissue Substitute, Open Approach
0RUM37Z	Supplement Left Elbow Joint with Autologous Tissue Substitute, Percutaneous Approach
0RUM3JZ	Supplement Left Elbow Joint with Synthetic Substitute, Percutaneous Approach
0RUM3KZ	Supplement Left Elbow Joint with Nonautologous Tissue Substitute, Percutaneous Approach
0RUM47Z	Supplement Left Elbow Joint with Autologous Tissue Substitute, Percutaneous Endoscopic Approach
0RUM4JZ	Supplement Left Elbow Joint with Synthetic Substitute, Percutaneous Endoscopic Approach
0RUM4KZ	Supplement Left Elbow Joint with Nonautologous Tissue Substitute, Percutaneous Endoscopic Approach
0SG0070	Fusion of Lumbar Vertebral Joint with Autologous Tissue Substitute, Anterior Approach, Anterior Column, Open Approach
0SG0071	Fusion of Lumbar Vertebral Joint with Autologous Tissue Substitute, Posterior Approach, Posterior Column, Open Approach
0SG007J	Fusion of Lumbar Vertebral Joint with Autologous Tissue Substitute, Posterior Approach, Anterior Column, Open Approach
0SG00A0	Fusion of Lumbar Vertebral Joint with Interbody Fusion Device, Anterior Approach, Anterior Column, Open Approach
0SG00AJ	Fusion of Lumbar Vertebral Joint with Interbody Fusion Device, Posterior Approach, Anterior Column, Open Approach
0SG00J0	Fusion of Lumbar Vertebral Joint with Synthetic Substitute, Anterior Approach, Anterior Column, Open Approach
0SG00J1	Fusion of Lumbar Vertebral Joint with Synthetic Substitute, Posterior Approach, Posterior Column, Open Approach
0SG00JJ	Fusion of Lumbar Vertebral Joint with Synthetic Substitute, Posterior Approach, Anterior Column, Open Approach
0SG00K0	Fusion of Lumbar Vertebral Joint with Nonautologous Tissue Substitute, Anterior Approach, Anterior Column, Open Approach
0SG00K1	Fusion of Lumbar Vertebral Joint with Nonautologous Tissue Substitute, Posterior Approach, Posterior Column, Open Approach
0SG00KJ	Fusion of Lumbar Vertebral Joint with Nonautologous Tissue Substitute, Posterior Approach, Anterior Column, Open Approach
0SG0370	Fusion of Lumbar Vertebral Joint with Autologous Tissue Substitute, Anterior Approach, Anterior Column, Percutaneous Approach
0SG0371	Fusion of Lumbar Vertebral Joint with Autologous Tissue Substitute, Posterior Approach, Posterior Column, Percutaneous Approach
0SG037J	Fusion of Lumbar Vertebral Joint with Autologous Tissue Substitute, Posterior Approach, Anterior Column, Percutaneous Approach
0SG03A0	Fusion of Lumbar Vertebral Joint with Interbody Fusion Device, Anterior Approach, Anterior Column, Percutaneous Approach
0SG03AJ	Fusion of Lumbar Vertebral Joint with Interbody Fusion Device, Posterior Approach, Anterior Column, Percutaneous Approach
0SG03J0	Fusion of Lumbar Vertebral Joint with Synthetic Substitute, Anterior Approach, Anterior Column, Percutaneous Approach
0SG03J1	Fusion of Lumbar Vertebral Joint with Synthetic Substitute, Posterior Approach, Posterior Column, Percutaneous Approach
0SG03JJ	Fusion of Lumbar Vertebral Joint with Synthetic Substitute, Posterior Approach, Anterior Column, Percutaneous Approach
0SG03K0	Fusion of Lumbar Vertebral Joint with Nonautologous Tissue Substitute, Anterior Approach, Anterior Column, Percutaneous Approach
0SG03K1	Fusion of Lumbar Vertebral Joint with Nonautologous Tissue Substitute, Posterior Approach, Posterior Column, Percutaneous Approach
0SG03KJ	Fusion of Lumbar Vertebral Joint with Nonautologous Tissue Substitute, Posterior Approach, Anterior Column, Percutaneous Approach
0SG0470	Fusion of Lumbar Vertebral Joint with Autologous Tissue Substitute, Anterior Approach, Anterior Column, Percutaneous Endoscopic Approach
0SG0471	Fusion of Lumbar Vertebral Joint with Autologous Tissue Substitute, Posterior Approach, Posterior Column, Percutaneous Endoscopic Approach
0SG047J	Fusion of Lumbar Vertebral Joint with Autologous Tissue Substitute, Posterior Approach, Anterior Column, Percutaneous Endoscopic Approach
0SG04A0	Fusion of Lumbar Vertebral Joint with Interbody Fusion Device, Anterior Approach, Anterior Column, Percutaneous Endoscopic Approach
0SG04AJ	Fusion of Lumbar Vertebral Joint with Interbody Fusion Device, Posterior Approach, Anterior Column, Percutaneous Endoscopic Approach
0SG04J0	Fusion of Lumbar Vertebral Joint with Synthetic Substitute, Anterior Approach, Anterior Column, Percutaneous Endoscopic Approach
0SG04J1	Fusion of Lumbar Vertebral Joint with Synthetic Substitute, Posterior Approach, Posterior Column, Percutaneous Endoscopic Approach
0SG04JJ	Fusion of Lumbar Vertebral Joint with Synthetic Substitute, Posterior Approach, Anterior Column, Percutaneous Endoscopic Approach
0SG04K0	Fusion of Lumbar Vertebral Joint with Nonautologous Tissue Substitute, Anterior Approach, Anterior Column, Percutaneous Endoscopic Approach
0SG04K1	Fusion of Lumbar Vertebral Joint with Nonautologous Tissue Substitute, Posterior Approach, Posterior Column, Percutaneous Endoscopic Approach
0SG04KJ	Fusion of Lumbar Vertebral Joint with Nonautologous Tissue Substitute, Posterior Approach, Anterior Column, Percutaneous Endoscopic Approach
0SG1070	Fusion of 2 or More Lumbar Vertebral Joints with Autologous Tissue Substitute, Anterior Approach, Anterior Column, Open Approach
0SG1071	Fusion of 2 or More Lumbar Vertebral Joints with Autologous Tissue Substitute, Posterior Approach, Posterior Column, Open Approach
0SG107J	Fusion of 2 or More Lumbar Vertebral Joints with Autologous Tissue Substitute, Posterior Approach, Anterior Column, Open Approach
0SG10A0	Fusion of 2 or More Lumbar Vertebral Joints with Interbody Fusion Device, Anterior Approach, Anterior Column, Open Approach
0SG10AJ	Fusion of 2 or More Lumbar Vertebral Joints with Interbody Fusion Device, Posterior Approach, Anterior Column, Open Approach
0SG10J0	Fusion of 2 or More Lumbar Vertebral Joints with Synthetic Substitute, Anterior Approach, Anterior Column, Open Approach

HAC 12: Surgical Site Infection-Certain Orthopedic Procedures of the Spine, Shoulder, and Elbow (continued)

Code	Description
0SG10J1	Fusion of 2 or More Lumbar Vertebral Joints with Synthetic Substitute, Posterior Approach, Posterior Column, Open Approach
0SG10JJ	Fusion of 2 or More Lumbar Vertebral Joints with Synthetic Substitute, Posterior Approach, Anterior Column, Open Approach
0SG10K0	Fusion of 2 or More Lumbar Vertebral Joints with Nonautologous Tissue Substitute, Anterior Approach, Anterior Column, Open Approach
0SG10K1	Fusion of 2 or More Lumbar Vertebral Joints with Nonautologous Tissue Substitute, Posterior Approach, Posterior Column, Open Approach
0SG10KJ	Fusion of 2 or More Lumbar Vertebral Joints with Nonautologous Tissue Substitute, Posterior Approach, Anterior Column, Open Approach
0SG1370	Fusion of 2 or More Lumbar Vertebral Joints with Autologous Tissue Substitute, Anterior Approach, Anterior Column, Percutaneous Approach
0SG1371	Fusion of 2 or More Lumbar Vertebral Joints with Autologous Tissue Substitute, Posterior Approach, Posterior Column, Percutaneous Approach
0SG137J	Fusion of 2 or More Lumbar Vertebral Joints with Autologous Tissue Substitute, Posterior Approach, Anterior Column, Percutaneous Approach
0SG13A0	Fusion of 2 or More Lumbar Vertebral Joints with Interbody Fusion Device, Anterior Approach, Anterior Column, Percutaneous Approach
0SG13AJ	Fusion of 2 or More Lumbar Vertebral Joints with Interbody Fusion Device, Posterior Approach, Anterior Column, Percutaneous Approach
0SG13J0	Fusion of 2 or More Lumbar Vertebral Joints with Synthetic Substitute, Anterior Approach, Anterior Column, Percutaneous Approach
0SG13J1	Fusion of 2 or More Lumbar Vertebral Joints with Synthetic Substitute, Posterior Approach, Posterior Column, Percutaneous Approach
0SG13JJ	Fusion of 2 or More Lumbar Vertebral Joints with Synthetic Substitute, Posterior Approach, Anterior Column, Percutaneous Approach
0SG13K0	Fusion of 2 or More Lumbar Vertebral Joints with Nonautologous Tissue Substitute, Anterior Approach, Anterior Column, Percutaneous Approach
0SG13K1	Fusion of 2 or More Lumbar Vertebral Joints with Nonautologous Tissue Substitute, Posterior Approach, Posterior Column, Percutaneous Approach
0SG13KJ	Fusion of 2 or More Lumbar Vertebral Joints with Nonautologous Tissue Substitute, Posterior Approach, Anterior Column, Percutaneous Approach
0SG1470	Fusion of 2 or More Lumbar Vertebral Joints with Autologous Tissue Substitute, Anterior Approach, Anterior Column, Percutaneous Endoscopic Approach
0SG1471	Fusion of 2 or More Lumbar Vertebral Joints with Autologous Tissue Substitute, Posterior Approach, Posterior Column, Percutaneous Endoscopic Approach
0SG147J	Fusion of 2 or More Lumbar Vertebral Joints with Autologous Tissue Substitute, Posterior Approach, Anterior Column, Percutaneous Endoscopic Approach
0SG14A0	Fusion of 2 or More Lumbar Vertebral Joints with Interbody Fusion Device, Anterior Approach, Anterior Column, Percutaneous Endoscopic Approach
0SG14AJ	Fusion of 2 or More Lumbar Vertebral Joints with Interbody Fusion Device, Posterior Approach, Anterior Column, Percutaneous Endoscopic Approach
0SG14J0	Fusion of 2 or More Lumbar Vertebral Joints with Synthetic Substitute, Anterior Approach, Anterior Column, Percutaneous Endoscopic Approach
0SG14J1	Fusion of 2 or More Lumbar Vertebral Joints with Synthetic Substitute, Posterior Approach, Posterior Column, Percutaneous Endoscopic Approach
0SG14JJ	Fusion of 2 or More Lumbar Vertebral Joints with Synthetic Substitute, Posterior Approach, Anterior Column, Percutaneous Endoscopic Approach
0SG14K0	Fusion of 2 or More Lumbar Vertebral Joints with Nonautologous Tissue Substitute, Anterior Approach, Anterior Column, Percutaneous Endoscopic Approach
0SG14K1	Fusion of 2 or More Lumbar Vertebral Joints with Nonautologous Tissue Substitute, Posterior Approach, Posterior Column, Percutaneous Endoscopic Approach
0SG14KJ	Fusion of 2 or More Lumbar Vertebral Joints with Nonautologous Tissue Substitute, Posterior Approach, Anterior Column, Percutaneous Endoscopic Approach
0SG3070	Fusion of Lumbosacral Joint with Autologous Tissue Substitute, Anterior Approach, Anterior Column, Open Approach
0SG3071	Fusion of Lumbosacral Joint with Autologous Tissue Substitute, Posterior Approach, Posterior Column, Open Approach
0SG307J	Fusion of Lumbosacral Joint with Autologous Tissue Substitute, Posterior Approach, Anterior Column, Open Approach
0SG30A0	Fusion of Lumbosacral Joint with Interbody Fusion Device, Anterior Approach, Anterior Column, Open Approach
0SG30AJ	Fusion of Lumbosacral Joint with Interbody Fusion Device, Posterior Approach, Anterior Column, Open Approach
0SG30J0	Fusion of Lumbosacral Joint with Synthetic Substitute, Anterior Approach, Anterior Column, Open Approach
0SG30J1	Fusion of Lumbosacral Joint with Synthetic Substitute, Posterior Approach, Posterior Column, Open Approach
0SG30JJ	Fusion of Lumbosacral Joint with Synthetic Substitute, Posterior Approach, Anterior Column, Open Approach
0SG30K0	Fusion of Lumbosacral Joint with Nonautologous Tissue Substitute, Anterior Approach, Anterior Column, Open Approach
0SG30K1	Fusion of Lumbosacral Joint with Nonautologous Tissue Substitute, Posterior Approach, Posterior Column, Open Approach
0SG30KJ	Fusion of Lumbosacral Joint with Nonautologous Tissue Substitute, Posterior Approach, Anterior Column, Open Approach
0SG3370	Fusion of Lumbosacral Joint with Autologous Tissue Substitute, Anterior Approach, Anterior Column, Percutaneous Approach
0SG3371	Fusion of Lumbosacral Joint with Autologous Tissue Substitute, Posterior Approach, Posterior Column, Percutaneous Approach
0SG337J	Fusion of Lumbosacral Joint with Autologous Tissue Substitute, Posterior Approach, Anterior Column, Percutaneous Approach
0SG33A0	Fusion of Lumbosacral Joint with Interbody Fusion Device, Anterior Approach, Anterior Column, Percutaneous Approach
0SG33AJ	Fusion of Lumbosacral Joint with Interbody Fusion Device, Posterior Approach, Anterior Column, Percutaneous Approach
0SG33J0	Fusion of Lumbosacral Joint with Synthetic Substitute, Anterior Approach, Anterior Column, Percutaneous Approach
0SG33J1	Fusion of Lumbosacral Joint with Synthetic Substitute, Posterior Approach, Posterior Column, Percutaneous Approach
0SG33JJ	Fusion of Lumbosacral Joint with Synthetic Substitute, Posterior Approach, Anterior Column, Percutaneous Approach
0SG33K0	Fusion of Lumbosacral Joint with Nonautologous Tissue Substitute, Anterior Approach, Anterior Column, Percutaneous Approach
0SG33K1	Fusion of Lumbosacral Joint with Nonautologous Tissue Substitute, Posterior Approach, Posterior Column, Percutaneous Approach
0SG33KJ	Fusion of Lumbosacral Joint with Nonautologous Tissue Substitute, Posterior Approach, Anterior Column, Percutaneous Approach
0SG3470	Fusion of Lumbosacral Joint with Autologous Tissue Substitute, Anterior Approach, Anterior Column, Percutaneous Endoscopic Approach
0SG3471	Fusion of Lumbosacral Joint with Autologous Tissue Substitute, Posterior Approach, Posterior Column, Percutaneous Endoscopic Approach
0SG347J	Fusion of Lumbosacral Joint with Autologous Tissue Substitute, Posterior Approach, Anterior Column, Percutaneous Endoscopic Approach
0SG34A0	Fusion of Lumbosacral Joint with Interbody Fusion Device, Anterior Approach, Anterior Column, Percutaneous Endoscopic Approach
0SG34AJ	Fusion of Lumbosacral Joint with Interbody Fusion Device, Posterior Approach, Anterior Column, Percutaneous Endoscopic Approach
0SG34J0	Fusion of Lumbosacral Joint with Synthetic Substitute, Anterior Approach, Anterior Column, Percutaneous Endoscopic Approach
0SG34J1	Fusion of Lumbosacral Joint with Synthetic Substitute, Posterior Approach, Posterior Column, Percutaneous Endoscopic Approach

Appendix K: Hospital Acquired Conditions

HAC 12: Surgical Site Infection-Certain Orthopedic Procedures of the Spine, Shoulder, and Elbow (continued)

Code	Description
0SG34JJ	Fusion of Lumbosacral Joint with Synthetic Substitute, Posterior Approach, Anterior Column, Percutaneous Endoscopic Approach
0SG34K0	Fusion of Lumbosacral Joint with Nonautologous Tissue Substitute, Anterior Approach, Anterior Column, Percutaneous Endoscopic Approach
0SG34K1	Fusion of Lumbosacral Joint with Nonautologous Tissue Substitute, Posterior Approach, Posterior Column, Percutaneous Endoscopic Approach
0SG34KJ	Fusion of Lumbosacral Joint with Nonautologous Tissue Substitute, Posterior Approach, Anterior Column, Percutaneous Endoscopic Approach
0SG704Z	Fusion of Right Sacroiliac Joint with Internal Fixation Device, Open Approach
0SG707Z	Fusion of Right Sacroiliac Joint with Autologous Tissue Substitute, Open Approach
0SG70JZ	Fusion of Right Sacroiliac Joint with Synthetic Substitute, Open Approach
0SG70KZ	Fusion of Right Sacroiliac Joint with Nonautologous Tissue Substitute, Open Approach
0SG734Z	Fusion of Right Sacroiliac Joint with Internal Fixation Device, Percutaneous Approach
0SG737Z	Fusion of Right Sacroiliac Joint with Autologous Tissue Substitute, Percutaneous Approach
0SG73JZ	Fusion of Right Sacroiliac Joint with Synthetic Substitute, Percutaneous Approach
0SG73KZ	Fusion of Right Sacroiliac Joint with Nonautologous Tissue Substitute, Percutaneous Approach
0SG744Z	Fusion of Right Sacroiliac Joint with Internal Fixation Device, Percutaneous Endoscopic Approach
0SG747Z	Fusion of Right Sacroiliac Joint with Autologous Tissue Substitute, Percutaneous Endoscopic Approach
0SG74JZ	Fusion of Right Sacroiliac Joint with Synthetic Substitute, Percutaneous Endoscopic Approach
0SG74KZ	Fusion of Right Sacroiliac Joint with Nonautologous Tissue Substitute, Percutaneous Endoscopic Approach
0SG804Z	Fusion of Left Sacroiliac Joint with Internal Fixation Device, Open Approach
0SG807Z	Fusion of Left Sacroiliac Joint with Autologous Tissue Substitute, Open Approach
0SG80JZ	Fusion of Left Sacroiliac Joint with Synthetic Substitute, Open Approach
0SG80KZ	Fusion of Left Sacroiliac Joint with Nonautologous Tissue Substitute, Open Approach
0SG834Z	Fusion of Left Sacroiliac Joint with Internal Fixation Device, Percutaneous Approach
0SG837Z	Fusion of Left Sacroiliac Joint with Autologous Tissue Substitute, Percutaneous Approach
0SG83JZ	Fusion of Left Sacroiliac Joint with Synthetic Substitute, Percutaneous Approach
0SG83KZ	Fusion of Left Sacroiliac Joint with Nonautologous Tissue Substitute, Percutaneous Approach
0SG844Z	Fusion of Left Sacroiliac Joint with Internal Fixation Device, Percutaneous Endoscopic Approach
0SG847Z	Fusion of Left Sacroiliac Joint with Autologous Tissue Substitute, Percutaneous Endoscopic Approach
0SG84JZ	Fusion of Left Sacroiliac Joint with Synthetic Substitute, Percutaneous Endoscopic Approach
0SG84KZ	Fusion of Left Sacroiliac Joint with Nonautologous Tissue Substitute, Percutaneous Endoscopic Approach
XRGA0R7	Fusion of Thoracolumbar Vertebral Joint using Custom-Made Anatomically Designed Interbody Fusion Device, Open Approach, New Technology Group 7
XRGA3R7	Fusion of Thoracolumbar Vertebral Joint using Custom-Made Anatomically Designed Interbody Fusion Device, Percutaneous Approach, New Technology Group 7
XRGA4R7	Fusion of Thoracolumbar Vertebral Joint using Custom-Made Anatomically Designed Interbody Fusion Device, Percutaneous Endoscopic Approach, New Technology Group 7
XRGB0R7	Fusion of Lumbar Vertebral Joint using Custom-Made Anatomically Designed Interbody Fusion Device, Open Approach, New Technology Group 7
XRGB3R7	Fusion of Lumbar Vertebral Joint using Custom-Made Anatomically Designed Interbody Fusion Device, Percutaneous Approach, New Technology Group 7
XRGB4R7	Fusion of Lumbar Vertebral Joint using Custom-Made Anatomically Designed Interbody Fusion Device, Percutaneous Endoscopic Approach, New Technology Group 7
XRGC0R7	Fusion of 2 or more Lumbar Vertebral Joints using Custom-Made Anatomically Designed Interbody Fusion Device, Open Approach, New Technology Group 7
XRGC3R7	Fusion of 2 or more Lumbar Vertebral Joints using Custom-Made Anatomically Designed Interbody Fusion Device, Percutaneous Approach, New Technology Group 7
XRGC4R7	Fusion of 2 or more Lumbar Vertebral Joints using Custom-Made Anatomically Designed Interbody Fusion Device, Percutaneous Endoscopic Approach, New Technology Group 7
XRGD0R7	Fusion of Lumbosacral Joint using Custom-Made Anatomically Designed Interbody Fusion Device, Open Approach, New Technology Group 7
XRGD3R7	Fusion of Lumbosacral Joint using Custom-Made Anatomically Designed Interbody Fusion Device, Percutaneous Approach, New Technology Group 7
XRGD4R7	Fusion of Lumbosacral Joint using Custom-Made Anatomically Designed Interbody Fusion Device, Percutaneous Endoscopic Approach, New Technology Group 7
XRGE058	Fusion of Right Sacroiliac Joint using Internal Fixation Device with Tulip Connector, Open Approach, New Technology Group 8
XRGE358	Fusion of Right Sacroiliac Joint using Internal Fixation Device with Tulip Connector, Percutaneous Approach, New Technology Group 8
XRGF058	Fusion of Left Sacroiliac Joint using Internal Fixation Device with Tulip Connector, Open Approach, New Technology Group 8
XRGF358	Fusion of Left Sacroiliac Joint using Internal Fixation Device with Tulip Connector, Percutaneous Approach, New Technology Group 8

HAC 13: Surgical Site Infection (SSI) Following Cardiac Implantable Electronic Device (CIED) Procedures

Secondary diagnosis not POA:

Code	Description
K68.11	Postprocedural retroperitoneal abscess
T81.40XA	Infection following a procedure, unspecified, initial encounter
T81.41XA	Infection following a procedure, superficial incisional surgical site, initial encounter
T81.42XA	Infection following a procedure, deep incisional surgical site, initial encounter
T81.43XA	Infection following a procedure, organ and space surgical site, initial encounter
T81.44XA	Sepsis following a procedure, initial encounter
T81.49XA	Infection following a procedure, other surgical site, initial encounter
T82.7XXA	Infection and inflammatory reaction due to other internal orthopedic prosthetic devices, implants and grafts, initial encounter

AND

Any of the following procedures:

Code	Description
02H40JZ	Insertion of Pacemaker Lead into Coronary Vein, Open Approach
02H40KZ	Insertion of Defibrillator Lead into Coronary Vein, Open Approach
02H40NZ	Insertion of Intracardiac Pacemaker into Coronary Vein, Open Approach
02H43JZ	Insertion of Pacemaker Lead into Coronary Vein, Percutaneous Approach
02H43KZ	Insertion of Defibrillator Lead into Coronary Vein, Percutaneous Approach
02H43MZ	Insertion of Cardiac Lead into Coronary Vein, Percutaneous Approach
02H43NZ	Insertion of Intracardiac Pacemaker into Coronary Vein, Percutaneous Approach
02H44JZ	Insertion of Pacemaker Lead into Coronary Vein, Percutaneous Endoscopic Approach
02H44KZ	Insertion of Defibrillator Lead into Coronary Vein, Percutaneous Endoscopic Approach
02H44NZ	Insertion of Intracardiac Pacemaker into Coronary Vein, Percutaneous Endoscopic Approach
02H60JZ	Insertion of Pacemaker Lead into Right Atrium, Open Approach
02H60KZ	Insertion of Defibrillator Lead into Right Atrium, Open Approach
02H60NZ	Insertion of Intracardiac Pacemaker into Right Atrium, Open Approach
02H63JZ	Insertion of Pacemaker Lead into Right Atrium, Percutaneous Approach
02H63KZ	Insertion of Defibrillator Lead into Right Atrium, Percutaneous Approach
02H63MZ	Insertion of Cardiac Lead into Right Atrium, Percutaneous Approach
02H63NZ	Insertion of Intracardiac Pacemaker into Right Atrium, Percutaneous Approach
02H64JZ	Insertion of Pacemaker Lead into Right Atrium, Percutaneous Endoscopic Approach
02H64KZ	Insertion of Defibrillator Lead into Right Atrium, Percutaneous Endoscopic Approach

HAC 13: Surgical Site Infection (SSI) Following Cardiac Implantable Electronic Device (CIED) Procedures (continued)

Code	Description
02H64NZ	Insertion of Intracardiac Pacemaker into Right Atrium, Percutaneous Endoscopic Approach
02H70JZ	Insertion of Pacemaker Lead into Left Atrium, Open Approach
02H70KZ	Insertion of Defibrillator Lead into Left Atrium, Open Approach
02H70NZ	Insertion of Intracardiac Pacemaker into Left Atrium, Open Approach
02H73JZ	Insertion of Pacemaker Lead into Left Atrium, Percutaneous Approach
02H73KZ	Insertion of Defibrillator Lead into Left Atrium, Percutaneous Approach
02H73MZ	Insertion of Cardiac Lead into Left Atrium, Percutaneous Approach
02H73NZ	Insertion of Intracardiac Pacemaker into Left Atrium, Percutaneous Approach
02H74JZ	Insertion of Pacemaker Lead into Left Atrium, Percutaneous Endoscopic Approach
02H74KZ	Insertion of Defibrillator Lead into Left Atrium, Percutaneous Endoscopic Approach
02H74NZ	Insertion of Intracardiac Pacemaker into Left Atrium, Percutaneous Endoscopic Approach
02HK0JZ	Insertion of Pacemaker Lead into Right Ventricle, Open Approach
02HK0KZ	Insertion of Defibrillator Lead into Right Ventricle, Open Approach
02HK0NZ	Insertion of Intracardiac Pacemaker into Right Ventricle, Open Approach
02HK3JZ	Insertion of Pacemaker Lead into Right Ventricle, Percutaneous Approach
02HK3KZ	Insertion of Defibrillator Lead into Right Ventricle, Percutaneous Approach
02HK3NZ	Insertion of Intracardiac Pacemaker into Right Ventricle, Percutaneous Approach
02HK4JZ	Insertion of Pacemaker Lead into Right Ventricle, Percutaneous Endoscopic Approach
02HK4KZ	Insertion of Defibrillator Lead into Right Ventricle, Percutaneous Endoscopic Approach
02HK4NZ	Insertion of Intracardiac Pacemaker into Right Ventricle, Percutaneous Endoscopic Approach
02HL0JZ	Insertion of Pacemaker Lead into Left Ventricle, Open Approach
02HL0KZ	Insertion of Defibrillator Lead into Left Ventricle, Open Approach
02HL0NZ	Insertion of Intracardiac Pacemaker into Left Ventricle, Open Approach
02HL3JZ	Insertion of Pacemaker Lead into Left Ventricle, Percutaneous Approach
02HL3KZ	Insertion of Defibrillator Lead into Left Ventricle, Percutaneous Approach
02HL3NZ	Insertion of Intracardiac Pacemaker into Left Ventricle, Percutaneous Approach
02HL4JZ	Insertion of Pacemaker Lead into Left Ventricle, Percutaneous Endoscopic Approach
02HL4KZ	Insertion of Defibrillator Lead into Left Ventricle, Percutaneous Endoscopic Approach
02HL4NZ	Insertion of Intracardiac Pacemaker into Left Ventricle, Percutaneous Endoscopic Approach
02HN0JZ	Insertion of Pacemaker Lead into Pericardium, Open Approach
02HN0KZ	Insertion of Defibrillator Lead into Pericardium, Open Approach
02HN0MZ	Insertion of Cardiac Lead into Pericardium, Open Approach
02HN3JZ	Insertion of Pacemaker Lead into Pericardium, Percutaneous Approach
02HN3KZ	Insertion of Defibrillator Lead into Pericardium, Percutaneous Approach
02HN3MZ	Insertion of Cardiac Lead into Pericardium, Percutaneous Approach
02HN4JZ	Insertion of Pacemaker Lead into Pericardium, Percutaneous Endoscopic Approach
02HN4KZ	Insertion of Defibrillator Lead into Pericardium, Percutaneous Endoscopic Approach
02HN4MZ	Insertion of Cardiac Lead into Pericardium, Percutaneous Endoscopic Approach
02PA0MZ	Removal of Cardiac Lead from Heart, Open Approach
02PA0NZ	Removal of Intracardiac Pacemaker from Heart, Open Approach
02PA3MZ	Removal of Cardiac Lead from Heart, Percutaneous Approach
02PA3NZ	Removal of Intracardiac Pacemaker from Heart, Percutaneous Approach
02PA4MZ	Removal of Cardiac Lead from Heart, Percutaneous Endoscopic Approach
02PA4NZ	Removal of Intracardiac Pacemaker from Heart, Percutaneous Endoscopic Approach
02PAXMZ	Removal of Cardiac Lead from Heart, External Approach
02WA0MZ	Revision of Cardiac Lead in Heart, Open Approach
02WA0NZ	Revision of Intracardiac Pacemaker in Heart, Open Approach
02WA3MZ	Revision of Cardiac Lead in Heart, Percutaneous Approach
02WA3NZ	Revision of Intracardiac Pacemaker in Heart, Percutaneous Approach
02WA4MZ	Revision of Cardiac Lead in Heart, Percutaneous Endoscopic Approach
02WA4NZ	Revision of Intracardiac Pacemaker in Heart, Percutaneous Endoscopic Approach
02WAXNZ	Revision of Intracardiac Pacemaker in Heart, External Approach
0JH604Z	Insertion of Pacemaker, Single Chamber into Chest Subcutaneous Tissue and Fascia, Open Approach
0JH605Z	Insertion of Pacemaker, Single Chamber Rate Responsive into Chest Subcutaneous Tissue and Fascia, Open Approach
0JH606Z	Insertion of Pacemaker, Dual Chamber into Chest Subcutaneous Tissue and Fascia, Open Approach
0JH607Z	Insertion of Cardiac Resynchronization Pacemaker Pulse Generator into Chest Subcutaneous Tissue and Fascia, Open Approach
0JH608Z	Insertion of Defibrillator Generator into Chest Subcutaneous Tissue and Fascia, Open Approach
0JH609Z	Insertion of Cardiac Resynchronization Defibrillator Pulse Generator into Chest Subcutaneous Tissue and Fascia, Open Approach
0JH60FZ	Insertion of Subcutaneous Defibrillator Lead into Chest Subcutaneous Tissue and Fascia, Open Approach
0JH60PZ	Insertion of Cardiac Rhythm Related Device into Chest Subcutaneous Tissue and Fascia, Open Approach
0JH634Z	Insertion of Pacemaker, Single Chamber into Chest Subcutaneous Tissue and Fascia, Percutaneous Approach
0JH635Z	Insertion of Pacemaker, Single Chamber Rate Responsive into Chest Subcutaneous Tissue and Fascia, Percutaneous Approach
0JH636Z	Insertion of Pacemaker, Dual Chamber into Chest Subcutaneous Tissue and Fascia, Percutaneous Approach
0JH637Z	Insertion of Cardiac Resynchronization Pacemaker Pulse Generator into Chest Subcutaneous Tissue and Fascia, Percutaneous Approach
0JH638Z	Insertion of Defibrillator Generator into Chest Subcutaneous Tissue and Fascia, Percutaneous Approach
0JH639Z	Insertion of Cardiac Resynchronization Defibrillator Pulse Generator into Chest Subcutaneous Tissue and Fascia, Percutaneous Approach
0JH63FZ	Insertion of Subcutaneous Defibrillator Lead into Chest Subcutaneous Tissue and Fascia, Percutaneous Approach
0JH63PZ	Insertion of Cardiac Rhythm Related Device into Chest Subcutaneous Tissue and Fascia, Percutaneous Approach
0JH804Z	Insertion of Pacemaker, Single Chamber into Abdomen Subcutaneous Tissue and Fascia, Open Approach
0JH805Z	Insertion of Pacemaker, Single Chamber Rate Responsive into Abdomen Subcutaneous Tissue and Fascia, Open Approach
0JH806Z	Insertion of Pacemaker, Dual Chamber into Abdomen Subcutaneous Tissue and Fascia, Open Approach
0JH807Z	Insertion of Cardiac Resynchronization Pacemaker Pulse Generator into Abdomen Subcutaneous Tissue and Fascia, Open Approach
0JH808Z	Insertion of Defibrillator Generator into Abdomen Subcutaneous Tissue and Fascia, Open Approach
0JH809Z	Insertion of Cardiac Resynchronization Defibrillator Pulse Generator into Abdomen Subcutaneous Tissue and Fascia, Open Approach
0JH80PZ	Insertion of Cardiac Rhythm Related Device into Abdomen Subcutaneous Tissue and Fascia, Open Approach
0JH834Z	Insertion of Pacemaker, Single Chamber into Abdomen Subcutaneous Tissue and Fascia, Percutaneous Approach
0JH835Z	Insertion of Pacemaker, Single Chamber Rate Responsive into Abdomen Subcutaneous Tissue and Fascia, Percutaneous Approach
0JH836Z	Insertion of Pacemaker, Dual Chamber into Abdomen Subcutaneous Tissue and Fascia, Percutaneous Approach
0JH837Z	Insertion of Cardiac Resynchronization Pacemaker Pulse Generator into Abdomen Subcutaneous Tissue and Fascia, Percutaneous Approach
0JH838Z	Insertion of Defibrillator Generator into Abdomen Subcutaneous Tissue and Fascia, Percutaneous Approach
0JH839Z	Insertion of Cardiac Resynchronization Defibrillator Pulse Generator into Abdomen Subcutaneous Tissue and Fascia, Percutaneous Approach
0JH83PZ	Insertion of Cardiac Rhythm Related Device into Abdomen Subcutaneous Tissue and Fascia, Percutaneous Approach
0JPT0FZ	Removal of Subcutaneous Defibrillator Lead from Trunk Subcutaneous Tissue and Fascia, Open Approach
0JPT0PZ	Removal of Cardiac Rhythm Related Device from Trunk Subcutaneous Tissue and Fascia, Open Approach

Appendix K: Hospital Acquired Conditions

HAC 13: Surgical Site Infection (SSI) Following Cardiac Implantable Electronic Device (CIED) Procedures (continued)

Code	Description
0JPT3FZ	Removal of Subcutaneous Defibrillator Lead from Trunk Subcutaneous Tissue and Fascia, Percutaneous Approach
0JPT3PZ	Removal of Cardiac Rhythm Related Device from Trunk Subcutaneous Tissue and Fascia, Percutaneous Approach
0JWT0FZ	Revision of Subcutaneous Defibrillator Lead in Trunk Subcutaneous Tissue and Fascia, Open Approach
0JWT0PZ	Revision of Cardiac Rhythm Related Device in Trunk Subcutaneous Tissue and Fascia, Open Approach
0JWT3FZ	Revision of Subcutaneous Defibrillator Lead in Trunk Subcutaneous Tissue and Fascia, Percutaneous Approach
0JWT3PZ	Revision of Cardiac Rhythm Related Device in Trunk Subcutaneous Tissue and Fascia, Percutaneous Approach
0JWTXFZ	Revision of Subcutaneous Defibrillator Lead in Trunk Subcutaneous Tissue and Fascia, External Approach
X2H63V9	Insertion of Dual-Chamber Intracardiac Pacemaker into Right Atrium, Percutaneous Approach, New Technology Group 9
X2HK3V9	Insertion of Dual-Chamber Intracardiac Pacemaker into Right Ventricle, Percutaneous Approach, New Technology Group 9

HAC 14: Iatrogenic Pneumothorax with Venous Catheterization

Secondary diagnosis not POA:
- J95.811 Postprocedural pneumothorax

AND

Any of the following procedures:

Code	Description
02H633Z	Insertion of Infusion Device into Right Atrium, Percutaneous Approach
02HK33Z	Insertion of Infusion Device into Right Ventricle, Percutaneous Approach
02HS33Z	Insertion of Infusion Device into Right Pulmonary Vein, Percutaneous Approach
02HS43Z	Insertion of Infusion Device into Right Pulmonary Vein, Percutaneous Endoscopic Approach
02HT33Z	Insertion of Infusion Device into Left Pulmonary Vein, Percutaneous Approach
02HT43Z	Insertion of Infusion Device into Left Pulmonary Vein, Percutaneous Endoscopic Approach
02HV33Z	Insertion of Infusion Device into Superior Vena Cava, Percutaneous Approach
02HV43Z	Insertion of Infusion Device into Superior Vena Cava, Percutaneous Endoscopic Approach
05H033Z	Insertion of Infusion Device into Azygos Vein, Percutaneous Approach
05H043Z	Insertion of Infusion Device into Azygos Vein, Percutaneous Endoscopic Approach
05H133Z	Insertion of Infusion Device into Hemiazygos Vein, Percutaneous Approach
05H143Z	Insertion of Infusion Device into Hemiazygos Vein, Percutaneous Endoscopic Approach
05H333Z	Insertion of Infusion Device into Right Innominate Vein, Percutaneous Approach
05H343Z	Insertion of Infusion Device into Right Innominate Vein, Percutaneous Endoscopic Approach
05H433Z	Insertion of Infusion Device into Left Innominate Vein, Percutaneous Approach
05H443Z	Insertion of Infusion Device into Left Innominate Vein, Percutaneous Endoscopic Approach
05H533Z	Insertion of Infusion Device into Right Subclavian Vein, Percutaneous Approach
05H543Z	Insertion of Infusion Device into Right Subclavian Vein, Percutaneous Endoscopic Approach
05H633Z	Insertion of Infusion Device into Left Subclavian Vein, Percutaneous Approach
05H643Z	Insertion of Infusion Device into Left Subclavian Vein, Percutaneous Endoscopic Approach
05HM33Z	Insertion of Infusion Device into Right Internal Jugular Vein, Percutaneous Approach
05HN33Z	Insertion of Infusion Device into Left Internal Jugular Vein, Percutaneous Approach
05HP33Z	Insertion of Infusion Device into Right External Jugular Vein, Percutaneous Approach
05HQ33Z	Insertion of Infusion Device into Left External Jugular Vein, Percutaneous Approach
0JH63XZ	Insertion of Vascular Access Device into Chest Subcutaneous Tissue and Fascia, Percutaneous Approach

_# Appendix L: Procedure Combination Tables

The tables below were developed to help simplify the relationship between ICD-10-PCS coding and MS-DRG assignment. The Centers for Medicare & Medicaid Services (CMS) has identified in the MS-DRG Definitions Manual certain procedure combinations that must occur in order to assign a specific MS-DRG. There are many factors influencing MS-DRG assignment, including principal and secondary diagnoses, MCC or CC use, sex of the patient, and discharge status. These tables should be used only as a guide. These tables were created based on the proposed, version 42, MS-DRG Grouper software and Definitions Manual files published with the fiscal 2025 IPPS proposed rule. To view the most current files, refer to the following:
https://www.cms.gov/Medicare/Medicare-Fee-for-Service-Payment/AcuteInpatientPPS/MS-DRG-Classifications-and-Software.

DRG 001-002 Heart Transplant or Implant of Heart Assist System

Heart Transplant

Replacement of Right Ventricle with Synthetic Substitue	Code also Replacement of Left Ventricle with Synthetic Substitute
02RK0JZ	02RL0JZ

Insertion with Removal of Heart Assist System

Type of Heart Assist System	Insertion into Heart by Approach	Code also Removal by Site and Approach	
		Heart	Thoracic Aorta, Descending
External, Biventricular	02HA[0,3,4]RS	02PA[0,3,4]RZ	02PW3RZ
External	02HA[0,4]RZ	02PA[0,3,4]RZ	02PW3RZ

Revision with Removal of Heart Assist System

Type of Heart Assist System	Revision in Heart by Approach	Code also Removal by Site and Approach	
		Heart	Thoracic Aorta, Descending
Implantable	02WA[0,3,4]QZ	02PA[0,3,4]RZ	02PW3RZ
External	02WA[0,3,4]RZ	02PA[0,3,4]RZ	02PW3RZ

Revision with Removal of Heart Assist System

Type of Heart Assist System	Revision in Thoracic Aorta, Descending by Approach	Code also Removal from Heart by Approach
External	02WW3RZ	02PA[0,3,4]RZ

Insertion of Heart Assist System and Conduit

Type of Heart Assist System	Insertion in Heart by Approach	Code also Insertion of Conduit by Site		
		Thoracic Aorta, Ascending	Axillary Artery, Right	Axillary Artery, Left
External	02HA0RZ	X2HX0F9	-	-
External	02HA3RZ	-	X2HL0F9	X2HM0F9

DRG 008 Simultaneous Pancreas/Kidney Transplant

Transplanted Body Part	Kidney Transplant by tissue type			Code also Pancreas Transplant by tissue type		
	Allogeneic	Syngeneic	Zooplastic	Allogeneic	Syngeneic	Zooplastic
Kidney, Right	0TY00Z0	0TY00Z1	0TY00Z2	0FYG0Z0	0FYG0Z1	0FYG0Z2
Kidney, Left	0TY10Z0	0TY10Z1	0TY10Z2			

DRG 019 Simultaneous Pancreas/Kidney Transplant with Hemodialysis

Transplanted Body Part	Kidney Transplant by tissue type			Code also Pancreas Transplant by tissue type			Code also Hemodialysis		
	Allogeneic	Syngeneic	Zooplastic	Allogeneic	Syngeneic	Zooplastic	< 6 Hours	6-18 Hours	> 18 Hours
Kidney, Right	0TY00Z0	0TY00Z1	0TY00Z2	0FYG0Z0	0FYG0Z1	0FYG0Z2	5A1D07Z	5A1D80Z	5A1D90Z
Kidney, Left	0TY10Z0	0TY10Z1	0TY10Z2						

Appendix L: Procedure Combination Tables

DRG 023-027 Craniotomy

Site of Neurostimulator Lead	Insertion of Lead by approach	Code also Insertion of Device by Type and Site						
		Neuro-stimulator Generator	Stimulator Multiple Array			Stimulator Multiple Array, Rechargeable		
		Skull	Chest	Back	Abdomen	Chest	Back	Abdomen
Brain	00H0[0,3,4]MZ	0NH00NZ	0JH6[0,3]DZ	0JH7[0,3]DZ	0JH8[0,3]DZ	0JH6[0,3]EZ	0JH7[0,3]EZ	0JH8[0,3]EZ
Cerebral Ventricle	00H6[0,3,4]MZ	0NH00NZ	0JH6[0,3]DZ	0JH7[0,3]DZ	0JH8[0,3]DZ	0JH6[0,3]EZ	0JH7[0,3]EZ	0JH8[0,3]EZ

DRG 028-030 Spinal Procedures

Generator Type	Insertion of Generator by Site			Code also Insertion of Neurostimulator Lead by Site	
	Chest	Abdomen	Back	Spinal Canal	Spinal Cord
Single Array	0JH6[0,3]BZ	0JH8[0,3]BZ	0JH7[0,3]BZ	00HU[0,3,4]MZ	00HV[0,3,4]MZ
Single Array, Rechargeable	0JH6[0,3]CZ	0JH8[0,3]CZ	0JH7[0,3]CZ	00HU[0,3,4]MZ	00HV[0,3,4]MZ
Multiple Array	0JH6[0,3]DZ	0JH8[0,3]DZ	0JH7[0,3]DZ	00HU[0,3,4]MZ	00HV[0,3,4]MZ
Multiple Array, Rechargeable	0JH6[0,3]EZ	—	0JH7[0,3]EZ	00HU[0,3,4]MZ	00HV[0,3,4]MZ
Multiple Array, Rechargeable	—	0JH8[0,3]EZ	—	00HU[0,3,4]MZ	00HV[0,3,4]MZ

DRG 040-042 Peripheral and Cranial Nerve and Other Nervous System Procedures

Insertion of Neurostimulator Generator and Lead

Insertion Single Array Generator, by Site		Code also Insertion of Lead by Site						
		Cranial Nerve	Peripheral Nerve	Azygos Vein	Innominate Vein, RT	Innominate Vein, LT	Stomach	Vagus Nerve
Chest	0JH6[0,3]BZ	00HE[0,3,4]MZ	01HY[0,3,4]MZ	05H0[0,3,4]MZ	05H3[0,3,4]MZ	05H4[0,3,4]MZ	0DH6[0,3,4]MZ	X0HQ3R8
Back	0JH7[0,3]BZ							
Abdomen	0JH8[0,3]BZ							

Insertion Single Array, Rechargeable Generator, by Site		Code also Insertion of Lead by Site						
		Cranial Nerve	Peripheral Nerve	Azygos Vein	Innominate Vein, RT	Innominate Vein, LT	Stomach	Vagus Nerve
Chest	0JH6[0,3]CZ	00HE[0,3,4]MZ	01HY[0,3,4]MZ	05H0[0,3,4]MZ	05H3[0,3,4]MZ	05H4[0,3,4]MZ	0DH6[0,3,4]MZ	X0HQ3R8
Back	0JH7[0,3]CZ							
Abdomen	0JH8[0,3]CZ							

Insertion Multiple Array Generator, by Site		Code also Insertion of Lead by Site						
		Cranial Nerve	Peripheral Nerve	Azygos Vein	Innominate Vein, RT	Innominate Vein, LT	Stomach	Vagus Nerve
Chest	0JH6[0,3]DZ	00HE[0,3,4]MZ	01HY[0,3,4]MZ	05H0[0,3,4]MZ	05H3[0,3,4]MZ	05H4[0,3,4]MZ	0DH6[0,3,4]MZ	X0HQ3R8
Back	0JH7[0,3]DZ							
Abdomen	0JH8[0,3]DZ							

Insertion Multiple Array, Rechargeable Generator, by Site		Code also Insertion of Lead by Site						
		Cranial Nerve	Peripheral Nerve	Azygos Vein	Innominate Vein, RT	Innominate Vein, LT	Stomach	Vagus Nerve
Chest	0JH6[0,3]EZ	00HE[0,3,4]MZ	01HY[0,3,4]MZ	05H0[0,3,4]MZ	05H3[0,3,4]MZ	05H4[0,3,4]MZ	0DH6[0,3,4]MZ	X0HQ3R8
Back	0JH7[0,3]EZ							
Abdomen	0JH8[0,3]EZ							

Insertion Stimulator Generator, by Site		Code also Insertion of Lead by Site						
		Cranial Nerve	Peripheral Nerve	Azygos Vein	Innominate Vein, RT	Innominate Vein, LT	Stomach	Vagus Nerve
Chest	0JH6[0,3]MZ	00HE[0,3,4]MZ	01HY[0,3,4]MZ	05H0[0,3,4]MZ	05H3[0,3,4]MZ	05H4[0,3,4]MZ	0DH6[0,3,4]MZ	X0HQ3R8
Back	0JH7[0,3]MZ							
Abdomen	0JH8[0,3]MZ							

DRG 242-244 Permanent Cardiac Pacemaker Implant
Insertion of Generator and Lead(s) Only

Generator Type	Insertion of Generator by Site		Code also Insertion of Lead by Site			
	Chest	Abdomen	Coronary Vein	Right Atrium (6)/ Left Atrium (7)	Right Ventricle (K)/ Left Ventricle (L)	Pericardium
Single Chamber	0JH6[0,3]4Z	0JH8[0,3]4Z	02H4[0,3,4][J,M]Z	02H[6,7][0,3,4][J,M]Z	02H[K,L][0,3,4][J,M]Z	02HN[0,3,4][J,M]Z
Single Chamber RR	0JH6[0,3]5Z	0JH8[0,3]5Z	02H4[0,3,4][J,M]Z	02H[6,7][0,3,4][J,M]Z	02H[K,L][0,3,4][J,M]Z	02HN[0,3,4][J,M]Z
Dual Chamber	0JH6[0,3]6Z	0JH8[0,3]6Z	02H4[0,3,4][J,M]Z	02H[6,7][0,3,4][J,M]Z	02H[K,L][0,3,4][J,M]Z	02HN[0,3,4][J,M]Z
Cardiac Resynch	0JH6[0,3]7Z	0JH8[0,3]7Z	02H4[0,3,4][J,M]Z	02H[6,7][0,3,4][J,M]Z	02H[K,L][0,3,4][J,M]Z	02HN[0,3,4][J,M]Z
Cardiac Rhythm Related	0JH6[0,3]PZ	0JH8[0,3]PZ	02H4[0,3,4][J,M]Z	02H[6,7][0,3,4][J,M]Z	02H[K,L][0,3,4][J,M]Z	02HN[0,3,4][J,M]Z

DRG 275-277 Cardiac Defibrillator Implant or Carotid Sinus Neurostimulator
Insertion of Generator with Insertion of Lead(s) into Coronary Vein, Atrium or Ventricle

Generator Type	Insertion of Generator by Site		Code also Insertion of Lead by Site				
	Chest	Abdomen	Coronary Vein	Atrium		Ventricle	
				Right	Left	Right	Left
Defibrillator	0JH6[0,3]8Z	0JH8[0,3]8Z	02H4[0,4]KZ	02H6[0,3,4]KZ	02H7[0,3,4]KZ	02HK[0,3,4]KZ	02HL[0,3,4]KZ
Cardiac Resynch Defibrillator Pulse Generator	0JH6[0,3]9Z	0JH8[0,3]9Z	02H4[0,3,4]KZ or 02H43[J,M]Z	02H6[0,3,4]KZ	02H7[0,3,4]KZ	02HK[0,3,4]KZ	02HL[0,3,4]KZ
Contractility Modulation Device	0JH6[0,3]AZ	0JH8[0,3]AZ	—	02H6[0,3,4]MZ	—	02HK[0,3,4]MZ	—

Insertion of Generator with Insertion of Lead(s) into Pericardium or Chest

Generator Type	Insertion of Generator by Site		Code also Insertion of Lead by Site and/or Type				
	Chest	Abdomen	Pericardium			Chest	
			Pacemaker	Defibrillator	Cardiac	Subcutaneous	Mediastinum
Defibrillator	0JH6[0,3]8Z	0JH8[0,3]8Z	02HN[0,3,4]JZ	02HN[0,3,4]KZ	02HN[0,3,4]MZ	0JH6[0,3]FZ	0WHC[0,3,4]GZ
Cardiac Resynch Defibrillator	0JH6[0,3]9Z	0JH8[0,3]9Z	02HN[0,3,4]JZ	02HN[0,3,4]KZ	02HN[0,3,4]MZ	0JH6[0,3]FZ	0WHC[0,3,4]GZ

Insertion of Generator with Insertion of Lead into Carotid Artery (BAROSTIM™ system)

Insertion of Generator by Site	Code also Insertion of Lead by Site	
Chest	Internal Carotid Artery, Right	Internal Carotid Artery, Left
0JH60MZ	03HK3MZ	03HL3MZ

DRG 326-328 Stomach, Esophageal and Duodenal Procedures

Site	Resection by Open Approach	Code also Resection of Pancreas by Open Approach
Duodenum	0DT90ZZ	0FTG0ZZ

DRG 344-346 Minor Small and Large Bowel Procedures

Site	Repair by Open Approach	Code also Repair by external approach of Abdominal Wall Stoma
Small Intestine	0DQ80ZZ	0WQFXZ2
Duodenum	0DQ90ZZ	0WQFXZ2
Jejunum	0DQA0ZZ	0WQFXZ2
Ileum	0DQB0ZZ	0WQFXZ2
Large Intestine	0DQE0ZZ	0WQFXZ2
Large Intestine, Right	0DQF0ZZ	0WQFXZ2
Large Intestine, Left	0DQG0ZZ	0WQFXZ2
Cecum	0DQH0ZZ	0WQFXZ2
Ascending Colon	0DQK0ZZ	0WQFXZ2
Transverse Colon	0DQL0ZZ	0WQFXZ2
Descending Colon	0DQM0ZZ	0WQFXZ2
Sigmoid Colon	0DQN0ZZ	0WQFXZ2

Appendix L: Procedure Combination Tables

DRG 456-458 Spinal Fusion Except Cervical with Spinal Curvature/Malignancy/Infection or Extensive Fusions

Fusion of Thoracic and Lumbar Vertebra, Anterior Column

2 to 7 Thoracic Vertebra		Code also 2 or more Lumbar Vertebra	
0RG[0,3,4][7,A,J,K]0	XRG70F3	0SG1[0,3,4][7,A,J,K]0	XRGC0F3

Fusion of Thoracic and Lumbar Vertebra, Posterior Column

2 to 7 Thoracic Vertebra			Code also 2 or more Lumbar Vertebra		
Posterior Approach	Anterior Approach	New Technology	Posterior Approach	Anterior Approach	New Technology
0RG7[0,3,4][7,J,K]1	0RG7[0,3,4][7,A,J,K]J	XRG7092 XRG70F3	0SG1[0,3,4][7,J,K]1	0SG1[0,3,4][7,A,J,K]J	XRGC092 XRGC0F3

DRG 461-462 Bilateral or Multiple Major Joint Procedures of Lower Extremity

For procedures to qualify as bilateral or multiple joint procedures, at least one replacement code or combination removal and replacement code from two different lower extremity sites from the following table(s) must be reported.

Examples: Left hip and right hip codes (bilateral); left hip and left knee codes (multiple); left hip and right ankle codes (multiple); left knee and right knee codes (bilateral); right hip removal and replacement, with right knee replacement

Hip, RT	Hip, LT	Knee, RT	Knee, LT	Ankle, RT	Ankle, LT
0SR9019	0SRB019	0SRC069	0SRD069	0SRF07Z	0SRG07Z
0SR901A	0SRB01A	0SRC06A	0SRD06A	0SRF0J9	0SRG0J9
0SR901Z	0SRB01Z	0SRC06Z	0SRD06Z	0SRF0JA	0SRG0JA
0SR9029	0SRB029	0SRC07Z	0SRD07Z	0SRF0JZ	0SRG0JZ
0SR902A	0SRB02A	0SRC0J9	0SRD0J9	0SRF0KZ	0SRG0KZ
0SR902Z	0SRB02Z	0SRC0JA	0SRD0JA		
0SR9039	0SRB039	0SRC0JZ	0SRD0JZ		
0SR903A	0SRB03A	0SRC0KZ	0SRD0KZ		
0SR903Z	0SRB03Z	0SRC0L9	0SRD0L9		
0SR9049	0SRB049	0SRC0LA	0SRD0LA		
0SR904A	0SRB04A	0SRC0LZ	0SRD0LZ		
0SR904Z	0SRB04Z	0SRC0M9	0SRD0M9		
0SR9069	0SRB069	0SRC0MA	0SRD0MA		
0SR906A	0SRB06A	0SRC0MZ	0SRD0MZ		
0SR906Z	0SRB06Z	0SRC0N9	0SRD0N9		
0SR907Z	0SRB07Z	0SRC0NA	0SRD0NA		
0SR90J9	0SRB0J9	0SRC0NZ	0SRD0NZ		
0SR90JA	0SRB0JA	0SRT07Z	0SRU07Z		
0SR90JZ	0SRB0JZ	0SRT0J9	0SRU0J9		
0SR90KZ	0SRB0KZ	0SRT0JA	0SRU0JA		
0SRA009	0SRE009	0SRT0JZ	0SRU0JZ		
0SRA00A	0SRE00A	0SRT0KZ	0SRU0KZ		
0SRA00Z	0SRE00Z	0SRV07Z	0SRW07Z		
0SRA019	0SRE019	0SRV0J9	0SRW0J9		
0SRA01A	0SRE01A	0SRV0JA	0SRW0JA		

Hip, RT	Hip, LT	Knee, RT	Knee, LT	Ankle, RT	Ankle, LT
0SRA01Z	0SRE01Z	0SRV0JZ	0SRW0JZ		
0SRA039	0SRE039	0SRV0KZ	0SRW0KZ		
0SRA03A	0SRE03A	0SPC0JZ	0SPD0JZ		
0SRA03Z	0SRE03Z				
0SRA07Z	0SRE07Z				
0SRA0J9	0SRE0J9				
0SRA0JA	0SRE0JA				
0SRA0JZ	0SRE0JZ				
0SRA0KZ	0SRE0KZ				
0SRR019	0SRS019				
0SRR01A	0SRS01A				
0SRR01Z	0SRS01Z				
0SRR039	0SRS039				
0SRR03A	0SRS03A				
0SRR03Z	0SRS03Z				
0SRR07Z	0SRS07Z				
0SRR0J9	0SRS0J9				
0SRR0JA	0SRS0JA				
0SRR0JZ	0SRS0JZ				
0SRR0KZ	0SRS0KZ				
0SU90BZ	0SUB0BZ				
0SUA0BZ	0SUE0BZ				
0SUR0BZ	0SUS0BZ				
0SP90JZ	0SPB0JZ				

Hip Procedure Combinations

Open Removal of Hip Spacer with Replacement

Removal of Spacer		Code also Replacement by Device Type					
		Metal	Metal on Poly	Ceramic	Ceramic on Poly	Oxidized Zirc on Poly	Synth Subst
Hip, RT	0SP908Z	0SR901[9,A,Z]	0SR902[9,A,Z]	0SR903[9,A,Z]	0SR904[9,A,Z]	0SR906[9,A,Z]	0SR90J[9,A,Z]
Hip, LT	0SPB08Z	0SRB01[9,A,Z]	0SRB02[9,A,Z]	0SRB03[9,A,Z]	0SRB04[9,A,Z]	0SRB06[9,A,Z]	0SRB0J[9,A,Z]

Open Removal of Hip Spacer with Replacement

Removal of Spacer		Code also Replacement by Device Type						
		Acetabular Surface				Femoral Surface		
		Poly	Metal	Ceramic	Synthetic	Metal	Ceramic	Synth
Hip, RT	0SP908Z	0SRA00[9,A,Z]	0SRA01[9,A,Z]	0SRA03[9,A,Z]	0SRA0J[9,A,Z]	0SRR01[9,A,Z]	0SRR03[9,A,Z]	0SRR0J[9,A,Z]
Hip, LT	0SPB08Z	0SRE00[9,A,Z]	0SRE01[9,A,Z]	0SRE03[9,A,Z]	0SRE0J[9,A,Z]	0SRS01[9,A,Z]	0SRS03[9,A,Z]	0SRS0J[9,A,Z]

Open Removal of Hip Liner with Replacement

Removal of Liner		Code also Replacement by Device Type					
		Metal	Metal on Poly	Ceramic	Ceramic on Poly	Oxidized Zirc on Poly	Synth Subst
Hip, RT	0SP909Z	0SR901[9,A,Z]	0SR902[9,A,Z]	0SR903[9,A,Z]	0SR904[9,A,Z]	0SR906[9,A,Z]	0SR90J[9,A,Z]
Hip, LT	0SPB09Z	0SRB01[9,A,Z]	0SRB02[9,A,Z]	0SRB03[9,A,Z]	0SRB04[9,A,Z]	0SRB06[9,A,Z]	0SRB0J[9,A,Z]

Open Removal of Hip Liner with Replacement

Removal of Liner		Code also Replacement by Device Type						
		Acetabular Surface				Femoral Surface		
		Poly	Metal	Ceramic	Synthetic	Metal	Ceramic	Synth
Hip, RT	0SP909Z	0SRA00[9,A,Z]	0SRA01[9,A,Z]	0SRA03[9,A,Z]	0SRA0J[9,A,Z]	0SRR01[9,A,Z]	0SRR03[9,A,Z]	0SRR0J[9,A,Z]
Hip, LT	0SPB09Z	0SRE00[9,A,Z]	0SRE01[9,A,Z]	0SRE03[9,A,Z]	0SRE0J[9,A,Z]	0SRS01[9,A,Z]	0SRS03[9,A,Z]	0SRS0J[9,A,Z]

Open Removal of Hip Resurfacing Device with Replacement

Removal of Resurfacing Device		Code also Replacement by Device Type					
		Metal	Metal on Poly	Ceramic	Ceramic on Poly	Oxidized Zirc on Poly	Synth Subst
Hip, RT	0SP90BZ	0SR901[9,A,Z]	0SR902[9,A,Z]	0SR903[9,A,Z]	0SR904[9,A,Z]	0SR906[9,A,Z]	0SR90J[9,A,Z]
Hip, LT	0SPB0BZ	0SRB01[9,A,Z]	0SRB02[9,A,Z]	0SRB03[9,A,Z]	0SRB04[9,A,Z]	0SRB06[9,A,Z]	0SRB0J[9,A,Z]

Open Removal of Hip Resurfacing Device with Replacement

Removal of Resurfacing Device		Code also Replacement by Device Type						
		Acetabular Surface				Femoral Surface		
		Poly	Metal	Ceramic	Synthetic	Metal	Ceramic	Synth
Hip, RT	0SP90BZ	0SRA00[9,A,Z]	0SRA01[9,A,Z]	0SRA03[9,A,Z]	0SRA0J[9,A,Z]	0SRR01[9,A,Z]	0SRR03[9,A,Z]	0SRR0J[9,A,Z]
Hip, LT	0SPB0BZ	0SRE00[9,A,Z]	0SRE01[9,A,Z]	0SRE03[9,A,Z]	0SRE0J[9,A,Z]	0SRS01[9,A,Z]	0SRS03[9,A,Z]	0SRS0J[9,A,Z]

Open Removal of Hip Articulating Spacer with Replacement

Removal of Articulating Spacer		Code also Replacement by Device Type					
		Metal	Metal on Poly	Ceramic	Ceramic on Poly	Oxidized Zirc on Poly	Synth Subst
Hip, RT	0SP90EZ	0SR901[9,A,Z]	0SR902[9,A,Z]	0SR903[9,A,Z]	0SR904[9,A,Z]	0SR906[9,A,Z]	0SR90J[9,A,Z]
Hip, LT	0SPB0EZ	0SRB01[9,A,Z]	0SRB02[9,A,Z]	0SRB03[9,A,Z]	0SRB04[9,A,Z]	0SRB06[9,A,Z]	0SRB0J[9,A,Z]

Open Removal of Hip Articulating Spacer with Replacement

Removal of Articulating Spacer		Code also Replacement by Device Type						
		Acetabular Surface				Femoral Surface		
		Poly	Metal	Ceramic	Synthetic	Metal	Ceramic	Synth
Hip, RT	0SP90EZ	0SRA00[9,A,Z]	0SRA01[9,A,Z]	0SRA03[9,A,Z]	0SRA0J[9,A,Z]	0SRR01[9,A,Z]	0SRR03[9,A,Z]	0SRR0J[9,A,Z]
Hip, LT	0SPB0EZ	0SRE00[9,A,Z]	0SRE01[9,A,Z]	0SRE03[9,A,Z]	0SRE0J[9,A,Z]	0SRS01[9,A,Z]	0SRS03[9,A,Z]	0SRS0J[9,A,Z]

Appendix L: Procedure Combination Tables

Open Removal of Hip Synthetic Substitute with Replacement

Removal of Synthetic Substitute		Code also Replacement by Device Type					
		Metal	Metal on Poly	Ceramic	Ceramic on Poly	Oxidized Zirc on Poly	Synth Subst
Hip, RT	0SP[9,A,R]0JZ	0SR901[9,A,Z]	0SR902[9,A,Z]	0SR903[9,A,Z]	0SR904[9,A,Z]	0SR906[9,A,Z]	0SR90J[9,A,Z]
Hip, LT	0SP[B,E,S]0JZ	0SRB01[9,A,Z]	0SRB02[9,A,Z]	0SRB03[9,A,Z]	0SRB04[9,A,Z]	0SRB06[9,A,Z]	0SRB0J[9,A,Z]

Open Removal of Hip Synthetic Substitute with Replacement

Removal of Synthetic Substitute		Code also Replacement by Device Type						
		Acetabular Surface				Femoral Surface		
		Poly	Metal	Ceramic	Synthetic	Metal	Ceramic	Synth
Hip, RT	0SP[9,A,R]0JZ	0SRA00[9,A,Z]	0SRA01[9,A,Z]	0SRA03[9,A,Z]	0SRA0J[9,A,Z]	0SRR01[9,A,Z]	0SRR03[9,A,Z]	0SRR0J[9,A,Z]
Hip, LT	0SP[B,E,S]0JZ	0SRE00[9,A,Z]	0SRE01[9,A,Z]	0SRE03[9,A,Z]	0SRE0J[9,A,Z]	0SRS01[9,A,Z]	0SRS03[9,A,Z]	0SRS0J[9,A,Z]

Percutaneous Endoscopic Removal of Hip Spacer with Open Replacement

Removal of Spacer		Code also Replacement by Device Type					
		Metal	Metal on Poly	Ceramic	Ceramic on Poly	Oxidized Zirc on Poly	Synth Subst
Hip, RT	0SP948Z	0SR901[9,A,Z]	0SR902[9,A,Z]	0SR903[9,A,Z]	0SR904[9,A,Z]	0SR906[9,A,Z]	0SR90J[9,A,Z]
Hip, LT	0SPB48Z	0SRB01[9,A,Z]	0SRB02[9,A,Z]	0SRB03[9,A,Z]	0SRB04[9,A,Z]	0SRB06[9,A,Z]	0SRB0J[9,A,Z]

Percutaneous Endoscopic Removal of Hip Spacer with Open Replacement

Removal of Spacer		Code also Replacement by Device Type						
		Acetabular Surface				Femoral Surface		
		Poly	Metal	Ceramic	Synthetic	Metal	Ceramic	Synth
Hip, RT	0SP948Z	0SRA00[9,A,Z]	0SRA01[9,A,Z]	0SRA03[9,A,Z]	0SRA0J[9,A,Z]	0SRR01[9,A,Z]	0SRR03[9,A,Z]	0SRR0J[9,A,Z]
Hip, LT	0SPB48Z	0SRE00[9,A,Z]	0SRE01[9,A,Z]	0SRE03[9,A,Z]	0SRE0J[9,A,Z]	0SRS01[9,A,Z]	0SRS03[9,A,Z]	0SRS0J[9,A,Z]

Percutaneous Endoscopic Removal of Hip Synthetic Substitute with Open Replacement

Removal of Synthetic Substitute		Code also Replacement by Device Type					
		Metal	Metal on Poly	Ceramic	Ceramic on Poly	Oxidized Zirc on Poly	Synth Subst
Hip, RT	0SP[9,A,R]4JZ	0SR901[9,A,Z]	0SR902[9,A,Z]	0SR903[9,A,Z]	0SR904[9,A,Z]	0SR906[9,A,Z]	0SR90J[9,A,Z]
Hip, LT	0SP[B,E,S]4JZ	0SRB01[9,A,Z]	0SRB02[9,A,Z]	0SRB03[9,A,Z]	0SRB04[9,A,Z]	0SRB06[9,A,Z]	0SRB0J[9,A,Z]

Percutaneous Endoscopic Removal of Hip Synthetic Substitute with Open Replacement

Removal of Synthetic Substitute		Code also Replacement by Device Type						
		Acetabular Surface				Femoral Surface		
		Poly	Metal	Ceramic	Synthetic	Metal	Ceramic	Synth
Hip, RT	0SP[9,A,R]4JZ	0SRA00[9,A,Z]	0SRA01[9,A,Z]	0SRA03[9,A,Z]	0SRA0J[9,A,Z]	0SRR01[9,A,Z]	0SRR03[9,A,Z]	0SRR0J[9,A,Z]
Hip, LT	0SP[B,E,S]4JZ	0SRE00[9,A,Z]	0SRE01[9,A,Z]	0SRE03[9,A,Z]	0SRE0J[9,A,Z]	0SRS01[9,A,Z]	0SRS03[9,A,Z]	0SRS0J[9,A,Z]

Knee Procedure Combinations

Removal of Knee Spacer with Replacement

Removal of Spacer		Code also Replacement by Type of Synthetic Substitute					
		Oxidized Zirc on Poly	Synthetic Substitute	Patello-femoral	Femoral Surface	Tibial Surface	Medial (L)/Lateral (M) Meniscus
Knee, RT	0SPC[0,3,4]8Z	0SRC06[9,A,Z]	0SRC0J[9,A,Z]	0SRC0N[9,A,Z]	0SRT0J[9,A,Z]	0SRV0J[9,A,Z]	XRRG0[L,M]8
Knee, LT	0SPD[0,3,4]8Z	0SRD06[9,A,Z]	0SRD0J[9,A,Z]	0SRD0N[9,A,Z]	0SRU0J[9,A,Z]	0SRW0J[9,A,Z]	XRRH0[L,M]8

Removal of Knee Liner with Replacement

Removal of Liner		Code also Replacement by Type of Synthetic Substitute						
		Oxidized Zirc on Poly	Synthetic Substitute	Medial (L)/Lateral (M) Unicondylar	Patello-femoral	Femoral Surface	Tibial Surface	Medial (L)/Lateral (M) Meniscus
Knee, RT	0SPC09Z	0SRC06[9,A,Z]	0SRC0J[9,A,Z]	0SRC0[L,M][9,A,Z]	0SRC0N[9,A,Z]	0SRT0J[9,A,Z]	0SRV0J[9,A,Z]	XRRG0[L,M]8
Knee, LT	0SPD09Z	0SRD06[9,A,Z]	0SRD0J[9,A,Z]	0SRD0[L,M][9,A,Z]	0SRD0N[9,A,Z]	0SRU0J[9,A,Z]	0SRW0J[9,A,Z]	XRRH0[L,M]8

Removal of Knee Articulating Spacer with Replacement

Removal of Articulating Spacer		Code also Replacement by Type of Synthetic Substitute				
		Oxidized Zirc on Poly	Synthetic Substitute	Femoral Surface	Tibial Surface	Medial (L)/ Lateral (M) Meniscus
Knee, RT	0SPC0EZ	0SRC06[9,A,Z]	0SRC0J[9,A,Z]	0SRT0J[9,A,Z]	0SRV0J[9,A,Z]	XRRG0[L,M]8
Knee, LT	0SPD0EZ	0SRD06[9,A,Z]	0SRD0J[9,A,Z]	0SRU0J[9,A,Z]	0SRW0J[9,A,Z]	XRRH0[L,M]8

Removal of Knee Patellar Surface with Replacement

Removal of Patellar Surface		Code also Replacement by Type of Synthetic Substitute					
		Oxidized Zirc on Poly	Synthetic Substitute	Patello-femoral	Femoral Surface	Tibial Surface	Medial (L)/Lateral (M) Meniscus
Knee, RT	0SPC[0,4]JC	0SRC06[9,A,Z]	0SRC0J[9,A,Z]	0SRC0N[9,A,Z]	0SRT0J[9,A,Z]	0SRV0J[9,A,Z]	XRRG0[L,M]8
Knee, LT	0SPD[0,4]JC	0SRD06[9,A,Z]	0SRD0J[9,A,Z]	0SRD0N[9,A,Z]	0SRU0J[9,A,Z]	0SRW0J[9,A,Z]	XRRH0[L,M]8

Removal of Knee Synthetic Substitute with Replacement

Removal of Synthetic Substitute		Code also Replacement by Type of Synthetic Substitute						
		Oxidized Zirc on Poly	Synthetic Substitute	Medial (L)/ Lateral (M) Unicondylar	Patello-femoral	Femoral Surface	Tibial Surface	Medial (L)/ Lateral (M) Meniscus
Knee, RT	0SPC[0,4]JZ	0SRC06[9,A,Z]	0SRC0J[9,A,Z]	0SRC0[L,M][9,A,Z]	0SRC0N[9,A,Z]	0SRT0J[9,A,Z]	0SRV0J[9,A,Z]	XRRG0[L,M]8
Knee, LT	0SPD[0,4]JZ	0SRD06[9,A,Z]	0SRD0J[9,A,Z]	0SRD0[L,M][9,A,Z]	0SRD0N[9,A,Z]	0SRU0J[9,A,Z]	0SRW0J[9,A,Z]	XRRH0[L,M]8

Removal of Knee Unicondylar Device with Replacement

Removal of Medial (L)/ Lateral (M) Unicondylar Device		Code also Replacement by Type of Synthetic Substitute					
		Oxidized Zirc on Poly	Synthetic Substitute	Medial Unicondylar	Femoral Surface	Tibial Surface	Medial (L)/Lateral (M) Meniscus
Knee, RT	0SPC[0,4][L,M]Z	0SRC06[9,A,Z]	0SRC0J[9,A,Z]	0SRC0L[9,A,Z]	0SRT0J[9,A,Z]	0SRV0J[9,A,Z]	XRRG0[L,M]8
Knee, LT	0SPD[0,4][L,M]Z	0SRD06[9,A,Z]	0SRD0J[9,A,Z]	0SRD0L[9,A,Z]	0SRU0J[9,A,Z]	0SRW0J[9,A,Z]	XRRH0[L,M]8

Removal of Knee Patellofemoral Device with Replacement

Removal of Patellofemoral Device		Code also Replacement by Type of Synthetic Substitute					
		Oxidized Zirc on Poly	Synthetic Substitute	Medial Unicondylar	Femoral Surface	Tibial Surface	Medial (L)/Lateral (M) Meniscus
Knee, RT	0SPC[0,4]NZ	0SRC06[9,A,Z]	0SRC0J[9,A,Z]	0SRC0L[9,A,Z]	0SRT0J[9,A,Z]	0SRV0J[9,A,Z]	XRRG0[L,M]8
Knee, LT	0SPD[0,4]NZ	0SRD06[9,A,Z]	0SRD0J[9,A,Z]	0SRD0L[9,A,Z]	0SRU0J[9,A,Z]	0SRW0J[9,A,Z]	XRRH0[L,M]8

Removal of Knee Femoral/Tibial Surface Device with Replacement

Removal of Femoral (T,U)/ Tibial (V,W) Surface		Code also Replacement by Type of Synthetic Substitute						
		Oxidized Zirc on Poly	Synthetic Substitute	Articulating Spacer	Patello-femoral	Femoral Surface	Tibial Surface	Medial (L)/Lateral (M) Meniscus
Knee, RT	0SP[T,V][0,4]JZ	0SRC06[9,A,Z]	0SRC0J[9,A,Z]	0SRC0EZ	0SRC0N[9,A,Z]	0SRT0J[9,A,Z]	0SRV0J[9,A,Z]	XRRG0[L,M]8
Knee, LT	0SP[U,W][0,4]JZ	0SRD06[9,A,Z]	0SRD0J[9,A,Z]	0SRD0EZ	0SRD0N[9,A,Z]	0SRU0J[9,A,Z]	0SRW0J[9,A,Z]	XRRH0[L,M]8

466-468 Revision of Hip or Knee Replacement

Hip Procedure Combinations

Open Removal of Hip Spacer with Replacement

Removal of Spacer		Code also Replacement by Device Type						
		Metal	Metal on Poly	Ceramic	Ceramic on Poly	Oxidized Zirc on Poly	Articulating Spacer	Synth Subst
Hip, RT	0SP908Z	0SR901[9,A,Z]	0SR902[9,A,Z]	0SR903[9,A,Z]	0SR904[9,A,Z]	0SR906[9,A,Z]	0SR90EZ	0SR90J[9,A,Z]
Hip, LT	0SPB08Z	0SRB01[9,A,Z]	0SRB02[9,A,Z]	0SRB03[9,A,Z]	0SRB04[9,A,Z]	0SRB06[9,A,Z]	0SRB0EZ	0SRB0J[9,A,Z]

Appendix L: Procedure Combination Tables

Open Removal of Hip Spacer with Replacement

Removal of Spacer		Code also Replacement by Device Type						
		Acetabular Surface				Femoral Surface		
		Poly	Metal	Ceramic	Synthetic	Metal	Ceramic	Synth
Hip, RT	0SP908Z	0SRA00[9,A,Z]	0SRA01[9,A,Z]	0SRA03[9,A,Z]	0SRA0J[9,A,Z]	0SRR01[9,A,Z]	0SRR03[9,A,Z]	0SRR0J[9,A,Z]
Hip, LT	0SPB08Z	0SRE00[9,A,Z]	0SRE01[9,A,Z]	0SRE03[9,A,Z]	0SRE0J[9,A,Z]	0SRS01[9,A,Z]	0SRS03[9,A,Z]	0SRS0J[9,A,Z]

Open Removal of Hip Spacer with Liner Insertion (supplement)

Removal of Spacer		Code also Supplement of Body Part by Site		
		Joint	Acetabular Surface	Femoral Surface
Hip, RT	0SP908Z	0SU909Z	0SUA09Z	0SUR09Z
Hip, LT	0SPB08Z	0SUB09Z	0SUE09Z	0SUS09Z

Open Removal of Hip Liner with Replacement

Removal of Liner		Code also Replacement by Device Type						
		Metal	Metal on Poly	Ceramic	Ceramic on Poly	Oxidized Zirc on Poly	Articulating Spacer	Synth Subst
Hip, RT	0SP909Z	0SR901[9,A,Z]	0SR902[9,A,Z]	0SR903[9,A,Z]	0SR904[9,A,Z]	0SR906[9,A,Z]	0SR90EZ	0SR90J[9,A,Z]
Hip, LT	0SPB09Z	0SRB01[9,A,Z]	0SRB02[9,A,Z]	0SRB03[9,A,Z]	0SRB04[9,A,Z]	0SRB06[9,A,Z]	0SRB0EZ	0SRB0J[9,A,Z]

Open Removal of Hip Liner with Replacement

Removal of Liner		Code also Replacement by Device Type						
		Acetabular Surface				Femoral Surface		
		Poly	Metal	Ceramic	Synthetic	Metal	Ceramic	Synth
Hip, RT	0SP909Z	0SRA00[9,A,Z]	0SRA01[9,A,Z]	0SRA03[9,A,Z]	0SRA0J[9,A,Z]	0SRR01[9,A,Z]	0SRR03[9,A,Z]	0SRR0J[9,A,Z]
Hip, LT	0SPB09Z	0SRE00[9,A,Z]	0SRE01[9,A,Z]	0SRE03[9,A,Z]	0SRE0J[9,A,Z]	0SRS01[9,A,Z]	0SRS03[9,A,Z]	0SRS0J[9,A,Z]

Open Removal of Hip Liner with Liner Insertion (supplement)

Removal of Liner		Code also Supplement of Body Part by Site		
		Joint	Acetabular Surface	Femoral Surface
Hip, RT	0SP909Z	0SU909Z	0SUA09Z	0SUR09Z
Hip, LT	0SPB09Z	0SUB09Z	0SUE09Z	0SUS09Z

Open Removal of Hip Resurfacing Device with Replacement

Removal of Resurfacing Device		Code also Replacement by Device Type						
		Metal	Metal on Poly	Ceramic	Ceramic on Poly	Oxidized Zirc on Poly	Articulating Spacer	Synth Subst
Hip, RT	0SP90BZ	0SR901[9,A,Z]	0SR902[9,A,Z]	0SR903[9,A,Z]	0SR904[9,A,Z]	0SR906[9,A,Z]	0SR90EZ	0SR90J[9,A,Z]
Hip, LT	0SPB0BZ	0SRB01[9,A,Z]	0SRB02[9,A,Z]	0SRB03[9,A,Z]	0SRB04[9,A,Z]	0SRB06[9,A,Z]	0SRB0EZ	0SRB0J[9,A,Z]

Open Removal of Hip Resurfacing Device with Replacement

Removal of Resurfacing Device		Code also Replacement by Device Type						
		Acetabular Surface				Femoral Surface		
		Poly	Metal	Ceramic	Synthetic	Metal	Ceramic	Synth
Hip, RT	0SP90BZ	0SRA00[9,A,Z]	0SRA01[9,A,Z]	0SRA03[9,A,Z]	0SRA0J[9,A,Z]	0SRR01[9,A,Z]	0SRR03[9,A,Z]	0SRR0J[9,A,Z]
Hip, LT	0SPB0BZ	0SRE00[9,A,Z]	0SRE01[9,A,Z]	0SRE03[9,A,Z]	0SRE0J[9,A,Z]	0SRS01[9,A,Z]	0SRS03[9,A,Z]	0SRS0J[9,A,Z]

Open Removal of Hip Resurfacing Device with Liner Insertion (supplement)

Removal of Resurfacing Device		Code also Supplement of Body Part by Site		
		Joint	Acetabular Surface	Femoral Surface
Hip, RT	0SP90BZ	0SU909Z	0SUA09Z	0SUR09Z
Hip, LT	0SPB0BZ	0SUB09Z	0SUE09Z	0SUS09Z

ICD-10-PCS 2025 — Appendix L: Procedure Combination Tables

Open Removal of Hip Articulating Spacer with Replacement

Removal of Articulating Spacer		Code also Replacement by Device Type					
		Metal	Metal on Poly	Ceramic	Ceramic on Poly	Oxidized Zirc on Poly	Synth Subst
Hip, RT	0SP90EZ	0SR901[9,A,Z]	0SR902[9,A,Z]	0SR903[9,A,Z]	0SR904[9,A,Z]	0SR906[9,A,Z]	0SR90J[9,A,Z]
Hip, LT	0SPB0EZ	0SRB01[9,A,Z]	0SRB02[9,A,Z]	0SRB03[9,A,Z]	0SRB04[9,A,Z]	0SRB06[9,A,Z]	0SRB0J[9,A,Z]

Open Removal of Hip Articulating Spacer with Replacement

Removal of Articulating Spacer		Code also Replacement by Device Type						
		Acetabular Surface				Femoral Surface		
		Poly	Metal	Ceramic	Synthetic	Metal	Ceramic	Synth
Hip, RT	0SP90EZ	0SRA00[9,A,Z]	0SRA01[9,A,Z]	0SRA03[9,A,Z]	0SRA0J[9,A,Z]	0SRR01[9,A,Z]	0SRR03[9,A,Z]	0SRR0J[9,A,Z]
Hip, LT	0SPB0EZ	0SRE00[9,A,Z]	0SRE01[9,A,Z]	0SRE03[9,A,Z]	0SRE0J[9,A,Z]	0SRS01[9,A,Z]	0SRS03[9,A,Z]	0SRS0J[9,A,Z]

Open Removal of Hip Articulating Spacer with Liner Insertion (supplement)

Removal of Articulating Spacer		Code also Supplement of Body Part by Site		
		Joint	Acetabular Surface	Femoral Surface
Hip, RT	0SP90EZ	0SU909Z	0SUA09Z	0SUR09Z
Hip, LT	0SPB0EZ	0SUB09Z	0SUE09Z	0SUS09Z

Open Removal of Hip Synthetic Substitute with Replacement

Removal of Synthetic Substitute		Code also Replacement by Device Type						
		Metal	Metal on Poly	Ceramic	Ceramic on Poly	Oxidized Zirc on Poly	Articulating Spacer	Synth Subst
Hip, RT	0SP[9,A,R]0JZ	0SR901[9,A,Z]	0SR902[9,A,Z]	0SR903[9,A,Z]	0SR904[9,A,Z]	0SR906[9,A,Z]	0SR90EZ	0SR90J[9,A,Z]
Hip, LT	0SP[B,E,S]0JZ	0SRB01[9,A,Z]	0SRB02[9,A,Z]	0SRB03[9,A,Z]	0SRB04[9,A,Z]	0SRB06[9,A,Z]	0SRB0EZ	0SRB0J[9,A,Z]

Open Removal of Hip Synthetic Substitute with Replacement

Removal of Synthetic Substitute		Code also Replacement by Device Type						
		Acetabular Surface				Femoral Surface		
		Poly	Metal	Ceramic	Synthetic	Metal	Ceramic	Synth
Hip, RT	0SP[9,A,R]0JZ	0SRA00[9,A,Z]	0SRA01[9,A,Z]	0SRA03[9,A,Z]	0SRA0J[9,A,Z]	0SRR01[9,A,Z]	0SRR03[9,A,Z]	0SRR0J[9,A,Z]
Hip, LT	0SP[B,E,S]0JZ	0SRE00[9,A,Z]	0SRE01[9,A,Z]	0SRE03[9,A,Z]	0SRE0J[9,A,Z]	0SRS01[9,A,Z]	0SRS03[9,A,Z]	0SRS0J[9,A,Z]

Percutaneous Endoscopic Removal of Hip Spacer with Open Replacement

Removal of Spacer		Code also Replacement by Device Type						
		Metal	Metal on Poly	Ceramic	Ceramic on Poly	Oxidized Zirc on Poly	Articulating Spacer	Synth Subst
Hip, RT	0SP948Z	0SR901[9,A,Z]	0SR902[9,A,Z]	0SR903[9,A,Z]	0SR904[9,A,Z]	0SR906[9,A,Z]	0SR90EZ	0SR90J[9,A,Z]
Hip, LT	0SPB48Z	0SRB01[9,A,Z]	0SRB02[9,A,Z]	0SRB03[9,A,Z]	0SRB04[9,A,Z]	0SRB06[9,A,Z]	0SRB0EZ	0SRB0J[9,A,Z]

Percutaneous Endoscopic Removal of Hip Spacer with Open Replacement

Removal of Spacer		Code also Replacement by Device Type						
		Acetabular Surface				Femoral Surface		
		Poly	Metal	Ceramic	Synthetic	Metal	Ceramic	Synth
Hip, RT	0SP948Z	0SRA00[9,A,Z]	0SRA01[9,A,Z]	0SRA03[9,A,Z]	0SRA0J[9,A,Z]	0SRR01[9,A,Z]	0SRR03[9,A,Z]	0SRR0J[9,A,Z]
Hip, LT	0SPB48Z	0SRE00[9,A,Z]	0SRE01[9,A,Z]	0SRE03[9,A,Z]	0SRE0J[9,A,Z]	0SRS01[9,A,Z]	0SRS03[9,A,Z]	0SRS0J[9,A,Z]

Percutaneous Endoscopic Removal of Hip Spacer with Open Liner Insertion (supplement)

Removal of Spacer		Code also Supplement of Body Part by Site		
		Joint	Acetabular Surface	Femoral Surface
Hip, RT	0SP948Z	0SU909Z	0SUA09Z	0SUR09Z
Hip, LT	0SPB48Z	0SUB09Z	0SUE09Z	0SUS09Z

Appendix L: Procedure Combination Tables

Percutaneous Endoscopic Removal of Hip Synthetic Substitute with Open Replacement

Removal of Synthetic Substitute		Code also Replacement by Device Type						
		Metal	Metal on Poly	Ceramic	Ceramic on Poly	Oxidized Zirc on Poly	Articulating Spacer	Synth Subst
Hip, RT	ØSP[9,A,R]4JZ	ØSR901[9,A,Z]	ØSR902[9,A,Z]	ØSR903[9,A,Z]	ØSR904[9,A,Z]	ØSR906[9,A,Z]	ØSR90EZ	ØSR90J[9,A,Z]
Hip, LT	ØSP[B,E,S]4JZ	ØSRB01[9,A,Z]	ØSRB02[9,A,Z]	ØSRB03[9,A,Z]	ØSRB04[9,A,Z]	ØSRB06[9,A,Z]	ØSRB0EZ	ØSRB0J[9,A,Z]

Percutaneous Endoscopic Removal of Hip Synthetic Substitute with Open Replacement

Removal of Synthetic Substitute		Code also Replacement by Device Type						
		Acetabular Surface				Femoral Surface		
		Poly	Metal	Ceramic	Synthetic	Metal	Ceramic	Synth
Hip, RT	ØSP[9,A,R]4JZ	ØSRA00[9,A,Z]	ØSRA01[9,A,Z]	ØSRA03[9,A,Z]	ØSRA0J[9,A,Z]	ØSRR01[9,A,Z]	ØSRR03[9,A,Z]	ØSRR0J[9,A,Z]
Hip, LT	ØSP[B,E,S]4JZ	ØSRE00[9,A,Z]	ØSRE01[9,A,Z]	ØSRE03[9,A,Z]	ØSRE0J[9,A,Z]	ØSRS01[9,A,Z]	ØSRS03[9,A,Z]	ØSRS0J[9,A,Z]

Percutaneous Endoscopic Removal of Hip Synthetic Substitute with Open Liner Insertion (supplement)

Removal of Synthetic Substitute		Code also Supplement of Body Part by Site		
		Joint	Acetabular Surface	Femoral Surface
Hip, RT	ØSP[9,A,R]4JZ	ØSU909Z	ØSUA09Z	ØSUR09Z
Hip, LT	ØSP[B,E,S]4JZ	ØSUB09Z	ØSUE09Z	ØSUS09Z

Knee Procedure Combinations

Removal of Knee Spacer with Replacement

Removal of Spacer		Code also Replacement by Type of Synthetic Substitute						
		Oxidized Zirc on Poly	Synthetic Substitute	Articulating Spacer	Patello-femoral	Femoral Surface	Tibial Surface	Medial (L)/Lateral (M) Meniscus
Knee, RT	ØSPC[0,3,4]8Z	ØSRC06[9,A,Z]	ØSRC0J[9,A,Z]	ØSRC0EZ	ØSRC0N[9,A,Z]	ØSRT0J[9,A,Z]	ØSRV0J[9,A,Z]	XRRG0[L,M]8
Knee, LT	ØSPD[0,3,4]8Z	ØSRD06[9,A,Z]	ØSRD0J[9,A,Z]	ØSRD0EZ	ØSRD0N[9,A,Z]	ØSRU0J[9,A,Z]	ØSRW0J[9,A,Z]	XRRH0[L,M]8

Removal of Knee Liner with Replacement

Removal of Liner		Code also Replacement by Type of Synthetic Substitute							
		Oxidized Zirc on Poly	Synthetic Substitute	Articulating Spacer	Medial (L)/Lateral (M) Unicondylar	Patello-femoral	Femoral Surface	Tibial Surface	Medial(L)/Lateral (M) Meniscus
Knee, RT	ØSPC09Z	ØSRC06[9,A,Z]	ØSRC0J[9,A,Z]	ØSRC0EZ	ØSRC0[L,M][9,A,Z]	ØSRC0N[9,A,Z]	ØSRT0J[9,A,Z]	ØSRV0J[9,A,Z]	XRRG0[L,M]8
Knee, LT	ØSPD09Z	ØSRD06[9,A,Z]	ØSRD0J[9,A,Z]	ØSRD0EZ	ØSRD0[L,M][9,A,Z]	ØSRD0N[9,A,Z]	ØSRU0J[9,A,Z]	ØSRW0J[9,A,Z]	XRRH0[L,M]8

Removal of Knee Articulating Spacer with Replacement

Removal of Articulating Spacer		Code also Replacement by Type of Synthetic Substitute				
		Oxidized Zirc on Poly	Synthetic Substitute	Femoral Surface	Tibial Surface	Medial (L)/Lateral (M) Meniscus
Knee, RT	ØSPC0EZ	ØSRC06[9,A,Z]	ØSRC0J[9,A,Z]	ØSRT0J[9,A,Z]	ØSRV0J[9,A,Z]	XRRG0[L,M]8
Knee, LT	ØSPD0EZ	ØSRD06[9,A,Z]	ØSRD0J[9,A,Z]	ØSRU0J[9,A,Z]	ØSRW0J[9,A,Z]	XRRH0[L,M]8

Removal of Knee Patellar Surface with Replacement

Removal of Patellar Surface		Code also Replacement by Type of Synthetic Substitute						
		Oxidized Zirc on Poly	Synthetic Substitute	Articulating Spacer	Patello-femoral	Femoral Surface	Tibial Surface	Medial (L)/Lateral (M) Meniscus
Knee, RT	ØSPC[0,4]JC	ØSRC06[9,A,Z]	ØSRC0J[9,A,Z]	ØSRC0EZ	ØSRC0N[9,A,Z]	ØSRT0J[9,A,Z]	ØSRV0J[9,A,Z]	XRRG0[L,M]8
Knee, LT	ØSPD[0,4]JC	ØSRD06[9,A,Z]	ØSRD0J[9,A,Z]	ØSRD0EZ	ØSRD0N[9,A,Z]	ØSRU0J[9,A,Z]	ØSRW0J[9,A,Z]	XRRH0[L,M]8

Removal of Knee Synthetic Substitute with Replacement

Removal of Synthetic Substitute		Code also Replacement by Type of Synthetic Substitute							
		Oxidized Zirc on Poly	Synthetic Substitute	Articulating Spacer	Medial (L)/ Lateral (M) Unicondylar	Patello-femoral	Femoral Surface	Tibial Surface	Medial (L)/ Lateral (M) Meniscus
Knee, RT	0SPC[0,4]JZ	0SRC06[9,A,Z]	0SRC0J[9,A,Z]	0SRC0EZ	0SRC0[L,M][9,A,Z]	0SRC0N[9,A,Z]	0SRT0J[9,A,Z]	0SRV0J[9,A,Z]	XRRG0[L,M]8
Knee, LT	0SPD[0,4]JZ	0SRD06[9,A,Z]	0SRD0J[9,A,Z]	0SRD0EZ	0SRD0[L,M][9,A,Z]	0SRD0N[9,A,Z]	0SRU0J[9,A,Z]	0SRW0J[9,A,Z]	XRRH0[L,M]8

Removal of Knee Unicondylar Device with Replacement

Removal of Medial (L)/ Lateral (M) Unicondylar Device		Code also Replacement by Type of Synthetic Substitute					
		Oxidized Zirc on Poly	Synthetic Substitute	Medial Unicondylar	Femoral Surface	Tibial Surface	Medial (L)/Lateral (M) Meniscus
Knee, RT	0SPC[0,4][L,M]Z	0SRC06[9,A,Z]	0SRC0J[9,A,Z]	0SRC0L[9,A,Z]	0SRT0J[9,A,Z]	0SRV0J[9,A,Z]	XRRG0[L,M]8
Knee, LT	0SPD[0,4][L,M]Z	0SRD06[9,A,Z]	0SRD0J[9,A,Z]	0SRD0L[9,A,Z]	0SRU0J[9,A,Z]	0SRW0J[9,A,Z]	XRRH0[L,M]8

Removal of Knee Patellofemoral Device with Replacement

Removal of Patellofemoral Device		Code also Replacement by Type of Synthetic Substitute					
		Oxidized Zirc on Poly	Synthetic Substitute	Medial Unicondylar	Femoral Surface	Tibial Surface	Medial (L)/Lateral (M) Meniscus
Knee, RT	0SPC[0,4]NZ	0SRC06[9,A,Z]	0SRC0J[9,A,Z]	0SRC0L[9,A,Z]	0SRT0J[9,A,Z]	0SRV0J[9,A,Z]	XRRG0[L,M]8
Knee, LT	0SPD[0,4]NZ	0SRD06[9,A,Z]	0SRD0J[9,A,Z]	0SRD0L[9,A,Z]	0SRU0J[9,A,Z]	0SRW0J[9,A,Z]	XRRH0[L,M]8

Removal of Knee Femoral/Tibial Surface Device with Replacement

Removal of Femoral (T,U)/ Tibial (V,W) Surface		Code also Replacement by Type of Synthetic Substitute							
		Oxidized Zirc on Poly	Synthetic Substitute	Articulating Spacer	Patello-femoral	Femoral Surface	Tibial Surface	Medial (L)/Lateral (M) Meniscus	
Knee, RT	0SP[T,V][0,4]JZ	0SRC06[9,A,Z]	0SRC0J[9,A,Z]	0SRC0EZ	0SRC0N[9,A,Z]	0SRT0J[9,A,Z]	0SRV0J[9,A,Z]	XRRG0[L,M]8	
Knee, LT	0SP[U,W][0,4]JZ	0SRD06[9,A,Z]	0SRD0J[9,A,Z]	0SRD0EZ	0SRD0N[9,A,Z]	0SRU0J[9,A,Z]	0SRW0J[9,A,Z]	XRRH0[L,M]8	

DRG 485-489 Knee Procedures

Joint	Removal of Liner by open approach	Code also Supplement of Tibial Surface by Site
Knee, RT	0SPC09Z	0SUV09Z
Knee, LT	0SPD09Z	0SUW09Z

DRG 515-517 Other Musculoskeletal System and Connective Tissue Procedures

Site	Reposition of Vertebra by percutaneous approach	Code also Supplement with Synthetic Substitute by Percutaneous Approach at site of Repositioned Vertebra
Cervical	0PS33ZZ	0PU33JZ
Coccyx	0QSS3ZZ	0QUS3JZ
Lumbar	0QS03ZZ	0QU03JZ
Sacrum	0QS13ZZ	0QU13JZ
Thoracic	0PS43ZZ	0PU43JZ

DRG 518-520 Back and Neck Procedures, Except Spinal Fusion, or Disc Devices/Neurostimulators

Generator Type	Insertion of Generator by Site			Code also Insertion Neurostimulator Lead by approach and Site	
	Chest	Abdomen	Back	Spinal Canal	Spinal Cord
Single Array	0JH6[0,3]BZ	0JH8[0,3]BZ	0JH7[0,3]BZ	00HU[0,3,4]MZ	00HV[0,3,4]MZ
Single Array, Rechargeable	0JH6[0,3]CZ	0JH8[0,3]CZ	0JH7[0,3]CZ	00HU[0,3,4]MZ	00HV[0,3,4]MZ
Multiple Array	0JH6[0,3]DZ	0JH8[0,3]DZ	0JH7[0,3]DZ	00HU[0,3,4]MZ	00HV[0,3,4]MZ
Multiple Array, Rechargeable	0JH6[0,3]EZ	—	0JH7[0,3]EZ	00HU[0,3,4]MZ	00HV[0,3,4]MZ
Multiple Array, Rechargeable	—	0JH8[0,3]EZ	—	00HU[0,3,4]MZ	00HV[0,3,4]MZ

Appendix L: Procedure Combination Tables

DRG 582-583 Mastectomy for Malignancy

Site	Resection by Open approach	Code also Resection of Lymph Nodes by Open approach by site			Code also Resection of Thorax Muscle by Open approach	
		Axillary	Internal Mammary	Thorax	Right	Left
Breast, Right	0HT0ZZ	07T50ZZ	07T80ZZ	07T70ZZ	0KTH0ZZ	—
Breast, Left	0HTU0ZZ	07T60ZZ	07T90ZZ	07T70ZZ	—	0KTJ0ZZ
Breast, Bilateral	0HTV0ZZ	07T50ZZ and 07T60ZZ	07T80ZZ and 07T90ZZ	07T70ZZ	0KTH0ZZ	0KTJ0ZZ

DRG 584-585 Breast Biopsy, Local Excision and Other Breast Procedures

Resection of Breast with Resection of Lymph Nodes and Thorax Muscle

Site	Resection by Open approach	Code also Resection of Lymph Nodes by Open approach by site			Code also Resection of Thorax Muscle by Open approach	
		Axillary	Internal Mammary	Thorax	Right	Left
Breast, Right	0HTT0ZZ	07T50ZZ	07T80ZZ	07T70ZZ	0KTH0ZZ	—
Breast, Left	0HTU0ZZ	07T60ZZ	07T90ZZ	07T70ZZ	—	0KTJ0ZZ
Breast, Bilateral	0HTV0ZZ	07T50ZZ and 07T60ZZ	07T80ZZ and 07T90ZZ	07T70ZZ	0KTH0ZZ	0KTJ0ZZ

Replacement of Breast Tissue

Site	Replacement by Percutaneous approach with Autologous Tissue	Code also Extraction of Subcutaneous Tissue by Percutaneous approach					
		Abdomen	Back	Buttock	Chest	Leg, Upper, Right	Leg, Upper, Left
Breast, Right	0HRT37Z	0JD83ZZ	0JD73ZZ	0JD93ZZ	0JD63ZZ	0JDL3ZZ	0JDM3ZZ
Breast, Left	0HRU37Z	0JD83ZZ	0JD73ZZ	0JD93ZZ	0JD63ZZ	0JDL3ZZ	0JDM3ZZ
Breast, Bilateral	0HRV37Z	0JD83ZZ	0JD73ZZ	0JD93ZZ	0JD63ZZ	0JDL3ZZ	0JDM3ZZ

DRG 628-630 Other Endocrine, Nutritional and Metabolic Procedures

Hip Procedure Combinations

Open Removal of Hip Spacer with Replacement

Removal of Spacer		Code also Replacement by Device Type					
		Metal	Metal on Poly	Ceramic	Ceramic on Poly	Oxidized Zirc on Poly	Synthetic Substitute
Hip, RT	0SP908Z	0SR901[9,A,Z]	0SR902[9,A,Z]	0SR903[9,A,Z]	0SR904[9,A,Z]	0SR906[9,A,Z]	0SR90J[9,A,Z]
Hip, LT	0SPB08Z	0SRB01[9,A,Z]	0SRB02[9,A,Z]	0SRB03[9,A,Z]	0SRB04[9,A,Z]	0SRB06[9,A,Z]	0SRB0J[9,A,Z]

Open Removal of Hip Spacer with Replacement

Removal of Spacer		Code also Replacement by Device Type						
		Acetabular Surface				Femoral Surface		
		Poly	Metal	Ceramic	Synthetic	Metal	Ceramic	Synthetic
Hip, RT	0SP908Z	0SRA00[9,A,Z]	0SRA01[9,A,Z]	0SRA03[9,A,Z]	0SRA0J[9,A,Z]	0SRR01[9,A,Z]	0SRR03[9,A,Z]	0SRR0J[9,A,Z]
Hip, LT	0SPB08Z	0SRE00[9,A,Z]	0SRE01[9,A,Z]	0SRE03[9,A,Z]	0SRE0J[9,A,Z]	0SRS01[9,A,Z]	0SRS03[9,A,Z]	0SRS0J[9,A,Z]

Open Removal of Hip Spacer with Liner Insertion (supplement)

Removal of Spacer		Code also Supplement of Body Part by Site		
		Joint	Acetabular Surface	Femoral Surface
Hip, RT	0SP908Z	0SU909Z	0SUA09Z	0SUR09Z
Hip, LT	0SPB08Z	0SUB09Z	0SUE09Z	0SUS09Z

Open Removal of Hip Liner with Replacement

Removal of Liner		Code also Replacement by Device Type					
		Metal	Metal on Poly	Ceramic	Ceramic on Poly	Oxidized Zirc on Poly	Synthetic Substitute
Hip, RT	0SP909Z	0SR901[9,A,Z]	0SR902[9,A,Z]	0SR903[9,A,Z]	0SR904[9,A,Z]	0SR906[9,A,Z]	0SR90J[9,A,Z]
Hip, LT	0SPB09Z	0SRB01[9,A,Z]	0SRB02[9,A,Z]	0SRB03[9,A,Z]	0SRB04[9,A,Z]	0SRB06[9,A,Z]	0SRB0J[9,A,Z]

Appendix L: Procedure Combination Tables

Open Removal of Hip Liner with Replacement

Removal of Liner			Code also Replacement by Device Type						
			Acetabular Surface				Femoral Surface		
			Poly	Metal	Ceramic	Synthetic	Metal	Ceramic	Synthetic
Hip, RT		ØSP9Ø9Z	ØSRAØØ[9,A,Z]	ØSRAØ1[9,A,Z]	ØSRAØ3[9,A,Z]	ØSRAØJ[9,A,Z]	ØSRRØ1[9,A,Z]	ØSRRØ3[9,A,Z]	ØSRRØJ[9,A,Z]
Hip, LT		ØSPBØ9Z	ØSREØØ[9,A,Z]	ØSREØ1[9,A,Z]	ØSREØ3[9,A,Z]	ØSREØJ[9,A,Z]	ØSRSØ1[9,A,Z]	ØSRSØ3[9,A,Z]	ØSRSØJ[9,A,Z]

Open Removal of Hip Liner with Liner Insertion (supplement)

Removal of Liner			Code also Supplement of Body Part by Site		
			Joint	Acetabular Surface	Femoral Surface
Hip, RT		ØSP9Ø9Z	ØSU9Ø9Z	ØSUAØ9Z	ØSURØ9Z
Hip, LT		ØSPBØ9Z	ØSUBØ9Z	ØSUEØ9Z	ØSUSØ9Z

Open Removal of Hip Resurfacing Device with Replacement

Removal of Resurfacing Device			Code also Replacement by Device Type					
			Metal	Metal on Poly	Ceramic	Ceramic on Poly	Oxidized Zirc on Poly	Synthetic Substitute
Hip, RT		ØSP9ØBZ	ØSR9Ø1[9,A,Z]	ØSR9Ø2[9,A,Z]	ØSR9Ø3[9,A,Z]	ØSR9Ø4[9,A,Z]	ØSR9Ø6[9,A,Z]	ØSR9ØJ[9,A,Z]
Hip, LT		ØSPBØBZ	ØSRBØ1[9,A,Z]	ØSRBØ2[9,A,Z]	ØSRBØ3[9,A,Z]	ØSRBØ4[9,A,Z]	ØSRBØ6[9,A,Z]	ØSRBØJ[9,A,Z]

Open Removal of Hip Resurfacing Device with Replacement

Removal of Resurfacing Device			Code also Replacement by Device Type						
			Acetabular Surface				Femoral Surface		
			Poly	Metal	Ceramic	Synthetic	Metal	Ceramic	Synthetic
Hip, RT		ØSP9ØBZ	ØSRAØØ[9,A,Z]	ØSRAØ1[9,A,Z]	ØSRAØ3[9,A,Z]	ØSRAØJ[9,A,Z]	ØSRRØ1[9,A,Z]	ØSRRØ3[9,A,Z]	ØSRRØJ[9,A,Z]
Hip, LT		ØSPBØBZ	ØSREØØ[9,A,Z]	ØSREØ1[9,A,Z]	ØSREØ3[9,A,Z]	ØSREØJ[9,A,Z]	ØSRSØ1[9,A,Z]	ØSRSØ3[9,A,Z]	ØSRSØJ[9,A,Z]

Open Removal of Hip Resurfacing Device with Liner Insertion (supplement)

Removal of Resurfacing Device			Code also Supplement of Body Part by Site		
			Joint	Acetabular Surface	Femoral Surface
Hip, RT		ØSP9ØBZ	ØSU9Ø9Z	ØSUAØ9Z	ØSURØ9Z
Hip, LT		ØSPBØBZ	ØSUBØ9Z	ØSUEØ9Z	ØSUSØ9Z

Open Removal of Hip Synthetic Substitute with Replacement

Removal of Synthetic Substitute			Code also Replacement by Device Type					
			Metal	Metal on Poly	Ceramic	Ceramic on Poly	Oxidized Zirc on Poly	Synthetic Substitute
Hip, RT		ØSP9ØJZ	ØSR9Ø1[9,A,Z]	ØSR9Ø2[9,A,Z]	ØSR9Ø3[9,A,Z]	ØSR9Ø4[9,A,Z]	ØSR9Ø6[9,A,Z]	ØSR9ØJ[9,A,Z]
Hip, LT		ØSPBØJZ	ØSRBØ1[9,A,Z]	ØSRBØ2[9,A,Z]	ØSRBØ3[9,A,Z]	ØSRBØ4[9,A,Z]	ØSRBØ6[9,A,Z]	ØSRBØJ[9,A,Z]

Open Removal of Hip Synthetic Substitute with Replacement

Removal of Synthetic Substitute			Code also Replacement by Device Type						
			Acetabular Surface				Femoral Surface		
			Poly	Metal	Ceramic	Synthetic	Metal	Ceramic	Synthetic
Hip, RT		ØSP9ØJZ	ØSRAØØ[9,A,Z]	ØSRAØ1[9,A,Z]	ØSRAØ3[9,A,Z]	ØSRAØJ[9,A,Z]	ØSRRØ1[9,A,Z]	ØSRRØ3[9,A,Z]	ØSRRØJ[9,A,Z]
Hip, LT		ØSPBØJZ	ØSREØØ[9,A,Z]	ØSREØ1[9,A,Z]	ØSREØ3[9,A,Z]	ØSREØJ[9,A,Z]	ØSRSØ1[9,A,Z]	ØSRSØ3[9,A,Z]	ØSRSØJ[9,A,Z]

Open Removal of Hip Acetabular/Femoral Surface with Replacement

Removal of Acetabular/Femoral Surface			Code also Replacement by Device Type					
			Metal	Metal on Poly	Ceramic	Ceramic on Poly	Oxidized Zirc on Poly	Synthetic Substitute
Hip, RT		ØSP[A,R]ØJZ	ØSR9Ø1[9,A,Z]	ØSR9Ø2[9,A,Z]	ØSR9Ø3[9,A,Z]	ØSR9Ø4[9,A,Z]	ØSR9Ø6[9,A,Z]	ØSR9ØJ[9,A,Z]
Hip, LT		ØSP[E,S]ØJZ	ØSRBØ1[9,A,Z]	ØSRBØ2[9,A,Z]	ØSRBØ3[9,A,Z]	ØSRBØ4[9,A,Z]	ØSRBØ6[9,A,Z]	ØSRBØJ[9,A,Z]

Appendix L: Procedure Combination Tables

Open Removal of Hip Acetabular/Femoral Surface with Replacement

Removal of Acetabular/Femoral Surface		Code also Replacement by Device Type							
		Acetabular Surface				Femoral Surface		
		Poly	Metal	Ceramic	Synthetic	Metal	Ceramic	Synthetic
Hip, RT	0SP[A,R]0JZ	0SRA00[9,A,Z]	0SRA01[9,A,Z]	0SRA03[9,A,Z]	0SRA0J[9,A,Z]	0SRR01[9,A,Z]	0SRR03[9,A,Z]	0SRR0J[9,A,Z]
Hip, LT	0SP[E,S]0JZ	0SRE00[9,A,Z]	0SRE01[9,A,Z]	0SRE03[9,A,Z]	0SRE0J[9,A,Z]	0SRS01[9,A,Z]	0SRS03[9,A,Z]	0SRS0J[9,A,Z]

Percutaneous Endoscopic Removal of Hip Spacer with Replacement

Removal of Spacer		Code also Replacement by Device Type					
		Metal	Metal on Poly	Ceramic	Ceramic on Poly	Oxidized Zirc on Poly	Synthetic Substitute
Hip, RT	0SP948Z	0SR901[9,A,Z]	0SR902[9,A,Z]	0SR903[9,A,Z]	0SR904[9,A,Z]	0SR906[9,A,Z]	0SR90J[9,A,Z]
Hip, LT	0SPB48Z	0SRB01[9,A,Z]	0SRB02[9,A,Z]	0SRB03[9,A,Z]	0SRB04[9,A,Z]	0SRB06[9,A,Z]	0SRB0J[9,A,Z]

Percutaneous Endoscopic Removal of Hip Spacer with Replacement

Removal of Spacer		Code also Replacement by Device Type							
		Acetabular Surface				Femoral Surface		
		Poly	Metal	Ceramic	Synthetic	Metal	Ceramic	Synthetic
Hip, RT	0SP948Z	0SRA00[9,A,Z]	0SRA01[9,A,Z]	0SRA03[9,A,Z]	0SRA0J[9,A,Z]	0SRR01[9,A,Z]	0SRR03[9,A,Z]	0SRR0J[9,A,Z]
Hip, LT	0SPB48Z	0SRE00[9,A,Z]	0SRE01[9,A,Z]	0SRE03[9,A,Z]	0SRE0J[9,A,Z]	0SRS01[9,A,Z]	0SRS03[9,A,Z]	0SRS0J[9,A,Z]

Percutaneous Endoscopic Removal of Hip Spacer with Liner Insertion (supplement)

Removal of Spacer		Code also Supplement of Body Part by Site		
		Joint	Acetabular Surface	Femoral Surface
Hip, RT	0SP948Z	0SU909Z	0SUA09Z	0SUR09Z
Hip, LT	0SPB48Z	0SUB09Z	0SUE09Z	0SUS09Z

Percutaneous Endoscopic Removal of Hip Synthetic Substitute with Replacement

Removal of Synthetic Substitute		Code also Replacement by Device Type					
		Metal	Metal on Poly	Ceramic	Ceramic on Poly	Oxidized Zirc on Poly	Synthetic Substitute
Hip, RT	0SP94JZ	0SR901[9,A,Z]	0SR902[9,A,Z]	0SR903[9,A,Z]	0SR904[9,A,Z]	0SR906[9,A,Z]	0SR90J[9,A,Z]
Hip, LT	0SPB4JZ	0SRB01[9,A,Z]	0SRB02[9,A,Z]	0SRB03[9,A,Z]	0SRB04[9,A,Z]	0SRB06[9,A,Z]	0SRB0J[9,A,Z]

Percutaneous Endoscopic of Hip Synthetic Substitute with Replacement

Removal of Synthetic Substitute		Code also Replacement by Device Type							
		Acetabular Surface				Femoral Surface		
		Poly	Metal	Ceramic	Synthetic	Metal	Ceramic	Synthetic
Hip, RT	0SP94JZ	0SRA00[9,A,Z]	0SRA01[9,A,Z]	0SRA03[9,A,Z]	0SRA0J[9,A,Z]	0SRR01[9,A,Z]	0SRR03[9,A,Z]	0SRR0J[9,A,Z]
Hip, LT	0SPB4JZ	0SRE00[9,A,Z]	0SRE01[9,A,Z]	0SRE03[9,A,Z]	0SRE0J[9,A,Z]	0SRS01[9,A,Z]	0SRS03[9,A,Z]	0SRS0J[9,A,Z]

Percutaneous Endoscopic Removal of Hip Synthetic Substitute with Liner Insertion (supplement)

Removal of Synthetic Substitute		Code also Supplement of Body Part by Site		
		Joint	Acetabular Surface	Femoral Surface
Hip, RT	0SP94JZ	0SU909Z	0SUA09Z	0SUR09Z
Hip, LT	0SPB4JZ	0SUB09Z	0SUE09Z	0SUS09Z

Percutaneous Endoscopic Removal of Hip Acetabular/Femoral Surface with Replacement

Removal of Acetabular/Femoral Surface		Code also Replacement by Device Type					
		Metal	Metal on Poly	Ceramic	Ceramic on Poly	Oxidized Zirc on Poly	Synthetic Substitute
Hip, RT	0SP[A,R]4JZ	0SR901[9,A,Z]	0SR902[9,A,Z]	0SR903[9,A,Z]	0SR904[9,A,Z]	0SR906[9,A,Z]	0SR90J[9,A,Z]
Hip, LT	0SP[E,S]4JZ	0SRB01[9,A,Z]	0SRB02[9,A,Z]	0SRB03[9,A,Z]	0SRB04[9,A,Z]	0SRB06[9,A,Z]	0SRB0J[9,A,Z]

Percutaneous Endoscopic of Hip Acetabular/Femoral Surface with Replacement

Removal of Acetabular/Femoral Surface		Code also Replacement by Device Type						
		Acetabular Surface				Femoral Surface		
		Poly	Metal	Ceramic	Synthetic	Metal	Ceramic	Synthetic
Hip, RT	0SP[A,R]4JZ	0SRA00[9,A,Z]	0SRA01[9,A,Z]	0SRA03[9,A,Z]	0SRA0J[9,A,Z]	0SRR01[9,A,Z]	0SRR03[9,A,Z]	0SRR0J[9,A,Z]
Hip, LT	0SP[E,S]4JZ	0SRE00[9,A,Z]	0SRE01[9,A,Z]	0SRE03[9,A,Z]	0SRE0J[9,A,Z]	0SRS01[9,A,Z]	0SRS03[9,A,Z]	0SRS0J[9,A,Z]

Percutaneous Endoscopic Removal of Hip Acetabular/Femoral Surface with Liner Insertion (supplement)

Removal of Acetabular/Femoral Surface		Code also Supplement of Body Part by Site		
		Joint	Acetabular Surface	Femoral Surface
Hip, RT	0SP[A,R]4JZ	0SU909Z	0SUA09Z	0SUR09Z
Hip, LT	0SP[E,S]4JZ	0SUB09Z	0SUE09Z	0SUS09Z

Knee Procedure Combinations

Removal of Knee Liner with Replacement

Removal of Liner		Code also Replacement by Device Type						
		Oxidized Zirc on Poly	Synthetic Substitute	Medial (L)/ Lateral (M) Unicondylar	Patello-femoral	Femoral Surface	Tibial Surface	Medial (L)/ Lateral (M) Meniscus
Knee, RT	0SPC09Z	0SRC06[9,A,Z]	0SRC0J[9,A,Z]	0SRC0[L,M][9,A,Z]	0SRC0N[9,A,Z]	0SRT0J[9,A,Z]	0SRV0J[9,A,Z]	XRRG0[L,M]8
Knee, LT	0SPD09Z	0SRD06[9,A,Z]	0SRD0J[9,A,Z]	0SRD0[L,M][9,A,Z]	0SRD0N[9,A,Z]	0SRU0J[9,A,Z]	0SRW0J[9,A,Z]	XRRH0[L,M]8

Removal of Knee Patellar Surface with Replacement

Removal of Patellar Surface		Code also Replacement of Surface Device	
		Femoral	Tibial
Knee, RT	0SPC[0,4]JC	0SRT0J[9,A,Z]	0SRV0J[9,A,Z]
Knee, LT	0SPD[0,4]JC	0SRU0J[9,A,Z]	0SRW0J[9,A,Z]

Removal of Knee Synthetic Substitute with Replacement

Removal of Synthetic Substitute		Code also Replacement of Surface Device	
		Femoral	Tibial
Knee, RT	0SPC[0,4]JZ	0SRT0J[9,A,Z]	0SRV0J[9,A,Z]
Knee, LT	0SPD[0,4]JZ	0SRU0J[9,A,Z]	0SRW0J[9,A,Z]

Removal of Knee Unicondylar Device with Replacement

Joint	Removal of Unicondylar Device		Code also Replacement of Surface Device	
	Medial	Lateral	Femoral	Tibial
Knee, RT	0SPC[0,4]LZ	0SPC[0,4]MZ	0SRT0J[9,A,Z]	0SRV0J[9,A,Z]
Knee, LT	0SPD[0,4]LZ	0SPD[0,4]MZ	0SRU0J[9,A,Z]	0SRW0J[9,A,Z]

Removal of Knee Patellofemoral Device with Replacement

Removal of Patellofemoral Device		Code also Replacement of Surface Device	
		Femoral	Tibial
Knee, RT	0SPC[0,4]NZ	0SRT0J[9,A,Z]	0SRV0J[9,A,Z]
Knee, LT	0SPD[0,4]NZ	0SRU0J[9,A,Z]	0SRW0J[9,A,Z]

Removal of Knee Femoral/Tibial Surface Device with Replacement

Joint	Removal of Surface Device		Code also Replacement of Surface Device	
	Femoral	Tibial	Femoral	Tibial
Knee, RT	0SPT[0,4]JZ	0SPV[0,4]JZ	0SRT0J[9,A,Z]	0SRV0J[9,A,Z]
Knee, LT	0SPU[0,4]JZ	0SPW[0,4]JZ	0SRU0J[9,A,Z]	0SRW0J[9,A,Z]

Appendix L: Procedure Combination Tables

DRG 662-664 Minor Bladder Procedure

Repair of Bladder	Code also Repair of Abdominal Wall	
	with Stoma	without Stoma
0TQB[0,3,4]ZZ	0WQFXZ2	0WQFXZZ

DRG 665-667 Prostatectomy

Site	Resection by approach				Code also Resection of Seminal Vesicles, Bilateral by approach	
	Open	Percutaneous Endoscopic	Via Natural or Artificial Opening	Via Natural or Artificial Opening Endoscopic	Open	Percutaneous Endoscopic
Prostate	0VT00ZZ	0VT04ZZ	0VT07ZZ	0VT08ZZ	0VT30ZZ	0VT34ZZ

DRG 707-708 Major Male Pelvic Procedures

Site	Resection by approach				Code also Resection of Seminal Vesicles, Bilateral by approach	
	Open	Percutaneous Endoscopic	Via Natural or Artificial Opening	Via Natural or Artificial Opening Endoscopic	Open	Percutaneous Endoscopic
Prostate	0VT00ZZ	0VT04ZZ	0VT07ZZ	0VT08ZZ	0VT30ZZ	0VT34ZZ

DRG 734-735 Pelvic Evisceration, Radical Hysterectomy and Radical Vulvectomy

Pelvic Evisceration

Resection by Site						
Bladder	Cervix	Fallopian Tubes, Bilateral	Ovaries, Bilateral	Urethra	Uterus	Vagina
0TTB0ZZ	0UTC0ZZ	0UT70ZZ	0UT20ZZ	0TTD0ZZ	0UT90ZZ	0UTG0ZZ

Radical Hysterectomy

Approach	Resection by Site		
	Cervix	Uterus	Uterine Support Structure
Vaginal	0UTC[7,8]ZZ	0UT9[7,8]ZZ	0UT4[7,8]ZZ
Abdominal, Endoscopic	0UTC4ZZ	0UT9[4,F]ZZ	0UT44ZZ
Abdominal, Open	0UTC0ZZ	0UT90ZZ	0UT40ZZ

Radical Vulvectomy

Resection by Site	Code also Excision of Inguinal Lymph Nodes by Approach	
Vulva	Right	Left
0UTM[0,X]ZZ	07BH[0,4]ZZ	07BJ[0,4]ZZ

Non-OR procedure combinations

Note: The following table identifies procedure combinations that are considered Non-OR even though one or more procedures of the combination are considered valid DRG OR procedures

Insertion with Removal of Intraluminal Device

Insertion of Intraluminal Device into Hepatobiliary Duct	Code also Removal of Intraluminal Device by Approach and Site			
	Via Natural or Artificial Opening		External	
	Hepatobiliary Duct	Pancreatic Duct	Hepatobiliary Duct	Pancreatic Duct
0FHB7DZ	0FPB[7,8]DZ	0FPD[7,8]DZ	0FPBXDZ	0FPDXDZ

Appendix M: Coding Exercises and Answers

Using the ICD-10-PCS tables construct the code that accurately represents the procedure performed.

Medical Surgical Section

Procedure	Code
1. Excision of malignant melanoma from skin of right ear	
2. Laparoscopy with excision of endometrial implant from left ovary	
3. Percutaneous needle core biopsy of right kidney	
4. EGD with excisional gastric biopsy	
5. Open endarterectomy of left common carotid artery	
6. Excision of basal cell carcinoma of lower lip	
7. Open excision of tail of pancreas	
8. Percutaneous biopsy of right gastrocnemius muscle	
9. Sigmoidoscopy with sigmoid polypectomy	
10. Open excision of lesion from right Achilles tendon	
11. Open resection of cecum	
12. Total excision of pituitary gland, open	
13. Explantation of left failed kidney, open	
14. Open left axillary total lymphadenectomy	
15. Laparoscopic-assisted vaginal hysterectomy	
16. Right total mastectomy, open	
17. Open resection of papillary muscle	
18. Total retropubic prostatectomy, open	
19. Laparoscopic cholecystectomy, hand-assisted	
20. Endoscopic bilateral total maxillary sinusectomy	
21. Amputation at right elbow level	
22. Right below-knee amputation, proximal tibia/fibula	
23. Fifth ray carpometacarpal joint amputation, left hand	
24. Right leg and hip amputation through ischium	
25. DIP joint amputation of right thumb	
26. Right wrist joint amputation	
27. Trans-metatarsal amputation of foot at left big toe	
28. Mid-shaft amputation, right humerus	
29. Left fourth toe amputation, mid-proximal phalanx	
30. Right above-knee amputation, distal femur	
31. Cryotherapy of wart on left hand	
32. Percutaneous radiofrequency ablation of right vocal cord lesion	
33. Left heart catheterization with laser destruction of arrhythmogenic focus, A-V node	
34. Cautery of nosebleed	
35. Transurethral endoscopic laser ablation of prostate	
36. Percutaneous cautery of oozing varicose vein, left calf	
37. Laparoscopy with destruction of endometriosis, bilateral ovaries	
38. Laser coagulation of right retinal vessel, percutaneous	
39. Thoracoscopic pleurodesis, left side	
40. Percutaneous insertion of Greenfield IVC filter	
41. Forceps total mouth extraction, upper and lower teeth	

Procedure	Code
42. Removal of left thumbnail	
43. Extraction of right intraocular lens without replacement, percutaneous	
44. Laparoscopy with needle aspiration of ova for in vitro fertilization	
45. Nonexcisional debridement of skin ulcer, right foot	
46. Open stripping of abdominal fascia, right side	
47. Hysteroscopy with D&C, diagnostic	
48. Liposuction for medical purposes, left upper arm	
49. Removal of tattered right ear drum fragments with tweezers	
50. Microincisional phlebectomy of spider veins, right lower leg	
51. Routine Foley catheter placement	
52. Incision and drainage of external anal abscess	
53. Percutaneous drainage of ascites	
54. Laparoscopy with left ovarian cystotomy and drainage	
55. Laparotomy and drain placement for liver abscess, right lobe	
56. Right knee arthrotomy with drain placement	
57. Thoracentesis of left pleural effusion	
58. Phlebotomy of left median cubital vein for polycythemia vera	
59. Percutaneous chest tube placement for right pneumothorax	
60. Endoscopic drainage of left ethmoid sinus	
61. External ventricular CSF drainage catheter placement via burr hole	
62. Removal of foreign body, right cornea	
63. Percutaneous mechanical thrombectomy, left brachial artery	
64. Esophagogastroscopy with removal of bezoar from stomach	
65. Foreign body removal, skin of left thumb	
66. Transurethral cystoscopy with removal of bladder stone	
67. Forceps removal of foreign body in right nostril	
68. Laparoscopy with excision of old suture from mesentery	
69. Incision and removal of right lacrimal duct stone	
70. Nonincisional removal of intraluminal foreign body from vagina	
71. Right common carotid endarterectomy, open	
72. Open excision of retained sliver, subcutaneous tissue of left foot	
73. Extracorporeal shockwave lithotripsy (ESWL), bilateral ureters	
74. Endoscopic retrograde cholangiopancreatography (ERCP) with lithotripsy of common bile duct stone	
75. Thoracotomy with crushing of pericardial calcifications	
76. Transurethral cystoscopy with fragmentation of bladder calculus	
77. Hysteroscopy with intraluminal lithotripsy of left fallopian tube calcification	
78. Division of right foot tendon, percutaneous	

Appendix M: Coding Exercises and Answers

Procedure	Code
79. Left heart catheterization with division of bundle of HIS	
80. Open osteotomy of capitate, left hand	
81. EGD with esophagotomy of esophagogastric junction	
82. Sacral rhizotomy for pain control, percutaneous	
83. Laparotomy with exploration and adhesiolysis of right ureter	
84. Incision of scar contracture, right elbow	
85. Frenulotomy for treatment of tongue-tie syndrome	
86. Right shoulder arthroscopy with coracoacromial ligament release	
87. Mitral valvulotomy for release of fused leaflets, open approach	
88. Percutaneous left Achilles tendon release	
89. Laparoscopy with lysis of peritoneal adhesions	
90. Manual rupture of right shoulder joint adhesions under general anesthesia	
91. Open posterior tarsal tunnel release	
92. Laparoscopy with freeing of left ovary and fallopian tube	
93. Liver transplant with donor matched liver	
94. Orthotopic heart transplant using porcine heart	
95. Right lung transplant, open, using organ donor match	
96. Transplant of large intestine, organ donor match	
97. Left kidney/pancreas organ bank transplant	
98. Replantation of avulsed scalp	
99. Reattachment of severed right ear	
100. Reattachment of traumatic left gastrocnemius avulsion, open	
101. Closed replantation of three avulsed teeth, lower jaw	
102. Reattachment of severed left hand	
103. Right open palmaris longus tendon transfer	
104. Endoscopic radial to median nerve transfer	
105. Fasciocutaneous flap closure of left thigh, open	
106. Transfer left index finger to left thumb position, open	
107. Percutaneous fascia transfer to fill defect, right neck	
108. Trigeminal to facial nerve transfer, percutaneous endoscopic	
109. Endoscopic left leg flexor hallucis longus tendon transfer	
110. Right scalp advancement flap to right temple	
111. Resection right breast with TRAM flap reconstruction, open	
112. Skin transfer flap closure of complex open wound, left lower back	
113. Open fracture reduction, right tibia	
114. Laparoscopy with gastropexy for malrotation	
115. Left knee arthroscopy with reposition of anterior cruciate ligament	
116. Open transposition of ulnar nerve	
117. Closed reduction with percutaneous internal fixation of right femoral neck fracture	
118. Trans-vaginal intraluminal cervical cerclage	
119. Cervical cerclage using Shirodkar technique	
120. Thoracotomy with banding of left pulmonary artery using extraluminal device	
121. Restriction of thoracic duct with intraluminal stent, percutaneous	

Procedure	Code
122. Craniotomy with clipping of cerebral aneurysm	
123. Nonincisional, transnasal placement of restrictive stent in right lacrimal duct	
124. Catheter-based temporary restriction of blood flow in abdominal aorta for treatment of cerebral ischemia	
125. Percutaneous ligation of esophageal vein	
126. Percutaneous embolization of left internal carotid-cavernous fistula	
127. Laparoscopy with bilateral occlusion of fallopian tubes using Hulka extraluminal clips	
128. Open suture ligation of failed AV graft, left brachial artery	
129. Percutaneous embolization of vascular supply, intracranial meningioma	
130. Percutaneous embolization of right uterine artery, using coils	
131. Open occlusion of left atrial appendage, using extraluminal pressure clips	
132. Percutaneous suture exclusion of left atrial appendage, via femoral artery access	
133. ERCP with balloon dilation of common bile duct	
134. PTCA of two coronary arteries, LAD with stent placement, RCA with no stent	
135. Cystoscopy with intraluminal dilation of bladder neck stricture	
136. Open dilation of old anastomosis, left femoral artery	
137. Dilation of upper esophageal stricture, direct visualization, with Bougie sound	
138. PTA of right brachial artery stenosis	
139. Transnasal dilation and stent placement in right lacrimal duct	
140. Hysteroscopy with balloon dilation of bilateral fallopian tubes	
141. Tracheoscopy with intraluminal dilation of tracheal stenosis	
142. Cystoscopy with dilation of left ureteral stricture, with stent placement	
143. Open gastric bypass with Roux-en-Y limb to jejunum	
144. Right temporal artery to intracranial artery bypass using Gore-Tex graft, open	
145. Tracheostomy formation with tracheostomy tube placement, percutaneous	
146. PICVA (percutaneous in situ coronary venous arterialization) of single coronary artery	
147. Open left femoral-popliteal artery bypass using cadaver vein graft	
148. Shunting of intrathecal cerebrospinal fluid to peritoneal cavity using synthetic shunt	
149. Colostomy formation, open, transverse colon to abdominal wall	
150. Open urinary diversion, left ureter, using ileal conduit to skin	
151. CABG of LAD using pedicled left internal mammary artery, open off-bypass	
152. Open pleuroperitoneal shunt, right pleural cavity, using synthetic device	
153. Percutaneous placement of ventriculoperitoneal shunt for treatment of hydrocephalus	
154. End-of-life replacement of spinal neurostimulator generator, multiple array, in lower abdomen	
155. Percutaneous insertion of spinal neurostimulator lead, lumbar spinal cord	

Procedure	Code
156. Percutaneous replacement of broken pacemaker lead in left atrium	
157. Open placement of dual chamber pacemaker generator in chest wall	
158. Percutaneous placement of venous central line in right internal jugular, with tip in superior vena cava	
159. Open insertion of multiple channel cochlear implant, left ear	
160. Percutaneous placement of Swan-Ganz catheter in pulmonary trunk	
161. Bronchoscopy with insertion of Low Dose, Pd-103 brachytherapy seeds, right lung	
162. Open insertion of interspinous process device into lumbar vertebral joint	
163. Open placement of bone growth stimulator, left femoral shaft	
164. Cystoscopy with placement of brachytherapy seeds in prostate gland	
165. Percutaneous insertion of Greenfield IVC filter	
166. Full-thickness skin graft to right lower arm, autograft (do not code graft harvest for this exercise)	
167. Excision of necrosed left femoral head with bone bank bone graft to fill the defect, open	
168. Penetrating keratoplasty of right cornea with donor matched cornea, percutaneous approach	
169. Excision of abdominal aorta with Gore-Tex graft replacement, open	
170. Total right knee arthroplasty with insertion of total knee prosthesis	
171. Tenonectomy with graft to right ankle using cadaver graft, open	
172. Mitral valve replacement using porcine valve, open	
173. Percutaneous phacoemulsification of right eye cataract with prosthetic lens insertion	
174. Transcatheter replacement of pulmonary valve using of bovine jugular vein valve	
175. Total left hip replacement using ceramic on ceramic prosthesis, without bone cement	
176. Aortic valve annuloplasty using ring, open	
177. Laparoscopic repair of left inguinal hernia with marlex plug	
178. Autograft nerve graft to right median nerve, percutaneous endoscopic (do not code graft harvest for this exercise)	
179. Exchange of liner in femoral component of previous left hip replacement, open approach	
180. Anterior colporrhaphy with polypropylene mesh reinforcement, open approach	
181. Implantation of CorCap cardiac support device, open approach	
182. Abdominal wall herniorrhaphy, open, using synthetic mesh	
183. Tendon graft to strengthen injured left shoulder using autograft, open (do not code graft harvest for this exercise)	
184. Onlay lamellar keratoplasty of left cornea using autograft, external approach	
185. Resurfacing procedure on right femoral head, open approach	
186. Exchange of drainage tube from right hip joint	
187. Tracheostomy tube exchange	
188. Change chest tube for left pneumothorax	

Procedure	Code
189. Exchange of cerebral ventriculostomy drainage tube	
190. Foley urinary catheter exchange	
191. Open removal of lumbar sympathetic neurostimulator lead	
192. Nonincisional removal of Swan-Ganz catheter from right pulmonary artery	
193. Laparotomy with removal of pancreatic drain	
194. Extubation, endotracheal tube	
195. Nonincisional PEG tube removal	
196. Transvaginal removal of brachytherapy seeds	
197. Transvaginal removal of extraluminal cervical cerclage	
198. Incision with removal of K-wire fixation, right first metatarsal	
199. Cystoscopy with retrieval of left ureteral stent	
200. Removal of nasogastric drainage tube for decompression	
201. Removal of external fixator, left radial fracture	
202. Trimming and reanastomosis of stenosed femorofemoral synthetic bypass graft, open	
203. Open revision of right hip replacement, with readjustment of prosthesis	
204. Adjustment of position, pacemaker lead in left ventricle, percutaneous	
205. External repositioning of Foley catheter to bladder	
206. Taking out loose screw and putting larger screw in fracture repair plate, left tibia	
207. Revision of totally implantable VAD port placement in chest wall, causing patient discomfort, open	
208. Thoracotomy with exploration of right pleural cavity	
209. Diagnostic laryngoscopy	
210. Exploratory arthrotomy of left knee	
211. Colposcopy with diagnostic hysteroscopy	
212. Digital rectal exam	
213. Diagnostic arthroscopy of right shoulder	
214. Endoscopy of maxillary sinus	
215. Laparotomy with palpation of liver	
216. Transurethral diagnostic cystoscopy	
217. Colonoscopy, discontinued at sigmoid colon	
218. Percutaneous mapping of basal ganglia	
219. Heart catheterization with cardiac mapping	
220. Intraoperative whole brain mapping via craniotomy	
221. Mapping of left cerebral hemisphere, percutaneous endoscopic	
222. Intraoperative cardiac mapping during open heart surgery	
223. Hysteroscopy with cautery of post-hysterectomy oozing and evacuation of clot	
224. Open exploration and ligation of post-op arterial bleeder, left forearm	
225. Control of post-operative retroperitoneal bleeding via laparotomy	
226. Reopening of thoracotomy site with drainage and control of post-op hemopericardium	
227. Arthroscopy with drainage of hemarthrosis at previous operative site, right knee	
228. Radiocarpal fusion of left hand with internal fixation, open	
229. Posterior approach spinal fusion at L1-L3 level with BAK cage interbody fusion device, open	

Appendix M: Coding Exercises and Answers

Procedure	Code
230. Intercarpal fusion of right hand with bone bank bone graft, open	
231. Sacrococcygeal fusion with bone graft from same operative site, open	
232. Interphalangeal fusion of left great toe, percutaneous pin fixation	
233. Suture repair of left radial nerve laceration	
234. Laparotomy with suture repair of blunt force duodenal laceration	
235. Perineoplasty with repair of old obstetric laceration, open	
236. Suture repair of right biceps tendon (upper arm) laceration, open	
237. Closure of abdominal wall stab wound	
238. Cosmetic face lift, open, no other information available	
239. Bilateral breast augmentation with silicone implants, open	
240. Cosmetic rhinoplasty with septal reduction and tip elevation using local tissue graft, open	
241. Abdominoplasty (tummy tuck), open	
242. Liposuction of bilateral thighs	
243. Creation of penis in female patient using tissue bank donor graft	
244. Creation of vagina in male patient using synthetic material	
245. Laparoscopic vertical (sleeve) gastrectomy	
246. Left uterine artery embolization with intraluminal biosphere injection	

Obstetrics

Procedure	Code
1. Abortion by dilation and evacuation following laminaria insertion	
2. Manually assisted spontaneous abortion	
3. Abortion by abortifacient insertion	
4. Bimanual pregnancy examination	
5. Extraperitoneal C-section, low transverse incision	
6. Fetal spinal tap, percutaneous	
7. Fetal kidney transplant, laparoscopic	
8. Open in utero repair of congenital diaphragmatic hernia	
9. Laparoscopy with total excision of tubal pregnancy	
10. Transvaginal removal of fetal monitoring electrode	

Placement

Procedure	Code
1. Placement of packing material, right ear	
2. Mechanical traction of entire left leg	
3. Removal of splint, right shoulder	
4. Placement of neck brace	
5. Change of vaginal packing	
6. Packing of wound, chest wall	
7. Sterile dressing placement to left groin region	
8. Removal of packing material from pharynx	
9. Placement of intermittent pneumatic compression device, covering entire right arm	
10. Exchange of pressure dressing to left thigh	

Administration

Procedure	Code
1. Peritoneal dialysis via indwelling catheter	
2. Transvaginal artificial insemination	
3. Infusion of total parenteral nutrition via central venous catheter	
4. Esophagogastroscopy with Botox injection into esophageal sphincter	
5. Percutaneous irrigation of knee joint	
6. Systemic infusion of recombinant tissue plasminogen activator (r-tPA) via peripheral venous catheter	
7. Transabdominal in vitro fertilization, implantation of donor ovum	
8. Autologous bone marrow transplant via central venous line	
9. Implantation of anti-microbial envelope with cardiac defibrillator placement, open	
10. Sclerotherapy of brachial plexus lesion, alcohol injection	
11. Percutaneous peripheral vein injection, glucarpidase	
12. Introduction of anti-infective envelope into subcutaneous tissue, open	

Measurement and Monitoring

Procedure	Code
1. Cardiac stress test, single measurement	
2. EGD with biliary flow measurement	
3. Right and left heart cardiac catheterization with bilateral sampling and pressure measurements	
4. Temperature monitoring, rectal	
5. Peripheral venous pulse, external, single measurement	
6. Holter monitoring	
7. Respiratory rate, external, single measurement	
8. Fetal heart rate monitoring, transvaginal	
9. Visual mobility test, single measurement	
10. Left ventricular cardiac output monitoring from pulmonary artery wedge (Swan-Ganz) catheter	
11. Olfactory acuity test, single measurement	

Extracorporeal or Systemic Assistance and Performance

Procedure	Code
1. Intermittent mechanical ventilation, 16 hours	
2. Intubated patient on mechanical ventilation, positioned prone for 14 hrs	
3. Cardiac countershock with successful conversion to sinus rhythm	
4. IPPB (intermittent positive pressure breathing) for mobilization of secretions, 22 hours	
5. Renal dialysis, 12 hours	
6. IABP (intra-aortic balloon pump) continuous	
7. Intraoperative cardiac pacing, continuous	
8. Intraoperative ECMO (extracorporeal membrane oxygenation), central	
9. Controlled mechanical ventilation (CMV), 45 hours	
10. Pulsatile compression boot with intermittent inflation	

Appendix M: Coding Exercises and Answers

Extracorporeal or Systemic Therapies

Procedure	Code
1. Donor thrombocytapheresis, single encounter	
2. Bili-lite phototherapy, series treatment	
3. Whole body hypothermia, single treatment	
4. Circulatory phototherapy, single encounter	
5. Shock wave therapy of plantar fascia, single treatment	
6. Antigen-free air conditioning, series treatment	
7. TMS (transcranial magnetic stimulation), series treatment	
8. Therapeutic ultrasound of peripheral vessels, single treatment	
9. Plasmapheresis, series treatment	
10. Extracorporeal electromagnetic stimulation (EMS) for urinary incontinence, single treatment	

Osteopathic

Procedure	Code
1. Isotonic muscle energy treatment of right leg	
2. Low velocity-high amplitude osteopathic treatment of head	
3. Lymphatic pump osteopathic treatment of left axilla	
4. Indirect osteopathic treatment of sacrum	
5. Articulatory osteopathic treatment of cervical region	

Other Procedures

Procedure	Code
1. Near infrared spectroscopy of leg vessels	
2. CT computer assisted sinus surgery	
3. Suture removal, abdominal wall	
4. Isolation after infectious disease exposure	
5. Robotic assisted open prostatectomy	
6. CSF extracted from LP shunt	

Chiropractic

Procedure	Code
1. Chiropractic treatment of lumbar region using long lever specific contact	
2. Chiropractic manipulation of abdominal region, indirect visceral	
3. Chiropractic extra-articular treatment of hip region	
4. Chiropractic treatment of sacrum using long and short lever specific contact	
5. Mechanically-assisted chiropractic manipulation of head	

Imaging

Procedure	Code
1. Noncontrast CT of abdomen and pelvis	
2. Intravascular ultrasound, left subclavian artery	
3. Fluoroscopic guidance for insertion of central venous catheter in SVC, low osmolar contrast	
4. Chest x-ray, AP/PA and lateral views	
5. Endoluminal ultrasound of gallbladder and bile ducts	
6. MRI of thyroid gland, contrast unspecified	
7. Esophageal videofluoroscopy study with oral barium contrast	
8. Portable x-ray study of right radius/ulna shaft, standard series	
9. Routine fetal ultrasound, second trimester twin gestation	
10. CT scan of bilateral lungs, high osmolar contrast with densitometry	
11. Fluoroscopic guidance for percutaneous transluminal angioplasty (PTA) of left common femoral artery, low osmolar contrast	

Nuclear Medicine

Procedure	Code
1. Tomo scan of right and left heart, unspecified radiopharmaceutical, qualitative gated rest	
2. Technetium pentetate assay of kidneys, ureters, and bladder	
3. Uniplanar scan of spine using technetium oxidronate, with first-pass study	
4. Thallous chloride tomographic scan of bilateral breasts	
5. PET scan of myocardium using rubidium	
6. Gallium citrate scan of head and neck, single plane imaging	
7. Xenon gas nonimaging probe of brain	
8. Upper GI scan, radiopharmaceutical unspecified, for gastric emptying	
9. Carbon 11 PET scan of brain with quantification	
10. Iodinated albumin nuclear medicine assay, blood plasma volume study	

Radiation Therapy

Procedure	Code
1. Plaque radiation of left eye, single port	
2. 8 MeV photon beam radiation to brain	
3. IORT of colon, 3 ports	
4. HDR brachytherapy of prostate using low dose palladium-103, unidirectional source	
5. Electron radiation treatment of right breast, with custom device	
6. Hyperthermia oncology treatment of pelvic region	
7. Contact radiation of tongue	
8. Heavy particle radiation treatment of pancreas, four risk sites	
9. LDR brachytherapy to spinal cord using iodine	
10. Whole body Phosphorus 32 administration with risk to hematopoietic system	

Physical Rehabilitation and Diagnostic Audiology

Procedure	Code
1. Bekesy assessment using audiometer	
2. Individual fitting of left eye prosthesis	
3. Physical therapy for range of motion and mobility, patient right hip, no special equipment	
4. Bedside swallow assessment using assessment kit	
5. Caregiver training in airway clearance techniques	
6. Application of short arm cast in rehabilitation setting	
7. Verbal assessment of patient's pain level	
8. Caregiver training in communication skills using manual communication board	
9. Group musculoskeletal balance training exercises, whole body, no special equipment	
10. Individual therapy for auditory processing using tape recorder	

Mental Health

Procedure	Code
1. Cognitive-behavioral psychotherapy, individual	
2. Narcosynthesis	
3. Light therapy	
4. ECT (electroconvulsive therapy), unilateral, single seizure	
5. Crisis intervention	
6. Neuropsychological testing	
7. Hypnosis	
8. Developmental testing	
9. Vocational counseling	
10. Family psychotherapy	

Substance Abuse Treatment

Procedure	Code
1. Naltrexone treatment for drug dependency	
2. Substance abuse treatment family counseling	
3. Medication monitoring of patient on methadone maintenance	
4. Individual interpersonal psychotherapy for drug abuse	
5. Patient in for alcohol detoxification treatment	
6. Group motivational counseling	
7. Individual 12-step psychotherapy for substance abuse	
8. Post-test infectious disease counseling for IV drug abuser	
9. Psychodynamic psychotherapy for drug dependent patient	
10. Group cognitive-behavioral counseling for substance abuse	

New Technology

Procedure	Code
1. Infusion of terlipressin via peripheral venous catheter	
2. Transcatheter dilation of right anterior tibial artery with Esprit™ stent	
3. Cranial reconstruction using Longeviti ClearFit® cranial implant	

Answers to Coding Exercises

Medical Surgical Section

Procedure	Code
1. Excision of malignant melanoma from skin of right ear	0HB2XZZ
2. Laparoscopy with excision of endometrial implant from left ovary	0UB14ZZ
3. Percutaneous needle core biopsy of right kidney	0TB03ZX
4. EGD with excisional gastric biopsy	0DB68ZX
5. Open endarterectomy of left common carotid artery	03CJ0ZZ
6. Excision of basal cell carcinoma of lower lip	0CB1XZZ
7. Open excision of tail of pancreas	0FBG0ZZ
8. Percutaneous biopsy of right gastrocnemius muscle	0KBS3ZX
9. Sigmoidoscopy with sigmoid polypectomy	0DBN8ZZ
10. Open excision of lesion from right Achilles tendon	0LBN0ZZ
11. Open resection of cecum	0DTH0ZZ
12. Total excision of pituitary gland, open	0GT00ZZ
13. Explantation of left failed kidney, open	0TT10ZZ
14. Open left axillary total lymphadenectomy	07T60ZZ (RESECTION is coded for cutting out a chain of lymph nodes.)
15. Laparoscopic-assisted vaginal hysterectomy	0UT9FZZ
16. Right total mastectomy, open	0HTT0ZZ
17. Open resection of papillary muscle	02TD0ZZ (The papillary muscle refers to the heart and is found in the *Heart and Great Vessels* body system.)
18. Total retropubic prostatectomy, open	0VT00ZZ
19. Laparoscopic cholecystectomy, hand-assisted	0FT44ZG
20. Endoscopic bilateral total maxillary sinusectomy	09TQ8ZZ, 09TR8ZZ
21. Amputation at right elbow level	0X6B0ZZ
22. Right below-knee amputation, proximal tibia/fibula	0Y6H0Z1 (The qualifier *High* here means the portion of the tib/fib closest to the knee.)
23. Fifth ray carpometacarpal joint amputation, left hand	0X6K0Z8 (A *complete* ray amputation is through the carpometacarpal joint.)
24. Right leg and hip amputation through ischium	0Y620ZZ (The *Hindquarter* body part includes amputation along any part of the hip bone.)
25. DIP joint amputation of right thumb	0X6L0Z3 (The qualifier *Low* here means through the distal interphalangeal joint.)
26. Right wrist joint amputation	0X6J0Z0 (Amputation at the wrist joint is considered a complete amputation of the hand.)
27. Trans-metatarsal amputation of foot at left big toe	0Y6N0Z9 (A *partial* amputation is through the shaft of the metatarsal bone.)
28. Mid-shaft amputation, right humerus	0X680Z2
29. Left fourth toe amputation, mid-proximal phalanx	0Y6W0Z1 (The qualifier *High* here means anywhere along the proximal phalanx.)
30. Right above-knee amputation, distal femur	0Y6C0Z3
31. Cryotherapy of wart on left hand	0H5GXZZ
32. Percutaneous radiofrequency ablation of right vocal cord lesion	0C5T3ZZ
33. Left heart catheterization with laser destruction of arrhythmogenic focus, A-V node	02583ZZ
34. Cautery of nosebleed	093K7ZZ
35. Transurethral endoscopic laser ablation of prostate	0V508ZZ
36. Percutaneous cautery of oozing varicose vein, left calf	0Y3J3ZZ
37. Laparoscopy with destruction of endometriosis, bilateral ovaries	0U524ZZ
38. Laser coagulation of right retinal vessel, percutaneous	085G3ZZ (The *Retinal Vessel* body-part values are in the *Eye* body system.)
39. Thoracoscopic pleurodesis, left side	0B5P4ZZ
40. Percutaneous insertion of Greenfield IVC filter	06H03DZ
41. Forceps total mouth extraction, upper and lower teeth	0CDWXZ2, 0CDXXZ2
42. Removal of left thumbnail	0HDQXZZ (No separate body-part value is given for thumbnail, so this is coded to *Fingernail*.)
43. Extraction of right intraocular lens without replacement, percutaneous	08DJ3ZZ
44. Laparoscopy with needle aspiration of ova for in vitro fertilization	0UDN4ZZ
45. Nonexcisional debridement of skin ulcer, right foot	0HDMXZZ
46. Open stripping of abdominal fascia, right side	0JD80ZZ
47. Hysteroscopy with D&C, diagnostic	0UDB8ZX
48. Liposuction for medical purposes, left upper arm	0JDF3ZZ (The *Percutaneous* approach is inherent in the liposuction technique.)
49. Removal of tattered right ear drum fragments with tweezers	09D77ZZ
50. Microincisional phlebectomy of spider veins, right lower leg	06DY3ZZ
51. Routine Foley catheter placement	0T9B70Z
52. Incision and drainage of external anal abscess	0D9QXZZ
53. Percutaneous drainage of ascites	0W9G3ZZ (This is drainage of the cavity and not the peritoneal membrane itself.)
54. Laparoscopy with left ovarian cystotomy and drainage	0U914ZZ
55. Laparotomy and drain placement for liver abscess, right lobe	0F9100Z
56. Right knee arthrotomy with drain placement	0S9C00Z
57. Thoracentesis of left pleural effusion	0W9B3ZZ (This is drainage of the pleural cavity)
58. Phlebotomy of left median cubital vein for polycythemia vera	059C3ZZ (The median cubital vein is a branch of the basilic vein)
59. Percutaneous chest tube placement for right pneumothorax	0W9930Z
60. Endoscopic drainage of left ethmoid sinus	099V4ZZ
61. External ventricular CSF drainage catheter placement via burr hole	009630Z

Answers to Coding Exercises

Procedure	Code
62. Removal of foreign body, right cornea	08C8XZZ
63. Percutaneous mechanical thrombectomy, left brachial artery	03C83ZZ
64. Esophagogastroscopy with removal of bezoar from stomach	0DC68ZZ
65. Foreign body removal, skin of left thumb	0HCGXZZ (There is no specific value for thumb skin, so the procedure is coded to *Hand*.)
66. Transurethral cystoscopy with removal of bladder stone	0TCB8ZZ
67. Forceps removal of foreign body in right nostril	09CKXZZ (Nostril is coded to the *Nasal mucosa and soft tissue* body-part value.)
68. Laparoscopy with excision of old suture from mesentery	0DCV4ZZ
69. Incision and removal of right lacrimal duct stone	08CX0ZZ
70. Nonincisional removal of intraluminal foreign body from vagina	0UCG7ZZ (The approach *External* is also a possibility. It is assumed here that since the patient went to the doctor to have the object removed, that it was not in the vaginal orifice.)
71. Right common carotid endarterectomy, open	03CH0ZZ
72. Open excision of retained sliver, subcutaneous tissue of left foot	0JCR0ZZ
73. Extracorporeal shockwave lithotripsy (ESWL), bilateral ureters	0TF6XZZ, 0TF7XZZ (The *Bilateral Ureter* body-part value is not available for the root operation FRAGMENTATION, so the procedures are coded separately.)
74. Endoscopic retrograde cholangiopancreatography (ERCP) with lithotripsy of common bile duct stone	0FF98ZZ (ERCP is performed through the mouth to the biliary system via the duodenum, so the approach value is *Via Natural or Artificial Opening Endoscopic*.)
75. Thoracotomy with crushing of pericardial calcifications	02FN0ZZ
76. Transurethral cystoscopy with fragmentation of bladder calculus	0TFB8ZZ
77. Hysteroscopy with intraluminal lithotripsy of left fallopian tube calcification	0UF68ZZ
78. Division of right foot tendon, percutaneous	0L8V3ZZ
79. Left heart catheterization with division of bundle of HIS	02883ZZ
80. Open osteotomy of capitate, left hand	0P8N0ZZ (The capitate is one of the carpal bones of the hand.)
81. EGD with esophagotomy of esophagogastric junction	0D948ZZ
82. Sacral rhizotomy for pain control, percutaneous	018R3ZZ
83. Laparotomy with exploration and adhesiolysis of right ureter	0TN60ZZ
84. Incision of scar contracture, right elbow	0HNDXZZ (The skin of the elbow region is coded to *Lower Arm*.)
85. Frenulotomy for treatment of tongue-tie syndrome	0CN7XZZ (The frenulum is coded to the body-part value *Tongue*.)

Procedure	Code
86. Right shoulder arthroscopy with coracoacromial ligament release	0MN14ZZ
87. Mitral valvulotomy for release of fused leaflets, open approach	02NG0ZZ
88. Percutaneous left Achilles tendon release	0LNP3ZZ
89. Laparoscopy with lysis of peritoneal adhesions	0DNW4ZZ
90. Manual rupture of right shoulder joint adhesions under general anesthesia	0RNJXZZ
91. Open posterior tarsal tunnel release	01NG0ZZ (The nerve released in the posterior tarsal tunnel is the tibial nerve.)
92. Laparoscopy with freeing of left ovary and fallopian tube	0UN14ZZ, 0UN64ZZ
93. Liver transplant with donor matched liver	0FY00Z0
94. Orthotopic heart transplant using porcine heart	02YA0Z2 (The donor heart comes from an animal [pig], so the qualifier value is *Zooplastic*.)
95. Right lung transplant, open, using organ donor match	0BYK0Z0
96. Transplant of large intestine, organ donor match	0DYE0Z0
97. Left kidney/pancreas organ bank transplant	0FYG0Z0, 0TY10Z0
98. Replantation of avulsed scalp	0HM0XZZ
99. Reattachment of severed right ear	09M0XZZ
100. Reattachment of traumatic left gastrocnemius avulsion, open	0KMT0ZZ
101. Closed replantation of three avulsed teeth, lower jaw	0CMXXZ1
102. Reattachment of severed left hand	0XMK0ZZ
103. Right open palmaris longus tendon transfer	0LX50ZZ
104. Endoscopic radial to median nerve transfer	01X64Z5
105. Fasciocutaneous flap closure of left thigh, open	0JXM0ZC (The qualifier identifies the body layers in addition to fascia included in the procedure.)
106. Transfer left index finger to left thumb position, open	0XXP0ZM
107. Percutaneous fascia transfer to fill defect, right neck	0JX43ZZ
108. Trigeminal to facial nerve transfer, percutaneous endoscopic	00XK4ZM
109. Endoscopic left leg flexor hallucis longus tendon transfer	0LXP4ZZ
110. Right scalp advancement flap to right temple	0HX0XZZ
111. Resection right breast with TRAM flap reconstruction, open	0HTT0ZZ, 0HRT076 (Code both the resection and the replacement per guideline B3.18)
112. Skin transfer flap closure of complex open wound, left lower back	0HX6XZZ
113. Open fracture reduction, right tibia	0QSG0ZZ
114. Laparoscopy with gastropexy for malrotation	0DS64ZZ
115. Left knee arthroscopy with reposition of anterior cruciate ligament	0MSP4ZZ
116. Open transposition of ulnar nerve	01S40ZZ
117. Closed reduction with percutaneous internal fixation of right femoral neck fracture	0QS634Z
118. Trans-vaginal intraluminal cervical cerclage	0UVC7DZ
119. Cervical cerclage using Shirodkar technique	0UVC7ZZ
120. Thoracotomy with banding of left pulmonary artery using extraluminal device	02VR0CZ

Procedure	Code
121. Restriction of thoracic duct with intraluminal stent, percutaneous	07VK3DZ
122. Craniotomy with clipping of cerebral aneurysm	03VG0CZ (The clip is placed lengthwise on the outside wall of the widened portion of the vessel.)
123. Nonincisional, transnasal placement of restrictive stent in right lacrimal duct	08VX7DZ
124. Catheter-based temporary restriction of blood flow in abdominal aorta for treatment of cerebral ischemia	04V03DJ
125. Percutaneous ligation of esophageal vein	06L33ZZ
126. Percutaneous embolization of left internal carotid-cavernous fistula	03LL3DZ
127. Laparoscopy with bilateral occlusion of fallopian tubes using Hulka extraluminal clips	0UL74CZ
128. Open suture ligation of failed AV graft, left brachial artery	03L80ZZ
129. Percutaneous embolization of vascular supply, intracranial meningioma	03LG3DZ
130. Percutaneous embolization of right uterine artery, using coils	04LE3DT
131. Open occlusion of left atrial appendage, using extraluminal pressure clips	02L70CK
132. Percutaneous suture exclusion of left atrial appendage, via femoral artery access	02L73ZK
133. ERCP with balloon dilation of common bile duct	0F798ZZ
134. PTCA of two coronary arteries, LAD with stent placement, RCA with no stent	02703DZ, 02703ZZ (A separate procedure is coded for each artery dilated, since the device value differs for each artery.)
135. Cystoscopy with intraluminal dilation of bladder neck stricture	0T7C8ZZ
136. Open dilation of old anastomosis, left femoral artery	047L0ZZ
137. Dilation of upper esophageal stricture, direct visualization, with Bougie sound	0D717ZZ
138. PTA of right brachial artery stenosis	03773ZZ
139. Transnasal dilation and stent placement in right lacrimal duct	087X7DZ
140. Hysteroscopy with balloon dilation of bilateral fallopian tubes	0U778ZZ
141. Tracheoscopy with intraluminal dilation of tracheal stenosis	0B718ZZ
142. Cystoscopy with dilation of left ureteral stricture, with stent placement	0T778DZ
143. Open gastric bypass with Roux-en-Y limb to jejunum	0D160ZA
144. Right temporal artery to intracranial artery bypass using Gore-Tex graft, open	031S0JG
145. Tracheostomy formation with tracheostomy tube placement, percutaneous	0B113F4
146. PICVA (percutaneous in situ coronary venous arterialization) of single coronary artery	02103D4
147. Open left femoral-popliteal artery bypass using cadaver vein graft	041L0KL
148. Shunting of intrathecal cerebrospinal fluid to peritoneal cavity using synthetic shunt	00160J6
149. Colostomy formation, open, transverse colon to abdominal wall	0D1L0Z4
150. Open urinary diversion, left ureter, using ileal conduit to skin	0T170ZC

Procedure	Code
151. CABG of LAD using pedicled left internal mammary artery, open off-bypass	02100Z9
152. Open pleuroperitoneal shunt, right pleural cavity, using synthetic device	0W190JG
153. Percutaneous placement of ventriculoperitoneal shunt for treatment of hydrocephalus	00163J6
154. End-of-life replacement of spinal neurostimulator generator, multiple array, in lower abdomen	0JH80DZ (Taking out of the old generator is coded separately to the root operation *Removal*)
155. Percutaneous insertion of spinal neurostimulator lead, lumbar spinal cord	00HV3MZ
156. Percutaneous replacement of broken pacemaker lead in left atrium	02H73JZ (Taking out the broken pacemaker lead is coded separately to the root operation *Removal*.)
157. Open placement of dual chamber pacemaker generator in chest wall	0JH606Z
158. Percutaneous placement of venous central line in right internal jugular, with tip in superior vena cava	02HV33Z
159. Open insertion of multiple channel cochlear implant, left ear	09HE06Z
160. Percutaneous placement of Swan-Ganz catheter in pulmonary trunk	02HP32Z (The Swan-Ganz catheter is coded to the device value *Monitoring Device* because it monitors pulmonary artery output.)
161. Bronchoscopy with insertion of Low Dose Pd-103 brachytherapy seeds, right lung	0BHK81Z, DB11BBZ
162. Open insertion of interspinous process device into lumbar vertebral joint	0SH00BZ
163. Open placement of bone growth stimulator, left femoral shaft	0QHY0MZ
164. Cystoscopy with placement of brachytherapy seeds in prostate gland	0VH081Z
165. Percutaneous insertion of Greenfield IVC filter	06H03DZ
166. Full-thickness skin graft to right lower arm, autograft (do not code graft harvest for this exercise)	0HRDX73
167. Excision of necrosed left femoral head with bone bank bone graft to fill the defect, open	0QR70KZ
168. Penetrating keratoplasty of right cornea with donor matched cornea, percutaneous approach	08R83KZ
169. Excision of abdominal aorta with Gore-Tex graft replacement, open	04R00JZ
170. Total right knee arthroplasty with insertion of total knee prosthesis	0SRC0JZ
171. Tenonectomy with graft to right ankle using cadaver graft, open	0LRS0KZ
172. Mitral valve replacement using porcine valve, open	02RG08Z
173. Percutaneous phacoemulsification of right eye cataract with prosthetic lens insertion	08RJ3JZ
174. Transcatheter replacement of pulmonary valve using of bovine jugular vein valve	02RH38Z
175. Total left hip replacement using ceramic on ceramic prosthesis, without bone cement	0SRB03A
176. Aortic valve annuloplasty using ring, open	02UF0JZ
177. Laparoscopic repair of left inguinal hernia with marlex plug	0YU64JZ
178. Autograft nerve graft to right median nerve, percutaneous endoscopic (do not code graft harvest for this exercise)	01U547Z

Answers to Coding Exercises

Procedure	Code
179. Exchange of liner in femoral component of previous left hip replacement, open approach	0SUS09Z (Taking out of the old liner is coded separately to the root operation *Removal*)
180. Anterior colporrhaphy with polypropylene mesh reinforcement, open approach	0JUC0JZ
181. Implantation of CorCap cardiac support device, open approach	02UA0JZ
182. Abdominal wall herniorrhaphy, open, using synthetic mesh	0WUF0JZ
183. Tendon graft to strengthen injured left shoulder using autograft, open (do not code graft harvest for this exercise)	0LU207Z
184. Onlay lamellar keratoplasty of left cornea using autograft, external approach	08U9X7Z
185. Resurfacing procedure on right femoral head, open approach	0SUR0BZ
186. Exchange of drainage tube from right hip joint	0S2YX0Z
187. Tracheostomy tube exchange	0B21XFZ
188. Change chest tube for left pneumothorax	0W2BX0Z
189. Exchange of cerebral ventriculostomy drainage tube	0020X0Z
190. Foley urinary catheter exchange	0T2BX0Z (This is coded to *Drainage Device* because urine is being drained.)
191. Open removal of lumbar sympathetic neurostimulator lead	01PY0MZ
192. Nonincisional removal of Swan-Ganz catheter from right pulmonary artery	02PYX2Z
193. Laparotomy with removal of pancreatic drain	0FPG00Z
194. Extubation, endotracheal tube	0BP1XDZ
195. Nonincisional PEG tube removal	0DP6XUZ
196. Transvaginal removal of brachytherapy seeds	0UPH71Z
197. Transvaginal removal of extraluminal cervical cerclage	0UPD7CZ
198. Incision with removal of K-wire fixation, right first metatarsal	0QPN04Z
199. Cystoscopy with retrieval of left ureteral stent	0TP98DZ
200. Removal of nasogastric drainage tube for decompression	0DP6X0Z
201. Removal of external fixator, left radial fracture	0PPJX5Z
202. Trimming and reanastomosis of stenosed femorofemoral synthetic bypass graft, open	04WY0JZ
203. Open revision of right hip replacement, with readjustment of prosthesis	0SW90JZ
204. Adjustment of position, pacemaker lead in left ventricle, percutaneous	02WA3MZ
205. External repositioning of Foley catheter to bladder	0TWBX0Z
206. Taking out loose screw and putting larger screw in fracture repair plate, left tibia	0QWH04Z
207. Revision of totally implantable VAD port placement in chest wall, causing patient discomfort, open	0JWT0WZ
208. Thoracotomy with exploration of right pleural cavity	0WJ90ZZ
209. Diagnostic laryngoscopy	0CJS8ZZ
210. Exploratory arthrotomy of left knee	0SJD0ZZ
211. Colposcopy with diagnostic hysteroscopy	0UJD8ZZ
212. Digital rectal exam	0DJD7ZZ
213. Diagnostic arthroscopy of right shoulder	0RJJ4ZZ
214. Endoscopy of maxillary sinus	09JY4ZZ
215. Laparotomy with palpation of liver	0FJ00ZZ
216. Transurethral diagnostic cystoscopy	0TJB8ZZ
217. Colonoscopy, discontinued at sigmoid colon	0DJD8ZZ
218. Percutaneous mapping of basal ganglia	00K83ZZ
219. Heart catheterization with cardiac mapping	02K83ZZ
220. Intraoperative whole brain mapping via craniotomy	00K00ZZ
221. Mapping of left cerebral hemisphere, percutaneous endoscopic	00K74ZZ
222. Intraoperative cardiac mapping during open heart surgery	02K80ZZ
223. Hysteroscopy with cautery of post-hysterectomy oozing and evacuation of clot	0W3R8ZZ
224. Open exploration and ligation of post-op arterial bleeder, left forearm	0X3F0ZZ
225. Control of post-operative retroperitoneal bleeding via laparotomy	0W3H0ZZ
226. Reopening of thoracotomy site with drainage and control of post-op hemopericardium	0W3D0ZZ
227. Arthroscopy with drainage of hemarthrosis at previous operative site, right knee	0Y3F4ZZ
228. Radiocarpal fusion of left hand with internal fixation, open	0RGP04Z
229. Posterior approach spinal fusion at L1-L3 level with BAK cage interbody fusion device, open	0SG10AJ
230. Intercarpal fusion of right hand with bone bank bone graft, open	0RGQ0KZ
231. Sacrococcygeal fusion with bone graft from same operative site, open	0SG507Z
232. Interphalangeal fusion of left great toe, percutaneous pin fixation	0SGQ34Z
233. Suture repair of left radial nerve laceration	01Q60ZZ (The approach value is *Open*, though the surgical exposure may have been created by the wound itself.)
234. Laparotomy with suture repair of blunt force duodenal laceration	0DQ90ZZ
235. Perineoplasty with repair of old obstetric laceration, open	0WQN0ZZ
236. Suture repair of right biceps tendon (upper arm) laceration, open	0LQ30ZZ
237. Closure of abdominal wall stab wound	0WQF0ZZ
238. Cosmetic face lift, open, no other information available	0W020ZZ
239. Bilateral breast augmentation with silicone implants, open	0HOV0JZ
240. Cosmetic rhinoplasty with septal reduction and tip elevation using local tissue graft, open	090K07Z
241. Abdominoplasty (tummy tuck), open	0W0F0ZZ
242. Liposuction of bilateral thighs	0J0L3ZZ, 0J0M3ZZ
243. Creation of penis in female patient using tissue bank donor graft	0W4N0K1
244. Creation of vagina in male patient using synthetic material	0W4M0J0
245. Laparoscopic vertical (sleeve) gastrectomy	0DB64Z3
246. Left uterine artery embolization with intraluminal biosphere injection	04LF3DU

Obstetrics

Procedure	Code
1. Abortion by dilation and evacuation following laminaria insertion	10A07ZW
2. Manually assisted spontaneous abortion	10E0XZZ (Since the pregnancy was not artificially terminated, this is coded to *Delivery* because it captures the procedure objective. The fact that it was an abortion will be identified in the diagnosis code.)
3. Abortion by abortifacient insertion	10A07ZX
4. Bimanual pregnancy examination	10J07ZZ
5. Extraperitoneal C-section, low transverse incision	10D00Z1
6. Fetal spinal tap, percutaneous	10903ZA
7. Fetal kidney transplant, laparoscopic	10Y04ZS
8. Open in utero repair of congenital diaphragmatic hernia	10Q00ZK (Diaphragm is classified to the *Respiratory* body system in the *Medical and Surgical* section.)
9. Laparoscopy with total excision of tubal pregnancy	10T24ZZ
10. Transvaginal removal of fetal monitoring electrode	10P073Z

Placement

Procedure	Code
1. Placement of packing material, right ear	2Y42X5Z
2. Mechanical traction of entire left leg	2W6MX0Z
3. Removal of splint, right shoulder	2W5AX1Z
4. Placement of neck brace	2W32X3Z
5. Change of vaginal packing	2Y04X5Z
6. Packing of wound, chest wall	2W44X5Z
7. Sterile dressing placement to left groin region	2W27X4Z
8. Removal of packing material from pharynx	2Y50X5Z
9. Placement of intermittent pneumatic compression device, covering entire right arm	2W18X7Z
10. Exchange of pressure dressing to left thigh	2W0PX6Z

Administration

Procedure	Code
1. Peritoneal dialysis via indwelling catheter	3E1M39Z
2. Transvaginal artificial insemination	3E0P7LZ
3. Infusion of total parenteral nutrition via central venous catheter	3E0436Z
4. Esophagogastroscopy with Botox injection into esophageal sphincter	3E0G8GC (Botulinum toxin is a paralyzing agent with temporary effects; it does not sclerose or destroy the nerve.)
5. Percutaneous irrigation of knee joint	3E1U38Z
6. Systemic infusion of recombinant tissue plasminogen activator (r-tPA) via peripheral venous catheter	3E03317
7. Transabdominal in vitro fertilization, implantation of donor ovum	3E0P3Q1
8. Autologous bone marrow transplant via central venous line	30243G0
9. Implantation of anti-microbial envelope with cardiac defibrillator placement, open	3E0102A
10. Sclerotherapy of brachial plexus lesion, alcohol injection	3E0T3TZ
11. Percutaneous peripheral vein injection, glucarpidase	3E033GQ
12. Introduction of anti-infective envelope into subcutaneous tissue, open	3E0102A

Measurement and Monitoring

Procedure	Code
1. Cardiac stress test, single measurement	4A02XM4
2. EGD with biliary flow measurement	4A0C85Z
3. Right and left heart cardiac catheterization with bilateral sampling and pressure measurements	4A023N8
4. Temperature monitoring, rectal	4A1Z7KZ
5. Peripheral venous pulse, external, single measurement	4A04XJ1
6. Holter monitoring	4A12X45
7. Respiratory rate, external, single measurement	4A09XCZ
8. Fetal heart rate monitoring, transvaginal	4A1H7CZ
9. Visual mobility test, single measurement	4A07X7Z
10. Left ventricular cardiac output monitoring from pulmonary artery wedge (Swan-Ganz) catheter	4A1239Z
11. Olfactory acuity test, single measurement	4A08X0Z

Extracorporeal or Systemic Assistance and Performance

Procedure	Code
1. Intermittent mechanical ventilation, 16 hours	5A1935Z
2. Intubated patient on mechanical ventilation, positioned prone for 14 hrs	5A09C5K
3. Cardiac countershock with successful conversion to sinus rhythm	5A2204Z
4. IPPB (intermittent positive pressure breathing) for mobilization of secretions, 22 hours	5A09358
5. Renal dialysis, 12 hours	5A1D80Z
6. IABP (intra-aortic balloon pump) continuous	5A02210
7. Intra-operative cardiac pacing, continuous	5A1223Z
8. Intraoperative ECMO (extracorporeal membrane oxygenation), central	5A15A2F
9. Controlled mechanical ventilation (CMV), 45 hours	5A1945Z
10. Pulsatile compression boot with intermittent inflation	5A02115 (This is coded to the function value *Cardiac Output*, because the purpose of such compression devices is to return blood to the heart faster.)

Extracorporeal or Systemic Therapies

Procedure	Code
1. Donor thrombocytapheresis, single encounter	6A550Z2
2. Bili-lite phototherapy, series treatment	6A601ZZ
3. Whole body hypothermia, single treatment	6A4Z0ZZ
4. Circulatory phototherapy, single encounter	6A650ZZ
5. Shock wave therapy of plantar fascia, single treatment	6A930ZZ
6. Antigen-free air conditioning, series treatment	6A0Z1ZZ
7. TMS (transcranial magnetic stimulation), series treatment	6A221ZZ

Answers to Coding Exercises

Procedure	Code
8. Therapeutic ultrasound of peripheral vessels, single treatment	6A750Z6
9. Plasmapheresis, series treatment	6A551Z3
10. Extracorporeal electromagnetic stimulation (EMS) for urinary incontinence, single treatment	6A210ZZ

Osteopathic

Procedure	Code
1. Isotonic muscle energy treatment of right leg	7W06X8Z
2. Low velocity-high amplitude osteopathic treatment of head	7W00X5Z
3. Lymphatic pump osteopathic treatment of left axilla	7W07X6Z
4. Indirect osteopathic treatment of sacrum	7W04X4Z
5. Articulatory osteopathic treatment of cervical region	7W01X0Z

Other Procedures

Procedure	Code
1. Near infrared spectroscopy of leg vessels	8E023DZ
2. CT computer assisted sinus surgery	8E09XBG (The primary procedure is coded separately.)
3. Suture removal, abdominal wall	8E0WXY8
4. Isolation after infectious disease exposure	8E0ZXY6
5. Robotic assisted open prostatectomy	8E0W0CZ (The primary procedure is coded separately.)
6. CSF extracted from LP shunt	8C01X6J

Chiropractic

Procedure	Code
1. Chiropractic treatment of lumbar region using long lever specific contact	9WB3XGZ
2. Chiropractic manipulation of abdominal region, indirect visceral	9WB9XCZ
3. Chiropractic extra-articular treatment of hip region	9WB6XDZ
4. Chiropractic treatment of sacrum using long and short lever specific contact	9WB4XJZ
5. Mechanically-assisted chiropractic manipulation of head	9WB0XKZ

Imaging

Procedure	Code
1. Noncontrast CT of abdomen and pelvis	BW21ZZZ
2. Intravascular ultrasound, left subclavian artery	B342ZZ3
3. Fluoroscopic guidance for insertion of central venous catheter in SVC, low osmolar contrast	B5181ZA
4. Chest x-ray, AP/PA and lateral views	BW03ZZZ
5. Endoluminal ultrasound of gallbladder and bile ducts	BF43ZZZ
6. MRI of thyroid gland, contrast unspecified	BG34YZZ
7. Esophageal videofluoroscopy study with oral barium contrast	BD11YZZ
8. Portable x-ray study of right radius/ulna shaft, standard series	BP0JZZZ
9. Routine fetal ultrasound, second trimester twin gestation	BY4DZZZ

Procedure	Code
10. CT scan of bilateral lungs, high osmolar contrast with densitometry	BB240ZZ
11. Fluoroscopic guidance for percutaneous transluminal angioplasty (PTA) of left common femoral artery, low osmolar contrast	B41G1ZZ

Nuclear Medicine

Procedure	Code
1. Tomo scan of right and left heart, unspecified radiopharmaceutical, qualitative gated rest	C226YZZ
2. Technetium pentetate assay of kidneys, ureters, and bladder	CT631ZZ
3. Uniplanar scan of spine using technetium oxidronate, with first-pass study	CP151ZZ
4. Thallous chloride tomographic scan of bilateral breasts	CH22SZZ
5. PET scan of myocardium using rubidium	C23GQZZ
6. Gallium citrate scan of head and neck, single plane imaging	CW1BLZZ
7. Xenon gas nonimaging probe of brain	C050VZZ
8. Upper GI scan, radiopharmaceutical unspecified, for gastric emptying	CD15YZZ
9. Carbon 11 PET scan of brain with quantification	C030BZZ
10. Iodinated albumin nuclear medicine assay, blood plasma volume study	C763HZZ

Radiation Therapy

Procedure	Code
1. Plaque radiation of left eye, single port	D8Y0FZZ
2. 8 MeV photon beam radiation to brain	D0011ZZ
3. IORT of colon, 3 ports	DDY5CZZ
4. HDR brachytherapy of prostate using low dose palladium-103, unidirectional source	DV10BB1
5. Electron radiation treatment of right breast, with custom device	DM013ZZ
6. Hyperthermia oncology treatment of pelvic region	DWY68ZZ
7. Contact radiation of tongue	D9Y57ZZ
8. Heavy particle radiation treatment of pancreas, four risk sites	DF034ZZ
9. LDR brachytherapy to spinal cord using iodine	D016B9Z
10. Whole body Phosphorus 32 administration with risk to hematopoietic system	DWY5GFZ

Physical Rehabilitation and Diagnostic Audiology

Procedure	Code
1. Bekesy assessment using audiometer	F13Z31Z
2. Individual fitting of left eye prosthesis	F0DZ8UZ
3. Physical therapy for range of motion and mobility, patient right hip, no special equipment	F07L0ZZ
4. Bedside swallow assessment using assessment kit	F00ZHYZ
5. Caregiver training in airway clearance techniques	F0FZ8ZZ
6. Application of short arm cast in rehabilitation setting	F0DZ7EZ (Inhibitory cast is listed in the equipment reference table under E, *Orthosis*.)
7. Verbal assessment of patient's pain level	F02ZFZZ

Procedure	Code
8. Caregiver training in communication skills using manual communication board	F0FZJMZ (Manual communication board is listed in the equipment reference table under M, *Augmentative/ Alternative Communication*.)
9. Group musculoskeletal balance training exercises, whole body, no special equipment	F07M6ZZ (Balance training is included in the motor treatment reference table under *Therapeutic Exercise*.)
10. Individual therapy for auditory processing using tape recorder	F09Z2KZ (Tape recorder is listed in the equipment reference table under *Audiovisual Equipment*.)

Mental Health

Procedure	Code
1. Cognitive-behavioral psychotherapy, individual	GZ58ZZZ
2. Narcosynthesis	GZGZZZZ
3. Light therapy	GZJZZZZ
4. ECT (electroconvulsive therapy), unilateral, single seizure	GZB0ZZZ
5. Crisis intervention	GZ2ZZZZ
6. Neuropsychological testing	GZ13ZZZ
7. Hypnosis	GZFZZZZ
8. Developmental testing	GZ10ZZZ
9. Vocational counseling	GZ61ZZZ
10. Family psychotherapy	GZ72ZZZ

Substance Abuse Treatment

Procedure	Code
1. Naltrexone treatment for drug dependency	HZ94ZZZ
2. Substance abuse treatment family counseling	HZ63ZZZ
3. Medication monitoring of patient on methadone maintenance	HZ81ZZZ
4. Individual interpersonal psychotherapy for drug abuse	HZ54ZZZ
5. Patient in for alcohol detoxification treatment	HZ2ZZZZ
6. Group motivational counseling	HZ47ZZZ
7. Individual 12-step psychotherapy for substance abuse	HZ53ZZZ
8. Post-test infectious disease counseling for IV drug abuser	HZ3CZZZ
9. Psychodynamic psychotherapy for drug dependent patient	HZ5CZZZ
10. Group cognitive-behavioral counseling for substance abuse	HZ42ZZZ

New Technology

Procedure	Code
1. Infusion of terlipressin via peripheral venous catheter	XW03367
2. Transcatheter dilation of right anterior tibial artery with Esprit™ stent	X27P3TA
3. Cranial reconstruction using Longeviti ClearFit® cranial implant	XNR80D9

Notes

Notes